A MANUAL FOR PEDIATRIC HOUSE OFFICERS

THE HARRIET LANE HANDBOOK

TWENTY-FIRST EDITION

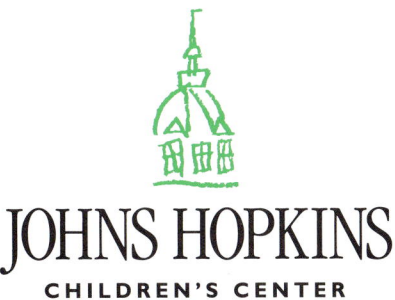

A MANUAL FOR PEDIATRIC HOUSE OFFICERS

THE HARRIET LANE HANDBOOK

TWENTY-FIRST EDITION

The Harriet Lane Service at
The Charlotte R. Bloomberg Children's Center of
The Johns Hopkins Hospital

EDITORS
HELEN K. HUGHES, MD, MPH
LAUREN K. KAHL, MD

ELSEVIER

ELSEVIER

1600 John F. Kennedy Blvd.
Ste 1800
Philadelphia, PA 19103-2899

THE HARRIET LANE HANDBOOK, 21ST EDITION
INTERNATIONAL EDITION
Copyright © 2018 by Elsevier, Inc. All rights reserved.

ISBN: 978-0-323-39955-5
ISBN: 978-0-323-47373-6

No part of this publication may be reproduced or transmitted in any form or by any means, electronic or mechanical, including photocopying, recording, or any information storage and retrieval system, without permission in writing from the publisher. Details on how to seek permission, further information about the Publisher's permissions policies and our arrangements with organizations such as the Copyright Clearance Center and the Copyright Licensing Agency, can be found at our website: www.elsevier.com/permissions.

This book and the individual contributions contained in it are protected under copyright by the Publisher (other than as may be noted herein).

Notices

Knowledge and best practice in this field are constantly changing. As new research and experience broaden our understanding, changes in research methods, professional practices, or medical treatment may become necessary.

Practitioners and researchers must always rely on their own experience and knowledge in evaluating and using any information, methods, compounds, or experiments described herein. In using such information or methods they should be mindful of their own safety and the safety of others, including parties for whom they have a professional responsibility.

With respect to any drug or pharmaceutical products identified, readers are advised to check the most current information provided (i) on procedures featured or (ii) by the manufacturer of each product to be administered, to verify the recommended dose or formula, the method and duration of administration, and contraindications. It is the responsibility of practitioners, relying on their own experience and knowledge of their patients, to make diagnoses, to determine dosages and the best treatment for each individual patient, and to take all appropriate safety precautions.

To the fullest extent of the law, neither the Publisher nor the authors, contributors, or editors, assume any liability for any injury and/or damage to persons or property as a matter of products liability, negligence or otherwise, or from any use or operation of any methods, products, instructions, or ideas contained in the material herein.

Previous editions copyrighted 2015, 2012, 2009, 2005, 2002, 2000, 1996, 1993, 1991, 1987, 1984, 1981, 1978, 1975, 1972, and 1969.

Library of Congress Cataloging-in-Publication Data

Names: Harriet Lane Service (Johns Hopkins Hospital), author. | Hughes, Helen (Helen Kinsman), editor. | Kahl, Lauren, editor.
Title: The Harriet Lane handbook : a manual for pediatric house officers / The Harriet Lane Service at The Charlotte R. Bloomberg Children's Center of The Johns Hopkins Hospital ; editors, Helen Hughes, Lauren Kahl.
Description: Twenty-first edition. | Philadelphia, PA : Elsevier, [2018] | Includes bibliographical references and index.
Identifiers: LCCN 2016048390 | ISBN 9780323399555 (pbk. : alk. paper) |
 ISBN 9780323473736 (international edition)
Subjects: | MESH: Pediatrics | Handbooks
Classification: LCC RJ48 | NLM WS 29 | DDC 618.92—dc23 LC record available at https://lccn.loc.gov/2016048390

Executive Content Strategist: Jim Merritt
Senior Content Development Specialist: Jennifer Ehlers
Publishing Services Manager: Patricia Tannian

Senior Project Manager: Cindy Thoms
Book Designer: Ashley Miner

Printed in United States of America

Last digit is the print number: 9 8 7 6 5 4 3 2

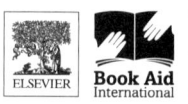

Working together
to grow libraries in
developing countries

www.elsevier.com • www.bookaid.org

To our families
Emily Fairchild, you are my selfless champion, cheerleader, and role model. Stephen Kinsman, thank you for giving me your unwavering support and infectious love of pediatrics. Andrew Hughes, you have given me a better life—and family—than I ever thought possible. Oliver, you are the light of my life.

Lorraine Kahl, my loving mother, thank you for your endless encouragement and example of insurmountable strength. Richard Kahl, my wonderful father, may everything I do be a reflection of you; I miss you every day. Richie Kahl, your resilience is an inspiration. Michael Untiet, thank you for your unconditional love and support that continues to challenge me and push me forward.

To our patients and their families
We will be forever grateful for the trust that you have placed in us.

To our residents
We are inspired daily by your hard work, resilience, and commitment to this noble profession.

To the consummate pediatricians and educators
George Dover and Julia McMillan

To our role model, teacher, and friend
Janet Serwint

And to
Tina Cheng,
Pediatrician-in-Chief,
The Johns Hopkins Hospital,
Fearless advocate for children, adolescents, and families

In loving memory of Dr. Idoreyin P. Montague

Preface

"Why this child? Why this disease? Why now?"

—Barton Childs, MD

The Harriet Lane Handbook was first developed in 1953 after Harrison Spencer (chief resident in 1950–1951) suggested that residents should write a pocket-sized "pearl book." As recounted by Henry Seidel, the first editor of *The Harriet Lane Handbook,* "Six of us began without funds and without [the] supervision of our elders, meeting sporadically around a table in the library of the Harriet Lane Home." The product of their efforts was a concise yet comprehensive handbook that became an indispensable tool for the residents of the Harriet Lane Home. Ultimately, Robert Cooke (department chief, 1956–1974) realized the potential of the handbook, and, with his backing, the fifth edition was published for widespread distribution by Year Book. Since that time, the handbook has been regularly updated and rigorously revised to reflect the most up-to-date information and clinical guidelines available. It has grown from a humble Hopkins resident "pearl book" to become a nationally and internationally respected clinical resource. Now translated into many languages, the handbook is still intended as an easy-to-use manual to help pediatricians provide current and comprehensive pediatric care.

Today, *The Harriet Lane Handbook* continues to be updated and revised *by* house officers *for* house officers. Recognizing the limit to what can be included in a pocket guide, additional information has been placed online and for use via mobile applications. This symbol throughout the chapters denotes online content in Expert Consult. The online-only content includes expanded text, tables, additional images, and other references.

In addition to including the most up-to-date guidelines, practice parameters, and references, we will highlight some of the most important improvements in the twenty-first edition of *The Harriet Lane Handbook:*

The **Procedures** chapter has been expanded, with increased online content dedicated to ultrasound and ultrasound-guided procedures.

The **Adolescent Medicine** chapter includes expanded information on sexually transmitted infections and pelvic inflammatory disease.

The **Dermatology** chapter includes new sections on nail disorders and disorders of pigmentation as well as an updated discussion of treatment for acne.

The **Fluids and Electrolytes** chapter has been restructured to aid in fluid and electrolyte calculations at the bedside.

The **Genetics** chapter has been expanded to include many more genetic conditions relevant to the pediatric house officer as well as a streamlined discussion of the relevant laboratory work-up for these conditions.

x   Preface

The **Microbiology and Infectious Disease** chapter includes expanded information related to fever of unknown origin, lymphadenopathy, and viral infections.

Medications listed in the **Formulary Adjunct** chapter have been moved to the **Formulary** for ease of reference.

The Harriet Lane Handbook, designed for pediatric house staff, was made possible by the extraordinary efforts of this year's senior resident class. It had been an honor to watch these fine doctors mature and refine their skills since internship. They have balanced their busy work schedules and personal lives while authoring the chapters that follow. We are grateful to each of them along with their faculty advisors, who selflessly dedicated their time to improve the quality and content of this publication. The high quality of this handbook is representative of our residents, who are the heart and soul of our department.

Chapter Title	Resident	Faculty Advisor
1. Emergency Management	Vanessa Ozomaro Jeffries, MD	Justin M. Jeffers, MD
2. Poisonings	Michael Hrdy, MD	Mitchell Goldstein, MD
3. Procedures	James H. Miller, MD	Erik Su, MD
	Matthew Moake, MD, PhD	Thuy L. Ngo, DO, MEd
4. Trauma, Burns, and Common Critical Care Emergencies	Amanda O'Halloran, MD	Branden Engorn, MD
		Lewis Romer, MD
		Melissa J Sacco, MD
		Dylan Stewart, MD
5. Adolescent Medicine	Kimberly M. Dickinson, MD, MPH	Krishna Upadhya, MD, MPH
		Renata Sanders, MD, MHS, ScM
6. Analgesia and Procedural Sedation	Jessica Berger, MD	Myron Yaster, MD
	Keri Borden Koszela, MD	
7. Cardiology	Madiha Raees, MD	Jane Crosson, MD
		William Ravekes, MD
		W. Reid Thompson, MD
8. Dermatology	Taisa Kohut, MD	Bernard Cohen, MD
	Angela Orozco, MD	
9. Development, Behavior, and Mental Health	Julia Thorn, MD	Emily Frosch, MD
		Alexander Hoon, MD, MPH
10. Endocrinology*	Jessica Jack, MD	David Cooke, MD
	Sarah Brunelli Young, MD, MS	
11. Fluids and Electrolytes	Candice M. Nalley, MD	Eric Balighian, MD
		Michael Barone, MD, MPH
12. Gastroenterology	Nina Guo, MD	Darla Shores, MD
	Ammarah Iqbal, MD, MPH	
13. Genetics: Metabolism and Dysmorphology	Christina Peroutka, MD	Joann Bodurtha, MD, MPH
		Ada Hamosh, MD, MPH
14. Hematology	Katherine Costa, MD	James Casella, MD
		Clifford Takemoto, MD
15. Immunology and Allergy	Jeremy Snyder, MD	Robert Wood, MD
		M. Elizabeth M. Younger, CRNP, PhD
16. Immunoprophylaxis	Alejandra Ellison-Barnes, MD	Ravit Boger, MD
17. Microbiology and Infectious Disease	Devan Jaganath, MD, MPH	Pranita D. Tamma, MD, MHS
	Rebecca G. Same, MD	

Chapter Title	Resident	Faculty Advisor
18. Neonatology	Jennifer Fundora, MD	Susan W. Aucott, MD
19. Nephrology	Riddhi Desai, MD, MPH	Jeffrey Fadrowski, MD, MHS
20. Neurology	Clare Stevens, MD	Thomas Crawford, MD
		Ryan Felling, MD, PhD
		Eric Kossoff, MD
		Christopher Oakley, MD
21. Nutrition and Growth	Brandon Smith, MD	Darla Shores, MD
	Jenifer Thompson, MS, RD, CSP	
22. Oncology	Chelsea Kotch, MD	Patrick Brown, MD
	Zarah Yusuf, MD	Nicole Arwood, PharmD, BCPPS
23. Palliative Care	Daniel Hindman, MD	Nancy Hutton, MD
		Matt Norvell, MDiv, MS, BCC
24. Pulmonology	Jason Gillon, MD	Laura Sterni, MD
25. Radiology	Kameron Lockamy Rogers, MD	Jane Benson, MD
26. Rheumatology	Nayimisha Balmuri, MD	Sangeeta Sule, MD, PhD
27. Blood Chemistries and Body Fluids	Helen K. Hughes, MD, MPH	Allison Chambliss, PhD
	Lauren K. Kahl, MD	Lori Sokoll, PhD
28. Biostatistics and Evidence-Based Medicine	Anirudh Ramesh, MD	Megan M. Tschudy, MD, MPH
29. Drug Dosages	Carlton K.K. Lee, PharmD, MPH	
30. Drugs in Renal Failure	Elizabeth A.S. Goswami, PharmD, BCPS, BCPPS	Carlton K.K. Lee, PharmD, MPH
	Helen K. Hughes, MD, MPH	

*A special thank you to Paula Neira, MSN, JD, RN, CEN, and Renata Sanders, MD, MPH, ScM, for their gracious time and efforts on the gender dysphoria section of this chapter.

The Formulary, which is undoubtedly the most popular handbook section, is complete, concise, and up to date thanks to the tireless efforts of Carlton K.K. Lee, PharmD, MPH. With each edition, he carefully updates, revises, and improves the section. His herculean efforts make the Formulary one of the most useful and cited pediatric drug reference texts available.

We are grateful and humbled to have the opportunity to build on the great work of the preceding editors: Drs. Henry Seidel, Harrison Spencer, William Friedman, Robert Haslam, Jerry Winkelstein, Herbert Swick, Dennis Headings, Kenneth Schuberth, Basil Zitelli, Jeffery Biller, Andrew Yeager, Cynthia Cole, Peter Rowe, Mary Greene, Kevin Johnson, Michael Barone, George Siberry, Robert Iannone, Veronica Gunn, Christian Nechyba, Jason Robertson, Nicole Shilkofski, Jason Custer, Rachel Rau, Megan Tschudy, Kristin Arcara, Jamie Flerlage, and Branden Engorn. Many of these previous editors continue to make important contributions to the education of the Harriet Lane house staff. As recent editors, Megan Tschudy, Jamie Flerlage, and Branden Engorn have been instrumental in helping us to navigate this process. We hope to live up to the legacy of these many outstanding clinicians, educators, and mentors.

An undertaking of this magnitude could not have been accomplished without the support and dedication of some extraordinary people. First, thanks to Kathy Mainhart, who is an invaluable asset to our program.

Without her guidance, we would all be lost. We are indebted to Dr. George Dover, whose tireless promotion of the Harriet Lane housestaff will be forever remembered – you will always have a home in our office. Thank you to Dr. Julia McMillan for your advocacy, wisdom, and kindness in our early days as editors. We owe much of the *Handbook*'s success to your expert leadership. To our new Department Director, Dr. Tina Cheng, we are so grateful for your mentorship and guidance – we can't wait to see your vision for the Children's Center take shape. Our special thanks go to our friends and mentors, Jeffrey Fadrowski and Thuy Ngo, for your unwavering support and timely reality checks. Finally, thank you to our program director, Janet Serwint, whose leadership and passion for education have enriched our lives, and the lives of hundreds of other Harriet Lane house staff. Your endless enthusiasm for pediatrics is inspiring to us all.

Residents	Interns
Ifunanya Agbim	Megan Askew
Suzanne Al-Hamad	Brittany Badesch
Madeleine Alvin	Samantha Bapty
Caren Armstrong	Jeanette Beaudry
Stephanie Baker	Victor Benevenuto
Mariju Baluyot	Eva Catenaccio
Justin Berk	Kristen Cercone
Alissa Cerny	Danielle deCampo
Kristen Coletti	Caroline DeBoer
John Creagh	Jonathan Eisenberg
Matthew DiGiusto	Amnha Elusta
Dana Furstenau	Lucas Falco
Zachary Gitlin	RaeLynn Forsyth
Meghan Kiley	Hanae Fujii-Rios
Keith Kleinman	Samuel Gottlieb
Theodore Kouo	Deborah Hall
Cecilia Kwak	Stephanie Hanke
Jasmine Lee-Barber	Brooke Krbec
Laura Livaditis	Marguerite Lloyd
Laura Malone	Nethra Madurai
Lauren McDaniel	Azeem Muritala
Matthew Molloy	Anisha Nadkarni
Joseph Muller	Chioma Nnamdi-Emetarom
Keren Muller	Maxine Pottenger
Robin Ortiz	Jessica Ratner
Chetna Pande	Harita Shah
Thomas Rappold	Soha Shah
Emily Stryker	Rachel Troch
Claudia Suarez-Makotsi	Jo Wilson
Jaclyn Tamaroff	Philip Zegelbone
	Lindy Zhang

Helen K. Hughes
Lauren K. Kahl

Contents

PART I Pediatric Acute Care

1. Emergency Management 2
   Vanessa Ozomaro Jeffries, MD

2. Poisonings 20
   Michael Hrdy, MD

3. Procedures 30
   James H. Miller, MD, and Matthew Moake, MD, PhD

4. Trauma, Burns, and Common Critical Care Emergencies 73
   Amanda O'Halloran, MD

PART II Diagnostic and Therapeutic Information

5. Adolescent Medicine 108
   Kimberly M. Dickinson, MD, MPH

6. Analgesia and Procedural Sedation 136
   Jessica Berger, MD, and Keri Borden Koszela, MD

7. Cardiology 156
   Madiha Raees, MD

8. Dermatology 203
   Taisa Kohut, MD, and Angela Orozco, MD

9. Development, Behavior, and Mental Health 229
   Julia Thorn, MD

10. Endocrinology 255
    Jessica Jack, MD, and Sarah Brunelli Young, MD, MS

11. Fluids and Electrolytes 290
    Candice M. Nalley, MD

12. Gastroenterology 316
    Nina Guo, MD, and Ammarah Iqbal, MD, MPH

13. Genetics: Metabolism and Dysmorphology 333
    Christina Peroutka, MD

14. Hematology 364
    Katherine Costa, MD

15. Immunology and Allergy 395
    Jeremy Snyder, MD

16. Immunoprophylaxis 412
    Alejandra Ellison-Barnes, MD

17. Microbiology and Infectious Disease 443
    Devan Jaganath, MD, MPH, and Rebecca G. Same, MD

18. Neonatology 490
    Jennifer Fundora, MD

- 19 Nephrology 516
  Riddhi Desai, MD, MPH
- 20 Neurology 548
  Clare Stevens, MD
- 21 Nutrition and Growth 570
  Brandon Smith, MD, and Jenifer Thompson, MS, RD, CSP
- 22 Oncology 607
  Chelsea Kotch, MD, and Zarah Yusuf, MD
- 23 Palliative Care 628
  Daniel Hindman, MD
- 24 Pulmonology 637
  Jason Gillon, MD
- 25 Radiology 663
  Kameron Lockamy Rogers, MD
- 26 Rheumatology 688
  Nayimisha Balmuri, MD

PART III Reference

- 27 Blood Chemistries and Body Fluids 708
  Helen K. Hughes, MD, MPH, and Lauren K. Kahl, MD
- 28 Biostatistics and Evidence-Based Medicine 721
  Anirudh Ramesh, MD

PART IV Formulary

- 29 Drug Dosages 732
  Carlton K.K. Lee, PharmD, MPH
- 30 Drugs in Renal Failure 1110
  Elizabeth A.S. Goswami, PharmD, BCPS, BCPPS, and Helen K. Hughes, MD, MPH

PART I

PEDIATRIC ACUTE CARE

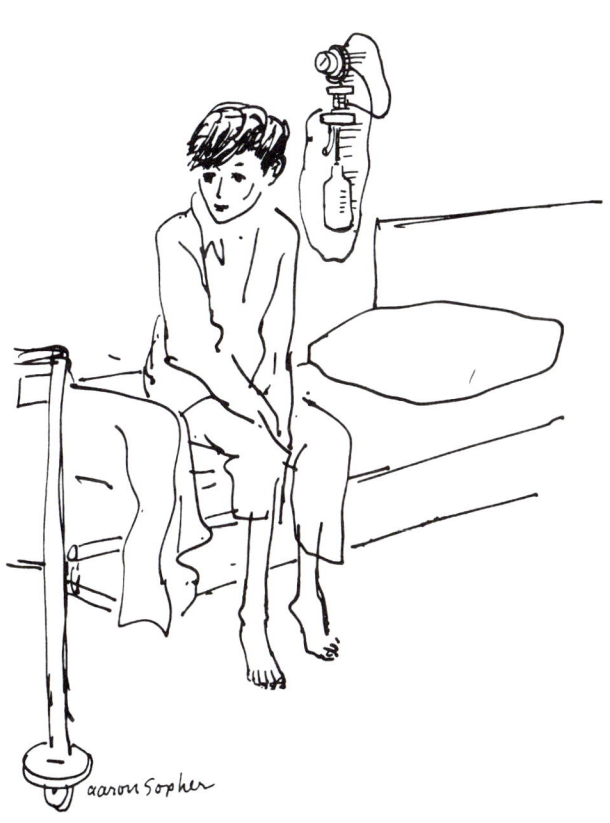

Chapter 1
Emergency Management
Vanessa Ozomaro Jeffries, MD

Pediatric emergency management begins with a general observational assessment—a brief assessment of a patient's general appearance, quality of breathing, and color can help one quickly identify the presence of a life threatening condition and determine next steps for intervention.[1] In the event of **sudden cardiac arrest**, providers should use the acronym C-A-B (circulation/chest compressions–airway–breathing), of which immediate chest compressions is the first step in management (see 2015 American Heart Association CPR guidelines). This section is presented in the C-A-B format to emphasize the importance of immediate, high-quality chest compressions in improving patient outcomes. The original A-B-C pathway remains the accepted method for rapid assessment and management of any critically ill patient.[2,6] If no imminent life threatening problem is identified, then one should proceed with a rapid primary assessment of the A, B, C, D, and Es. The history, physical exam, and laboratory studies should closely follow.

I. CIRCULATION[2-9]

A. Assessment

1. **Perfusion:**
a. Assess pulse: If infant/child is unresponsive and not breathing (gasps do not count as breathing), healthcare providers **may take up to 10 seconds** to feel for pulse (brachial in infants, carotid/femoral in children).[2]
    (1) **If pulseless**, immediately begin chest compressions (see Circulation, B.1).
    (2) **If pulse**, begin A-B-C pathway of evaluation.
b. Assess capillary refill (<2 s = normal, 2 to 5 s = delayed, and >5 s suggests shock), mentation, and urine output (if urinary catheter in place).
2. **Rate/rhythm:** Assess for bradycardia, tachycardia, abnormal rhythm, or asystole. Generally, bradycardia requiring chest compressions is <60 beats/min; tachycardia of >220 beats/min suggests tachyarrhythmia rather than sinus tachycardia.
3. **Blood pressure (BP):** Hypotension is a late manifestation of circulatory compromise. Can be calculated in children >1 year with following formula:

$$\text{Hypotension} = \text{Systolic BP} < [70 + (2 \times \text{age in years})]$$

TABLE 1.1
MANAGEMENT OF CIRCULATION[3-5]

	Infants	Prepubertal Children	Adolescents/Adults
Location	1 fingerbreadth below intermammary line	2 fingerbreadths below intermammary line	Lower half of sternum
Rate	100–120 per minute	—	—
Depth*	1½ inches (4 cm)	2 inches (5 cm)	2–2.4 inches (5 cm)
Compressions: Ventilation†	15:2 (2 rescuers) 30:2 (1 rescuer)	15:2 (2 rescuers) 30:2 (1 rescuer)	30:2 (1 or 2 rescuers)

*Depth of compressions should be at least one-third of anteroposterior diameter of the chest. Depth values are approximations for most infants and children.
†If intubated, give one breath every 6–8 seconds (8–10/min) without interrupting chest compressions. If there is return of spontaneous circulation, give one breath every 3–5 seconds.

B. Management (Table 1.1)[3,4]

1. **Chest compressions**
   a. Press hard (see Table 1.1 for age-specific depth of compression) and fast (100–120 per minute) on backboard base and allow full recoil and minimal interruption.
   b. For infants, two-thumb technique with hands encircling chest is preferred. Use two-finger technique for infants if only single rescuer available.
   c. Use end-tidal CO_2 to estimate effectiveness (<20 mmHg indicates inadequate compressions).
2. **Use of automated external defibrillator (AED):** To determine whether rhythm is shockable, use an AED/defibrillator. In infants aged <1 year, a manual defibrillator is preferred. If not available, use available AED. Pediatric dose attenuator preferred (if available).
3. **Resuscitation with poor perfusion and shock:**
   a. Optimize oxygen delivery with supplemental O_2.
   b. Support respirations to reduce work of patient.
   c. Place intraosseous (IO) access immediately if in arrest and/or if intravenous (IV) access not obtained within 90 seconds.
   d. Resuscitation fluids are isotonic crystalloids (lactated Ringer's solution or normal saline).
      (1) Give up to three 20-mL/kg boluses each within 5 minutes for a total of 60 mL/kg in the first 15 minutes after presentation; reassess patient and check for hepatomegaly after each bolus. The 2015 AHA guidelines recommend extreme caution with administration of bolus IV fluids, especially if critical care resources are not available.
      (2) 5- to 10-mL/kg bolus in patients with known or suspected cardiac insufficiency.
      (3) Consider inotropic support (see Chapter 4 for shock management).

(4) Consider colloids such as albumin, plasma, or packed red blood cells if poor response to crystalloids.
e. Identify type of shock: Hypovolemia, cardiogenic (congenital heart disease, myocarditis, cardiomyopathy, arrhythmia), distributive (sepsis, anaphylaxis, neurogenic), obstructive [pulmonary embolus (PE), cardiac tamponade, tension pneumothorax].
f. Pharmacotherapy (see inside front cover and consider stress-dose corticosteroids and/or antibiotics if applicable.)

II. AIRWAY[7-10]

A. Assessment

1. **Assess airway patency; think about obstruction:** Head tilt/chin lift (or jaw thrust if injury suspected) to open airway. Avoid overextension in infants, as this may occlude airway.
2. **Assess for spontaneous respiration:** If no spontaneous respirations, begin ventilating via rescue breaths, bag-mask, or endotracheal tube.
3. **Assess adequacy of respirations:**
a. Look for chest rise.
b. Recognize signs of distress (grunting, stridor, tachypnea, flaring, retractions, accessory muscle use, wheezes).

B. Management[7-17]

1. **Equipment**
a. Bag-mask ventilation may be used indefinitely if ventilating effectively (look at chest rise). Cricoid pressure (Sellick maneuver) can be used to minimize gastric inflation and aspiration; however, excessive use should be avoided as to not obstruct the trachea.
b. If available, consider $EtCO_2$ as measure of effective ventilation.
c. Use oral or nasopharyngeal airway in patients with obstruction:
   (1) Oral: Unconscious patients—measure from corner of mouth to mandibular angle.
   (2) Nasal: Conscious patients—measure from tip of nose to tragus of ear.
d. Laryngeal mask airway: Simple way to secure an airway (no laryngoscopy needed), especially in difficult airways; does not prevent aspiration.
2. **Intubation:** Indicated for (impending) respiratory failure, obstruction, airway protection, pharmacotherapy, or need for likely prolonged support
a. Equipment: **SOAP-ME** (**S**uction, **O**xygen, **A**irway Supplies, **P**harmacology, **M**onitoring **E**quipment)
   (1) Laryngoscope blade:
      (a) Miller (straight blade):
         (i) #00–1 for premature to 2 months
         (ii) #1 for 3 months to 3 years
         (iii) #2 for >3 years

(b) Macintosh (curved blade):
    (i) #2 for >2 years
    (ii) #3 for >8 years
(2) Endotracheal tube (ETT): Both cuffed and uncuffed ETT are acceptable, but cuffed is preferred in certain populations (i.e., poor lung compliance, high airway resistance, glottic air leak, or between ages 1–2 years)
    (a) Size determination:
        (i) Cuffed ETT (mm) = (age/4) + 3.5
        (ii) Uncuffed ETT (mm) = (age/4) + 4
        (iii) Use length-based resuscitation tape to estimate
    (b) Approximate depth of insertion in cm = ETT size × 3
    (c) Stylet should not extend beyond the distal end of the ETT
    (d) Attach end-tidal CO_2 monitor as confirmation of placement and effectiveness of chest compressions if applicable
(3) Nasogastric tube (NGT): To decompress the stomach; measure from nose to angle of jaw to xiphoid for depth of insertion
b. Rapid sequence intubation (RSI) recommended for aspiration risk:
    (1) Preoxygenate with nonrebreather at 100% O_2 for minimum of 3 minutes:
        (a) Do not use positive-pressure ventilation (PPV) unless patient effort is inadequate
        (b) Children have less oxygen/respiratory reserve than adults, owing to higher oxygen consumption and lower functional residual capacity
    (2) See Fig. 1.1 and Table 1.2 for drugs used for RSI (adjunct, sedative, paralytic). Important considerations in choosing appropriate agents include clinical scenario, allergies, presence of neuromuscular disease, anatomic abnormalities, or hemodynamic status.
    (3) For patients who are difficult to mask ventilate or have difficult airways, consider sedation without paralysis and the assistance of subspecialists (anesthesiology and otolaryngology).
c. Procedure (attempts should not exceed 30 seconds):
    (1) Preoxygenate with 100% O_2.
    (2) Administer intubation medications (see Fig. 1.1 and Table 1.1).
    (3) Use of cricoid pressure to prevent aspiration during bag-valve-mask ventilation and intubation is optional. (Note: No benefit of cricoid pressure has been demonstrated. Do not continue if it interferes with ventilation or speed of intubation.)
    (4) Use scissoring technique to open mouth.
    (5) Hold laryngoscope blade in left hand. Insert blade into right side of mouth, sweeping tongue to the left out of line of vision.
    (6) Advance blade to epiglottis. With straight blade, lift up, directly lifting the epiglottis to view cords. With curved blade, place tip in vallecula, elevate the epiglottis to visualize the vocal cords.

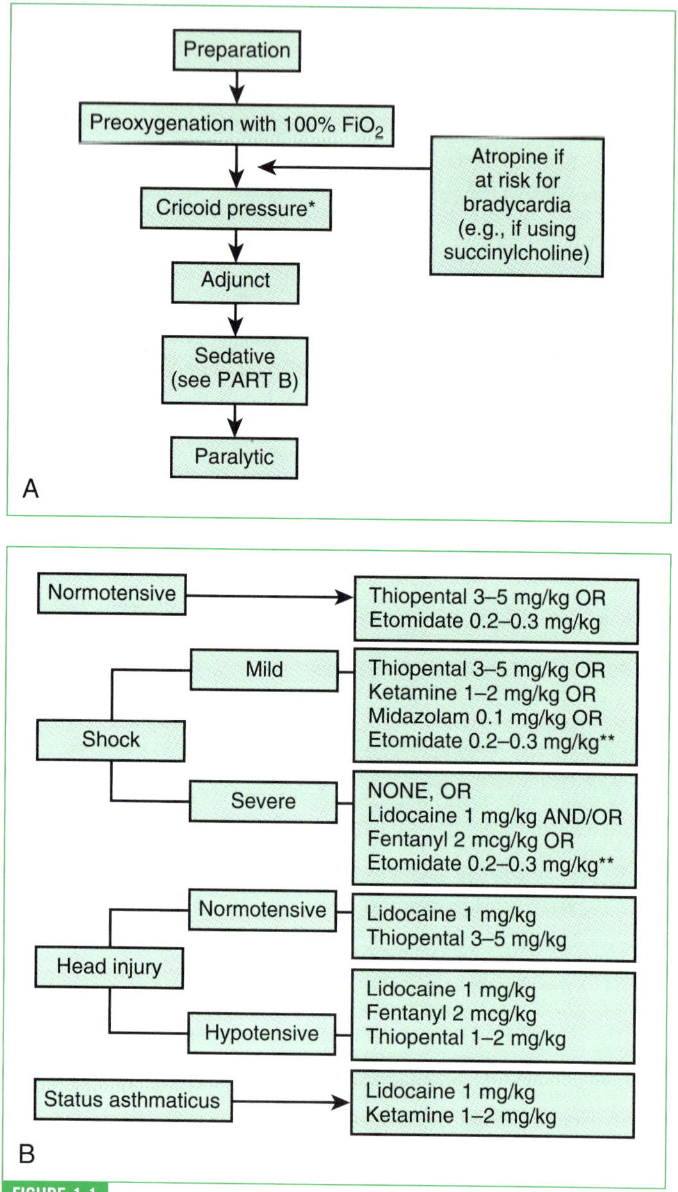

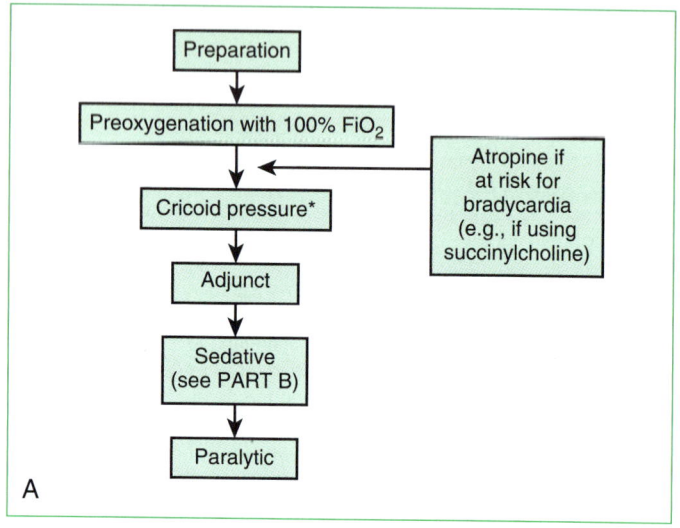

FIGURE 1.1

A, Treatment algorithm for intubation. **B,** Sedation options. *No benefit of cricoid pressure has been demonstrated. Do not continue if it interferes with ventilation or speed of intubation. **Do not use routinely in patients with septic shock. (*Modified from Nichols DG, Yaster M, Lappe DG, et al., eds. Golden Hour: The Handbook of Advanced Pediatric Life Support. St Louis: Mosby; 1996:29.*)

TABLE 1.2
RAPID-SEQUENCE INTUBATION MEDICATIONS

Drug	Dose	Comments
ADJUNCTS (FIRST)		
Atropine (vagolytic)	0.02 mg/kg IV/IO Adult dose: 0.5–1.0 mg; max: 3 mg	+ Vagolytic; prevents bradycardia and reduces oral secretions − Tachycardia, pupil dilation eliminates ability to examine cardiovascular and neurologic status (i.e., pupillary reflexes) No minimum dose when using as premedication for intubation **Indication:** High risk of bradycardia (i.e., succinylcholine use)
Lidocaine (optional anesthetic)	1 mg/kg IV/IO; max 100 mg/dose	+ Blunts ICP spike, decreased gag/cough; controls ventricular arrhythmias **Indication:** Good premedication for shock, arrhythmia, elevated ICP, and status asthmaticus
SEDATIVE-HYPNOTIC (SECOND)		
Thiopental (barbiturate)	3–5 mg/kg IV/IO if normotensive 1–2 mg/kg IV/IO if hypotensive	+ Decreases O_2 consumption and cerebral blood flow − Vasodilation and myocardial depression; may increase oral secretions, cause bronchospasm/laryngospasm (not to be used for asthma) **Indication:** Drug of choice for increased ICP
Ketamine (NMDA receptor antagonist)	1–2 mg/kg IV/IO or 4–10 mg/kg IM	+ Bronchodilation; catecholamine release may benefit hemodynamically unstable patients − May increase BP, HR, and oral secretions; may cause laryngospasm; contraindicated in eye injuries; likely insignificant rise in ICP **Indication:** Drug of choice for asthma
Midazolam (benzodiazepine)	0.05–0.1 mg/kg IV/IO Max total dose of 10 mg	+ Amnestic and anticonvulsant properties − Respiratory depression/apnea, hypotension, and myocardial depression **Indication:** Mild shock
Fentanyl (opiate)	1–3 mcg/kg IV/IO **NOTE:** Fentanyl is dosed in mcg/kg, not mg/kg	+ Fewest hemodynamic effects of all opiates − Chest wall rigidity with high dose or rapid administration; cannot use with MAOIs **Indication:** Shock
Etomidate (imidazole/hypnotic)	0.2–0.3 mg/kg IV/IO	+ Cardiovascular neutral; decreases ICP − Exacerbates adrenal insufficiency by inhibiting 11-beta-hydroxylase **Indication:** Patients with severe shock, especially cardiac patients. (Do not use routinely in patients with septic shock)

Continued

TABLE 1.2
RAPID-SEQUENCE INTUBATION MEDICATIONS—cont'd

Drug	Dose	Comments
Propofol (sedative-hypnotic)	2 mg/kg IV/IO	+ Extremely quick onset and short duration; blood pressure lowering; good antiemetic − Hypotension and profound myocardial depression; contraindicated in patients with egg allergy **Indication:** Induction agent for general anesthesia
PARALYTICS (NEUROMUSCULAR BLOCKERS) (THIRD)		
Succinylcholine (depolarizing)	1–2 mg/kg IV/IO 2–4 mg/kg IM	+ Quick onset (30–60 s), short duration (3–6 min) make it an ideal paralytic − Irreversible; bradycardia in <5 years old or with rapid doses; increased risk of malignant hyperthermia; contraindicated in burns, massive trauma/muscle injury, neuromuscular disease, myopathies, eye injuries, renal insufficiency
Vecuronium (nondepolarizing)	0.1 mg/kg IV/IO	+ Onset 70–120 s; cardiovascular neutral − Duration 30–90 min; must wait 30–45 min to reverse with glycopyrrolate and neostigmine **Indication:** When succinylcholine contraindicated or when longer term paralysis desired
Rocuronium (nondepolarizing)	0.6–1.2 mg/kg IV/IO	+ Quicker onset (30–60 s), shorter acting than vecuronium; cardiovascular neutral − Duration 30–60 min; may reverse in 30 min with glycopyrrolate and neostigmine

+, Potential advantages; −, potential disadvantages or cautions; BP, blood pressure; HR, heart rate; ICP, intracranial pressure; IM, intramuscular; IO, intraosseous infusion; IV, intravenous; MAOI, monoamine oxidase inhibitor; NMDA, N-methyl-D-aspartate.

(7) If possible, have another person hand over the tube, maintaining direct visualization, and pass through cords until black marker reaches the level of the cords.
(8) Hold ETT firmly against the lip until tube is securely taped.
(9) Verify ETT placement: observe chest wall movement, auscultation in both axillae and epigastrium, end-tidal CO_2 detection (there will be a false-negative response if there is no effective pulmonary circulation), improvement in oxygen saturation, chest radiograph, and repeat direct laryngoscopy to visualize ETT.
(10) If available, in-line continuous CO_2 detection should be used.
(11) If patient is in cardiac arrest, continue chest compressions as long as possible during intubation process to minimize interruptions in compressions.

III. BREATHING[2,7,8,18]

A. Assessment
Once airway is secured, continually reevaluate ETT positioning (listen for breath sounds). Acute respiratory failure may signify **D**isplacement of the ETT, **O**bstruction, **P**neumothorax, or **E**quipment failure (DOPE).

B. Management
1. **Mouth-to-mouth or mouth-to-nose breathing:** provide two slow breaths (1 sec/breath) initially. For newborns, apply one breath for every three chest compressions. In infants and children, apply two breaths after 30 compressions (one rescuer) or two breaths after 15 compressions (two rescuers). Breaths should have adequate volume to cause chest rise.
2. **Bag-mask ventilation** is used at a rate of 20 breaths/min (30 breaths/min in infants) using the E-C technique:
a. Use nondominant hand to create a C with thumb and index finger over top of mask. Ensure a good seal, but *do not* push down on mask. Hook remaining fingers around the mandible (*not* the soft tissues of the neck), with the fifth finger on the angle creating an E, and lift the mandible up toward the mask.
b. Assess chest expansion and breath sounds.
c. Decompress stomach with orogastric or NGT with prolonged bag-mask ventilation.
3. **Endotracheal intubation:** See prior section.

IV. ALLERGIC EMERGENCIES (ANAPHYLAXIS)[19,20]

A. Definition
1. **A rapid-onset immunoglobulin (Ig) E–mediated systemic allergic reaction involving multiple organ systems, including two or more of the following:**
a. **Cutaneous/mucosal** (flushing, urticaria, pruritus, angioedema); seen in 90%
b. **Respiratory** (laryngeal edema, bronchospasm, dyspnea, wheezing, stridor, hypoxemia); seen in ≈70%
c. **Gastrointestinal (GI)** (vomiting, diarrhea, nausea, crampy abdominal pain); seen in ≈40% to 50%
d. **Circulatory** (tachycardia, hypotension, syncope); seen in ≈30% to 40%
2. **Initial reaction may be delayed for several hours AND symptoms may recur up to 72 hours after initial recovery.** Patients should therefore be observed for a minimum of 6 to 24 hours for late-phase symptoms.

B. Initial Management
1. **Remove/stop exposure to precipitating antigen.**
2. **Epinephrine** = mainstay of therapy. While performing ABCs, immediately give intramuscular (IM) epinephrine, 0.01 mg/kg

(0.01 mL/kg) of 1:1000 subcutaneously (SQ) or IM (maximum dose 0.5 mg). Repeat every 5 minutes as needed. Site of choice is lateral aspect of the thigh, owing to its vascularity.
3. **Establish airway**, and give O_2 and PPV as needed.
4. Obtain IV access, Trendelenburg position with head 30 degrees below feet, administer fluid boluses followed by cardiac inotropes as needed (see Chapter 4).
5. **Histamine-1 receptor antagonist** such as diphenhydramine, 1 to 2 mg/kg via IM, IV, or oral (PO) route (maximum dose, 50 mg). Also consider a histamine-2 receptor antagonist (e.g., ranitidine).
6. **Corticosteroids** help prevent the late phase of the allergic response. Administer methylprednisolone in a 2-mg/kg IV bolus, followed by 2 mg/kg/day IV or IM, divided every 6 hours, or prednisone, 2 mg/kg PO once daily.
7. **Albuterol** 2.5 mg for <30 kg, 5 mg for >30 kg, for bronchospasm or wheezing. Repeat every 15 minutes as needed.
8. **Racemic epinephrine** 0.5 mL of 2.25% solution inhaled for signs of upper airway obstruction.
9. Patient should be discharged with an **Epi-Pen** (>30 kg), **Epi-Pen Junior** (<30 kg), or comparable injectable epinephrine product with specific instructions on appropriate use, as well as an anaphylaxis action plan.

V. RESPIRATORY EMERGENCIES[21]

The hallmark of upper airway obstruction is stridor, whereas lower airway obstruction is characterized by cough, wheeze, and a prolonged expiratory phase.

A. Asthma[22-25]

Lower airway obstruction resulting from triad of inflammation, bronchospasm, and increased secretions:
1. **Assessment:** Respiratory rate (RR), work of breathing, O_2 saturation, heart rate (HR), peak expiratory flow, alertness, color.
2. **Initial management:**
a. Give O_2 to keep saturation >95%.
b. Administer inhaled β-agonists: metered-dose inhaler or nebulized albuterol as often as needed.
c. Ipratropium bromide.
d. Steroids:
   (1) Severe illness: methylprednisolone, 2 mg/kg IV/IM bolus, then 2 mg/kg/day divided every 6 hours
   (2) Mild-to-moderate illness: prednisone/prednisolone 2 mg/kg (max 60 mg) PO every 24 hours for 5 days OR dexamethasone 0.6 mg/kg (max 16 mg) every 24 hours for 2 days
   (3) Systemic steroids require a minimum of 2–4 hours to take effect

e. If air movement is still poor despite maximizing above therapy:
   (1) Epinephrine: 0.01 mg/kg (0.01 mL/kg) of 1:1000 SQ or IM (maximum dose 0.5 mg)
      (a) Bronchodilator, vasopressor, and inotropic effects
      (b) Short acting (~15 min) and should be used as temporizing rather than definitive therapy
   (2) Terbutaline:
      (a) 0.01 mg/kg SQ (maximum dose 0.4 mg) every 15 minutes for up to three doses
      (b) IV terbutaline—consider if no response to second dose of SQ (see Further Management section for dosing)
         (i) Limited by cardiac intolerance. Monitor continuous 12-lead electrocardiogram, cardiac enzymes, urinalysis (UA), and electrolytes.
      (c) Consider in severely ill patients or in patients who are uncooperative with inhaled beta agonists
   (3) Magnesium sulfate: 25 to 75 mg/kg/dose IV or IM (maximum 2 grams) infused over 20 minutes
      (a) Smooth muscle relaxant; relieves bronchospasm
      (b) Many clinicians advise giving a saline bolus prior to administration, because hypotension may result
      (c) Contraindicated if patient already has significant hypotension or renal insufficiency
3. **Further management:** If incomplete or poor response, consider obtaining an arterial blood gas value
   NOTE: A normalizing Pco_2 is often a sign of impending respiratory failure.
a. Maximize and continue initial treatments.
b. Terbutaline 2 to 10 mcg/kg IV load, followed by continuous infusion of 0.1 to 0.4 mcg/kg/min titrated to effect in increments of 0.1 to 0.2 mcg/kg/min every 30 minutes depending on clinical response. Infusion should be started with lowest possible dose; doses as high as 10 mcg/kg/min have been used. Use appropriate cardiac monitoring in intensive care unit (ICU), as above.
c. A helium (≥70%) and oxygen mixture may be of some benefit in the critically ill patient, but is more useful in upper airway edema. Avoid use in the hypoxic patient.
d. Noninvasive positive-pressure ventilation (e.g., BiPAP) may be used in patients with impending respiratory failure, both as a temporizing measure and to avoid intubation, but requires a cooperative patient with spontaneous respirations.
e. Methylxanthines (e.g., aminophylline) may be considered in the ICU setting but have significant side effects and have not been shown to affect intubation rates or length of hospital stay.
4. **Intubation** of those with acute asthma is potentially dangerous, and should be reserved for impending respiratory arrest.

a. Indications for endotracheal intubation include deteriorating mental status, severe hypoxemia, and respiratory or cardiac arrest.
b. Intubation can increase airway hyper-responsiveness and obstruction
c. Use lidocaine as adjunct and ketamine for sedative (see Fig. 1.1 and Table 1.1).
d. Consider using an inhaled anesthetic such as isoflurane.
5. Hypotension: Result of air trapping, hyperinflation, and therefore decreased pulmonary venous return. See Section I.B.3 for management. Definitive treatment is reducing lower airway obstruction.

B. Upper Airway Obstruction[26-29]

Upper airway obstruction is most commonly caused by foreign body aspiration or infection.
1. **Epiglottitis:** Most often affects children between 2 and 7 years, but may occur at any age. This is a true emergency involving cellulitis and edema of the epiglottis, aryepiglottic folds, and hypopharynx.
a. Patient is usually febrile, anxious, and toxic appearing, with sore throat, drooling, respiratory distress, stridor, tachypnea, and *tripod positioning* (sitting forward supported by both arms, with neck extended and chin thrust out). Any agitation of the child may cause complete obstruction, so avoid invasive procedures/evaluation until airway is secured.
b. Unobtrusively give O_2 (blow-by). Nothing by mouth, monitor with pulse oximetry, allow parent to hold patient.
c. Summon epiglottitis team (most senior pediatrician, anesthesiologist, intensive care physician, and otolaryngologist in hospital).
d. Management options:
   (1) If unstable (unresponsive, cyanotic, bradycardic) → emergently intubate
   (2) If stable with high suspicion → take patient to operating room for laryngoscopy and intubation under general anesthesia
   (3) If stable with moderate or low suspicion → obtain lateral neck radiographs to confirm
e. After airway is secure, obtain cultures of blood and epiglottic surface. Begin antibiotics to cover *Haemophilus influenzae* type B, *Streptococcus pneumoniae,* group A streptococci, *Staphylococcus aureus*.
f. Epiglottitis may also be caused by thermal injury, caustic ingestion, or foreign body.
2. **Croup (laryngotracheobronchitis):** Most common in infants 6 to 36 months. Croup is a common syndrome involving inflammation of the subglottic area; presents with fever, barking cough, and stridor. Patients rarely appear toxic, as in epiglottitis.
a. Mild (no stridor at rest): Treat with minimal disturbance, cool mist, hydration, antipyretics, and consider steroids.

b. Moderate to severe (stridor at rest with/without respiratory distress).
    (1) Racemic epinephrine. After administering, observe for a minimum of 2 to 4 hours, owing to potential for rebound obstruction. Hospitalize if more than one nebulization required.
    (2) Dexamethasone, 0.3 to 0.6 mg/kg IV, IM, or PO once. Effect lasts 2 to 3 days. Alternatively, nebulized budesonide may be used, although little data exist to support its use, and some studies find it inferior to dexamethasone.
    (3) A helium (≥70%) and oxygen mixture may decrease resistance to turbulent gas flow through a narrowed airway.
    (4) The efficacy of mist therapy is not established.
c. If a child fails to respond as expected to therapy, consider other etiologies (e.g., retropharyngeal abscess, bacterial tracheitis, subglottic stenosis, epiglottitis, foreign body). Obtain airway radiography, computed tomography (CT), and evaluation by otolaryngology or anesthesiology.
3. **Foreign-body aspiration (FBA):** Occurs most often in children aged 6 months to 3 years old. It frequently involves hot dogs, candy, peanuts, grapes, or balloons. Most events are unwitnessed, so suspect this in children with sudden-onset choking, stridor, or wheezing.
a. If FBA is suspected and patient is stable, obtain bilateral lateral decubitus chest X-ray to assess for hyperinflation, atelectasis, and/or mediastinal shift.
b. If there is high index of suspicion and patient is stable (i.e., forcefully coughing, well-oxygenated), removal of the foreign body by bronchoscopy or laryngoscopy should be attempted in a controlled environment. A normal chest X-ray does not rule out FBA.
c. If the patient is unable to speak, moves air poorly, or is cyanotic:
    (1) Infant: Place infant over arm or rest on lap. Give five back blows between the scapulae. If unsuccessful, turn infant over and give five chest thrusts (*not* abdominal thrusts).
    (2) Child: Perform five abdominal thrusts (Heimlich maneuver) from behind a sitting or standing child.
    (3) After back, chest, and/or abdominal thrusts, open mouth using tongue–jaw lift and remove foreign body if visualized. Do not attempt blind finger sweeps. Magill forceps may be used to retrieve objects in the posterior pharynx. Ventilate if unconscious, and repeat sequence as needed.
    (4) If there is complete airway obstruction and the patient cannot be ventilated by bag-valve mask or ETT, consider percutaneous (needle) cricothyrotomy.[8]

VI. NEUROLOGIC EMERGENCIES

A. Altered States of Consciousness[30]

1. **Assessment:** Range of mental status includes alert, confused, disoriented, delirious, lethargic, stuporous, and comatose.

> **BOX 1.1**
> **DIFFERENTIAL DIAGNOSIS OF ALTERED LEVEL OF CONSCIOUSNESS**
>
> **I. Structural Causes**
>
> Vascular—e.g., cerebrovascular accident, cerebral vein thrombosis
> Increased intracranial pressure—e.g., hydrocephalus, tumor, abscess, cyst, subdural empyema, pseudotumor cerebri
> Trauma (intracranial hemorrhage, diffuse cerebral swelling, shaken baby syndrome)
>
> **II. Medical Causes**
>
> Anoxia
> Hypothermia/hyperthermia
> Metabolic—e.g., inborn errors of metabolism, diabetic ketoacidosis, hyperammonemia, uremia, hypoglycemia, electrolyte abnormality
> Infection—e.g., sepsis, meningitis, encephalitis, subdural empyema
> Seizure/postictal state
> Toxins/ingestions
> Psychiatric/psychogenic

Modified from Avner J. Altered states of consciousness. Pediatr Rev. 2006;27:331-337.

a. History: Consider structural versus medical causes (Box 1.1). Obtain history of trauma, ingestion, infection, fasting, drug use, diabetes, seizure, or other neurologic disorder.
b. Examination: Assess HR, BP, respiratory pattern, Glasgow Coma Scale (Table 1.3), temperature, pupillary response, fundoscopy [a late finding, absence of papilledema does not rule out increased intracranial pressure (ICP)], rash, abnormal posturing, and focal neurologic signs.
2. **Acute traumatic head injury:**[31]
a. Assess pupillary response:
    (1) Blown pupil: Elevate head of bed, hyperventilate, maintain BP, administer hypertonic saline and/or mannitol
b. Head imaging: see Trauma, Burns, Critical Care Emergencies chapter for PECARN head imaging criteria[32]
3. **Management of coma:**
a. **A**irway (with cervical spine immobilization), **B**reathing, **C**irculation, **D**-stick, **O**xygen, **N**aloxone, **T**hiamine (ABC DON'T)
    (1) Naloxone, 0.1 mg/kg IV, IM, SQ, or ETT (maximum dose, 2 mg). Repeat as necessary, given short half-life (in case of opiate intoxication)
    (2) Thiamine, 100 mg IV (before starting glucose in adolescents, in case of alcoholism or eating disorder)
    (3) $D_{25}W$, 2 to 4 mL/kg IV bolus if hypoglycemia is present
b. Laboratory tests: Consider complete blood cell count, electrolytes, liver function tests, NH_3, lactate, toxicology screen (serum and urine;

TABLE 1.3
COMA SCALES

Glasgow Coma Scale		Modified Coma Scale for Infants	
Activity	Best Response	Activity	Best Response
EYE OPENING			
Spontaneous	4	Spontaneous	4
To speech	3	To speech	3
To pain	2	To pain	2
None	1	None	1
VERBAL			
Oriented	5	Coo/babbles	5
Confused	4	Irritable	4
Inappropriate words	3	Cries to pain	3
Nonspecific sounds	2	Moans to pain	2
None	1	None	1
MOTOR			
Follows commands	6	Normal, spontaneous movements	6
Localizes pain	5	Withdraws to touch	5
Withdraws to pain	4	Withdraws to pain	4
Abnormal flexion	3	Abnormal flexion	3
Abnormal extension	2	Abnormal extension	2
None	1	None	1

Data from Jennet B, Teasdale G. Aspects of coma after severe head injury. Lancet. *1977;1:878* and James HE. Neurologic evaluation and support in the child with an acute brain insult. Pediatr Ann. *1986;15:16.*

always include salicylate and acetaminophen levels), blood gas, serum osmolality, prothrombin time (PT)/partial thromboplastin time, and blood/urine culture. If patient is an infant or toddler, consider assessment of plasma amino acids, urine organic acids, and other appropriate metabolic workup

c. If meningitis or encephalitis are suspected, consider lumbar puncture (LP) and start antibiotics and acyclovir
d. Request emergency head CT after ABCs are stabilized; consider neurosurgical consultation and electroencephalogram (EEG) if indicated
e. If ingestion is suspected, airway must be protected before GI decontamination (see Chapter 2)
f. Monitor Glasgow Coma Scale and reassess frequently (see Table 1.3).

B. Status Epilepticus[33,34]

See Chapter 20 for nonacute evaluation and management of seizures.

1. **Assessment:** Common causes of childhood seizures include electrolyte abnormalities, hypoglycemia, fever, subtherapeutic anticonvulsant levels, central nervous system (CNS) infections, trauma, toxic ingestion, and metabolic abnormalities. Consider specific patient history, such as shunt malfunction in patient with ventriculoperitoneal

TABLE 1.4
ACUTE MANAGEMENT OF SEIZURES

Time (min)	Intervention
0–5	Stabilize patient Assess airway, breathing, circulation, and vital signs. Administer oxygen. Obtain IV or IO access. Consider hypoglycemia, thiamine deficiency, intoxication (dextrose, thiamine, naloxone may be given immediately if suspected) Obtain laboratory studies: consider glucose, electrolytes, calcium, magnesium, blood gas, CBC, BUN, creatinine, LFTs, toxicology screen, anticonvulsant levels, blood culture (if infection is suspected) Initial screening history and physical examination
5–15	Begin pharmacotherapy: Lorazepam (Ativan), 0.05–0.1 mg/kg IV/IM, max dose 2 mg Or Diazepam (Valium), 0.2–0.5 mg/kg IV (0.5 mg/kg rectally); max dose <5 y/o: 5 mg, >5 y/o: 10 mg May repeat lorazepam or diazepam 5–10 min after initial dose
15–25	If seizure persists, load with one of the following: 1. Fosphenytoin* 15–20 mg PE/kg IV/IM at 3 mg PE/kg/min via peripheral IV line (maximum 150 mg PE/min). If given IM, may require multiple dosing sites 2. Phenytoin[†] 15–20 mg/kg IV at rate not to exceed 1 mg/kg/min via central line 3. Phenobarbital 15–20 mg/kg IV at rate not to exceed 1 mg/kg/min
25–40	If seizure persists: Levetiracetam 20–30 mg/kg IV at 5 mg/kg/min; or valproate 20 mg/kg IV at 5 mg/kg/min May give phenobarbital at this time if still seizing at 5 minutes and (fos)phenytoin previously used Additional phenytoin or fosphenytoin 5 mg/kg after 12 hr for goal serum level of 10 mg/L Additional phenobarbital 5 mg/kg/dose every 15–30 min (maximum total dose of 30 mg/kg; be prepared to support respirations)
40–60	If seizure persists,[‡] consider pentobarbital, midazolam, or general anesthesia in intensive care unit. Avoid paralytics.

*Fosphenytoin dosed as phenytoin equivalent (PE).
[†]Phenytoin may be contraindicated for seizures secondary to alcohol withdrawal or most ingestions (see Chapter 2).
[‡]Pyridoxine 100 mg IV in infants with persistent initial seizure
BUN, Blood urea nitrogen; CBC, complete blood cell count; CT, computed tomography; EEG, electroencephalogram; LFTs, liver function tests; IM, intramuscular; IO, intraosseous; IV, intravenous
Modified from Abend, NS, Dlugos, DJ. Treatment of refractory status epilepticus: literature review and a proposed protocol. Pediatr Neurol. 2008;38:377.

shunt. Less common causes include vascular, neoplastic, and endocrine diseases.
2. **Acute management of seizures** (Table 1.4): If CNS infection is suspected, give antibiotics and/or acyclovir early.

3. **Diagnostic workup:** When stable, workup may include CT or magnetic resonance imaging, EEG, and LP.

REFERENCES

1. Dieckman R, Brownstein D, Gausche-Hill M. The pediatric assessment triangle: a novel approach for the rapid evaluation of children. *Pediatr Emerg Care.* 2010;26:312-315.
2. Berg MD, Schexnayder SM, Chameides L, et al. Part 13: Pediatric basic life support: 2010 American Heart Association guidelines for cardiopulmonary resuscitation and emergency cardiovascular care. *Circulation.* 2010;122(18 suppl 3):S862-S875.
3. Atkins DL, Berger S, Duff JP, et al. Part 11: Pediatric basic life support and cardiopulmonary resuscitation quality: 2015 American Heart Association guidelines update for cardiopulmonary resuscitation and emergency cardiovascular care. *Circulation.* 2015;132(18 suppl 2):S519-S525.
4. Stevenson AG, McGowan J, Evans AL, et al. CPR for children: one hand or two? *Resuscitation.* 2005;64:205-208.
5. Field JM, Hazinski MF, Sayre MR, et al. Part 1: executive summary: 2010 American Heart Association guidelines for cardiopulmonary resuscitation and emergency cardiovascular care. *Circulation.* 2010;122(18 suppl 3):S640-S656.
6. De Caen AR, Berg MD, Chameides L, et al. Part 12: Pediatric advanced life support: 2015 American Heart Association guidelines update for cardiopulmonary resuscitation and emergency cardiovascular care. *Circulation.* 2015;132(18 suppl 2):S526-S542.
7. American Heart Association. Pediatric advanced life support. *Pediatrics.* 2006;117:e1005-e1028.
8. Nichols DG, Yaster M, Lappe DG, et al., eds. *Golden Hour: The Handbook of Advanced Pediatric Life Support.* St Louis: Mosby; 1996.
9. Chameides LC, Samson RA, Schexnayder SM, et al., eds. *Pediatric Advanced Life Support Provider Manual.* Dallas: American Heart Association, Subcommittee on Pediatric Resuscitation; 2011.
10. Sagarin MJ, Barton ED, Chng YM, et al. Airway management by US and Canadian emergency medicine residents: a multicenter analysis of more than 6,000 endotracheal intubation attempts. *Ann Emerg Med.* 2005;46:328-336.
11. American Heart Association. Pharmacology. In: *Pediatric Advanced Life Support Provider Manual.* Dallas: American Heart Association, Subcommittee on Pediatric Resuscitation; 2006:228.
12. Sagarin MJ, Chiang V, Sakles JC, et al. Rapid sequence intubation for pediatric emergency airway management. *Pediatr Emerg Care.* 2002;18:417-423.
13. Zelicof-Paul A, Smith-Lockridge A, Schnadower D, et al. Controversies in rapid sequence intubation in children. *Curr Opin Pediatr.* 2005;17:355-362.
14. Sivilotti ML, Filbin MR, Murray HE, et al. Does the sedative agent facilitate emergency rapid sequence intubation? *Acad Emerg Med.* 2003;10:612-620.
15. Perry J, Lee J, Wells G. Rocuronium versus succinylcholine for rapid sequence induction intubation. *Cochrane Database Syst Rev.* 2003;(1):CD002788.
16. Trethewy CE, Burrows JM, Clausen D, Doherty SR. Effectiveness of cricoid pressure in preventing gastric aspiration during rapid sequence intubation in the emergency department: study protocol for a randomised controlled trial. *Trials.* 2012;13:17.

17. Ahmed Z, Zestos M, Chidiac E, Lerman J. A survey of cricoid pressure use among pediatric anesthesiologists. *Paediatr Anaesth*. 2009;19(2):183-187.
18. Berg RA, Sanders AB, Kern KB, et al. Adverse hemodynamic effects of interrupting chest compressions for rescue breathing during cardiopulmonary resuscitation for ventricular fibrillation cardiac arrest. *Circulation*. 2001;104:2465-2470.
19. Sampson HA, Munoz-Furlong A. Second symposium on the definition and management of anaphylaxis: summary report—Second National Institute of Allergy and Infectious Disease/Food Allergy and Anaphylaxis Network symposium. *J Allergy Clin Immunol*. 2006;117:391-397.
20. Lee JM, Greenes DS. Biphasic anaphylactic reactions in pediatrics. *Pediatrics*. 2000;106:762-766.
21. Luten RC, Kissoon N. The difficult pediatric airway. In: Walls RM, ed. *Manual of Emergency Management*. 2nd ed. Philadelphia: Williams & Wilkins; 2004:236.
22. National Asthma Education and Prevention Program. *Expert Panel Report III: Guidelines for the Diagnosis and Management of Asthma*. Bethesda, MD: National Heart, Lung and Blood Institute; 2007.
23. Keeney GE, Gray MP, Morrison AK, et al. Dexamethasone for acute asthma exacerbations in children: a meta-analysis. *Pediatrics*. 2014;133(3):493-499.
24. Carroll CL, Schramm CM. Noninvasive positive pressure ventilation for the treatment of status asthmaticus in children. *Ann Allergy Asthma Immunol*. 2006;96:454-459.
25. Mitra A, Bassler D, Goodman K, et al. Intravenous aminophylline for acute severe asthma in children over two years receiving inhaled bronchodilators. *Cochrane Database Syst Rev*. 2005;(2):CD001276.
26. Cherry JD. Croup (laryngitis, laryngotracheitis, spasmodic croup, laryngotracheobronchitis, bacterial tracheitis, and laryngotracheobronchopneumonitis). In: Feigin RD, Cherry JD, Demmler H, et al., eds. *Textbook of Pediatric Infectious Diseases*. 6th ed. Philadelphia: Saunders; 2009:254.
27. Alberta Medical Association. Guideline for the diagnosis and management of croup. Alberta Clinical Practice Guidelines 2008. Published on the Alberta Medical Association Practice Guideline Website.
28. McMillan JA, Feigin RD, DeAngelis C, et al. Epiglottitis. In: *Oski's Pediatrics: Principles and Practice*. 4th ed. Philadelphia: Lippincott Williams & Wilkins; 2006.
29. Beharloo F, Veyckemans F, Francis C, et al. Tracheobronchial foreign bodies. Presentation and management in children and adults. *Chest*. 1999;115:1357-1362.
30. Avner J. Altered states of consciousness. *Pediatr Rev*. 2006;27:331-338.
31. Kochanek PM, Carney N, Adelson PD, et al. American Academy of Pediatrics–Section on Neurological Surgery, American Association of Neurological Surgeons/Congress of Neurological Surgeons, Child Neurology Society, European Society of Pediatric and Neonatal Intensive Care, Neurocritical Care Society, Pediatric Neurocritical Care Research Group, Society of Critical Care Medicine, Paediatric Intensive Care Society UK, Society for Neuroscience in Anesthesiology and Critical Care, World Federation of Pediatric Intensive and Critical Care Societies. Guidelines for the acute medical management of severe traumatic brain injury in infants, children, and adolescents–second edition. *Pediatr Crit Care Med*. 2012;13(suppl 1):S1-S82.

32. Kupperman N, Holmes F, Dayan P, et al. Identification of children at very low risk of clinically-important brain injuries after head trauma: a prospective cohort study. *Lancet*. 2009;374(9696):1160-1170.
33. Abend NS, Dlugos DJ. Treatment of refractory status epilepticus: literature review and a proposed protocol. *Pediatr Neurol*. 2008;38:377-390.
34. Wheless JW. Treatment of status epilepticus in children. *Pediatr Ann*. 2004;33:376-383.

Chapter 2
Poisonings

Michael Hrdy, MD

See additional content on Expert Consult

Whenever ingestion is suspected, contact local poison control at 1-800-222-1222.

I. WEB RESOURCES

- American Association of Poison Control Centers: http://www.aapcc.org/
- American Academy of Clinical Toxicology: http://www.clintox.org/index.cfm
- Centers for Disease Control and Prevention, Section on Environmental Health: http://www.cdc.gov/nceh

II. INITIAL EVALUATION

A. History

1. **Exposure history**
   a. Obtain history from witnesses and/or close contacts.
   b. Route, timing, and number of exposures (acute, chronic, or repeated ingestion), prior treatments or decontamination efforts.[1,2]
2. **Substance identification**
   a. Attempt to identify exact name of substance ingested and constituents, including product name, active ingredients, possible contaminants, expiration date, concentration, and dose.
   b. Consult local poison control for pill identification: 1-800-222-1222.
3. **Quantity of substance ingested**
   a. Attempt to estimate the missing volume of liquid or the number of missing pills from a container.
4. **Environmental information**
   a. Accessible items in the house or garage; open containers; spilled tablets; household members taking medications, visitors to the house, herbs, or other complementary medicines.[2]

B. Laboratory Findings

1. **Toxicology screens**: Includes amphetamines, barbiturates, cocaine, ethanol, and opiates (Table 2.1).
   a. If a particular type of ingestion is suspected, verify that the agent is included in the toxicology test.[2]
   b. When obtaining a urine toxicology test, consider measuring both aspirin and acetaminophen blood levels because these are common analgesic ingredients in many medications.[2]

TABLE 2.1
URINE TOXICOLOGY SCREEN*

Agent	Time Detectable in Urine
Amphetamines	2–4 days; up to 15 days
Benzodiazepines	3 days (if short-term use); 4–6 weeks (if >1 year use)
Buprenorphine	3–4 days
Cannabinoids	2–7 days (occasional use); 21–30 days (chronic use)
Cocaine	12 hours (parent form); 12–72 hours (metabolites)
Codeine	2–6 days
Ethanol	2–4 hours; up to 24 hours†
Heroin	2–4 days
Hydromorphone	2–4 days
3,4-Methylenedioxymethamphetamine (MDMA)	3–4 days
Methadone	Up to 3 days
Methamphetamine	2–5 days (depends on urine pH)
Morphine	2–4 days (up to 14 days)
Phencyclidine (PCP)	2–8 days (occasional use); 30 days (regular use)

The length of detection of drugs of abuse in urine varies. The above periods of detection should only be considered rough estimates and depend upon the individual's metabolism, physical condition, fluid intake, and frequency and quantity of ingestion.[6]
*Recognize drugs not detected by routine toxicology screens
†If test measures metabolite ethyl glucoride, test may be positive for up to 80 hours.

c. Gas chromatography or gas mass spectroscopy can distinguish medications that may cause a false-positive toxicology screen.[3,4]

C. Clinical Diagnostic Aids (Table EC 2.A)

III. TOXIDROMES

See Table 2.2.

IV. INGESTION AND ANTIDOTES

See Table 2.3.

A. In General, the Following Are Guidelines of Supportive Care for the Management of Ingestions.

1. **For hypotension,** patients often require aggressive fluid resuscitation or vasopressors.
2. **Treat hyperpyrexia with cooling measures.**
3. **For ingestions that cause seizure,** treat with benzodiazepines unless otherwise specified.
4. **Selective decontamination with activated charcoal.**[5]
a. Most effective when used within first hour after ingestion
b. Substances not commonly absorbed: Electrolytes, iron, alcohols, most water-based compounds
c. Contraindications: Unprotected airway, disrupted gastrointestinal tract, increased risk of aspiration

TABLE 2.2
TOXIDROMES

Drug Class	Signs and Symptoms	Causative Agents
Anticholinergic: "Mad as a hatter, red as a beet, blind as a bat, hot as a hare, dry as a bone."	Delirium, psychosis, paranoia, dilated pupils, thirst, hyperthermia, ↑HR, urinary retention	Antihistamines, phenothiazines, scopolamine, tricyclic antidepressants
Cholinergic: Muscarinic	Salivation, lacrimation, urination, defecation, ↑HR emesis, bronchospasm	Organophosphates
Cholinergic: Nicotinic	Muscle fasciculations, paralysis, ↑HR, ↑BP	Tobacco, black widow venom, insecticides
Opiates	Sedation, constricted pupils, hypoventilation, ↓BP	Opioids
Sympathomimetics	Agitation, dilated pupils, ↑HR, ↓BP, moist skin	Amphetamines, cocaine, albuterol, caffeine, PCP
Sedative/hypnotic	Depressed mental status, normal pupils, ↓BP	Benzodiazepines, barbiturates
Serotonergic	Confusion, flushing, ↑HR, shivering, hyperreflexia, muscle rigidity, clonus	SSRIs (alone or in combination with other meds, including MAOIs, tramadol, and TCAs)

5. **Hemodialysis** may be indicated to remove a drug/toxin regardless of renal function or in cases of renal impairment.
6. Consult local poison control for further management at 1-800-222-1222.

V. ACETAMINOPHEN OVERDOSE[6-10]

Metabolites are hepatotoxic. Reactive intermediates can cause liver necrosis.

A. Four Phases of Intoxication:

1. **Phase 1 (first 24 hr):** nonspecific symptoms such as nausea, malaise, vomiting
2. **Phase 2 (24 to 72 hr):** above symptoms resolve, right upper quadrant pain and hepatomegaly develop. Increase in liver function tests, bilirubin levels, and prothrombin time
3. **Phase 3 (72 to 96 hr):** return of nonspecific symptoms as well as evidence of liver failure (e.g., jaundice, hypoglycemia, coagulopathy)
4. **Phase 4 (4 days to 2 weeks):** recovery or death

B. Treatment Criteria

1. **Serum acetaminophen** concentration above the possible toxicity line on the Rumack–Matthew nomogram (Fig. 2.1)
2. **History of ingesting more than 200 mg/kg or 10 g** (whichever is less) and serum concentration not available or time of ingestion not known

TABLE 2.3
COMMONLY INGESTED AGENTS[6]

Ingested Agent	Signs and Symptoms	Antidote[6]
Acetaminophen	See Section V	
Amphetamine	See sympathomimetics toxidrome in Table 2.2	Supportive care (see above)
Anticholinergics[1]	See anticholinergic toxidrome in Table 2.2	**Physostigmine:** See formulary for dosing
Anticholinesterase (insecticides, donepezil, mushrooms)	See cholinergic:muscarinic and cholinergic:nicotinic toxidrome in Table 2.2	**Atropine:** See formulary for dosing
Antihistamines[14]	See anticholinergic toxidrome in Table 2.2; paradoxical CNS stimulation, dizziness, seizures, prolonged QT[15]	Supportive care (see above)
Benzodiazepines[16,17]	Coma, dysarthria, ataxia, drowsiness, hallucinations, confusion, agitation, bradycardia, hypotension, respiratory depression	**Flumazenil:** See Formulary for dosing
β-blockers[18-20]	Coma, seizures, altered mental status, hallucinations, bradycardia, AV conduction block,[15] congestive heart failure, hypotension, respiratory depression, bronchospasm, hypoglycemia	**Glucagon:** See Formulary for dosing; see **insulin/dextrose** treatment in calcium channel blockers
Calcium channel blockers[19,20]	Seizures, coma, dysarthria, lethargy, confusion, bradycardia, AV conduction block, widened QRS,[15] hypotension, pulmonary edema, hyperglycemia, flushing	**CaCl (10%):** See formulary for dosing **CaGluc (10%):** See formulary for dosing **Glucagon:** See formulary for dosing **Insulin/dextrose:** 1 U/kg bolus → infuse at 0.1–1 U/kg/hr; give with D25W 0.25 g/kg bolus → 0.5 g/kg/hr infusion
Clonidine[20]	Symptoms resemble an opioid toxidrome. CNS depression, coma, lethargy, hypothermia, miosis, bradycardia, profound hypotension, respiratory depression	See opioid antidote
Cocaine[21]	See sympathomimetics toxidrome in Table 2.2	Supportive care (see above)
Detergent pods[22,23]	Vomiting, sedation, aspiration, respiratory distress	Supportive care (see above)
Ecstasy[21]	Hallucinations, teeth grinding, hyperthermia, seizures	Supportive care (see above)

Continued

TABLE 2.3

COMMONLY INGESTED AGENTS[6]—cont'd

Ingested Agent	Signs and Symptoms	Antidote[6]
Ethanol[1,24]	See sedative/hypnotic toxidrome in Table 2.2	Supportive care (see above)
Ethylene glycol/methanol[1,24]	Similar to ethanol; additionally, blurry or double vision, metabolic acidosis, abdominal pain	**Fomepizole:** See formulary for dosing. Alternatively, if not available, can use ethanol (see formulary for dosing), but requires more monitoring than fomepizole
Iron[25,26]	Vomiting, diarrhea, ↓BP, lethargy, renal failure	**Deferoxamine:** See formulary for dosing
Lead	See Section VI	
Nicotine	Vomiting and nicotinic toxidrome in Table 2.2	Supportive care (see above)
NSAIDs	Nausea, vomiting, epigastric pain, headache, GI hemorrhage, renal failure	Supportive care (see above)
Opioids	See opioid toxidrome in Table 2.2	**Naloxone:** See formulary for dosing
Organophosphates	See cholinergic:muscarinic toxidrome in Table 2.2	If muscle fasciculations, respiratory depression, coma, use **Pralidoxime:** see formulary for dosing. **Atropine:** used for muscarinic effects (see anticholinesterase)
Salicylates[24]	GI upset, tinnitus, tachypnea, hyperpyrexia, dizziness, lethargy, dysarthria, seizure, coma, cerebral edema	Supportive care (see above)
Serotonin syndrome	Seizures, muscle rigidity, myoclonus, hyperpyrexia, flushing, rhabdomyolysis	**Cyproheptadine:** See formulary for dosing; *for agitation:* **Diazepam:** See formulary for dosing
Sulfonylureas[24]	Fatigue, dizziness, agitation, confusion, tachycardia, diaphoresis	**Dextrose:** 0.5–1 g/kg (2–4 mL/kg of D25W) *After euglycemia achieved:* **Octreotide:** 1–2 mcg/kg SQ Q6–12 hr if rebound hypoglycemia after dextrose
Synthetic cannabinoids[27]	Agitation, altered sensorium, tachycardia, hypertension, vomiting, mydriasis, hypokalemia	Supportive care (see above)
TCA[28,29]	Seizures, delirium, widened QRS possibly leading to ventricular arrhythmias,[15] hypotension	*For wide QRS complex:* **NaHCO$_3$:** 1–2 mEq/kg IV; goal serum pH 7.45–7.55, *For torsades:* **MgSO$_4$:** 50 mg/kg IV over 5–15 min (max dose 2 grams)
Warfarin	Bleeding	**Phytonadione/Vitamin K$_1$:** See formulary for dosing

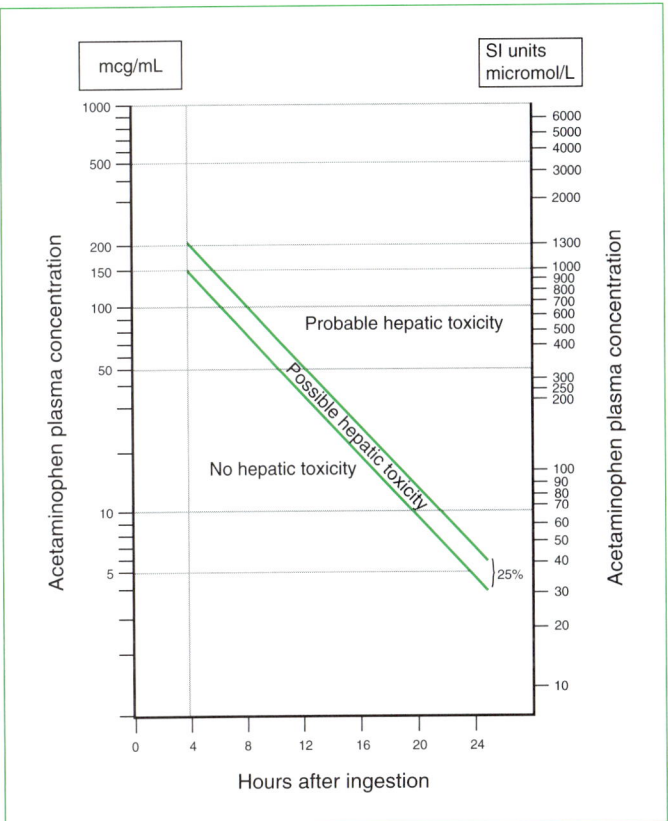

FIGURE 2.1
Semilogarithmic plot of plasma acetaminophen levels versus time. This nomogram is valid for use after acute ingestions of acetaminophen. The need for treatment cannot be extrapolated based on a level before 4 hours. *(Data from Pediatrics 55:871, 1975 and Micromedex.)*

C. Antidotes: *N*-Acetylcysteine (See Formulary for Detailed Dosing Instructions).

1. **PO:** 140 mg/kg loading dose followed by 70 mg/kg Q4 hr for 17 doses (18 total doses including loading dose).
2. **IV:** 150 mg/kg *N*-acetylcysteine IV over 60 minutes followed by 12.5 mg/kg/hr × 4 hours followed by 6.25 mg/kg/hr × 16 hours for a total of 21 hours of infusion. Some patients may require more than 21 hours of *N*-acetylcysteine administration.

3. **Liver failure:** Treat patients in liver failure with *N*-acetylcysteine IV at the same dose as above. Continue 6.25 mg/kg/hr infusion until resolution of encephalopathy, decreasing aminotransferases, and improvement in coagulopathy.

VI. LEAD POISONINGS[11-13]

A. **Etiologies:** paint, dust, soil, drinking water, cosmetics, cookware, toys, and caregivers with occupations and/or hobbies utilizing lead-containing materials or substances*
B. **Definition:** Center for Disease Control and Prevention (CDC) defines an elevated blood lead level (BLL) as ≥5 mcg/dL[11]
C. **Overview of Symptoms by BLL:**
   1. **BLL >40 mcg/dL:** irritability, vomiting, abdominal pain, constipation, and anorexia
   2. **BLL >70 mcg/dL:** lethargy, seizure, and coma. **NOTE:** Children may be asymptomatic with lead levels >100 mcg/dL
D. **Management** (Tables 2.4 and 2.5)
   1. Chelation therapy
      a. **Routine indication: BLL ≥46 mcg/dL**
      b. **Overview of antidotes:**
         1) **Succimer:** 10 mg/kg/dose or 350 mg/m²/dose PO Q8 hr × 5 days then Q12 hr × 14 days (see formulary for details)

---

*Children aged 1 to 5 years are at greatest risk of lead poisoning.

TABLE 2.4
MANAGEMENT OF LEAD POISONING[11]

Blood Lead Levels (BLL)	Recommended Guidelines
≥5 and <10 mcg/dL	1. Provide education about reducing environmental lead exposure and reducing dietary lead absorption* 2. Perform environmental assessment in homes built before 1978 3. Follow repeat blood lead testing guidelines (see Table 2.5)
≥10 and ≤45 mcg/dL	1. As above for BLL ≥5 and <10 mcg/dL 2. Environmental investigation and lead hazard reduction 3. Complete history and exam 4. Iron level, complete blood cell count (CBC), abdominal radiography (if ingestion is suspected) with bowel decontamination if indicated 5. Neurodevelopmental monitoring
BLL ≥45 and ≤69 mcg/dL	1. As above for BLL ≤45 mcg/dL 2. Check free erythrocyte protoporphyrin 3. Administer chelation therapy (see section VI.D.)
BLL ≥70 mcg/dL	1. As above for BLL ≥45 mcg/dL 2. Hospitalize and commence chelation therapy

*Iron, calcium, and vitamin C help minimize absorption of lead.

TABLE 2.5
REPEAT BLOOD LEAD TESTING GUIDELINES[11]

If Screening BLL is:	Time Frame of Confirmation of Screening BLL	Follow-Up Testing (After Confirmatory Testing)	Later Follow-Up Testing After BLL Declining
≥5–9 mcg/dL	1–3 months	3 months	6–9 months
10–19 mcg/dL	1 week–1 month*	1–3 months	3–6 months
20–24 mcg/dL	1 week–1 month*	1–3 months	1–3 months
25–44 mcg/dL	1 week–1 month*	2 weeks–1 month	1 month
45–59 mcg/dL	48 hours	As soon as possible	
60–69 mcg/dL	24 hours		
>70 mcg/dL	Urgently		

*The higher the blood lead level (BLL) on the screening test, the more urgent the need for confirmatory testing.

   2) **Edetate (EDTA) calcium disodium:** 1000 mg/m^2/24 hr IV infusion as an 8–24 hr infusion OR intermittent dosing divided Q12 hr × 5 days. May repeat course as needed after 2–4 days of no EDTA. Please see formulary for detailed dosing. Warning: Do not mistake edetate disodium for edetate calcium disodium. Edetate calcium disodium is the correct medicine used for the treatment of lead poisoning.
   3) **D-penicillamine:** Due to possible severe adverse events, this is a third-line agent, and should only be given in consultation with an expert in pediatric lead poisoning. Do not give D-penicillamine to patients with a penicillin allergy.
 c. **Nonroutine indications:** patient with encephalopathy
   1) **Give Dimercaprol (BAL):** 4 mg/kg/dose IM Q4 hr × 2–7 days; immediately after second dose of dimercaprol, give EDTA 1500 mg/m^2/day IV as a continuous infusion for 8–24 hours or two divided doses × 5 days. Please see the formulary for detailed dose instructions.

REFERENCES

1. Nelson L, Lewin N, Howland MA, et al. *Goldfrank's Toxicologic Emergencies*. 9th ed. New York: McGraw-Hill; 2010.
2. Dart RC, Rumack BH. Poisoning. In: Hay WW, Levin MJ, Sondheimer JM, et al., eds. *Current Pediatric Diagnosis and Treatment*. 19th ed. New York: McGraw-Hill; 2009:313-338.
3. Hoppe-Roberts JM. Poisoning mortality in United States: comparison of national mortality statistics and poison control center reports. *Ann Emerg Med*. 2000;35(5):440-448.
4. Reisfield GM, Goldberger BA, Bertholf RL. 'False-positive' and 'false-negative' test results in clinical urine drug testing. *Bioanalysis*. 2009;1(5):937-952.
5. Fleisher GR, Ludwig S, et al., eds. *Textbook of Pediatric Emergency Medicine*. 6th ed. Philadelphia, PA: Lippincott Williams & Wilkins; 2010.

6. POISINDEX® System [Internet database]. Greenwood Village, CO: Thomson Reuters (Healthcare) Inc. Updated periodically.
7. Hanhan UA. The poisoned child in the pediatric intensive care unit. *Pediatr Clin North Am.* 2008;55:669-686.
8. White M, Liebelt EL. Update on antidotes for pediatric poisonings. *Pediatr Emerg Care.* 2006;22:740-749.
9. Calello D, Osterhoudt KC, Henretig FM. New and novel antidotes in pediatrics. *Pediatr Emerg Care.* 2006;22:523-530.
10. Kanter MZ. Comparison of oral and IV acetylcysteine in the treatment of acetaminophen poisoning. *Am J Health Syst Pharm.* 2006;63:1821-1827.
11. Advisory Committee on Childhood Lead Poisoning Prevention of the Centers for Disease Control and Prevention. Low level lead exposure harms children: A renewed call for primary prevention. <http://www.cdc.gov/nceh/lead/ACCLPP/Final_Document_030712.pdf>. Published January 2012.
12. American Academy of Pediatrics, Committee on Environmental Health. Lead exposure in children: prevention, detection, and management. *Pediatrics.* 2005;116:1036-1046.
13. Davoli CT, Serwint JR, Chisolm JJ. Asymptomatic children with venous lead levels >100 mcg/dL. *Pediatrics.* 1996;98:965-968.
14. Scharman EJ, Erdman AR, Wax PM, et al. Diphenhydramine and dimenhydrinate poisoning: An evidence-based consensus guideline for out-of-hospital management. *Clin Toxicol (Phila).* 2006;44:205-223.
15. Delk C, Holstege CP, Brady WJ. Electrocardiographic abnormalities associated with poisoning. *Am J Emerg Med.* 2007;25:672-687.
16. Isbister GK, O'Regan L, Sibbritt D, et al. Alprazolam is relatively more toxic than other benzodiazepines in overdose. *Br J Clin Pharmacol.* 2004;58(1):88-95.
17. Thomson JS. Use of flumazenil in benzodiazepine overdose. *Emerg Med J.* 2006;23:162.
18. Love JN, Howell JM, Klein-Schwartz W, et al. Lack of toxicity from pediatric beta-blocker exposure. *Hum Exp Toxicol.* 2006;25:341-346.
19. Shepard G. Treatment of poisoning caused by beta-adrenergic and calcium-channel blockers. *Am J Health Syst Pharm.* 2006;63(19):1828-1835.
20. DeWitt CR, Waksman JC. Pharmacology, pathophysiology and management of calcium channel blocker and beta-blocker toxicity. *Toxicol Rev.* 2004;23:223-238.
21. Kaul P. Substance abuse. In: Hay WW, Levin MJ, Sondheimer JM, et al., eds. *Current Pediatric Diagnosis and Treatment.* 19th ed. New York: McGraw-Hill; 2009:137-151.
22. Sebastian T, Shirron KC, Conklin LS. Detergent pod ingestions in young children: a case series. *Clin Pediatr.* 2014;53(11):1091-1093.
23. Beuhler MC, Gala PK, Wolfe HA, et al. Laundry detergent "pod" ingestions: a case series and discussion of recent literature. *Pediatr Emerg Care.* 2013;29:743-747.
24. Henry K, Harris CR. Deadly ingestions. *Pediatr Clin North Am.* 2006;53:293-315.
25. Aldridge MD. Acute iron poisoning: What every pediatric intensive care unit nurse should know. *Dimens Crit Care Nurs.* 2007;26:43-48.
26. Manoguerra AS, Erdman AR, Booze LL, et al. Iron ingestion: an evidence-based consensus guideline for out-of-hospital management. *Clin Toxicol (Phila).* 2005;43:553-570.

27. Hermanns-Clausen M, Kneisel S, Szabo B, et al. Acute toxicity due to the confirmed consumption of synthetic cannabinoids: clinical and laboratory findings. *Addiction*. 2012;108:534-544.
28. Miller J. Managing antidepression overdoses. *Emerg Med Serv*. 2004;33:113-119.
29. Rosenbaum TG, Kou M. Are one or two dangerous? Tricyclic antidepressant exposure in toddlers. *J Emerg Med*. 2005;28:169-174.

Chapter 3
Procedures
James H. Miller, MD, and Matthew Moake, MD, PhD

See additional content on Expert Consult

I. GENERAL GUIDELINES

A. Consent
Before performing any procedure, it is crucial to obtain informed consent from the parent or guardian by explaining the procedure, the indications, any risks involved, and any alternatives. Obtaining consent should not impede life-saving emergency procedures. Requirements for verbal and/or written consent vary between institutions.

B. Risks
1. **All invasive procedures involve pain, risk for infection and bleeding, and injury to neighboring structures.** Specific complications are listed by procedure.
2. **Sedation and analgesia should be planned in advance, and the risks of such explained to the parent and/or patient as appropriate.** In general, 1% lidocaine buffered with sodium bicarbonate is adequate for local analgesia. See Chapter 6 for Analgesia and Procedural Sedation guidelines. Also see the "AAP Guidelines for Monitoring and Management of Pediatric Patients During and After Sedation for Diagnostic and Therapeutic Procedures."[1]
3. **Universal precautions should be followed for all patient contact that exposes the healthcare provider to blood, amniotic fluid, pericardial fluid, pleural fluid, synovial fluid, cerebrospinal fluid (CSF), semen, vaginal secretions, urine, saliva, or any other bodily fluids.**
4. **Proper sterile technique is essential to achieving good wound closure, decreasing transmittable diseases, and preventing wound contamination.**
5. **Videos are available for some procedures via *New England Journal of Medicine's* "Videos in Clinical Medicine."** Links to videos will be available on Expert Consult.

II. ULTRASOUND FOR PROCEDURES

A. Introduction to Ultrasound
Ultrasound has become an increasingly important bedside diagnostic and procedural aid. Ultrasound can improve visualization of subcutaneous structures noninvasively during procedures and improve precision. Ultrasound caveats important for certain procedures are noted below, where applicable. Please see expert consult for expanded information.

B. Ultrasound Basics

1. **Probe Selection**
   a. Linear transducers use high frequencies to produce high resolution images and are primarily used for procedures in pediatrics. A wide area of contact at the skin surface facilitates needle placement in procedures.
   b. Curvilinear transducers use low to midrange frequencies and permit deep structure visualization. Though they provide a wide area of skin contact to facilitate procedures near concave and convex surfaces, larger curvilinear probes are difficult to use in small children.
   c. There are a variety of other probes (phased-array, microconvex) that generate sector shaped images but are predominantly used for diagnostic purposes.
   d. Do not clean probes with chlorhexidine, isopropyl alcohol, or alcohol-containing cleaners as they will damage the probe. Consult your ultrasound machine's instructions on optimal cleaning materials.
   e. Take care not to drop probes or to let their cables be damaged. Do not use a probe with cracked transducer housing.

2. **Image Optimization**
   a. Ensure adequate contact by using enough ultrasound gel and applying comfortable pressure on the skin.
   b. Gain: Increase to optimize imaging of target. Decrease to reduce brightness of artifacts obscuring target.
   c. Frequency: Increase to improve image resolution of shallow structures. Decrease to improve imaging of deep structures.
   d. Depth: Adjust to visualize structure of interest and at least a centimeter of tissue below that structure.

III. VASCULAR ACCESS AND SAMPLING

A. Heelstick and Fingerstick[2]

1. **Indications:** Blood sampling in infants for laboratory studies less affected by hemolysis.
2. **Complications:** Infection, bleeding, osteomyelitis.
3. **Procedure:**
   a. Warm heel or finger.
   b. Clean with alcohol.
   c. Puncture heel using a lancet on the lateral part of the heel, avoiding the posterior area.
   d. Puncture finger using a lancet on the palmar lateral surface of the finger near the tip.
   e. Wipe away the first drop of blood, and then collect the sample using a capillary tube or container.
   f. Alternate between squeezing blood from the leg toward the heel (or from the hand toward the finger) and then releasing the pressure for several seconds.

B. Peripheral Intravenous Access

1. **Indications:** Blood sampling and access to peripheral venous circulation to deliver fluid, medications, or blood products.
2. **Complications:** Thrombosis, infection.
3. **Procedure:**
   a. Choose an intravenous (IV) access site.
   b. Apply tourniquet around the extremity proximal to this site.
   c. Prepare site with alcohol or chlorhexidine.
   d. Insert IV catheter, bevel up, at an angle almost parallel to the skin, advancing until a *flash* of blood is seen in the catheter hub. Advance the plastic catheter only, remove the needle, and secure the catheter.
   e. After removing tourniquet, attach a syringe and apply gentle negative pressure to withdraw blood for serum sampling. Then, attach T connector filled with saline to the catheter, flush with normal saline (NS) to ensure patency of the IV line.
4. **Ultrasound-Guided Procedure:**
   a. With ultrasound, identify a vein that does not appear to branch or to be tortuous. Perform this by sliding the probe along the course of the vessel and identifying its direction and branching. The saphenous veins in the calves, veins in the forearms, antecubital areas, inside of the upper arms, and external jugular veins are areas where ultrasound guidance can help.
   b. Prepare the site, and in the case of limb vessels, place a tourniquet proximal to the insertion site.
   c. Image the vessel with a linear probe placed transverse to the vessel. An ideal vessel appears less than 1 cm below the skin surface. Deeper vessels are prone to through-and-through perforation of the vessel. Infiltration around deeper vessels is also a risk, as a shorter length of catheter resides in the vessel after insertion.
   d. Insert the needle into the skin at a shallow (usually <30-degree) angle to the skin at the midline of the probe near where it contacts the skin. With the probe visualizing the vessel transversely, slowly advance the needle and follow the tip of the needle by sliding the probe away from you. Advance the ultrasound probe until the needle punctures the vessel wall.
   e. Proceed with cannulation of the vessel and secure the intravenous catheter per standard procedure.
5. **A video on peripheral IV placement is available on the *New England Journal of Medicine's* website.**
6. **A video on ultrasound-guided peripheral IV placement is available on the *New England Journal of Medicine's* website.**

C. External Jugular Puncture and Catheterization[3]

1. **Indications:** Blood sampling in patients with inadequate peripheral vascular access or during resuscitation.
2. **Complications:** Infection, bleeding, pneumothorax.

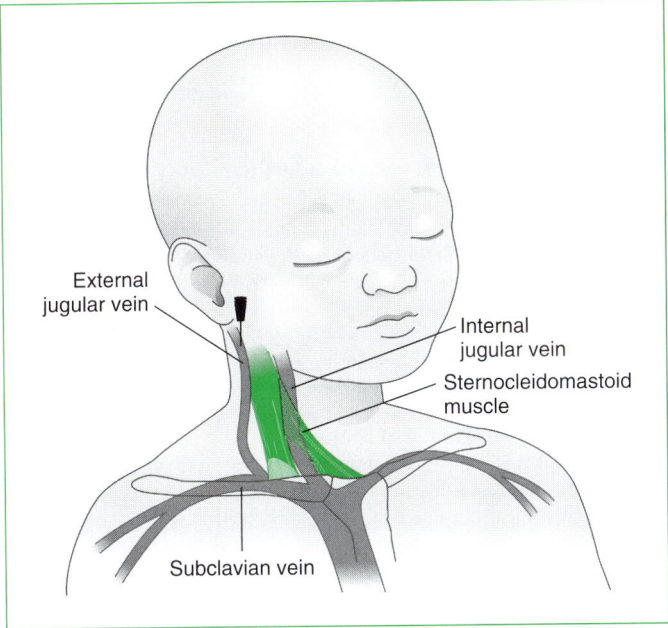

FIGURE 3.1

External jugular cannulation. *(From Dieckmann R, Fiser D, Selbst S.* Pediatric Emergency and Critical Care Procedures. *St. Louis: Mosby; 1997.)*

3. **Procedure:** (Fig. 3.1)
a. Restrain patient securely and place with head turned away from side of cannulation. Position with towel roll under shoulders or with head over side of bed to extend neck and accentuate the posterior margin of the sternocleidomastoid muscle on the side of venipuncture.
b. Prepare area in a sterile fashion.
c. The external jugular vein will distend if its most proximal segment is occluded or if the child cries. The vein runs from the angle of the mandible to the posterior border of the lower third of the sternocleidomastoid muscle.
d. With continuous negative suction on the syringe, insert the needle at about a 30-degree angle to the skin. Continue as with any peripheral venipuncture.
e. Apply a sterile dressing, and put pressure on the puncture site for 5 minutes.
f. Catheterization (see Fig 3.1): Place patient in the 15- to 20-degree Trendelenberg position. Turn the head 45 degrees to the contralateral side. Enter the vein at the point where it crosses the

sternocleidomastoid muscle. Proceed with peripheral catheter placement as described in Section III.B.d.

D. Radial Artery Puncture and Catheterization[3,4]

1. **Indications:** Arterial blood sampling or frequent blood gas and continuous blood pressure monitoring in an intensive care setting.
2. **Complications:** Infection, bleeding, occlusion of artery by hematoma or thrombosis, ischemia if ulnar circulation is inadequate.
3. **Procedure:**
a. Before the procedure, test adequacy of ulnar blood flow with the Allen test: Clench the hand while simultaneously compressing ulnar and radial arteries. The hand will blanch. Release pressure from the ulnar artery, and observe the flushing response. Procedure is safe to perform if the entire hand flushes.
b. Locate the radial pulse. It is optional to infiltrate the area over the point of maximal impulse with lidocaine. Avoid infusion into the vessel by aspirating before infusing. Prepare the site in a sterile fashion.
c. Puncture: Insert a butterfly needle attached to a syringe at a 30-to 60-degree angle over the point of maximal impulse. Blood should flow freely into the syringe in a pulsatile fashion. Suction may be required for plastic tubes. Once the sample is obtained, apply firm, constant pressure for 5 minutes and then place a pressure dressing on the puncture site.
d. Catheter placement: Secure the patient's hand to an arm board. Leave the fingers exposed to observe any color changes. Prepare the wrist with sterile technique and infiltrate over the point of maximal impulse with 1% lidocaine. Insert an IV catheter with its needle at a 30-degree angle to the horizontal until a flash of blood is seen in the catheter hub. Advance the plastic catheter and remove the needle. Alternatively, pass the needle and catheter through the artery to transfix it, and then withdraw the needle. Very slowly, withdraw the catheter until free flow of blood is noted, then advance the catheter and secure in place using sutures or tape. Seldinger technique, see section IIF (Fig. 3.2) using a guidewire can also be used. Apply a sterile dressing and infuse heparinized isotonic fluid (per protocol) at a minimum of 1 mL/hr. A pressure transducer may be attached to monitor blood pressure.
e. Suggested size of arterial catheters based on weight:
   (1) Infant (<10 kg): 24 G or 2.5 Fr, 2.5 cm
   (2) Child (10–40 kg): 22 G or 2.4 Fr, 2.5 cm
   (3) Adolescent (>40 kg): 20 G
4. **Ultrasound-Guided Procedure**
a. Use the linear probe. After the sterile field has been prepped, apply gel to the probe and place within a sterile cover. Place the ultrasound probe transverse to the artery on the radial, posterior tibial, or dorsalis pedis pulse. Identify the artery, which will appear pulsatile with some compression. Once the artery has been identified, center the probe

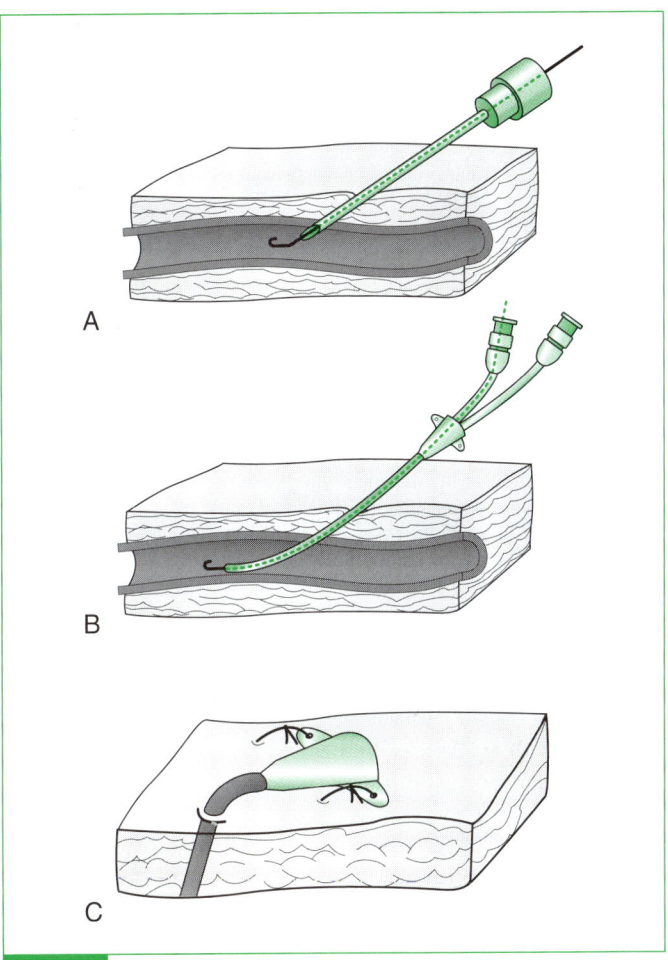

FIGURE 3.2

Seldinger technique. **A,** Guidewire is placed through introducer needle into lumen of vein. **B,** Catheter is advanced into vein lumen along guidewire. **C,** Hub of catheter is secured to skin with suture. *(Modified from Fuhrman B, Zimmerman J. Pediatric Critical Care. 4th ed. Philadelphia: Mosby; 2011.)*

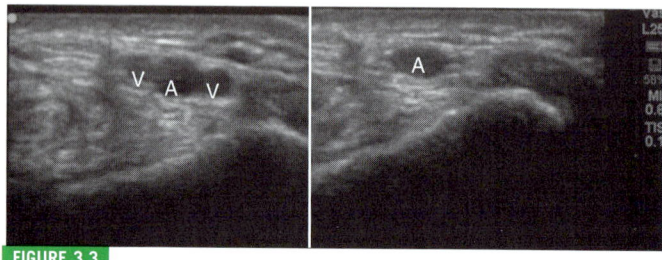

FIGURE 3.3
Ultrasound transverse view of radial artery. In the left image, the radial artery is seen in cross section with veins on either side. On the right image, pressure has been applied and the veins are collapsed while the artery remains patent. A-artery, V-vein. *(From Weiner MM, Geldard P, Mittnacht AJC. Ultrasound guided vascular access: a comprehensive review. J Cardiothorac Vasc Anesth. 2013;27(2):345-360.)*

over the vessel (Fig. 3.3). Insert the needle into the skin at a 45-degree angle at the midline of the probe near where it contacts the skin. With the probe visualizing the vessel transversely, slowly advance the needle and follow the tip of the needle by sliding the probe away. Advance the ultrasound probe until the needle punctures the vessel wall. Proceed with the rest of the procedure after vessel puncture, as described above.

5. **Videos on arterial puncture and radial artery catheterization are available on the *New England Journal of Medicine's* website.**
6. **A video on ultrasound-guided radial artery catheterization is available on the *New England Journal of Medicine's* website.**

E. Posterior Tibial and Dorsalis Pedis Artery Puncture[4]

1. **Indications:** Arterial blood sampling when radial artery puncture is unsuccessful or inaccessible.
2. **Complications:** Infection, bleeding, ischemia if circulation is inadequate.
3. **Procedure (see Section IIID for technique):**
a. Posterior tibial artery: Puncture the artery posterior to medial malleolus while holding the foot in dorsiflexion.
b. Dorsalis pedis artery: Puncture the artery at dorsal midfoot between first and second toes while holding the foot in plantar flexion.

F. Central Venous Catheter Placement[3,5–7]

1. **Indications:** To obtain emergency access to central venous circulation, monitor central venous pressure, deliver high-concentration parenteral nutrition or prolonged IV therapy, or infuse blood products or large volumes of fluid.
2. **Complications:** Infection, bleeding, arterial or venous perforation, pneumothorax, hemothorax, thrombosis, catheter fragment in circulation, air embolism.

3. **Ultrasound guidance:** Has become standard practice to facilitate placement of internal jugular vein central venous catheters. It has been shown to reduce insertion time as well as complication rates when effectively implemented in certain anatomic areas.[8]
4. **Access sites:**
a. Subclavian vein: Risks include pleural injury, pneumothorax, hemothorax, or pleural infusion causing hydrothorax as well as subclavian artery injury. The artery below the clavicle is not compressible and therefore inadvertent puncture is life threatening in patients with a coagulopathy.
b. Internal jugular vein: Avoid in the case of contralateral internal jugular occlusion and ipsilateral internalized cerebral ventriculostomy shunt. It is technically very difficult in patients with cervical collars and tracheostomies and discouraged in these cases if another route is readily available.
c. Femoral vein: Discouraged in severe pelvic trauma.
5. **Procedure:** Seldinger technique (see Fig. 3.2)
a. Secure patient, prepare site, and drape according to the following guidelines for sterile technique[7]:
   (1) Wash hands.
   (2) Wear hat, mask, eye shield, sterile gloves, and sterile gown.
   (3) Prep procedure site for 30 seconds (chlorhexidine), and allow to dry for an additional 30 seconds (in groin, scrub for 2 minutes, and allow to dry for 1 minute).
   (4) Use sterile technique to drape the site and the patient completely from bedrail to bedrail.
   (5) Flush catheter with sterile saline; some institutions protocolize heparinized saline for this.
   (6) Attach slip-tip syringe to puncture needle.
b. Insert needle at a 30-to 45-degree angle, applying negative pressure to the syringe to locate vessel.
c. When there is blood return, insert a guidewire through the needle into the vein. Watch for cardiac ectopy.
d. Remove the needle, firmly holding the guidewire.
e. Slip a catheter that has already been flushed with sterile saline over the wire into the vein. Use a twisting motion, if necessary. The entry site may be enlarged with a small skin incision or dilator. Pass the entire catheter over the wire until the hub is at the skin surface. Slowly remove the wire, ensure blood flow through the catheter, and secure the catheter by suture.
f. Apply a sterile dressing over the site.
g. For internal jugular and subclavian vessels, obtain a chest radiograph to confirm placement and rule out pneumothorax.
6. **Approach:**
a. Internal jugular (Fig. 3.4): Place patient in the 15- to 20-degree Trendelenburg position. Place a towel roll under the shoulders running

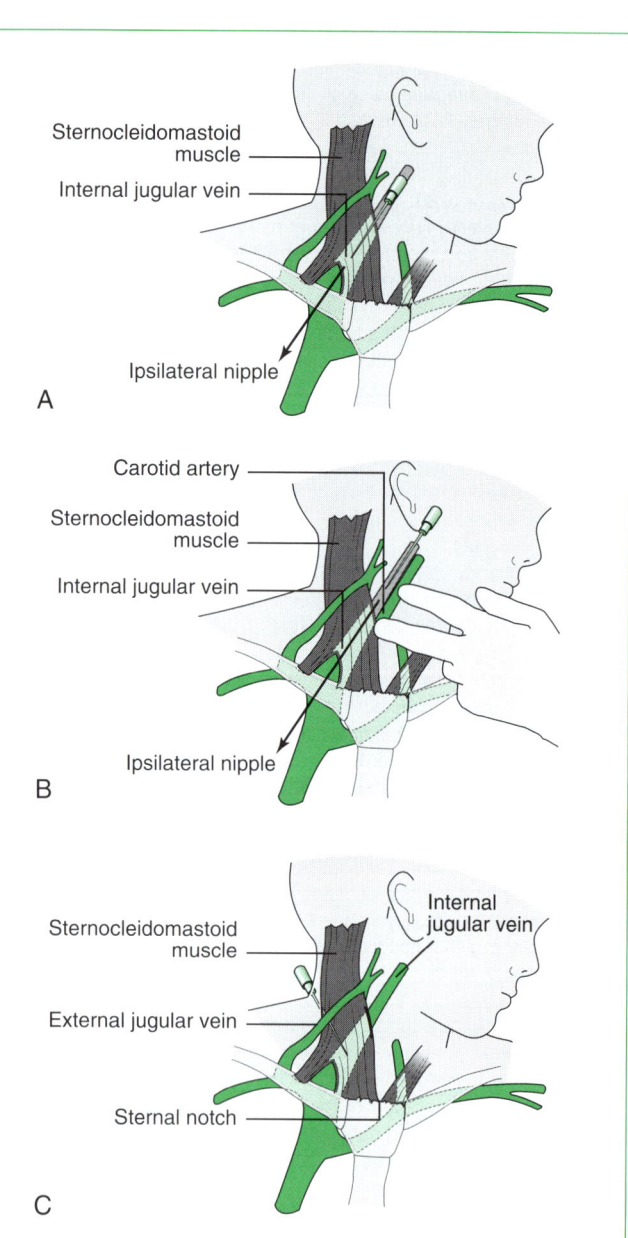

FIGURE 3.4

Approaches to the internal jugular vein. Patient is supine in slight Trendelenburg position, with neck extended over a shoulder roll and head rotated away from side of approach. **A,** Middle approach. Introducer needle enters at apex of a triangle formed by the heads of the sternocleidomastoid muscle and clavicle and is directed toward the ipsilateral nipple at an angle of approximately 30 degrees with the skin. **B,** Anterior approach. Carotid pulse is palpated and may be slightly retracted medially. Introducer needle enters along anterior margin of sternocleidomastoid about halfway between sternal notch and mastoid process and is directed toward the ipsilateral nipple. **C,** Posterior approach. Introducer needle enters at the point where external jugular vein crosses posterior margin of sternocleidomastoid and is directed under its head toward sternal notch. *(Modified from Fuhrman B, Zimmerman J.* Pediatric Critical Care. *4th ed. Philadelphia: Mosby; 2011.)*

---

laterally so that the patient's neck is safely hyperextended as long as such a position is clinically safe. Turn head away from the site of line placement.
(1) Ultrasound-guided approach: Generally recommended for internal jugular access. Use the linear probe. After the sterile field has been prepped, apply gel to the probe and place within a sterile cover. Orient the ultrasound probe transverse to the neck veins near the carotid pulse. Identify the internal jugular vein (IJ), which will usually be lateral and anterior to the carotid artery. With downward pressure from the probe, the IJ will usually be compressible while the carotid artery will be pulsatile. An important caveat is that a patient with jugular venous distention from right ventricular dysfunction may demonstrate a pulsatile IJ, though it will likely be more compressible than the carotid artery. Once the IJ has been identified, center the probe over the vessel (Fig. 3.5A). Insert the needle into the skin at a 30- to 45-degree angle at the midline of the probe near where it contacts the skin. Take care not to puncture the sterile cover of the probe. With the probe visualizing the vessel transversely, slowly advance the needle and follow the tip of the needle by sliding the probe away from you. Remember that the course of the vessel is towards the ipsilateral nipple. Advance the ultrasound probe until the needle punctures the vessel wall. Proceed with the Seldinger technique after venipuncture, as described above. The ultrasound can be placed parallel to the vessel to view the guidewire, if desired (Fig. 3.5B).
(2) Landmark approach: Palpate the sternal and clavicular heads of the sternocleidomastoid muscle, and enter at the apex of the triangle formed. An alternative landmark for puncture is halfway between the sternal notch and the tip of the mastoid process.

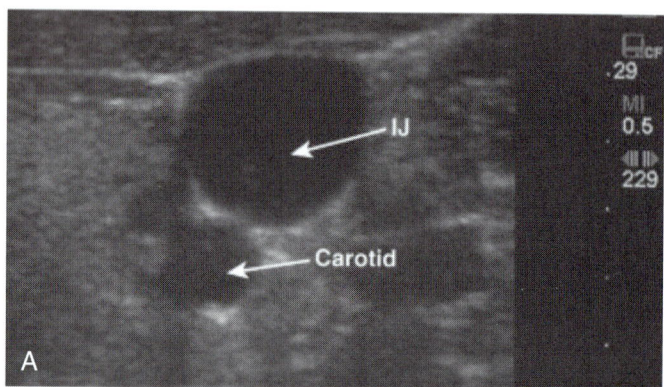

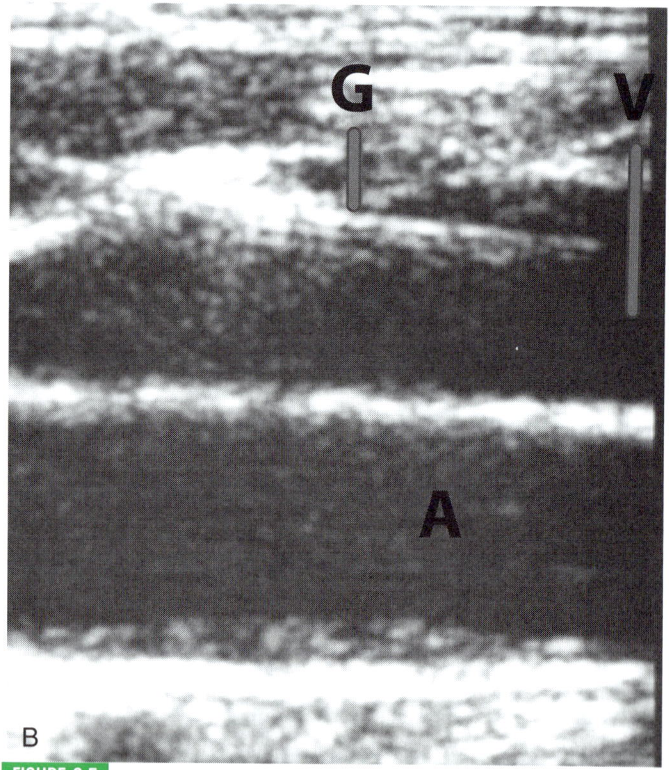

FIGURE 3.5

A, Ultrasound transverse view of internal jugular vein and carotid artery. In this short axis view, the internal jugular vein (IJ) is seen anterior and lateral to the carotid artery. The artery is often smaller and pulsatile while the IJ is usually larger and compressible. Just anterior to the IJ is the sternocleidomastoid muscle. **B,** Ultrasound longitudinal view of internal jugular vein. The internal jugular vein (V) is superficial to the carotid artery (A). The guidewire can be seen as a bright, hyperechoic line (G) crossing the wall of the vein and then remaining in the lumen of the jugular vein. (**B,** *From* Adams J. Emergency Medicine: Clinical Essentials. *Philadelphia: Elsevier; 2013:50-54.e1.*) From *Grevstad U, Gregersen P, Rasmussen LS. Intravenous access in the emergency patient.* Curr Anaesth Crit Care. *2009;20(3):120-127.*)

Insert the needle at a 30- to 45-degree angle to the skin, and aim laterally towards the ipsilateral nipple. When blood flow is obtained, continue with the Seldinger technique. The right side is preferable because of a straight course for the catheter to the right atrium, absence of thoracic duct, and lower pleural dome. The internal jugular vein usually runs lateral to the carotid artery.

b. Subclavian vein (Fig. 3.6): Position child in the Trendelenburg position with a towel roll running cranial to caudad under the thoracic spine to support the sternum vertically above the level of the shoulders. Insert the needle just lateral to the proximal angle of the clavicle, were the medial third and lateral two-thirds of the clavicle meet. Aim the needle under the distal third of the clavicle, slightly cephalad toward the sternal notch. The path of the needle must pass under the clavicle. When blood flow is obtained, continue with the Seldinger technique. If access is not obtained in three attempts another vessel should be accessed.

c. Femoral vein (Fig. 3.7): Position the child securely with the hip flexed and abducted. Locate the femoral pulse just distal to the inguinal crease. In infants, the vein is 5–6 mm *medial* to the arterial pulse. In adolescents, the vein is usually 10–15 mm *medial* to the pulse. Palpate the femoral artery with the hand that is not performing the venipuncture. Insert the needle medial to the pulse. The needle should enter the skin 2–3 cm distal to the inguinal ligament at a 30- to 45-degree angle. Avoid entering the abdomen. When blood flow is obtained, continue with the Seldinger technique.

(1) Ultrasound-guided approach: Apply the linear probe transversely to the femoral vessels distal to the inguinal ligament. Placing it over the femoral pulse helps localize the vessels. Identify the femoral vein, which is medial to the femoral artery (Fig. 3.8).

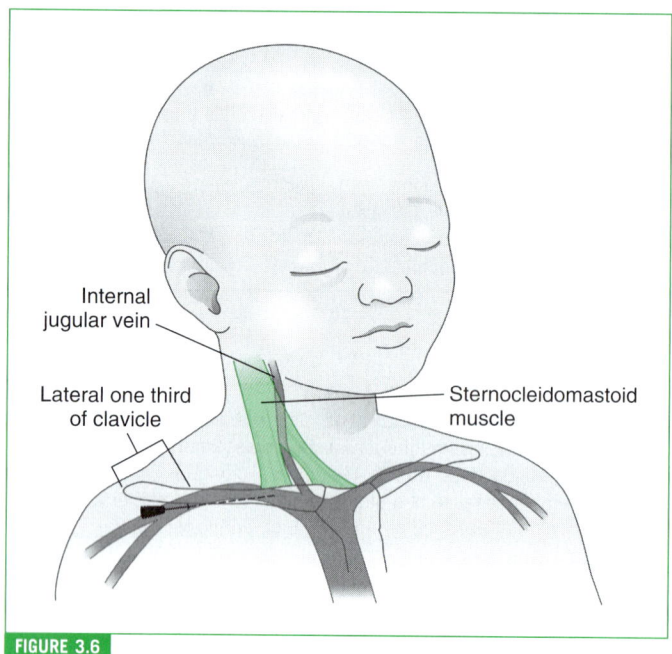

FIGURE 3.6

Subclavian vein cannulation. *(From Dieckmann R, Fiser D, Selbst S.* Pediatric Emergency and Critical Care Procedures. *St. Louis: Mosby; 1997.)*

Insert the needle into the skin at a 30-to 45-degree angle at the midline of the probe near where it contacts the skin. Take care not to puncture the sterile cover of the probe. With the probe visualizing the vessel transversely, slowly advance the needle and follow the tip of the needle by sliding the probe away from you. Remember that the course of the vessel is towards the umbilicus. Advance the ultrasound probe until the needle punctures the vessel wall. Proceed with the Seldinger technique after venipuncture, as described above. Place the ultrasound probe down and take care not to let it fall off of the bed. The ultrasound can be placed longitudinally over the vessel to view the guidewire, if desired.

7. **Videos on femoral venous and subclavian venous catheter placement are available on the *New England Journal of Medicine's* website.**
8. **A video on ultrasound-guided internal jugular catheterization is available on the *New England Journal of Medicine's* website.**

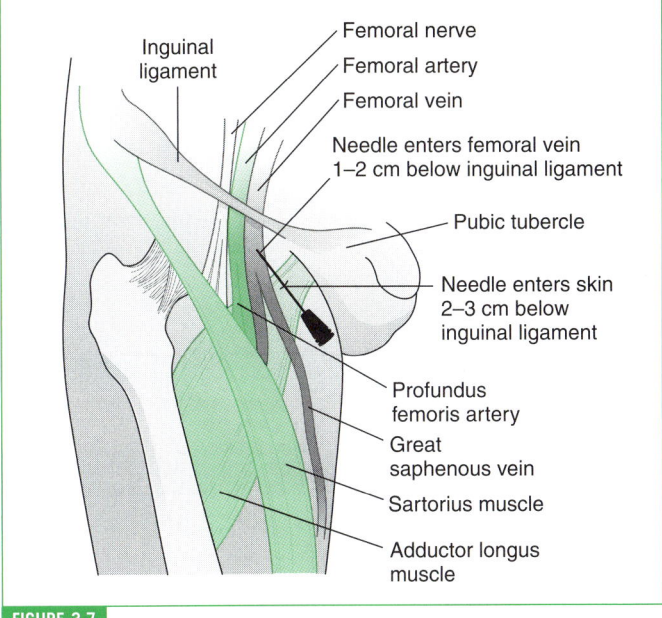

FIGURE 3.7

Femoral vein cannulation with anatomy. *(Modified from Dieckmann R, Fiser D, Selbst S. Pediatric Emergency and Critical Care Procedures. St. Louis: Mosby; 1997.)*

G. Intraosseous (IO) Access[3,4] (Fig. 3.9)

1. **Indications:** Obtain emergency access in children during life-threatening situations. This is very useful during cardiopulmonary arrest, shock, burns, and life-threatening status epilepticus. IO line can be used to infuse medications, blood products, or fluids. The IO needle should be removed once adequate vascular access has been established.
2. **Complications:**
a. Complications are rare, particularly with the correct technique. Frequency of complications increases with prolonged infusions.
b. Complications include extravasation of fluid from incomplete or through and through cortex penetration, infection, bleeding, osteomyelitis, compartment syndrome, fat embolism, fracture, epiphyseal injury.
3. **Sites of entry (in order of preference):**
a. Anteromedial surface of the proximal tibia, 2 cm below and 1–2 cm medial to the tibial tuberosity on the flat part of the bone (see Fig. 3.9).

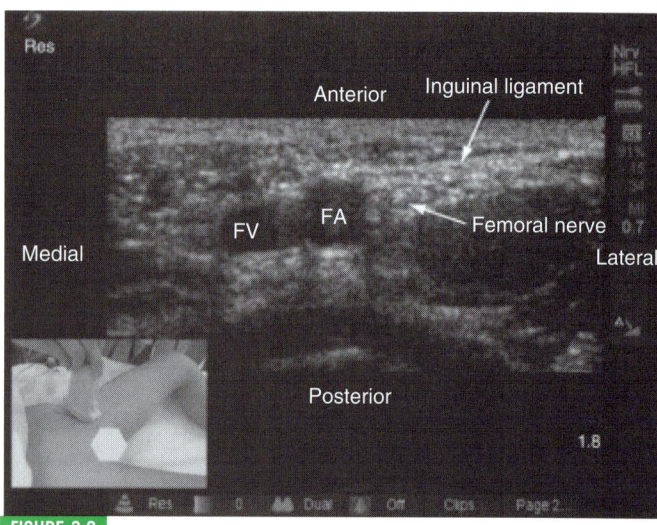

FIGURE 3.8

Ultrasound transverse view of femoral vein and artery. In this transverse image of the thigh, the femoral vein (FV) is medial to the femoral artery (FA) and nerve. The inguinal ligament can also be seen more superficially in this image. In practice, cannulation of the femoral vein should take place distal to the inguinal ligament. Inset shows ultrasound probe position on thigh for related image. *(From A. Karmakar MK, Kwok WH. Practice of Anesthesia for Infants and Children. 2013;880-908.e3.)*

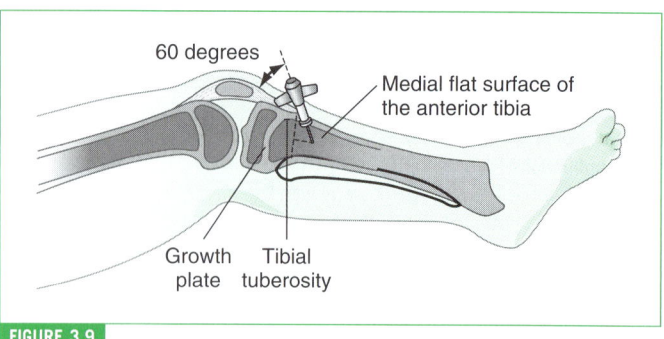

FIGURE 3.9

Intraosseous needle placement using standard anterior tibial approach. Insertion point is in the midline on medial flat surface of anterior tibia, 1–3 cm (2 fingerbreadths) below tibial tuberosity. *(From Dieckmann R, Fiser D, Selbst S. Pediatric Emergency and Critical Care Procedures. St. Louis: Mosby; 1997.)*

b. Distal femur 3 cm above the lateral condyle in the midline.
c. Medial surface of the distal tibia 1–2 cm above the medial malleolus (may be a more effective site in older children).
d. Proximal humerus, 2 cm below the acromion process into the greater tubercle with the arm held in adduction and internal rotation.
e. Anterosuperior iliac spine at a 90-degree angle to the long axis of the body.

4. **Procedure:**
a. Prepare the selected site in a sterile fashion.
b. If the child is conscious, anesthetize the puncture site down to the periosteum with 1% lidocaine (optional in emergency situations).
c. Choose between a manual IO or drill-powered IO insertion device:
   (1) For manual IO needle: Insert a 15- to 18-gauge IO needle perpendicular to the skin at an angle away from the epiphyseal plate, and advance to the periosteum. With a boring rotary motion, penetrate through the cortex until there is a decrease in resistance, indicating that you have reached the marrow. The needle should stand firmly without support. Secure the needle carefully.
   (2) For drill-powered IO needle: Enter skin with the needle perpendicular to the skin, as with the manual needle, and press the needle until you meet the periosteum. Apply easy pressure while gently depressing the drill trigger until you feel a "pop" or a sudden decrease in resistance. Remove the drill while holding the needle steady to ensure stability prior to securing the needle. Use an EZ-IO AD for patients >40 kg, and use EZ-IO PD for patients >6 kg and <40 kg.
d. Remove the stylet and attempt to aspirate marrow. (Note that it is not necessary to aspirate marrow). Flush with crystalloid solution. Observe for fluid extravasation. Marrow can be sent to determine glucose levels, chemistries, blood types and cross-matches, hemoglobin levels, blood gas analyses, and cultures.
e. Attach standard IV tubing. Any crystalloid, blood product, or drug that may be infused into a peripheral vein may also be infused into the IO space, but increased pressure (through pressure bag or push) may be necessary for infusion. There is a high risk for obstruction if continuous high-pressure fluids are not flushed through the IO needle.

5. **A video on IO catheter placement is available on the *New England Journal of Medicine's* website.**

H. Umbilical Artery (UA) and Umbilical Vein (UV) Catheterization[3]

1. **Indications:** Vascular access (via UV), blood pressure monitoring (via UA), or blood gas monitoring (via UA) in critically ill neonates.
2. **Complications:** Infection, bleeding, hemorrhage, perforation of vessel, thrombosis with distal embolization, ischemia or infarction of lower

extremities, bowel, or kidney, arrhythmia if catheter is in the heart, air embolus.
3. **Caution:** UA catheterization should never be performed if omphalitis or peritonitis is present. It is contraindicated in the presence of possible necrotizing enterocolitis or intestinal hypoperfusion.
4. **Line placement:**
a. Arterial line: Low line vs. high line.
   (1) Low line: Tip of catheter should lie just above the aortic bifurcation between L3 and L5. This avoids renal and mesenteric arteries near L1, possibly decreasing the incidence of thrombosis or ischemia.
   (2) High line: Tip of catheter should be above the diaphragm between T6 and T9. A high line may be recommended in infants weighing less than 750 g, in whom a low line could easily slip out.
b. UV catheters should be placed in the inferior vena cava above the level of the ductus venosus and the hepatic veins and below the level of the right atrium.
c. Catheter length: Determine the length of catheter required using either a standardized graph based on shoulder-umbilical length or the birth weight (BW) regression formula below:
   (1) UAC Low Line (cm) = BW (kg) x 7
   (2) UAC High Line (cm) = (3 x BW (kg)) + 9
   (3) UVC Length (cm) = 0.5 x UAC high line (cm) +1.
5. **Procedure for UA line** (Fig. 3.10)**:**
a. Determine the length of the catheter to be inserted for either high (T6–T9) or low (L3–L5) position.
b. Restrain infant. Maintain the infant's temperature during the procedure. Prepare and drape the umbilical cord and adjacent skin using sterile technique.
c. Flush the catheter with sterile saline solution before insertion. Ensure that there are no air bubbles in the catheter or attached syringe.
d. Place sterile umbilical tape around the base of the cord. Cut through the cord horizontally about 1.5–2 cm from the skin; tighten the umbilical tape to prevent bleeding.
e. Identify the one large, thin-walled umbilical vein and two smaller, thick-walled arteries. Use one tip of open, curved forceps to gently probe and dilate one artery. Use both points of closed forceps, and dilate artery by allowing forceps to open gently.
f. Grasp the catheter 1 cm from its tip with toothless forceps and insert the catheter into the lumen of the artery. Aim the tip toward the feet and gently advance the catheter to the desired distance. *Do not force.* If resistance is encountered, try loosening umbilical tape, applying steady and gentle pressure, or manipulating the angle of the umbilical cord to the skin. Often the catheter cannot

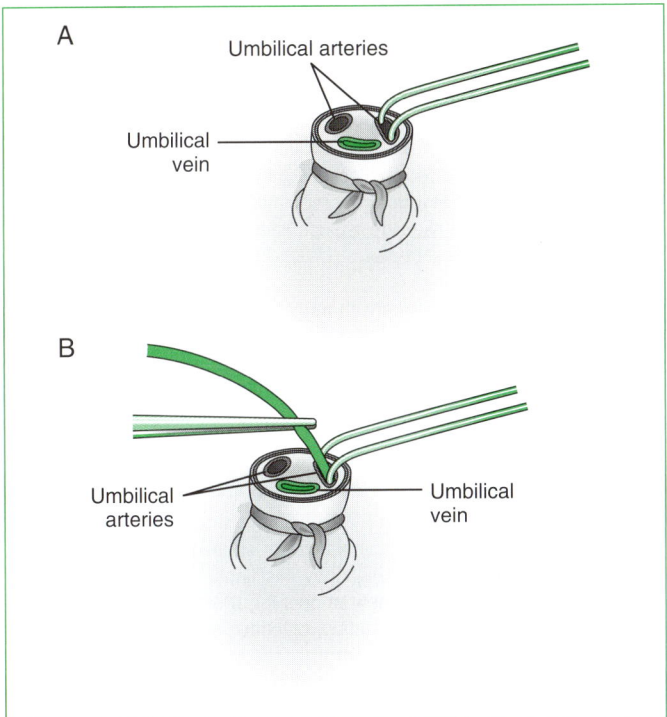

FIGURE 3.10

Placement of umbilical arterial catheter. **A,** Dilating lumen of umbilical artery. **B,** Insertion of umbilical artery catheter. *(From Dieckmann R, Fiser D, Selbst S.* Pediatric Emergency and Critical Care Procedures. *St. Louis: Mosby; 1997.)*

    be advanced because of the creation of a "false luminal tract." There should be good blood return when the catheter enters the iliac artery.
g. Confirm catheter tip position with x-ray or ultrasound. Secure catheter with a suture through the cord, a marker tape, and a tape bridge. The catheter may be pulled back but *not* advanced once the sterile field is broken.
h. Ultrasound confirmation (see Expert Consult).
i. Observe for complications: Blanching or cyanosis of lower extremities, perforation, thrombosis, embolism, or infection. If any complications occur, the catheter should be removed.
j. Use isotonic fluids containing heparin per institutional policy. Never use hypoosmolar fluids in the UA.

6. **Procedure for UV line** (see Fig. 3.10)**:**
   a. Determine the desired length and follow steps "a" through "d" for UA catheter placement.
   b. Isolate the thin-walled umbilical vein, clear thrombi with forceps, and insert catheter, aiming the tip toward the right shoulder. Gently advance the catheter to the desired distance. *Do not force.* If resistance is encountered, try loosening the umbilical tape, applying steady and gentle pressure, or manipulating the angle of the umbilical cord to the skin. Resistance is commonly met at the abdominal wall and again at the portal system. *Do not* infuse anything into the liver.
   c. Confirm catheter tip position with x-ray or ultrasound. Secure catheter as described in step "g" for UA placement.
   d. Ultrasound confirmation of UVC (See Expert Consult).
7. **A video on UV/UA line placement is available on the *New England Journal of Medicine's* website.**

IV. BODY FLUID SAMPLING

A. Lumbar Puncture[3,4]

1. **Indications:** Examination of spinal fluid for suspected infection, inflammatory disorder, or malignancy, instillation of intrathecal chemotherapy, or measurement of opening pressure.
2. **Complications:** Local pain, infection, bleeding, spinal fluid leak, hematoma, spinal headache, and acquired epidermal spinal cord tumor (caused by implantation of epidermal material into the spinal canal if no stylet is used on skin entry).
3. **Cautions and contraindications:**
   a. Increased intracranial pressure (ICP): Before lumbar puncture (LP), perform a funduscopic examination. Presence of papilledema, retinal hemorrhage, or clinical suspicion of increased ICP should prompt further evaluation and may be a contraindication to the procedure. A sudden drop in spinal canal fluid pressure by rapid release of CSF may cause fatal herniation. If LP is to be performed, proceed with extreme caution. Computed tomography (CT) may be indicated before LP if there is suspected intracranial bleeding, focal mass lesion, or increased ICP. A normal CT scan does not rule out increased ICP but usually excludes conditions that may put the patient at risk for herniation. Decision to obtain CT should not delay appropriate antibiotic therapy, if indicated.
   b. Bleeding diathesis: Platelet count >50,000/mm^3 is desirable before LP, and correction of any clotting factor deficiencies can minimize the risk for bleeding and subsequent cord or nerve root compression.
   c. Overlying skin infection may result in inoculation of CSF with organisms.

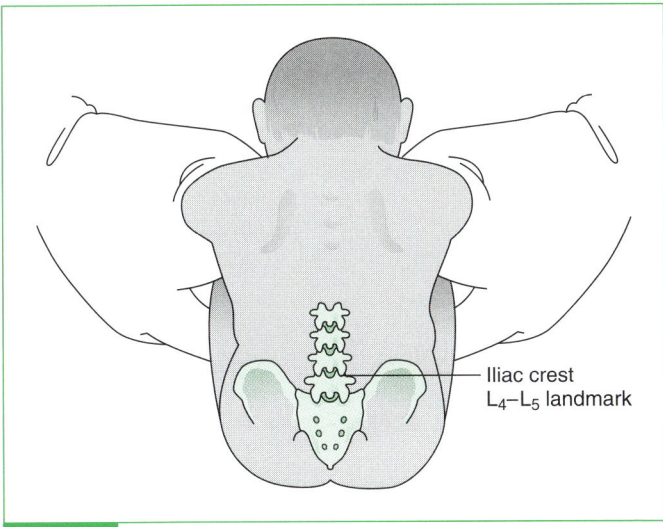

FIGURE 3.11

Lumbar puncture site in sitting position. *(From Dieckmann R, Fiser D, Selbst S. Pediatric Emergency and Critical Care Procedures. St. Louis: Mosby; 1997.)*

d. LP should be deferred in unstable patients, and appropriate therapy should be initiated, including antibiotics, if indicated.

4. **Procedure:**
a. Apply local anesthetic cream if sufficient time is available.
b. Position child in either the sitting position (Fig. 3.11) or lateral recumbent position (Fig. 3.12), with hips, knees, and neck flexed. Keep shoulders and hips aligned (perpendicular to the examining table in recumbent position) to avoid rotating the spine. *Do not* compromise a small infant's cardiorespiratory status with positioning.
c. Locate the desired intervertebral space (either L3-4 or L4-5) by drawing an imaginary line between the top of the iliac crests. Alternatively, ultrasound can be used to mark the intervertebral space (see Expert Consult).
d. Ultrasound marking (See Expert Consult)
e. Prepare the skin in a sterile fashion. Drape conservatively to make monitoring the infant possible. Use a 20G to 22G spinal needle with stylet (1.5 or 3.5 inch depending on the size of the child). A smaller-gauge needle will decrease the incidence of spinal headache and CSF leak.
f. Overlying skin and interspinous tissue can be anesthetized with 1% lidocaine using a 25G needle.

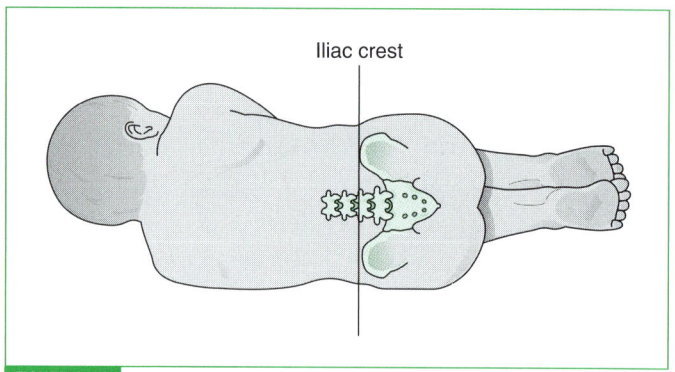

FIGURE 3.12

Lumbar puncture site in lateral (recumbent) position. *(From Dieckmann R, Fiser D, Selbst S.* Pediatric Emergency and Critical Care Procedures. *St. Louis: Mosby; 1997.)*

    g. Puncture the skin in the midline just caudad to the palpated spinous process, angling slightly cephalad towards the umbilicus. Advance several millimeters at a time, and withdraw stylet frequently to check for CSF flow. Needle may be advanced without the stylet once it is completely through the skin. In small infants, one may *not* feel a change in resistance or "pop" as the dura is penetrated.

    h. If resistance is met initially (you hit bone), withdraw needle to just under the skin surface and redirect the angle of the needle slightly.

    i. Send CSF for appropriate studies (see Chapter 27 for normal values). Send the first tube for culture and Gram stain, the second tube for measurement of glucose and protein levels, and the last tube for cell count and differential. An additional tube can be collected for viral cultures, polymerase chain reaction (PCR), or CSF metabolic studies, if indicated. If subarachnoid hemorrhage or traumatic tap is suspected, send the first and fourth tubes for cell count, and ask the laboratory to examine the CSF for xanthochromia.

    j. Accurate measurement of CSF pressure can be made only with the patient lying quietly on his or her side in an unflexed position. It is not a reliable measurement in the sitting position. Once the free flow of spinal fluid is obtained, attach the manometer and measure CSF pressure. Opening pressure is recorded as the level at which CSF is steady.

5. **A video on lumbar punctures is available on the *New England Journal of Medicine's* website.**

Chapter 3 Procedures 51

B. Needle Decompression, Chest Tube Placement, and Thoracentesis[3,6]

1. **Indications:** Evacuation of a pneumothorax, hemothorax, chylothorax, large pleural effusion, or empyema for diagnostic or therapeutic purposes.
2. **Complications:** Infection, bleeding, pneumothorax, hemothorax, pulmonary contusion or laceration, puncture of diaphragm, spleen, or liver, or bronchopleural fistula.
3. **Procedure: Needle decompression.**
a. Preferably prepare and drape the skin as clean as possible as this is often performed in an emergency. Sterility is optimal.
b. Insert a large-bore angiocatheter (14–22-gauge based on patient size) into the anterior second intercostal space in the midclavicular line. Insert needle over superior aspect of rib margin to avoid neurovascular structures.
c. When pleural space is entered, withdraw needle and attach catheter to a three-way stopcock and syringe, and aspirate air. The stopcock is used to stop air flow through the catheter when sufficient evacuation has been performed.
d. Subsequent insertion of a chest tube is often necessary for ongoing release of air. It is advised not to completely evacuate chest prior to placement of chest tube to avoid pleural injury.
4. **A video on needle decompression of spontaneous pneumothorax is available on the *New England Journal of Medicine's* website.**
5. **Procedure (Fig. 3.13): Chest tube insertion.**
a. See inside front cover for chest tube sizes.
b. Position child supine or with affected side up and arm restrained overhead.
c. Point of entry is the third to fifth intercostal space in the mid- to anterior axillary line, usually at the level of the nipple (avoid breast tissue).
d. Prepare skin and drape in a sterile fashion.
e. Patient may require sedation (see Chapter 6). Locally anesthetize skin, subcutaneous tissue, periosteum of rib, chest wall muscles, and pleura with 1% lidocaine.
f. Make a sterile 1- to 3-cm incision one intercostal space below desired insertion point, and bluntly dissect with a hemostat through tissue layers until the superior portion of the rib is reached, avoiding the neurovascular bundle on the inferior portion of the rib.
g. Push hemostat over the top of the rib, through pleura, and into pleural space. Enter the pleural space cautiously and not deeper than 1 cm. Spread hemostat to open, place chest tube in clamp, and guide through entry site to desired distance.
h. For pneumothorax, insert tube anteriorly toward the apex. For pleural effusion, direct tube inferiorly and posteriorly.
i. Secure chest tube with sutures, first suturing a "purse string" of continuous running sutures encircling approximately a square

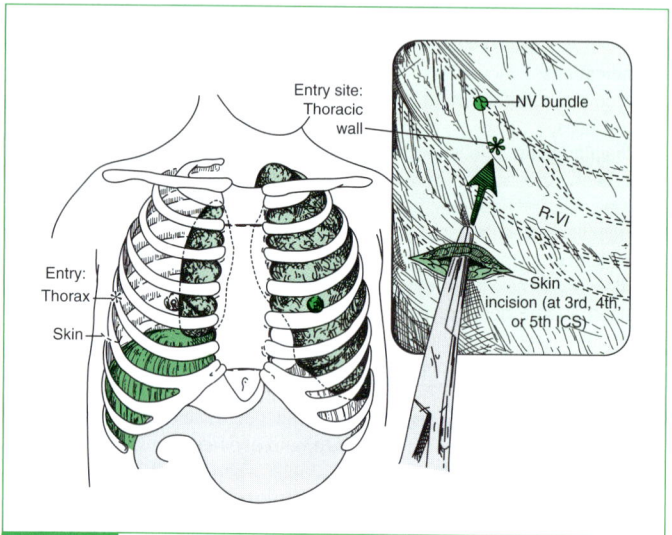

FIGURE 3.13

Technique for insertion of chest tube. ICS, Intercostal space; NV, neurovascular; R-VI, sixth rib. *(Modified from Fleisher G, Ludwig S.* Pediatric Emergency Medicine. *3rd ed. Baltimore: Williams & Wilkins; 2000.)*

centimeter around the site of insertion. This is placed such that an equal length emerges both from where the purse string enters and exits the skin. The pursestring is tightened with a surgical knot at the skin. Then wrap both free ends of suture multiple times around the tube in opposite directions, tying after at least 7 wraps have been performed to form a braided or "ballerina slipper" pattern on the tube. Make sure that the wraps are closely placed and tight around the insertion site near where the drain enters the skin. This improves retention of the tube should it accidentally be pulled. An additional anchor is recommended by securely taping the chest tube to the chest several inches caudad from the insertion site to the patient's flank.

j. Attach to a drainage system with 20–30 cm H_2O or water seal.
k. Apply a sterile occlusive dressing with petroleum gauze at the insertion site.
l. Confirm position and function with chest radiograph.
6. **A video on chest tube insertion is available on the *New England Journal of Medicine's* website.**
7. **Procedure: Thoracentesis (Fig. 3.14)**
a. Confirm fluid in pleural space by clinical examination and radiographs or ultrasonography.

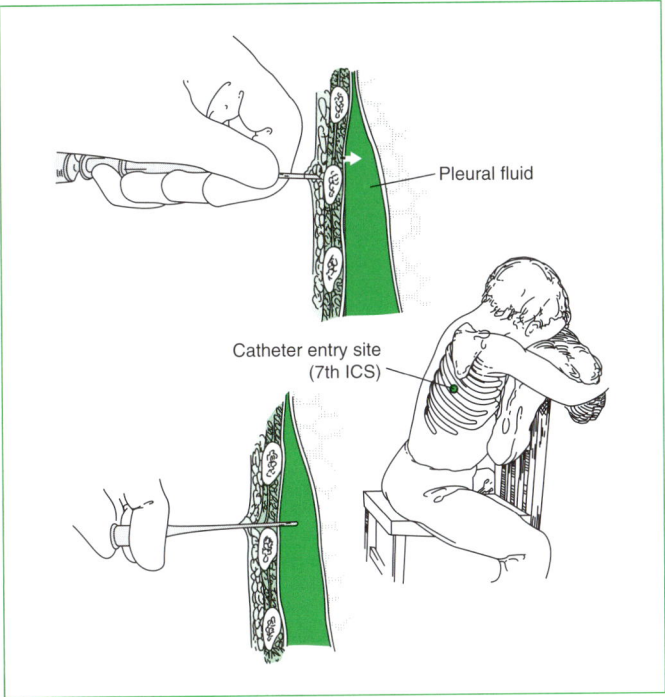

FIGURE 3.14

Thoracentesis. ICS, Intercostal space. *(Modified from Fleisher G, Ludwig S.* Pediatric Emergency Medicine. *3rd ed. Baltimore: Williams & Wilkins; 2000.)*

(1) A curvilinear or linear probe can be used.
(2) Proceed with preparation and draping of the patient per the normal procedure described.
(3) Place a sterile probe cover over the ultrasound probe.
(4) Apply the probe parallel to the spine on the affected hemithorax below the axilla or scapula depending on the positioning of the patient. Starting inferiorly at the lower ribs, move the probe cephalad until the pleural effusion is visualized. The pleural effusion will appear dark while lung tissue will appear bright (Fig. 3.15). Confirmation of the effusion space can be performed with the probe placed parallel inside the intercostal space to remove the obscuring effects of ribs.
(5) Identify a rib space suitable for thoracentesis based on distance from lung tissue and other structures and mark site. Ensure that the diaphragm (a bright, hyperechoic line that moves with

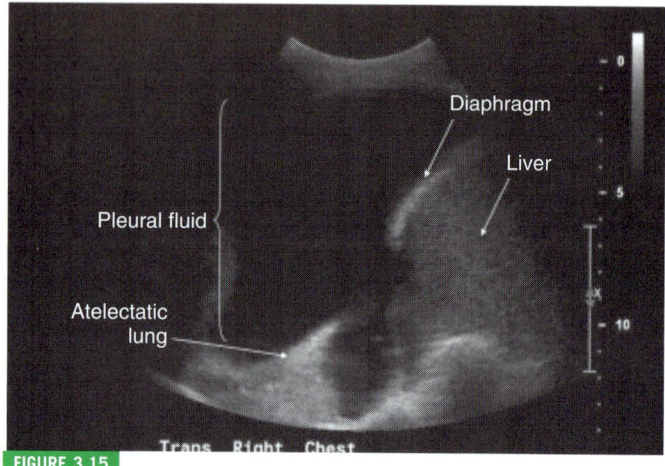

FIGURE 3.15

Ultrasound of pleural effusion. A longitudinal view of the thorax demonstrating a right sided pleural effusion. The black fluid collection is the pleural effusion; at the base of the image atelectatic lung is visualized deep to the effusion. The diaphragm and liver are also in view and labeled. Care should be taken to select a rib space that avoids the moving diaphragm and a large pocket of pleural fluid that avoids lung tissue. *(From Broder J. Diagnostic Imaging for the Emergency Physician. Philadelphia: Elsevier 2011;185-296.)*

      respiration on ultrasound) does not move into the area to be instrumented during respiration prior to selecting site.
   (6) This site can be marked for insertion for the procedure. A variation of this process is to identify the site prior to preparation and draping. If marking is performed before draping, the patient should not be moved before needle insertion.
   (7) The procedure should then proceed with needle insertion, as described below.
b. If possible, place child in sitting position leaning over table; otherwise place supine.
c. Point of entry is usually in the seventh intercostal space and posterior axillary line.
d. Prepare and drape area in a sterile fashion.
e. Anesthetize skin, subcutaneous tissue, rib periosteum, chest wall, and pleura with 1% lidocaine.
f. Advance an 18- to 22-gauge IV catheter or large-bore needle attached to a syringe onto the rib, and then "walk" over the superior aspect into the pleural space while providing steady negative pressure; often a popping sensation is perceived. *Be careful not to advance too far into the pleural cavity.* If an IV or drainage catheter (with Seldinger

guidewire) is used, the soft catheter may be advanced into the pleural space, aiming towards the patient's spine.
g. Attach syringe and stopcock device to remove fluid for diagnostic studies and therapeutic reasons (see Chapter 27 for evaluation of pleural fluid).
h. After removing needle or catheter, place an occlusive dressing over the site and obtain a chest radiograph to rule out pneumothorax.
8. **A video on thoracentesis is available on the *New England Journal of Medicine's* website.**

C. Pericardiocentesis[3,6]

1. **Indications:** To obtain pericardial fluid in cardiac tamponade emergently or nonemergently for diagnostic or therapeutic purposes.
2. **Complications:** Bleeding, infection, puncture of myocardium, cardiac dysrhythmia, hemopericardium or pneumopericardium, pneumothorax, hemothorax, cardiac arrest, death.
3. **Procedure** (Fig. 3.16)**:**
a. Unless contraindicated, provide sedation and/or analgesia for the patient. Monitor electrocardiogram (ECG).
b. Ultrasound is sometimes used to visualize a pericardial effusion for planning a nonemergent pericardiocentesis. Typically the apical four chamber view is used for this. The details of the use of ultrasound for this procedure are beyond the scope of this text.
c. Place patient head inclined at a 30-degree angle (reverse Trendelenburg). Have patient secured.
d. Prepare and drape puncture site in a sterile fashion. A drape across the upper chest may obscure important landmarks.
e. Anesthetize puncture site with 1% lidocaine.
f. Insert an 18- or 20-gauge needle with attached 20-cc syringe just to the left of the xiphoid process, 1 cm inferior to the bottom rib at about a 45-degree angle to the skin. A sterile ECG attachment is sometimes available and can be attached for monitoring needle position. The trajectory of the needle should be towards the patient's left shoulder.
g. Gently aspirate while advancing the needle towards the patient's left shoulder until pericardial fluid is obtained. Monitor ECG for any changes that suggest penetration of the myocardium.
h. Gently and slowly remove the fluid. Rapid withdrawal of pericardial fluid can result in shock or myocardial insufficiency.
i. Send fluid for appropriate laboratory studies (see Chapter 27).
j. Whenever possible this is best performed under echocardiographic guidance.
4. **A video on pericardiocentesis is available on the *New England Journal of Medicine's* website.**

D. Paracentesis[4]

1. **Indications:** Percutaneous removal of intraperitoneal fluid for diagnostic or therapeutic purposes.

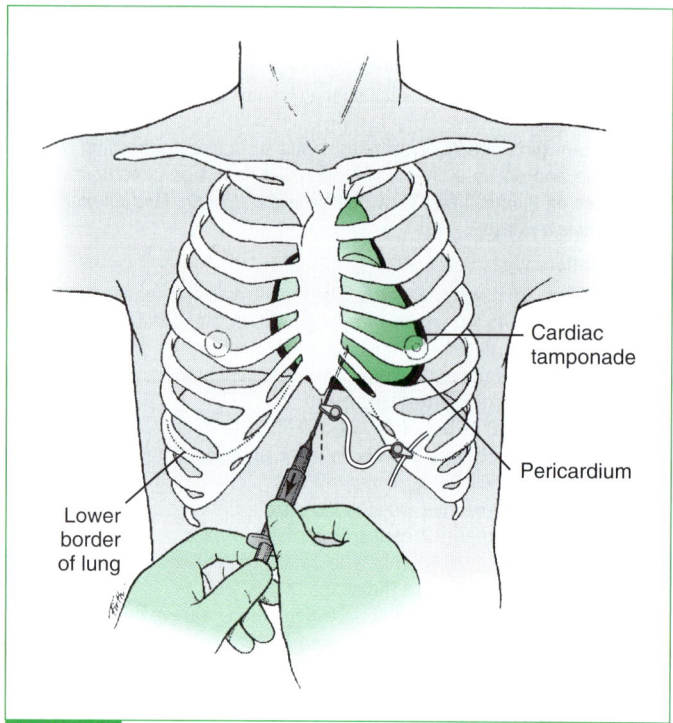

FIGURE 3.16

Insertion of needle for pericardiocentesis at junction of xiphoid and left costal margin, aiming toward left shoulder. *(Modified from Brundage SI, Scott BG, Karmy-Jones R, et al. Pericardiocentesis and pericardial window. In: Shoemaker WC, Velmahos BC, Demetriades D, eds. Procedures and Monitoring for the Critically Ill. Philadelphia: Saunders; 2002. p. 57.)*

2. **Complications:** Bleeding, infection, puncture of viscera.
3. **Cautions:**
a. *Do not* remove a large amount of fluid too rapidly; hypovolemia and hypotension may result from rapid fluid shifts.
b. Avoid scars from previous surgery; localized bowel adhesions increase the chance of entering a viscus in these areas.
c. Urinary bladder should be empty to avoid perforation.
d. Never perform paracentesis through an area of cellulitis.
e. Insertion should be performed either midline below the umbilicus or lateral to the rectus muscles to avoid puncturing the inferior epigastric arteries.

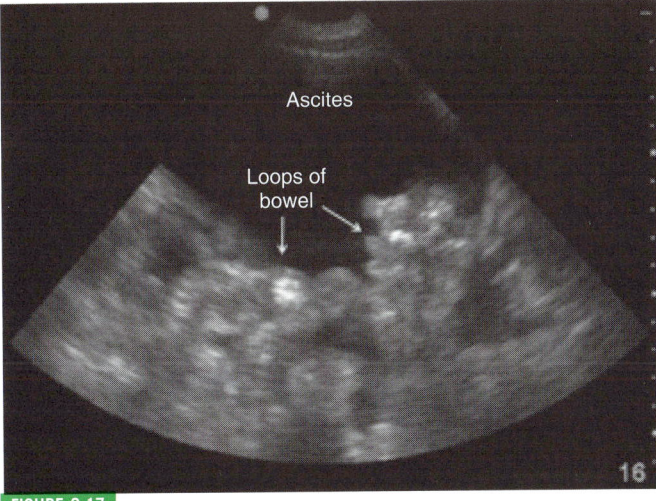

FIGURE 3.17

Ultrasound of ascites for abdominal paracentesis. This view of the abdomen demonstrates ascites (black) with loops of bowel noted deeper. Care must be taken to ensure adequate distance between the bowel wall and abdominal wall prior to marking the site of paracentesis. *(From Hatch, N, Wu, T. Advanced ultrasound procedures.* Crit Care Clin. *2014;30[2]. 309-325.)*

4. **Procedure:**
   a. Prepare and drape abdomen in a sterile fashion.
   b. With patient in supine position, place a linear or curvilinear ultrasound probe in the area where the puncture will be performed in the midline, right, or left lower quadrant.
      (1) Identify an ascites pocket, which will appear dark (Fig. 3.17).
      (2) Ensure a distance of at least 2 cm between bowel and peritoneal wall.
      (3) Look for the inferior epigastric vessels along the peritoneal wall. More advanced users with expertise in Doppler imaging can use this to help identify them. These vessels should be avoided and tend to lay along the lateral margins of the rectus abdominis muscles. Therefore, they are often easier to identify with the probe oriented transverse to the spine.
      (4) Mark site and continue with paracentesis as described below.
   c. Anesthetize the puncture site with 1% lidocaine.
   d. With patient in semisupine, sitting, or lateral decubitus position, insert a 16- to 22-gauge IV catheter attached to a syringe at the marked site. If ultrasound is unavailable, insert needle in the midline, 2 cm

below umbilicus. In neonates, insert just lateral to rectus muscle in the right or left lower quadrants, a few centimeters above the inguinal ligament.
e. Aiming cephalad, insert needle at a 45-degree angle while one hand pulls the skin caudally until entering the peritoneal cavity. This creates a "Z-track" when the skin is released and the needle removed. Apply continuous negative pressure.
f. Once fluid appears in the syringe, remove introducer needle and leave catheter in place. Attach a stopcock and aspirate slowly until an adequate amount of fluid has been obtained for studies or symptomatic relief.
g. If, on entering the peritoneal cavity, air is aspirated, withdraw the needle immediately. Aspirated air suggests entrance into a hollow viscus, especially if the patient does not have pneumoperitoneum (penetration of a hollow viscus during paracentesis does not frequently lead to complications). Repeat paracentesis with sterile equipment. The aspiration of bright red blood is suspicious for arterial puncture. Management of hemoperitoneum in this patient population may result in a surgical emergency depending on whether the patient manifests vital sign instability.
h. Send fluid for appropriate laboratory studies (see Chapter 27).
5. **A video on paracentesis is available on the *New England Journal of Medicine's* website.**

E. Urinary Bladder Catheterization[4]

1. **Indications:** To obtain urine for urinalysis and sterile culture and to accurately monitor hydration status.
2. **Complications:** Hematuria, infection, trauma to urethra or bladder, intravesical knot of catheter (rarely occurs).
3. **Caution:** Catheterization is contraindicated in pelvic fractures, known trauma to the urethra, or blood at the meatus.
4. **Procedure:**
a. Infant/child should not have voided within 1 hour of procedure.
b. Prepare the urethral opening using sterile technique.
c. In males, apply gentle traction to the penis to straighten the urethra. In uncircumcised male infants, expose the meatus with gentle retraction of the foreskin. The foreskin has to be retracted only far enough to visualize the meatus.
d. In girls, the urethral orifice may be difficult to visualize, but it is usually immediately anterior to the vaginal orifice.
e. Gently insert a lubricated catheter into the urethra. Slowly advance catheter until resistance is met at the external sphincter. Continued pressure will overcome this resistance, and the catheter will enter the bladder. Only a few centimeters of advancement are required to reach the bladder in girls. In boys, insert a few centimeters longer than the shaft of the penis.

f. Carefully remove the catheter once specimen is obtained, and cleanse skin of iodine.

g. If indwelling Foley catheter is inserted, inflate balloon with sterile water or saline as indicated on bulb, then connect catheter to drainage tubing attached to urine drainage bag. Secure catheter tubing to inner thigh.

5. **Videos on catheterization of the male urethra and catheterization of the female urethra are available on the *New England Journal of Medicine's* website.**

F. Suprapubic Bladder Aspiration[3]

1. **Indications:** To obtain urine in a sterile manner for urinalysis and culture in children younger than 2 years (avoid in children with genitourinary tract anomalies, coagulopathy, or intestinal obstruction). This bypasses distal urethra, thereby minimizing risk for contamination.
2. **Complications:** Infection (cellulitis), hematuria (usually microscopic), intestinal perforation.
3. **Procedure** (Fig. 3.18)**:**
a. Anterior rectal pressure in girls or gentle penile pressure in boys may be used to prevent urination during the procedure. Child should not have voided within 1 hour of procedure.
b. Restrain child in the supine, frog-leg position. Prepare suprapubic area in a sterile fashion.
c. The site for puncture is 1–2 cm above the symphysis pubis in the midline. Use a syringe with a 22-gauge, 1-inch needle, and puncture at a 10- to 20- degree angle to the perpendicular, aiming slightly caudad.
d. Ultrasound guidance (see Expert Consult).
e. Gently exert suction as the needle is advanced until urine enters syringe. The needle should not be advanced more than 3 cm. Aspirate urine with gentle suction.
f. Remove needle, cleanse skin of iodine, and apply a sterile bandage.
4. **A video of suprapubic bladder aspiration is available on the *New England Journal of Medicine's* website.**

G. Knee Arthrocentesis[3]

1. **Indications:** Evaluation of fluid for the diagnosis of disease, including infectious, inflammatory, and crystalline disease, and removal of fluid for relief of pain and/or functional limitation.
2. **Contraindications:** Bleeding diathesis, local fracture, overlying skin infection.
3. **Complications:** Pain, bleeding, infection.
4. **Procedure:** Place child supine on exam table with knee in full extension, with use of a padded roll underneath the knee for support, if unable to fully extend. The lateral or medial approach

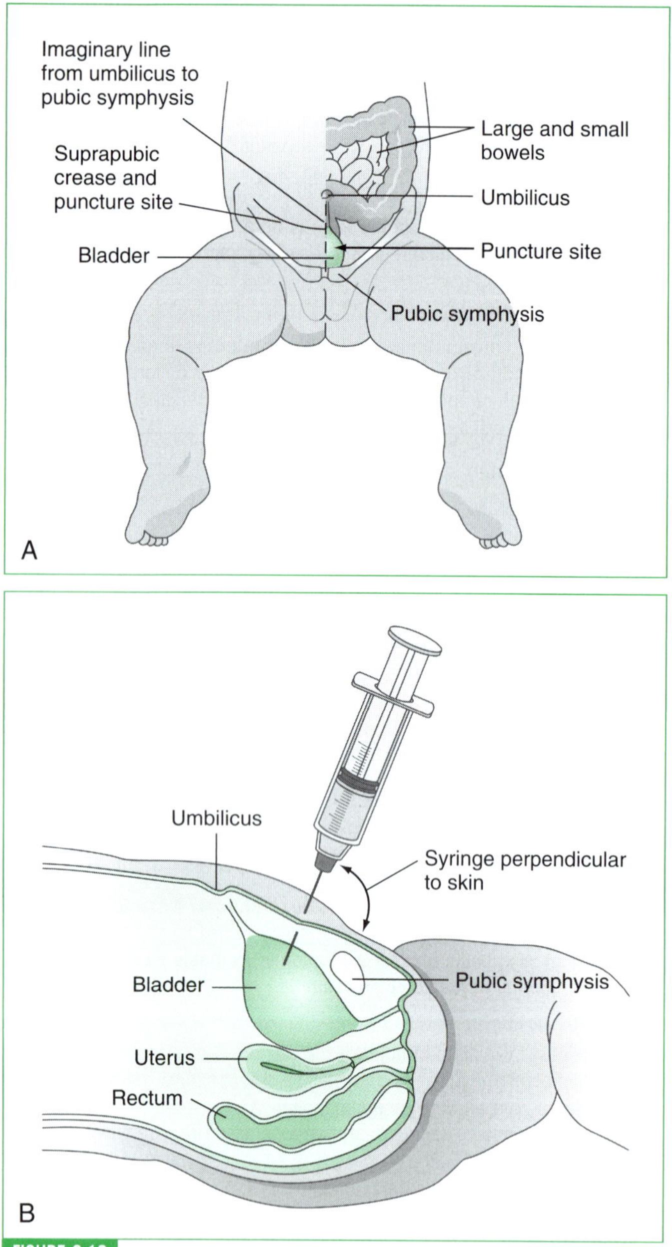

FIGURE 3.18

Landmarks for suprapubic bladder aspiration. (*Modified from Dieckmann R, Fiser D, Selbst S. Pediatric Emergency and Critical Care Procedures. St. Louis: Mosby; 1997.*)

can be made, with the lateral approach preferred to avoid the vastus medialis muscle. The puncture point should be at the posterior margin of the patella in both cases. Prep the overlying skin in a sterile fashion, and once cleaned, numb the area using 1% lidocaine with a small gauge needle. Then, using an 18-gauge needle attached to a syringe, puncture the skin at a 10- to 20- degree downward angle, and advance under continuous syringe suction until fluid is withdrawn, indicating entry into the joint space. In large effusions, several syringes may be needed for complete fluid removal if so desired, and the needle may have to be redirected to access pockets of fluid. Upon completion, withdraw the needle and cover the wound with a sterile gauze dressing. Synovial fluid can then be sent for studies as indicated.
5. **A video on knee arthrocentesis is available on the *New England Journal of Medicine's* website.**

H. Soft Tissue Aspiration[9]

1. **Indications:** Cellulitis that is unresponsive to initial standard therapy, recurrent cellulitis or abscesses, immunocompromised patients in whom organism recovery is necessary and may affect antimicrobial therapy.
2. **Complications:** Pain, infection, bleeding.
3. **Procedure:**
a. Select site to aspirate at the point of maximal inflammation (more likely to increase recovery of causative agent than leading edge of erythema or center).[9]
b. Cleanse area in a sterile fashion.
c. Local anesthesia with 1% lidocaine is optional.
d. Fill tuberculin syringe with 0.1–0.2 mL of *nonbacteriostatic* sterile saline, and attach to needle.
e. Using 18- or 20-gauge needle (22-gauge for facial cellulitis), advance to appropriate depth and apply negative pressure while withdrawing needle.
f. Send fluid from aspiration for Gram stain and cultures. If no fluid is obtained, needle can be streaked on agar plate. Consider acid-fast bacillus (AFB) and fungal stains in immunocompromised patients.

I. Incision and Drainage (I & D) of Abscess[3]

1. **Indications:** Diagnostic and therapeutic drainage of soft tissue abscess.
2. **Complications:** Inadequate abscess drainage, local tissue injury, pain, scar formation, and in rare cases fistula formation. Consider specialized surgical evaluation for abscesses in cosmetically or anatomically sensitive areas such as the face, breast, or the anogenital region.

3. **Ultrasound Identification:** Ultrasound imaging can be used to differentiate cellulitis from abscess.
a. Use a linear probe and place the probe over the area of interest and scan it systematically such that the entire area of interest is examined.
b. Cellulitis characteristics on ultrasound
    (1) Increased edema, tissue may appear slightly darker, and will have distorted, indistinct margins.
    (2) Areas may have a "cobblestone" appearance caused by edema (Fig. 3.19).
c. Abscess Characteristics
    (1) Dark fluid collection distinct from surrounding tissue (see Fig. 3.19).
    (2) Often round or oval in shape.
4. **Procedure:** Consider procedural sedation based upon the child's expected tolerance of the procedure and the location/size/complexity of the abscess. Apply topical anesthetic cream to the abscess to numb superficial epidermis. Prep the overlying skin in a sterile fashion, and once cleaned, numb the area using 1% lidocaine and a small gauge needle, performing first a circumferential field block of the abscess area followed by direct injection to the planned incision site. Incise the skin over the abscess down to the superficial fascia using a scalpel

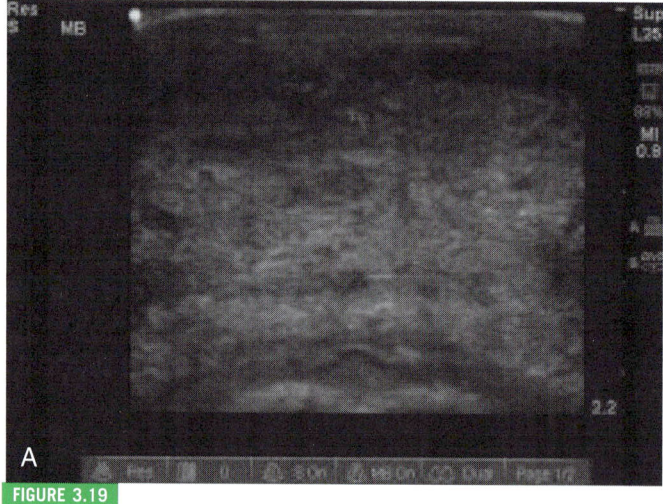

FIGURE 3.19

Ultrasound characteristics of soft tissue cellulitis and abscess. **A,** Cellulitis characterized by bright (hyperechoic) tissue due to edema and inflammation in the tissue.

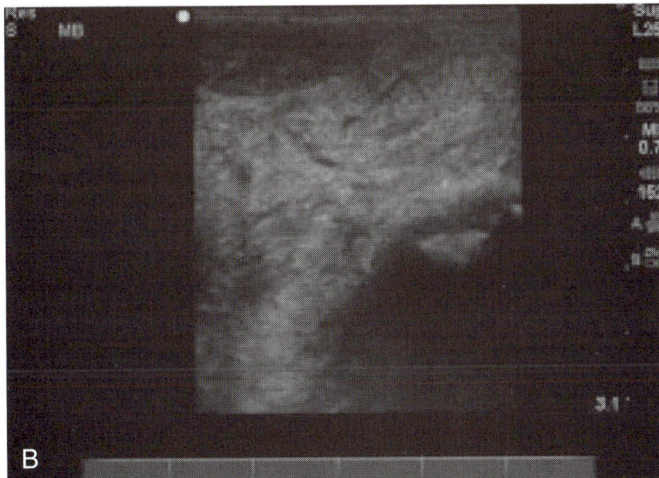

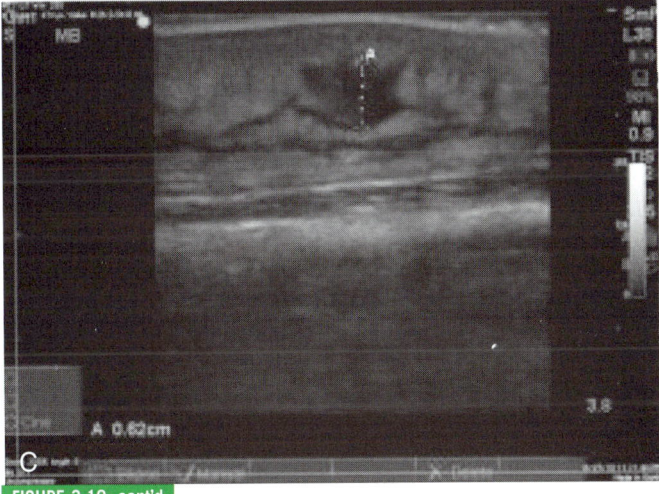

FIGURE 3.19, cont'd
B, This image demonstrates the classic "cobblestone" appearance which is a later ultrasound finding in cellulitis. **C,** A black (anechoic) rounded structure is noted in the soft tissue, which is characteristic of a soft tissue abscess. Some abscesses may appear dark gray depending on the characteristics of the fluid within the abscess. *(From Leeson K, Leeson B. Pediatric ultrasound: applications in the emergency department.* Emerg Med Clin North Am. *2013;31(3):809-829.)*

blade cutting parallel to the natural crease of the skin, if present. Using hemostats, bluntly widen and undermine the incision to break up any septated or loculated fluid collections. Vigorously irrigate the wound using sterile NS to improve removal of purulent material. If desired, introduce a sterile packing strip into the wound using the hemostats, making sure to fill in an outside to inside pattern without overfilling. Leave a 2- to 3-cm tail outside the wound to facilitate removal and cover the wound with an absorbent dressing. Packing material should be removed in 1–2 days with a minimum of daily dressing changes until healed.
5. **A video on I & D of Abscesses is available on the *New England Journal of Medicine's* website.**

V. IMMUNIZATION AND MEDICATION ADMINISTRATION[4]

NOTE: Please see Chapter 16, "Immunoprophylaxis," and Chapter 29, "Drug Dosages," for relevant vaccines and medications and their appropriate administration routes.

A. Subcutaneous Injections

1. **Indications:** Immunizations and other medications.
2. **Complications:** Bleeding, infection, allergic reaction, lipohypertrophy or lipoatrophy after repeated injections.
3. **Procedure:**
a. Locate injection site: Upper outer arm or outer aspect of upper thigh.
b. Cleanse skin with alcohol.
c. Insert 0.5-inch, 25- or 27-gauge needle into subcutaneous layer at a 45-degree angle to the skin. Aspirate for blood, and then inject medication.

B. Intramuscular Injections

1. **Indications:** Immunizations and other medications.
2. **Complications:** Bleeding, infection, allergic reaction, nerve injury.
3. **Cautions:**
a. Avoid intramuscular (IM) injections in a child with a bleeding disorder or thrombocytopenia.
b. Maximum volume to be injected is 0.5 mL in a small infant, 1 mL in an older infant, 2 mL in a school-aged child, and 3 mL in an adolescent.
4. **Procedure:**
a. Locate injection site: Anterolateral upper thigh (vastus lateralis muscle) in smaller child or outer aspect of upper arm (deltoid) in older one. The dorsal gluteal region is less commonly used because of risk for nerve or vascular injury. To find the ventral gluteal site, form a triangle by placing your index finger on the anterior iliac spine and your middle finger on the most superior aspect of the iliac crest. The injection should occur in the middle of the triangle formed by the two fingers and the iliac crest.

b. Cleanse skin with alcohol.
c. Pinch muscle with free hand and insert 1-inch, 23- or 25-gauge needle until hub is flush with skin surface. For deltoid and ventral gluteal muscles, needle should be perpendicular to skin. For anterolateral thigh, needle should be at a 45-degree angle to the long axis of the thigh. Aspirate for blood, and then inject medication.

VI. BASIC LACERATION REPAIR[3]

A. Suturing

1. **Basic Suture Techniques** (Fig. 3.20):
a. Simple interrupted: Basic closure of most uncomplicated wounds.
b. Horizontal mattress: Provides eversion of wound edges.
c. Vertical mattress: For added strength in areas of thick skin or areas of skin movement; provides eversion of wound edges.
d. Running intradermal: For cosmetic closures.
e. Deep dermal: For bringing together deeper portions of wounds with dissolving sutures to allow improved approximation and closure of superficial surfaces.
2. **Procedure:**
a. See Table 3.1 for sutures material, size, and time for removal.
b. **NOTE:** Lacerations of the face, lips, hands, genitalia, mouth, or periorbital area may require consultation with a specialist. Ideally, lacerations at increased risk for infection (areas with poor blood supply, contaminated, or crush injury) should be sutured within 6 hours of injury. Clean wounds in cosmetically important areas may be closed up to 24 hours after injury in the absence of significant contamination or devitalization. In general, bite wounds should not be sutured except in areas of high cosmetic importance (face). The longer the sutures are left in place, the greater the scarring and potential for infection. Sutures in cosmetically sensitive areas should be removed as soon as possible. Sutures in high tension areas (e.g., extensor surfaces) should stay in longer.
c. Prepare child for procedure with appropriate sedation, analgesia, and restraint.
d. Anesthetize the wound with topical anesthetic or with lidocaine mixed with bicarbonate (with or without epinephrine) by injecting the anesthetic into the subcutaneous tissues (see Formulary).
e. Forcefully irrigate the wound with copious amounts of sterile NS. Use at least 100 mL per 1 cm of wound. This is the most important step in preventing infection.
f. Prepare and drape the patient for a sterile procedure.
g. Debride the wound when indicated. Probe for foreign bodies as indicated. Consider obtaining a radiograph if a radiopaque foreign body was involved in the injury.
h. Select suture type for percutaneous closure (see Table 3.1).

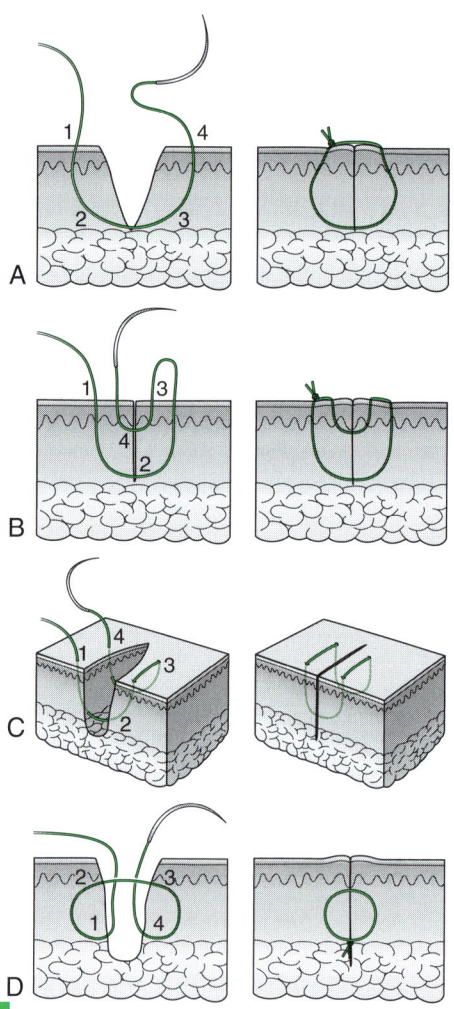

FIGURE 3.20

A–D, Suture techniques. (A) Simple interrupted. (B) Vertical mattress. (C) Horizontal mattress. (D) Deep dermal. *(Modified from Srivastava D, Taylor RS. Suturing Technique and Other Closure Materials. In: Robinson JK, Hanke CW, Siegel DM, et al., eds. Surgery of the Skin. 3rd ed. Elsevier: Philadelphia, PA; 2015:193-213.)*

TABLE 3.1
GUIDELINES FOR SUTURE MATERIAL, SIZE, AND REMOVAL

Body Region	Monofilament* (for Superficial Lacerations)	Absorbable† (for Deep Lacerations)	Duration (Days)
Scalp	5–0 or 4–0	4–0	5–7
Face	6–0	5–0	3–5
Eyelid	7–0 or 6–0	—	3–5
Eyebrow	6–0 or 5–0	5–0	3–5
Trunk	5–0 or 4–0	3–0	5–7
Extremities	5–0 or 4–0	4–0	7–10
Joint surface	4–0	—	10–14
Hand	5–0	5–0	7
Foot sole	4–0 or 3–0	4–0	7–10

*Examples of monofilament nonabsorbable sutures: Nylon, polypropylene. Good for the outermost layer of skin. Use 4–5 throws per knot. Polypropylene is good for scalp, eyebrows.
†Examples of absorbable sutures: Polyglycolic acid and polyglactin 910 (Vicryl). Good for deeper, subcuticular layers.

    i. Match layers of injured tissues. Carefully match the depth of the bite taken on each side of the wound when suturing. Take equal bites from both wound edges. Apply slight thumb pressure on the wound edge as the needle is entering the opposite side. Pull the sutures to approximate wound edges, but not too tightly to avoid tissue necrosis. In delicate areas, sutures should be approximately 2 mm apart and 2 mm from the wound edge. Larger bites are acceptable where cosmesis is less important.[3]

    j. When suturing is complete, apply topical antibiotic and sterile dressing. If laceration is in proximity of a joint, splinting of the affected area to limit mobility often speeds healing and prevents wound separation.

    k. Check wounds at 48–72 hours in cases where wounds are of questionable viability, if wound was packed, or for patients prescribed prophylactic antibiotics. Change dressing at checkup.

    l. For hand lacerations, close skin only; do not use subcutaneous stitches. Elevate and immobilize the hand. Consider consulting a hand or plastics specialist.

    m. Consider the need for tetanus prophylaxis (see Chapter 16, Table 16.3, for guidelines).

3. **A video on basic laceration repair is available on the *New England Journal of Medicine's* website.**

B. Skin Staples

1. **Indications:**

a. Best for scalp, trunk, extremities.
b. More rapid application than sutures but can be more painful to remove.
c. Lower rates of wound infection.

2. **Contraindications:**
a. Not for areas that require meticulous cosmesis.
b. Avoid in patients who require magnetic resonance imaging (MRI) or computed tomography (CT).
3. **Procedure:**
a. Apply topical anesthetic as above. Injection of lidocaine is not routinely employed when using staples.
b. Clean and irrigate wound as with suturing.
c. Appose wound edges, press stapler firmly against skin at center of apposed edges, and staple.
d. Apply antibiotic ointment and sterile bandage.
e. Left in place for the same length of time as sutures (see Table 3.1).
f. To remove, use staple remover.

C. Tissue Adhesives[10]

1. **Indications:**
a. For use with superficial lacerations with clean edges.
b. Excellent cosmetic results, ease of application, and reduced patient anxiety.
c. Lower rates of wound infection.
2. **Contraindications:**
a. Not for use in areas under large amounts of tension (e.g., hands, joints).
b. Use caution with areas near the eye or over areas with hair such as the eyebrow.
3. **Procedure:**
a. Use pressure to achieve hemostasis and clean the wound as explained previously.
b. Hold together wound edges.
c. Apply adhesive dropwise along the wound surface, avoiding applying adhesive to the inside of the wound. Hold in place for 20–30 seconds.
d. If the wound is malaligned, remove the adhesive with forceps and reapply. Petroleum jelly or similar substance can aid in removal of skin adhesive.
e. Adhesive will slough off after 7–10 days.
f. Antibiotic ointments or other creams/lotions should not be applied to the adhesive as this can cause premature loosening of the glue and subsequent wound dehiscence.

VII. MUSCULOSKELETAL PROCEDURES

A. Basic Splinting[3]

1. **Indications:** to provide short-term stabilization of limb injuries while accommodating swelling associated with acute injuries.
2. **Complications:** pressure sores, dermatitis, neurovascular impairment.

3. **Procedure:**
   a. Determine style of splint needed.
   b. Measure and cut fiberglass or plaster to appropriate length. If using plaster, upper-extremity splints require 8–10 layers, and lower-extremity splints require 12–14 layers.
   c. Pad extremity with cotton roll padding, taking care to overlap each turn by 50%. In prepackaged fiberglass splints, additional padding is not generally required. Bony prominences may require additional padding. Place cotton between digits if they are in a splint.
   d. Immerse plaster slabs into room temperature water until bubbling stops. Smooth out wet plaster slab, avoiding any wrinkles. Fiberglass splints will harden when exposed to air; however, application of a small amount of room temperature water can accelerate this process.
   e. Position splint over extremity and mold to desired contour. Wrap with an elastic bandage to hold molded splint onto extremity in position of function. Continue to hold desired form of splint upon extremity until fully hardened.
   f. **NOTE:** Plaster becomes hot while drying. Using warm water will decrease drying time. This may result in inadequate time to mold splint. Turn edge of the splint back on itself to produce a smooth surface. Take care to cover the sharp edges of fiberglass.
   g. Use crutches or slings as indicated.
   h. The need for orthopedic referral should be individually assessed.
   i. Emergent orthopedic consultation is required when there is concern for neurovascular compromise or compartment syndrome of the affected extremity.
4. **Postsplint Care:**
   a. Standard rest, ice, and elevation of affected extremity should be performed.
   b. Avoid weight bearing on splinted extremity.
   c. Do not get splint wet. Splints can be wrapped in water-resistant items such as a plastic bag or a specially designed splint bag to allow for showering. Use a hair dryer in instances where the splint has accidentally gotten wet.
   d. Do not stick items such as a pen or clothes hanger to scratch inside the splint.
   e. If areas in or distal to the splint develop numbness, tingling, increased pain, turn blue or pale, or become swollen, you should loosen the elastic bandage of the splint. Seek immediate medical care if this does not quickly (<30 minutes) resolve these symptoms.
5. **A video on basic splinting techniques is available on the *New England Journal of Medicine's* website.**

B. Selected Splints and Indications (Fig. 3.21)

See Expert Consult for description of specific splints.

C. Radial Head Subluxation (Nursemaid's Elbow) Reduction

1. **Presentation:** Commonly occurs in children aged 1–4 years with a history of inability to use an arm after it was pulled. Child presents with affected arm held at the side in pronation, with elbow slightly flexed.
2. **Caution:** Rule out a fracture clinically before doing procedure. Consider radiograph if mechanism of injury or history is atypical.
3. **Procedure:**
a. Support the elbow with one hand, and place your thumb laterally over the radial head at the elbow. With your other hand, grasp the child's hand in a handshake position or at the wrist.
b. Quickly and deliberately supinate and externally rotate the forearm, and simultaneously flex the elbow. Alternatively, hyperpronation alone may be used. You may feel a click as reduction occurs.
c. Most children will begin to use the arm within 15 minutes, some immediately after reduction. If reduction occurs after a prolonged period of subluxation, it may take the child longer to recover use of the arm. In this case, the arm should be immobilized with a posterior splint.
d. If procedure is unsuccessful, consider obtaining a radiograph. Maneuver may be repeated if needed.
4. **A video on reduction of nursemaid's elbow is available on the *New England Journal of Medicine's* website.**

D. Finger/Toe Dislocation Reduction[3]

1. **Indications:** Interphalangeal and metacarpophalangeal/metatarsophalangeal dislocations.
2. **Complications:** Fracture of phalanges, entrapment of neurovascular structures.
3. **Cautions:** Volar dislocations and dorsal dislocations with interposition of the volar plate or entrapment of the metacarpal/metatarsal head often cannot be performed using closed reduction.
4. **Procedure:** Evaluate for neurovascular compromise in the affected digit. Perform radiographs to evaluate for possible fracture. Consider procedural sedation or a digital block prior to procedure. Grasp the extremity proximal to fracture to allow for stabilization. Grasp the tip of the distal digit and apply longitudinal traction, with the joint typically slipping into place. Alternatively, grasp the distal phalanx and mildly hyperextend to accentuate the deformity while applying longitudinal traction. After reduction, again evaluate neurovascular status and obtain radiographs to ensure proper position and to further evaluate for fracture. Immobilize the joint using a padded splint using full extension for distal interphalangeal joints and 20–30 degrees of flexion for proximal interphalangeal joints.

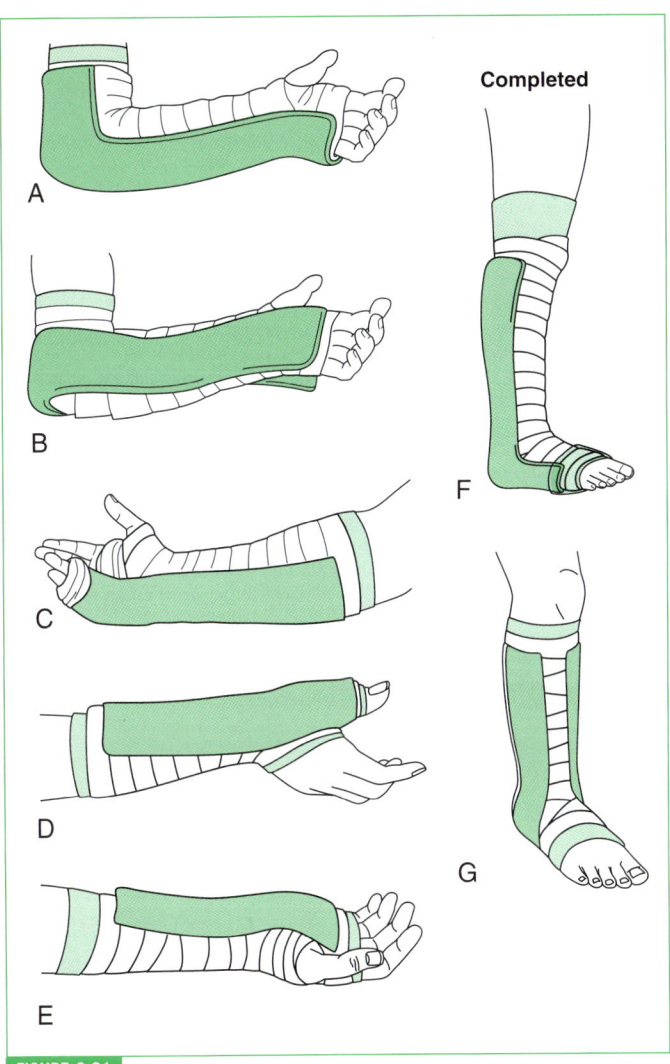

FIGURE 3.21

Selected splint types. Light green layer is stockinette, white layer is cotton roll, dark green layer is the splint. (A) Long arm posterior splint. (B) Sugar tong forearm splint. (C) Ulnar gutter splint. (D). Thumb spica splint. (E) Volar splint. (F) Posterior ankle splint. (G) Ankle stirrup splint.

REFERENCES

1. AAP guidelines for monitoring and management of pediatric patients during and after sedation for diagnostic and therapeutic procedures: an update. *Pediatrics.* 2006;118:2587-2602.
2. Barone MA. Pediatric procedures. In: *Oski's Pediatrics: Principles and Practice.* Philadelphia: Lippincott Williams & Wilkins; 4th edition, 2006:2671-2687.
3. Fleisher G, Ludwig S. *Textbook of Pediatric Emergency Medicine.* 6th ed. Baltimore: Williams & Wilkins; 2010. pp1-2000
4. Dieckmann R, Fiser D, Selbst S. *Illustrated Textbook of Pediatric Emergency and Critical Care Procedures.* St. Louis: Mosby; 1997. pp1-796
5. Jain A, Haines L. Ultrasound-guided critical care procedures. In: *Critical Care Emergency Medicine.* New York: McGraw-Hill; 2012.
6. Nichols DG, Yaster M, Lappe DG, et al. *Golden Hour: The Handbook of Advanced Pediatric Life Support.* 2nd ed. St. Louis: Mosby; 1996.
7. Berenholtz SM, Pronovost PJ, Lipsett PA, et al. Eliminating catheter-related bloodstream infections in the intensive care unit. *Crit Care Med.* 2004;32:2014-2020.
8. Brass P, Hellmich M, Kolodziej L, et al. Ultrasound guidance versus anatomical landmarks for internal jugular vein catheterization. *Cochrane Database Syst Rev.* 2015;1:CD006962.
9. Howe PM, Eduardo Fajardo J, Orcutt MA. Etiologic diagnosis of cellulitis: comparison of aspirates obtained from the leading edge and the point of maximal inflammation. *Pediatr Infect Dis J.* 1987;6:685-686.
10. Hines EQ, Klein BL, Cohen JS. Glue adhesives for repairing minor skin lacerations. Contemporary Pediatrics Online. December 31, 2012.

Chapter 4
Trauma, Burns, and Common Critical Care Emergencies
Amanda O'Halloran, MD

See additional content on Expert Consult

I. WEB RESOURCES
- The Pediatric Critical Care Medicine Website: http://pedsccm.org/
- Pediatric Trauma Society: http://www.pediatrictraumasociety.org/
- Centers for Disease Control and Prevention Guidelines: HEADS UP to Youth Sports: http://www.cdc.gov//headsup/youthsports/index.html
- Orthopedic Trauma Association: Pediatrics Core Curriculum. http://ota.org/education/resident-resources/core-curriculum/pediatrics/
- American Burn Association: http://www.ameriburn.org/
- Centers for Disease Control Prevention of Child Maltreatment: http://www.cdc.gov/ViolencePrevention/childmaltreatment/index.html

II. TRAUMA: OVERVIEW[1]

A. Primary Survey
The primary survey includes assessment of the ABCs (airway, breathing, circulation) via the algorithm CAB: Circulation, Airway, and Breathing.[2] See Chapter 1 for a complete algorithm.
NOTE: The CAB sequence is currently in use by the American Heart Association as part of the Pediatric Advanced Life Support algorithm. The Advanced Trauma Life Support algorithm developed by the American College of Surgeons continues to support the ABC sequence in the primary survey.

B. Secondary Survey
Procedures used in a secondary survey are listed in Table 4.1, and include assessment of neurologic status using the quick screen **AVPU** (**A**lert, **V**ocal stimulation response, **P**ainful stimulation response, **U**nresponsive) or Glasgow Coma Scale (GCS). Remove all patient clothing and perform a thorough head-to-toe examination. Remember to keep the child warm during the examination.

C. AMPLE History
Obtain an **AMPLE** history: **A**llergies, **M**edications, **P**ast illnesses, **L**ast meal, **E**vents preceding injury.

TABLE 4.1
SECONDARY SURVEY

Organ System	Secondary Survey
HEAD	Scalp/skull injury Raccoon eyes: periorbital ecchymoses; suggests orbital roof fracture Battle sign: ecchymoses behind pinna; suggests mastoid fracture Cerebrospinal fluid leak from ears/nose or hemotympanum suggests basilar skull fracture Pupil size, symmetry, and reactivity: Unilateral dilation of one pupil suggests compression of cranial nerve (CN) III and possible impending herniation; bilateral dilation of pupils is ominous and suggests bilateral CN III compression or severe anoxia and ischemia Corneal reflex Fundoscopic examination for papilledema as evidence of increased pressure Hyphema
NECK	Cervical spine tenderness, deformity, injury Trachea midline Subcutaneous emphysema Hematoma Bruit
CHEST	Clavicle deformity, tenderness Breath sounds, heart sounds Chest wall symmetry, paradoxical movement, rib deformity/fracture Petechiae over chest/head suggest traumatic asphyxia
ABDOMEN	Serial examinations to evaluate tenderness, distention, ecchymosis Shoulder pain suggests referred subdiaphragmatic process Orogastric aspirates with blood or bile suggest intraabdominal injury Splenic laceration suggested by left upper quadrant rib tenderness, flank pain, and/or flank ecchymoses ("seatbelt sign")
PELVIS	Tenderness, symmetry, deformity, stability
GENITOURINARY	Laceration, ecchymoses, hematoma, bleeding Rectal tone, blood, displaced prostate Blood at urinary meatus suggests urethral injury; do not catheterize

TABLE 4.1	
SECONDARY SURVEY—cont'd	
Organ System	Secondary Survey
BACK	Log-roll patient to evaluate spine for step-off along spinal column Tenderness Open or penetrating wound
EXTREMITIES	Neurovascular status: Pulse, perfusion, pallor, paresthesias, paralysis, pain Deformity, crepitus, pain Motor/sensory examination Compartment syndrome: Pain out of proportion to expected; distal pallor/pulselessness
NEUROLOGIC	Quick screen: **A**lert, **V**ocal stimulation response, **P**ainful stimulation response, **U**nresponsive (AVPU) or Glasgow Coma Scale
SKIN	Capillary refill, perfusion Lacerations, abrasions, contusion

III. SPECIFIC TRAUMATIC INJURIES

A. Minor Closed Head Trauma[3]

1. **Head injury can be caused by penetrating trauma, blunt force, rotational acceleration, or acceleration-deceleration injury.** Closed head trauma (CHT) can lead to depressed or nondepressed skull fracture, epidural or subdural hematoma, cerebral contusion, brain edema, increased intracranial pressure (ICP), brain herniation, concussion (mild to moderate diffuse brain injury), diffuse axonal injury (DAI), and/or coma.
2. **Evaluation:**
a. Physical examination [after CAB and cervical spine (C-spine) immobilization]:
   (1) Assign GCS score (see Chapter 1).
   (2) Obtain vital signs; pay special attention to Cushing triad (hypertension, bradycardia, irregular respiratory pattern) as an indication of increased ICP.
   (3) Perform neurologic examination as part of secondary survey (see Table 4.1).
   (4) If severe symptoms or vital sign changes are present, or if major CHT, follow procedures for emergency management of increased ICP and coma (see Section IV.B).
   (5) Rule out possible drug or alcohol ingestion/use as etiology of altered mental status.

b. Associated symptoms: Altered level or loss of consciousness (LOC), amnesia (before, during, or after the event), mental status change, behavior change, seizure activity, vomiting, headache, gait disturbance, visual change, or lethargy since event
c. Mechanism of injury:
    (1) Linear forces: Less likely to cause LOC; more commonly lead to skull fractures, intracranial hematoma, or cerebral contusion
    (2) Rotational forces: Commonly cause LOC; occasionally associated with DAI
    (3) Suspect abuse if mechanism of injury is not consistent with sustained injuries
3. **Management**[4]:
a. Evaluate C-spine (see Section III.B)
b. Consider if noncontrast computed tomography (CT) scan of head is indicated (Box 4.1)[5,6]
    (1) Most cases may be observed initially in the emergency department (ED) without neuroimaging.
    (2) Vomiting or brief LOC is not an absolute indication for head CT.

BOX 4.1
PECARN CLINICAL DECISION RULE FOR DETERMINING WHETHER HEAD CT IS NEEDED IN THE SETTING OF MINOR CLOSED HEAD TRAUMA[5]

	High Risk for ciTBI: Obtain head CT if any of the below criteria are present	Lower Risk for ciTBI: Consider head CT vs. observation
<2 YEARS OLD	• GCS ≤14 • Other signs of AMS • Palpable skull fracture	• LOC ≥5 s • Occipital, parietal, or temporal hematoma • Not acting normally • Severe mechanism of injury
≥2 YEARS OLD	• GCS ≤14 • Other signs of AMS • Signs of basilar skull fracture	• LOC • Vomiting • Severe mechanism of injury • Severe headache

Severe mechanism of injury is defined as: (1) Motorvehicle collision (MVC) with patient ejection, death of another passenger, or rollover, (2) pedestrian struck by motor vehicle without helmet, (3) falls > 3 feet (<2 years old) or falls > 5 feet (≥2 years old), or (4) head struck by high-impact object.
AMS, altered mental status; CT, computed tomography; ciTBI, clinically important traumatic brain injury; GCS, Glasgow Coma Scale; LOC, loss of consciousness
Modified from Kuppermann N, Holmes JF, Dayan PS, et al. Identification of children at very low risk of clinically-important brain injuries after head trauma: a prospective cohort study. Lancet. 2009;374:1160-1170

c. Observe patient:
   Monitor for 4–6 hours to detect delayed signs/symptoms of intracranial injury. A symptom-free lucid period can precede variable degrees of acute-onset mental status change with epidural bleeds.
d. Disposition
   (1) For stable patients, recommend continued observation at home and counsel parents on indications to have the patient re-evaluated by medical staff.
   (2) Consider hospitalizing patients with the following symptoms:
      (a) Depressed or declining level of consciousness or prolonged unconsciousness (GCS 8–12)
      (b) Focal neurologic deficit
      (c) Increasing headache, persistent vomiting, or seizures
      (d) Cerebrospinal fluid otorrhea or rhinorrhea, hemotympanum, mastoid ecchymosis (Battle sign), or periorbital ecchymosis (raccoon eyes)
      (e) Linear skull fracture crossing the groove of the middle meningeal artery, a venous sinus of the dura, or the foramen magnum
      (f) Depressed or compound skull fracture, or fracture into the frontal sinus
      (g) Bleeding disorder or a patient on anticoagulation therapy
      (h) Intoxication, illness, or injury obscuring the neurologic state
      (i) Suspected nonaccidental trauma
      (j) Patient is unable to return to ED for reassessment, or if there are concerns about caregiver reliability
e. Concussions in sports-related injuries[7,8]:
   (1) Definition: Trauma-induced alteration of consciousness that may or may not cause LOC. Often without neurologic signs/symptoms or neuroimaging changes at the time of evaluation.
   (2) Immediate signs: Change in playing ability, confusion, slowing, memory disturbance, incoordination, headache, dizziness, nausea, vomiting, and LOC.
   (3) Postconcussive symptoms: Headaches, fatigue, sleep disturbance, nausea/vomiting, vision changes, tinnitus, balance problems, emotional/behavioral changes, sensitivity to light or sound, and cognitive changes.
   (4) Evaluation: Evaluate CAB and risk for C-spine injury. Include history of prior concussions. Perform complete neurologic examination, including mental status assessment. Routine neuroimaging is not recommended.
   (5) Management
      (a) Return to play only if: no signs or symptoms during rest or exertion, normal neurologic examination, and neuroimaging normal (if obtained).

(b) Consider need for cognitive rest.
(c) Consider neuropsychologic testing if history of multiple injuries or if recovery is not progressing as expected.
(6) Refer to Centers for Disease Control and Prevention Guidelines: HEADS UP to Youth Sports: http://www.cdc.gov//headsup/youthsports/index.html.[9]

B. Cervical Spine Injuries[3,10,11]

1. **Incidence and mechanism**
a. 1.5% of pediatric trauma patients.
b. Mechanism: Severe, blunt trauma. Most commonly MVC but also falls, diving-related injuries, acceleration-deceleration injuries, and some sports (i.e., football, horseback riding, wrestling).
2. **Immobilize C-spine immediately until injury can be excluded.**[12,13]
a. Ideally immobilized by first responder.
b. Children aged <8 years may need support under the neck/shoulders to maintain neutral position and avoid neck flexion due to size of occiput. Neutral position is with gaze preference perpendicular to backboard.
3. **Clinically clearing the C-spine**[10]:
a. Consider *not* obtaining radiographs if the following are present and the patient is ≥8 years old:
   (1) Low-risk mechanism of injury
   (2) No predisposing factors to C-spine injury (e.g., Down syndrome)
   (3) Alert without change in mental status or intoxication
   (4) Normal complete neurologic exam and no neurologic symptoms
   (5) No painful distracting injuries
   (6) No pain with midline neck palpation and no neck pain
   (7) Normal active and passive range of motion (only evaluate after determining no midline pain on palpation)
4. **Radiographic studies:**
a. Minimum: Posteroanterior (PA) and lateral views (including C7). Oblique and flexion/extension films can be helpful, but should not be obtained routinely.
b. Consider CT scan if radiographs are inadequate to exclude bony injury. If magnetic resonance imaging (MRI) is easily available and will not require sedation, consider obtaining an MRI instead of CT scan. Keep in mind that MRI has lower sensitivity for detecting bony injuries.[14]
c. Spinal cord injury without radiographic abnormality (SCIWORA): Neurologic symptoms persist with no radiographic abnormality. Consider MRI to visualize soft tissue, spinal cord.
d. See Chapter 25 for reading C-spine films and evaluation of SCIWORA.

C. Blunt Thoracic and Abdominal Trauma[15,16]

1. **Anatomic considerations in children:** Pliable rib cage, solid organs proportionally larger than those of adults, underdeveloped abdominal musculature

2. **Common injuries:**
   a. Thoracic: Pneumothorax, hemothorax, pulmonary contusion, fractures, damage to major blood vessels, heart, or diaphragm
   b. Intraabdominal injury (IAI): Damage to spleen, liver, kidneys, pancreas, genitourinary (GU) system, or major blood vessels; hematomas or perforations within the gastrointestinal (GI) tract
3. **Evaluation:**
   a. Careful history and physical examination
   b. Laboratory studies:
      (1) Type and cross-match
      (2) Thoracic injury: Complete blood cell count (CBC), pulse oximetry; consider arterial blood gas (ABG)
      (3) Abdominal injury: CBC (follow serial hemoglobin values), electrolytes, liver function tests, amylase, lipase, urinalysis
   c. Radiologic evaluation:
      (1) Chest radiograph. Consider chest CT with intravenous (IV) contrast if abnormal radiographs or mechanism with severe deceleration injury.
      (2) Abdominal CT with IV contrast: Gold standard for IAI diagnosis. Routine oral contrast *not* indicated; high false-negative rate for hollow viscous injury.
      (3) Focused Assessment with Sonography for Trauma (FAST): Moderate sensitivity for abdominal free fluid. Should not be used alone for IAI evaluation but can be useful combined with exam findings and labs (e.g., LFTs). Consider sonography when coexisting injuries (e.g., neurologic or significant orthopedic) prevent CT scan.
4. **Emergency treatment:**
   a. If significant trauma is suspected or diagnosed, consult a pediatric surgeon.
   b. Tension pneumothorax:
      (1) Signs: Marked respiratory distress, distended neck veins, contralateral tracheal deviation, diminished breath sounds, compromised systemic perfusion, trauma arrest
      (2) Treatment: Needle decompression then chest tube placement directed toward lung apex (see Chapter 3)
   c. Open pneumothorax (also known as "sucking chest wound"): Allows free flow of air between atmosphere and hemithorax. Cover defect with occlusive dressing (i.e., petroleum jelly gauze), give positive-pressure ventilation, and insert chest tube (see Chapter 3).
   d. Hemothorax: Provide fluid resuscitation, followed by placement of a chest tube directed posteriorly and inferiorly.
   e. Abdominal trauma: Penetrating trauma requires surgical evaluation and exploration. Nonoperative management may be possible in blunt trauma, even in the presence of intraabdominal bleeding. Bleeding from injured spleen, kidneys, or liver is often self-limited. The decision

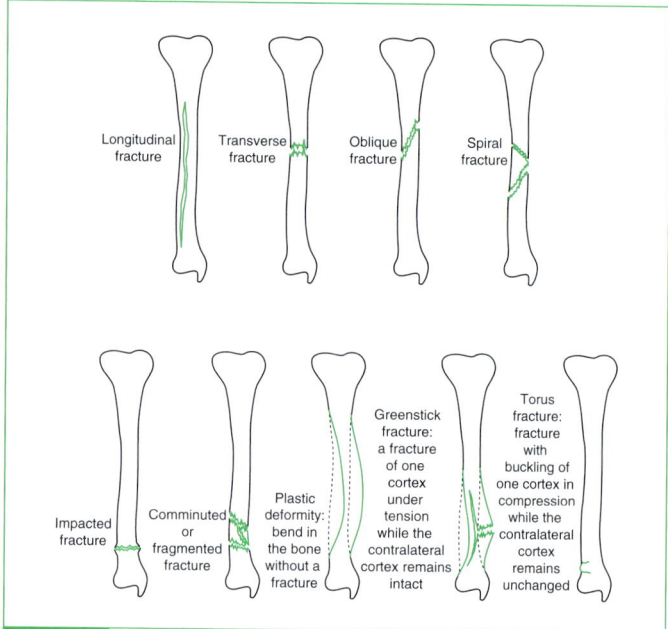

FIGURE 4.1

Fracture patterns unique to children. *(Modified from Ogden JA. Skeletal injury in the child. 3rd ed. Philadelphia: WB Saunders; 2000.)*

to pursue operative vs. nonoperative management should be made by a surgeon.

D. Orthopedic/Long Bone Trauma[17,18,19]

1. **Fractures:** Some fracture patterns are unique to children (Fig. 4.1). Growth plate injuries are classified by the Salter-Harris classification (see Chapter 25, Table 25.2). Because ligaments are stronger than bones or growth plates in children, dislocations and sprains are relatively uncommon, whereas growth plate disruption and bone avulsion are more common. For basic splinting techniques, see Chapter 3.
2. **Compartment syndrome**[18]: Elevated muscle compartment pressure (due to space limitation by surrounding fascia) impairs blood flow, resulting in nerve and muscle damage.
a. Common causes include crush injury, fractures (most commonly tibial), burns, infections (necrotizing fasciitis), or hemorrhage.
b. Marked by **6 P**s: **P**ain (earliest symptom), **P**aresthesias, **P**allor, **P**oikilothermia, **P**aralysis, **P**ulselessness.

(1) Unremitting pain, even after appropriate analgesia, is the most sensitive sign.
(2) Pain with passive muscle stretch is a strong indicator.
c. Intercompartmental pressure measurement: Normal = 10 mmHg; symptoms occur with pressures 20–30 mmHg.
d. Management: Emergency fasciotomy within 6 hours of onset; absolutely indicated if pressure >30 mmHg.
e. Complications: Rhabdomyolysis. Follow-up urinalysis, creatine kinase (CK), electrolytes (risk for hyperkalemia). Consider fluid resuscitation, urine alkalinization (goal urine pH > 6.5), or mannitol (0.25–0.5 g/kg with a maximum single dose of 12.5 grams). Monitor osmolal gap closely if mannitol is administered.

IV. COMMON CRITICAL CARE EMERGENCIES[20]

A. Hypertensive Crisis[21,22]

1. **Definitions**
a. Hypertensive emergency: Acutely elevated blood pressure (BP) (usually significantly greater than 99% for age and gender) with evidence of end-organ damage (neurologic, renal, ocular, hepatic, or cardiovascular impairment).
b. Hypertensive urgency: Acute significant BP elevation without end-organ damage. Often with minor symptoms (headache, vomiting, blurred vision).
c. For BP normal values based on age, height, and weight, see Tables 7.1 and 7.2 and Figs. 7.2 and 7.3.
d. Etiologies: Usually secondary. Renal disease (parenchymal and renovascular), endocrine disease, cathecholamine-producing tumors, ingestions, medication or medication withdrawal, elevated ICP.

2. **Presentation and evaluation**
a. Presentation: Encephalopathy, focal neurologic deficits (e.g., facial palsy), headaches, seizures, vision changes, papilledema, retinal hemorrhage, tachycardia, gallop, rales, abnormal pulses, jugular venous distention (JVD), cushingoid appearance, nausea/vomiting
b. Examination: Four-extremity BP measurements with appropriate cuff, visual acuity, fundoscopic exam, thyroid exam, heart and lung auscultation, abdominal palpation, complete neurologic and mental status assessment
c. Initial studies: CBC, electrolytes, urinalysis, BUN, creatinine, chest radiograph, electrocardiogram
d. Subsequent studies: Consider echocardiogram, abdominal and renal ultrasound, head CT, urine catecholamines, thyroid and adrenal testing, toxicology screen, renin level
e. Consult nephrology and/or cardiology

3. **Management:**
a. **Rule out elevated ICP as the cause before lowering BP.**

b. Goal: Reduce BP by ≤25% in the first 8 hours after presentation. Reduce to ≤90% for age over the next 24–48 hours.
c. Hypertensive emergency
   (1) Initial: IV bolus of labetalol or hydralazine (IM hydralazine if unable to obtain IV access). Repeat the bolus if needed.
   (2) ICU management: Nicardipine or labetalol continuous infusion with intraarterial line monitoring. Transition to oral medication once stable.
   (3) See Table 4.2 for hypertensive emergency medications.
d. Hypertensive urgency
   (1) See Table 4.3 for hypertensive urgency medications. Oral route is often adequate. Use of sublingual nifedipine is *not* recommended; a precipitous uncontrolled fall in BP may result.
   See Expert Consult for additional management considerations.

B. Increased Intracranial Pressure[23,24,25]

See Chapter 20 for evaluation and management of hydrocephalus.
1. **Assessment:**
a. Causes: Traumatic brain injury (TBI) (most common), meningitis, encephalitis, hemorrhage or hematoma, central nervous system (CNS) tumor, intracranial abscess, hypoxic ischemic encephalopathy (HIE).
b. History: Trauma, prior shunt or other neurologic surgical or medical condition, vomiting (especially morning vomiting), fever, headache, neck pain, unsteadiness, seizure, vision change, gaze preference, and change in mental status. In infants, ask about irritability, vomiting, poor feeding, developmental regression, and lethargy.
c. Physical examination:
   (1) Evaluate vital signs for Cushing triad (hypertension, bradycardia, irregular respiratory pattern) as a sign of increasing ICP.
   (2) Thorough neurologic examination: Attention to photophobia, pupillary response/symmetry, papilledema, cranial nerve dysfunction (especially paralysis of upward gaze or abduction), bulging fontanelle, neck stiffness, neurologic deficit, abnormal posturing, ataxia, altered mental status, or evidence of trauma.
   (3) Laboratory studies: CBC, electrolytes, glucose, toxicology screen, blood culture. Lumbar puncture is contraindicated due to herniation risk if the cause is obstructive.
2. **Management:**
a. Cerebral perfusion pressure (CPP) = mean arterial pressure (MAP) − ICP
   (1) Adequate CPP is critical. Maintain BP and volume.
   (2) Consider epinephrine or phenylephrine infusion to maintain blood pressure if needed.
   (3) Goal minimum CPP in severe TBI is age-dependent[26]
      (a) 0–5 years of age: Above 40 mmHg
      (b) 6–17 years of age: Above 50 mmHg
      (c) Adult: Above 50-60 mmHg

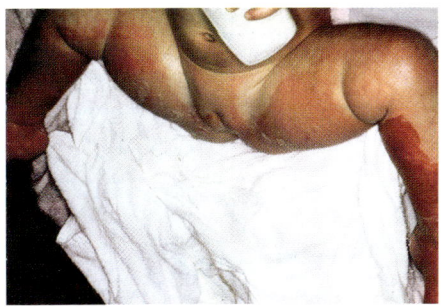

FIGURE 4.6
Infant who has been burned when immersed in hot water: lower extremities and buttocks. *(From Zitelli B, Davis H. Atlas of pediatric physical diagnosis. 5th ed. St. Louis: Mosby; 2008.)*

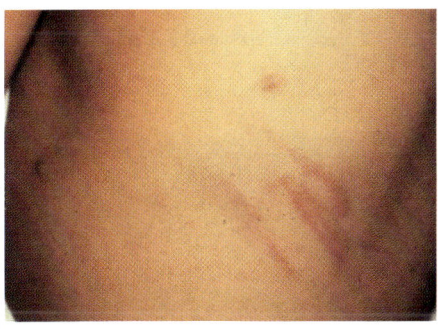

FIGURE 4.7
Child who has been beaten with a looped cord. *(From Zitelli B, Davis H. Atlas of pediatric physical diagnosis. 5th ed. St. Louis: Mosby; 2008.)*

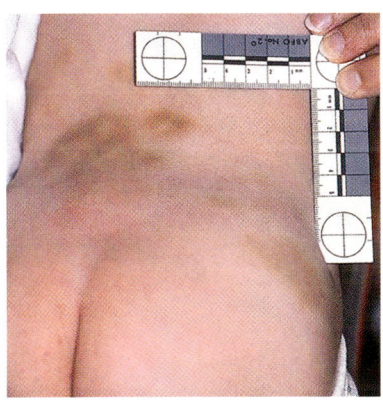

FIGURE 4.8
Child with suspicious bruising on lower back. *(From Zitelli B, Davis H. Atlas of pediatric physical diagnosis. 5th ed. St. Louis: Mosby; 2008.)*

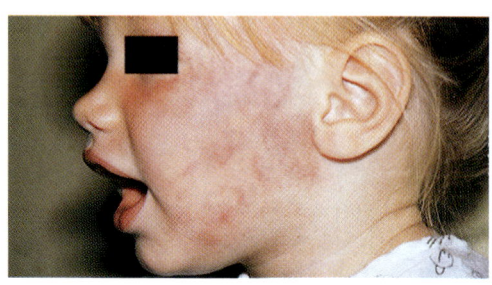

FIGURE 4.9
Toddler slapped in the face with linear hand marks visible. *(From Zitelli B, Davis H. Atlas of pediatric physical diagnosis. 5th ed. St. Louis: Mosby; 2008.)*

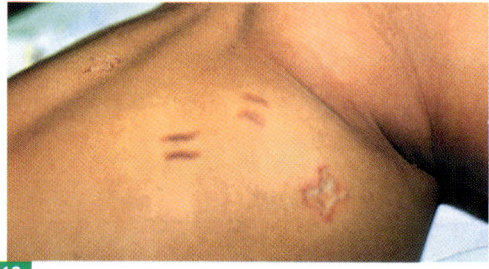

FIGURE 4.10
Skin burned with hot cigarette lighter. *(From Zitelli B, Davis H. Atlas of pediatric physical diagnosis. 5th ed. St. Louis: Mosby; 2008.)*

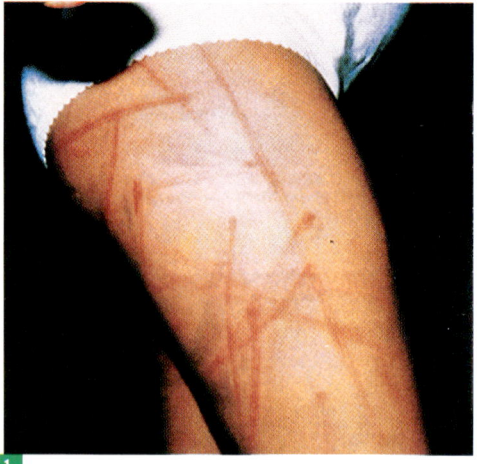

FIGURE 4.11
Child beaten with a switch. *(From Zitelli B, Davis H. Atlas of pediatric physical diagnosis. 5th ed. St. Louis: Mosby; 2008.)*

TABLE 4.2
INJECTABLE MEDICATIONS FOR HYPERTENSIVE EMERGENCY*

Drug	Onset and Peak Effect	Duration	Dosing Frequency	Comments and Adverse Effects
INTERMITTENT DOSING				
Hydralazine (arteriole vasodilator)	Onset: 5–30 min Peak: 20–40 min	2–6 hr	4–6 hr	May be given IV or IM May cause reflex tachycardia, prolonged hypotension, nausea, headache, lupus-like syndrome, or peripheral neuritis Adjust dosing for renal disease.
Enalapril (ACE inhibitor)	Onset: 15 min Peak: 1–4 hr	6 hr (but up to 24 hr is possible)	Infants and children: 8–24 hr Adolescents: 6 hr	May cause AKI, hyperkalemia, or cholestatic jaundice
CONTINUOUS INTRAVENOUS INFUSIONS				
Labetalol (α-, β-blocker)	Onset: 2–5 min Peak: 5–15 min	2–4 hr	An IV bolus dose can be given before starting a continuous infusion. Repeated bolus doses have been given to adults as frequently as every 10 minutes.	ICU setting strongly recommended. Can cause hyperkalemia, bronchospasm
Nicardipine (dihydropyridine channel blocker)	Onset: 1–2 min Peak: 50% of the effect is seen within 45 min	Effects decrease within 30 min–50 hr after stopping the infusion (50% of effect within first 30 min)	Titrate infusion dose every 15–30 minutes until goal BP is achieved.	ICU setting strongly recommended May cause reflex tachycardia, peripheral edema, headache, nausea, vomiting. Decreased clearance with hepatic dysfunction

*See formulary for dosing.

ACE, angiotensin-converting enzyme; AKI, acute kidney injury; BP, blood pressure; ICU, Intensive care unit; IM, intramuscular; IV, intravenous.

Modified from Baracco R, Mattoo TK. Pediatric hypertensive emergencies. Curr Hypertens Rep. 2014; 6:456. Additional information obtained from the following: Lexicomp Online, 2016 and Micromedex, 2016.

TABLE 4.3
ENTERAL MEDICATIONS FOR HYPERTENSIVE URGENCY*

Drug	Onset and Peak Effect	Duration	Dosing Frequency	Comments and Adverse Effects
Clonidine (decreased peripheral vascular resistance)	Onset: 30–60 min Peak: 2–4 hr	6–10 hr	Initial: 8–12 hr Dosing can later be increased to every 6 hr	Monitor for bradycardia and use cautiously with arrhythmias. Can cause rebound hypertension.
Minoxidil (potassium channel opener, vasodilator)	Onset: 30 min Peak: 2–8 hr	2–5 days	Initial: 24 hr Dosing can later be increased to every 12 hr	Contraindicated in pheochromocytoma. Can cause sinus tachycardia. Black box warning includes pericardial effusion/cardiac tamponade.
Labetalol (α-, β-blocker)	Onset: 20 min–2 hr Peak: 1–4 hr	8–24 hr (dose-dependent)	12 hr	Use cautiously in pheochromocytoma. Avoid in asthma.

*See Formulary for dosing.
Modified from Baracco R, Mattoo TK. Pediatric hypertensive emergencies. Curr Hypertens Rep. 2014;16:456. Additional information obtained from the following: Lexicomp Online, 2016 and Micromedex, 2016.

  b. See Fig. 4.2 for acute management of increased ICP while neurosurgical intensive care is being arranged.
  c. Other therapies and considerations
    (1) Consider neurology consult for prophylactic seizure control to reduce incidence of early posttraumatic seizures in children with TBI. Prophylactic antiepileptic drugs are not indicated for prevention of late posttraumatic seizures.[26]
    (2) In space-occupying lesions (tumors, abscesses), consider dexamethasone to reduce cerebral edema (in consultation with a neurosurgeon). Otherwise, corticosteroids are not recommended for children with TBI.
    (3) Maintain normothermia (avoid hyper- or hypothermia).[26]

C. Shock[27,28]
1. **Definition:** Physiologic state characterized by inadequate oxygen and nutrient delivery to meet tissue demands.
a. Compensated shock: Body maintains perfusion to vital organs. Clinical suspicion is important, as blood pressure changes are a late finding. Tachycardia is often the most sensitive vital sign change.

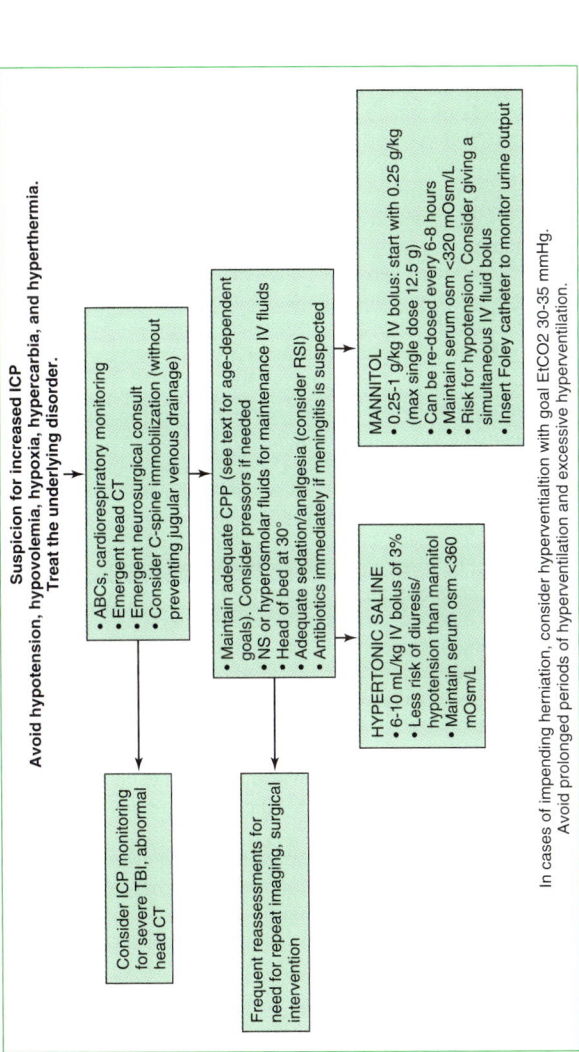

FIGURE 4.2

Emergency management of elevated intracranial pressure (ICP). CPP, cerebral perfusion pressure; CT, computed tomography; NS, normal saline; RSI, rapid sequence intubation; TBI, traumatic brain injury. Modified from (1) Roosevelt GE, Paradis NA. Cerebral Resuscitation. Pediatric Emergency Medicine. 2008;94-105 and (2) Kochanek PM, Carney N, Adelson P, Det al. Guidelines for the Acute Management of Severe Traumatic Brain Injury in Infants, Children, and Adolescents—Second Edition. Pediatr Crit Care Med. 2012;13:1.

b. Decompensated shock: Poor perfusion, tachycardia, hypotension, altered mental status, and oliguria/anuria.
2. **Types (and causes) of shock** (see Table EC 4.A for associated hemodynamics, including expected heart rate, preload, contractility, and systemic vascular resistance):
a. Cardiogenic shock (myocarditis, congestive heart disease, arrhythmias, etc.): Characterized by signs of decreased cardiac output and fluid overload; hepatomegaly, JVD, gallop, rales.
b. Hypovolemic shock (hemorrhagic and nonhemorrhagic) See Table EC 4.B for characterization of shock based on percentage of blood volume loss
c. Distributive shock (including septic, anaphylactic, and neurogenic shock)
d. Obstructive shock (including cardiac tamponade, tension pneumothorax, massive pulmonary embolism)
3. **Management:** Always treat the underlying cause.
a. Distributive and hypovolemic shock: See Fig. 4.3 for acute management.
b. Cardiogenic shock:
   (1) When concerned for cardiogenic shock, evaluation needs to include ECG, chest x-ray, and echocardiogram.
   (2) Dehydration and fluid resuscitation: Dehydration is often present but must be treated judiciously. In cardiogenic shock, stroke volume and ability to tolerate fluid administration are limited by fluid overload that may result in stretching of myocardial fibers beyond the point of optimal contraction.
      (a) Perform targeted physical exam, including evaluation of liver edge, respiratory status, and heart rate before initiating fluid resuscitation.
      (b) If no signs of fluid overload are present and dehydration is suspected, small fluid boluses (5–10 cc/kg) can be given slowly with frequent re-evaluation.
      (c) Discontinue fluid resuscitation with signs of fluid overload: elevation or no change in heart rate, worsening hepatomegaly, worsening respiratory status, or rales.
   (3) Optimizing preload and afterload are crucial. Consider noninvasive ventilation (CPAP or BiPAP) or inotropic medications (i.e., milrinone).
   (4) Arrange for pediatric intensive care. Diuretics and inotropes may be indicated.
c. Obstructive shock: Management is directed at the primary etiology.
d. Anaphylaxis: See Chapter 1 for additional information on management.

Initial management:

- Early recognition based on vital sign and physical examination changes is key
- Establish access via large-bore IV or IO
- Start high-flow oxygen via facemask or nasal cannula, even in the absence of respiratory distress

First 5–15 minutes:

- Rapidly push 20 mL/kg isotonic saline
  - Each 20 mL/kg should be given in 5 minutes or less
  - Many patients require total of 60 mL/kg. Some may require up to 200 mL/kg within the first hour of shock
  - Continue until perfusion improves or signs of fluid overload such as rales or hepatomegaly develop
  - Consider PRBC transfusion for hemorrhagic shock
- Correct hypoglycemia and hypocalcemia
- Start broad-spectrum IV antibiotics

At 15 minutes without reversal of shock:

- Start inotrope via second IV/IO access site.
  - Cold shock—dopamine 5 to 20 mcg/kg/min
  - Warm shock—norepinephrine 0.05 to 2 mcg/kg/min
- Consider securing airway with early intubation and mechanical ventilation
  - Goal $ScvO_2$ ≥70%

At 60 minutes without reversal of shock:

- Give hydrocortisone 2 mg/kg (max 100 mg) in patients at risk for adrenal insufficiency or unresponsive to pressors
- Transfer to pediatric intensive care unit

Note:

It is very important to prepare for each step in advance so that the recommended interventions can be completed within 1 hour of recognizing shock.

FIGURE 4.3

Emergency management of pediatric hypovolemic/distributive shock—the first hour. *(From Brierley J, Carcillo JA, Choong K, et al. Clinical practice parameters for hemodynamic support of pediatric and neonatal septic shock: 2007 update from The American College of Critical Care Medicine. Crit Care Med. 2009; 37: 666-688.)*

D. Pulmonary Hypertension[29,30]

1. **Definition**
a. Increased PA pressures:
   (1) Mean PA pressure >25 mmHg at rest or >30 mmHg with exercise
   OR
   (2) Echocardiogram indicating systolic PA pressure ≥½ systemic systolic pressure
b. With or without acute and/or chronic right ventricular failure

2. **Causes**
a. Common causes include bronchopulmonary dysplasia, chronic lung disease, and congenital heart disease
b. Other causes include chronic hypoxia (e.g., patients with cystic fibrosis), chronic airway obstruction, vasculitic abnormalities (e.g., patients with sickle cell disease or connective tissue disease), and idiopathic or sporadic

3. **Presentation and evaluation**
a. Presentation
   (1) Presentation of pulmonary hypertensive crisis is similar to cold shock: tachycardia, hypotension, cool extremities, poor perfusion, altered mental status. **Patients with acute pulmonary hypertensive crisis will also have a bounding right ventricle, loud holosystolic murmur, and palpably engorged liver edge. A gallop, peripheral edema, or JVD may also be present.**
   (2) Acute presentation with crisis is often prompted by intercurrent viral respiratory illness, aspiration, or periprocedural anesthesia.
b. Evaluation
   (1) Acute evaluation includes physical exam, continuous ECG and pulse oximetry, chest x-ray, echocardiogram, CBC, complete metabolic panel, magnesium and phosphate levels, urinalysis, pro-brain natriuretic peptide, and ABG.
   (2) Cardiac catheterization with pressure measurements remains the diagnostic gold standard (mostly used in non-emergency situations). Six-minute walk tests may be appropriate for serial follow-up for older patients.

4. **Management of acute pulmonary hypertensive crisis**
a. **Immediate consultation with an experienced pediatric pulmonary hypertension specialist is essential.**
b. Sedative or anesthetic agents that decrease systemic vascular resistance should be avoided, as this will drop preload delivery to the acutely ailing right ventricle.
c. Supplemental oxygen: May decrease pulmonary vasoconstriction.
d. Inhaled medications (nitric oxide, prostanoids): Inhaled nitric oxide (iNO) may be given via nasal cannula (simple or high-flow) and

causes vasodilation. Monitor closely for rebound pulmonary hypertension and methemoglobinemia.
   e. Sildenafil: Potentiates the effects of iNO. Given orally or by gastric tube.
   f. Careful fluid resuscitation: 5–10 mL/kg fluid boluses with frequent reassessment for signs of fluid overload. Avoid hypovolemia as it can worsen cardiac output.
   g. Avoid bradycardia: Cardiac output may become heart rate dependent due to poor left ventricular filling. Consider early administration of a chronotrope.
   h. Maintain normal blood pH: Acidosis causes pulmonary vasoconstriction. Fluid boluses and/or sodium bicarbonate may be needed to maintain normal blood pH. Remedy hypercarbia as necessary.
5. **Chronic therapy**
   a. One or more pulmonary vasodilators may be required long-term to lower pulmonary vascular resistance, mitigate symptoms, and prolong survival.
   b. Serial clinical evaluations, echocardiograms, measurements of brain natriuretic peptide, 6-minute walk tests, and cardiac catheterizations will be needed to monitor therapy.
   c. Lung transplantation will be a consideration for selected patients.

E. Respiratory Failure[31]

1. **Definition:** Failure of the lungs to exchange oxygen and/or carbon dioxide. Causes include the following:
   a. Neurologic: Muscle weakness, altered sensorium, CNS impairment
   b. Obstruction: Foreign body, inflammation
   c. Parenchymal disease: Pneumonia, pulmonary edema, acute respiratory distress syndrome (ARDS), asthma
   d. Mechanical: Abnormal chest wall, trauma
2. **Management:**
   a. Noninvasive positive-pressure ventilation
   b. Intubation and mechanical ventilation (see Chapter 1 for discussion of intubation)
3. **Types of ventilatory support:**
   a. Volume limited:
      (1) Delivers a preset tidal volume to a patient, regardless of pressure required.
      (2) Risk for barotrauma reduced by pressure alarms and pressure pop-off valves that limit peak inspiratory pressure (PIP).
   b. Pressure limited:
      (1) Gas flow is delivered to the patient until a preset pressure is reached and then held for the set inspiratory time (reduces the risk for barotrauma).

(2) Useful for neonatal and infant ventilatory support (<10 kg), where the volume of gas being delivered is small in relation to the volume of compressible air in the ventilator circuit, which makes reliable delivery of a set tidal volume difficult.
  c. High-frequency ventilation
     See additional content on Expert Consult.[33]

4. **Respiratory and ventilator parameters:**
a. PIP: Peak pressure attained during the respiratory cycle
b. Positive end-expiratory pressure (PEEP): Airway pressure maintained between inspiratory and expiratory phases; prevents alveolar collapse during expiration, decreases work of reinflation, and improves gas exchange
c. Rate (intermittent mandatory ventilation): Number of mechanical breaths delivered per minute
d. Inspired oxygen concentration (FiO_2): Fraction of oxygen present in inspired gas
e. Inspiratory time (Ti): Length of time spent in the inspiratory phase of the respiratory cycle
f. Tidal volume (V_T): Volume of gas delivered during inspiration
g. Mean airway pressure: ($\overline{PAW}$): Average pressure over entire respiratory cycle

5. **Modes of operation:**
a. Noninvasive positive-pressure ventilation[32]: Respiratory support provided through face mask or nasal prongs for children with mild to moderate respiratory distress. Requires very close monitoring for worsening of respiratory status that would require endotracheal intubation and mechanical ventilation.
   (1) Contraindications: Severe respiratory disease, hemodynamic instability, high aspiration risk, inability to maintain proper seal, facial injuries, need for airway protection (e.g., epiglottitis, burns)
   (2) CPAP: Delivers airflow (with set FiO_2) to maintain a set airway pressure
   (3) BiPAP: Delivers airflow to maintain set pressures for inspiration and expiration
   (4) Heated humidified high-flow nasal cannula (HHFNC)[33]
       (a) Generally > 1 liter per minute (LPM) in neonates and > 6 LPM in children.
       (b) Evidence suggests that HHFNC can reduce the risk of intubation in neonates and in children with bronchiolitis.
       (c) Reevaluate for improvement in respiratory status and heart rate after 60–90 minutes of HHFNC or sooner as needed based on clinical status.
b. Intermittent mandatory ventilation (IMV): A preset number of breaths are delivered each minute. Patient can take breaths on his or her own, but the ventilator may cycle on during a patient breath.

c. Synchronized IMV (SIMV): Similar to IMV, but the ventilator synchronizes delivered breaths with inspiratory effort and allows the patient to finish expiration before cycling on. More comfortable for patient than IMV.
d. Assist control ventilation (AC): Every inspiratory effort by the patient triggers a ventilator-delivered breath at the set V_T. Ventilator-initiated breaths are delivered when the spontaneous rate falls below the backup rate.
e. Pressure support ventilation: Inspiratory effort opens a valve, allowing airflow at a preset positive pressure. Patient determines rate and inspiratory time. May be used in combination with other modes of operation. Determine effectiveness of ventilation by monitoring tidal volumes.

6. **Initial ventilator settings:**
a. Volume limited:
   (1) Rate: Approximately normal range for age (see Table 24.1)
   (2) V_T: Approximately 8–10 mL/kg
   (3) Minute ventilation (V_E) × $PaCO_2$ = constant (for volume-limited ventilation)
   (4) Ti: Generally use inspiration-to-expiration ratio of 1:2. More prolonged expiratory phases are required for obstructive diseases to avoid air trapping
   (5) FiO_2: Selected to maintain targeted oxygen saturation and partial pressure of arterial oxygen (PaO_2)
b. Pressure limited:
   (1) Rate: Approximately normal range for age (see Table 24.1).
   (2) PEEP: Start with 3–5 cm H_2O and increase as clinically indicated. Monitor for decreases in cardiac output with increasing PEEP.
   (3) PIP: Set at pressure required to produce adequate chest wall movement (approximate this using hand-ventilating and manometry).
   (4) FiO_2: Selected to maintain targeted oxygen saturation and PaO_2.
c. HFOV: See additional content on Expert Consult.
d. High-frequency jet ventilator: See additional content on Expert Consult.

7. **Further ventilator management:**
a. Follow patient closely with pulse oximetry, end-tidal carbon dioxide measurements, and clinical assessment. Confirm findings with ABGs and adjust ventilator parameters as indicated (Table 4.4).
b. In cases of ARDS or other condition of poor compliance or air leaks, permissive hypercapnia and V_T of 5 mL/kg should be used to avoid barotrauma.
c. Parameters for initiating high-frequency ventilation:
   (1) Oxygenation index (OI) >40 (see Section IV.F.4 for calculation of OI)

TABLE 4.4
EFFECTS OF VENTILATOR SETTING CHANGES

Ventilator Setting Changes	Typical Effects on Blood Gases	
	Paco$_2$	Pao$_2$
↑ PIP	↓	↑
↑ PEEP	↑	↑
↑ Rate (IMV)	↓	Minimal ↑
↑ I:E ratio	No change	↑
↑ Fio$_2$	No change	↑
↑ Flow	Minimal ↓	Minimal ↑
↑ Power (in HFOV)	↓	No change
↑ PAW (in HFOV)	Minimal ↓	↑

Fio$_2$, Fraction of inspired oxygen; HFOV, high-frequency oscillatory ventilation; I:E, inspiratory/expiratory ratio; IMV, intermittent mechanical ventilation; Paco$_2$, partial pressure of carbon dioxide; Pao$_2$, partial pressure of arterial oxygen; PAW, mean airway pressure; PEEP, positive end-expiratory pressure; PIP, peak inspiratory pressure.

    (2) Inability to provide adequate oxygenation or ventilation with conventional ventilator
8. **Determining extubation readiness**[34]
a. No validated tools or techniques that are more reliable or predictive than clinical judgment.
b. At a minimum, all patients should have a spontaneous breathing test (extubation readiness trial) with minimal pressure support (PS) or a T-piece.
c. Upper airway obstruction is predicted to cause up to 37% of failed pediatric extubations.
    (1) Serial measurements of air leak around endotracheal tube are often used to help predict extubation readiness or postextubation stridor. Many providers use air leak <30 cm H$_2$O as helpful in predicting extubation success.
    (2) Air leak around endotracheal tube <20 cm H$_2$O can help predict postextubation stridor, especially in children aged more than 7 years.
d. Negative inspiratory force (NIF) measurements
    (1) No standardized approach
    (2) NIF measurements >20–25 cm H$_2$O may correlate with successful weaning and extubation

F. Critical Care Reference Data
1. **Minute ventilation (V$_E$):**

$$V_E = \text{Respiratory rate} \times \text{Tidal volume (V}_T\text{)}$$

2. **Alveolar gas equation:**

$$PAO_2 = PiO_2 - (PaCO_2/R)$$
$$PiO_2 = FiO_2 \times (PB - 47 \text{ mmHg})$$

Chapter 4 Trauma, Burns, and Common Critical Care Emergencies 93

a. Pi_{O_2} = partial pressure of inspired O_2 minus 150 mmHg at sea level on room air
b. R = respiratory exchange quotient (CO_2 produced/O_2 consumed) = 0.8
c. Pa_{CO_2} = partial pressure of alveolar CO_2 minus partial pressure of arterial CO_2 (Pa_{CO_2})
d. P_B = atmospheric pressure = 760 mmHg at sea level. Adjust for high-altitude environment
e. Water vapor pressure = 47 mmHg
f. Pa_{O_2} = partial pressure of O_2 in the alveoli

3. **Alveolar-arterial oxygen gradient (A-a gradient):**

$$A - a\ gradient = PA_{O_2} - Pa_{O_2}$$

a. Obtain ABG, measuring Pa_{O_2} and Pa_{CO_2} with patient on 100% Fi_{O_2} for at least 15 minutes
b. Calculate the PA_{O_2} and then the A-a gradient
c. The larger the gradient, the more serious the respiratory compromise. A normal gradient is 20–65 mmHg on 100% O_2 or 5–20 mmHg on room air.

4. **Oxygenation Index (OI):**

$$OI = \frac{mean\ airway\ pressure\ (cm\ H_2O) \times Fi_{O_2} \times 100}{Pa_{O_2}}$$

a. OI >35 for 5–6 hours is one criterion for extracorporeal membrane oxygenation (ECMO)
See more critical care reference data on Expert Consult.

G. Status Asthmaticus (see Chapter 1)

H. Status Epilepticus (see Chapter 1)

V. ANIMAL BITES[35]

A. Wound Considerations

1. **High infection risk:** Puncture wounds, crush injury, bites over hand, foot, genitalia, or joint surface, bites from a cat or human, wounds in asplenic or immunocompromised patients, wounds with care delayed >12 hours
2. **Special considerations:**
a. Deep bites: Possibility of foreign body or fracture—consider radiographs (especially for hand or scalp)
b. Periorbital bites: Possibility of corneal abrasion, lacrimal duct involvement, or other ocular damage—consider ophthalmologic evaluation
c. Hand: Site most prone to infection—follow for development of osteomyelitis.
d. Nose: Evaluate for cartilage injury.
e. Animal species (Table 4.5)

TABLE 4.5
ANIMAL BITES

Animal	Common Organism(s)	Special Considerations
DOG	Staphylococcus aureus Pasteurella multocida Streptococcus spp. Capnocytophaga canimorsus Anaerobes	Crush injury
CAT	P. multocida S. aureus Moraxella catarrhalis Bartonella henselae	Deep puncture wound Often associated with fulminant infection, abscess, and/or osteomyelitis Slow to respond to treatment
HUMAN	Streptococcus viridans S. aureus Anaerobes Eikenella corrodens Hepatitis B and C HIV (rare, associated with blood in biter's saliva)	Consider child abuse, especially if intercanine distance > 3 cm High infection and complication rate
RODENT	Streptobacillus moniliformis Spirillum minus	Low incidence of secondary infection Rat-bite fever—occurs rarely

3. **Management**
  a. Wound hygiene:
    (1) Irrigate with copious amounts (at least 100 mL/cm of laceration) of sterile saline using high-pressure syringe irrigation. Do not irrigate puncture wounds. Do not soak the wound. Do not use alcohol or peroxide to clean.
    (2) Debride devitalized tissue and evaluate for foreign bodies.
    (3) Consider surgical debridement/exploration for extensive wounds, wounds involving metacarpophalangeal joints, and cranial bites by a large animal.
    (4) Culture only if evidence of infection is present.
  b. Closure:
    (1) Avoid closing wounds with high infection risk (see Section V.A). Exception: Cat bites on the face or scalp may be closed.
    (2) Wounds that involve tendons, joints, deep fascia, or major vasculature should be evaluated by a plastic or hand surgeon and, if indicated, closed in the operating room.
    (3) Suturing: When indicated, closure should be done with minimal simple interrupted nylon sutures that are as superficial as possible. Loosely approximate wound edges. Use prophylactic antibiotics.
      (a) Head and neck: Can usually be safely sutured (with exceptions noted) after copious irrigation and wound debridement if within 6–8 hours of injury and no signs of infection. Facial wounds often require primary closure for

cosmetic reasons; good vascular supply lowers infection risk.
- (b) Hands: In large wounds, subcutaneous dead space should be closed with minimal absorbable sutures, with delayed cutaneous closure in 3–5 days if there is no evidence of infection.
- c. Imaging: Obtain if bite is extensive, on the hand or closed fist, and after a "mauling" injury. Imaging can reveal fracture, air in joint space, or a foreign body in the wound.
- d. Infection
  - (1) Prophylactic antibiotics are indicated in cases of high infection risk, as listed in Section V.A. See Chapter 17 for appropriate antibiotic therapies and treatment course.
  - (2) Subtle pain and tenderness may be the first sign of infection. Wounds that subsequently become infected may require drainage and debridement, possibly under anesthesia. Adjust antibiotic therapy according to Gram stain and culture results.
- e. Rabies and tetanus prophylaxis:
  - (1) Tetanus: See Chapter 16 for prophylaxis guidelines for nonclean wounds.
  - (2) Rabies: Always give postexposure prophylaxis when animal is a skunk, raccoon, bat, fox, woodchuck, or other carnivore. For further details, see Chapter 16.
- f. Disposition:
  - (1) Outpatient care: Obtain careful follow-up of all bite wounds within 24–48 hours, especially those requiring surgical closure. Extremity wounds, especially of the hands, should be immobilized in position of function and kept elevated. Wounds should be kept clean and dry.
  - (2) Inpatient care: Consider hospitalization for observation and parenteral antibiotics for significant human bites, immunocompromised or asplenic hosts, deep or severe infections, bites associated with systemic complaints, bites with significant functional or cosmetic morbidity, and/or unreliable follow-up or care by parent/guardian.

VI. BURNS[3,26,36]

A. Evaluation of Pediatric Burns (Tables 4.6 and 4.7)

NOTE: Depending on the extent and type of burn, severity may progress over the first 48–72 hours after injury; complete daily assessment as necessary. Consider early referral to a pediatric burn center.

B. Burn Mapping

Calculate total body surface area (TBSA) burned (Fig. 4.4): based only on percentage of partial- and full-thickness burns.

96 Part I Pediatric Acute Care

TABLE 4.6
THERMAL INJURY

Type of Burn	Description/Comment
FLAME	Most common type of burn worldwide; when clothing burns, the heat exposure is prolonged, and the severity increased.
SCALD/CONTACT	Most common type of burn in the US; mortality for full-thickness scald burns is similar to that in flame burns when total body surface area involved is equivalent; see Fig. 4.4
CHEMICAL	Tissue is damaged by protein coagulation or liquefaction rather than hyperthermic activity
ELECTRICAL	Injury is often extensive, involving skeletal muscle and other tissues in addition to the skin damage. Extent of damage may not be initially apparent. The tissues with the least resistance are most heat sensitive; bone offers the most resistance, nerve tissue the least. Cardiac arrest due to passage of current through the heart can occur.
INHALATION	Present in 30% of victims of major flame burns and increases mortality. Consider when there is evidence of fire in enclosed space. Signs include singed nares, facial burns, charred lips, carbonaceous secretions, posterior pharynx edema, hoarseness, cough, or wheezing.
COLD INJURY/FROSTBITE	Freezing results in direct tissue injury. Toes, fingers, ears, and nose are commonly involved. Initial treatment includes rewarming in tepid (105°–110°F) water for 20–40 minutes. Excision of tissue should not be done until complete demarcation of nonviable tissue has occurred.

C. Emergency Management of Pediatric Burns[37]

1. **Acute stabilization:**
a. Airway and breathing
   (1) Inhalation injury: Assume carbon monoxide poisoning with severe and/or closed-space burns.
      (a) Physical examination: Symptoms may be delayed after injury. Signs and symptoms that may predict acute inhalational injury include cough, facial burns, inflamed nares, soot in nares, stridor, sputum production, wheezing, and altered mental status.
      (b) Evaluation: Chest radiograph, ABGs with co-oximetry, and bedside spirometry. **NOTE:** Use co-oximetry instead of pulse oximetry to measure oxyhemoglobin. 12-lead ECG to evaluate for myocardial ischemia or infarction.
   (2) Management
      (a) Consider early intubation for >30% TBSA burned, stridor, signs of inhalation injury or upper airway obstruction.
      NOTE: Upper airway obstruction progresses rapidly with thermal or chemical burns to the face, nares, or oropharynx.

TABLE 4.7
BURN CLASSIFICATION*

SUPERFICIAL	Injury to epidermis only. Characterized by erythema, pain: includes sunburn or minor scalds. Patients with only superficial burns do not usually require intravenous fluid replacement. Not included in estimate of surface area burned. Generally heals on its own without scarring in 3–5 days.
SUPERFICIAL PARTIAL THICKNESS	Damages but does not destroy epidermis and dermis. Characterized by intense pain, blisters, pink to cherry-red skin, moist and weepy. Nails, hair, sebaceous glands, and nerves intact. Can progress to deep partial- or full-thickness burn. Spontaneous re-epithelialization in 2–3 weeks.
DEEP PARTIAL THICKNESS	Injury to epidermis and dermis. Characterized by intense pain, dry and white in color. Can result in disruption of nails, hair, sebaceous glands. May cause scarring; skin grafting usually required.
FULL THICKNESS	Injury involves all layers of skin, characterized by charred black color, ± dry or white areas. Pain may be intense or absent, depending on nerve ending involvement. Causes scarring; skin grafting required.

*See Fig. EC 4.A for images of burn classifications.

     (b) Administer humidified 100% supplemental oxygen through a nonrebreather mask until carboxyhemoglobin (COHb) level is <10%. Elimination half-life of COHb is dependent on PaO_2 (consider hyperbaric O_2 if pH is <7.4 and COHb is elevated). Make decisions based on PaO_2 rather than pulse oximetry.
     (c) Give aerosolized bronchodilators as needed. Avoid corticosteroid use for airway edema unless needed.
     (d) Observe for a minimum of 24 hours.
  b. Circulation:
    (1) Start formulaic fluid resuscitation (Fig. 4.5): IV fluid resuscitation with lactated Ringer solution or injection for burns >20% BSA or with any evidence of smoke inhalation.
    (2) Consider central venous access for burns >25% BSA.
    (3) Consider adding colloid to IV fluids after 12 hours (albumin 1 g/kg/day) if urine output remains poor.
    (4) Withhold potassium from IV fluids generally for the first 48 hours because of a large release of potassium from damaged tissues.
  c. Exposure: Remove clothes to stop the burning process. Cool water may be used to cool the patient, but then immediately wrap them in dry clean blankets to prevent hypothermia.

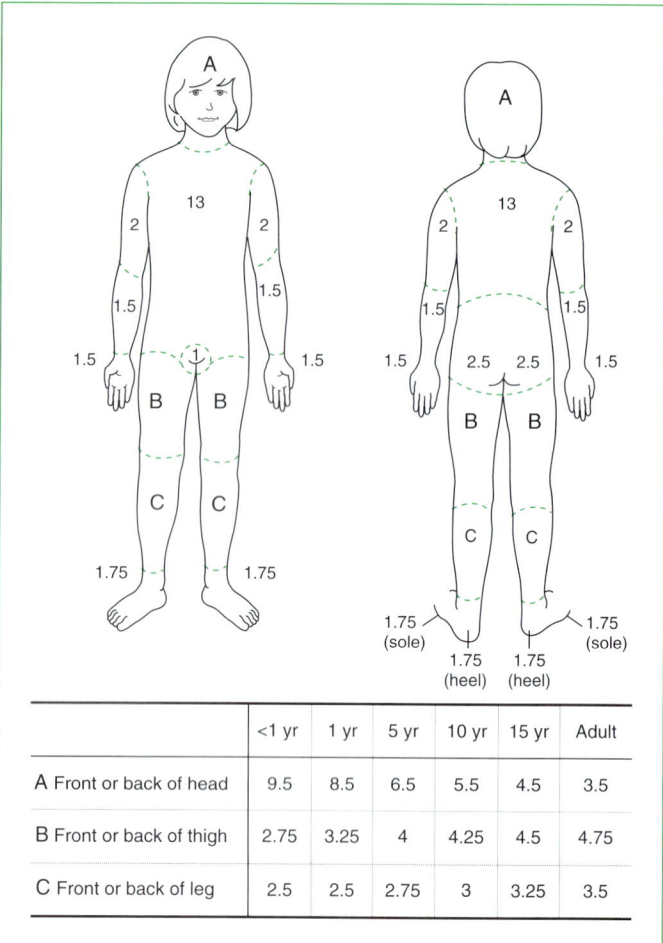

FIGURE 4.4

Burn assessment chart. All numbers are percentages. *(From Barkin RM, Rosen P. Emergency pediatrics: a guide to ambulatory care. 6th ed. St. Louis: Mosby; 2003.)*

2. **Secondary survey and special considerations:** Full head-to-toe assessment.
a. Consider associated traumatic injuries.
b. Electrical injury can produce deep tissue damage, intravascular thrombosis, cardiac and respiratory arrest, cardiac arrhythmias, and fractures secondary to muscle contraction. Look for exit site in electrical injury.

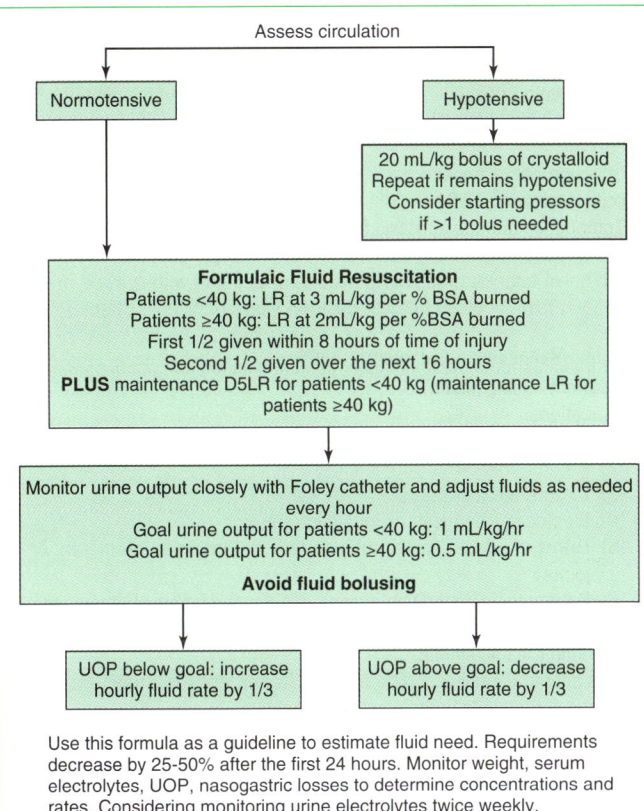

FIGURE 4.5

Formulaic fluid resuscitation for pediatric burns. Initiate formulaic fluid resuscitation for pediatric patients with burns totaling greater than 20% of TBSA.

   c. Chemical burns: Wash away or neutralize chemicals; brush dry chemical away and flush with copious warmed water.
   d. Assess for signs of compartment syndrome frequently after fluid resuscitation has begun.
   e. GI:
      (1) Place gastric tube for decompression.
      (2) Begin prophylaxis for Curling stress ulcers with histamine-2 receptor blocker, proton-pump inhibitor, and/or antacid.
      (3) Place a postpyloric enteral feeding tube and begin feeds as soon as it is safe to do so.

f. Eye: Ophthalmologic evaluation as necessary. Use topical ophthalmic antibiotics if abrasions are present.
g. GU: Consider Foley catheter to monitor urine output during fluid resuscitation phase.
h. Pain management: IV opioid therapy often necessary for pain control.
i. Infection risk: Consider early pediatric infectious disease consult for burns involving TBSA >25%.
j. Tetanus immunoprophylaxis for patients with < three prior tetanus toxoid doses (including DTaP, DT, Td, or Tdap); patients with unknown tetanus prophylaxis history; or patients with ≥ three prior tetanus toxoid doses, but last dose >5 years prior (see Chapter 16).

D. Further Management of Pediatric Burns
1. **Inpatient management:**
a. Indications:
   (1) Any partial-thickness burn >10% TBSA
   (2) Any full-thickness burn
   (3) Circumferential burns
   (4) Electrical, chemical, or inhalation injury
   (5) Burns of critical areas, such as face, hands, feet, perineum, or joints
   (6) Patient with underlying chronic illness, suspicion of abuse, or unsafe home environment
2. **Outpatient management:**
a. Indications: If burn is <10% total TBSA and does not meet previous criteria for inpatient management.
b. Management:
   (1) Clean with warm saline or mild soap and water. Debride open wounds and necrotic tissue.
   (2) Apply topical antibacterial agent such as bacitracin or silver-impregnated dressings; cover with nonadherent dressing (Box EC 4.A).
   (3) Dressing changes: If using bacitracin, clean daily as mentioned previously, then change dressing. Premedicate with pain medication 30 minutes before each dressing change. If using silver-impregnated dressings, daily changes are not needed and the dressings may stay in place until follow-up.
   (4) Oral antibiotics are not indicated.
   (5) Follow-up within 1 week at a pediatric burn center is highly recommended.

E. Burn Prevention:
Install smoke detectors outside every bedroom and on each floor, install carbon monoxide detectors, and keep water heater temperature set at <49°C (<120°F). Measure bath water temperature before use.

VII. CHILD ABUSE[3,38,39]

A. Introduction
A multidisciplinary approach is warranted in cases of suspected abuse and neglect. The multidisciplinary team should include medical providers, law enforcement, social service workers, and prosecutors. Although particular populations are especially vulnerable (children with special healthcare needs and infants), all children could be abused, so an approach to evaluating injuries should be applied uniformly.

B. Evaluation and Management
The medical professional should suspect, diagnose, treat, report, and document all cases of child abuse, neglect, or maltreatment. It is the role of the physician to report any suspected case of abuse, regardless of whether there is proof of abuse.

1. **Suspect:** Increase suspicion if there is inappropriate parental response, inadequate history of injury, a mechanism inconsistent with physical findings, evidence of neglect or failure to thrive, evidence of disturbed emotions or expressions in a child, prior history of suspicious events, or parental substance abuse.

NOTE: A delay in seeking medical attention may increase suspicion of abuse, but this alone does not necessarily indicate abuse.

2. **Diagnose:** Attempt to correlate all physical findings with history; photodocument if possible (Figs. 4.6 to 4.11, color insert).
a. Physical exam
   (1) Skin findings
      (a) Bruises: Shape of bruises is important. Be suspicious of bruises in protected areas (chest, abdomen, back, buttocks).
         i. Inflicted: Located in unusual places, patterned, multiple bruises or bruises in different stages of healing, bruises that do not fit the history and developmental stage
         ii. Accidental: Usually located at bony surfaces such as shins, cheek, or forehead; bruises are in the same stage of healing; history fits the bruise
      (b) Bites: Shape, size, and location are important. Intercanine distance of >3 cm is suggestive of human bites, which generally crush more than lacerate
      (c) Burns: Signs concerning for child maltreatment include multiple burn sites, well-demarcated edges, stocking/glove distributions, absence of splash marks, symmetrically burned buttocks and/or lower legs, mirror image burns of extremities, symmetrical involvement of palms or soles, spared inguinal or other flexural creases, central sparing over buttocks or perineum, parent denial that the lesion is a burn, parent attributing the cause of the burn to a sibling, and delay in seeking medical attention

(2) Ophthalmologic exam
  (a) Evaluation for retinal hemorrhages should be performed by an ophthalmologist using dilated indirect ophthalmoscopy.
  (b) Retinoschisis or retinal hemorrhages that are too numerous to count, multilayered, or continue to the periphery of the retina are virtually pathognomonic for abusive head trauma.
(3) Genital exam
  (a) If sexual abuse is suspected to have occurred within 72 hours for a child younger than age 12 years or within 120 hours for a child older than 12 years, defer interview and GU examination at presenting facility and urgently involve a multidisciplinary team with expertise in evaluation of sexual abuse if available. Avoid collection of laboratory specimens without input from this team. Nonacute examinations falling outside of the above time windows should be deferred to a child advocacy center.
  (b) Genital examination should be performed by trained forensic specialist, owing to anatomic variability (especially of hymen).
  (c) Normal genital examination does not rule out abuse; 95% of examinations are normal in cases of abuse.

b. Other Studies and Considerations
  (1) See Section III. A. and IV. B. if head trauma is suspected.
  (2) See Section III. C. if blunt thoracic or abdominal trauma is suspected. Duodenal hematomas are suspicious for nonaccidental blunt trauma; may lead to upper GI obstruction.
  (3) Fractures:
    (a) Certain fracture types are suspicious for nonaccidental trauma (Table 4.8).
    (b) Skeletal survey is suggested to evaluate suspicious bony trauma in any child; these studies are mandatory for children aged <2 years (see Chapter 25 for components).
    (c) Bone scan may be indicated to identify early or difficult-to-detect fractures.
  (4) Noncontrast head CT is useful for visualizing intracranial hemorrhage but unreliable for detection of skull fractures.
  (5) MRI may identify lesions not detected by CT (e.g., posterior fossa injury and diffuse axonal injury).

3. **Treat:** Medical stabilization is primary goal. Prevention of further injuries is the long-term goal.
4. **Report:** All healthcare providers are required by law to report suspected child maltreatment to the local police and/or child welfare agency. Suspicion supported by objective evidence is the criterion for reporting, and should first be discussed with not only the entire medical team but also the family. The professional who makes such reports is immune from any civil or criminal liability.

TABLE 4.8
SKELETAL INJURY IN NONACCIDENTAL TRAUMA

SKELETAL INJURY	Correlate mechanism of injury with physical finding; rule out any underlying bony pathology.
LONG BONES	Classic fracture is the epiphyseal/metaphyseal fracture, seen as a "bucket handle" or "corner" fracture at the end of long bones. Often secondary to jerking/shaking of a child's limb but can also be caused by natural shearing forces. Spiral fractures may be suspicious of abuse but can be seen with rotational forces (e.g., "toddler's fracture" of tibia).
RIBS	Posterior nondisplaced rib fractures are usually due to severe squeezing of the rib cage. May not be visible on plain film until callus formation.
SKULL	Fractures >3 mm wide, complex fractures, bilateral fractures, and nonparietal fractures suggest forces greater than those sustained from minor household trauma.

5. **Document:** Carefully and legibly document the following: reported and suspected history and mechanisms of injury, any history given by the victim in his or her own words (use quotation marks), information provided by other providers or services, and physical examination findings, including drawings of injuries and details of dimensions, color, shape, and texture. Always consider early use of police crime laboratory photography to document injuries.

REFERENCES

1. Marx J, Hockberger R, Walls R. *Rosen's Emergency Medicine: Concepts and Clinical Practice*. 7th ed. St Louis: Mosby; 2009.
2. Atkins DL, Berger S, Duff JP, et al. Part 11: Pediatric Basic Life Support and Cardiopulmonary Resuscitation Quality: 2015 American Heart Association Guidelines Update for Cardiopulmonary Resuscitation and Emergency Cardiovascular Care. *Circulation*. 2015;132(18 suppl 2):S519-S525.
3. Fleisher GR, Ludwig S, eds. *Textbook of Pediatric Emergency Medicine*. 5th ed. Philadelphia: Lippincott Williams & Wilkins; 2006.
4. Mehta S. Neuroimaging for paediatric minor closed head injuries. *Paediatr Child Health*. 2007;12:482-484.
5. Kuppermann N, Holmes JF, Dayan PS, et al. Identification of children at very low risk of clinically-important brain injuries after head trauma: a prospective cohort study. *Lancet*. 2009;374:1160-1170.
6. Easter JS, Bakes K, Dhaliwal J, et al. Comparison of PECARN, CATCH, and CHALICE rules for children with minor head injury: a prospective cohort study. *Ann Emerg Med*. 2014;64(2):145-152.
7. Kirkwood MW, Yeates KO, Wilson PE. Pediatric sport-related concussion: a review of the clinical management of an oft-neglected population. *Pediatrics*. 2006;117:1359-1371.
8. Halstead ME, Walter KD, the Council on Sports Medicine and Fitness. Clinical Report—Sport-Related Concussion in Children and Adolescents. *Pediatrics*. 2010;126:3.

9. "HEADS UP to Youth Sports." Centers for Disease Control and Prevention, National Center for Injury Prevention and Control, Division of Unintentional Injury Prevention. 2015. http://www.cdc.gov//headsup/youthsports/index.html.
10. Viccellio P, Simon H, Pressman BD, et al. A prospective multicenter study of cervical spine injury in children. *Pediatrics*. 2001;108(2):e20.
11. Patel JC, Tepas JJ, Mollitt DL, et al. Pediatric cervical spine injuries: defining the disease. *J Pediatr Surg*. 2001;36(2):373-376.
12. Nypaver M, Treloar D. Neutral cervical spine positioning in children. *Ann Emerg Med*. 1994;23:208-211.
13. Schriger DL, Larmon B, LeGassick T, et al. Spinal immobilization on a flat backboard: does it result in neutral position of the cervical spine? *Ann Emerg Med*. 1991;20:8-10.
14. Tat ST, Mejia MJ, Freishtat RJ. Imaging, clearance, and controversies in pediatric cervical spine trauma. *Pediatr Emerg Care*. 2014;30:911-915.
15. Sanchez J, Paidas C. Childhood trauma: now and in the new millennium. *Surg Clin North Am*. 1999;79:1503-1535.
16. Schonfeld D, Lee LK. Blunt abdominal trauma in children. *Curr Opin Pediatr*. 2012;24:314-318.
17. Green NE. *Skeletal Trauma in Children*. 3rd ed. Philadelphia: WB Saunders; 2003.
18. Canale ST. *Campbell's Operative Orthopedics*. 10th ed. St Louis: Mosby; 2003.
19. Offiah A, van Rijn RR, Perez-Rossello JM, et al. Skeletal imaging of child abuse (non-accidental injury). *Pediatr Radiol*. 2009;39:461-470.
20. Nichols DG, Yaster M, Lappe DG, et al. *Golden Hour: The Handbook of Advanced Pediatric Life Support*. 2nd ed. St Louis: Mosby; 1996.
21. Baracco R, Mattoo TK. Pediatric hypertensive emergencies. *Curr Hypertens Rep*. 2014;16:456.
22. Brady T. Hypertension. *Pediatr Rev*. 2012;33(12):541-552.
23. Kochanek P, Carney N, Adelson PD, et al. Guidelines for the acute medical management of severe traumatic brain injury in infants, children, and adolescents-second edition. *Pediatr Crit Care Med*. 2012;13(Suppl 1):S1-S82.
24. Roosevelt GE, Paradis NA. Cerebral Resuscitation. Pediatric Emergency Medicine. 2008:94-105.
25. Rogers M. *Textbook of Pediatric Intensive Care*. 4th ed. Baltimore: Williams & Wilkins; 2008.
26. Hardcastle N, Benzon HA, Vavilala MS. Update on the 2012 guidelines for the management of pediatric traumatic brain injury—information for the anesthesiologist. *Paediatr Anaesth*. 2014;24:703-710.
27. Brierley J, Carcillo JA, Choong K, et al. Clinical practice parameters for hemodynamic support of pediatric and neonatal septic shock: 2007 update from The American College of Critical Care Medicine. *Crit Care Med*. 2009;37:666-688.
28. Biban P, Gaffuri M, Spaggiari S, et al. Early recognition and management of septic shock in children. *Pediatr Rep*. 2012;4:e13.
29. Hawkins A, Tulloh R. Treatment of pediatric pulmonary hypertension. *Vasc Health Risk Manag*. 2009;5:509-524.
30. Collaco JM, Romer LH, Stuart BD, et al. Frontiers in pulmonary hypertension in infants and children with bronchopulmonary dysplasia. *Pediatr Pulmonol*. 2012;47(11):1042-1053.
31. Mesiano G, Davis GM. Ventilatory strategies in the neonatal and paediatric intensive care units. *Paediatr Respir Rev*. 2008;9:281-288.

32. Essouri S, Carroll C. Noninvasive support and ventilation for pediatric Acute Respiratory Distress Syndrome: proceedings from the Pediatric Acute Lung Injury Consensus Conference. *Pediatr Crit Care Med.* 2015;16(5 Suppl 1):S102-S110.
33. Lee JH, Rehder KJ, Williford L, et al. Use of high flow nasal cannula in critically ill infants, children, and adults: a critical review of the literature. *Intensive Care Med.* 2013;39:247-257.
34. Newth CJL, Venkataraman S, Willson D, et al. Weaning and Extubation Readiness in Pediatric Patients. *Pediatr Crit Care Med.* 2009;10(1):1-11.
35. Thomas N, Brook I. Animal bite-associated infections: microbiology and treatment. *Expert Rev Anti Infect Ther.* 2011;9:215-226.
36. Barkin RM, Rosen P. *Emergency Pediatrics: A Guide to Ambulatory Care.* 6th ed. St Louis: Mosby; 2003.
37. Ahrenholz DH, Cope N, Dimick AR, et al. Practice Guidelines for Burn Care. American Burn Assocation. *J Burn Care and Rehab.* 2001.
38. Kellogg N. The evaluation of sexual abuse in children. *Pediatrics.* 2005;116:506-512.
39. Sato Y. Imaging of nonaccidental head injury. *Pediatr Radiol.* 2009;39(suppl 2):S230-S235.

PART II

DIAGNOSTIC AND THERAPEUTIC INFORMATION

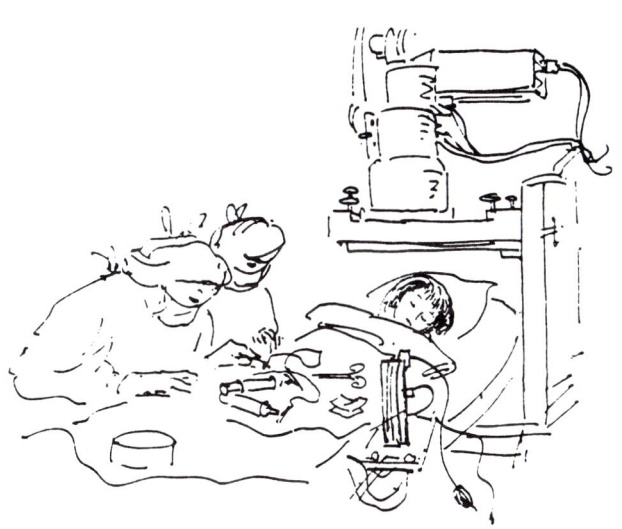

Chapter 5
Adolescent Medicine
Kimberly M. Dickinson, MD, MPH

See additional content on Expert Consult

I. WEB RESOURCES

A. Websites for Clinicians
- American Academy of Pediatrics (AAP) on adolescent health: http://www2.aap.org/sections/adolescenthealth/
- Centers for Disease Control and Prevention (CDC) on contraception: http://www.cdc.gov/reproductivehealth/unintendedpregnancy/contraception.htm
- CDC on sexually transmitted infection treatment guidelines: http://www.cdc.gov/std/tg2015
- Society for Adolescent Medicine: http://www.adolescenthealth.org

B. Websites for Patients
- Drug abuse: http://www.teens.drugabuse.gov
- Sexual health: http://www.ashastd.org, http://www.stayteen.org
- Young women's health: http://www.youngwomenshealth.org

II. INTRODUCTION TO ADOLESCENT HEALTH

A. Pubertal Development[1-6]
1. **Female breast development** (Fig. 5.1)
2. **Male genital development** (Table 5.1; also see Table 10.24 for testicular volumes)
3. **Female and male pubic hair development** (Table 5.2)
4. **Gynecomastia in males**
  a. Generally occurs in middle to late stages of puberty.
  b. Etiology: Breast growth stimulated by estradiol.
  c. Prevalence: Occurs in 50% of boys (50% unilateral, 50% bilateral).
  d. Clinical course: Regression usually occurs over a 2-year period.
  e. Physical examination: With the patient supine, the breast is palpated, looking for glandular or fibroglandular breast tissue beneath the nipple and areola, compared to the lateral breast tissue in order to distinguish true gynecomastia from adiposity, pseudogynecomastia, or a pathologic etiology. A testicular examination should also be performed.
  f. Treatment: Often no treatment is necessary. Severe or nonregressing cases may warrant surgical referral.

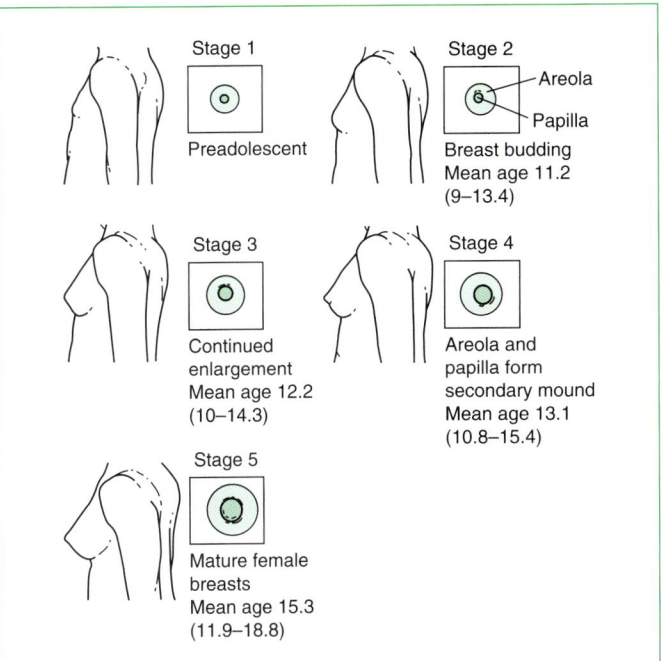

FIGURE 5.1

Tanner stages of breast development in females. *(Modified from Johnson TR, Moore WM. Children Are Different: Developmental Physiology. 2nd ed. Columbus, Ohio, Ross Laboratories, 1978. Mean age and range [2 standard deviations around mean] from Joffe A. Introduction to adolescent medicine. In McMillan JA, DeAngelis CD, Feigin RD, et al., eds. Oski's Pediatrics: Principles and Practice. 4th ed. Philadelphia: Lippincott Williams & Wilkins; 2006:549-550.)*

5. **Precocious puberty**[7]**:** The onset of secondary sexual characteristics before age 8 in girls and age 9 in boys.
6. **Delayed puberty**[8]**:** Lack of breast development by age 13 in girls and lack of secondary sexual development by age 14 in boys (see Fig. 10.5 for more information on the approach to a child with delayed puberty).

B. Psychosocial and Medicosocial History

1. Psychosocial Development of Adolescents[9]: Progression through adolescence is characterized by cognitive, psychosocial, and emotional developments, which help adolescents to establish their identity and autonomy (Table EC 5.A on Expert Consult).

TABLE 5.1
GENITAL DEVELOPMENT (MALE)

Stage	Comment (±2 Standard Deviations Around Mean Age)
1	Pre-pubertal
2	Enlargement of scrotum and testes; skin of scrotum reddens and changes in texture; little or no enlargement of penis; mean age 11.4 yr (9.5–13.8 yr)
3	Enlargement of penis, first mainly in length; further growth of testes and scrotum; mean age 12.9 yr (10.8–14.9 yr)
4	Increased size of penis with growth in breadth and development of glans; further enlargement of testes and scrotum and increased darkening of scrotal skin; mean age 13.8 yr (11.7–15.8 yr)
5	Genitalia adult in size and shape; mean age 14.9 yr (13–17.3 yr)

Data from Joffe A. Introduction to adolescent medicine. In McMillan JA, DeAngelis CD, Feigin RD, et al, eds. Oski's Pediatrics: Principles and Practice. 4th ed. Philadelphia: Lippincott Williams & Wilkins; 2006:546-557.

TABLE 5.2
PUBIC HAIR TANNER STAGING

Tanner Stage	Appearance
1	No hair
2	Sparse, downy hair at base of symphysis pubis
3	Sparse, coarse hair across symphysis pubis
4	Adult hair quality, fills in pubic triangle, no spread to thighs
5	Adult quality and distribution including spread to medial thighs

Data from Alario AJ, Birnkrant JD. "Sexual Maturation and Tanner Staging." Practical Guide To The Care Of The Pediatric Patient. 2nd ed. St. Louis: Mosby; 2007:798-800.

2. HEADSSS[10-12]: A brief instrument that screens for psychosocial factors, which impact adolescent mental and physical health (Box 5.1).

III. ADOLESCENT HEALTH MAINTENANCE

Bright Futures Guidelines for the Health Supervision of Adolescents[13] (Box EC 5.B on Expert Consult)

A. Confidentiality

Adolescents are concerned about the confidentiality of their interactions with healthcare providers. Laws governing a minor's ability to consent to healthcare vary by state and the type of service. More current information can be found at the Guttmacher Institute's website (http://www.guttmacher.org/statecenter/spibs/spib_OMCL.pdf).

B. Chief Complaint

Hidden Agenda: Adolescents may have a chief complaint that obscures their real concern at their visit. At the beginning of a consultation, open-ended questions ("What brings you in today?" or "Is there anything else concerning you?") can help to reveal the actual reason for the visit.

BOX 5.1
HEADSSS ASSESSMENT

(H)OME: Household composition, family dynamics and relationships, living and sleeping arrangements, recent changes, any periods of homelessness, running away from home

(E)DUCATION/EMPLOYMENT/EATING: School performance, attendance, suspensions; attitude toward school; favorite, most difficult, best subjects; special educational needs; goals for the future; afterschool job or other work history (see Section III.C, Review of Systems, for eating/nutrition questions)

(A)CTIVITIES: Friendships with same or opposite sex, ages of friends, best friend, dating, recreational activities, physical activity, sports participation, hobbies, and interests

(D)RUGS: Personal use of tobacco, alcohol, illicit drugs, anabolic steroids; peer substance use; family substance use and attitudes; if personal use, determine frequency, quantity, binge, injury with use; consider use of **CRAFFT** questionnaires (Box 5.2)

(S)EXUALITY: See Box EC 5.A for the "Five Ps" of the sexual history; additional helpful information includes age at first sexual act, number of lifetime and current partners, ages of partners, recent change in partners; knowledge of emergency contraception and sexually transmitted infection/human immunodeficiency virus (STI/HIV) prevention; prior testing for STI/HIV, prior pregnancies, abortions; ever fathered a child; history of nonconsensual intimate physical contact or sex; pain/discomfort with sex

(S)UICIDE/DEPRESSION: Feelings about self, both positive and negative; history of depression or other mental health problems; sleep problems (difficulty getting to sleep, early waking); changes in appetite or weight; anhedonia; irritability; anxiety; current or prior suicidal thoughts or attempts; other self-harming or injurious behavior

(S)AFETY: Feeling unsafe at home, at school, or in the community; bullying; guns in the home; weapon carrying, what kinds of weapons; fighting; arrests; gang membership, seatbelt use

C. Review of Systems (Areas of Emphasis With an Adolescent)

1. **Nutrition:** Dietary habits, including skipped meals, special diets, purging methods, recent weight gain or loss
2. **Cardiac:** Syncopal or presyncopal events, chest pain on exercise, history of heart murmur
3. **Respiratory:** Wheezing/asthma, dyspnea during exercise
4. **Neurologic:** History of significant head trauma/concussion, numbness, tingling, seizures
5. **Dermatologic:** Acne, moles, rashes, warts
6. **Genitourinary:** Dysuria, urgency, frequency, discharge, bleeding
7. **Gynecologic:** Menarche, last menstrual period, frequency/regularity, longest interval between periods, duration, dysmenorrhea, menometrorrhagia, reproductive life plan
8. **Psychiatric:** Assessment for symptoms or feelings of depression

D. Family History

Including psychiatric disorders, suicide, alcoholism or substance abuse, and chronic medical conditions or familial risk factors (hypertension, diabetes, cholesterol, thrombosis, family history of sudden cardiac death or congenital heart disease, stroke, cancer, asthma, tuberculosis, HIV).

E. Medical History

Includes information about chronic conditions/medications (including illicit and performance-enhancing agents), hospitalizations/surgeries, allergies (especially those associated with anaphylaxis or respiratory compromise), congenital heart disease, seizure disorders, and immunization status.

Note: See Chapter 7 and Table EC 7.D for further information about exercise restrictions with cardiac disease.

F. Adolescent Physical Examination (Most Pertinent Aspects)[3,4,14]

Whenever possible, examine the patient in a gown to ensure a complete and thorough examination.

Note: Pre-Participation Examination (PPE) is an opportunity to screen for risk factors that are related to participation in sports. However, it is also an opportunity to deliver preventative services, as this may be a young person's only visit during adolescence.

1. **Vital signs:** Height, weight (calculate body mass index [BMI]), and blood pressure with percentiles should be measured and **trended at each visit**
2. **Vision/Hearing screening:** Assess for visual acuity, pupil equality, use of corrective lenses, hearing loss
3. **Dentition and gums:** Tobacco use, enamel erosion from induced vomiting, need for dental care
4. **Skin:** Acne (type and distribution of lesions) (See Tables 8.1, 8.2, and 8.3 for treatment guidelines), atypical nevi, acanthosis nigricans, scars, rashes, evidence of contagious infections (varicella, impetigo, scabies, tinea corporis, molloscum contagiosum), piercings and tattoos
5. **Thyroid:** Size, nodules
6. **Cardiac:** Rate and rhythm, pulses (radial/femoral), auscultation for murmurs both standing and supine (See Table 7.3 for a list of innocent heart murmurs)
7. **Spine:** Routine screening for idiopathic scoliosis is not recommended. However, clinicians should be prepared to evaluate scoliosis if it is discovered or the patient or parents express concern.
8. **Musculoskeletal Exam:** a detailed description is available in Fig. EC 5.A on Expert Consult.
9. **Breasts:** Sexual maturity rating for females (see Fig. 5.1), masses (females), gynecomastia (males)
10. **Abdomen:** Hepatosplenomegaly (contraindication for contact sports), abdominal pain/tenderness

11. **Genitalia:** Consider the use of a chaperone. For both male and female genital examinations, there should be an explanation before the examination and normal findings should be commented on. Nongenital parts of the body should be examined first and painful areas should be examined last. Lengthy discussion should be avoided while the patient is undressed and in a compromising position.
    a. Male[15]:
       (1) External examination: Visual inspection for sexual maturity rating for hair (Tanner stage; see Table 5.1), and examination of the penis, urethral meatus, and perianal region. Assess for pubic lice, signs of STIs (warts, ulcers, erosions, discharge), and inguinal hernias.
       (2) Genital examination for sexual maturity rating for testicles (see Table 10.24) and identification of masses, hydroceles, and varicoceles. If there are signs of proctitis (i.e., dysuria or pelvic pain), a digital rectal examination should be performed in all men 18 years and older.
    b. Female[16-17]:
       (1) External examination: Visual inspection for sexual maturity rating for hair (Tanner stage; see Table 5.2), and examination of the urethral meatus, vaginal introitus, and perianal region. Assess for lice, signs of STI (warts, ulcers, erosions, discharge), rashes, and evidence of trauma.
       (2) Internal examination (pelvic examination): **Should be performed when the patient is symptomatic (pelvic pain, vaginal discharge, menstrual disorders) or has an acute concern. It is not routinely recommended for healthy asymptomatic women under 21 years of age.** Indications include vaginal discharge (assess cervix for mucopurulent discharge, friability, large ectropion, foreign body), lower abdominal or pelvic pain, urinary symptoms in sexually active females, menstrual disorders (amenorrhea, abnormal vaginal bleeding, or dysmenorrhea refractory to medical therapy), consideration of intrauterine device or diaphragm, and suspected or reported sexual abuse or rape (refer to a specialized center if not appropriately trained and equipped to document evidence of trauma and collect forensic specimens).

G. Screening Laboratory Tests and Procedures

1. **A lack of research and evidence for screening examinations in adolescence** has led to variability in guidelines for topics such as screening for dyslipidemia, iron-deficiency anemia, diabetes, and tuberculosis. Updated guidelines that have been issued by various organizations may be accessed at the listed sites. The recommendations that follow are largely based on CDC guidelines:
a. Bright Futures: http://brightfutures.aap.org

b. CDC: http://www.cdc.gov/healthyyouth/index.htm
c. U.S. Preventive Services Task Force (USPSTF): https://www.uspreventiveservicestaskforce.org
d. The American Congress of Obstetricians and Gynecologists (ACOG): http://acog.org

2. **Adolescents may legally consent to medical care for STIs without parental notification** in all 50 states and Washington, D.C.; however, providers should be aware of barriers to confidentiality related to medical billing and explanation of benefits by insurance companies. The Guttmacher Organization provides an overview of minors' consent laws, including STI treatment (http://www.guttmacher.org/statecenter/spibs/spib_MASS.pdf).

3. **Sexually transmitted infections, screening guidelines, and treatment recommendations for sexually active adolescents.**[18-22]
   a. HIV: Begin routine yearly screening with opt-out consent starting at age 13. Screen all high-risk individuals at least annually and screen more frequently based on risk. Screen all individuals who seek STI testing. Re-screen for HIV 3–4 months after the diagnosis of a STI. Screening (antibody) tests will not pick up acute infections. If there is concern regarding recent exposure, ribonucleic acid (RNA) testing should be ordered. All pregnant women should be screened at their first prenatal visit. Several point-of-care rapid HIV-1 antibody tests provide results in minutes to hours. These tests have sensitivity and specificity rates similar to standard enzyme immunoassay (EIA). In routine care, a negative rapid antibody test result does not need confirmation; however, as with EIAs, positive results should be confirmed with a more specific test, such as a Western blot or immunofluorescent assay. See Chapter 17 for more information on HIV pre-exposure prophylaxis and treatment.
   b. Syphilis: Routine screening is recommended at least annually for persons at risk, although certain groups, including young men who have sex with men (YMSM) or those with HIV, should be tested every 6 months. All pregnant women should be screened at their first prenatal visit. Clinical and serologic evaluation should be performed at 6 and 12 months after treatment in order to ensure appropriate reduction in titers. See Table 5.3 for information on treatment.
   c. Chlamydia and Gonorrhea:
      (1) *Chlamydia trachomatis* (CT): Routine screening should be carried out in sexually active females < 25 years of age. For males, screening is especially recommended in high prevalence communities and/or settings (e.g., STI clinics, adolescent clinics, and correctional facilities). For sexually active YMSM, tests should be performed at least annually at the sites of contact (urethra and rectum), and every 3–6 months in increased risk cases.

TABLE 5.3
SEXUALLY TRANSMITTED AND GENITOURINARY INFECTIONS: GUIDELINES FOR MANAGEMENT*

Infection	Clinical Diagnosis	Empiric Therapy	Comments
CHLAMYDIA INFECTIONS	Uncomplicated urethritis, endocervicitis, or proctitis	Azithromycin 1 g PO once **OR** Doxycycline 100 mg PO BID for 7 days *Alt: erythromycin PO QID* **OR** *fluoroquinolone for 7 days*	Consider empirical treatment for gonorrhea secondary to common co-infection. See below for instructions for therapy for sexual partners.
	Chlamydia infection in pregnancy	Azithromycin 1 g PO once **OR** Amoxicillin 500 mg PO TID for 7 days **OR** Erythromycin PO QID for 7 days	Repeat testing (3 weeks posttreatment) to document chlamydial eradication is in all pregnant patients.
GONORRHEA INFECTIONS	Uncomplicated infection of the cervix, urethra, rectum, or pharynx	Ceftriaxone 250 mg IM once **PLUS** Azithromycin 1 g PO	Dual treatment is recommended for gonorrhea secondary to organism resistance.
	Epididymitis	Ceftriaxone 250 mg IM once **PLUS** Doxycycline 100 mg PO BID for 10 days	For MSM, add a fluoroquinolone for 10 days.
	Disseminated gonococcal infections	Ceftriaxone 1 g IV/IM daily *Alt: cefotaxime 1g IV Q8 hours*	Can switch to cefixime 400 mg PO BID 24–48 hours after clinical improvement. Total therapy course: 7 days.
PELVIC INFLAMMATORY DISEASE		**Outpatient:** Ceftriaxone 250 mg IM once **PLUS** Doxycycline 100 mg PO BID for 14 days ± metronidazole 500 mg PO BID x 14 days	

Continued

TABLE 5.3
SEXUALLY TRANSMITTED AND GENITOURINARY INFECTIONS: GUIDELINES FOR MANAGEMENT*—cont'd

Infection	Clinical Diagnosis	Empiric Therapy	Comments
		Inpatient: Regimen A (2 g Cefotetan IV Q12 hr **OR** 2 g Cefoxitin IV Q6 hr) **PLUS** doxycycline 100 mg IV Q12 hr **OR Regimen B:** clindamycin 900 mg IV Q8 hr **PLUS** gentamicin 2 mg/kg loading dose, then 1.5 mg/kg IV Q8 hr maintenance (or single daily dosing)	Switch to oral therapy 24 hours after clinical improvement to complete 14 days of treatment with doxycycline BID or clindamycin QID.
SYPHILIS	Primary, secondary, or early latent syphilis (<1 year duration)	Benzathine PCN G 50,000 U/kg (max 2.4 million units) IM (single dose) Alt: doxycycline 100 mg PO BID for 14 days **OR** tetracycline 500 mg PO QID for 14 days	Data is limited for penicillin alternatives
	Late syphilis (>1 year duration); tertiary syphilis	Benzathine PCN G 50,000 U/kg (max 2.4 million units) IM Q1 week for 3 weeks Alt: doxycycline 100 mg PO BID for 28 days **OR** tetracycline 500 mg PO QID for 28 days	
HERPES (GENITAL, NONNEONATAL)		Acyclovir or Valacyclovir	See formulary for treatment for initial infection and recurrence

*Patients should be instructed to refer their partners for diagnosis, testing, and treatment. For dosing for children aged≤ 8 years or weighing <45 kg or for additional alternative regimens, please refer to the CDC Treatment Guidelines, 2015: http://www.cdc.gov/std/tg2015/.
PCN G, penicillin G.

Pharyngeal screening is not recommended for the general public. All pregnant women under 25 years of age should be screened. Testing for cure is recommended at 3–4 weeks for all pregnant women. All persons should be retested 3 months after treatment due to high reinfection rates.
- (2) *Neisseria gonorrhoeae* (GC): Routine screening should be performed in sexually active females < 25 years of age. For sexually active YMSM, screening should be performed at least annually at the sites of contact (urethra, rectum, or pharynx), and every 3–6 months in high-risk cases. Testing for cure is required for extra-genital infections, particularly pharyngeal gonorrhea, if they are treated with alternative therapies; this is due to a high rate of resistance. All pregnant women under 25 years of age should be screened. Retesting should be performed 3 months after treatment due to high reinfection rates.
- (3) Method of screening:
    - Females: Self- or provider-collected vaginal nucleic acid amplification test (NAAT) is the preferred method to screen for CT/GC; self-collected specimens may have higher patient acceptability. **Vaginal swabs are as sensitive and specific as cervical swabs, and both are more accurate than urine samples.**
    - Males: Urine NAAT is preferred.
- d. Vaginal Infections, Genital Ulcers, and Warts
    - (1) Diagnostic features of vaginal infections (Table 5.4) can assist in differentiating normal vaginal discharge from bacterial vaginosis, trichomoniasis, and yeast vaginitis.
    - (2) Diagnostic features of various genital lesions, as well as management of warts and ulcers, are presented in Table 5.5.
- e. Other STIs:
    - (1) Routine screening of asymptomatic adolescents is not recommended for other STIs, e.g., trichomoniasis, herpes simplex virus (HSV), hepatitis B and C viruses (HBV, HCV), and human papillomavirus (HPV). However, if a woman tests positive for trichomoniasis, she should be retested 3 months after treatment.
    - (2) Refer to the CDC guidelines for specific additional recommendations for STI screening in YMSM and HIV-positive adolescents who might require more thorough and frequent evaluations.
    - (3) Advise patients to refrain from intercourse until 7 days after full therapy is complete, the partner is treated, and all visible lesions have resolved.

Text continued on p. 122

TABLE 5.4
DIAGNOSTIC FEATURES AND MANAGEMENT OF VAGINAL INFECTIONS

	No Infection/ Physiologic Leukorrhea	Vulvovaginal Candidiasis	Trichomoniasis	Bacterial Vaginosis**
Etiology	—	*Candida albicans* and other yeasts	*Trichomonas vaginalis*	*Gardnerella vaginalis*, anaerobic bacteria, mycoplasma
Typical symptoms	None	Vulvar itching, irritation, ↑ discharge	Malodorous frothy discharge, vulvar itching	Malodorous, slightly ↑ discharge
Discharge				
Amount	Variable; usually scant	Scant to moderate	Profuse	Moderate
Color*	Clear or white	White	Yellow-green	Usually white or gray
Consistency	Nonhomogenous	Clumped; adherent plaques	Homogenous	Homogenous, low viscosity; smoothly coats vaginal walls
Vulvar/vaginal inflammation	No	Yes	Yes	No
pH of vaginal fluid†	Usually < 4.5	Usually < 4.5	Usually > 5.0	Usually > 4.5
Amine ("fishy") odor with 10% potassium hydroxide (KOH)	None	None	May be present	Present, positive "whiff-amine" test

Microscopy[‡]	Normal epithelial cells; *Lactobacillus* predominates	Leukocytes, epithelial cells, yeast, mycelia, or pseudomycelia in 40%–80% of cases	Leukocytes; motile trichomonads seen in 50%–70% of symptomatic patients, less often if asymptomatic	Clue cells, few leukocytes; *Lactobacillus* outnumbered by profuse mixed flora (nearly always including *G. vaginalis* plus anaerobes)
Usual treatment (see Formulary)	None	Fluconazole 150 mg PO once OR intravaginal azole cream	Metronidazole 2 g PO once	Metronidazole 500 mg PO BID for 7 days **OR** Metronidazole Gel 0.75% (5 g) intravaginally daily for 5 days **OR** Clindamycin Cream 2% 5 g intravaginally for 7 days
Management of sex partners	None	None	Treatment recommended	None

NOTE: Refer to Formulary for dosing information.

*Color of discharge is determined by examining vaginal discharge against the white background of a swab.

**Despite more sensitive and specific laboratory tests, cost and practicality make the Amsel criteria the best in-office method to diagnose Bacterial Vaginosis. To diagnose BV, at least 3 criteria must be present: 1. Homogenous, thin, gray/white discharge 2. Vaginal pH >4.5, 3. Positive whiff-amine test 4. Clue cells on wet mount

[†]pH determination is not useful if blood is present.

[‡]To detect fungal elements, vaginal fluid is digested with 10% KOH before microscopic examination; to examine for other features, fluid is mixed (1:1) with physiologic saline.

From Workowski KA, Berman S. *Sexually transmitted diseases treatment guidelines, 2010.* MMWR Recomm Rep. *2010;59 (RR-12):1-110.*

TABLE 5.5
DIAGNOSTIC FEATURES AND MANAGEMENT OF GENITAL ULCERS AND WARTS

Infection	Clinical Presentation	Presumptive Diagnosis	Definitive Diagnosis	Treatment/Management of Sex Partners
Genital herpes	Grouped vesicles, painful shallow ulcers to mild clinical manifestation (redness, pain, excoriations). HSV-2 more common cause of genital lesions	Tzanck preparation with multinucleated giant cells	HSV PCR	No known cure. Prompt initiation of therapy shortens duration of first episode. For severe recurrent disease, initiate therapy at start of prodrome or within 1 day. Transmission can occur during asymptomatic periods. See Formulary for dosing of acyclovir, famciclovir, or valacyclovir.
Chancroid	Etiology: *Haemophilus ducreyi* Painful genital ulcer; tender, suppurative inguinal adenopathy	No evidence of *Treponema pallidum* (syphilis) on dark-field microscopy or serologic testing; negative HSV	Use of special media (not widely available in United States); sensitivity < 80%	Single dose: Azithromycin 1 g orally **OR** Ceftriaxone 250 mg IM. Partners should be examined and treated, regardless of whether symptoms are present, or if they have had sex within 10 days preceding onset of patient's symptoms. Syphilis is a common co-pathogen with chancroid.
Primary syphilis	Indurated, well-defined, usually single painless ulcer or chancre; nontender inguinal adenopathy	Nontreponemal serologic test: VDRL, RPR, or STS	Treponemal serologic test: FTA-ABS or MHA-TP; darkfield microscopy or direct fluorescent antibody tests of lesion exudates or tissue	Parenteral penicillin G (see Table 5.3 for preparation(s), dosage, and length of treatment.) Treat presumptively for persons exposed within 3 months preceding the diagnosis of primary syphilis in a sex partner or who were exposed >90 days preceding the diagnosis and in whom serologic tests may not be immediately available or follow-up is uncertain.

HPV infection (genital warts)	Single or multiple soft, fleshy, papillary or sessile, painless growths around anus, vulvovaginal area, penis, urethra, or perineum; no inguinal adenopathy	Typical clinical presentation	Papanicolaou smear revealing typical cytological changes	Treatment does not eradicate infection. Goal: Removal of exophytic warts. Exclude cervical dysplasia before treatment. 1. **Patient-administered therapies include:** podofilox gel or imiquimod cream (contraindicated in pregnancy). 2. **Clinician-applied therapies include:** bichloracetic or trichloroacetic acid, surgical removal, and cryotherapy with liquid nitrogen or cryoprobe. Podofilox, imiquimod, and podophyllin are contraindicated in pregnancy. Period of communicability unknown.

NOTE: Chancroid, lymphogranuloma venereum (LGV), and granuloma inguinale should be considered in the differential diagnosis of genital ulcers if the clinical presentation is atypical and tests for herpes and syphilis are negative.

FTA-ABS, Fluorescent treponemal antibody absorbed; HPV, human papillomavirus; HSV, herpes simplex virus; IM, intramuscular; MHA-TP, micro-hemagglutination assay for antibody to *Treponema pallidum*; RPR, rapid plasma reagin; STS, serologic test for syphilis; VDRL, Venereal Disease Research Laboratory.

Modified from Workowski KA, Berman S. *Sexually transmitted diseases treatment guidelines, 2010.* MMWR Recomm Rep. *2010;59 (RR-12):1-110.*

(4) In heterosexual men and women with Chlamydia or gonorrhea for whom health department partner-management strategies are impractical or unavailable and whose providers are concerned about partners' access to prompt clinical evaluation and treatment, expedited partner therapy may be an option depending on local and state laws.

4. **Pelvic inflammatory disease:** Acute infection of the upper genital tract, occurring most often in women aged 15–25 years.
a. Differential diagnosis is broad and includes endometriosis, tubo-ovarian abscess, ovarian cyst, ectopic pregnancy, acute surgical abdomen, inflammatory bowel disease (IBD), pyelonephritis, dysmenorrhea, septic/threatened abortion.
b. Microbiology: *N. gonorrhoeae* and *C. trachomatis* are the most commonly identified pathogens, additional pathogens include *Mycoplasma genitalium*. Often polymicrobial in nature.
c. Workup: Pelvic and bimanual examination, gonorrhea/chlamydia (GC/CT) and HIV testing, human chorionic gonadotropin (hCG), wet preparation, erythrocyte sedimentation rate (ESR), C-reactive protein (CRP), and urinalysis/urine culture (UA/UCx) if clinically indicated. Consider a complete blood cell count (CBC) with differential and pelvic ultrasound if the patient is ill-appearing, has an adnexal mass on bimanual examination, or is not improving after antibiotics.
d. Minimum diagnostic criteria: Uterine, adnexal, or cervical motion tenderness without other identifiable causes. One or more of the following additional criteria enhances specificity: fever (>38.3°C), mucopurulent vaginal or cervical discharge, leukocytes on saline microscopy, increased ESR or CRP, laboratory documentation of chlamydial or gonorrhea infection.
e. Treatment: Empirical treatment is indicated for all sexually active females if minimum diagnostic criteria are met and no other cause for symptoms is identified. See Table 5.3 and the CDC STD Treatment Guidelines for most up-to-date information and alternative regimens (www.cdc.gov/std/tg2015/pid.htm).
f. Admission criteria: Cannot exclude acute surgical abdomen, presence of tubo-ovarian abscess, pregnancy, immunodeficiency, severe illness (nausea, vomiting, anorexia), inability to tolerate or follow outpatient oral regimen, failure to respond to appropriate outpatient therapy, or follow-up cannot be ensured.

5. **Cervical cancer cytologic analysis** [Papanicolaou (Pap) smear][23]
a. *Immunocompetent:* Regardless of age of sexual debut, cervical cancer screening with Pap smear should not begin until a woman is 21 years old. The risk of adverse pregnancy outcomes outweighs benefits of screening and treatment, given the low rate of cervical cancer and high rate of resolution of HPV infections. Subsequent tests should be done every 3 years. Cytologic evaluation only should be used, HPV testing is only recommended if cytology

is abnormal (ASC-US or higher). HPV testing is indicated until age 30.
b. *HIV+ or immunosuppressed (e.g., organ transplant recipient, systemic lupus erythematosus patient, poorly controlled diabetic):* Every 6 months in first year after HIV diagnosis or after sexual debut if immunosuppressed; thereafter, annually. Immunosuppressed adolescents with abnormal cytologic results should be referred for further management.

6. **Health Maintenance**[13]
a. Immunizations: See Table 5.6 for recommendations on common immunizations given during adolescence. Refer to Chapter 16 for dosing, route, and formulation.
b. Cholesterol screening: *All* children should undergo cholesterol screening once between ages 9–11 years and once between ages 17–21 years.
c. Diabetes screening: Consider screening for type 2 diabetes in children who have a BMI >85% for age and sex who also have other risk factors including family history.[24]
d. Selective screening for tuberculosis, anemia, and vision and hearing abnormalities if patient screens positive on risk screening questions.

IV. SEXUAL HEALTH

A. Sexual Orientation[25-26]

Sexual orientation is a composition of sexual attraction, behavior, and identity. Sexual attraction is an enduring pattern of sexual/romantic feelings. Sexual behavior describes the pattern of sexual activity in which a person participates. Sexual identity is the conception of self, based on attraction, behavior, and/or membership in social group through shared sexual orientation. Adolescents may explore a variety of sexual activities (penile-vaginal, anal, or oral intercourse) that do not reflect their sexual identity or orientation (e.g., heterosexual, homosexual, bisexual). Sexual attraction does not always mirror sexual behavior. Conversely, adolescents may self-identify with a particular sexual orientation but not be sexually active.

B. Gender Identity

Gender is comprised of gender identity, gender expression, and natal or biological gender. Gender identity is an individual's self-awareness as male or female. Gender expression relates to the mannerisms, personal traits, clothing choices, etc., that serve to communicate a person's identity as they relate to a particular societal gender role. Natal sex refers to the sex karyotype (XX, XY, XO, XXY, etc.) and sex phenotype (external genitals, gonads, internal sex organs) with which a person was born.
1. **Transgender:** An individual whose gender identity (internal sense) or gender expression (behavior, etc.) differs from the natal sex assigned at birth.

TABLE 5.6

RECOMMENDED IMMUNIZATIONS FOR PRETEENS AND ADOLESCENTS

Vaccinations	When to Administer	Special Considerations
Influenza	Yearly	Contraindicated in patients with severe egg protein allergy or who have a history of Guillain-Barré syndrome
Meningococcal vaccine (MCV4)	1st dose age 11–12 and booster at age 16 or before entering college	Adolescents with HIV should receive 3 doses. 2nd dose 2 months apart during age 11–12 plus booster at age 16. Safe in pregnancy.
Tdap (Tetanus, diphtheria, pertussis)	Age 11–12. Td booster (no pertussis coverage) should be given every 10 years. Give Tdap as booster if patient did not previously receive Tdap.	Pregnant women should receive booster during every third trimester of pregnancy. Tdap (not Td) contraindicated in patients who had seizures within 1 week of childhood DTP or DTap administration.
Hepatitis B (HBV)	All unvaccinated adolescents at risk for hepatitis should be vaccinated. See CDC's Hepatitis B VIS for more information.	Patients require 3-dose series. 2nd dose given 4 weeks after 1st dose and 3rd dose given 5 months after 2nd dose. Wait 28 days after immunization prior to donating blood.
Human Papillomavirus (HPV)	Age 11–12. May be given as early as age 9. Recommended for females through age 26 and for males through age 21.	Patients require 3-dose series. 2nd dose given 1–2 months after 1st dose. 3rd dose given 6 months after 1st dose. Not recommended for pregnant women.
Hepatitis A (HAV)	Consider in high-risk patients who did not receive routine vaccination as children. See CDC's Hepatitis A VIS for more information.	Contraindicated in patients with latex allergy. Can be considered during pregnancy.
Varicella (Chickenpox)	People 13 years of age and older (who have never had chickenpox or received chickenpox vaccine) should get two doses of the varicella vaccine at least 28 days apart.	Pregnant women should not receive until after delivery. Women should not get pregnant for 1 month after getting chickenpox vaccine. Contraindicated in highly immunocompromised patients.

Adapted from the Center for Disease Control and Prevention's Vaccine Information Statements (VIS). Available at http://www.cdc.gov/vaccines/hcp/vis/.

2. **Gender nonconforming:** Gender expression by an individual that does not match masculine and feminine gender norms.
3. **Gender identity is unrelated to sexual orientation**. Transgender or transvestite individuals may feel themselves to be heterosexual, homosexual, or bisexual.

C. Contraception[27-28]

The U.S. Department of Health and Human Services requires contraception be covered by insurance plans without a co-pay.
1. **Special considerations in adolescents**
a. Barriers may include confidentiality concerns, fear of pelvic examination, and fear of side effects (e.g., weight gain, bleeding, etc.).
b. Adherence and continuation rates in adolescents are superior with long-acting reversible contraception (LARC) methods such as the intrauterine device and etonogestrel implant.
c. **Counseling should include discussion of need for barrier method to prevent STIs**, as well as tips for increasing adherence.
2. **Methods of contraception** (Fig. 5.2). Methods displayed in order of effectiveness.
3. **Contraception selection and initiation:**
a. Selecting a contraceptive method: Please refer to the CDC Medical Eligibility Criteria (http://www.cdc.gov/reproductivehealth/unintendedpregnancy/usmec.htm) for any relative or absolute contraindications for each hormonal contraceptive method based on an individual's medical comorbidities and the CDC's Selected Practice Recommendations (http://www.cdc.gov/reproductivehealth/unintendedPregnancy/USSPR.htm) for minimum requirements to start each method.
   (1) To appropriately start a hormonal method, the basic medical history should include assessment of clotting risk, blood pressure, pregnancy status, and any other pertinent medical comorbidities.
   (2) Related to clotting symptoms for a person on a combined method, a mnemonic to remember the more serious complications of combined hormonal contraception is **ACHES:**
      (a) **A**bdominal pain (pelvic vein or mesenteric vein thrombosis, pancreatitis)
      (b) **C**hest pain (pulmonary embolism)
      (c) **H**eadaches (thrombotic or hemorrhagic stroke, retinal vein thrombosis)
      (d) **E**ye symptoms (thrombotic or hemorrhagic stroke, retinal vein thrombosis)
      (e) **S**evere leg pain (thrombophlebitis of the lower extremities)
   (3) To support adherence and continuation, use a patient-centered approach, review method effectiveness, and provide anticipatory guidance regarding side effects of each method when assisting an adolescent in selecting a new contraceptive method. Many

BIRTH CONTROL GUIDE

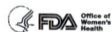

Medicines To Help You

Most Effective ↑

Methods	Number of pregnancies expected per 100 women*	Use	Some Risks
Sterilization Surgery for Women	less than 1	Onetime procedure Permanent	• Pain • Bleeding • Infection or other complications after surgery • Ectopic (tubal) pregnancy
Surgical Sterilization Implant for Women	less than 1	Onetime procedure Waiting period before it works Permanent	• Mild to moderate pain after insertion • Ectopic (tubal) pregnancy
Sterilization Surgery for Men	less than 1	Onetime procedure Waiting period before it works Permanent	• Pain • Bleeding • Infection
Implantable Rod	less than 1	Inserted by a healthcare provider Lasts up to 3 years	• Changes in bleeding patterns • Weight gain • Breast and abdominal pain
IUD Copper	less than 1	Inserted by a healthcare provider Lasts up to 10 years	• Cramps • Bleeding • Pelvic inflammatory disease • Infertility • Tear or hole in the uterus
IUD w/ Progestin	less than 1	Inserted by a healthcare provider Lasts up to 3-5 years	• Irregular bleeding • No periods • Abdominal/pelvic pain • Ovarian cysts
Shot/Injection	6	Need a shot every 3 months	• Bone loss • Bleeding between periods • Weight gain • Nervousness • Abdominal discomfort • Headaches
Oral Contraceptives (Combined Pill) "The Pill"	9	Must swallow a pill every day	• Nausea • Breast Tenderness • Headache • Rare: high blood pressure, blood clots, heart attack, stroke
Oral Contraceptives (Progestin only) "The MiniPill"	9	Must swallow a pill every day	• Irregular bleeding • Headache • Breast tenderness • Nausea • Dizziness
Oral Contraceptives Extended/Continuous Use "The Pill"	9	Must swallow a pill every day	• Risks are similar to other oral contraceptives (combined) • Light bleeding or spotting between periods
Patch	9	Put on a new patch each week for 3 weeks (21 total days). Don't put on a patch during the fourth week.	• Exposure to higher average levels of estrogen than most oral contraceptives
Vaginal Contraceptive Ring	9	Put the ring into the vagina yourself. Keep the ring in your vagina for 3 weeks and then take it out for one week.	• Vaginal discharge • Discomfort in the vagina • Mild irritation • Risks are similar to oral contraceptives (combined)
Diaphragm with Spermicide	12	Must use every time you have sex.	• Irritation • Allergic reactions • Urinary tract infection • Toxic shock
Sponge with Spermicide	12-24	Must use every time you have sex.	• Irritation • Allergic reactions • Hard time removing • Toxic shock
Cervical Cap with Spermicide	17-23	Must use every time you have sex.	• Irritation • Allergic reactions • Abnormal Pap test • Toxic shock
Male Condom	18	Must use every time you have sex. Except for abstinence, latex condoms are the best protection against HIV/AIDS and other STIs.	• Allergic reactions
Female Condom	21	Must use every time you have sex. May give some protection against STIs.	• Irritation • Allergic reactions
Spermicide Alone	28	Must use every time you have sex.	• Irritation • Allergic reactions • Urinary tract infection
Emergency Contraception – If your primary method of birth control fails			
Plan B Plan B One Step Next Choice	7 out of every 8 women who would have gotten pregnant will not become pregnant after taking Plan B, Plan B One-Step, or Next Choice	Swallow the pills within 3 days after having unprotected sex.	• Nausea • Vomiting • Abdominal pain • Fatigue • Headache
Ella	6 or 7 out of every 10 women who would have gotten pregnant will not become pregnant after taking Ella.	Swallow the pill within 5 days after having unprotected sex.	• Headache • Nausea • Abdominal pain • Menstrual pain • Tiredness • Dizziness

Least Effective

*effectiveness of the different methods during typical/actual use (including sometimes using a method in a way that is not correct or not consistent)   http://www.fda.gov/birthcontrol

FIGURE 5.2

Comparing effectiveness of family planning methods. *(From World Health Organization Department of Reproductive Health and Research [WHO/RHR] and Johns Hopkins Bloomberg School of Public Health/Center for Communication Programs [CCP], Knowledge for Health Project. Family Planning: A Global Handbook for Providers (2011 Update). Baltimore, Geneva: CCP and WHO; 2011.)* Available at: http://www.fda.gov/downloads/ForConsumers/ByAudience/ForWomen/FreePublications/UCM356451.pdf.)

websites including http://www.bedsider.org help young adults make educated decisions regarding their reproductive options.
  b. Quick start: Defined as starting a method of contraception on the day of the visit (not waiting until a new menstrual cycle begins). Anyone can use the quick start method. Fig. 5.3 shows principles of quick-start contraception regimens. See CDC recommendations on how to be reasonably certain a patient is not pregnant.[32]
4. **Description and patient use instructions for various contraceptive methods**
  a. **Intrauterine Device (IUD):** Long-acting reversible contraception, inserted into the uterus by a trained medical provider. Increased risk of pelvic infection with placement, but the absolute risk of infection is low and exists only within the first 3 weeks after placement. Return to fertility is rapid after removal. Among the most effective forms of birth control.
    (1) Copper: hormone-free, may be used for up to 10 years.
    (2) Progestin-containing: two types with differing amounts of progestin that may be used for 3–5 years depending on the type. May lead to decreased menstrual flow or amenorrhea.
  b. **Subdermal Implant**: Progestin-only, long-acting reversible contraception. Matchstick-sized, and newer models are radio-opaque. Maximum duration of action is 3 years. Return to fertility is rapid after removal. May be less effective for women who are overweight or obese.
    (1) Placed by a trained medical provider. A 4-cm rod inserted under the skin in the medial aspect of the upper arm, using local anesthetic.
    (2) Removal requires a small incision. Must replace every 3 years.
  c. **Depot medroxyprogesterone acetate (DMPA [Depo-Provera]) injection:** Progestin-only method, with duration of action for 3 months. Typical use failure rate of 6%. Effects are not quickly reversible, may take up to 9 months for ovulation to return. Menstrual irregularity is common, but often resolves after several cycles. Patient should be encouraged to receive adequate calcium and vitamin D due to association with decrease in bone mineral density with this form of contraception.
    (1) Initial injection within first 5 days after onset of menses (or quick start; see Fig. 5.3).
    (2) Reinjection every 11–13 weeks [depending on whether injection is intramuscular (IM) or subcutaneous (SQ)]. Timeliness is important.
    (3) If bleeding is bothersome, consider a 7–10 day course of conjugated estrogen.
    (4) Per FDA black box warning, should not be used for longer than 2 consecutive years unless other forms of birth control are inadequate, due to concern for loss of bone mineral density. Bone density returns after discontinuation of DMPA. In practice, however, for many adolescent the benefits of effective

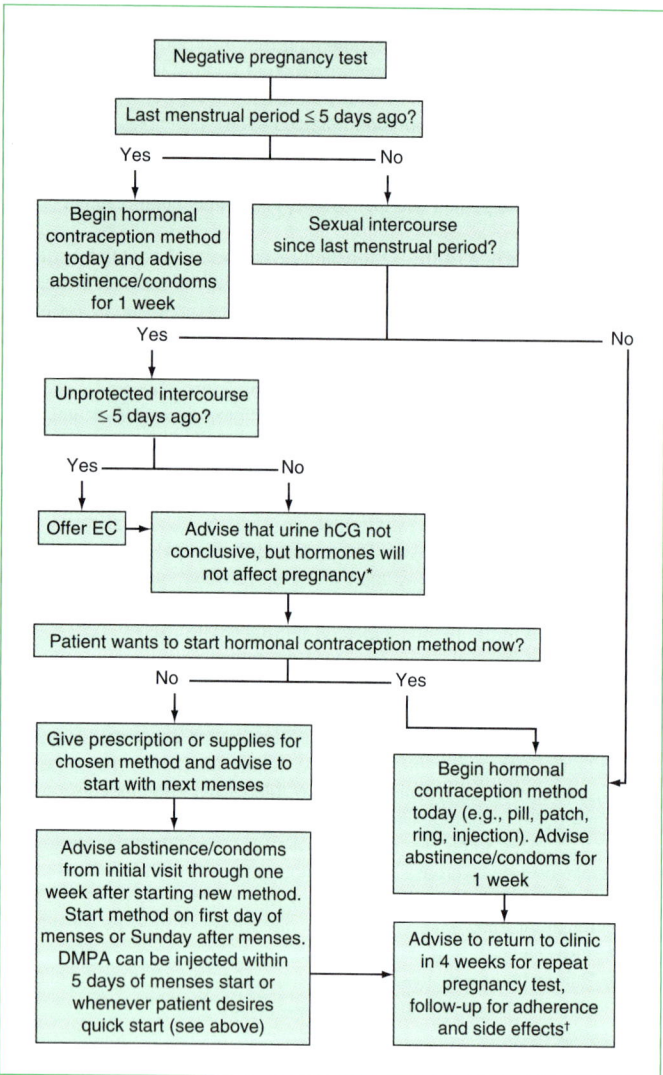

FIGURE 5.3

Algorithm for quick start initiation of contraception. EC, Emergency contraception; hCG, human chorionic gonadotropin.*Pregnancy tests may take 2–3 weeks after sex to be accurate.†Consider pregnancy test at second depot medroxyprogesterone acetate (DMPA [Depo-Provera]) injection if quick-start regimen was used and patient failed 4-week follow-up visit. *(Modified from Zieman M, Hatcher RA, Cwiak C, et al. A Pocket Guide to Managing Contraception. Tiger, Georgia: Bridging the Gap Foundation; 2010:142.)*

contraception outweigh the risks associated with loss of bone mineral density and DMPA can be used beyond this time period.
d. **Combined hormonal oral contraceptive pills (OCPs):** Commonly referred to as the "pill", a combination of estrogen and progestin that must be taken every day to prevent pregnancy. Typical failure rates are approximately 8% and may be higher in teens. Known to improve dysmenorrhea and are first-line therapy for endometriosis. Newer formulations exist, known as extended-cycle regimens, which reduce the number of menstrual cycles per year. **Progestin-only pills or the "mini-pill"** can be used for those with contraindications to estrogen-containing formulations, but are more sensitive to timing, require daily use, and have no pill-free interval.
   (1) One pill per day. If using progestin-only pills, the recommendation is to take at the same time each day.
   (2) The first pill should be taken either on the day of the visit (quick start) or between the first and seventh day after the start of the menstrual period (most commonly Sunday).
   (3) Some pill packs have 28 pills, others have 21 pills. When the 28-day pack is empty, immediately start taking pills from a new pack. When the 21-day pack is empty, wait 1 week (7 days), then begin taking pills from a new pack.
   (4) If you vomit within 30 minutes of taking a pill, take another pill or use a backup method if you have sex during the next 7 days.
   (5) If you forget to take a pill, take it as soon as you remember, even if it means taking two pills in 1 day.
   (6) If you forget to take two or more pills, take two pills every day until you are back on schedule. Use a backup method (e.g., condoms) or do not have sex for 7 days.
   (7) If you miss two or more menstrual periods, go to a clinic for a pregnancy test.
   (8) If you feel nauseous on the pills, consider changing the time of day you take them.
e. **Transdermal (patch) contraceptive:** Contains estrogen and progestin, greater exposure to estrogen than with other methods, may have more estrogen-related side effects. May be less effective in women who weigh more than 90 kg.
   (1) Apply within 1–5 days after the onset of menses (first day is preferred) or quick start. Place on upper arm, upper back, abdomen or buttock but not over chest or breast area. Do not place on irritated skin. Wear only one patch at a time.
   (2) Replace weekly for 3 weeks. Allow 1 week without patch for menses, then restart cycle.
   (3) Rotate location of patch to avoid skin irritation.
   (4) If patch falls off, put on new patch as soon as possible and use a backup method of contraception.

f. **Vaginal ring**: Flexible latex-free ring that contains estrogen and progestin. May be used continuously (avoiding period week) by replacing with a new ring every 4 weeks (or the same day every month) to help reduce pelvic pain and dysmenorrhea. This method requires user comfort with insertion and removal. Screen for comfort with this method by asking if the adolescent is comfortable using tampons. Patient may experience increased vaginal discharge or irritation.
   (1) Place ring in vagina for 3 weeks.
   (2) Remove ring for 1 week for withdrawal bleeding.
   (3) Place new ring in vagina for 3 weeks.
   (4) If ring is expelled, rinse with water and reinsert; backup contraception is needed if ring is out for >3 hours.
g. **Barrier methods**: Require placement prior to sexual intercourse. Include cervical sponge, cervical cap, cervical shield, diaphragm (these methods are used in conjunction with spermicide), as well as female and male condoms.
h. **Fertility awareness-based methods of pregnancy prevention**: Involves following a woman's menstrual cycle to help prevent pregnancy. More information available at: http://irh.org/standard-days-method/

5. **Emergency contraception (EC)**[29]: Used to prevent pregnancy following unprotected sex. Use of oral emergency contraception will not disrupt an established pregnancy.
a. Methods:
   (1) Progestin only: Levonorgestrel 1.5 mg orally (PO) once (brand name "Plan B One Step" or "Next Choice" with older formulation). "Plan B" consisting of two 0.75-mg tablets that patients should be instructed to take together, regardless of packet instructions. Most efficacious within 72 hours of coitus but effective through 120 hours. Effectiveness decreases every 24 hours.
   (2) Selective progesterone receptor modulator: Ulipristal (UPA) (brand name "Ella"). 30 mg PO once. Equally effective for up to 120 hours.
   (3) Combined hormonal: Known as the "Yuzpe method," involves counseling patients to take two doses of OCPs, with each dose containing at least 100 mcg of ethinyl estradiol and at least 500 mcg of levonorgestrel (either 8 total tablets: 4 at a time, 12 hours apart, or for more precise instructions for a particular combination pill; refer to http://www.ecprinceton.edu). Most effective in first 72 hours. Consider prescribing an antiemetic, such as metoclopramide or meclizine, for use 1 hour before first dose.
   (4) Copper intrauterine device (IUD) may be inserted within 5 days of coitus.
b. Mechanism of action: Mixed hormonal or progestin-only methods work by interfering with or delaying ovulation and do not interfere with established pregnancy. UPA, likewise, works by delaying ovulation.

c. Guidelines and instructions for use:
   (1) Counseling about EC should be a routine part of anticipatory guidance for all female and male adolescents.
   (2) Levonorgestrel methods are available over the counter—no prescription necessary—however cost may be a barrier for OTC access. UPA requires a prescription regardless of patient age.
   (3) When prescribing EC, it is important to know which pharmacies stock EC. Advance prescriptions should be considered for all teens aged 16 and younger, regardless of current sexual activity.
   (4) EC should be taken as soon as possible; there is a linear relationship between efficacy and the time from intercourse to treatment. If patient experiences emesis within 3 hours of taking EC, another dose should be taken as soon as possible.
   (5) If using progestin or mixed hormonal EC, taking the EC dose should not be delayed for pregnancy test, given diminishing efficacy over time to dosing.
   (6) Discuss proper use of regular, reliable birth control for the future, especially for patients frequently using EC.
   (7) May be combined with other ongoing methods of birth control.
      (a) OCPs may be started immediately after progestin-only or combined hormonal EC dosing has been completed. DMPA may be given the same day.
      (b) Patient should abstain from sexual intercourse or use barrier contraception for 7 days (14 if using UPA) or until her next menses, whichever comes first.
   (8) No absolute limit of EC frequency during a cycle.
   (9) Perform pregnancy test if no menses within 3 weeks of progestin-only or combined hormonal methods, or if menses more than 1 week late with UPA.
   (10) Advise patients to schedule a primary care medical visit after EC usage (pregnancy test and appropriate STI testing or treatment).
d. Contraindications:
   (1) For progestin-only regimens: Pregnancy, given lack of efficacy with potential for side effects; no evidence of teratogenicity.
   (2) For UPA: Pregnancy, given potential for first-trimester fetal loss; no evidence of teratogenicity.
   (3) For estrogen-containing regimens: Same as those for OCPs, but use over time has shown that such stringent restrictions for single use are unnecessary. History of previous thrombosis is not a contraindication for single use, but progestin-only methods are preferred.

D. Follow-Up Recommendations:

Two or three follow-up visits per year to monitor patient compliance, blood pressure, side effects, and satisfaction with chosen birth control option.

V. MENTAL HEALTH

A. Anxiety and Depression

Please refer to Disorders of Mental Health, Chapter 9, Section VIII. Confidentiality regarding mental health issues in adolescents is extremely important, and should be maintained except for in life-threatening situations. The Patient Health Quesionnaire-2 (PHQ-2) is an important initial screening tool for depression, which elicits responses relevant to mood (feeling down, depressed, or hopeless) and anhedonia (little interest or pleasure in doing things). Patients who screen positive should then be screened with the PHQ-9 to determine if they meet criteria for a depressive disorder.[30]

B. Suicidal Ideation[31]

1. **Suicide is a leading cause of mortality among adolescents.** Risk factors include male sex, American Indian/Alaska Native racial background, bisexual or homosexual orientation, isolation or living alone, history of acute stressor or recent loss, family history of suicide, personal or family history of suicide attempt, personal or parental mental health problems, physical or sexual abuse, substance use, and firearms in the home (even if properly stored and secured).
2. **Screening questions for suicidal ideation are best asked after initial questioning regarding stressors, mood, and depressive symptoms.** Remember that irritability, vague or multiple somatic complaints, and behavioral problems may indicate depression in an adolescent.
3. **In addition to risk factors above,** assessment of suicidal risk should also include whether the adolescent has a plan, the potential lethality of the plan, access to means to carry out the plan, and whether the plan has ever been attempted.
4. **Any adolescent with risk factors and a suicide plan should be considered an imminent risk and not be allowed to leave the office.** Providers should contact local crisis support resources and undertake immediate consultation with a mental health professional; potential courses of action must be individualized but include same-day mental health appointment, transfer to a psychiatric emergency room, and psychiatric hospitalization.
5. **Any adolescent with risk factors but no suicide plan or preparation should be considered moderate risk.** He or she should be provided with an immediate plan for behavioral health treatment, information about emergency resources, and ideas for coping strategies.

C. School Problems

Please refer to Chapter 9 for more information on learning disabilities (Medical Evaluation of Developmental Disorders) and attention deficit hyperactivity disorder (ADHD).

> **BOX 5.2**
> **CRAFFT QUESTIONNAIRE**[32]
>
> **C**—Have you ever ridden in a **C**AR driven by someone (or yourself) who was "high" or had been using alcohol or drugs?
> **R**—Do you ever use alcohol or drugs to **R**ELAX, feel better about yourself, or fit in?
> **A**—Do you ever use alcohol/drugs while you are **A**LONE?
> **F**—Do your family or **F**RIENDS ever tell you that you should cut down on your drinking or drug use?
> **F**—Do you ever **F**ORGET things you did while using alcohol or drugs?
> **T**—Have you gotten into **T**ROUBLE while you were using alcohol or drugs?
> **NOTE:** Answering yes to two or more questions is a positive screen.

D. Substance Use[32]

1. **Spectrum of substance use behavior:** Ranges from experimentation to limited use to dependence.
2. **Drugs of abuse and acute toxidromes:** See Chapter 2.
3. **Screening, brief intervention, and referral to treatment**
   a. **S**ubstance use screening: Any alcohol, marijuana, other drugs in the past 12 months? If yes, administer full CRAFFT questionnaire (Box 5.2). If no, administer only "Car" question (Have you ever ridden in a car with a driver who had used alcohol or drugs?)
   b. **B**rief **I**ntervention: stratify risk based on responses to screening questions.
      (1) Low risk (abstinent): Reinforce decisions with praise and anticipatory guidance regarding riding in a car with a driver under the influence.
      (2) Yes to "Car" question: Counsel, encourage safety plan, consider Contract for Life (http://www.sadd.org/contract.htm).
      (3) Moderate risk (CRAFFT negative): Advise to stop using the substance, educate regarding health risks of continued use, praise personal attributes.
      (4) High risk (CRAFFT ≥ 2): Conduct in-depth assessment using motivational enhancement techniques, conduct brief negotiated interview, or refer as appropriate.
   c. **R**eferral to **T**reatment: Further evaluation by a specialist in mental health/addiction can guide referral to an appropriate level of care.
4. **Levels of care**
   a. Substance use treatment may be delivered in a variety of settings, ranging from outpatient therapy to partial hospital to inpatient or residential treatment.
   b. Considerations for detoxification: Medical management of symptoms of withdrawal, particularly pertinent to teens dependent on alcohol,

opioids, or benzodiazepines. **NOTE:** Detoxification is not equivalent to substance abuse treatment; once acute withdrawal symptoms have been managed, engage patient in a treatment program.

VI. TRANSITIONING ADOLESCENTS INTO ADULT CARE[33]

All adolescents, particularly those with special healthcare needs or chronic conditions, benefit from careful attention to the process of transitioning to adult care. Resources for how to approach and organize the transition process including guidance on transition readiness and planning are available at http://www.gottransition.org/.

REFERENCES

1. Kulin H, Muller J. The biological aspects of puberty. *Pediatr Rev.* 1996;17(3):75-86.
2. Bordini B, Rosenfield RL. Normal Pubertal Development: Part II: Clinical Aspects of Puberty. *Pediatr Rev.* 2011;32(7):281-292.
3. Joffe A. Introduction to adolescent medicine. In: McMillan JA, DeAngelis CD, Feigan RD, et al., eds. *Oski's Pediatrics: Principles and Practice*. 4th ed. Philadelphia: Lippincott Williams & Wilkins; 2006: 546-557.
4. Neinstein LS, et al. *Adolescent Health Care: A Practical Guide*. Philadelphia: Wolters Kluwer Health/Lippincott Williams & Wilkins; 2007.
5. Rosen D. Physiologic growth and development during adolescence. *Pediatr Rev.* 2004;25(6):194-200.
6. Alario AJ, Birnkrant JD. "Sexual Maturation and Tanner Staging." *Practical Guide To The Care Of The Pediatric Patient*. 2nd ed. St. Louis: Mosby; 2007:798-800. Print.
7. Muir A. Precocious puberty. *Pediatr Rev.* 2006;27(10):373-381.
8. Kaplowitz PB. Delayed puberty. *Pediatr Rev.* 2005;31(5):189-195.
9. Sanders RA. Adolescent psychosocial, social, and cognitive development. *Pediatr Rev.* 2013;34(8):354-359.
10. Goldenring JM, Rosen DS. Getting into adolescent heads: an essential update. *Contemp Pediatr.* 2004;21(1):64-90.
11. Fishman M, Bruner A, Adger H. Substance abuse among children and adolescents. *Pediatr Rev.* 1997;18(11):397-398.
12. Knight JR, Sherritt L, Shrier LA, et al. Validity of the CRAFFT substance abuse screening test among adolescent clinic patients. *Arch Pediatr Adolesc Med.* 2002;156:607-614.
13. American Academy of Pediatrics. Recommendations for Preventative Pediatric Health Care. Bright Future/American Academy of Pediatrics. Available at http://www.aap.org/en-us/presional-resources/practice-support/Periodicity/periodicity%20Schedule_FINAL.pdf. May 2015.
14. Frye S. Care of the student athlete. *Contemp Pediatrics.* 2015;32(8):30-35.
15. Marcell AV, et al. Male adolescent sexual and reproductive health care. *Pediatrics.* 2011;128(6):e1658-e1676.
16. Kaskowitz A, Quint E. A practical overview of managing adolescent gynecologic conditions in the pediatric office. *Pediatr Rev.* 2014;35(9):371-381.
17. American College of Obstetricians and Gynecologists. Well-woman visit. Committee Opinion No. 534. *Obstet Gynecol.* 2014;120:421-424.

18. Branson BM, Handsfield H, Lampe MA, et al. Revised recommendations for HIV testing of adults, adolescents, and pregnant women in health care settings. *MMWR Recomm Rep*. 2006;55:1-12.
19. Moyer VA & U.S. Preventive Services Task Force. Screening for HIV: U.S. Preventive Services Task Force recommendation statement. *Ann Intern Med*. 2013;159:51-60.
20. Committee on Pediatric AIDS, Emmanueal PJ, Martinez J. American Academy of Pediatrics. Adolescents and HIV infection: the pediatrician's role in promoting routine testing. *Pediatrics*. 2011;128(5):1023-1029.
21. Workowski KA, Bolan GA. Sexually transmitted diseases treatment guidelines, 2015. *MMWR Recomm Rep*. 2015;64(RR3):1-137.
22. Centers for Disease Control and Prevention. 2015 Sexually Transmitted Infection Guidelines: Emerging Issues. Available at http://www.cdc.gov/std/tg2015/emerging.htm.
23. American College of Obstetricians and Gynecologists. ACOG Committee Opinion No. 463: Cervical cancer in adolescents: screening, evaluation, and management. *Obstet Gynecol*. 2010;116:469-472.
24. American Diabetes Association. Consensus Statement: Type 2 diabetes in children and adolescents. *Diabetes Care*. 2000;23(3):381-389.
25. Frankowski BL. Committee on Adolescence. Sexual orientation and adolescents. *Pediatrics*. 2004;113(6):1827-1832.
26. Tulloch T, Kaufman M. Adolescent sexuality. *Pediatr Rev*. 2015;34(1):29-37.
27. Upadhya KK. Contraception for adolescents. *Pediatr Rev*. 2013;34(9):384-394.
28. Zurawin RK, Ayensu-Coker L. Innovations in contraception: a review. *Clin Obstet Gynecol*. 2007;50(2):425-439.
29. Committee on Adolescence. Emergency contraception. *Pediatrics*. 2012;130(6):1174-1182.
30. Arroll B, et al. Screening for depression in primary care with two verbally asked questions: cross sectional study. *BMJ*. 2003;327(7424):1144-1146.
31. Shain BM. Suicide and suicide attempts in adolescents. *Pediatrics*. 2007;120:669-676.
32. Committee on Substance Abuse. Substance use screening, brief intervention, and referral to treatment for pediatricians. *Pediatrics*. 2011;128(5):e1330-e1340.
33. American Academy of Pediatrics. Clinical Report—Supporting the health care transition from adolescence to adulthood in the medical home. *Pediatrics*. 2011;128(1):182-200.

Chapter 6
Analgesia and Procedural Sedation

Jessica Berger, MD, and Keri Borden Koszela, MD

See additional content on Expert Consult

I. WEB RESOURCES

- International Association for the Study of Pain: http://childpain.org/
- American Pain Society: http://www.ampainsoc.org/
- American Society of Anesthesiologists: http://www.asahq.org/

II. PAIN ASSESSMENT

A. Infant[1]

1. **Physiologic responses seen primarily in acute pain; subsides with continuing/chronic pain.** Characterized by oxygen desaturation, crying, diaphoresis, flushing or pallor, and increases in blood pressure, heart rate, and respiratory rate.
2. **Behavioral response** (Table 6.1):
a. Observe characteristics and duration of cry, facial expressions, visual tracking, body movements, and response to stimuli.
b. Neonatal Infant Pain Scale (NIPS): Behavioral assessment tool for the preterm neonate and full-term neonate up to 6 weeks after birth.
c. FLACC scale (Table 6.2): Measures and evaluates pain interventions by quantifying pain behaviors, including **F**acial expression, **L**eg movement, **A**ctivity, **C**ry, and **C**onsolability, with scores ranging from 0–10.[2] Revised FLACC scale is reliable in children with cognitive impairment.[3]

B. Preschooler

In addition to physiologic and behavioral responses, the **FACES** pain scale revised can be used to assess pain intensity in children as young as 3 years of age (Fig. 6.1).

C. School-Age and Adolescent

Evaluate physiologic and behavioral responses; ask about description, location, and character of pain. Starting at age 7, children can use the standard subjective pain rating scale, in which 0 is no pain and 10 is the worst pain ever experienced.

Chapter 6 Analgesia and Procedural Sedation

TABLE 6.1
DEVELOPMENTAL RESPONSES TO PAIN

Stage	Age	Response
Infant	<6 mo	No expression of anticipatory fear. Level of anxiety reflects that of the parent.
	6–18 mo	Anticipatory fear of painful experiences begins to develop.
Preschooler	18–24 mo	Verbalization. Children express pain with words such as "hurt" and "boo-boo."
	3 yr	Localization and identification of external causes. Children more reliably assess their pain but continue to depend on visual cues for localization and are unable to understand a reason for pain.
School-age child	5–7 yr	Cooperation. Children have improved understanding of pain and ability to localize it and cooperate.

Data from Yaster M, et al. Cognitive Development Aspects of Pain in School-Age Children. Pain In Infants, Children, and Adolescents. 1993;65-74.

TABLE 6.2
FLACC PAIN ASSESSMENT TOOL

FACE
0—No particular expression or smile
1—Occasional grimace or frown, withdrawn, disinterested
2—Frequent to constant frown, quivering chin, clenched jaw

LEGS
0—Normal position or relaxed
1—Uneasy, restless, tense
2—Kicking or legs drawn up

ACTIVITY
0—Lying quietly, normal position, moves easily
1—Squirming, shifting back and forth, tense
2—Arched, rigid, or jerking

CRY
0—No cry (awake or asleep)
1—Moans or whimpers, occasional complaint
2—Crying steadily, screams or sobs, frequent complaints

CONSOLABILITY
0—Content, relaxed
1—Reassured by occasional touching, hugging, or being talked to; distractible
2—Difficult to console or comfort

Modified from Manworren R, Hynan L. Clinical validation of FLACC: preverbal patient pain scale. Pediatr Nurs. 2003;29:140-146.

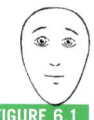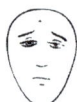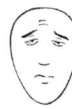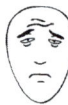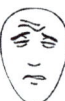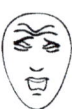

FIGURE 6.1

FACES pain scale revised. *(From Hicks CL, von Baeyer CL, Spafford PA, et al. The Faces Pain Scale-Revised: toward a common metric in pediatric pain measurement. Pain. 2001;93:173-183; with instructions and translations as found on http://www.usask.ca/childpain/fpsr/. This Faces Pain Scale-Revised has been reproduced with permission of the International Association for the Study of Pain (IASP). The figure may not be reproduced for any other purpose without permission.)*

III. ANALGESICS[1,4]

A. Safety

1. Due to the danger of acetaminophen toxicity when using combined opioid-acetaminophen products (such as hydrocodone-acetaminophen or oxycodone-acetaminophen), it is preferable to avoid combined products, and to prescribe opioids and acetaminophen separately.[5]
2. **Codeine is no longer recommended for use in children due to risk of overdose and unpredictable analgesic effects. As of 2013, the FDA issued a black-box warning for use of codeine after tonsillectomy and adenoidectomy (T&A).** Over-metabolism occurs in approximately 3%–5% of the population, and can potentially lead to catastrophic overdose, particularly in children for whom T&A is performed to manage a history of sleep apnea.[6] Approximately 10% of codeine is converted to morphine in the liver. Codeine has little to no analgesic effect in newborns and in the estimated 10% of the U.S. population in which hepatic conversion does not occur.[5]
3. **Meperidine is no longer recommended for use in children due to risk of neurotoxicity.** Meperidine is metabolized to normeperidine, a slowly eliminated active metabolite that can accumulate in the setting of renal dysfunction or multiple doses leading to neurotoxic adverse effects, including agitation, tremors, myoclonus, and seizures.[7] It also has catastrophic interactions with MAO inhibitors.
4. **Tramadol** is an opioid pain reliever (with additional effects on multiple nonopioid receptors). Similar to **codeine**, tramadol may be over-metabolized in some children to O-desmethyltramadol, an active opiate metabolite, with potentially fatal respiratory depression. Use of the drug in children is considered off-label at this time.[8]

B. Nonopioid Analgesics

Weak analgesics with antipyretic activity are commonly used to manage mild to moderate pain of nonvisceral origin. Nonopioid analgesics can be administered alone or in combination with opiates. Drugs, routes of administration, and specific comments are as follows:

1. **Acetaminophen [by mouth (PO)/per rectum (PR)/intravenous (IV)]:** Weak analgesic with no anti-inflammatory activity, no platelet inhibition, or

gastrointestinal (GI) irritation. Hepatotoxicity can occur with high doses.
2. **Aspirin (PO/PR):** Associated with platelet inhibition and GI irritation. Avoid in pediatrics, owing to risk of Reye syndrome.
3. **Choline magnesium trisalicylate (PO):** No platelet inhibition. Also associated with Reye syndrome.
4. **Nonsteroidal anti-inflammatory drugs (NSAIDs):** Ibuprofen (PO/IV), ketorolac [IV/intramuscular (IM)/PO/intranasal (IN)], naproxen (PO), diclofenac (PO/IV), and celecoxib (PO).
    a. Especially useful for sickle cell, bony, rheumatic, and inflammatory pain.
    b. Associated with GI symptoms (epigastric pain, gastritis, GI bleeding). Concurrent histamine-2-receptor blocker is recommended with prolonged use. The selective cyclooxygenase-2 (COX-2) inhibitor, celecoxib is associated with fewer GI symptoms than nonselective NSAIDs.[9]
    c. Other adverse effects include interference with platelet aggregation, bronchoconstriction, hypersensitivity reactions, and azotemia. May interfere with bone healing. Should be avoided in patients with severe renal disease, dehydration, or heart failure.
    NOTE: Ketorolac is a potent analgesic (0.5 mg/kg IV is equivalent to 0.05 mg/kg morphine).
    See the quick reference to analgesic drugs in Table EC 6.A on Expert Consult.

C. Opioids (Table 6.3)

1. **Produce analgesia by binding to mu receptors in the brain and spinal cord.**
2. **Most flexible and widely used analgesics for moderate and severe pain.**
3. **Side effects:** Pruritus, nausea, vomiting, constipation, urine retention, and (rarely) respiratory depression and hypotension.
4. **Morphine:** Gold standard in this drug class.
5. Long-acting opioids (methadone, extended-release tablets and patches) are not recommended for acute pain.
6. Although opioids are essential for the treatment of moderate to severe pain, we recommend caution in the quantity that is dispensed. It is safest to dispense no more than is needed, and usually no more than a 5–7 day supply.

D. Local Anesthetics[4,10,11,12]

Administered topically or subcutaneously into peripheral nerves (e.g., digital nerve, penile nerve block) or centrally (epidural/spinal). They act by temporarily blocking nerve conduction at the sodium channel.
1. **For all local anesthetics, 1% solution = 10 mg/mL**
2. **Topical local anesthetics** (Table 6.4)[13]

TABLE 6.3
COMMONLY USED OPIATES

Drug	Route; Equi-analgesic Doses (mg/kg/dose)*	Onset (min)	Duration (hr)	Side Effects	Comments
Fentanyl	IV: 0.001 Transdermal: 0.001 Transmucosal: 0.01	1–2 12 15	0.5–1 2–3	• Pruritus • Bradycardia • Chest wall rigidity with doses >5 mcg/kg (but can occur at all doses); treat with naloxone or neuromuscular blockade	Rarely causes cardiovascular instability (relatively safer in hypovolemia, congenital heart disease, or head trauma). Respiratory depressant effect much longer (4 hr) than analgesic effect. Levels of unbound drug are higher in newborns. Most commonly used opioid for short, painful procedures, but transdermal route is more effective in chronic pain situations.
Hydromorphone	IV/SQ: 0.015 PO: 0.02–0.1	5–10 30–60	3–4		Less sedation, nausea, and pruritus than morphine.
Methadone	IV: 0.1 PO: 0.1	5–10 30–60	4–24 4–24		Initial dose may produce analgesia for 3–4 hr; duration of action is increased with repeated dosing. Useful for neuropathic pain and opioid weaning due to unique mechanism of NMDA blockade.
Morphine	IV: 0.1 IM/SQ: 0.1–0.2 PO: 0.3–0.5	5–10 10–30 30–60	3–4 4–5 4–5	• Seizures in neonates • Can cause significant histamine release	The gold standard against which all other opioids are compared. Available in sustained-release form for chronic pain.
Oxycodone	PO: 0.1	30–60	3–4		Available in sustained-release form for chronic pain. Much less nauseating than codeine.

*NOTE: For larger patients approaching adult sizes, see formulary for adult dosing.

IM, Intramuscular; IV, intravenous; PO, by mouth; SQ, subcutaneous

Data from Yaster M, Cote C, Krane E, et al. Pediatric Pain Management and Sedation Handbook. St Louis: Mosby; 1997:29-50; FDA Drug Safety Communication: Safety review update of codeine use in children; new Boxed Warning and Contraindication on use after tonsillectomy and/or adenoidectomy. 02-2013. http://www.fda.gov/Drugs/DrugSafety/ucm339112.htm; Jenco M. FDA issues warning on tramadol use in those under age 17. AAP News. 22 Sept 2015.

TABLE 6.4
COMMONLY USED TOPICAL LOCAL ANESTHETICS

	Components	Indications	Peak Effect	Duration*	Cautions†
EMLA	Lidocaine 2.5% Prilocaine 2.5%	Intact skin only Venipuncture, circumcision, LP, abscess drainage, BMA	60 min	90 min	Methemoglobinemia: not for use in patients predisposed to methemoglobinemia (e.g., G6PD deficiency, some medications) Infants <3 mo of age: use sparingly (up to 1 g is safe)
LMX	Lidocaine 4%	Same as EMLA	30 min	60 min	Same as EMLA
LET	Lidocaine 4% Epinephrine 0.1% Tetracaine 0.5% Can be mixed with cellulose to create a gel	Safe for nonintact skin Lacerations Not for use in contaminated wounds	30 min	45 min	Vasoconstriction: contraindicated in areas supplied by end arteries (e.g., pinna, nose, penis, digits) Avoid contact with mucous membranes
Viscous lidocaine	Lidocaine 2% May be mixed with Maalox and Benadryl elixir in a 1:1:1 ratio for palatability	Safe for nonintact skin Mucous membranes (e.g., urethral catheter placement, mucositis)	10 min	30 min	Overuse can lead to life-threatening toxicity Not to be used for teething

*Approximate
†Maximum lidocaine dose is 5 mg/kg.
BMA, Bone marrow aspiration; EMLA, eutectic mixture of local anesthetics; G6PD, glucose-6-phosphate dehydrogenase; LP, lumbar puncture
Data from Krauss B, Green SM. Sedation and analgesia for procedures in children. N Engl J Med. 2000;342:938–945; Zempsky W, Cravero J. Relief of pain and anxiety in pediatric patients in emergency medical systems. Pediatrics. 2004;114:1348-1356.

TABLE 6.5
COMMONLY USED INJECTABLE LOCAL ANESTHETICS[1,10]

Agent	Concentration (%)(1% solution = 10 mg/mL)	Max dose (mg/kg)	Onset (min)	Duration (hr)
Lidocaine	0.5–2	5	3	0.5–2
Lidocaine with epinephrine	0.5–2	7	3	1–3
Bupivicaine	0.25–0.75	2.5	15	2–4
Bupivicaine with epinephrine	0.25–0.75	3	15	4–8

NOTE: Max volume = (max mg/kg × weight in kg)/(% solution × 10)
Data from St Germain Brent A. The management of pain in the emergency department. Pediatr Clin North Am. 2000;47:651-679; Yaster M, Cote C, Krane E, et al. Pediatric Pain Management and Sedation Handbook. St Louis: Mosby; 1997:51-72.

3. **Injectable local anesthetics** (Table 6.5):
  a. Infiltration of the skin at the site: Used for painful procedures such as wound closure, IV line placement, or lumbar puncture.
  b. To reduce stinging from injection, use a small needle (27- to 30-gauge). Alkalinize anesthetic: Add 1 mL (1 mEq) sodium bicarbonate to 9 mL lidocaine (or 29 mL bupivacaine), use lowest concentration of anesthetic available, warm solution (between 37° and 42° C), inject anesthetic slowly, and rub skin at injection site first.
  c. To enhance efficacy and duration, add epinephrine to decrease vascular uptake. **Never use local anesthetics with epinephrine in areas supplied by end arteries (e.g., pinna, digits, nasal tip, penis).**
  d. Toxicity: Central nervous system (CNS) and cardiac toxicity are of greatest concern. CNS symptoms are seen before cardiovascular collapse. Progression of symptoms: Perioral numbness, dizziness, auditory disturbances, muscular twitching, unconsciousness, seizures, coma, respiratory arrest, cardiovascular collapse. It is important to calculate the volume limit of the local anesthetic and always draw up less than the maximum volume (see Formulary for maximum doses). Lipid emulsion therapy and possibly cardiopulmonary bypass may be required for systemic toxicity. If concerned for systemic toxicity, please contact an anesthesiologist and/or call poison control at 1-800-222-1222.

NOTE: Bupivicaine is associated with more severe cardiac toxicity than lidocaine.

E. NONPHARMACOLOGIC MEASURES OF PAIN RELIEF[14,15]

1. **Sucrose for neonates (Sweet Ease):**
  a. Indications: Procedures such as heel sticks, immunizations, venipuncture, IV line insertion, arterial puncture, insertion of a Foley catheter, and lumbar puncture in neonates and infants. Strongest evidence exists for infants aged 0–1 month,[14] but more recent evidence suggests efficacy up to 12 months.[15]

b. Procedure: administer up to 2 mL of 24% sucrose into the infant's mouth by syringe or from a nipple/pacifier ~ 2 minutes before procedure.
   NOTE: Effective doses in very low-birth-weight infants may be as low as 0.05–0.1 mL of 24% sucrose, and in term neonates may be as high as 2 mL of 24% sucrose.
c. May be given for more than one procedure within a relatively short period of time but should not be administered more than twice in 1 hour.
   NOTE: Studies have suggested potential adverse neurocognitive effects with many repeated doses.[15]
d. Effectiveness has been most often studied with adjunctive pacifier/nipple and parental holding, which may contribute to stress/pain alleviation.
e. Avoid use if patient is under nothing by mouth (NPO) restrictions.
2. **Parental presence.**
3. **Distraction with toys.**
4. **Child life specialists strongly encouraged.**

IV. PATIENT-CONTROLLED ANALGESIA

A. Definition

Patient-controlled analgesia (PCA) is a device that enables a patient to receive continuous (basal) opioids and/or self-administer small supplemental doses (bolus) of analgesics on an as-needed basis. In children younger than 6 years (or physically/mentally handicapped), a family member, caregiver, or nurse may administer doses (i.e., surrogate PCA, PCA by proxy, or parent/nurse-controlled analgesia).

B. Indications

Moderate to severe pain of acute or chronic nature. Commonly used in sickle cell disease, post-surgery, post-trauma, burns, and cancer. Also for preemptive pain management (e.g., to facilitate dressing changes).

C. Routes of Administration

IV, SQ, or epidural

D. Agents (Table 6.6)

TABLE 6.6
ORDERS FOR PATIENT-CONTROLLED ANALGESIA

Drug	Basal Rate (mcg/kg/hr)	Bolus Dose (mcg/kg)	Lockout Period (min)	Boluses (hr)	Max Dose (mcg/kg/hr)
Morphine	10–30	10–30	6–10	4–6	100–150
Hydromorphone	3–5	3–5	6–10	4–6	15–20
Fentanyl	0.5–1	0.5–10	6–10	2–3	2–4

Data from Yaster M, Cote C, Krane E, et al. Pediatric Pain Management and Sedation Handbook. St Louis: Mosby; 1997:100.

E. Adjuvants

1. Low-dose naloxone (Narcan) infusion (1 mcg/kg/hr) reduces incidence of pruritus and nausea.
2. Low-dose ketamine infusion (0.1 mg/kg/hr) helpful in oncology mucositis, visceral pain, and neuropathic pain due to mechanism of NMDA blockade. May be used with or as an alternative to methadone.

F. Complications

1. **Pruritus, nausea, constipation, urine retention, excessive drowsiness, and respiratory depression.**

V. OPIOID TAPERING[4]

A. Indications

Because of the development of dependence and the potential for withdrawal, a tapering schedule is required if the patient has received frequent opioid analgesics for >5–10 days.

B. Withdrawal

1. **See Box 18.1 for symptoms of opioid withdrawal.**
2. **Onset of signs and symptoms:** 6–12 hours after the last dose of morphine and 36–48 hours after the last dose of methadone.
3. **Duration:** 7–14 days, with a peak intensity reached within 2–4 days.

C. Guidelines

1. **Conversion:** All drugs should be converted to a single equi-analgesic member of that group (Table 6.7).
2. **PCA wean:** Drug dosing should be changed from continuous/intermittent IV infusion to PO bolus therapy around the clock. If the patient is on PCA, the first PO dose should be administered, then the basal infusion should be stopped 30–60 minutes later.

TABLE 6.7
RELATIVE POTENCIES AND EQUIVALENCE OF OPIOIDS

Drug	Morphine Equivalence Ratio	IV Dose (mg/kg)	Equivalent PO Dose (mg/kg)
Methadone	0.25–1*	0.1	0.1
Morphine	1	0.1	0.3–0.5
Hydromorphone	5–7	0.015	0.02–0.1
Fentanyl	80–100	0.001	NA

NOTE: Removing a transdermal fentanyl patch does not stop opioid uptake from the skin; fentanyl will continue to be absorbed for 12–24 hr after patch removal (fentanyl 25-mcg patch administers 25 mcg/hr of fentanyl).
*Morphine-to-methadone conversion in the tolerant/dependent patient is variable. We recommend starting at the lowest conversion ratio, 0.25.
IV, intravenous; NA, not applicable; PO, by mouth
From Yaster M, Cote C, Krane E, et al. Pediatric Pain Management and Sedation Handbook. St Louis: Mosby; 1997:40.

Bolus doses should be retained, but reduced by 25%–50%. PCA should be discontinued if no boluses are required in the next 6 hours. If the patient continues to experience pain, considering increasing PO dose or adding adjuvant analgesic (e.g., NSAID).
3. **Slow dose decrease:** During an intermittent IV/PO wean, the total daily dose should be decreased by 10%–20% of the original dose every 1–2 days (e.g., to taper a morphine dose of 40 mg/day, decrease the daily dose by 4–8 mg every 1–2 days).
4. **Oral regimen:** If not done previously, IV dosing should be converted to equivalent PO administration 1–2 days before discharge, and titration should be continued as outlined previously.
5. **Adjunctive therapy:** α_2-Agonists (e.g., clonidine, dexmedetomidine).
a. Clonidine in combination with an opioid has been shown to decrease the length of time needed for opioid weaning in neonatal abstinence syndrome, with few short-term side effects. Long-term safety has yet to be thoroughly investigated.[16]
b. Limited data exist evaluating the use of oral clonidine in iatrogenic opioid abstinence syndrome in critically ill patients, but both transdermal clonidine and dexmedetomidine have shown promise.[17]
c. Several studies have examined the use of clonidine in treating opioid dependence, but insufficient data exist to support its routine use outside of the neonatal setting.[18]

D. Examples (Box 6.1)

VI. PROCEDURAL SEDATION[1,4,10,11,12,19]

A. Definitions

1. **Mild sedation (anxiolysis):** Intent is anxiolysis with maintenance of consciousness. Practically, obtained when a single drug is given once at a low dose. Mild sedation can easily progress to deep sedation and general anesthesia.
2. **Moderate sedation:** Formerly known as *conscious sedation*, i.e., a controlled state of depressed consciousness during which airway reflexes and airway patency are maintained. Patient responds appropriately to age-appropriate commands (e.g., "Open your eyes") and light touch. Practically, obtained any time a combination of a sedative-hypnotic and an analgesic is used. Moderate sedation can easily progress to deep sedation and general anesthesia.
3. **Deep sedation:** A controlled state of depressed consciousness during which airway reflexes and airway patency may not be maintained, and the child is unable to respond to physical or verbal stimuli. In practice, deep sedation is required for most painful procedures in children. The following IV drugs always produce deep sedation: propofol, etomidate, thiopental, and methohexital. Deep sedation can progress to general anesthesia.

> **BOX 6.1**
>
> **EXAMPLES OF OPIOID TAPERING**
>
> **Example 1**
>
> Patient on morphine patient-controlled analgesia (PCA) to be converted to oral (PO) morphine with home weaning.
> For example: morphine PCA basal rate = 2 mg/hr, average bolus rate = 0.5 mg/hr
> Step 1: Calculate daily dose: basal + bolus = (2 mg/hr × 24 hr) + (0.5 mg/hr × 24 hr) = 60 mg intravenous (IV) morphine
> Step 2: Convert according to drug potency: morphine IV/morphine oral = approx. 3:1 potency; 3 × 60 mg = 180 mg PO morphine
> Step 3: Prescribe 90 mg BID or 60 mg TID; wean 10%–20% of original dose (30 mg) every 1–2 days
>
> **Example 2**
>
> Patient on morphine PCA to be converted to transdermal fentanyl. Morphine PCA basal rate = 2 mg/hr. No boluses.
> Step 1: Convert according to drug potency: fentanyl/morphine = approx. 100:1 potency; 2 mg/hr morphine = 2000 mcg/hr morphine = 20 mcg/hr fentanyl
> Step 2: Prescribe 25-mcg fentanyl patch (delivers 25 mcg/hr fentanyl)
> Step 3: Stop IV morphine 8 hr after patch is applied; prescribe second patch at 72 hr
> Step 4: Prescribe as-needed (PRN) IV morphine with caution

Data from Yaster M, Cote C, Krane E, et al. Pediatric Pain Management and Sedation Handbook. St Louis: Mosby; 1997:29-50.

4. **Dissociative sedation:** Unique state of sedation achieved with ketamine. Deep level of depressed consciousness; however, airway reflexes and patency are generally maintained.

See the Quick Reference to Sedative-Hypnotic Drugs in Table EC 6.A.

B. Preparation

1. The patient should be **NPO** for solids and clear liquids[20] (Table 6.8 shows current American Society of Anesthesiologists recommendations).
   See Fig. EC 6.A on Expert Consult for more information on fasting recommendations.
2. **Written informed consent**
3. **Focused patient history:**
   a. Allergies and medications.
   b. Airway (asthma, acute respiratory disease, reactive airway disease), airway obstruction (mediastinal mass, history of noisy breathing, obstructive sleep apnea), craniofacial abnormalities (e.g., Pfeiffer, Crouzon, Apert, Pierre Robin syndromes), and recent upper respiratory infection (URI), which suggests increased risk of

TABLE 6.8
FASTING RECOMMENDATIONS FOR ANESTHESIA

Food Type	Minimum Fasting Period (hr)
Clear liquids	2
Breast milk	4
Nonhuman milk, formula	6
Solids	8

Data from Practice guidelines for preoperative fasting and the use of pharmacologic agents to reduce the risk of pulmonary aspiration: application to healthy patients undergoing elective procedures. A report by the American Society of Anesthesiologists Task Force on Preoperative Fasting and Use of Pharmacological Agents to Reduce the Risk of Pulmonary Aspiration (Online). http://anesthesiology.pubs.asahq.org/article.aspx?articleid=1933410

laryngospasm. Of note, there is no formal recommendation as to whether surgery should be cancelled in the setting of a viral illness, nor is there a consensus as to when it may be safe to reschedule after a URI. Many anesthesiologists recommend waiting 1–2 weeks, although others may wait as long as 4–6 weeks.[21]

c. Aspiration risk (neuromuscular disease, esophageal disease, altered mental status, obesity, and pregnancy)
d. Prematurity, comorbidities, and adverse reactions to sedatives and anesthesia

4. **Physical examination:** With specific attention to head, ears, eyes, nose, and throat (HEENT), lungs, cardiac examination, and neuromuscular function. Assess ability to open mouth and extend neck. If risk for moderate sedation is too high, an anesthesia consultation and general anesthesia should be considered. See Fig. EC 6.B on Expert Consult for the Mallampati classification system, which is used to assess the airway for the likelihood of difficult direct laryngoscopy and intubation.
5. **Determine American Society of Anesthesiologists Physical Status Classification:** See Table EC 6.B on Expert Consult. Class I and II patients are generally good candidates for mild, moderate, or deep sedation outside of the operating room.[20]
6. **Have an emergency plan ready:** Make sure qualified backup personnel and equipment are close by.
7. **Personnel:** Two providers are required. One provider should perform the procedure, and a separate provider should monitor the patient during sedation and recovery.
8. **Ensure IV access**.
9. **Have airway/intubation equipment available** (see Chapter 1).
10. **Medications to have available:** Those for rapid sequence intubation (see Chapter 1) or emergencies (e.g., epinephrine, atropine).
11. **Antagonist *(reversal)* agents** should be readily available (e.g., naloxone, flumazenil).

C. Monitoring

1. **Vital signs:** Baseline vital signs (including pulse oximetry) should be obtained. Heart rate, oxygen saturation, and respiratory rate should be continuously monitored, and blood pressure monitored intermittently. Vital signs should be recorded at least every 5 minutes until the patient returns to the pre-sedation level of consciousness.

NOTE: Complications most often occur 5–10 minutes after administration of IV medication and immediately after a procedure is completed (when the stimuli associated with the procedure are removed).[12]

NOTE: Pulse oximetry measures oxygen saturation not ventilation. Desaturation occurs within 1–2 minutes of apnea and may not occur for several minutes if supplemental oxygen is being administred by any route (e.g. nasal cannula, blow by, or face mask). Impedance plethysmography may fail to detect airway obstruction.[22]

2. **Airway:** Airway patency and adequacy of ventilation should be frequently assessed through capnography, auscultation, or direct visualization.

D. Pharmacologic Agents

1. **Goal of sedation:** To tailor drug combinations to provide levels of analgesia, sedation-hypnosis, and anxiolysis that are deep enough to facilitate the procedure but shallow enough to avoid loss of airway reflexes.
2. **CNS, cardiovascular, and respiratory depression** are potentiated by combining sedative drugs and/or opioids and by rapid drug infusion. Titration to the desired effect should be performed.
3. **Common sedative/hypnotic agents (Box 6.2).** Also see Tables 6.3 and 6.9 for more information on opiates and barbiturates/benzodiazepines.
4. Reversal agents:
a. Naloxone: Opioid antagonist. See Box 6.3 for Narcan administration protocol.
b. Flumazenil: Benzodiazepine antagonist. See Formulary for dosing details.

E. Discharge Criteria[12]

1. **Airway is patent and cardiovascular function is stable.**
2. **Easy arousability; intact protective reflexes (swallow and cough, gag reflex).**
3. **Ability to talk and sit up unaided** (if age appropriate).
4. **Alternatively, for very young or intellectually disabled children**, goal is to return as close as possible to pre-sedation level of responsiveness.
5. **Adequate hydration.**
6. **Recovery after sedation protocols** varies but typically ranges from 60–120 minutes.

F. Examples of Sedation Protocols (Tables 6.10 and 6.11)

Text continued on p. 154

BOX 6.2
PROPERTIES OF COMMON SEDATIVE-HYPNOTIC AGENTS

Sedating Antihistamines (Diphenhydramine, Hydroxyzine)

- Mild sedative-hypnotics with antiemetic and antipruritic properties; used for sedation and treatment of opiate side effects
- No anxiolytic or analgesic effects

Barbiturates

- Contraindicated in patients with porphyria; suitable only for nonpainful procedures
- No anxiolytic or analgesic effects

Benzodiazepines

- Reversible with flumazenil
- + Anxiolytic effects; no analgesic effects

Opioids

- Reversible with naloxone
- + Analgesic effects; no anxiolytic effects

Ketamine[1,10-13]

- Phencyclidine derivative that causes potent dissociative anesthesia, analgesia, and amnesia
- Nystagmus indicates likely therapeutic effect
- Vocalizations/movement may occur even with adequate sedation
- Results in "dissociative sedation" by any route
- Onset: IV, 0.5–2 min; IM, 5–10 min; PO/PR, 20–45 min
- Duration: IV, 20–60 min; IM, 30–90 min; PO/PR, 60–120+ min
- ***CNS effects:*** Increased ICP, emergence delirium with auditory, visual, and tactile hallucinations
- ***Cardiovascular effects:*** Inhibits catecholamine reuptake, causing increased HR, BP, SVR, PVR, direct myocardial depression
- ***Respiratory effects:*** Bronchodilation (useful in asthmatics), increased secretions (can result in laryngospasm), maintenance of ventilatory response to hypoxia, relative maintenance of airway reflexes
- ***Other effects:*** Increased muscle tone, myoclonic jerks, increased IOP, nausea, emesis
- ***Contraindications:*** Increased ICP, increased IOP, hypertension, preexisting psychotic disorders

Propofol

- For the purpose of deep sedation or general anesthesia, give 0.5–1 mg/kg IV bolus, followed by 50–100 mcg/kg/min infusion
- Rapid onset and brief recovery (5–15 min), antiemetic and euphoric
- Caution: Respiratory depression, apnea, hypotension
- + Anxiolytic. No analgesic effects

Continued

> **BOX 6.2**
> **PROPERTIES OF COMMON SEDATIVE-HYPNOTIC AGENTS—cont'd**
>
> **Dexmedetomidine***
>
> - Give 0.5–2 mcg/kg IV load over 10 min, followed by 0.2–1 mcg/kg/hr infusion.
> - Extremely rapid onset and brief recovery (5–15 min).
> - Does not cause respiratory depression or apnea.
> - + Anxiolytic and analgesic effects.
> - Dexmedetomidine can also be given intranasally (1–2 mcg/kg). It will take 30–60 min to attain natural sleep, and patients will briefly awaken with stimulation. Can cause hypotension and bradycardia. Increased cost compared with other medications.
>
> **Dexmedetomidine and Ketamine**
>
> - Most effective regimen appears to be use of bolus dose of both agents, dexmedetomidine (1 mcg/kg) and ketamine (1–2 mg/kg), to initiate sedation.
> - This can then be followed by a dexmedetomidine infusion (1–2 mcg/kg/hr) with supplemental bolus doses of ketamine (0.5–1 mg/kg) as needed.
>
> **Nitrous Oxide**
>
> - Inhaled, pleasant-smelling gas delivered as a mixture with oxygen.
> - +Amnestic, anxiolytic, and analgesic effects.
> - Extremely rapid onset and recovery.
> - Efficacy similar to midazolam for minor procedures such as venipuncture, intravenous catheter placement, laceration repair, or lumbar puncture.[23]
> - Due to risk for delivery of hypoxic gas mixture, avoid concentrations higher than 70% (30% oxygen).
> - Must be given in combination with other sedative drugs for more painful procedures.

*These examples reflect commonly used current protocols at the Johns Hopkins Children's Center; variations are found at other institutions. See Formulary for dosing recommendations.

BP, Blood pressure; CNS, central nervous system; HR, heart rate; ICP, intracranial pressure; IM, intramuscular; IOP, intraocular pressure; IV, intravenous; PO, oral; PR, rectal; PVR, pulmonary vascular resistance; SVR, systemic vascular resistance

Data from Yaster M, Cote C, Krane E, et al. Pediatric Pain Management and Sedation Handbook. *St Louis: Mosby; 1997:376-382;* St Germain Brent A. The management of pain in the emergency department. Pediatr Clin North Am. 2000;47:651-679; and Cote CJ, Lerman J, Todres ID, et al. A Practice of Anesthesia for Infants and Children. *Philadelphia: WB Saunders, 2001.*

TABLE 6.9
COMMONLY USED BENZODIAZEPINES* AND BARBITURATES[1,5,14]

Drug Class	Duration of Action	Drug	Route	Onset (min)	Duration (hr)	Comments
Benzodiazepines	Short	Midazolam (Versed)	IV IM/IN PO/PR	1–3 5–10 10–30	1–2	• Has rapid and predictable onset of action, short recovery time • Causes amnesia • Results in mild depression of hypoxic ventilatory drive
	Intermediate	Diazepam (Valium)	IV (painful) PR PO	1–3 7–15 30–60	0.25–1 2–3 2–3	• Poor choice for procedural sedation • Excellent for muscle relaxation or prolonged sedation • Painful on IV injection • Faster onset than midazolam
	Long	Lorazepam (Ativan)	IV IM PO	1–5 10–20 30–60	3–4 3–6 3–6	• Poor choice for procedural sedation • Ideal for prolonged anxiolysis, seizure treatment
Barbiturates	Short	Methohexital	PR[†]	5–10	1–1.5	• PR form used as sedative for nonpainful procedures
	Intermediate	Pentobarbital	IV IM PO/PR	1–10 5–15 15–60	1–4 2–4 2–4	• Predictable sedation and immobility for nonpainful procedures • Minimal respiratory depression when used alone • Associated with slow wake up and agitation

*Use IV solution for PO, PR, and IN administration. Rectal diazepam gel (Diastat) is also available.

[†]IV administration produces general anesthesia; only PR should be used for sedation.

IM, Intramuscular; IN, intranasal; IV, intravenous; PO, by mouth; PR, per rectum

Data from Yaster M, Cote C, Krane E, et al. Pediatric Pain Management and Sedation Handbook. St Louis: Mosby, 1997:345-374; St Germain Brent A. The management of pain in the emergency department. Pediatr Clin North Am. 2000;47:651-679; and Cote CJ, Lerman J, Todres ID, et al. A Practice of Anesthesia for Infants and Children. Philadelphia: WB Saunders; 2001.

BOX 6.3
NALOXONE (NARCAN) ADMINISTRATION*

Indications: Patients Requiring Naloxone (Narcan) Usually Meet All of the Following Criteria

- Unresponsive to physical stimulation
- Shallow respirations or respiratory rate <8 breaths/min[†]
- Pinpoint pupils

Procedure

1. **Stop opioid administration** (as well as other sedative drugs), start the **ABCs** (**A**irway, **B**reathing, **C**irculation), and call for **HELP**.
2. **Dilute naloxone:**
   a. If child >40 kg: Mix 0.4 mg (1 ampule) of naloxone with 9 mL of normal saline (final concentration 0.04 mg/mL = 40 mcg/mL)
   b. If child < 40 kg, dilute 0.1 mg (one-fourth ampule) in 9 mL of normal saline to make 0.01 mg/mL solution = 10 mcg/mL
3. **Administer and observe response:** Administer dilute naloxone *slowly* (1–2 mcg/kg/dose IV over 2 min). Observe patient response.
4. **Titrate to effect:** Within 1–2 min, patient should open eyes and respond. If not, continue until a total dose of 10 mcg/kg is given. If no response is obtained, evaluate for other cause of sedation/respiratory depression.
5. **Discontinue naloxone administration:** Discontinue naloxone as soon as patient responds (e.g., takes deep breaths when directed).
6. **Caution:** Another dose of naloxone may be required within 30 min of first dose (duration of action of naloxone is shorter than that of most opioids).
7. **Monitor patient:** Assign a staff member to monitor sedation/respiratory status and remind patient to take deep breaths as necessary.
8. **Alternative analgesia:** Provide nonopioids for pain relief. Resume opioid administration at half the original dose when the patient is easily aroused and respiratory rate is >9 breaths/min.

*Naloxone administration for patients being treated for pain. Higher doses may be necessary for patients found in the community or those with signs of cardiopulmonary failure. Please see formulary for additional dosing.
[†]Respiratory rates that require naloxone vary according to infant's/child's usual rate.
Modified from McCaffery M, Pasero C. Pain: Clinical Manual. St Louis: Mosby, 1999:269-270.

TABLE 6.10

EXAMPLES OF SEDATION PROTOCOLS*

Protocol/Doses	Comments
Ketamine (1 mg/kg/dose IV × 1–3 doses)	Lowest rates of adverse events when ketamine used alone[‡]
Ketamine + midazolam + atropine ("ketazolam") **IV route:** Ketamine 1 mg/kg/dose × 1–3 doses Midazolam 0.05 mg/kg × 1 dose Atropine 0.02 mg/kg × 1 dose **IM route:** combine (use smallest volume possible) Ketamine 1.5–2 mg/kg Midazolam 0.15–0.2 mg/kg Atropine 0.02 mg/kg	Atropine = antisialagogue Midazolam = counter emergence delirium
Midazolam + fentanyl Midazolam 0.1 mg/kg IV × 3 doses PRN Fentanyl 1 mcg/kg IV × 3 doses PRN	High likelihood of respiratory depression Infuse fentanyl no more frequently than Q3 min

*These examples reflect commonly used current protocols at the Johns Hopkins Children's Center; variations are found at other institutions.
[‡]Green, SM, Roback MG, Krauss B, et al. Predictors of emesis and recovery agitation with emergency department ketamine sedation: an individual-patient data meta-analysis of 8,282 children. *Ann Emerg Med.* 2009;54:171-180.
Modified from Yaster M, Cote C, Krane E, et al. Pediatric Pain Management and Sedation Handbook. *St Louis: Mosby; 1997.*

TABLE 6.11

SUGGESTED ANALGESIA AND SEDATION PROTOCOLS

Pain Threshold	Procedure	Suggested Choices
Nonpainful	CT/MRI/EEG/ECHO	Midazolam*
Mild	Phlebotomy/IV	EMLA
	LP	EMLA (± midazolam)
	Pelvic exam	Midazolam
	Minor laceration, well vascularized	LET
	Minor laceration, not well vascularized	Lidocaine
Moderate	BM aspiration	EMLA (± midazolam)
	Arthrocentesis	Lidocaine (local) for cooperative child or ketamine[†] for uncooperative child
	Fracture reduction	Ketamine
	Major laceration	Ketamine or fentanyl + midazolam
	Burn debridement	Ketamine or fentanyl + midazolam
	Long procedures (>30 min)	Consider general anesthesia
Severe	Fracture reduction	Ketamine
	Long procedures (>30 min)	Consider general anesthesia

*Caution for antiepileptics for EEG.
[†]Ketamine should not be chosen with head injury or open globe eye injury.
BM, Bone marrow; CT, computed tomography; ECHO, echocardiogram; EEG, electroencephalogram; EMLA, eutectic mixture of local anesthetics; LP, lumbar puncture; LET, lidocaine, epinephrine, tetracaine; MRI, magnetic resonance imaging
Modified from Yaster M, Cote C, Krane E, et al. Pediatric Pain Management and Sedation Handbook. *St Louis: Mosby, 1997:551-552.*

REFERENCES

1. Yaster M, Cote C, Krane E, et al. *Pediatric Pain Management and Sedation Handbook*. St Louis: Mosby; 1997.
2. Manworren R, Hynan L. Clinical validation of FLACC: preverbal patient pain scale. *Pediatr Nurs*. 2003;29:140-146.
3. Malviya S, Voepel-Lewis T. The revised FLACC observational pain tool: improved reliability and validity for pain assessment in children with cognitive impairment. *Paediatr Anaesth*. 2006;16:258-265.
4. Yaster M, Maxwell LG. Pediatric regional anesthesia. *Anesthesiology*. 1989;70:324-338.
5. George JA, Park PS, Hunsberger J, et al. An Analysis of 34,218 Pediatric Outpatient Controlled Substance Prescriptions. *Anesth Analg*. 2016; 122(3):807-813.
6. FDA Drug Safety Communication: Safety review update of codeine use in children; new Boxed Warning and Contraindication on use after tonsillectomy and/or adenoidectomy. 02-2013. http://www.fda.gov/Drugs/DrugSafety/ucm339112.htm.
7. Benner KW, Durham SH. Meperidine restriction in a pediatric hospital. *J Pediatr Pharmacol Ther*. 2011;16(3):185-190.
8. Jenco M. FDA issues warning on tramadol use in those under age 17. *AAP News*. Sept 2015;22.
9. Essex MN, Zhang RY, Berger MF, et al. Safety of celecoxib compared with placebo and non-selective NSAIDs: cumulative meta-analysis of 89 randomized controlled trials. *Expert Opin Drug Saf*. 2013;12(4):465-477.
10. St Germain Brent A. The management of pain in the emergency department. *Pediatr Clin North Am*. 2000;47:651-679.
11. Krauss B, Green S. Procedural sedation and analgesia in children. *Lancet*. 2006;367:766-780.
12. Krauss B, Green SM. Sedation and analgesia for procedures in children. *N Engl J Med*. 2000;342:938-945.
13. Zempsky W, Cravero J. Relief of pain and anxiety in pediatric patients in emergency medical systems. *Pediatrics*. 2004;114:1348-1356.
14. Stevens B, Yamada J, Ohlsson A. Sucrose for analgesia in newborn infants undergoing painful procedures (review). *Cochrane Database Syst Rev*. 2010;(1):CD00106.
15. Harrison D, Stevens B, Bueno M, et al. Efficacy of sweet solutions for analgesia in infants between 1 and 12 months of age: a systematic review. *Arch Dis Child*. 2010;95:406-413.
16. Agthe AG, Kim GR, Mathias KB, et al. Clonidine as an adjunct therapy to opioids for neonatal abstinence syndrome: a randomized, controlled trial. *Pediatrics*. 2009;123:e849-e856.
17. Honey BL, Benefield RJ, Miller JL, et al. α2-Receptor agonists for treatment and prevention of iatrogenic opioid abstinence syndrome in critically ill patients. *Ann Pharmacother*. 2009;43:1506-1511.
18. Gowing L, Farrell M, Ali R, et al. Alpha-2 adrenergic agonists for the management of opioid withdrawal (review). *Cochrane Database Syst Rev*. 2009;(3):CD002024.
19. Cote CJ, Lerman J, Todres ID. *A Practice of Anesthesia for Infants and Children*. 4th ed. Philadelphia: WB Saunders; 2008.
20. American Academy of Pediatrics Committee on Drugs. Guidelines for monitoring and management of pediatric patients during and after sedation

for diagnostic and therapeutic procedures: an update. *Pediatrics.* 2006;118:2587-2602.
21. Tait AR, Malviya S. Anesthesia for the child with an upper respiratory infection: still a dilemma? *Anesth Analg.* 2005;100:59-65.
22. Practice guidelines for sedation and analgesia by non-anesthesiologists. *Anesthesiology.* 2002;96:1004-1017.
23. Tobias JD. Applications of nitrous oxide for procedural sedation in the pediatric population. *Pediatr Emerg Care.* 2013;29(2):245-265.

Chapter 7
Cardiology
Madiha Raees, MD

See additional content on Expert Consult

I. WEB RESOURCES
- http://www.pted.org
- http://www.murmurlab.org

II. PHYSICAL EXAMINATION

A. Heart Rate
Refer to Table 7.4 for normal heart rate (HR) by age.

B. Blood Pressure

1. **Blood pressure:**
a. Normal blood pressure values [systolic blood pressure (SBP), diastolic blood pressure (DBP)] by age[1,2]: Tables 7.1 and 7.2; Figs. 7.1, 7.2, and 7.3.
   For normal blood pressure values that are not found within the aforementioned tables, please refer to Appendix B of The Fourth Report on the Diagnosis, Evaluation, and Treatment of High Blood Pressure in Children and Adolescents on how to calculate Z-scores and percentiles.[2]
   For normal blood pressure values in preterm infants, see Table EC 7.A on Expert Consult.
2. **Pulse pressure = systolic pressure–diastolic pressure.**
a. Wide pulse pressure (>40 mmHg): Differential diagnosis includes aortic insufficiency, arteriovenous fistula, patent ductus arteriosus, thyrotoxicosis, and warm shock.
b. Narrow pulse pressure (<25 mmHg): Differential diagnosis includes aortic stenosis, pericardial effusion, pericardial tamponade, pericarditis, significant tachycardia, and cold shock.
3. **Mean arterial pressure (MAP)**
a. MAP = diastolic pressure + (pulse pressure/3) OR 1/3 systolic pressure + 2/3 diastolic pressure
b. Preterm infants and newborns: Normal MAP = gestational age in weeks + 5
4. **Abnormalities in blood pressure**
a. Four-limb blood pressure measurements can be used to assess for coarctation of the aorta. Because of the possibility of an aberrant right

Text continued on p. 163

TABLE 7.1
BLOOD PRESSURE LEVELS FOR THE 50TH, 90TH, 95TH, AND 99TH PERCENTILES OF BLOOD PRESSURE FOR GIRLS AGED 1–17 YEARS BY PERCENTILES OF HEIGHT[2]

Age, yr	BP Percentile[†]	SBP, mmHg Percentile of Height*							DBP, mmHg Percentile of Height*						
		5th	10th	25th	50th	75th	90th	95th	5th	10th	25th	50th	75th	90th	95th
1	50th	83	84	85	86	88	89	90	38	39	39	40	41	41	42
	90th	97	97	98	100	101	102	103	52	53	53	54	55	55	56
	95th	100	101	102	104	105	106	107	56	57	57	58	59	59	60
	99th	108	108	109	111	112	113	114	64	64	65	65	66	67	67
2	50th	85	85	87	88	89	91	91	43	44	44	45	46	46	47
	90th	98	99	100	101	103	104	105	57	58	58	59	60	61	61
	95th	102	103	104	105	107	108	109	61	62	62	63	64	65	65
	99th	109	110	111	112	114	115	116	69	69	70	70	71	72	72
3	50th	86	87	88	89	91	92	93	47	48	48	49	50	50	51
	90th	100	100	102	103	104	106	106	61	62	62	63	64	64	65
	95th	104	104	105	107	108	109	110	65	66	66	67	68	68	69
	99th	111	111	113	114	115	116	117	73	73	74	74	75	76	76
4	50th	88	88	90	91	92	94	94	50	50	51	52	52	53	54
	90th	101	102	103	104	106	107	108	64	64	65	66	67	67	68
	95th	105	106	107	108	110	111	112	68	68	69	70	71	71	72
	99th	112	113	114	115	117	118	119	76	76	76	77	78	79	79
5	50th	89	90	91	93	94	95	96	52	53	53	54	55	55	56
	90th	103	103	105	106	107	109	109	66	67	67	68	69	69	70
	95th	107	107	108	110	111	112	113	70	71	71	72	73	73	74
	99th	114	114	116	117	118	120	120	78	78	79	79	80	81	81

Continued

TABLE 7.1
BLOOD PRESSURE LEVELS FOR THE 50TH, 90TH, 95TH, AND 99TH PERCENTILES OF BLOOD PRESSURE FOR GIRLS AGED 1–17 YEARS BY PERCENTILES OF HEIGHT—cont'd

Age, yr	BP Percentile[†]	SBP, mmHg — Percentile of Height[*]							DBP, mmHg — Percentile of Height[*]						
		5th	10th	25th	50th	75th	90th	95th	5th	10th	25th	50th	75th	90th	95th
6	50th	91	92	93	94	96	97	98	54	54	55	56	56	57	58
	90th	104	105	106	108	109	110	111	68	68	69	70	70	71	72
	95th	108	109	110	111	113	114	115	72	72	73	74	74	75	76
	99th	115	116	117	119	120	121	122	80	80	80	81	82	83	83
7	50th	93	93	95	96	97	99	99	55	56	56	57	58	58	59
	90th	106	107	108	109	111	112	113	69	70	70	71	72	72	73
	95th	110	111	112	113	115	116	116	73	74	74	75	76	76	77
	99th	117	118	119	120	122	123	124	81	81	82	82	83	84	84
8	50th	95	95	96	98	99	100	101	57	57	57	58	59	60	60
	90th	108	109	110	111	113	114	114	71	71	71	72	73	74	74
	95th	112	112	114	115	116	118	118	75	75	75	76	77	78	78
	99th	119	120	121	122	123	125	125	82	82	83	83	84	85	86
9	50th	96	97	98	100	101	102	103	58	58	58	59	60	61	61
	90th	110	110	112	113	114	116	116	72	72	72	73	74	75	75
	95th	114	114	115	117	118	119	120	76	76	76	77	78	79	79
	99th	121	121	123	124	125	127	127	83	83	84	84	85	86	87
10	50th	98	99	100	102	103	104	105	59	59	59	60	61	62	62
	90th	112	112	114	115	116	118	118	73	73	73	74	75	76	76
	95th	116	116	117	119	120	121	122	77	77	77	78	79	80	80
	99th	123	123	125	126	127	129	129	84	84	85	86	86	87	88
11	50th	100	101	102	103	105	106	107	60	60	60	61	62	63	63
	90th	114	114	116	117	118	119	120	74	74	74	75	76	77	77
	95th	118	118	119	121	122	123	124	78	78	78	79	80	81	81
	99th	125	125	126	128	129	130	131	85	85	86	87	87	88	89

Chapter 7 Cardiology

Age	BP Percentile	SBP (Height %ile)							DBP (Height %ile)						
		5th	10th	25th	50th	75th	90th	95th	5th	10th	25th	50th	75th	90th	95th
12	50th	102	103	104	105	107	108	109	61	61	61	61	62	64	64
	90th	116	116	117	119	120	121	122	75	75	75	76	76	78	78
	95th	119	120	121	123	124	125	126	79	79	79	79	80	82	82
	99th	127	127	128	130	131	132	133	86	86	87	88	88	89	90
13	50th	104	105	106	107	109	110	110	62	62	62	63	63	65	65
	90th	117	118	119	121	122	123	124	76	76	76	77	78	79	79
	95th	121	122	123	124	126	127	128	80	80	80	81	81	83	83
	99th	128	129	130	132	133	134	135	87	87	88	89	89	90	91
14	50th	106	106	107	109	110	111	112	63	63	63	64	65	66	66
	90th	119	120	121	122	124	125	125	77	77	77	78	78	80	80
	95th	123	123	125	126	127	129	129	81	81	81	82	83	84	84
	99th	130	131	132	133	135	136	136	88	88	89	90	90	91	92
15	50th	107	108	109	110	111	113	113	64	64	64	65	66	67	67
	90th	120	121	122	123	125	126	127	78	78	78	79	79	81	81
	95th	124	125	127	127	129	130	131	82	82	82	83	83	85	85
	99th	131	132	134	135	136	137	138	89	89	89	90	91	92	93
16	50th	108	108	110	111	112	114	114	64	64	64	65	66	67	68
	90th	121	122	123	124	126	127	128	78	78	79	79	80	81	82
	95th	125	126	127	128	130	131	132	82	82	83	83	84	85	86
	99th	132	133	134	135	137	138	139	90	90	90	91	91	93	93
17	50th	108	109	110	111	113	114	115	65	65	65	66	67	67	68
	90th	122	122	123	125	126	127	128	78	79	79	80	80	81	82
	95th	125	126	127	129	130	131	132	82	83	83	84	85	85	86
	99th	133	133	134	136	137	138	139	90	90	91	91	92	93	93

DBP, diastolic blood pressure; SBP, systolic blood pressure.
*Height percentile determined by standard growth curves
†Blood pressure percentile determined by a single measurement
Adapted from the National High Blood Pressure Education Program Working Group on High Blood Pressure in Children and Adolescents. The fourth report on the diagnosis, evaluation, and treatment of high blood pressure in children and adolescents. Pediatrics. 2004;114(2 Suppl):555-576.

TABLE 7.2
BLOOD PRESSURE LEVELS FOR THE 50TH, 90TH, 95TH, AND 99TH PERCENTILES OF BLOOD PRESSURE FOR BOYS AGED 1–17 YEARS BY PERCENTILES OF HEIGHT[2]

Age, yr	BP Percentile[†]	SBP, mmHg Percentile of Height[*]							DBP, mmHg Percentile of Height[*]						
		5th	10th	25th	50th	75th	90th	95th	5th	10th	25th	50th	75th	90th	95th
1	50th	80	81	83	85	87	88	89	34	35	36	37	38	39	39
	90th	94	95	97	99	100	102	103	49	50	51	52	53	53	54
	95th	98	99	101	103	104	106	106	54	54	55	56	57	58	58
	99th	105	106	108	110	112	113	114	61	62	63	64	65	66	66
2	50th	84	85	87	88	90	92	92	39	40	41	42	43	44	44
	90th	97	99	100	102	104	105	106	54	55	56	57	58	58	59
	95th	101	102	104	106	108	109	110	59	59	60	61	62	63	63
	99th	109	110	111	113	115	117	117	66	67	68	69	70	71	71
3	50th	86	87	89	91	93	94	95	44	44	45	46	47	48	48
	90th	100	101	103	105	107	108	109	59	59	60	61	62	63	63
	95th	104	105	107	109	110	112	113	63	63	64	65	66	67	67
	99th	111	112	114	116	118	119	120	71	71	72	73	74	75	75
4	50th	88	89	91	93	95	96	97	47	48	49	50	51	51	52
	90th	102	103	105	107	109	110	111	62	63	64	65	66	66	67
	95th	106	107	109	111	112	114	115	66	67	68	69	70	71	71
	99th	113	114	116	118	120	121	122	74	75	76	77	78	78	79
5	50th	90	91	93	95	96	98	98	50	51	52	53	54	55	55
	90th	104	105	106	108	110	111	112	65	66	67	68	69	69	70
	95th	108	109	110	112	114	115	116	69	70	71	72	73	74	74
	99th	115	116	118	120	121	123	123	77	78	79	80	81	81	82

Chapter 7 Cardiology

Age (Year)	BP Percentile	SBP (mmHg) by Percentile of Height							DBP (mmHg) by Percentile of Height						
		5%	10%	25%	50%	75%	90%	95%	5%	10%	25%	50%	75%	90%	95%
6	50th	91	92	94	96	98	99	100	53	53	54	55	56	57	57
	90th	105	106	108	110	111	113	113	68	68	69	70	71	72	72
	95th	109	110	112	114	115	117	117	72	72	73	74	75	76	76
	99th	116	117	119	121	123	124	125	80	80	81	82	83	84	84
7	50th	92	94	95	97	99	100	101	55	55	56	57	58	59	59
	90th	106	107	109	111	113	114	115	70	70	71	72	73	74	74
	95th	110	111	113	115	117	118	119	74	74	75	76	77	78	78
	99th	117	118	120	122	124	125	126	82	82	83	84	85	86	86
8	50th	94	95	97	99	100	102	102	56	57	58	59	60	60	61
	90th	107	109	110	112	114	115	116	71	72	72	73	74	75	76
	95th	111	112	114	116	118	119	120	75	76	77	78	79	79	80
	99th	119	120	122	123	125	127	127	83	84	85	86	87	87	88
9	50th	95	96	98	100	102	103	104	57	58	59	60	61	61	62
	90th	109	110	112	114	115	117	118	72	73	73	74	75	76	77
	95th	113	114	116	118	119	121	121	76	77	78	79	80	81	81
	99th	120	121	123	125	127	128	129	84	85	86	87	88	88	89
10	50th	97	98	100	102	103	105	106	58	58	59	60	61	61	62
	90th	111	112	114	115	117	119	119	73	73	74	75	76	77	78
	95th	115	116	117	119	121	122	123	77	78	79	80	81	81	82
	99th	122	123	125	127	128	130	130	85	86	86	88	88	89	90
11	50th	99	100	102	104	105	107	107	59	59	60	61	61	62	63
	90th	113	114	115	117	119	120	121	74	74	75	76	77	78	78
	95th	117	118	119	121	123	124	125	78	78	79	80	81	81	82
	99th	124	125	127	129	130	132	132	86	86	87	88	89	89	90
12	50th	101	102	104	106	108	109	110	59	60	60	61	62	63	63
	90th	115	116	118	120	121	123	123	74	75	75	76	77	78	79
	95th	119	120	122	123	125	127	127	78	79	80	81	82	82	83
	99th	126	127	129	131	133	134	135	86	87	88	89	90	90	91

Continued

TABLE 7.2
BLOOD PRESSURE LEVELS FOR THE 50TH, 90TH, 95TH, AND 99TH PERCENTILES OF BLOOD PRESSURE FOR BOYS AGED 1–17 YEARS BY PERCENTILES OF HEIGHT—cont'd

Age, yr	BP Percentile[†]	SBP, mmHg Percentile of Height[*]							DBP, mmHg Percentile of Height[*]						
		5th	10th	25th	50th	75th	90th	95th	5th	10th	25th	50th	75th	90th	95th
13	50th	104	105	106	108	110	111	112	60	60	61	62	63	64	64
	90th	117	118	120	122	124	125	126	75	75	76	77	78	79	79
	95th	121	122	124	126	128	129	130	79	79	80	81	82	83	83
	99th	128	130	131	133	135	136	137	87	87	88	89	90	91	91
14	50th	106	107	109	111	113	114	115	60	61	62	63	64	65	65
	90th	120	121	123	125	126	128	128	75	76	77	78	79	79	80
	95th	124	125	127	128	130	132	132	80	80	81	82	83	84	84
	99th	131	132	134	136	138	139	140	87	88	89	90	91	92	92
15	50th	109	110	112	113	115	117	117	61	62	63	64	65	66	66
	90th	122	124	125	127	129	130	131	76	77	78	79	80	80	81
	95th	126	127	129	131	133	134	135	81	81	82	83	84	85	85
	99th	134	135	136	138	140	142	142	88	89	90	91	92	93	93
16	50th	111	112	114	116	118	119	120	63	63	64	65	66	67	67
	90th	125	126	128	130	131	133	134	78	78	79	80	81	82	82
	95th	129	130	132	134	135	137	137	82	83	83	84	85	86	87
	99th	136	137	139	141	143	144	145	90	90	91	92	93	94	94
17	50th	114	115	116	118	120	121	122	65	66	66	67	68	69	70
	90th	127	128	130	132	134	135	136	80	80	81	82	83	84	84
	95th	131	232	134	136	138	139	140	84	85	86	87	87	88	89
	99th	139	140	141	143	145	146	147	92	93	93	94	95	96	97

DBP, diastolic blood pressure; SBP, systolic blood pressure.
[*]Height percentile determined by standard growth curves
[†]Blood pressure percentile determined by a single measurement

Adapted from the National High Blood Pressure Education Program Working Group on High Blood Pressure in Children and Adolescents: The fourth report on the diagnosis, evaluation, and treatment of high blood pressure in children and adolescents. Pediatrics 2004;114(2 Suppl):555-576.

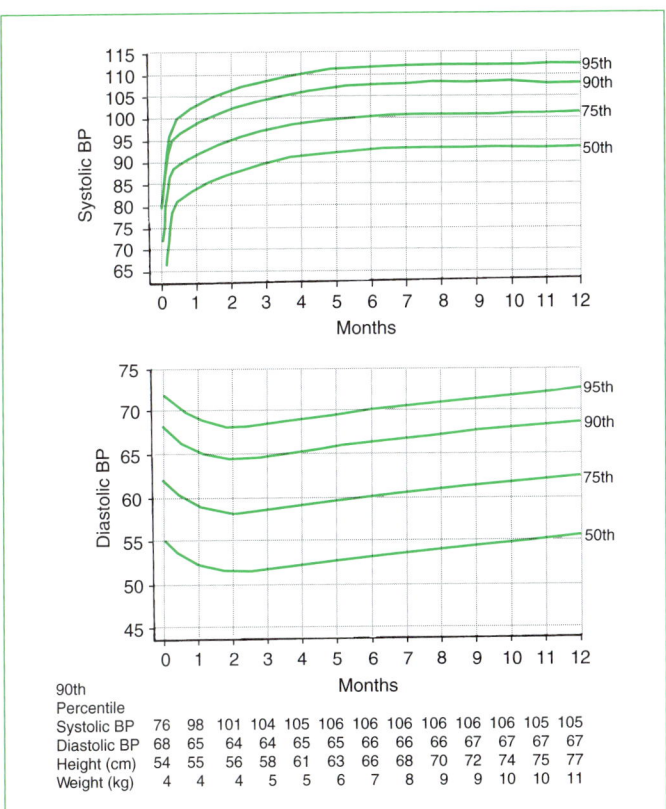

FIGURE 7.1

Age-specific percentiles of blood pressure (BP) measurements in boys from birth to 12 months of age; Korotkoff phase IV (K4) used for diastolic BP (DBP). *(From Task Force on Blood Pressure Control in Children. Report of the Second Task Force on Blood Pressure Control in Children. Pediatrics. 1987;79:1-25.)*

subclavian artery, blood pressure must be measured in both the right and left arms.
b. Pulsus paradoxus: Exaggeration of the normal drop in SBP seen with inspiration. Determine SBP at the end of exhalation and then during inhalation; if the difference is >10 mmHg, consider pericardial effusion, tamponade, pericarditis, severe asthma, or restrictive cardiomyopathies.

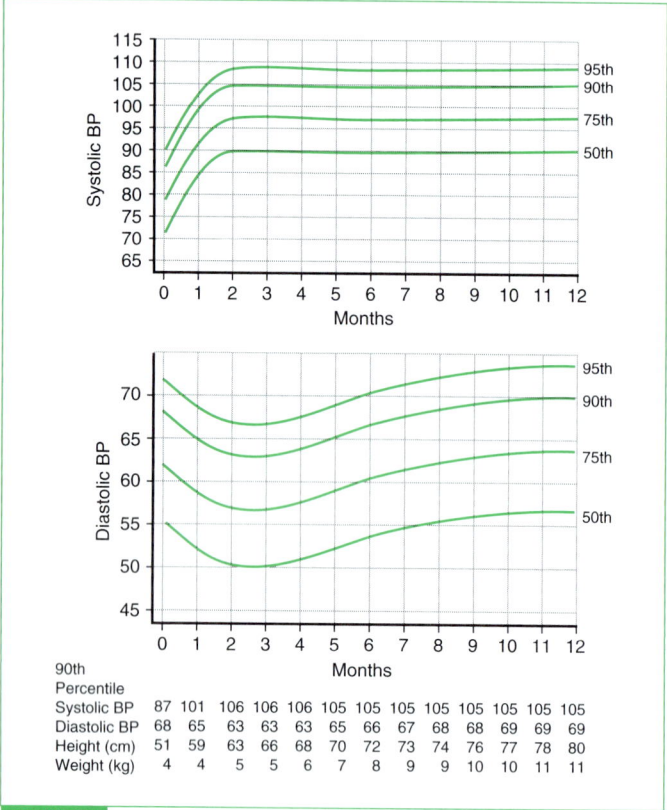

FIGURE 7.2

Age-specific percentile of blood pressure (BP) measurements in girls from birth to 12 months of age; Korotkoff phase IV (K4) used for diastolic BP (DBP). *(From Task Force on Blood Pressure Control in Children. Report of the Second Task Force on Blood Pressure Control in Children. Pediatrics. 1987;79:1-25.)*

C. Heart Sounds

1. **S_1:** Associated with closure of mitral and tricuspid valves; heard best at the apex or left lower sternal border (LLSB)
2. **S_2:** Associated with closure of pulmonary and aortic valves; heard best at the left upper sternal border (LUSB), and has normal physiologic splitting that increases with inspiration
3. **S_3:** Heard best at the apex or LLSB
4. **S_4:** Heard at the apex

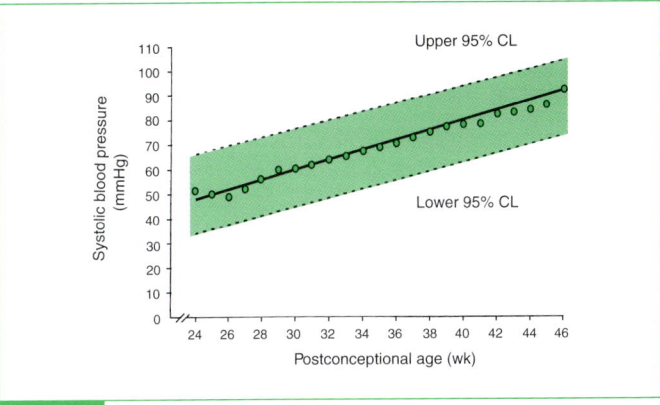

FIGURE 7.3
Linear regression of the mean systolic blood pressure (SBP) based on post-conceptional age (gestational age in weeks plus weeks after delivery). CL, Confidence limit. *(Data from Zubrow AB, Hulman S, Kushner H, et al. Determinants of blood pressure in infants admitted to neonatal intensive care units: a prospective multicenter study. Philadelphia Neonatal Blood Pressure Study Group. J Perinatol. 1995;15(6): 470-479.)*

D. Systolic and Diastolic Sounds
See Box 7.1 for abnormal heart sounds.[3]

E. Murmurs[4]
More information is available at http://www.murmurlab.org. The clinical characteristics are summarized in Table 7.3.[3]

1. **Grading of heart murmurs:** Intensified by states of higher cardiac output (e.g., anemia, anxiety, fever, exercise).[3]
a. Grade I: Barely audible
b. Grade II: Soft but easily audible
c. Grade III: Moderately loud but not accompanied by a thrill
d. Grade IV: Louder, associated with a thrill
e. Grade V: Audible with a stethoscope barely on the chest
f. Grade VI: Audible with a stethoscope off the chest
2. **Benign heart murmurs:**
a. Caused by a disturbance of the laminar flow of blood; frequently produced as the diameter of the blood's pathway decreases and velocity increases.
b. Present in >80% of children sometime during childhood, most commonly beginning at age 3 to 4 years.
c. Accentuated in high-output states, especially with fever and anemia.

BOX 7.1
SUMMARY OF ABNORMAL HEART SOUNDS

- **Widely split S_1:** Ebstein anomaly, RBBB
- **Widely split and fixed S_2:** Right ventricular volume overload (e.g., ASD, PAPVR), pressure overload (e.g., PS), electrical delay in RV contraction (e.g., RBBB), early aortic closure (e.g., MR), occasionally heard in normal child
- **Narrowly split S_2:** Pulmonary hypertension, AS, delay in LV contraction (e.g., LBBB), occasionally heard in normal child
- **Single S_2:** Pulmonary hypertension, one semilunar valve (e.g., pulmonary atresia, aortic atresia, truncus arteriosus), P2 not audible (e.g., TGA, TOF, severe PS), severe AS, occasionally heard in normal child
- **Paradoxically split S_2:** Severe AS, LBBB, Wolff-Parkinson-White syndrome (type B)
- **Abnormal intensity of P2:** Increased P2 (e.g., pulmonary hypertension), decreased P2 (e.g., severe PS, TOF, TS)
- **S_3:** Occasionally heard in healthy children or adults or may indicate dilated ventricles (e.g., large VSD, CHF)
- **S_4:** Always pathologic; decreased ventricular compliance
- **Ejection click:** Heard with stenosis of the semilunar valves, dilated great arteries in the setting of pulmonary or systemic hypertension, idiopathic dilation of the PA, TOF, persistent truncus arteriosus
- **Midsystolic click:** Heard at the apex in mitral valve prolapse
- **Diastolic opening snap:** Rare in children; associated with TS/MS

AS, Aortic stenosis; ASD, atrial septal defect; CHF, congestive heart failure; LBBB, left bundle-branch block; MR, mitral regurgitation; MS, mitral stenosis; PA, pulmonary artery; PAPVR, partial anomalous pulmonary venous return; PS, pulmonary stenosis; RBBB, right bundle-branch block; RV, right ventricular; TGA, transposition of the great arteries; TOF, tetralogy of Fallot; TS, tricuspid stenosis; VSD, ventricular septal defect.
Modified from Park MK. Pediatric Cardiology for Practitioners. 5th ed. St Louis: Elsevier; 2008:25.

d. Normal electrocardiogram (ECG) and radiographic findings.
NOTE: ECG and chest radiograph are not routinely used or cost-effective screening tools for distinguishing benign from pathologic murmurs.
3. **A murmur is likely to be pathologic when one or more of the following are present:** symptoms; cyanosis; a systolic murmur that is loud (grade ≥ 3/6), harsh, pansystolic, or long in duration; diastolic murmur; abnormal heart sounds; presence of a click; abnormally strong or weak pulses
4. **Systolic and diastolic heart murmurs** (Box 7.2)

III. ELECTROCARDIOGRAPHY

A. Basic Electrocardiography Principles

1. **Lead placement** (Fig. 7.4)
2. **ECG complexes**
a. P wave: Represents atrial depolarization
b. QRS complex: Represents ventricular depolarization

TABLE 7.3
COMMON INNOCENT HEART MURMURS

Type (Timing)	Description of Murmur	Age Group
Classic vibratory murmur (Still's murmur; systolic)	Maximal at LMSB or between LLSB and apex Grade 2–3/6 in intensity Low-frequency vibratory, twanging string, groaning, squeaking, or musical	3–6 yr; occasionally in infancy
Pulmonary ejection murmur (systolic)	Maximal at LUSB Early to midsystolic Grade 1–3/6 in intensity Blowing in quality	8–14 yr
Pulmonary flow murmur of newborn (systolic)	Maximal at LUSB Transmits well to left and right chest, axilla, and back Grade 1–2/6 in intensity	Premature and full-term newborns Usually disappears by 3–6 mo
Venous hum (continuous)	Maximal at right (or left) supraclavicular and infraclavicular areas Grade 1–3/6 in intensity Inaudible in supine position Intensity changes with rotation of head and disappears with compression of jugular vein	3–6 yr
Carotid bruit (systolic)	Right supraclavicular area over carotids Grade 2–3/6 in intensity Occasional thrill over carotid	Any age

LLSB, Left lower sternal border; LMSB, left middle sternal border; LUSB, left upper sternal border
From Park MK. Pediatric Cardiology for Practitioners. 5th ed. St Louis: Elsevier; 2008:36.

  c. T wave: Represents ventricular repolarization
  d. U wave: May follow the T wave and represents late phases of ventricular repolarization
3. **Systematic approach for evaluating ECGs** (Table 7.4 shows normal ECG parameters)[3,5]:
a. Rate
   (1) Standardization: Paper speed is 25 mm/sec. One small square = 1 mm = 0.04 sec. One large square = 5 mm = 0.2 sec. Amplitude standard: 10 mm = 1 mV
   (2) Calculation: HR (beats per minute) = 60 divided by the average R-R interval in seconds, or 1500 divided by the R-R interval in millimeters
b. Rhythm
   (1) Sinus rhythm: Every QRS complex is preceded by a P wave, normal PR interval [although PR interval may be prolonged, as in

> ### BOX 7.2
> ### SYSTOLIC AND DIASTOLIC HEART MURMURS
>
> **I RUSB**
>
> Aortic valve stenosis (supravalvar, subvalvar)
> *Aortic regurgitation*
>
> **II LUSB**
>
> Pulmonary valve stenosis
> Atrial septal defect
> Pulmonary ejection murmur, innocent
> Pulmonary flow murmur of newborn
> Pulmonary artery stenosis
> Aortic stenosis
> Coarctation of the aorta
> Patent ductus arteriosus
> Partial anomalous pulmonary venous return (PAPVR)
> Total anomalous pulmonary venous return (TAPVR)
> *Pulmonary regurgitation*
>
> **III LLSB**
>
> Ventricular septal defect, including atrioventricular septal defect
> Vibratory innocent murmur (Still's murmur)
> HOCM (IHSS)
> Tricuspid regurgitation
> Tetralogy of Fallot
> *Tricuspid stenosis*
>
> **IV Apex**
>
> Mitral regurgitation
> Vibratory innocent murmur (Still's murmur)
> Mitral valve prolapse
> Aortic stenosis
> HOCM (IHSS)
> *Mitral stenosis*

Murmurs listed by the location at which they are best heard. *Diastolic murmurs are in italics.* HOCM, Hypertrophic obstructive cardiomyopathy; IHSS, idiopathic hypertrophic subaortic stenosis; LLSB, left lower sternal border; LUSB, left upper sternal border; RUSB, right upper sternal border
From Park MK. Pediatric Cardiology for Practitioners. 5th ed. St Louis: Elsevier; 2008:30.

      first-degree atrioventricular (AV) block], and normal P-wave axis (upright P in leads I and aVF).

   (2) There is normal respiratory variation of the R-R interval without morphologic changes of the P wave or QRS complex.

  c. Axis: The direction of the QRS in leads I and aVF should be observed, the quadrant determined, and comparison made with age-matched normal values (Fig. 7.5; see Table 7.4).

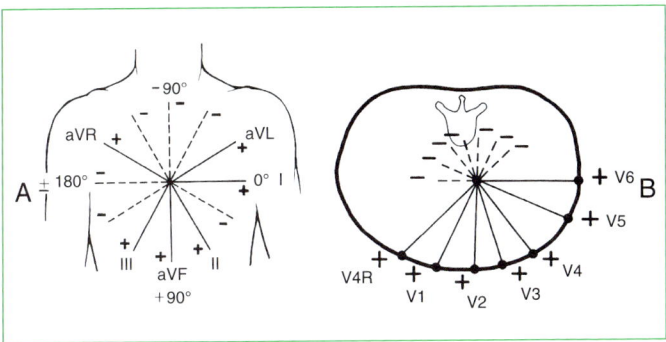

FIGURE 7.4
A. Hexaxial reference system, **B.** Horizontal reference system. *(Modified from Park MK, Guntheroth WG. How to Read Pediatric ECGs. 4th ed. Philadelphia: Elsevier; 2006:3.)*

d. Intervals (PR, QRS, QTc): See Table 7.4 for normal PR and QRS intervals. The QTc is calculated using the Bazett formula:
QTc = QT *(sec)* measured/$\sqrt{R-R}$
(the average of three measurements taken from the same lead)
The R-R interval should extend from the R wave in the QRS complex where QT to the preceding R wave is measured. Normal values for QTc are:
(1) 0.44 sec is 97th percentile for infants 3–4 days old[6]
(2) ≤0.45 sec in all males aged >1 week and in prepubescent females
(3) ≤0.46 sec for postpubescent females

e. P-wave size and shape: A normal P wave should be <0.10 sec in children and <0.08 sec in infants, with an amplitude of <0.3 mV (3 mm in height, with normal standardization).

f. R-wave progression: In general, there is a normal increase in R-wave size and a decrease in S-wave size from leads V_1 to V_6 (with dominant S waves in the right precordial leads and dominant R waves in the left precordial leads), representing dominance of left ventricular forces. However, newborns and infants have a normal dominance of the right ventricle.

g. Q waves: Normal Q waves are usually <0.04 sec in duration and <25% of the total QRS amplitude. Q waves are <5 mm deep in the left precordial leads and aVF, and ≤8 mm deep in lead III for children aged <3 years.

h. ST-segment (Fig. 7.6): ST-segment elevation or depression of >1 mm in the limb leads and >2 mm in the precordial leads is consistent with myocardial ischemia or injury. **NOTE:** J-depression is an upsloping of the ST segment and a normal variant.

TABLE 7.4
NORMAL PEDIATRIC ELECTROCARDIOGRAM (ECG) PARAMETERS

Age	Heart Rate (bpm)	QRS Axis*	PR interval (sec)*	QRS Duration (sec)†	Lead V₁ R-Wave Amplitude (mm)†	Lead V₁ S-Wave Amplitude (mm)†	Lead V₁ R/S Ratio	Lead V₆ R-Wave Amplitude (mm)†	Lead V₆ S-Wave Amplitude (mm)†	Lead V₆ R/S Ratio
0–7 days	95–160 (125)	+30 to 180 (110)	0.08–0.12 (0.10)	0.05 (0.07)	13.3 (25.5)	7.7 (18.8)	2.5	4.8 (11.8)	3.2 (9.6)	2.2
1–3 wk	105–180 (145)	+30 to 180 (110)	0.08–0.12 (0.10)	0.05 (0.07)	10.6 (20.8)	4.2 (10.8)	2.9	7.6 (16.4)	3.4 (9.8)	3.3
1–6 mo	110–180 (145)	+10 to +125 (+70)	0.08–0.13 (0.11)	0.05 (0.07)	9.7 (19)	5.4 (15)	2.3	12.4 (22)	2.8 (8.3)	5.6
6–12 mo	110–170 (135)	+10 to +125 (+60)	0.10–0.14 (0.12)	0.05 (0.07)	9.4 (20.3)	6.4 (18.1)	1.6	12.6 (22.7)	2.1 (7.2)	7.6
1–3 yr	90–150 (120)	+10 to +125 (+60)	0.10–0.14 (0.12)	0.06 (0.07)	8.5 (18)	9 (21)	1.2	14 (23.3)	1.7 (6)	10
4–5 yr	65–135 (110)	0 to +110 (+60)	0.11–0.15 (0.13)	0.07 (0.08)	7.6 (16)	11 (22.5)	0.8	15.6 (25)	1.4 (4.7)	11.2
6–8 yr	60–130 (100)	−15 to +110 (+60)	0.12–0.16 (0.14)	0.07 (0.08)	6 (13)	12 (24.5)	0.6	16.3 (26)	1.1 (3.9)	13
9–11 yr	60–110 (85)	−15 to +110 (+60)	0.12–0.17 (0.14)	0.07 (0.09)	5.4 (12.1)	11.9 (25.4)	0.5	16.3 (25.4)	1.0 (3.9)	14.3
12–16 yr	60–110 (85)	−15 to +110 (+60)	0.12–0.17 (0.15)	0.07 (0.10)	4.1 (9.9)	10.8 (21.2)	0.5	14.3 (23)	0.8 (3.7)	14.7
>16 yr	60–100 (80)	−15 to +110 (+60)	0.12–0.20 (0.15)	0.08 (0.10)	3 (9)	10 (20)	0.3	10 (20)	0.8 (3.7)	12

*Normal range and (mean).
†Mean and (98th percentile).
Data from Park MK. Pediatric Cardiology for Practitioners. 5th ed. St Louis: Elsevier; 2008 and Davignon A, et al. Normal ECG standards for infants and children. Pediatr Cardiol. 1979;1:123-131.

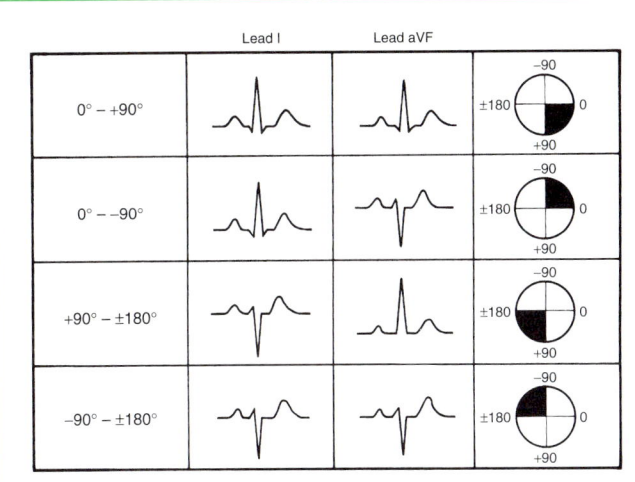

FIGURE 7.5
Location of quadrants of the mean QRS axis from leads I and aVF. *(From Park MK, Guntheroth WG. How to Read Pediatric ECGs. 4th ed. Philadelphia: Elsevier; 2006:17.)*

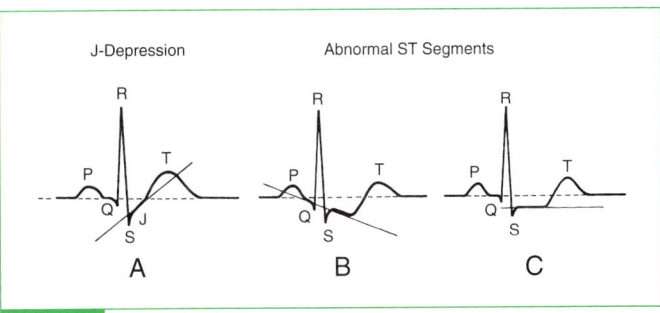

FIGURE 7.6
Nonpathologic (nonischemic) and pathologic (ischemic) ST and T changes. **A.** Characteristic nonischemic ST-segment alteration called J-depression (note that ST slope is upward), **B–C.** Ischemic or pathologic ST-segment alterations, **B.** Downward slope of ST segment, **C.** Horizontal segment is sustained. *(From Park MK, Guntheroth WG. How to Read Pediatric ECGs. 4th ed. Philadelphia: Elsevier; 2006:107.)*

i. T wave:
   (1) Inverted T waves in V_1 and V_2 can be normal in children up to adolescence (Table 7.5).
   (2) Tall, peaked T waves may be seen in hyperkalemia.
   (3) Flat or low T waves may be seen in hypokalemia, hypothyroidism, normal newborns, and myocardial/pericardial ischemia and inflammation.
j. Hypertrophy/enlargement
   (1) Atrial enlargement (Fig. 7.7)
   (2) Ventricular hypertrophy: Diagnosed by QRS axis, voltage, and R/S ratio (Box 7.3; see also Table 7.4)

B. ECG Abnormalities

1. **Nonventricular arrhythmias** (Table 7.6; Figs. 7.8 and 7.9)[7]
2. **Ventricular arrhythmias** (Table 7.7; Fig. 7.10)

TABLE 7.5
NORMAL T-WAVE AXIS

Age	V_1, V_2	AVF	I, V_5, V_6
Birth–1 day	±	+	±
1–4 days	±	+	+
4 days to adolescent	−	+	+
Adolescent to adult	+	+	+

+, T wave positive; −, T wave negative; ±, T wave normally either positive or negative

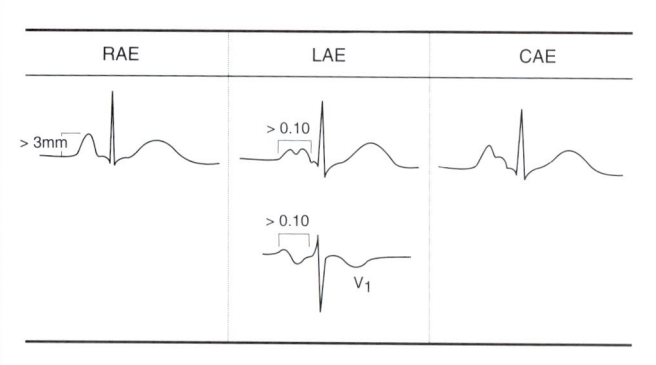

FIGURE 7.7
Criteria for atrial enlargement. CAE, Combined atrial enlargement; LAE, left atrial enlargement; RAE, right atrial enlargement. *(From Park MK. Pediatric Cardiology for Practitioners. 5th ed. St Louis: Elsevier; 2008:53.)*

> **BOX 7.3**
>
> **VENTRICULAR HYPERTROPHY CRITERIA**
>
> **Right Ventricular Hypertrophy (RVH) Criteria**
>
> **Must Have at Least One of the Following:**
>
> Upright T wave in lead V_1 after 3 days of age to adolescence
> Presence of Q wave in V_1 (QR or QRS pattern)
> Increased right and anterior QRS voltage (with normal QRS duration):
>   R in lead V_1, >98th percentile for age
>   S in lead V_6, >98th percentile for age
> Right ventricular strain (associated with inverted T wave in V_1 with tall R wave)
>
> **Left Ventricular Hypertrophy (LVH) Criteria**
>
> Left ventricular strain (associated with inverted T wave in leads V_6, I, and/or aVF)
>
> **Supplemental Criteria:**
>
> Left axis deviation (LAD) for patient's age
> Volume overload (associated with Q wave >5 mm and tall T waves in V_5 or V_6)
> Increased QRS voltage in left leads (with normal QRS duration):
>   R in lead V_6 (and I, aVL, V_5), >98th percentile for age
>   S in lead V_1, >98th percentile for age

3. **Nonventricular conduction disturbances** (Fig. 7.11 and Table 7.8)[8]
4. **Ventricular conduction disturbances** (Table 7.9)

C. ECG Findings Secondary to Electrolyte Disturbances, Medications, and Systemic Illnesses (Table 7.10)[7,9]

D. Long QT

1. Diagnosis:
a. In general, QTc is similar in males and females from birth until late adolescence (0.37–0.44 sec).
b. In adults, prolonged QTc is >0.45 sec for males and >0.45–0.46 sec for females.
c. In approximately 10% of cases, patients may have a normal QTc on ECG. Patients may also have a family history of long QT associated with unexplained syncope, seizure, or cardiac arrest, without prolongation of QTc on ECG.
d. Treadmill exercise testing may prolong the QTc and will sometimes induce arrhythmias.
2. **Complications:** Associated with ventricular arrhythmias (torsades de pointes), syncope, and sudden death.

Text continued on p. 179

TABLE 7.6
NONVENTRICULAR ARRHYTHMIAS

Name/Description	Cause	Treatment
SINUS		
TACHYCARDIA		
Normal sinus rhythm with HR >95th percentile for age (usually infants: <220 beats/min and children: <180 beats/min)	Hypovolemia, shock, anemia, sepsis, fever, anxiety, CHF, PE, myocardial disease, drugs (e.g., β-agonists, albuterol, caffeine, atropine)	Address underlying cause
BRADYCARDIA		
Normal sinus rhythm with HR <5th percentile for age	Normal (especially in athletic individuals), increased ICP, hypoxia, hyperkalemia, hypercalcemia, vagal stimulation, hypothyroidism, hypothermia, drugs (e.g., opioids, digoxin, β-blockers), long QT	Address underlying cause; if symptomatic, refer to inside back cover for bradycardia algorithm
SUPRAVENTRICULAR*		
PREMATURE ATRIAL CONTRACTION (PAC)		
Narrow QRS complex; ectopic focus in atria with abnormal P-wave morphology	Digitalis toxicity, medications (e.g., caffeine, theophylline, sympathomimetics), normal variant	Treat digitalis toxicity; otherwise no treatment needed
ATRIAL FLUTTER		
Atrial rate 250–350 beats/min; characteristic saw-tooth or flutter pattern with variable ventricular response rate and normal QRS complex	Dilated atria, previous intra-atrial surgery, valvular or ischemic heart disease, idiopathic in newborns	Synchronized cardioversion or overdrive pacing; treat underlying cause
ATRIAL FIBRILLATION		
Irregular; atrial rate 350–600 beats/min, yielding characteristic fibrillatory pattern (no discrete P waves) and irregular ventricular response rate of about 110–150 beats/min with normal QRS complex	Wolff-Parkinson-White syndrome and those listed previously for atrial flutter (except not idiopathic), alcohol exposure, familial	Synchronized cardioversion; then may need anticoagulation pretreatment

TABLE 7.6
NONVENTRICULAR ARRHYTHMIAS—cont'd

Name/Description	Cause	Treatment
SVT		
Sudden run of three or more consecutive premature supraventricular beats at >220 beats/min (infant) or >180 beats/min (child), with narrow QRS complex and absent/abnormal P wave; either sustained (>30 sec) or nonsustained	Most commonly idiopathic but may be seen in congenital heart disease (e.g., Ebstein anomaly, transposition)	Vagal maneuvers, adenosine; if unstable, need immediate synchronized cardioversion (0.5 J/kg up to 1 J/kg). Consult cardiologist. See "Tachycardia with Poor Perfusion" or "Tachycardia with Adequate Perfusion" algorithms in the back of the book.
I. *AV Reentrant:* Presence of accessory bypass pathway, in conjunction with AV node, establishes cyclic pattern of reentry independent of SA node; most common cause of nonsinus tachycardia in children (see Wolff-Parkinson-White syndrome, Table 7.9 and Fig. 7.9)		
II. *Junctional:* Automatic focus; simultaneous depolarization of atria and ventricles yields invisible P wave or retrograde P wave	Cardiac surgery, idiopathic	Adjust for clinical situation; consult cardiology
III. *Ectopic atrial tachycardia:* Rapid firing of ectopic focus in atrium	Idiopathic	AV nodal blockade, ablation
NODAL ESCAPE/JUNCTIONAL RHYTHM		
Abnormal rhythm driven by AV node impulse, giving normal QRS complex and invisible P wave (buried in preceding QRS or T wave) or retrograde P wave (negative in lead II, positive in aVR); seen in sinus bradycardia	Common after surgery of atria	Often requires no treatment. If rate is slow enough, may require pacemaker.

*Abnormal rhythm resulting from ectopic focus in atria or AV node, or from accessory conduction pathways. Characterized by different P-wave shape and abnormal P-wave axis. QRS morphology usually normal. See Figs. 7.8 and 7.9.[6]

AV, Atrioventricular; CHF, congestive heart failure; HR, heart rate; ICP, intracranial pressure; PE, pulmonary embolism; SA, sinoatrial; SVT, supraventricular tachycardia.

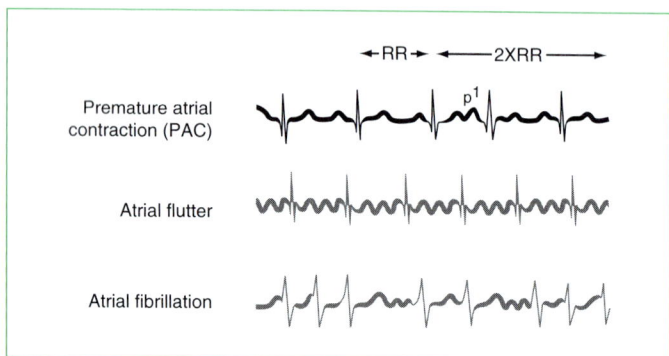

FIGURE 7.8

Supraventricular arrhythmias. p¹, Premature atrial contraction. *(From Park MK, Guntheroth WG. How to Read Pediatric ECGs. 4th ed. Philadelphia: Elsevier; 2006:129.)*

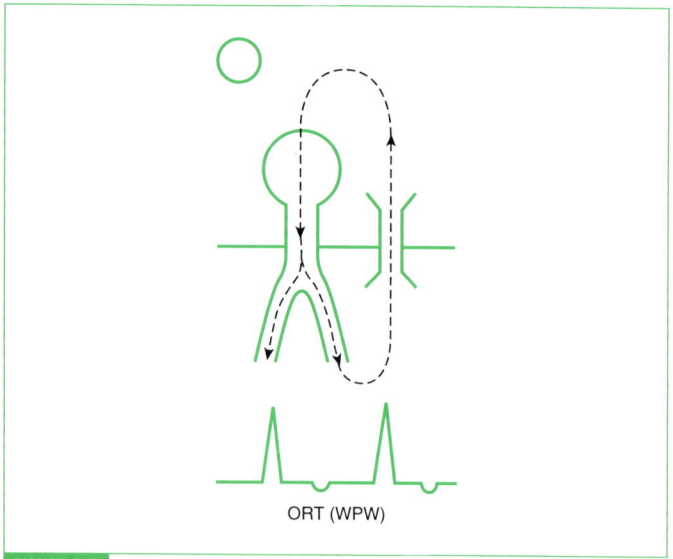

FIGURE 7.9

Supraventricular tachycardia pathway: Mechanism for orthodromic reciprocating tachycardia (ORT) [i.e., Wolff-Parkinson-White (WPW)]. The diagram shows sinoatrial (SA) node (upper left circle), with atrioventricular (AV) node (above horizontal line) and bundle branches crossing to the ventricle (below horizontal line). *(Adapted from Walsh EP. Cardiac arrhythmias. In: Fyler DC, ed. Nadas' Pediatric Cardiology. Philadelphia: Hanley & Belfus; 1992:384.)*

TABLE 7.7
VENTRICULAR ARRHYTHMIAS

Name/Description	Cause	Treatment
PREMATURE VENTRICULAR CONTRACTION (PVC)		
Ectopic ventricular focus causing early depolarization. Abnormally wide QRS complex appears prematurely, usually with full compensatory pause. May be unifocal or multifocal. **Bigeminy:** Alternating normal and abnormal QRS complexes. **Trigeminy:** Two normal QRS complexes followed by an abnormal one. **Couplet:** Two consecutive PVCs.	Myocarditis, myocardial injury, cardiomyopathy, long QT, congenital and acquired heart disease, drugs (catecholamines, theophylline, caffeine, anesthetics), MVP, anxiety, hypokalemia, hypoxia, hypomagnesemia. Can be normal variant.	None. More worrisome if associated with underlying heart disease or syncope, if worse with activity, or if they are multiform (especially couplets). Address underlying cause, rule out structural heart disease.
VENTRICULAR TACHYCARDIA		
Series of three or more PVCs at rapid rate (120–250 beats/min), with wide QRS complex and dissociated, retrograde, or no P wave	See causes of PVCs (70% have underlying cause).	See "Tachycardia with Poor Perfusion" and "Tachycardia with Adequate Perfusion" algorithms in back of handbook.
VENTRICULAR FIBRILLATION		
Depolarization of ventricles in uncoordinated asynchronous pattern, yielding abnormal QRS complexes of varying size and morphology with irregular, rapid rate. Rare in children.	Myocarditis, MI, postoperative state, digitalis or quinidine toxicity, catecholamines, severe hypoxia, electrolyte disturbances, long QT	Requires immediate defibrillation. See algorithm for "Asystole and Pulseless Arrest" at back of book.

MI, Myocardial infarction; MVP, mitral valve prolapse

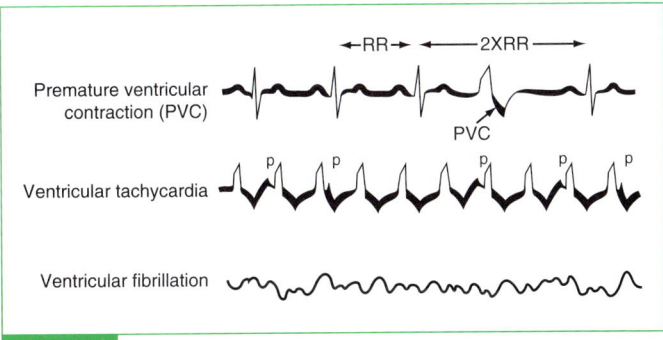

FIGURE 7.10

Ventricular arrhythmias. p, p wave; RR, R-R interval; PVC, premature ventricular contraction. *(From Park MK, Guntheroth WG. How to Read Pediatric ECGs. 4th ed. Philadelphia: Elsevier; 2006:138.)*

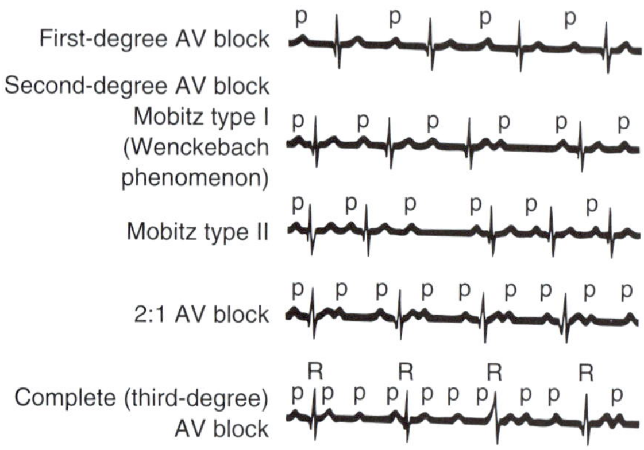

FIGURE 7.11

Conduction blocks. p, p wave; R, QRS complex. *(From Park MK, Guntheroth WG. How to Read Pediatric ECGs. 4th ed. Philadelphia: Elsevier; 2006:141.)*

TABLE 7.8

NONVENTRICULAR CONDUCTION DISTURBANCES

Name/Description*	Cause	Treatment
FIRST-DEGREE HEART BLOCK		
Abnormal but asymptomatic delay in conduction through AV node, yielding prolongation of PR interval	Acute rheumatic fever, tickborne (i.e., Lyme) disease, connective tissue disease, congenital heart disease, cardiomyopathy, digitalis toxicity, postoperative state, normal children	No specific treatment except address the underlying cause
SECOND-DEGREE HEART BLOCK: MOBITZ TYPE I (WENCKEBACH)		
Progressive lengthening of PR interval until a QRS complex is not conducted. Common finding in asymptomatic teenagers.	Myocarditis, cardiomyopathy, congenital heart disease, postoperative state, MI, toxicity (digitalis, β-blocker), normal children, Lyme disease, lupus	Address underlying cause, or none needed
SECOND-DEGREE HEART BLOCK: MOBITZ TYPE II		
Loss of conduction to ventricle without lengthening of the PR interval. May progress to complete heart block.	Same as for Mobitz type I	Address underlying cause; may need pacemaker
THIRD-DEGREE (COMPLETE) HEART BLOCK		
Complete dissociation of atrial and ventricular conduction, with atrial rate faster than ventricular rate. P wave and PP interval regular; RR interval regular and much slower.	Congenital due to maternal lupus or other connective tissue disease	If bradycardic and symptomatic, consider pacing; see bradycardia algorithm at back of book.

*High-degree AV block: Conduction of atrial impulse at regular intervals, yielding 2:1 block (two atrial impulses for each ventricular response), 3:1 block, etc.
AV, Atrioventricular; MI, myocardial infarction.

TABLE 7.9
VENTRICULAR CONDUCTION DISTURBANCES

Name/Description	Criteria	Causes/Treatment
RIGHT BUNDLE-BRANCH BLOCK (RBBB)		
Delayed right bundle conduction prolongs RV depolarization time, leading to wide QRS.	1. Prolonged or wide QRS with terminal slurred R' (m-shaped RSR' or RR') in V_1, V_2, aVR 2. Wide and slurred S wave in leads I and V_6	ASD, surgery with right ventriculotomy, occasionally seen in normal children
LEFT BUNDLE-BRANCH BLOCK (LBBB)		
Delayed left bundle conduction prolongs septal and LV depolarization time, leading to wide QRS with loss of usual septal signal; there is still a predominance of left ventricle forces. Rare in children.	1. Wide negative QRS complex in lead V_1 with loss of septal R wave 2. Wide R or RR' complex in lead V_6 with loss of septal Q wave	Hypertension, ischemic or valvular heart disease, cardiomyopathy
WOLFF-PARKINSON-WHITE (WPW)		
Atrial impulse transmitted via anomalous conduction pathway to ventricles, bypassing AV node and normal ventricular conduction system. Leads to early and prolonged depolarization of ventricles. Bypass pathway is a predisposing condition for SVT.	1. Shortened PR interval 2. Delta wave 3. Wide QRS	Acute management of SVT if necessary, as previously described; consider ablation of accessory pathway if recurrent SVT. All patients need cardiology referral.

ASD, Atrial septal defect; LV, left ventricle; RV, right ventricle; SVT, supraventricular tachycardia.

3. **Management:**
a. Congenital long QT is managed with β-blockers and/or defibrillators, and rarely requires cardiac sympathetic denervation or cardiac pacemakers.
b. Acquired long QT is managed by treatment of arrhythmias, discontinuation of precipitating drugs, and correction of metabolic abnormalities.

E. Hyperkalemia:
ECG changes dependent on the serum K+ level; however, the ECG may be normal with serum K+ levels between 2.5 and 6 mEq/L.
1. **Serum K^+ < 2.5 mEq/L:** Depressed ST segment, diphasic T wave
2. **Serum K^+ > 6 mEq/L:** Tall T wave
3. **Serum K^+ > 7.5 mEq/L:** Long PR interval, wide QRS, tall T wave
4. **Serum K^+ > 9 mEq/L:** Absent P wave, sinusoidal

TABLE 7.10
SYSTEMIC EFFECTS ON ELECTROCARDIOGRAM

	Short QT	Long QT-U	Prolonged QRS	ST-T Changes	Sinus Tachycardia	Sinus Bradycardia	AV Block	Ventricular Tachycardia	Miscellaneous
CHEMISTRY									
Hyperkalemia			X	X			X	X	Low-voltage Ps; peaked Ts
Hypokalemia		X		X					
Hypercalcemia	X					X	X		
Hypocalcemia		X			X		X	X	
Hypermagnesemia							X		
Hypomagnesemia		X							
DRUGS									
Digitalis	X			X		T	X	T	
Phenothiazines		T						T	
Phenytoin	X						X		
Propranolol	X					X	T		
Tricyclic antidepressants		T	T	T	T		T	T	
Verapamil						X	X		

MISCELLANEOUS

Condition							Notes
CNS injury	X					X	
Friedreich ataxia		X	X	X		X	Atrial flutter
Duchenne muscular dystrophy			X		X		Atrial flutter
Myotonic dystrophy	X	X	X			X	
Collagen vascular disease		X				X	X
Hypothyroidism				X			Low voltage
Hyperthyroidism	X	X	X			X	
Lyme disease	X					X	
Holt-Oram, maternal lupus						X	

CNS, Central nervous system; T, present only with drug toxicity; X, present

Data from Garson A Jr. The Electrocardiogram in Infants and Children: A Systematic Approach. Philadelphia: Lea & Febiger; 1983:172 and Walsh EP. Cardiac arrhythmias. In: Fyler DC, Nadas A, eds. Pediatric Cardiology. Philadelphia: Hanley & Belfus; 1992:141-143.

F. Myocardial Infarction (MI) in Children

1. **Etiology:** Anomalous origin or aberrant course of a coronary artery, Kawasaki disease, congenital heart disease (presurgical and postsurgical), and dilated cardiomyopathy. Less often associated with hypertension, lupus, myocarditis, cocaine ingestion, and use of adrenergic drugs (e.g., β-agonists used for asthma). Rare in children.
2. **Frequent ECG findings in children with acute MI**[10,11] (Fig. 7.12):
a. New-onset wide Q waves (>0.035 sec) seen within first few hours (persist over several years).
b. ST-segment elevation (>2 mm) seen within first few hours.
c. Diphasic T waves seen within first few days (becoming sharply inverted, then normalizing over time).
d. Prolonged QTc interval (>0.44 sec) with abnormal Q waves.
e. Deep, wide Q waves in leads I, aVL, or V_6 without Q waves in II, III, aVF, suggest anomalous origin of the left coronary artery.
3. **Other criteria:**
a. Elevated creatine kinase (CK)/MB fraction: Not specific for acute MI in children.
b. Cardiac troponin I: More sensitive indicator of early myocardial damage in children.[11] Becomes elevated within hours of cardiac injury, persists for 4–7 days is specific for cardiac injury.

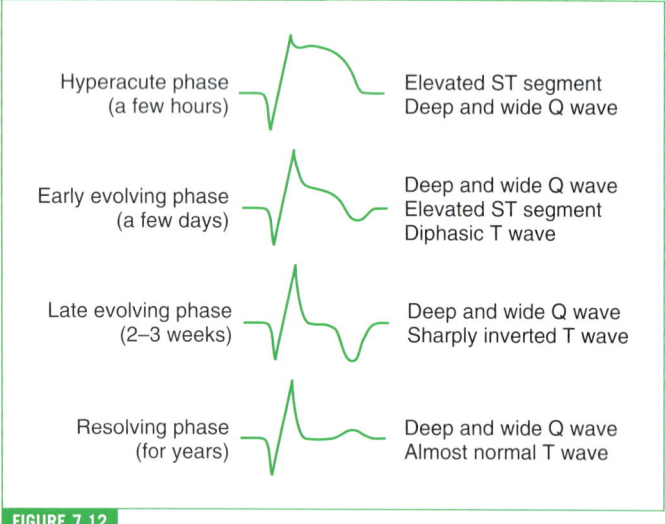

FIGURE 7.12

Sequential changes during myocardial infarction (MI). *(From Park MK, Guntheroth WG. How to Read Pediatric ECGs. 4th ed. Philadelphia: Elsevier; 2006:115.)*

IV. IMAGING

A. Chest Radiograph
Please see Chapter 25 for more information on chest radiography.
1. **Evaluate the heart:**
a. Size: Cardiac shadow should be <50% of thoracic width (i.e., maximal width between inner margins of ribs, as measured on a posteroanterior radiograph during inspiration).
b. Shape: Can aid in diagnosis of chamber/vessel enlargement and some congenital heart diseases (Fig. 7.13).
c. Situs (levocardia, mesocardia, dextrocardia).
2. **Evaluate the lung fields:**
a. Decreased pulmonary blood flow: Seen in pulmonary or tricuspid stenosis/atresia, tetralogy of Fallot (TOF), and pulmonary hypertension (peripheral pruning).
b. Increased pulmonary blood flow is seen as increased pulmonary vascular markings (PVMs) with redistribution from the bases to the apices of the lungs and extension to lateral lung fields (see Tables 7.12 and 7.13).
c. Venous congestion, or congestive heart failure (CHF): Increased central PVMs, interstitial and alveolar pulmonary edema (air bronchograms), septal lines, and pleural effusions (see Tables 7.12 and 7.13).

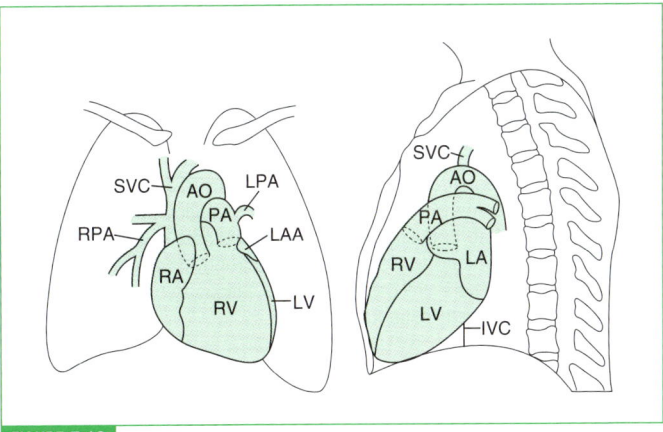

FIGURE 7.13
Radiological contours of the heart. AO, Aorta; IVC, inferior vena cava; LA, left atrium; LAA, left atrial appendage; LPA, left pulmonary artery; LV, left ventricle; PA, pulmonary artery; RA, right atrium; RPA, right pulmonary artery; RV, right ventricle; SVC, superior vena cava.

3. **Evaluate the trachea:**
Usually bends slightly to the right above the carina in normal patients with a left-sided aortic arch. A perfectly straight or left-bending trachea suggests a right aortic arch, which may be associated with other defects (e.g., TOF, truncus arteriosus, vascular rings, chromosome 22 microdeletion).
4. **Skeletal anomalies:**
a. Rib notching (e.g., from collateral vessels in patients aged >5 years with coarctation of the aorta)
b. Sternal abnormalities (e.g., Holt-Oram syndrome, pectus excavatum in Marfan, Ehlers-Danlos, and Noonan syndromes)
c. Vertebral anomalies (e.g., VATER/VACTERL syndrome: **V**ertebral anomalies, **A**nal atresia, **T**rach**e**oesophageal fistula, **R**adial and **R**enal, **C**ardiac, and **L**imb anomalies)

B. Echocardiography

1. **Approach:**
a. Transthoracic echocardiography (TTE) does not require general anesthesia and is simpler to perform than transesophageal echocardiography (TEE); however, it does have limitations in some patients (e.g., uncooperative and obese patients, or those with suspected endocarditis).
b. TEE uses an ultrasound transducer on the end of a modified endoscope to view the heart from the esophagus and stomach, allowing for better imaging of intracardiac structures. TEE also allows for better imaging in obese and intraoperative patients, and is useful for visualizing very small lesions, such as some vegetations.
2. **Shortening fraction (FS):**
Very reliable index of left ventricular function. Normal values range from 30%–45%, depending on age.[12]
For more information on echocardiography see Expert Consult, Chapter 7.

C. Cardiac Catheterization[13,14]

1. Performed in pediatric patients for both diagnostic and interventional purposes, including pressure measurements, angiography, embolization of abnormal vessels, dilation of atretic valves and vessels, device closure of cardiac defects, and electrophysiology procedures to mention a few. There are potential complications to be aware of when caring for a post-cath patient:
a. Common: arrhythmias (SVT, AV block, bradycardia, etc.), vascular complications (thrombosis, perforation, decreased/absent pulses), intervention-related (balloon rupture, device embolization, etc.), and bleeding.
b. Other complications include myocardial/vessel staining, cardiac perforation, cardiac tamponade, air embolus, infection, allergic reaction, cardiac arrest, and death.
See Fig. EC 7.A for a diagram of normal pressure values.

V. CONGENITAL HEART DISEASE

A. Pulse Oximetry Screening for Critical Congenital Heart Disease

1. **To be done as late as possible but before discharge from nursery, preferably >24 hours of life due to decreased false-positive rate.** Recommended to use the right hand and one foot, either in parallel or direct sequence.
2. **The screening result would be considered positive if:**
   a. Any oxygen saturation measure is <90%.
   b. Oxygen saturation is <95% in both extremities on 3 measures, each separated by 1 hour.
   c. There is a >3% absolute difference in oxygen saturation between the right hand and foot on three measures, each separated by 1 hour.

B. Common Syndromes Associated With Cardiac Lesions (Table 7.11)

C. Acyanotic Lesions (Table 7.12)

D. Cyanotic Lesions (Table 7.13)

A hyperoxia test is used to evaluate the etiology of cyanosis in neonates. A baseline arterial blood gas (ABG) with saturation at $FiO_2 = 0.21$ is obtained. Then, the infant is placed in an oxygen hood at $FiO_2 = 1$ for a minimum of 10 min, and the ABG is repeated. In cardiac disease, there

TABLE 7.11
MAJOR SYNDROMES ASSOCIATED WITH CARDIAC DEFECTS

Syndrome	Dominant Cardiac Defect
CHARGE	TOF, truncus arteriosus, aortic arch abnormalities
DiGeorge	Aortic arch anomalies, TOF, truncus arteriosus, VSD, PDA
Trisomy 21	Atrioventricular septal defect, VSD
Marfan	Aortic root dilation, mitral valve prolapse
Loeys-Dietz	Aortic root dilation with higher risk of rupture at smaller dimensions
Noonan	Supravalvular pulmonic stenosis, LVH
Turner	COA, bicuspid aortic valve, aortic root dilation as a teenager
Williams	Supravalvular aortic stenosis, pulmonary artery stenosis
FAS	Occasional: VSD, PDA, ASD, TOF
IDM	TGA, VSD, COA, cardiomyopathy
VATER/VACTERL	VSD
VCFS	Truncus arteriosus, TOF, pulmonary atresia with VSD, TGA, interrupted aortic arch

ASD, Atrial septal defect; CHARGE, a syndrome of associated defects including **C**oloboma of the eye, **H**eart anomaly, choanal **A**tresia, **R**etardation, and **G**enital and **E**ar anomalies; COA, coarctation of aorta; FAS, fetal alcohol syndrome; IDM, infant of diabetic mother; LVH, left ventricular hypertrophy; PDA, patent ductus arteriosus; TGA, transposition of the great arteries; TOF, tetralogy of Fallot; VATER/VACTERL, association of **V**ertebral anomalies, **A**nal atresia, **C**ardiac anomalies, **T**racheo**e**sophageal fistula, **R**enal/radial anomalies, **L**imb defects; VCFS, velocardiofacial syndrome; VSD, ventricular septal defect.
Adapted from Park MK. Pediatric Cardiology for Practitioners. 5th ed. St Louis: Elsevier; 2008:10-12.

TABLE 7.12
ACYANOTIC CONGENITAL HEART DISEASE

Lesion Type	% of CHD/Examination Findings	ECG Findings	Chest Radiograph Findings
Ventricular septal defect (VSD)	2–5/6 holosystolic murmur, loudest at the LLSB, ± systolic thrill ± apical diastolic rumble with large shunt With large VSD and pulmonary hypertension, S_2 may be narrow	Small VSD: Normal Medium VSD: LVH ± LAE Large VSD: BVH ± LAE, pure RVH	May show cardiomegaly and increased PVMs, depending on amount of left-to-right shunting
Atrial septal defect (ASD)	Wide, fixed split S_2 with grade 2–3/6 SEM at the LUSB May have mid-diastolic rumble at LLSB	Small ASD: Normal Large ASD: RAD and mild RVH or RBBB with RSR′ in V_1	May show cardiomegaly with increased PVMs if hemodynamically significant ASD
Patent ductus arteriosus (PDA)	40%–60% in VLBW infants 1–4/6 continuous "machinery" murmur loudest at LUSB Wide pulse pressure	Small–moderate PDA: Normal or LVH Large PDA: BVH	May have cardiomegaly and increased PVMs, depending on size of shunt (see Chapter 18, Section IX.A, for treatment)
Atrioventricular septal defects	Most occur in Down syndrome Hyperactive precordium with systolic thrill at LLSB and loud S_2 ± grade 3–4/6 holosystolic regurgitant murmur along LLSB ± systolic murmur of MR at apex ± mid-diastolic rumble at LLSB or at apex ± gallop rhythm	Superior QRS axis RVH and LVH may be present	Cardiomegaly with increased PVMs
Pulmonary stenosis (PS)	Ejection click at LUSB with valvular PS—click intensity varies with respiration, decreasing with inspiration and increasing with expiration S_2 may split widely with P_2 diminished in intensity SEM (2–5/6) ± thrill at LUSB with radiation to back and sides	Mild PS: Normal Moderate PS: RAD and RVH Severe PS: RAE and RVH with strain	Normal heart size with normal to decreased PVMs

TABLE 7.12
ACYANOTIC CONGENITAL HEART DISEASE—cont'd

Lesion Type	% of CHD/Examination Findings	ECG Findings	Chest Radiograph Findings
Aortic stenosis (AS)	Systolic thrill at RUSB, suprasternal notch, or over carotids Ejection click that does not vary with respiration if valvular AS Harsh SEM (2–4/6) at second RICS or third LICS, with radiation to neck and apex ± early diastolic decrescendo murmur due to AR Narrow pulse pressure if severe stenosis	Mild AS: Normal Moderate–severe AS: LVH ± strain	Usually normal
Coarctation of aorta may present as: 1. Infant in CHF 2. Child with HTN 3. Child with murmur	Male/female ratio of 2:1 2–3/6 SEM at LUSB, radiating to left interscapular area Bicuspid valve is often associated, so may have systolic ejection click at apex and RUSB BP in lower extremities will be lower than in upper extremities. Pulse oximetry discrepancy of >5% between upper and lower extremities is also suggestive of coarctation.	*In infancy:* RVH or RBBB *In older children:* LVH	Marked cardiomegaly and pulmonary venous congestion. Rib notching from collateral circulation usually not seen in children younger than 5 years because collaterals not yet established.

AR, Aortic regurgitation; ASD, atrial septal defect; BP, blood pressure; BVH, biventricular hypertrophy; CDG, congenital disorders of glycosylation; CHD, congenital heart disease; CHF, congestive heart failure; HTN, hypertension; LAE, left atrial enlargement; LICS, left intercostal space; LLSB, left lower sternal border; LUSB, left upper sternal border; LVH, left ventricular hypertrophy; MR, mitral regurgitation; PVM, pulmonary vascular markings; RAD, right axis deviation; RAE, right atrial enlargement; RBBB, right bundle-branch block; RICS, right intercostal space; RUSB, right upper sternal border; RVH, right ventricular hypertrophy; SEM, systolic ejection murmur; VLBW, very low birth weight (i.e. <1500 g); VSD, ventricular septal defect.

will not be a significant change in PaO$_2$ following the oxygen challenge test. A PaO$_2$ of >200 after exposure to FiO$_2$ of 1.0 is considered normal, and >150 indicates pulmonary rather than cardiac disease. **Note:** Pulse oximetry is not useful for following changes in oxygenation once saturation has reached 100% (approximately a PaO$_2$ of >90 mmHg).[12-17]

1. See Table EC 7.B for interpretation of oxygen challenge test (hyperoxia test).
2. Table 7.14 shows acute management of hypercyanotic spells in TOF.

TABLE 7.13
CYANOTIC CONGENITAL HEART DISEASE

Lesion	Examination Findings	ECG Findings	Chest Radiograph Findings
Tetralogy of Fallot: 1. Large VSD 2. RVOT obstruction 3. RVH 4. Overriding aorta Degree of RVOT obstruction will determine whether there is clinical cyanosis. If PS is mild, there will be a left-to-right shunt, and child will be acyanotic. Increased obstruction leads to increased right-to-left shunting across VSD, and child will be cyanotic.	Loud SEM at LMSB and LUSB and a loud, single S_2 ± thrill at LMSB and LLSB. *Tet spells:* Occur in young infants. As RVOT obstruction increases or systemic resistance decreases, right-to-left shunting across VSD occurs. May present with tachypnea, increasing cyanosis, and decreasing murmur. See Table 7.14 for treatment.	RAD and RVH	Boot-shaped heart with normal heart size ± decreased PVMs
Transposition of great arteries	Nonspecific. Extreme cyanosis. Loud, single S_2. No murmur unless there is associated VSD or PS.	RAD and RVH (due to RV acting as systemic ventricle). Upright T wave in V_1 after age 3 days may be only abnormality.	Classic finding: "egg on a string" with cardiomegaly; possible increased PVMs
Tricuspid atresia: Absent tricuspid valve and hypoplastic RV and PA. Must have ASD, PDA, or VSD to survive.	Single S_2 + grade 2–3/6 systolic regurgitation murmur at LLSB if VSD is present. Occasional PDA murmur.	Superior QRS axis; RAE or CAE and LVH	Normal or slightly enlarged heart size; may have boot-shaped heart
Total anomalous pulmonary venous return Instead of draining into LA, pulmonary veins drain into the following locations. Must have ASD or PFO for survival: *Supracardiac (most common):* SVC *Cardiac:* Coronary sinus or RA *Subdiaphragmatic:* IVC, portal vein, ductus venosus, or hepatic vein *Mixed type*	Hyperactive RV impulse, quadruple rhythm, S_2 fixed and widely split, 2–3/6 SEM at LUSB, and mid-diastolic rumble at LLSB	RAD, RVH (RSR' in V_1). May see RAE	Cardiomegaly and increased PVMs; classic finding is "snowman in a snowstorm," but this is rarely seen until after age 4 months.

TABLE 7.13
CYANOTIC CONGENITAL HEART DISEASE—cont'd

Lesion	Examination Findings	ECG Findings	Chest Radiograph Findings
OTHER			
Cyanotic CHDs that occur at a frequency of <1% each include pulmonary atresia, Ebstein anomaly, truncus arteriosus, single ventricle, and double outlet right ventricle			

ASD, Atrial septal defect; CAE, common atrial enlargement; ECG, electrocardiogram; IVC, inferior vena cava; LA, left atrium; LLSB, left lower sternal border; LMSB, left midsternal border; LUSB, left upper sternal border; LVH, left ventricular hypertrophy; PA, pulmonary artery; PDA, patent ductus arteriosus; PFO, patent foramen ovale; PVM, pulmonary vascular markings; PS, pulmonary stenosis; RA, right atrium; RAD, right-axis deviation; RAE, right atrial enlargement; RV, right ventricle; RVH, right ventricular hypertrophy; RVOT, right ventricular outflow tract; SEM, systolic ejection murmur; SVC, superior vena cava; VSD, ventricular septal defect.

TABLE 7.14
TREATMENT OPTIONS FOR TET SPELLS

Treatment	Rationale
INITIAL OPTIONS	
Calm child	Decreases PVR
Encourage knee-chest position	Decreases venous return and increases SVR
Oxygen	Reduces hypoxemia, decreases PVR
IV fluids	Provides volume resuscitation
Morphine (morphine sulfate 0.1–0.2 mg/kg SQ or IM)	Decreases venous return, decreases PVR, relaxes infundibulum. Do *not* try to establish IV access initially; use SQ route.
IF THERE IS NO RESPONSE TO INITIAL MEASURES	
Phenylephrine (0.02 mg/kg IV)	Increases SVR
Propranolol (0.15–0.25 mg/kg slow IV push)	Has negative inotropic effect on infundibular myocardium; may block drop in SVR
Ketamine (0.25–1 mg/kg IV)	Increases SVR and sedates
OTHER	
Correct anemia	Increases delivery of oxygen to tissues
Correct pathologic tachyarrhythmias	May abort hypoxic spell
Infuse glucose	Avoids hypoglycemia from increased utilization and depletion of glycogen stores

IM, Intramuscular; IV, intravenous; PVR, peripheral venous resistance; SQ, subcutaneous; SVR, systemic vascular resistance
From Park MK. Pediatric Cardiology for Practitioners. 5th ed. St Louis: Elsevier; 2008:239.

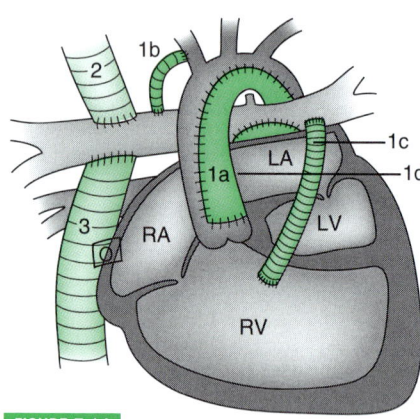

FIGURE 7.14

Schematic diagram of cardiac shunts, including the modified Blalock-Taussig (BT), Sano modification, bidirectional Glenn, and Fontan shunts.

E. Surgeries and Other Interventions (Fig. 7.14)

1. **Atrial septostomy:** Creates an intra-atrial opening to allow for mixing or shunting between atria of systemic and pulmonary venous blood. Used for transposition of the great arteries (TGA) and hypoplastic left heart syndrome (HLHS) with restrictive atrial septum; less commonly, used for tricuspid, mitral, aortic, and pulmonary atresia, and sometimes total anomalous pulmonary venous return. Most commonly performed percutaneously with a balloon-tipped catheter (Rashkind procedure).
2. **Palliative systemic–to–pulmonary artery shunts,** such as the Blalock-Taussig shunt [subclavian artery to pulmonary artery (PA)]: Use systemic arterial flow to increase pulmonary blood flow in cardiac lesions with impaired pulmonary perfusion (e.g., TOF, hypoplastic right heart, tricuspid atresia, pulmonary atresia).
3. **Palliative superior vena cava–to–pulmonary artery shunts,** such as the Glenn shunt or the hemi-Fontan [superior vena cava to the right pulmonary artery (RPA)]: Directs a portion of the systemic venous return directly into the pulmonary blood flow as an intermediate step to a Fontan procedure. This procedure is usually performed outside the neonatal period, when there is lower pulmonary vascular resistance.
4. **The Fontan procedure:** Performed after the Glenn shunt; involves anastomosis of the right atria and/or inferior vena cava to pulmonary arteries via conduits or creating a right atrial tunnel; separates

systemic and pulmonary circulations in patients with functionally single ventricles (tricuspid atresia, HLHS).
5. **The Norwood procedure:** Used for HLHS.
a. Stage 1 (neonatal period): To provide systemic blood flow, anastomosis of the proximal main pulmonary artery (MPA) is made to the aorta with aortic arch reconstruction and patch closure of the distal MPA. To provide pulmonary blood flow, a modified right Blalock-Taussig shunt (subclavian artery to RPA) or Sano modification (RV to PA conduit) is performed. An atrialseptal defect is created if needed to decompress the left atrium and allow for adequate left-to-right flow. Expected O_2 saturations: 75%–85%.
b. Stage 2 (3–6 months of age): Bidirectional Glenn shunt or hemi-Fontan to reduce volume overload of single right ventricle. Expected O_2 saturations: 80%–85%.
c. Modified Fontan (age 18 mo–4 yr): Needed to completely separate systemic and pulmonary circulations. Restores normal O_2 saturation, with an expected O_2 saturation >92%.
6. **Arterial switch procedure**: Used for repair TGA. Connects the aorta to left ventricle and pulmonary artery to right ventricle. Procedure also involves reconnecting coronary arteries to aorta.
7. **Ross procedure:** Pulmonary root autograft for aortic stenosis; autologous pulmonary valve replaces aortic valve, and aortic or pulmonary allograft replaces pulmonary valve.

VI. ACQUIRED HEART DISEASE
A. Endocarditis
1. **Common causative organisms:** Approximately 70% of endocarditis is caused by streptococcal species (*Streptococcus viridans,* enterococci), 20% by staphylococcal species (*Staphylococcus aureus, Staphylococcus epidermidis*), and 10% by other organisms (*Haemophilus influenzae,* gram-negative bacteria, fungi).
2. **Clinical findings** include a new heart murmur, recurrent fever, splenomegaly, petechiae, fatigue, Osler nodes (tender nodules at the fingertips), Janeway lesions (painless hemorrhagic areas on the palms or soles), splinter hemorrhages, and Roth spots (retinal hemorrhages).

B. Bacterial Endocarditis Prophylaxis
See Table 7.15 for antibiotic choices and Box 7.4 for cardiac conditions requiring prophylaxis.[18]
1. **All dental procedures** that involve treatment of gingival tissue, the periapical region of the teeth, or oral mucosal perforation
2. **Invasive procedures** that involve incision or biopsy of respiratory mucosa, such as tonsillectomy and adenoidectomy
3. **Not recommended** for genitourinary or gastrointestinal tract procedures; solely for bacterial endocarditis prevention

TABLE 7.15
PROPHYLACTIC REGIMENS FOR DENTAL AND RESPIRATORY TRACT PROCEDURES

Drug	Dosing* (not to exceed adult dose)
Amoxicillin[†]	Adult: 2 g; Child: 50 mg/kg PO
Ampicillin	Adult: 2 g; Child: 50 mg/kg IM/IV
Cefazolin or ceftriaxone[‡]	Adult: 1 g; Child: 50 mg/kg IM/IV
Cephalexin[‡]	Adult: 2 g; Child: 50 mg/kg PO
Clindamycin	Adult: 600 mg; Child: 20 mg/kg PO/IM/IV
Azithromycin/clarithromycin	Adult: 500 mg; Child: 15 mg/kg PO

*Oral (PO) medications should be given 1 hour before procedure; intramuscular/intravenous (IM/IV) medications should be given within 30 min prior to procedure.
[†]Standard general prophylaxis
[‡]Cephalosporins should not be used in persons with intermediate-type hypersensitivity reaction to penicillins or ampicillin.
Adapted from Wilson W, Taubert KA, Gewitz M, et al. Prevention of infective endocarditis: Guidelines from the American Heart Association: A guideline from the American Heart Association Rheumatic Fever, Endocarditis, and Kawasaki Disease Committee, Council on Cardiovascular Disease in the Young, and the Council on Clinical Cardiology, Council on Cardiovascular Surgery and Anesthesia, and the Quality of Care and Outcomes Research Interdisciplinary Working Group. Circulation. 2007;116(15):1736-1754.

BOX 7.4
CARDIAC CONDITIONS FOR WHICH ANTIBIOTIC PROPHYLAXIS IS RECOMMENDED FOR DENTAL, RESPIRATORY TRACT, INFECTED SKIN, SKIN STRUCTURES, OR MUSCULOSKELETAL TISSUE PROCEDURES

- Prosthetic cardiac valve
- Previous bacterial endocarditis
- Congenital heart disease (CHD)—Limited to the following conditions[1]
  - Unrepaired cyanotic defect, including palliative shunts and conduits
  - Completely repaired CHD with prosthetic material/device (placed by surgery or catheterization), during first 6 months after procedure[2]
  - Repaired CHD with residual defects at or adjacent to the site of prosthetic patch or device (which inhibit endothelialization)
  - Cardiac transplantation patients who develop cardiac valvulopathy

[1]Conditions associated with the highest risk of adverse outcome from endocarditis.
[2]Endothelialization process of prosthetic material occurs within 6 months after the procedure.
Data from Wilson W, Taubert KA, Gewitz M, et al. Prevention of infective endocarditis: Guidelines from the American Heart Association: A guideline from the American Heart Association Rheumatic Fever, Endocarditis, and Kawasaki Disease Committee, Council on Cardiovascular Disease in the Young, and the Council on Clinical Cardiology, Council on Cardiovascular Surgery and Anesthesia, and the Quality of Care and Outcomes Research Interdisciplinary Working Group. Circulation. 2007;116(15):1736-1754.

C. Myocardial Disease

1. **Dilated cardiomyopathy:** End result of myocardial damage, leading to atrial and ventricular dilation with decreased systolic contractile function of the ventricles.
  a. Etiology: Infectious, toxic (alcohol, anthracyclines), metabolic (hypothyroidism, muscular dystrophy), immunologic, collagen vascular disease, nutritional deficiency (kwashiorkor, beriberi)
  b. Symptoms: Fatigue, weakness, shortness of breath
  c. Examination: Look for signs of CHF (e.g., tachycardia, tachypnea, rales, cold extremities, jugular venous distention, hepatomegaly, peripheral edema, S_3 gallop, displacement of point of maximal impulse to the left and inferiorly).
  d. Chest radiograph: Generalized cardiomegaly, pulmonary congestion
  e. ECG: Sinus tachycardia, left ventricular hypertrophy (LVH), possible atrial enlargement, arrhythmias, conduction disturbances, and ST-segment and T-wave changes
  f. Echocardiography: Enlarged ventricles (increased end-diastolic and end-systolic dimensions) with little or no wall thickening; decreased shortening fraction
  g. Treatment: Management of CHF [digoxin, diuretics, vasodilation, angiotensin-converting enzyme (ACE) inhibitors, and rest]. Anticoagulants should be considered to decrease the risk of thrombus formation. Cardiac transplant may eventually be required.

2. **Hypertrophic cardiomyopathy:** Abnormality of myocardial cells leading to significant ventricular hypertrophy, particularly of left ventricle, with small to normal ventricular dimensions. Increased contractile function but impaired filling secondary to stiff ventricles. The most common type is asymmetrical septal hypertrophy, also called *idiopathic hypertrophic subaortic stenosis*, with varying degrees of obstruction. A 4%–6% incidence of sudden death in children and adolescents with hypertrophic obstructive cardiomyopathy.
  a. Etiology: Genetic (autosomal dominant, 60% of cases) or sporadic (40% of cases)
  b. Symptoms: Easy fatigability, anginal pain, shortness of breath, occasional palpitations
  c. Examination: Usually in adolescents or young adults; signs include left ventricular heave, sharp upstroke of arterial pulse, murmur of mitral regurgitation, midsystolic ejection murmur along left midsternal border (LMSB) that increases in intensity in the standing position (in patients with midcavity left ventricular obstruction).
  d. Chest radiograph: Globular-shaped heart with left ventricular enlargement
  e. ECG: LVH, prominent Q waves (septal hypertrophy), ST-segment and T-wave changes, arrhythmias
  f. Echocardiography: Extent and location of hypertrophy, obstruction, increased contractility

g. Treatment: Moderate restriction of physical activity, administration of negative inotropes (β-blocker, calcium channel blocker) to help improve filling, and subacute bacterial endocarditis prophylaxis. If at increased risk for sudden death, may consider implantable defibrillator. If symptomatic with subaortic obstruction, may benefit from myectomy.
3. **Restrictive cardiomyopathy:** Myocardial or endocardial disease (usually infiltrative or fibrotic), resulting in stiff ventricular walls with restriction of diastolic filling but normal contractile function. Results in atrial enlargement. Associated with a high mortality rate. Very rare in children.
a. Etiology: Scleroderma, amyloidosis, sarcoidosis, mucopolysaccharidosis
b. Treatment: Supportive, poor prognosis. Diuretics, anticoagulants, calcium channel blockers, a pacemaker for heart block, cardiac transplantation if severe.
4. **Myocarditis:** Inflammation of myocardial tissue
a. Etiology: Viral (Coxsackie virus, echovirus, adenovirus, poliomyelitis, mumps, measles, rubella, cytomegalovirus, HIV, arbovirus, influenza); bacterial, rickettsial, fungal, or parasitic infection; immune-mediated disease (Kawasaki disease, acute rheumatic fever); collagen vascular disease; toxin-induced.
b. Symptoms: Nonspecific and inconsistent, depending on severity of disease. Variably anorexia, lethargy, emesis, lightheadedness, cold extremities, shortness of breath.
c. Examination: Look for signs of CHF (tachycardia, tachypnea, jugular venous distention, rales, gallop, hepatomegaly); occasionally a soft systolic murmur or arrhythmia may be noted.
d. Chest radiograph: Variable cardiomegaly and pulmonary edema
e. ECG: Low QRS voltages throughout (<5 mm), ST-segment and T-wave changes (e.g., decreased T-wave amplitude), prolongation of QT interval, arrhythmias (especially premature contractions, first- or second-degree AV block)
f. Laboratory tests: CK, troponin
g. Echocardiography: Enlargement of heart chambers, impaired left ventricular function
h. Treatment: Bed rest, diuretics, inotropes (dopamine, dobutamine, milrinone), digoxin, gamma globulin (2 g/kg over 24 hours), ACE inhibitors, possibly steroids. May require heart transplantation if no improvement ($\approx$20%–25% of cases).

D. Pericardial Disease

1. **Pericarditis:** Inflammation of visceral and parietal layers of pericardium
a. Etiology: Viral (especially echovirus, Coxsackie virus B), tuberculosis, bacterial, uremic, neoplastic, collagen vascular, post-MI or post-pericardiotomy, radiation-induced, drug-induced (e.g., procainamide, hydralazine), or idiopathic

b. Symptoms: Chest pain (retrosternal or precordial, radiating to back or shoulder, pleuritic in nature, alleviated by leaning forward, aggravated by supine position), dyspnea
c. Examination: Pericardial friction rub, distant heart sounds, fever, tachypnea
d. ECG: Diffuse ST-segment elevation in almost all leads (representing inflammation of adjacent myocardium); PR-segment depression
e. Treatment: Often self-limited. Treat underlying condition and provide symptomatic treatment with rest, analgesia, and antiinflammatory drugs

2. **Pericardial effusion:** Accumulation of excess fluid in pericardial sac
a. Etiology: Associated with acute pericarditis (exudative fluid) or serous effusion resulting from increased capillary hydrostatic pressure (e.g., CHF), decreased plasma oncotic pressure (e.g., hypoproteinemia), and increased capillary permeability (transudative fluid).
b. Symptoms: Can present with no symptoms, dull ache in left chest, abdominal pain, or symptoms of cardiac tamponade (see later).
c. Examination: Muffled distant heart sounds, dullness to percussion of posterior left chest (secondary to atelectasis from large pericardial sac), hemodynamic signs of cardiac compression
d. Chest radiograph: Globular symmetrical cardiomegaly
e. ECG: Decreased voltage of QRS complexes, electrical alternans (variation of QRS axis with each beat secondary to swinging of heart within pericardial fluid)
f. Echocardiography shows extent and location of hypertrophy, obstruction, increased contractility.
g. Treatment: Address underlying condition. Observe if asymptomatic; use pericardiocentesis if there is sudden increase in volume or hemodynamic compromise. Nonsteroidal antiinflammatory drugs (NSAIDs) or steroids may be of benefit, depending on etiology.

3. **Cardiac tamponade:** Accumulation of pericardial fluid under high pressure, causing compression of cardiac chambers, limiting filling, and decreasing stroke volume and cardiac output.
a. Etiology: Same as pericardial effusion; most commonly associated with viral infection, neoplasm, uremia, and acute hemorrhage.
b. Symptoms: Dyspnea, fatigue, cold extremities
c. Examination: Jugular venous distention, hepatomegaly, peripheral edema, tachypnea, rales (from increased systemic and pulmonary venous pressure), hypotension, tachycardia, pulsus paradoxus (decrease in SBP by >10 mmHg with each inspiration), decreased capillary refill (from decreased stroke volume and cardiac output), quiet precordium, and muffled heart sounds
d. ECG: Sinus tachycardia, decreased voltage, electrical alternans
e. Echocardiography: Right ventricular collapse in early diastole, right atrial/left atrial collapse in end-diastole and early systole

f. Treatment: Pericardiocentesis with temporary catheter left in place if necessary (see Fig. 3.12); pericardial window or stripping if it is a recurrent condition

E. Kawasaki Disease[19]

Acute febrile vasculitis of unknown etiology, common in children aged <8 years, and is the leading cause of acquired childhood heart disease in developed countries.

1. **Etiology:** Unknown; thought to be immune regulated in response to infectious agents or environmental toxins.
2. **Diagnosis:**
a. Typical Kawasaki disease: Based on clinical criteria. These include high fever lasting 5 days or more, plus at least 4 of the following 5 criteria:
    (1) Bilateral, painless, bulbar conjunctival injection without exudate
    (2) Erythematous mouth and pharynx, strawberry tongue, or red cracked lips
    (3) Polymorphous exanthem (may be morbilliform, maculopapular, or scarlatiniform)
    (4) Swelling of hands and feet with erythema of palms and soles
    (5) Cervical lymphadenopathy (>1.5 cm in diameter), usually single and unilateral
b. Atypical/incomplete Kawasaki disease: A suspicion of Kawasaki disease but with fewer of the criteria required for diagnosis. Even without all criteria, there is a risk for coronary artery abnormalities.
    (1) More often seen in infants. Echocardiography should be considered in any infant <6 months with fever >7 days duration, laboratory evidence of systemic inflammation, and no other explanation for the febrile illness.
    (2) See Fig. 7.15 for evaluation of incomplete Kawasaki disease.
    (3) Supplemental laboratory criteria: Albumin ≤3.0 g/dL, anemia for age, elevation of alanine aminotransferase, platelets after 7 days ≥ 450,000/mm^3, white blood cell count ≥15,000/mm^3, and urine white blood cells/hpf ≥10.
3. **Other clinical findings:** Often associated with extreme irritability, abdominal pain, diarrhea, vomiting. Also seen are arthritis and arthralgias, hepatic enlargement, jaundice, acute acalculous distention of the gallbladder, carditis, aseptic meningitis (50% of those undergoing LP).
4. **Laboratory findings:** Leukocytosis with left shift, neutrophils with vacuoles or toxic granules, elevated C-reactive protein (CRP) or erythrocyte sedimentation rate (ESR) (seen acutely), thrombocytosis (after first week, peaking at 3 weeks), normocytic and normochromic anemia, sterile pyuria (33%), increased transaminases (40%), hyperbilirubinemia (10%).

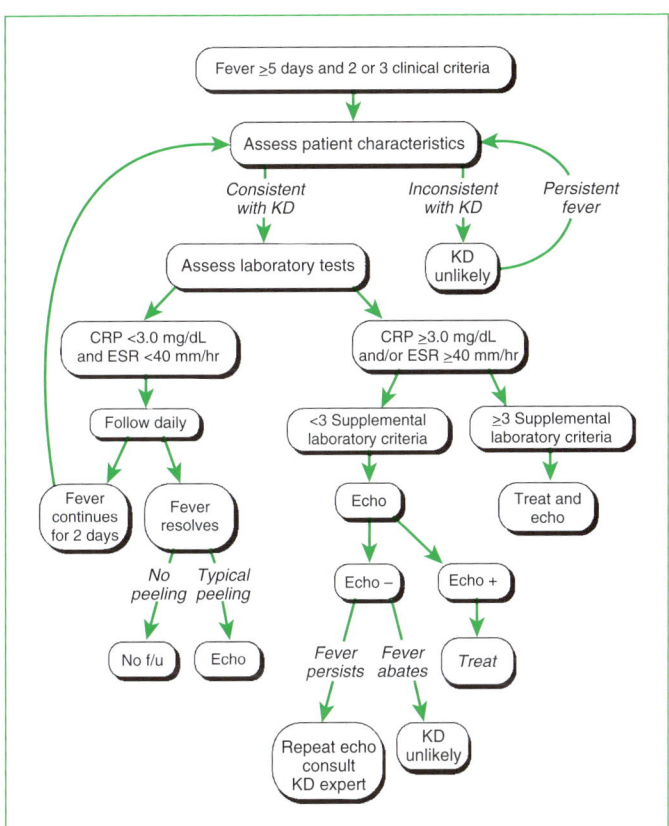

FIGURE 7.15

Evaluation of incomplete Kawasaki disease (KD). CRP, C-reactive protein; echo, echocardiogram; ESR, erythrocyte sedimentation rate; f/u, follow-up. *(From Newburger JW, Takahashi M, Gerber MA, et al. Diagnosis, treatment, and long-term management of Kawasaki disease, Council on Cardiovascular Disease in the Young, American Heart Association.. Circulation. 2004;110(17):2747-2771.)*

5. **Subacute phase (11–25 days after onset of illness):** Resolution of fever, rash, and lymphadenopathy. Often, desquamation of the fingertips or toes and thrombocytosis occur.
   Cardiovascular complications: If untreated, 20%–25% develop coronary artery aneurysms and dilation in subacute phase (peak prevalence occurs about 2–4 weeks after onset of disease; rarely appears after 6 weeks) and are at risk for coronary thrombosis acutely and coronary stenosis chronically. Carditis; aortic, mitral, and tricuspid

regurgitation; pericardial effusion; CHF; MI; left ventricular dysfunction; and ECG changes may also occur.

6. **Convalescent phase:** ESR, CRP, and platelet count return to normal. Those with coronary artery abnormalities are at increased risk for MI, arrhythmias, and sudden death.
7. **Management** (see also Table EC 7.C)[19]
a. Intravenous immunoglobulin (IVIG)
   (1) Shown to reduce incidence of coronary artery dilation to <3% and decrease duration of fever if given in the first 10 days of illness. Current recommended regimen is a single dose of IVIG, 2 g/kg over 10–12 hours.
   (2) Some 10% of patients treated with IVIG fail to respond (persistent or recurrent fever ≥36 hr after IVIG completion). Retreat with second dose.
b. Aspirin is recommended for both its antiinflammatory and antiplatelet effects. The American Heart Association (AHA) recommends initial high-dose aspirin (80–100 mg/kg/day divided in four doses) until 48–72 hours after defervescence. Given with IVIG. Then continue with low-dose aspirin (3–5 mg/kg/day as a single daily dose) for 6–8 weeks or until platelet count and ESR are normal (if there are no coronary artery abnormalities) or indefinitely if coronary artery abnormalities persist.
c. Dipyridamole, 4 mg/kg divided in three doses, is sometimes used as an alternative to aspirin, particularly if symptoms of influenza or varicella arise while on aspirin (concern for Reye syndrome).
d. Follow-up: Serial echocardiography is recommended to assess coronary arteries and left ventricular function (at time of diagnosis, at 2 weeks, at 6–8 weeks, and at 12 months [optional]). More frequent intervals and long-term follow-up are recommended if abnormalities are seen on echocardiography. Cardiac catheterization may be necessary.

F. Rheumatic Heart Disease

1. **Etiology:** Believed to be an immunologically mediated delayed sequela of group A streptococcal pharyngitis
2. **Clinical findings:** History of streptococcal pharyngitis 1–5 weeks before onset of symptoms. Often with pallor, malaise, easy fatigability
3. **Diagnosis:** Jones criteria (Box 7.5)
4. **Management:** Penicillin, bed rest, salicylates, supportive management of CHF (if present) with diuretics, digoxin, morphine

G. Lyme Disease

1. **Etiology:** Following infection with *Borrelia burgdorferi*
2. **Clinical symptoms:** About 8%–10% of patients will get AV block. Other possible cardiac symptoms include myocarditis and pericarditis.

> **BOX 7.5**
>
> **GUIDELINES FOR DIAGNOSIS OF INITIAL ATTACK OF RHEUMATIC FEVER (JONES CRITERIA)**
>
> | Major Manifestations | Minor Manifestations |
> |---|---|
> | Carditis | Clinical findings: |
> | Polyarthritis | Arthralgia |
> | Chorea | Fever |
> | Erythema marginatum | Laboratory findings: |
> | Subcutaneous nodule | Elevated acute phase reactants (erythrocyte sedimentation rate, C-reactive protein) |
> | | Prolonged PR interval |
>
> **Plus**
>
> **Supporting Evidence of Antecedent Group a Streptococcal Infection**
>
> Positive throat culture or rapid streptococcal antigen test
> Elevated or rising streptococcal antibody titer

NOTE: If supported by evidence of preceding group A streptococcal infection, the presence of two major manifestations or of one major and two minor manifestations indicates a high probability of acute rheumatic fever.

VII. EXERCISE RECOMMENDATIONS FOR CONGENITAL HEART DISEASE

See Table EC 7.D for exercise recommendations for congenital heart disease.[20]

VIII. LIPID MONITORING RECOMMENDATIONS

A. Screening of Children and Adolescents[21]

1. **Universal screening** of nonfasting, non-HDL cholesterol in children 9–11 years old (prior to onset of puberty) and again in individuals 17–21 years.
2. **Targeted screening** should occur in children 2–8 years old and adolescents 12–16 years old, with two fasting lipid profiles (between 2 weeks and 3 months apart, results averaged) for the following risk factors:
a. Moderate or high-risk medical condition including history of prematurity, very low birth weight, congenital heart disease (repaired or nonrepaired), recurrent urinary tract infections, known renal or urologic malformations, family history of congenital renal disease, solid organ transplant, malignancy or bone marrow transplant, treatment with drugs known to raise blood pressure, other systemic illness associated with hypertension (e.g., neurofibromatosis, tuberous sclerosis), evidence of elevated intracranial pressure.
b. Have other cardiovascular risk factors including diabetes, hypertension, body mass index ≥95th percentile, smoke cigarettes.

c. Have a family history of early cardiovascular disease (CVD) or severe hypercholesterolemia
   (1) Parent or grandparent who is <55 years old (males) or <65 years old (females) and has suffered an MI or sudden death, undergone a coronary artery procedure, or who has evidence of coronary atherosclerosis, peripheral vascular disease, or cerebrovascular disease
   (2) Parent with total cholesterol ≥240 mg/dL or known dyslipidemia

B. Goals for Lipid Levels in Childhood

1. **Total cholesterol**
a. Acceptable (<170 mg/dL): Repeat measurement in 3–5 years
b. Borderline (170–199 mg/dL): Repeat cholesterol and average with previous measurement. If <170 mg/dL, repeat in 3–5 years. If ≥ 170 mg/dL, obtain lipoprotein analysis
c. High (≥200 mg/dL): Obtain lipoprotein analysis
2. **Low-density lipoprotein (LDL) cholesterol**
a. Acceptable (<110 mg/dL)
b. Borderline (110–129 mg/dL)
c. High (≥130 mg/dL)

C. Management of Hyperlipidemia[21]

1. **Normal and borderline elevated LDL levels:** Education, risk factor intervention, including diet, smoking cessation, and an exercise program. For borderline levels, reevaluate in 1 year. For abnormal nonfasting levels, repeat fasting lipid profiles.
2. **High LDL levels:** Examine for secondary causes (liver, thyroid, renal disorders) and familial disorders. Initiate a low-fat, low-cholesterol diet; reevaluate in 6 months. **Note:** For LDL cholesterol >250 mg/dL or triglyceridemia >500 mg/dL, refer directly to a lipid specialist.
3. **Drug therapy:** Should be considered in children aged >10 years after failure of a 6- to 12-month diet therapy trial, as follows:
a. LDL >190 mg/dL without other CVD risk factors
b. LDL >160 mg/dL with risk factors (diabetes, obesity, hypertension, positive family history of premature CVD)
c. LDL >130 mg/dL in children with diabetes mellitus
d. Bile acid sequestrants and statins are the usual first-line drugs for treatment in children
4. **Persistently high triglycerides (>150 mg/dL) and reduced HDL (<35 mg/dL):** Evaluate for secondary causes (diabetes, alcohol abuse, renal or thyroid disease). Treatment is diet and exercise.

IX. CARDIOVASCULAR SCREENING

A. Sports[22]

There is no established or mandated preparticipation sports screening. There is a recommended history and physical examination screening from the AHA. Routine ECGs are not required unless there is suspicion of underlying cardiac disease (Box EC 7.A).

B. Attention–Deficit/Hyperactivity Disorder (ADHD)
1. **Obtain a good patient and family history as well as physical examination.**
2. **There is not an increased risk of sudden cardiac death in children without cardiac disease taking ADHD medications.** There is no consensus on universal ECG screening. ECGs should be obtained in those who screen with positive answers on history, polypharmacy, tachycardia while on medications, and history of significant cardiac disease. If a patient has significant heart disease or concern for cardiac disease, have patient evaluated by a pediatric cardiologist.

REFERENCES

1. Zubrow AB, Hulman S, Kushner H, et al. Determinants of blood pressure in infants admitted to neonatal intensive care units: a prospective multicenter study. Philadelphia Neonatal Blood Pressure Study Group. *J Perinatol.* 1995;15:470-479.
2. National High Blood Pressure Education Program Working Group on High Blood Pressure in Children and Adolescents. The fourth report on the diagnosis, evaluation, and treatment of high blood pressure in children and adolescents. *Pediatrics.* 2004;114(2 Suppl 4th Report):555-576.
3. Park MK. *Pediatric Cardiology for Practitioners.* 5th ed. St Louis: Mosby; 2008.
4. Sapin SO. Recognizing normal heart murmurs: a logic-based mnemonic. *Pediatrics.* 1997;99:616-619.
5. Davignon A, Rautaharju P, Boisselle E, et al. Normal ECG standards for infants and children. *Pediatr Cardiol.* 1979;1:123-131.
6. Schwartz PJ, Stramba-Badiale M, Segantini A, et al. Prolongation of the QT interval and the sudden infant death syndrome. *N Engl J Med.* 1998;338:1709-1714.
7. Garson A Jr. *The Electrocardiogram in Infants and Children: A Systematic Approach.* Philadelphia: Lea & Febiger; 1983.
8. Park MK, Guntheroth WG. *How to Read Pediatric ECGs.* 4th ed. Philadelphia: Mosby; 2006.
9. Walsh EP. Cardiac arrhythmias. In: Fyler DC, Nadas A, eds. *Pediatric Cardiology.* Philadelphia: Hanley & Belfus; 1992:384.
10. Towbin JA, Bricker JT, Garson A Jr. Electrocardiographic criteria for diagnosis of acute myocardial infarction in childhood. *Am J Cardiol.* 1992;69:1545-1548.
11. Hirsch R, Landt Y, Porter S, et al. Cardiac troponin I in pediatrics: normal values and potential use in assessment of cardiac injury. *J Pediatr.* 1997;130:872-877.
12. Colan SD, Parness IA, Spevak PJ, et al. Developmental modulation of myocardial mechanics: age- and growth-related alterations in afterload and contractility. *J Am Coll Cardiol.* 1992;19:619-629.
13. Stanger P, Heymann MA, Tarnoff H, et al. Complications of cardiac catheterization of neonates, infants, and children. *Circulation.* 1974;50: 595-608.

14. Vitiello R, McCrindle BW, Nykanen D, et al. Complications associated with pediatric cardiac catheterization. *J Am Coll Cardiol*. 1998;32(5):1433-1440.
15. Lees MH. Cyanosis of the newborn infant: recognition and clinical evaluation. *J Pediatr*. 1970;77:484-498.
16. Kitterman JA. Cyanosis in the newborn infant. *Pediatr Rev*. 1982;4:13-24.
17. Jones RW, Baumer JH, Joseph MC, et al. Arterial oxygen tension and response to oxygen breathing in differential diagnosis of heart disease in infancy. *Arch Dis Child*. 1976;51:667-673.
18. Wilson W, Taubert KA, Gewitz M, et al. Prevention of infective endocarditis: guidelines from the American Heart Association: a guideline from the American Heart Association Rheumatic Fever, Endocarditis, and Kawasaki Disease Committee, Council on Cardiovascular Disease in the Young, and the Council on Clinical Cardiology, Council on Cardiovascular Surgery and Anesthesia, and the Quality of Care and Outcomes Research Interdisciplinary Working Group. *Circulation*. 2007;116:1736-1754.
19. Newburger JW, Takahashi M, Gerber MA, et al. Diagnosis, treatment, and long-term management of Kawasaki disease. *Circulation*. 2004;110:2747-2771.
20. Maron BJ, Zipes DP. Introduction: eligibility recommendations for competitive athletes with cardiovascular abnormalities. *J Am Coll Cardiol*. 2005;45:1318-1321.
21. Expert Panel on Integrated Guidelines for Cardiovascular Health and Risk Reduction in Children and Adolescents: summary report. *Pediatrics*. 2011;128(Suppl 5):S213-S256.
22. Maron BJ, Thompson PD, Ackerman MJ, et al. Recommendations and considerations related to preparticipation screening for cardiovascular abnormalities in competitive athletes: 2007 update: a scientific statement from the American Heart Association Council on Nutrition, Physical Activity, and Metabolism: endorsed by the American College of Cardiology Foundation. *Circulation*. 2007;115:1643-1655.

Chapter 8
Dermatology

Taisa Kohut, MD, and Angela Orozco, MD

See additional content on Expert Consult

I. EVALUATION AND CLINICAL DESCRIPTIONS OF SKIN FINDINGS

A. Primary Skin Lesions (Fig. 8.1A)

1. **Macule:** Small flat lesion with altered color (<1 cm)
2. **Patch:** Large macule (>1 cm), also used to describe large macule with scale
3. **Papule:** Elevated, well-circumscribed lesion (<1 cm)
4. **Plaque:** Large papule (>1 cm)
5. **Nodule:** Mass located in dermis or subcutaneous fat (may be solid or soft)
6. **Tumor:** Large nodule
7. **Vesicle:** Blister with transparent fluid
8. **Bulla:** Large vesicle
9. **Wheal:** Erythematous, well-circumscribed, raised, edematous lesion that appears and disappears quickly

B. Secondary Skin Lesions (See Fig. 8.1B)

1. **Scale:** Small, thin plate of horny epithelium
2. **Pustule:** Well-circumscribed elevated lesion filled with pus
3. **Crust:** Exudative mass consisting of blood, scale, and pus from skin erosions or ruptured vesicles/papules
4. **Ulcer:** Erosion of dermis and cutis, with clearly defined edges
5. **Scar:** Formation of new connective tissue after damage to epidermis and cutis, leaving permanent change in skin
6. **Excoriation:** Surface marks, often linear secondary to scratching
7. **Fissure:** Linear skin crack with inflammation and pain

II. VASCULAR ANOMALIES[1]

A. Benign Vascular Tumors

1. Hemangiomas (Fig. 8.2, color plates)
a. **Pathogenesis:** Benign vascular tumor with a phase of rapid proliferation followed by phase of spontaneous involution. Most occur within 2 days to 2 months of life. Undergo rapid growth phase in first few months, with 80% peaking by 3 months. Many begin to regress by 6 months, with a rate of 10% complete involution per year (i.e., 50% or more completely involute by 5 years).
b. **Clinical presentation:** Newborns may demonstrate pale macules with threadlike telangiectasias that later develop into hemangiomas. Often,

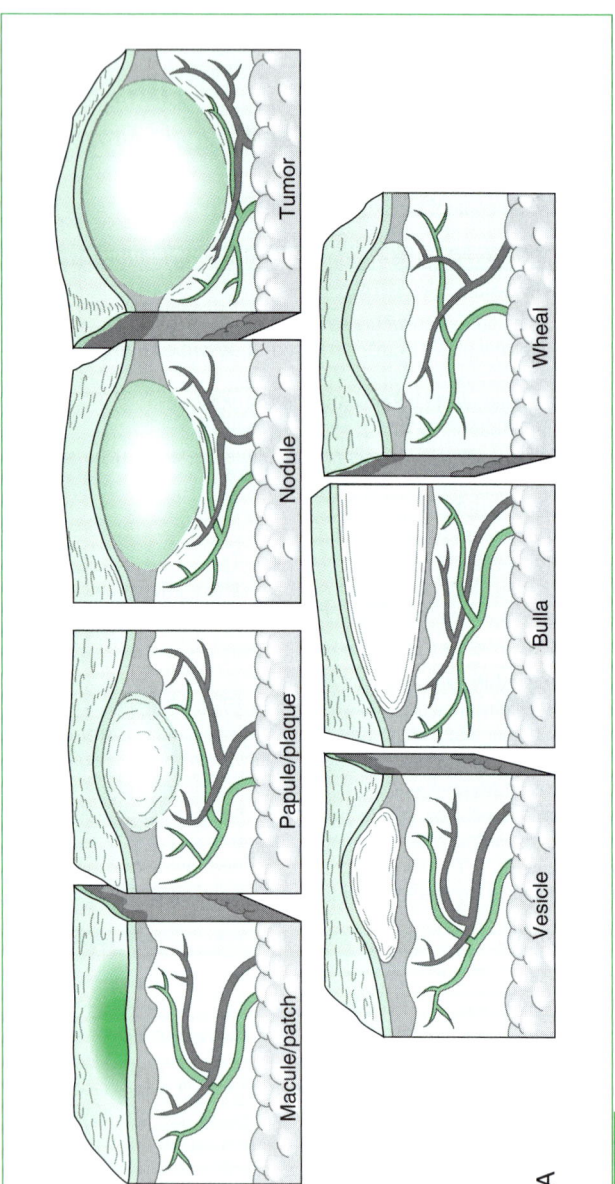

FIGURE 8.1
Pattern diagnosis. **A,** Primary skin lesions.

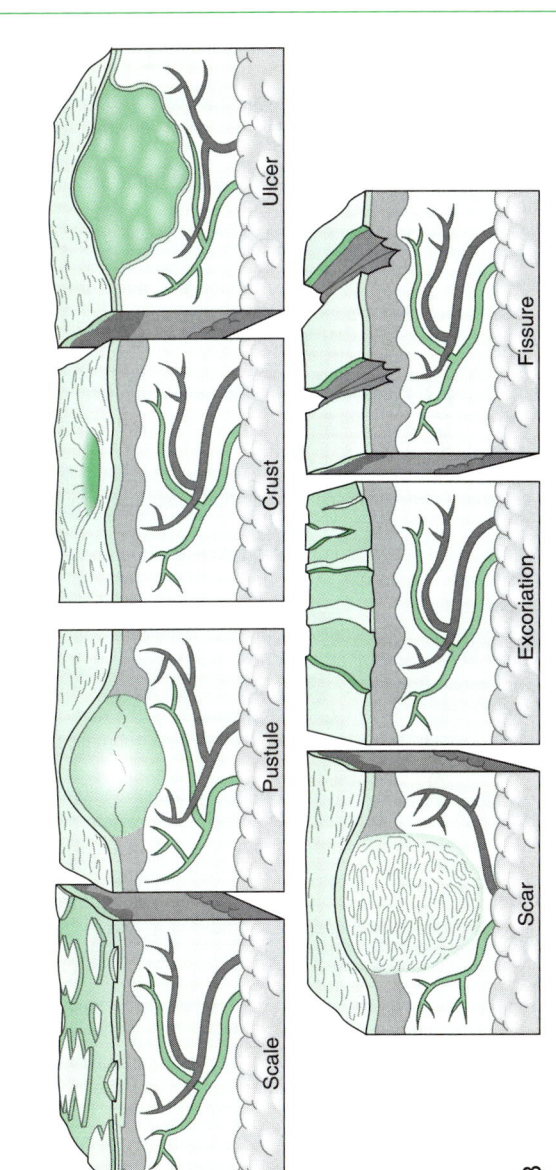

FIGURE 8.1, cont'd
B, Secondary skin lesions. *(From Cohen BA. Pediatric Dermatology. 2nd ed. St Louis: Mosby; 1999:5.)*

there are both superficial and deep components, but can present as only superficial. After involution, can have residual skin changes including scarring and atrophy.
- (1) Superficial: Bright red papule, nodule, plaque.
- (2) Deep: Firm, rubbery nodule/tumor, often with overlying blue-purple discoloration.
- (3) Size: Range from a few millimeters to many centimeters.

c. **Complications**
- (1) Ulceration: Most common complication. Can be extremely painful and will scar.
- (2) Bleeding: Usually minimal, can be stopped with direct pressure
- (3) Visual obstruction: From periorbital hemangiomas, especially involving upper medial eyelid. Require evaluation by an ophthalmologist.
- (4) Airway obstruction: Seen with airway hemangiomas. Infants with lesions in a beard distribution (i.e., chin, lower lip, mandible, anterior neck) are at greater risk. May have hoarseness, stridor, cough, and cyanosis.
- (5) Otitis externa: From ear hemangiomas that obstruct the auditory canal
- (6) Deformation/destruction of important cosmetic structures: From especially large lesions (i.e., ear, nasal septum, vermillion border)

d. **Associated syndromes**
- (1) PHACES syndrome: **P**osterior cranial fossa malformations (as well as multiple other cerebral arteriovenous anomalies), large segmental facial **H**emangiomas, **A**rterial lesions, **C**ardiovascular anomalies (aortic coarctation, other anomalies of the aortic and mesenteric vessels), **E**ye anomalies, **S**ternal cleft anomalies/supraumbilical raphes[2]
- (2) Lumbar (sacral, pelvis) syndrome: **L**ower body hemangioma, **U**rogenital anomalies, **U**lceration, **M**yelopathy, **B**ony deformities, **A**norectal malformations, **A**rterial anomalies, and **R**enal anomalies. Require evaluation with magnetic resonance imaging.

e. **Diagnosis:** Usually diagnosed clinically. Atypical clinical findings, growth pattern, and equivocal imaging should prompt tissue biopsy to exclude other neoplasms or unusual vascular malformations.

f. **Treatment**
- (1) Most require no intervention. Decision to treat should be based on location, size, pattern, age of patient, and risk of complications. Photo documentation is used to follow the growth and regression process.
- (2) Treatment of clinically significant infantile hemangiomas
    - A. Propranolol (Hemangeol)[3]
        - (a) Nonselective β-adrenergic blocker given orally; should be initiated under careful supervision of a pediatric dermatologist or other practitioner experienced in management.

(b) Patients should be clinically screened for cardiac disease. Electrocardiogram and/or echocardiogram are not required but obtained only when indicated (e.g., heart murmur, suspected cardiac/other vascular anomalies).

(c) Contraindications include: premature infants <5 weeks corrected age; weight less than 2 kg; history of bronchospasm or asthma; bradycardia, decompensated heart failure, greater than 1st degree heart block, BP < 50/30 mmHg.

(d) For dosing details, please see reference 3 and the Formulary.

(3) Steroids: No randomized trials comparing propranolol and systemic oral corticosteroids exist, but retrospective data suggest propranolol is more effective and has fewer adverse effects.

(4) Topical timolol: Efficacy noted in superficial hemangiomas and treatment duration >3 months.

B. Pyogenic Granuloma (Lobular Capillary Hemangioma)
(Fig. 8.3, Color Plates)

1. **Clinical presentation:** Benign vascular tumor, appears as small bright red papule that grows over several weeks to months into sessile or pedunculated papule with a "collarette" or scale. Usually no bigger than 1 cm. Can bleed profusely with minor trauma and can ulcerate. Rarely spontaneously regresses. Seen in all ages; average age of diagnosis, 6 months to 10 years. Located on head and neck, sometimes in oral mucosa
2. **Management:** Treatment usually required, given frequent bleeding and ulceration.
a. Shave excision or curettage with cautery of base: Recommended for pedunculated lesions.
b. Surgical excision: May be necessary for large or unusual lesions, but recurrence rates are high.
c. Laser therapy: Can be used for small pyogenic granulomas but may require two to three treatments.

C. For More Information Regarding Vascular Tumors and Vascular Malformations, Please See: http://issva.org Homepage and Select Classification[1]

III. INFECTIONS

A. Viral
1. Warts
a. **Clinical presentation:**
    (1) Common warts: Skin-colored, rough, minimally scaly papules and nodules found most commonly on the hands, although can occur anywhere on the body. Can be solitary or multiple, range from a few millimeters to several centimeters, and may form large

plaques or a confluent linear pattern secondary to autoinoculation. May be persistent in immunocompromised patients.
- (2) Flat warts: Occur over the hands, arms, and face; usually <2 mm wide. Often present in clusters.
- (3) Plantar warts: Occur on soles of feet. Can be painful; appear as inward-growing, hyperkeratotic plaques and papules. Trauma on weight-bearing surfaces results in small black dots (petechiae from thrombosed vessels on the surface of the wart).

b. **Treatment**[4]**:**
- (1) Spontaneous resolution occurs in >75% of warts in otherwise healthy individuals within 3 years. No treatment clearly better than placebo, except for topical salicylic acid.
- (2) Keratolytics (i.e., topical salicylates): Work by removing excess scales within and around warts and by triggering an inflammatory reaction. Particularly effective in combination with adhesive tape occlusion; response may take 4–6 months.
- (3) Destructive techniques: Not more effective than placebo. Can be painful and cause scarring, so not recommended in children.

2. *Molluscum contagiosum* (Fig. 8.4, color plates)
a. **Pathogenesis:** Caused by large DNA poxvirus. Spread by skin-to-skin contact.
b. **Clinical presentation:** Dome-shaped, often umbilicated, translucent to white papules that range from 1 mm to 1 cm. May be pruritic and can be surrounded with erythema, resembling eczema. Can occur anywhere except palms and soles, most commonly on the trunk and intertriginous areas. Can occur in the genital area and lower abdomen when obtained as a sexually transmitted infection.
c. **Treatment:** Most spontaneously resolve within a few months and do not require intervention. Treatment may cause scarring and not more effective than placebo. Recurrences common. Monitor for secondary bacterial infection.

3. Reactive erythema (Fig. 8.5; Figs. 8.6 to 8.12, color plates)
a. **Clinical presentation:** Group of disorders characterized by erythematous patches, plaques, and nodules that vary in size, shape, and distribution.
b. **Etiology:** Represent cutaneous reaction patterns triggered by endogenous and environmental factors.

B. Parasitic Infestations

1. Scabies (Fig. 8.13, color plates)
a. **Pathogenesis:** Caused by the mite *Sarcoptes scabiei*. Spread by skin-to-skin contact and through fomites; can live for 2 days away from a human host. Female mites burrow under the skin at a rate of 2 mm/day and lay eggs as they tunnel (up to 25 eggs).
b. **Clinical presentation:** Initial lesion is a small, erythematous papule that is easy to overlook. Can have burrows (elongated, edematous

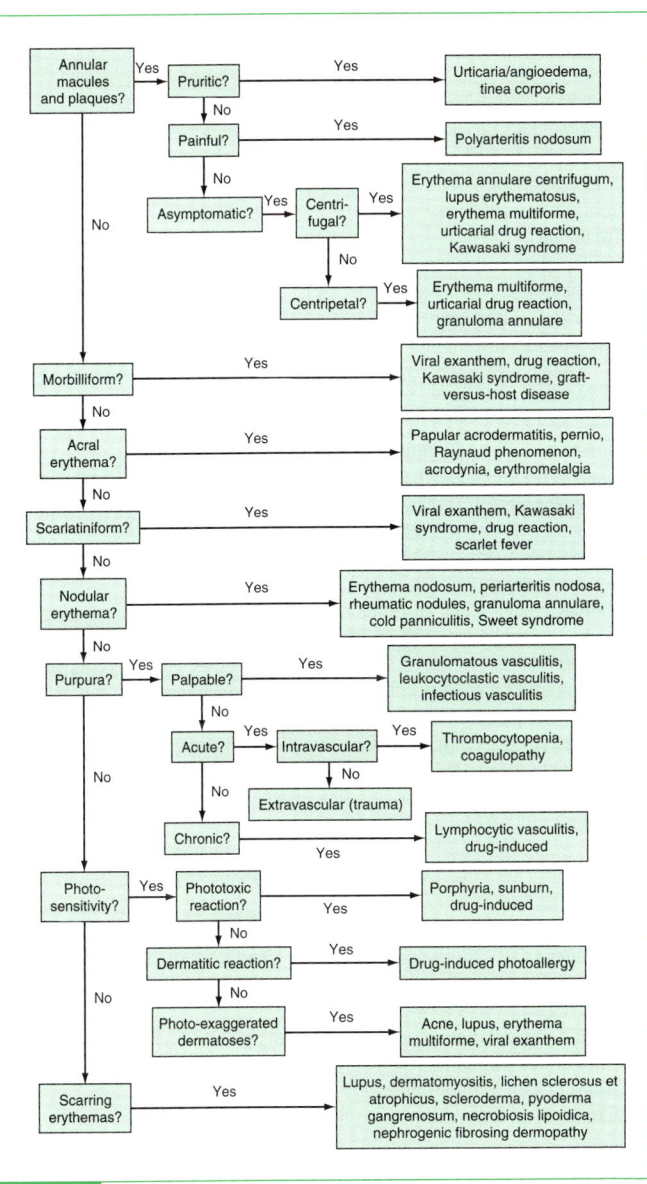

FIGURE 8.5
Reactive erythema. *(Modified from Cohen BA. Atlas of Pediatric Dermatology. 3rd ed. St Louis: Mosby; 2005:97.)*

papulovesicles, often with a pustule at the advancing border), which are pathognomonic. Most commonly located in interdigital webs, wrist folds, elbows, axilla, buttocks, and belt line. Burrows are most dramatic in patients who are unable to scratch (e.g., infants). Disseminated eczematous eruption results in generalized severe pruritus, especially at night. Can become nodular, particularly in intertriginous areas, or be susceptible to superinfection due to frequent excoriations.

c. **Treatment**[5]:
  (1) Permethrin cream: 5% cream applied to affected areas of skin, including under fingernails, face, and scalp. Rinse off after 8–14 hours. Can repeat in 7–10 days.
  (2) Ivermectin (off-label use): 200 mcg/kg oral dose; can repeat in 2 weeks. Efficacy comparable to permethrin cream.

C. Fungal (Figs. 8.14 to 8.17, Color Plates)

1. Tinea capitis (see **Section IV**)
2. Tinea versicolor (see Fig. 8.14, color plates)
a. **Pathogenesis:** Caused by *Malassezia* (previously *Pityrosporum*), a lipid-dependent yeast. Exacerbated by hot/humid weather, hyperhidrosis, topical skin oil use. Not associated with poor hygiene. Not contagious.
b. **Clinical presentation:** Macules or patches that are hypopigmented, hyperpigmented, or erythematous. Hypopigmented areas tend to be more prominent in the summer because affected areas do not tan. Lesions often have a fine scale and can be mildly pruritic but are usually asymptomatic.
c. **Diagnosis:** Potassium hydroxide (KOH) microscopy reveals hyphae and yeast cells that appear like "spaghetti and meatballs."
d. **Treatment:** Topical antifungals (miconazole, oxiconazole, ketoconazole) or selenium sulfide are effective. Given the risk of hepatotoxicity, oral azole antifungals are reserved for resistant or widespread disease (oral terbinafine not effective). Pigmentation changes may take months to resolve despite successful treatment.
3. Tinea corporis[6] (see Fig. 8.15, color plates)
a. **Pathogenesis:** Can be spread through direct contact and fomites, especially in sports where there is close contact (e.g., wrestling).
b. **Clinical presentation:** Pruritic, erythematous, annular patch, or plaque with central clearing and a scaly raised border. Typically affects glabrous skin (smooth and bare).
c. **Diagnosis:** Usually diagnosed clinically, but a KOH preparation or fungal culture can be used to help guide diagnosis.
d. **Treatment:** Topical antifungals (terbinafine, azole antifungals) until the lesion resolves, plus 1–2 additional weeks. Widespread eruption may require oral antibiotics.

D. Bacterial

1. Impetigo
a. **Pathogenesis:** Contagious bacterial infection of the skin, most commonly caused by *Staphylococcus aureus*, with a minority of cases caused by group A β-hemolytic *Streptococcus*. Methicillin-resistant *S. aureus* impetigo in the community and hospital settings is on the rise.
b. **Clinical presentation:**
   (1) Nonbullous impetigo: Papules that evolve into erythematous pustules or vesicles that break and form thick, honey-colored crusts and plaques. Commonly overlying any break to skin barrier. Usually found on face and extremities.
   (2) Bullous impetigo: Painless vesicles that evolve into flaccid bullae with clear/yellow fluid that turns darker; often leaves a yellow/brown crust when bullae rupture. Seen more in infants and young children. Caused by exfoliative toxin A from *S. aureus*.

IV. HAIR LOSS: DIAGNOSIS AND TREATMENT (Figs. 8.17 to 8.21, Color Plates)

A. Tinea Capitis (see Fig. 8.17, Color Plates)

1. **Pathogenesis:** Mostly caused by *Trichophyton tonsurans* (but *Trichophyton violeum* and *Trichophyton sudanese* are clinically similar), sometimes *Microsporum canis*. Can be spread through contact and fomites.
2. **Epidemiology:** Usually occurs in young children aged 1–10 years. African-American children more commonly affected, perhaps owing to the structure of their hair, but any age and ethnicity can be affected.
3. **Clinical presentation:**
a. Black dot tinea capitis: Most common. Slowly growing, erythematous, scaling patches. These areas develop alopecia, and black dots are visible on scalp where hair has broken off.
b. Gray patch ("seborrheic dermatitis") tinea capitis: Erythematous, scaling, well-demarcated patch that grows centrifugally. Hair breaks off a few millimeters above the scalp and takes on a gray/frosted appearance.
c. Kerion (see Fig. 8.18, color plates): Complication of tinea capitis or tinea corporis. Type IV delayed hypersensitivity reaction to fungal infection. Appears as raised, boggy/spongy lesions, often tender and covered with exudate. Can be associated with posterior cervical lymphadenopathy.
4. **Diagnosis:** Can be made clinically, since oral antifungal therapy is indicated, but tinea capitis should be confirmed by examining a KOH preparation under direct microscopic examination or culture of broken-off and surrounding hair.

5. **Treatment**[6]: First-line therapy includes oral griseofulvin for 10–12 weeks (which should be taken with fatty foods for improved absorption) and terbinafine, which is administered for 6 weeks. Topical antifungals will not be curative. All family members, particularly other children, should be examined carefully for subtle infection and treated. Selenium sulfide 2.5% shampoo may shorten the period of shedding of fungal organisms and reduce infection of unaffected family members.

B. Alopecia Areata (see Fig. 8.19, Color Plates)

1. **Clinical presentation:** Chronic inflammatory (probably autoimmune) disease that starts with small bald patches and normal-appearing underlying skin. New lesions may demonstrate subtle erythema and be pruritic. Bald patches may enlarge to involve large areas of the scalp or other hair-bearing areas. Many experience good hair regrowth within 1–2 years, although most will relapse. A minority progress to total loss of all scalp (alopecia totalis) and/or body hair (alopecia universalis).
2. **Diagnosis:** Usually clinical diagnosis. Biopsy is necessary in rare cases.
3. **Treatment**[7]: First-line therapy is topical and occasionally intralesional steroids. Minoxidil, anthralin, contact sensitization, and ultraviolet light therapy are second line. No evidence-based data that any therapy is better than placebo, so treatments with significant risk of toxicity should be avoided, particularly in children. Older children, adolescents, and young adults with longstanding localized areas of hair loss have the best prognosis.

C. Telogen Effluvium (See Fig. 8.20, Color Plates)

1. **Pathogenesis:** Most common cause of diffuse hair loss, usually after stressful state (major illnesses or surgery, pregnancy, severe weight loss). Mature hair follicles switch prematurely to the telogen (resting) state, with shedding within 3 months.
2. **Clinical presentation:** Diffuse hair thinning 3 months after a stressful event. May not be clinically obvious to an outsider until more than 20% of hair is lost.
3. **Treatment:** Self-limited, regrowth usually occurs over the next few months.

D. Traction Alopecia (See Fig. 8.21, Color Plates)

1. **Pathogenesis:** Result of hairstyles that apply tension for long periods of time.
2. **Clinical presentation:** Noninflammatory linear areas of hair loss at margins of hairline, part line, or scattered regions, depending on hairstyling procedures used.
3. **Treatment:** Avoidance of styling products or styles that result in traction. If traction remains for long periods, condition may progress to permanent scarring hair loss.

E. Trichotillomania

1. **Pathogenesis:** Alopecia due to compulsive urge to pull out one's own hair, resulting in irregular areas of incomplete hair loss. Alopecia notable mainly on the scalp; can involve eyebrows and eyelashes. Onset is usually after age 10 and should be distinguished from hair pulling in younger children that resolves without treatment in most cases.
2. **Clinical presentation:** Characterized by hair of differing lengths; area of hair loss can be unusual in shape.
3. **Treatment:** Many cases require behavioral modification. Adolescents may benefit from psychiatric evaluation; condition can be associated with anxiety, depression, and obsessive-compulsive disorder.

V. ACNE VULGARIS

A. Pathogenesis

1. **Blockade of follicular opening from hyperkeratinization**
2. **Increased sebum production**
3. **Proliferation of *Propionibacterium acnes***
4. **Inflammation**
5. **Risk factors:** Androgens, family history, and stress. No strong evidence that dietary habits affect acne.

B. Clinical Presentation

1. **Noninflammatory lesions**
   a. Closed comedo (whitehead): Accumulation of sebum and keratinous material, resulting in white/skin-colored papules without surrounding erythema.
   b. Open comedo (blackhead): Dilated follicles packed with keratinocytes, oils, and melanin.
2. **Inflammatory lesions:** Papules, pustules, nodules, cysts. Typically appear later in the course of acne and vary from 1- to 2-mm micropapules to nodules >5 mm. Nodulocystic presentations are more likely to lead to permanent scarring and/or hyperpigmentation.

C. Classification: Used to Estimate Severity, but Not Always Practical In A Clinical Setting

1. **Mild:** <20 comedones, <15 inflammatory lesions, or total <30
2. **Moderate:** 20–100 comedones, 15–50 inflammatory lesions, or total 30–125
3. **Severe:** >100 comedones, >50 inflammatory lesions, >5 cysts, or total >125
4. **Clinician should also consider** the number of skin areas involved and extent in each area (e.g., face, back, chest; occasionally arms, legs, scalp)

D. Treatment[8,9,10] (Table 8.1)

1. **Skin care:** Gentle nonabrasive cleaning. Avoid picking or popping lesions. Vigorous scrubbing and abrasive cleaners can worsen acne.
2. **Topical retinoids** (Table 8.2): First-line therapy for mild to moderate acne. Normalize follicular keratinization and decrease inflammation. A pea-sized amount should be applied to cover the entire face. Can cause irritation and dryness of skin. Retinoids should probably be used at a different time of day than benzoyl peroxide (BPO) to minimize risk of irritation, especially when therapy is initiated. Three topical retinoids (tretinoin, adapalene, and tazarotene) are available by prescription in the United States.
3. **Topical antimicrobials:**
  a. Erythromycin and clindamycin. Avoid topical antibiotics as monotherapy. Topical BPO should be added to optimize efficacy.
  b. BPO: Oxidizing agent with antibacterial and mild anticomedolytic properties. Reduces emergence of less sensitive *P. acnes* variants when used with topical antibiotics. Can bleach hair, clothing, towels. Washes may be most convenient formulation, because they can be rinsed off in the shower.
  c. Dapsone: Has antimicrobial and anti-inflammatory effects. Most effective against inflammatory lesions. Efficacy enhanced when combined with topical retinoid as compared with BPO.
4. **Oral antibiotics** (Table 8.3): First line for moderate to severe inflammatory acne. Avoid oral antibiotics as monotherapy, owing to increased antibiotic resistance. Use with BPO and/or topical retinoids. Try to limit length of therapy, and reassess clinically at 6–12 weeks
  a. Tetracycline derivatives (tetracycline, doxycycline, and minocycline) commonly used for children older than 8 years.
  b. Alternatives for children younger than 8 years and those with tetracycline allergies include erythromycin, azithromycin, and trimethoprim/sulfamethoxazole.
  c. Side effects: photosensitivity and "pill esophagitis" with doxycycline and drug hypersensitivity syndrome, Stevens-Johnson syndrome, or lupus like syndrome with minocycline.
5. **Hormonal therapy:** Good alternative for pubertal females who have sudden onset of moderate to severe acne and have not responded to conventional first-line therapy. Should not be used as monotherapy. Reduces sebum production and androgen levels.
  a. Combination oral contraceptives: Ortho Tri-Cyclen, Estrostep, and Yaz
  b. Spironolactone: antiandrogen; overall role and appropriate age of initiation not yet fully determined
6. **Oral isotretinoin:** Reserved for patients with severe nodular, cystic, or scarring acne who do not respond to traditional therapy. Should be managed by a dermatologist. Significantly decreases sebum

TABLE 8.1
PEDIATRIC TREATMENT RECOMMENDATION FOR MILD, MODERATE, AND SEVERE ACNE

	Initial Treatment*	Inadequate Response	Additional Treatment Considerations
Mild acne (comedonal or inflammatory/mixed lesions)	Benzoyl peroxide (BPO) or topical retinoid **OR** Topical combination therapy: BPO + Antibiotic or Retinoid + BPO or Retinoid + Antibiotic + BPO	Add BPO or retinoid if not already prescribed OR change topical retinoid concentration, type and/or formulation OR change topical combination therapy	Previous treatment/history Costs Vehicle selection Ease of use Managing expectations/side effects Psychological impact Active scarring Regimen complexity Assess adherence
Moderate acne (comedonal or inflammatory/mixed lesions)	Topical combination therapy: Retinoid + BPO or Retinoid + (BPO + Antibiotic) or (Retinoid + Antibiotic) + BPO **OR** Oral Antibiotic + Topical Retinoid + BPO or Topical Retinoid + Antibiotic + BPO	Change topical retinoid concentration, type and/or formulation and/or change topical combination therapy OR add or change oral antibiotic. Females: consider hormonal therapy. Consider oral isotretinoin (dermatology referral).	Previous treatment/history Costs Vehicle selection Ease of use Managing expectations/side effects Psychological impact Active scarring Regimen complexity Assess adherence
Severe acne (inflammatory/Mixed and/or nodular lesions)	Combination therapy: Oral Antibiotic + Topical Retinoid + BPO +/– Topical Antibiotic	Consider changing oral antibiotic AND consider oral isotretinoin. Females: consider hormonal therapy. Strongly consider referral to dermatology.	Previous treatment/history Costs Vehicle selection Ease of use Managing expectations/side effects Psychological impact Active scarring Regimen complexity Assess adherence: consider change of topical retinoid

*Topical dapsone may be considered as a single therapy or in place of a topical antibiotic. Topical fixed-combination prescriptions available.

Data from Eichenfield LF, Krakowski AC, Piggott C, et al. Evidence-based recommendations for the diagnosis and treatment of pediatric acne. Pediatrics. 2013;131:S163-S186.

TABLE 8.2
FORMULATIONS AND CONCENTRATIONS OF TOPICAL RETINOIDS

Retinoid	Formulation[a]	Strength (%)	Pregnancy Category
TRETINOIN	Cream	0.025, 0.05, 0.1	C
	Gel	0.01, 0.025	
	Gel (micronized)	0.05	
	Microsphere gel	0.04, 0.1	
	Polymerized cream	0.025	
	Polymerized gel	0.025	
ADAPALENE	Cream	0.1	C
	Gel	0.1, 0.3	
	Solution	0.1	
	Lotion	0.1	
TAZAROTENE	Gel	0.05, 0.1	X
	Cream	0.05, 0.1	

[a]Numerous generic retinoids are available. Branded products are available under the following trade names: Atralin, Avita, and Retin-A Micro for tretinoin; Differin for adapalene; and Tazorac for tazarotene.

Data from Eichenfield LF, Krakowski AC, Piggott C, et al. Evidence-based recommendations for the diagnosis and treatment of pediatric acne. Pediatrics. 2013;131:S163-S186, Table 4.

production, inflammation, *P. acnes*, and can diminish scarring. Most patients have complete resolution of their acne after 16–20 weeks of use.

a. Side effects:
   (1) Teratogenicity: Patients and physicians are mandated by the FDA to comply with iPledge, a computerized risk management program designed to eliminate fetal exposure to isotretinoin. Female patients of child-bearing potential must use two forms of birth control and routinely get pregnancy tests.
   (2) Hepatoxicity, hyperlipidemia, and bone marrow suppression. A complete blood cell count, fasting lipid profile, and liver function tests should be obtained before initiation of therapy and repeated at 4 and 8 weeks.
   (3) Three other significant and controversial groups of adverse effects described in drug's package insert: bone effects, inflammatory bowel disease, and mood changes.

VI. COMMON NEONATAL DERMATOLOGIC CONDITIONS (Fig. 8.22; Figs. 8.23 to 8.31, Color Plates)

A. Erythema Toxicum Neonatorum (See Fig. 8.23, Color Plates)

Most common rash of full-term infants; incidence declines with lower birth weight and prematurity. Appears as small erythematous macules and papules that evolve into pustules on erythematous bases. Rash occurs most often by 24–48 hours of life but can be present at birth or emerge as late as 2–3 weeks. Self-limited, resolves within 5–7 days; recurrences possible. Pustular fluid reveals eosinophils.

TABLE 8.3
ORAL ANTIBIOTICS USED FOR TREATMENT OF MODERATE TO SEVERE ACNE VULGARIS

Antibiotic	Potential Adverse Effects	Comments
DOXYCYCLINE	Pill esophagitis; photosensitivity; staining of forming tooth enamel (<8 years of age); vaginal candidiasis	Take with large glass of water and maintain upward position ~1 hr; optimize photoprotection; avoid in children without permanent teeth
ERYTHROMYCIN	GI upset; drug-drug interactions	High prevalence of antibiotic resistant *Propionibacterium acnes*
TETRACYCLINE	Fixed drug eruption; GI symptoms; staining of forming tooth enamel (<8 years of age); vaginal candidiasis	Ingest on empty stomach preferable; absorption decreased if taken with iron, calcium, dairy products; avoid in children without permanent teeth
MINOCYCLINE (IMMEDIATE RELEASE)	Cutaneous and/or mucosal hyperpigmentation; DHS (systemic, within first 1–2 mo); LLS; SJS; vestibular toxicity (within first few days); staining of forming tooth enamel (<8 years of age); vaginal candidiasis	Can be taken with meals; warn patient about dizziness/vertigo; avoid in children without permanent teeth; monitor for pigmentary changes on skin
MINOCYCLINE EXTENDED RELEASE TABLETS	Same as above although above side effects reported predominantly with immediate release formulations; lower incidence of acute vestibular side effects with weight–based dosing	Less accumulation of drug over time due to pharmokinetic properties of extended release formulation, may correlate with decreased hyperpigmentation
TRIMETHOPRIM/SULFAMETHOXAZOLE	Severe cutaneous eruptions (TEN, SJS); bone marrow suppression; drug eruptions; fixed drug eruption	Not recommended as first or second–line agent for acne

DHS, Drug hypersensitivty syndrome; GI, gastrointestinal; LLS, lupus like syndrome; SJS, Stephens-Johnson syndrome; TEN, toxic epidermal necrolysis.
Modified from Eichenfield LF, Krakowski AC, Piggott C, et al. Evidence-based recommendations for the diagnosis and treatment of pediatric acne. Pediatrics. *2013;131:S163-S186, Table 5.*

B. Transient Neonatal Pustular Melanosis (See Figs. 8.24 and 8.25, Color Plates)

More commonly affects full-term infants with darker pigmentation. At birth, appears as small pustules on nonerythematous bases that rupture and leave erythematous/hyperpigmented macules with a collarette of

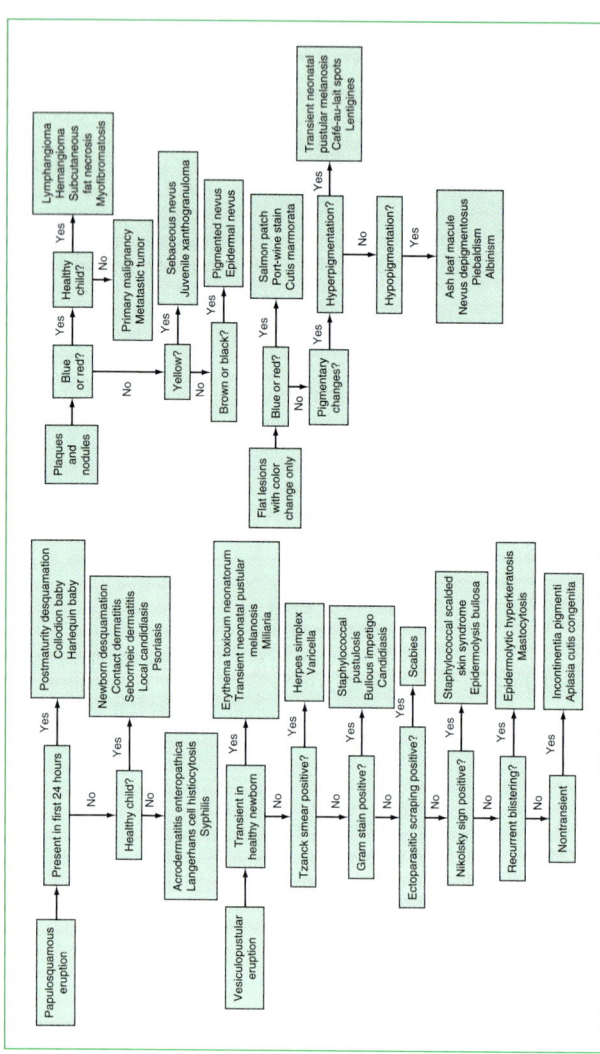

FIGURE 8.22
Evaluation of neonatal rashes. *(Modified from Cohen BA. Atlas of Pediatric Dermatology. 3rd ed. St Louis: Mosby; 2005:62.)*

scale. Self-limited; macules fade over weeks to months. Pustular fluid reveals neutrophils.

C. Miliaria (Heat Rash, Prickly Heat) (See Fig. 8.26, Color Plates)

Common newborn rash associated with warmer climates, incubator use, or occlusion with clothes/dressings. Appears as small erythematous papules or pustules usually on face, scalp, or intertriginous areas. Due to obstruction of eccrine sweat ducts in the stratum corneum. Rash resolves when infant is placed in cooler environment or tight clothing/dressings are removed.

D. Milia (See Fig. 8.27, Color Plates)

Common newborn rash. Appears as 1- to 3-mm white/yellow papules, frequently found on nose and face; due to retention of keratin and sebaceous materials in pilosebaceous follicles. Self-limited, resolves within first few weeks of life.

E. Neonatal Acne (See Fig. 8.28, Color Plates)

Seen in 20% of infants. Appears as inflammatory papules or pustules without comedones, usually on face and scalp. Secondary to effect of maternal and endogenous androgens on infant's sebaceous glands. Peaks around 1 month, resolves within a few months, usually without intervention. Does not increase risk of acne as an adolescent.

F. Seborrheic Dermatitis (Cradle Cap) (See Figs. 8.29 and 8.30, Color Plates)

Common rash characterized by erythematous plaques with greasy yellow scales. Located in areas rich with sebaceous glands, such as scalp, cheeks, ears, eyebrows, intertriginous areas, diaper area. Unknown etiology. Can be seen in newborns, more commonly in infants aged 1–4 months. Self-limited and resolves within a few weeks to months. Can remove scales on scalp with soft brush/fine comb. In more severe cases, antifungal shampoos or low-potency topical steroid can shorten the course.

G. Congenital Dermal Melanocytosis (Previously Known as Mongolian Spots)

Most common pigmented lesion of newborns, usually seen in babies with darker skin tone. Appear as blue/gray macules without definite disappearance of dermal melanocytes. Spots typically fade within first few years of life, with majority resolved by age 10 years. Can be mistaken for child abuse thus accurate documentation at newborn and well-child visits is important. Should be differentiated from other pigmented lesions (e.g., blue nevi, nevus of Ota, nevus of Ito).

H. Diaper Candidiasis (See Fig. 8.31, Color Plates)

Very common diaper rash, characterized by a red, raised rash with small raised and infected areas around the periphery called *satellite lesions*. Etiology is usually irritation or seborrheic dermatitis that can become secondarily infected with *Candida*. Commonly seen in infancy during periods of diaper wearing. Can be minimized by keeping diaper area clean, as dry as possible, with frequent diaper changes and use of topical agents such as powders. Treatment with topical nystatin, miconazole, or clotrimazole is sufficient.

VII. AUTOIMMUNE AND ALLERGIC LESIONS (Figs. 8.32 to 8.41, Color Plates)

A. Autoimmune Bullous Diseases

1. **Very rare in children** but should be considered if bullous lesions do not respond to standard therapy. Suspicion for any of the following should warrant referral to a dermatologist for diagnosis and management.
2. **Pemphigus vulgaris** (see Fig. 8.32, color plates):
   a. Pathogenesis: IgG autoantibodies to adhesion molecules desmoglein-1 and desmoglein-3, which interrupts integrity of epidermis and/or mucosa and results in extensive blister formation.
   b. Clinical presentation: Flaccid bullae that start in the mouth and spread to face, scalp, trunk, extremities, and other mucosal membranes. Positive Nikolsky sign. Ruptured blisters are painful and prone to secondary infection. Can lead to impaired oral intake if there is significant oral mucosal involvement.
   c. Treatment: Immunosuppressants (systemic glucocorticoids, rituximab, intravenous immunoglobulin).
3. **Pemphigus foliaceus:**
   a. Pathogenesis: IgG autoantibodies to desmoglein-1. Antibodies bind to the same antigen as in bullous impetigo and staphylococcal scalded skin syndrome, so lesions are superficial and rupture easily. Can be triggered by certain drugs, including thiol compounds and penicillins
   b. Clinical presentation: Scaling, crusting erosions on erythematous base that appear on face, scalp, trunk, and back. No mucosal involvement. Lesions are more superficial than in pemphigus vulgaris.
   c. Treatment: Immunosuppressants
4. **Bullous pemphigoid:**
   a. Pathogenesis: Autoantibodies to the epithelial basement membrane that results in an inflammatory cascade and causes separation of epidermis from dermis and epithelium from subepithelium
   b. Clinical presentation: Prodrome of inflammatory lesions that progresses into large (1–3 cm), tense, extremely pruritic bullae on trunk, flexural regions, and intertriginous areas. A minority have oral mucosal lesions. Negative Nikolsky sign
   c. Treatment: Immunosuppressants
5. **Dermatitis herpetiformis:**
   a. Pathogenesis: Strong genetic predisposition and link to gluten intolerance/celiac disease. IgA deposits found in dermal papillae.

b. Clinical presentation: Symmetric, intensely pruritic papulovesicles clustered on extensor surfaces.
c. Treatment: Dapsone, strict gluten-free diet.

B. Contact Dermatitis

1. **Irritant dermatitis:** Exposure to physical, chemical, or mechanical irritants to the skin. Top two causes in children are dry skin dermatitis and diaper dermatitis.
2. **Allergic dermatitis** (see Fig. 8.33, color plates):
a. Pathogenesis: T-cell–mediated immune reaction in response to an environmental trigger that comes into contact with the skin. After initial exposure causes sensitization, an allergic response occurs with subsequent exposures.
b. Allergens: Common antigens are *Toxicodendron* spp. (poison ivy, poison oak, poison sumac). Also nickel, cobalt, gold, dyes, formaldehyde.
c. Clinical presentation: Pruritic erythematous dermatitis that can progress to a chronic stage involving scaling, lichenification, and pigmentary changes. Initial reaction occurs after a sensitization period of 7–10 days in susceptible individuals. Antigen reexposure causes a more rapid reactivation reaction.
    (1) Poison ivy (see Fig. 8.34, color plates): Exposure to urushiol, the allergenic substance in poison ivy, causes streaks of erythematous papules, pustules, and vesicles. Highly pruritic, can become edematous, especially if rash is on face or genitals. In extreme cases, anaphylaxis can occur.
3. **Diagnosis:** Careful history taking. Patch testing may also be helpful.
4. **Treatment:**
a. Remove causative agent. For poison ivy contact, remove clothing and wash skin with mild soap and water as soon as possible.
b. Mild dermatitis: Topical steroids.
c. Widespread or severe dermatitis: Systemic steroids for 2–3 weeks. There is no role for short courses of steroids (e.g., Medrol dose pack), because eruption will flare when drug is stopped.

C. Atopic Dermatitis (Eczema) (See Figs 8.35 to 8.39)

1. **Pathogenesis:** Due to impaired skin barrier function from combination of genetic and environmental factors, including a defect in filaggrin, a protein essential for keratinization and epidermal homeostasis. An inadequate skin barrier leads to transepidermal water loss. Can be associated with elevated serum E.
2. **Epidemiology**[11]**:** Affects up to 20% of children in the United States, the vast majority with onset before age 5 years. Many with other comorbidities including asthma, allergic rhinitis, and food allergies. Eczema resolves or improves in over 75% of patients by adulthood.
3. **Clinical presentation:** Dry, pruritic skin with acute changes including erythema, vesicles, crusting, and chronic changes, including

lichenification, scaling, and postinflammatory hypopigmentation or hyperpigmentation.
a. Infantile form: Erythematous, scaly lesions on the cheeks, scalp, and extensor surfaces. Diaper area usually spared
b. Childhood form: Lichenified plaques in flexural areas
c. Adolescence: More localized and lichenified skin changes. May be predominantly on hands and feet

4. **Treatment**[11]:
a. Lifestyle: Avoiding triggers, including products with alcohol, fragrances, and astringents, sweat, allergens, and excessive bathing. Bathing time should be <5 minutes, skin should be patted dry (not rubbed) afterward and followed by rapid application of an emollient.
b. Skin hydration: Frequent use of bland lubricants with low or no water content (e.g., petroleum jelly, Vaseline, Aquaphor). Lotions have high water and low oil content and can actually worsen dry skin.
c. Antihistamines: Used primarily for sedating effects. Also helpful in children with concomitant environmental allergies or hives
d. Treatment for inflammation:
  (1) Topical steroids[12] (Table 8.4)
    (a) Low- and medium-potency steroid ointments once or twice daily for 7 days for eczema flares. Severe flares may require a higher-potency steroid for a longer duration of therapy, followed by a taper to lower-potency steroids. Use of topical steroids in areas where skin is thin (i.e., groin, axilla, face, under breasts) should generally be avoided, although can consider short duration of low-potency steroid for these areas. Topical lubricant can be applied over steroid.
  (2) Topical calcineurin inhibitors: Tacrolimus ointment, pimecrolimus cream
    (a) Second-line therapy; should be used in consultation with a dermatologist. In 2006, the FDA placed a "black box" warning on these medications because of possible increased risk of cancer, although no data confirm this as yet, and long-term safety studies are pending.[13]

5. **Complications**[14]:
a. Bacterial superinfection: Usually *S. aureus*, sometimes group A *Streptococcus*. Depending on extent of infection, can be treated with topical mupirocin to systemic antibiotics. Can also take diluted bleach baths once to twice a week (mix 1/4 to 1/2 cup of bleach in full tub of lukewarm water and soak for 10 minutes, then rinse off with fresh water).
b. Eczema herpeticum superinfection with herpes simplex virus-1 or -2, can cause severe systemic infection. Presents as vesiculopustular lesions with central punched-out erosions that do not respond to oral antibiotics. Must be treated systemically with acyclovir/valacyclovir. Should be evaluated by ophthalmologist if there is concern for eye involvement.

TABLE 8.4
RELATIVE POTENCIES OF TOPICAL CORTICOSTEROIDS

Class	Drug	Dosage form(s)	Strength (%)
I. VERY HIGH POTENCY	Augmented betamethasone dipropionate	Ointment	0.05
	Clobetasol propionate	Cream, foam, ointment	0.05
	Diflorasone diacetate	Ointment	0.05
	Halobetasol propionate	Cream, ointment	0.05
II. HIGH POTENCY	Amcinonide	Cream, lotion, ointment	0.1
	Augmented betamethasone dipropionate	Cream	0.05
	Betamethasone propionate	Cream, foam, ointment, solution	0.05
	Desoximetasone	Cream, ointment	0.25
	Desoximetasone	Gel	0.05
	Diflorasone diacetate	Cream	0.05
	Fluocinonide	Cream, gel, ointment, solution	0.05
	Halcinonide	Cream, ointment	0.1
	Mometasone furoate	Ointment	0.1
	Triamcinolone acetonide	Cream, ointment	0.5
III–IV. MEDIUM POTENCY	Betamethasone valerate	Cream, foam, lotion, ointment	0.1
	Clocortolone pivalate	Cream	0.1
	Desoximetasone	Cream	0.05
	Fluocinolone acetonide	Cream, ointment	0.025
	Flurandrenolide	Cream, ointment	0.05
	Fluticasone propionate	Cream	0.05
	Fluticasone propionate	Ointment	0.005
	Mometasone furoate	Cream	0.1
	Triamcinolone acetonide	Cream	0.1
V. LOWER-MEDIUM POTENCY	Hydrocortisone butyrate	Cream, ointment, solution	0.1
	Hydrocortisone probutate	Cream	0.1
	Hydrocortisone valerate	Cream, ointment	0.2
	Prednicarbate	Cream	0.1
VI: LOW POTENCY	Alclometasone dipropionate	Cream, ointment	0.05
	Desonide	Cream, gel, foam, ointment	0.05
	Fluocinonide acetonide	Cream, solution	0.01
VII. LOWEST POTENCY	Dexamethasone	Cream	0.1
	Hydrocortisone	Cream, lotion, ointment, solution	0.25, 0.5, 1
	Hydrocortisone acetate	Cream, ointment	0.5–1

Modified from Eichenfield LF, Tom WL, Berger TG, et al. Guidelines of care for the management of atopic dermatitis. Section 2. Management and treatment of atopic dermatitis with topical therapies. J Am Acad Dernatol. 2014;71(1):116-132, Table V.

D. Papular Urticaria (See Fig. 8.40, Color Plates)

1. **Pathogenesis:** Caused by insect bite-induced hypersensitivity (IBIH), usually from fleas, mosquitos, or bedbugs. Due to delayed type IV hypersensitivity reactions.
2. **Clinical presentation/epidemiology:** Summarized by the SCRATCH principles.[15]

Symmetric eruption: Exposed areas and scalp commonly affected. Spares diaper region, palms, and soles.

Cluster: Appear as "meal clusters" or "breakfast, lunch, and dinner" which are linear or triangular groupings of lesions. Associated with bedbugs and fleas.

Rover not required: A remote animal exposure or lack of pet at home does not rule out IBIH.

Age: Tends to peak by age 2 years. Not seen in newborn period. Most tend to develop tolerance by age 10.

Target lesions: Characteristic of IBIH, especially in darkly pigmented patients. Also, **T**ime: emphasize chronic nature of eruption and need for patience and watchful waiting.

Confused pediatrician/parent: Diagnosis often met with disbelief by parent and/or referring pediatrician.

Household: Because of the nature of the hypersensitivity, usually only affects one family member in the household.

3. **Management (the 3 Ps):**

Prevention: Wear protective clothing, use insect repellent when outside, launder bedding and mattress pads for bedbugs, and maximize flea control for pets.

Pruritis control: Topical steroids or antihistamines may be of some benefit.

Patience: IBIH can be frustrating because of its persistent, recurrent nature. Ensure patients that their symptoms will resolve and they will eventually develop tolerance.

VIII. NAIL DISORDERS[16]

A. Acquired Nail Disorders

1. Paronychia: Red, tender swelling of proximal or lateral nail folds (Figs. EC 8.A and EC 8.B)
a. Acute form: Caused by bacterial invasion after trauma to cuticle
   (1) Clinical features: Exquisite pain, sudden swelling, and abscess formation around one nail.
   (2) Treatment: Responds quickly to drainage of abscess and warm tap-water soaks; occasionally anti-staphylococcal antibiotics required.
b. Chronic form: May involve one or several nails, history of frequent exposure to water (i.e., thumb-sucking); causative organisms *Candida* species, usually *C. albicans*.
   (1) Clinical features: Mild tenderness, small amount of pus may sometimes be expressed, nail maybe discolored or dystrophic.

(2) Treatment: resolved with topical antifungal agents and water avoidance; heals without scarring when thumb-sucking ends.
2. Nail dystrophy: distortion and discoloration of normal nail-plate structure; often traumatic or inflammatory causes (Figs. EC 8.C to EC 8.H).
a. Onychomycosis: a result of dermatophyte fungal infection, unusual before puberty.
b. Complications of trauma: Subungal hematoma, i.e., brown-black nail discoloration following crush injury, usually resolves without treatment; large painful blood collections may be drained. Must differentiate from melanoma and melanonychia.
c. Complications of underlying dermatosis: nail psoriasis, atopic nails
3. Nail changes and systemic disease (Figs. EC 8.I and EC 8.J)
a. Clubbing: complication of chronic lung or heart disease.
b. Beau lines: transverse, white lines/grooves that move distally with nail growth; due to growth arrest from systemic illness, medications, or toxins.

B. Congenital/Hereditary Nail Disorders

1. Isolated nail disorders (Figs. EC 8.K and 8.L)
a. Congenital nail dystrophy: clubbing and spooning (koilonychia), maybe autosomal dominant with no other anomalies
b. Congenital ingrown toenails: most self-limiting
2. Genodermatosis and systemic disease (Figs. EC 8.M and EC 8.N)
a. Periungal fibromas: arise in proximal nail groove, common finding in tuberous sclerosis
b. Congenital nail hypoplasia: can occur with intrauterine exposure to anticonvulsants, alcohol, and warfarin

IX. DISORDERS OF PIGMENTATION[17]

A. Hyperpigmentation

1. Epidermal melanosis: most lesions appear tan or light brown
a. Café au lait spots (Fig. EC 8.O): discrete tan macules that appear at birth or during childhood in 10%–20% of normal individuals, sizes vary from freckles to patches, may involve any site on skin
   (1) Diagnostic marker for NF-1 if: six or more lesions each >5 mm in diameter in someone aged <15 years.
b. Freckles (ephelides): reddish-tan and brown macules on sun-exposed surfaces, usually 2–3 mm in diameter.
   (1) Prevention: photoprotection may decrease reoccurrence during spring/summer months
   (2) Independent risk factor for melanoma in adulthood
c. Acanthosis nigricans (Figs. EC 8.P and EC 8.Q): brown-to-black hyperpigmentation with velvety or warty skin in intertriginous areas
   (1) Idiopathic form: most common variant; occurs in obese individuals with insulin resistance at risk for type II diabetes, may decrease after puberty with weight reduction

2. Dermal melanosis: Slate-gray, dark brown, or bluish green lesions.
a. Postinflammatory hyperpigmentation (Fig. EC 8.R): Most common cause of increased pigmentation.
   (1) Pathogenesis: Follows inflammatory processes in the skin like diaper dermatitis, insect bites, drug reactions and traumatic injuries.
   (2) Clinical features: Lesions localized, follow distribution of resolving disorder; more prominent in darkly pigmented children.
   (3) Treatment: None indicated, lesions fade over several months.
b. Acquired nevomelanocytic nevi (aka: pigmented nevi or moles) (Fig. EC 8.S)
   (1) Pathogenesis: Develop in early childhood as flat lesions called junctional nevi, then develop into compound nevi when nevus cells migrate into the dermis and lesions enlarge and become papular.
   (2) Clinical features: Increase in darkness, size, and number during puberty; generally do not exceed 5 mm and retain regularity in color, texture and symmetry; on sun-exposed areas.
   (3) Treatment: Excision unnecessary as long as appearance is unremarkable.
   (4) Changes associated with development of melanoma: Changes in size, shape, or border contours; changes in surfaces characteristics; changes in color; burning, itching, or redness.
c. Melanomas (Fig. EC 8.T)
   (1) Pathogenesis: May occur de novo or within acquired or congenital nevi.
   (2) Epidemiology: High lifetime risk in those with family history of malignant melanomas and presence of multiple, large, and irregularly pigmented, bordered, and textured nevi.
   (3) Management: Children in high-risk families must be carefully observed for atypical nevi development especially in adolescence; changing nevi with unusual appearance must be biopsied.
d. Spitz nevus (aka spindle and epithelial cell nevus) (Fig. EC 8.U): Innocent nevomelanocytic nevus often confused with malignant melanoma.
   (1) Clinical features: Rapidly growing, dome-shaped, red papules or nodules on face or lower extremities.
   (2) Management: Observe if features of innocent acquired nevus are present; biopsy if early rapid growth of lesion.

B. Hypopigmentation and Depigmentation

1. Localized hypopigmentation
a. Hypopigmented macules (Fig. EC 8.V)
   (1) Epidemiology: 0.1% of normal newborns have a single hypopigmented macule; but may be a marker for tuberous sclerosis as 70%–90% of those affected have such macules on the trunk at birth.

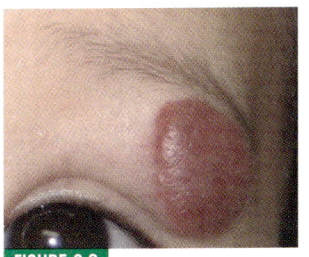

FIGURE 8.2
Infantile hemangioma. *(From Cohen BA. Atlas of Pediatric Dermatology. 3rd ed. St Louis: Mosby; 2005:126.)*

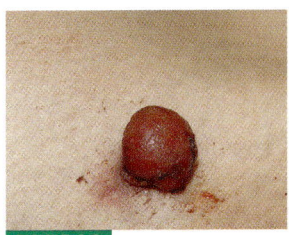

FIGURE 8.3
Pyogenic granuloma. *(From Cohen BA. Dermatology Image Atlas. Available at http://www.dermatlas.org/, 2001.)*

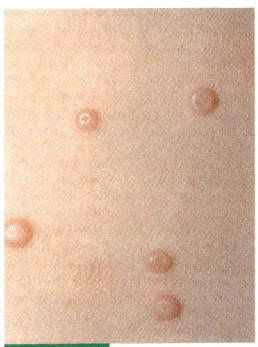

FIGURE 8.4
Molluscum contagiosum. *(From Cohen BA. Atlas of Pediatric Dermatology. 3rd ed. St Louis: Mosby; 2005:126.)*

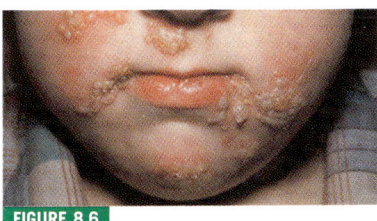

FIGURE 8.6
Herpetic gingivostomatitis. *(Modified from Cohen BA. Atlas of Pediatric Dermatology. 3rd ed. St Louis: Mosby; 2005:103.)*

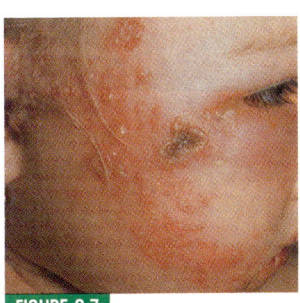

FIGURE 8.7
Herpes zoster. *(From Cohen BA. Atlas of Pediatric Dermatology. 3rd ed. St Louis: Mosby; 2005:106.)*

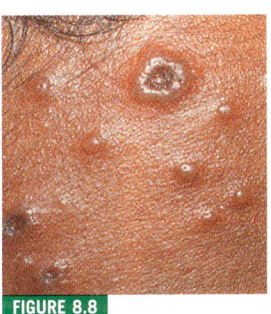

FIGURE 8.8
Varicella. *(From Cohen BA. Atlas of Pediatric Dermatology. 3rd ed. St Louis: Mosby; 2005:104.)*

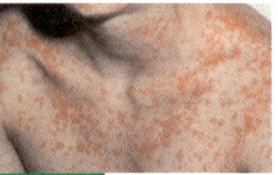

FIGURE 8.9
Measles. *(From Cohen BA. Atlas of Pediatric Dermatology. 3rd ed. St Louis: Mosby; 2005:166.)*

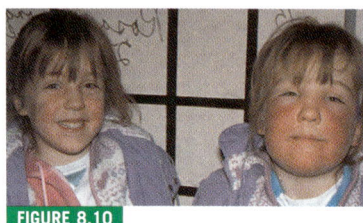

FIGURE 8.10
Fifth disease. *(From Cohen BA. Atlas of Pediatric Dermatology. 3rd ed. St Louis: Mosby; 2005:167.)*

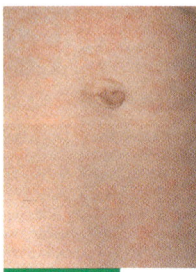

FIGURE 8.11
Roseola. *(From Cohen BA. Atlas of Pediatric Dermatology. 3rd ed. St Louis: Mosby; 2005:168.)*

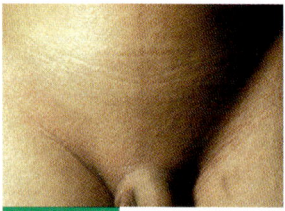

FIGURE 8.12
Scarlet fever. *(From Cohen BA. Dermatology Image Atlas. Available at http://www.dermatlas.org/, 2001.)*

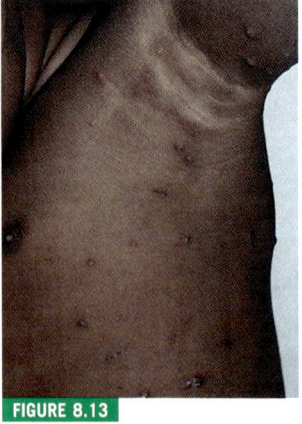

FIGURE 8.13
Scabies. *(From Cohen BA. Atlas of Pediatric Dermatology. 3rd ed. St Louis: Mosby; 2005:126.)*

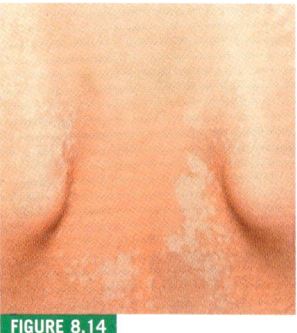

FIGURE 8.14
Tinea versicolor. *(From Cohen BA. Atlas of Pediatric Dermatology. St Louis: Mosby; 1993.)*

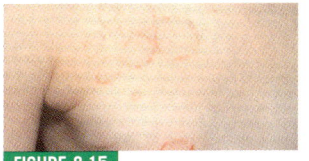

FIGURE 8.15
Tinea corporis. *(From Cohen BA. Atlas of Pediatric Dermatology. 3rd ed. St Louis: Mosby; 2005:94.)*

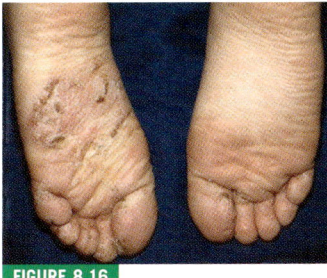

FIGURE 8.16
Tinea pedis. *(From Cohen BA. Dermatology Image Atlas. Available at http://www.dermatlas.org/, 2001.)*

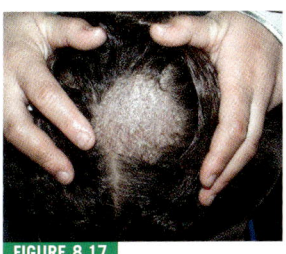

FIGURE 8.17
Tinea capitis. *(From Cohen BA. Atlas of Pediatric Dermatology. 3rd ed. St Louis: Mosby; 1993.)*

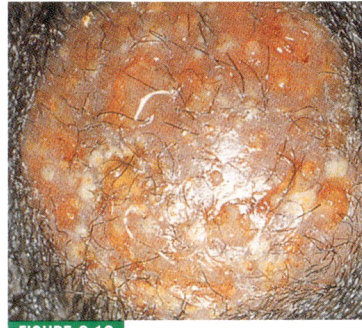

FIGURE 8.18
Kerion. *(From Cohen BA. Atlas of Pediatric Dermatology. 3rd ed. St Louis: Mosby; 2005:207.)*

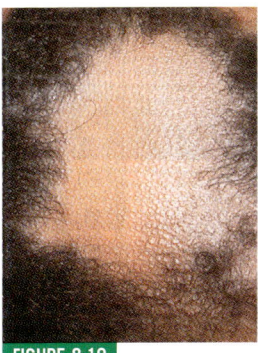

FIGURE 8.19
Alopecia areata. *(From Cohen BA. Atlas of Pediatric Dermatology. 3rd ed. St Louis: Mosby; 2005:208.)*

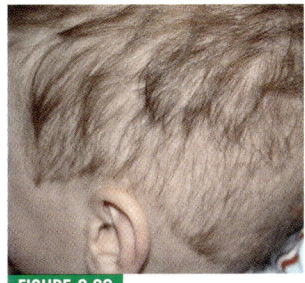

FIGURE 8.20
Telogen effluvium. *(From Cohen BA. Dermatology Image Atlas. Available at http://www.dermatlas.org/, 2001.)*

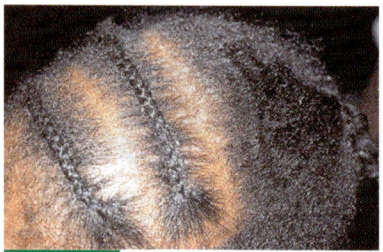

FIGURE 8.21
Traction alopecia. (From Cohen BA. Atlas of Pediatric Dermatology. 3rd ed. St Louis: Mosby; 2005:209.)

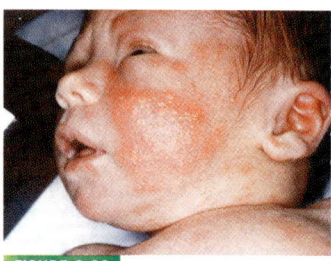

FIGURE 8.23
Erythema toxicum neonatorum. (From Cohen BA. Pediatric Dermatology. 2nd ed. St Louis: Mosby; 1999:18.)

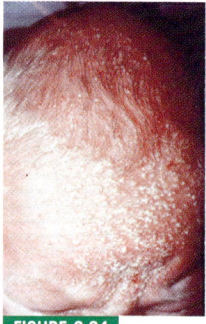

FIGURE 8.24
Transient neonatal pustular melanosis. (From Cohen BA. Atlas of Pediatric Dermatology. 3rd ed. St Louis: Mosby; 2005:20.)

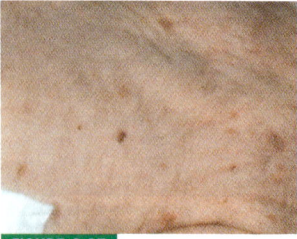

FIGURE 8.25
Hyperpigmentation from resolving transient neonatal pustular melanosis. (From Cohen BA. Atlas of Pediatric Dermatology. 3rd ed. St Louis: Mosby; 2005:20.)

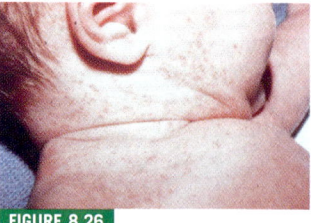

FIGURE 8.26
Miliaria rubra. (From Cohen BA. Atlas of Pediatric Dermatology. 3rd ed. St Louis: Mosby; 2005:22.)

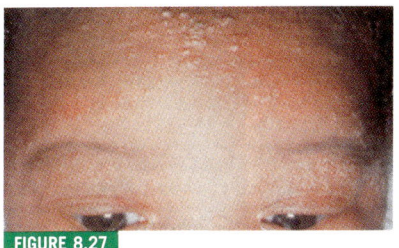

FIGURE 8.27
Milia. *(From Cohen BA. Atlas of Pediatric Dermatology. 3rd ed. St Louis: Mosby; 2005:22.)*

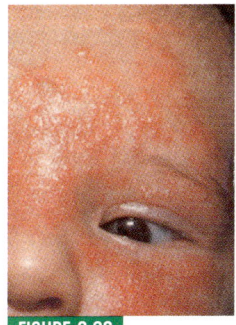

FIGURE 8.28
Neonatal acne. *(From Cohen BA. Atlas of Pediatric Dermatology. 3rd ed. St Louis: Mosby; 2005:23.)*

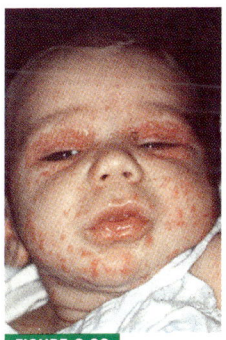

FIGURE 8.29
Seborrheic dermatitis. *(From Cohen BA. Atlas of Pediatric Dermatology. 3rd ed. St Louis: Mosby; 2005:33.)*

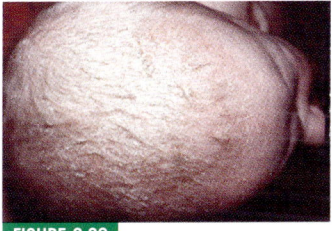

FIGURE 8.30
Seborrheic dermatitis. *(From Cohen BA. Atlas of Pediatric Dermatology. 3rd ed. St Louis: Mosby; 2005:33.)*

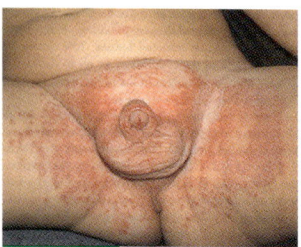

FIGURE 8.31
Diaper candidiasis. *(From Cohen BA. Atlas of Pediatric Dermatology. 3rd ed. St Louis: Mosby; 2005:34.)*

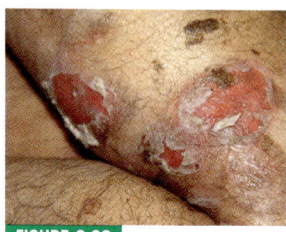

FIGURE 8.32
Pemphigus vulgaris. *(From Cohen BA. Dermatology Image Atlas. Available at http://www.dermatlas.org/, 2001.)*

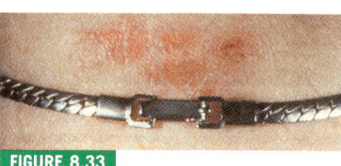

FIGURE 8.33
Allergic contact dermatitis. *(From Cohen BA. Atlas of Pediatric Dermatology. 3rd ed. St Louis: Mosby; 2005:75.)*

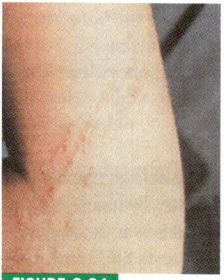

FIGURE 8.34
Poison ivy. *(From Cohen BA. Dermatology Image Atlas. Available at http://www.dermatlas.org/, 2001.)*

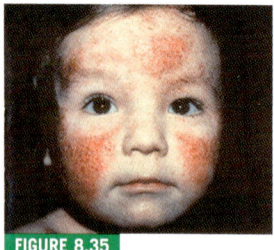

FIGURE 8.35
Infantile eczema. *(From Cohen BA. Atlas of Pediatric Dermatology. 3rd ed. St Louis: Mosby; 2005:79.)*

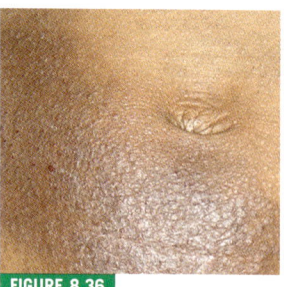

FIGURE 8.36
Childhood eczema. *(From Cohen BA. Dermatology Image Atlas. Available at http://www.dermatlas.org/, 2001.)*

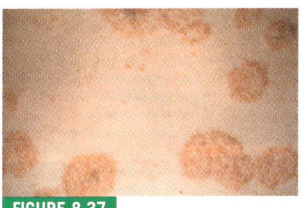

FIGURE 8.37
Nummular eczema. *(From Cohen BA. Atlas of Pediatric Dermatology. 3rd ed. St Louis: Mosby; 2005:80.)*

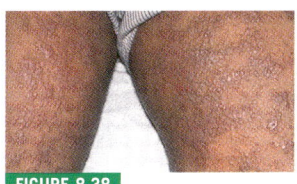

FIGURE 8.38
Follicular eczema. *(From Cohen BA. Atlas of Pediatric Dermatology. 3rd ed. St Louis: Mosby; 2005:80.)*

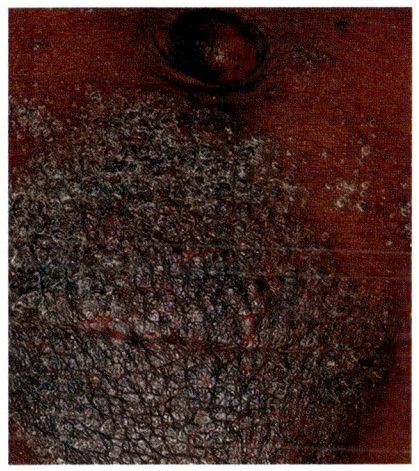

FIGURE 8.39
Childhood eczema with lesion in suprapubic area. *(From Cohen BA. Atlas of Pediatric Dermatology. 3rd ed. St Louis: Mosby; 2005.)*

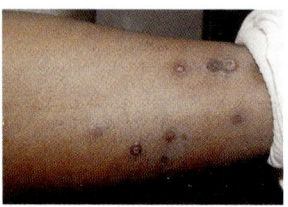

FIGURE 8.40
Papular urticaria. *(From Cohen BA. Dermatology Image Atlas. Available at http://www.dermatlas.org/, 2001.)*

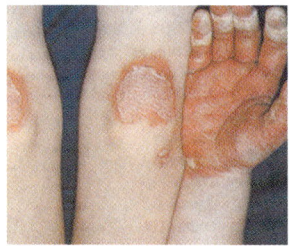

FIGURE 8.41
Psoriasis. *(From Cohen BA. Atlas of Pediatric Dermatology. 3rd ed. St Louis: Mosby; 2005:67.)*

(2) Clinical features: Minority are lancet or ash-leaf shaped, but may be round, oval, dermatomal, segmental or irregularly shaped; vary from pinpoint confetti spots to large patches >10 cm; trunk involvement most common.
(3) Diagnosis: Wood lamp helpful in lightly pigmented children.
(4) Management: In those where systemic disease is suspected, close observation for other cutaneous findings and systemic symptoms is indicated.

b. Postinflammatory hypopigmentation (Fig. EC 8.W)
   (1) Pathogenesis: May appear after an inflammatory skin condition.
   (2) Clinical features: Patches usually variable in size and irregularly shaped; concomitant hyperpigmentation also common; seen in association with primary lesions of underlying disorder (such as atopic dermatitis).

2. Diffuse hypopigmentation
a. Albinism: Heterogeneous group of inherited disorders manifested by generalized hypopigmentation or depigmentation of skin, eyes, and hair.

C. Dyspigmentation

1. Blaschkoid dyspigmentation[18]: Congenital hypopigmentation and hyperpigmentation along the lines of Blaschko (Fig. EC 8.X)
a. Patterns of hyper- or hypopigmentation: Whorl shape on trunk, V-shape on the back, waves on the vertex scalp.
b. Pathogenesis: Blaschko lines occur due to genetic mosaicism.
c. Children unlikely to have or develop serious extracutaneous involvement.

REFERENCES

1. ISSVA Classification of Vascular Anomalies. International Society for the Study of Vascular Anomalies. Available at: http://issva.org/classification. Accessed April 2014.
2. Hartemink DA, Chiu YE, Drolet BA, et al. PHACES syndrome: a review. *Int J Pediatr Otorhinolaryngol*. 2009;73:181-187.
3. FDA, Pierre Fabre Pharmaceuticals. *Hemangeol*. March 2014. Available at: http://www.accessdata.fda.gov/drugsatfda_docs/label/2014/205410s000lbl.pdf. Accessed October 2015.
4. Kwok CS, Gibbs S, Bennett C. Topical treatment for cutaneous warts. *Cochrane Database Syst Rev*. 2012;(9):CD001781.
5. Hicks MI, Elston DM. Scabies. *Dermatol Ther*. 2009;22:279-292.
6. Andrews MD, Burns M. Common tinea infections in children. *Am Fam Physician*. 2008;77:1415-1420.
7. Alkhalifah A, Alsantali A, Wang E, et al. Alopecia areata update: part II. Treatment. *J Am Acad Dermatol*. 2010;62:191-202.
8. Zaenglein AL, Thiboutot DM. Expert committee recommendations for acne management. *Pediatrics*. 2006;118:1188-1199.
9. Archer CB, Cohen SN, Baron SE. Guidance on the diagnosis and clinical management of acne. *Clin Exp Dermatol*. 2012;37(suppl 1):1-6.

10. Eichenfield LF, Krakowski AC, Piggott C, et al. Evidence-based recommendations for the diagnosis and treatment of pediatric acne. *Pediatrics*. 2013;131(Suppl 3):S163-S186.
11. McAleer MA, Flohr C, Irvine AD. Management of difficult and severe eczema in childhood. *BMJ*. 2012;345:e4770.
12. Eichenfield LF, Tom WL, Berger TG, et al. Guidelines of care for the management of atopic dermatitis. Section 2. Management and treatment of atopic dermatitis with topical therapies. *J Am Acad Dernatol*. 2014;71(1):116-132.
13. Patel TS, Greer SC, Skinner RB Jr. Cancer concerns with topical immunomodulators in atopic dermatitis: overview of data and recommendations to clinicians. *Am J Clin Dermatol*. 2007;8:189-194.
14. Boquniewicz M, Leung DY. Recent insights into atopic dermatitis and implications for management of infectious complications. *J Allergy Clin Immunol*. 2010;125:4-13.
15. Hernandez RG, Cohen BA. Insect bite-induced hypersensitivity and the SCRATCH p16. rinciples: a new approach to papular urticaria. *Pediatrics*. 2006;118:e189-e196.
16. Cohen BA. Disorders of the Hair and Nails. In: *Pediatric Dermatology*. 4th ed. Philadelphia: Elsevier; 2013:211-239.
17. Cohen BA. Disorders in Pigmentation. In: *Pediatric Dermatology*. 4th ed. Philadelphia: Elsevier; 2013:48-68.
18. Cohen J, Shahrokh K, Cohen B. Analysis of 36 Cases of Blaschkoid dyspigmentation: reading between the lines of Blaschko. *Pediatr Dermatol*. 2014;31(4):471-476.

Chapter 9
Development, Behavior, and Mental Health
Julia Thorn, MD

See additional content on Expert Consult

I. WEB RESOURCES

- Attention deficit/hyperactivity disorder (ADHD): www.chadd.org
- ADHD Medication Guide: www.ADHDMedicationGuide.com
- American Academy of Pediatrics (AAP)—Developmental and Behavioral Pediatrics: www.dbpeds.org
- Autism Speaks: www.autismspeaks.org
- Bright Futures: www.brightfutures.org
- Cerebral Palsy Foundation: www.yourcpf.org
- Child and Adolescent Psychiatry Practice Parameters: www.aacap.org
- Disability Programs and Services: www.disability.gov
- Individuals with Disabilities Education Act (IDEA): idea.ed.gov
- Intellectual Disability: aaidd.org
- Mental health patient and provider handouts: www.nimh.nih.gov
- National Center for Learning Disabilities: www.ncld.org
- National Dissemination Center for Children with Disabilities (NICHCY) legacy resources: http://www.parentcenterhub.org/nichcy-resources/
- National Early Childhood Technical Assistance Center: www.ectacenter.org
- Reach Out and Read: www.reachoutandread.org

II. DEVELOPMENTAL DEFINITIONS[1]

A. Developmental Streams

1. **Gross Motor Skills:** Descriptions of posture and locomotion—in general, how a child moves from one location to another
2. **Fine-Motor and Visual-Motor Problem-Solving Skills:** Upper extremity and hand manipulative abilities and hand-eye coordination. Require an intact motor substrate and a given level of nonverbal cognitive ability
3. **Language:** The ability to understand and communicate with another person. The best predictor of intellectual performance, in the absence of a communication disorder or significant hearing impairment.
4. **Personal-Social Skills:** Communicative in origin, and represent the cumulative impact of language comprehension and problem-solving skills
5. **Adaptive Skills:** Skills concerned with self-help or activities of daily living

B. Developmental Quotient (DQ)

1. **A calculation that reflects the rate of development** in any given stream, and represents the percentage of normal development present at the time of testing. DQ = (developmental age/chronologic age) × 100
2. **Two separate developmental assessments** over time are more predictive of later abilities than a single assessment
3. In contrast to DQ, intelligence quotient has statistical reliability and validity

C. Abnormal Development

1. **Delay**
   a. Performance significantly below average (DQ < 70) in a given area of development. May occur in a single stream or several streams ("global developmental delay").
2. **Deviancy**
   a. Atypical development within a single stream, such as developmental milestones occurring out of sequence. Deviancy does not necessarily imply abnormality but should alert one to the possibility that problems may exist.
   Example: An infant who rolls at an early age may have abnormally increased tone.
   b. Deviancy may also denote emergence of a presentation that is not typically part of the developmental sequence.
   Example: A toddler showing no interest in peers.
3. **Dissociation**
   a. A substantial difference in the rate of development between two or more streams.
   Example: Increased motor delay relative to cognition seen in some children with cerebral palsy.

III. GUIDELINES FOR NORMAL DEVELOPMENT AND BEHAVIOR

A. Developmental Milestones (Table 9.1)

1. Developmental assessment is based on the premise that milestone acquisition occurs at a specific rate in an orderly and sequential manner.

B. Reach Out and Read Milestones of Early Literacy (Table 9.2)

C. Age-Appropriate Behavioral Issues in Infancy and Early Childhood (Table 9.3)

IV. DEVELOPMENTAL SCREENING AND EVALUATION

A. Developmental Surveillance and Screening Guidelines

1. **Developmental *surveillance* should be included in every well-child visit, and any concerns should be addressed immediately with formal screening.** Five components:

Text continued on p. 235

TABLE 9.1
DEVELOPMENTAL MILESTONES

Age	Gross Motor	Visual–Motor/Problem-Solving	Language	Social/Adaptive
1 mo	Raises head from prone position	Visually fixes, follows to midline, has tight grasp	Alerts to sound	Regards face
2 mo	Holds head in midline, lifts chest off table	No longer clenches fists tightly, follows object past midline	Smiles socially (after being stroked or talked to)	Recognizes parent
3 mo	Supports on forearms in prone position, holds head up steadily	Holds hands open at rest, follows in circular fashion, responds to visual threat	Coos (produces long vowel sounds in musical fashion)	Reaches for familiar people or objects, anticipates feeding
4 mo	Rolls over, supports on wrists, shifts weight	Reaches with arms in unison, brings hands to midline	Laughs, orients to voice	Enjoys looking around
6 mo	Sits unsupported, puts feet in mouth in supine position	Unilateral reach, uses raking grasp, transfers objects	Babbles, ah-goo, razz, lateral orientation to bell	Recognizes that someone is a stranger
9 mo	Pivots when sitting, crawls well, pulls to stand, cruises	Uses immature pincer grasp, probes with forefinger, holds bottle, throws objects	Says "mama, dada" indiscriminately, gestures, waves bye-bye, understands "no"	Starts exploring environment, plays gesture games (e.g., pat-a-cake)
12 mo	Walks alone	Uses mature pincer grasp, can make a crayon mark, releases voluntarily	Uses two words other than "mama, dada" or proper nouns, jargoning (runs several unintelligible words together with tone or inflection), one-step command with gesture	Imitates actions, comes when called, cooperates with dressing

Continued

TABLE 9.1
DEVELOPMENTAL MILESTONES—cont'd

Age	Gross Motor	Visual–Motor/Problem-Solving	Language	Social/Adaptive
15 mo	Creeps up stairs, walks backward independently	Scribbles in imitation, builds tower of two blocks in imitation	Uses 4–6 words, follows one-step command without gesture	15–18 mo: uses spoon and cup
18 mo	Runs, throws objects from standing without falling	Scribbles spontaneously, builds tower of three blocks, turns two or three pages at a time	Mature jargoning (includes intelligible words), 7–10 word vocabulary, knows five body parts	Copies parent in tasks (sweeping, dusting), plays in company of other children
24 mo	Walks up and down steps without help	Imitates stroke with pencil, builds tower of seven blocks, turns pages one at a time, removes shoes, pants, etc.	Uses pronouns (I, you, me) inappropriately, follows two-step commands, 50-word vocabulary, uses two-word sentences	Parallel play
3 yr	Can alternate feet going up steps, pedals tricycle	Copies a circle, undresses completely, dresses partially, dries hands if reminded, unbuttons	Uses minimum of 250 words, three-word sentences, uses plurals, knows all pronouns, repeats two digits	Group play, shares toys, takes turns, plays well with others, knows full name, age, gender
4 yr	Hops, skips, alternates feet going down steps	Copies a square, buttons clothing, dresses self completely, catches ball	Knows colors, says song or poem from memory, asks questions	Tells "tall tales," plays cooperatively with a group of children
5 yr	Skips alternating feet, jumps over low obstacles	Copies triangle, ties shoes, spreads with knife	Prints first name, asks what a word means	Plays competitive games, abides by rules, likes to help in household tasks

From Caputo AJ, Biehl RF. Functional developmental evaluation: prerequisite to habilitation. Pediatr Clin North Am. 1973;20:3; Capute AJ, Accardo PJ. Linguistic and auditory milestones during the first two years of life: a language inventory for the practitioner. Clin Pediatr. 1978;17:847; and Capute AJ, Shapiro BK, Wachtel RC, et al. The Clinical Linguistic and Auditory Milestone Scale (CLAMS): identification of cognitive defects in motor delayed children. Am J Dis Child. 1986;140:694. Rounded norms from Capute AJ, Palmer FB, Shapiro BK, et al. Clinical Linguistic and Auditory Milestone Scale: prediction of cognition in infancy. Dev Med Child Neurol. 1986;28:762.

TABLE 9.2
REACH OUT AND READ MILESTONES OF EARLY LITERACY

Age	Motor	Cognitive
6–12 mo	Reaches for books, turns pages with help	Looks at pictures, pats pictures
12–18 mo	Carries book, holds book with help, turns several board pages at a time	Points to pictures with a single finger, points to specific items on page, gives book to adult
18–24 mo	Turns one board page at a time	Repeats and retells parts of known stories
24–36 mo	Begins to turn paper pages	Looks at favorite books on own, repeats and retells whole phrases and stories, associates pictures with text of story
3 yr	Turns paper pages easily	Growing attention span, recites favorite stories, begins to identify single letters
4 yr and older	Writes name	Uses past tense and plurals, answers "what will happen next?"

From Reach Out and Read National Center: www.reachoutandread.org.

TABLE 9.3
AGE-APPROPRIATE BEHAVIORAL ISSUES IN INFANCY AND EARLY CHILDHOOD

Age	Behavioral Issue	Symptoms	Guidance
1–3 mo	Colic	Paroxysms of fussiness/crying, 3+ hr per day, 3+ days per wk, may pull knees up to chest, pass flatus	Crying usually peaks at 6 wk and resolves by 3–4 mo. Prevent overstimulation; swaddle infant; use white noise, swing, or car rides to soothe. Avoid medication and formula changes. Encourage breaks for the primary caregiver.
3–4 mo	Trained night feeding	Night awakening	Comfort quietly, avoid reinforcing behavior (i.e., avoid night feeds). Do not play at night. Introducing cereal or solid food does not reduce awakening. Develop a consistent bedtime routine. Place baby in bed while drowsy and not fully asleep.

Continued

TABLE 9.3

AGE-APPROPRIATE BEHAVIORAL ISSUES IN INFANCY AND EARLY CHILDHOOD—cont'd

Age	Behavioral Issue	Symptoms	Guidance
9 mo	Stranger anxiety/separation anxiety	Distress when separated from parent or approached by a stranger	Use a transitional object (e.g., special toy, blanket); use routine or ritual to separate from parent; may continue until 24 mo but can reduce in intensity.
	Developmental night waking	Separation anxiety at night	Keep lights off. Avoid picking child up or feeding. May reassure verbally at regular intervals or place a transitional object in crib.
12 mo	Aggression	Biting, hitting, kicking in frustration	Say "no" with negative facial cues. Begin time out (1 minute per year of age). No eye contact or interaction, place in a nonstimulating location. May restrain child gently until cooperation is achieved.
	Need for limit setting	Exploration of environment, danger of injury	Avoid punishing exploration or poor judgment. Emphasize child-proofing and distraction.
18 mo	Temper tantrums	Occur with frustration, attention-seeking rage, negativity/refusal	Try to determine cause, react appropriately (i.e., help child who is frustrated, ignore attention-seeking behavior). Make sure child is in a safe location.
24 mo	Toilet training	Child needs to demonstrate readiness: shows interest, neurologic maturity (i.e., recognizes urge to urinate or defecate), ability to walk to bathroom and undress self, desire to please/imitate parents, increasing periods of daytime dryness	Age range for toilet training is usually 2–4 yr. Give guidance early; may introduce potty seat but avoid pressure or punishment for accidents. Wait until the child is ready. Expect some periods of regression, especially with stressors.

TABLE 9.3
AGE-APPROPRIATE BEHAVIORAL ISSUES IN INFANCY AND EARLY CHILDHOOD—cont'd

Age	Behavioral Issue	Symptoms	Guidance
24–36 mo	New sibling	Regression, aggressive behavior	Allow for special time with parent, 10–20 min daily of one-on-one time exclusively devoted to the older sibling(s). Child chooses activity with parent. No interruptions. May not be taken away as punishment.
36 mo	Nightmares	Awakens crying, may or may not complain of bad dream	Reassure child, explain that he or she had a bad dream. Leave bedroom door open, use a nightlight, demonstrate there are no monsters under the bed. Discuss dream the following day. Avoid scary movies or television shows.
	Night terrors	Agitation, screaming 1–2 h after going to bed. Child may have eyes open but not respond to parent. May occur at same time each night	May be familial, not volitional. *Prevention:* For several nights, awaken child 15 min before terrors typically occur. Avoid overtiredness. *Acute:* Be calm; speak in soft, soothing, repetitive tones; help child return to sleep. Protect child against injury.

From Dixon SD, Stein MT. Encounters with Children: Pediatric Behavior and Development. St Louis: Mosby, 2000.

a. Eliciting and attending to the parent's concerns: "Do you have any concerns about your child's development? Behavior? Learning?"
b. Maintaining a developmental history: "What changes have you seen in your child's development since our last visit?"; "How old would you say your child acts?"
c. Making accurate and informed observations of the child
d. Identifying the presence of risk and protective factors
e. Documenting the process and findings
2. **Standardized developmental *screening* should be administered at 9-month, 18-month, and 30-month well-child visits**, in the absence of developmental concerns. If a 30-month visit is not possible, this screening can be done at the 24-month visit.
3. **See full American Academy of Pediatrics (AAP) guideline for developmental screening algorithm**[2]

B. Commonly Used Developmental Screening and Assessment Tools

1. **Appropriate screening tests vary with age and suspected diagnosis.** Several developmental screening and assessment tools are available, such as the **Ages and Stages Questionnaire** (ASQ) and **Capute Scales** (Table 9.4).
   a. **Goodenough–Harris Draw-a-Person Test:** Give the child a pencil and a sheet of blank paper. Instruct the child to "draw a person; draw the best person you can." Use scoring guidelines to assess drawing and compare with norms for age (Box EC 9.A on Expert Consult).
   b. **Gesell figures** (Fig. 9.1): Ask the child to copy various shapes
   c. **Gesell block skills** (Fig. EC 9.A): Ask the child to reproduce block structures as built by the examiner
2. Significant delay, deviancy, dissociation, or developmental "red flags" (Table 9.5) on surveillance or screening merit referrals for:
   a. Developmental and appropriate subspecialist evaluations
   b. Early intervention services for children aged 0 to 3 years (see Section VII, Developmental Referral and Intervention)

V. MEDICAL EVALUATION OF DEVELOPMENTAL DISORDERS

A. History

1. **Prenatal and birth:** Prenatal genetic screening, perception of fetal movement, pregnancy complications, toxins/teratogens, gestational age, birthweight, days in hospital, complications, newborn screen
2. **Past medical problems:** Trauma, infection, medication
3. **Developmental history:** Timing of milestone achievement, delayed skills, loss of skills (regression)
4. **Behavioral history:** Social skills, eye contact, affection, hyperactivity, impulsivity, inattention, distractibility, self-regulation, perseveration, worries/avoidance, stereotypies, peculiar habits
5. **Educational history:** Need for special services, grade retention, established educational plans
6. **Family history:** Developmental disabilities, late talkers or walkers, poor school performance, ADHD, seizures, tics, recurrent miscarriage, stillbirth, neonatal death, congenital malformations, mental illness, parental consanguinity. A three-generation pedigree should be constructed (see Chapter 13),

B. Physical Examination

1. **General:** Height, weight, head circumference, dysmorphic features, cardiac murmurs, midline defects, hepatosplenomegaly, skin exam
2. **Age-directed neurologic examination:** Cranial nerves, tone, strength, postural reactions, functional abilities, reflexes (including primitive reflexes for infants; Tables EC 9.A and 9.B)

TABLE 9.4
DEVELOPMENTAL AND MENTAL HEALTH SCREENING TESTS BY DIAGNOSIS

Symptoms or Diagnosis Evaluated	Screening Test	Age	Administration Time	Completed by	Comments	Weblink
DEVELOPMENT						
Cognitive/motor development	Ages and Stages Questionnaire (ASQ)	4–60 mo	10–15 min	Parent	Increased time efficiency (can fill out while waiting) Document milestones that are difficult to assess in the office	http://www.agesandstages.com
Developmental and behavioral problems	Parents' Evaluation of Developmental Status (PEDS)	0–8 yr	2–10 min	Parent	May also be useful as a surveillance tool	http://www.pedstest.com
Language, problem-solving development	Capute Scales: Clinical Linguistic and Auditory Milestone Scale (CLAMS); Clinical Adaptive Test (CAT)	3–36 mo	15–20 min	Clinician	Give quantitative DQs for language (CLAMS) and visual-motor problem-solving (CAT) abilities	http://www.brookespublishing.com/resource-center/screening-and-assessment/the-capute-scales/
Autism spectrum disorders	Modified Checklist for Autism in Toddlers, Revised with Follow-Up (M-CHAT-R/F)	16–30 mo	5–10 min	Parent	Positive screens require clinician follow-up	www.m-chat.org
	Communication and Symbolic Behavior Scales and Developmental Profile (CSBS DP; Infant Toddler Checklist)	6–24 mo	5–10 min	Parent	The Infant Toddler Checklist is a one-page questionnaire that is part of a larger standardized screening tool (CSBS DP) Can be used in patients as young as 6 months	www.brookespublishing.com/checklist.pdf
	Childhood Autism Screening Test (CAST)	4–11 yr	10 min	Parent	Only screening tool evaluated in preschool population	http://www.autismresearchcentre.com/project_9_cast

Continued

TABLE 9.4
DEVELOPMENTAL AND MENTAL HEALTH SCREENING TESTS BY DIAGNOSIS—cont'd

Symptoms or Diagnosis Evaluated	Screening Test	Age	Administration Time	Completed by	Comments	Weblink
MENTAL HEALTH						
General psychosocial screening	Pediatric Symptom Checklist (PSC)	4–16 yr	<5 min	Parent or child/adolescent	Assesses attention, externalizing, and internalizing symptoms	http://www.massgeneral.org/psychiatry/services/psc_home.aspx
Attention deficit/hyperactivity disorder (ADHD)	Vanderbilt Diagnostic Rating Scales	6–12 yr	10 min	Parent Teachers	Separate scales for functioning in different domains (home, school)	http://www.nichq.org/childrens-health/adhd/resources/vanderbilt-assessment-scales
ADHD plus other domains	Conners' Rating Scales-Revised	3–17 yr	20 min	Parent or patient if 12–17 years Teacher	Six distinct scales that assess oppositionality, cognitive problems/inattention, hyperactivity, anxiety/shyness, perfectionism, social problems, and psychosomatic problems	www.mhs.com/conners3
Anxiety	Self-Report for Childhood Anxiety Related Emotional Disorders (SCARED)	8+ yr	5 min	Parent Patient	Separate scales for parent and patient Does not assess for OCD, PTSD Multiple subscales of anxiety	http://www.midss.org/content/screen-child-anxiety-related-disorders-scared
	Spence Children's Anxiety Scale	2.5–12 yr	5–10 min	Parent or patient if 8–12 years		http://www.scaswebsite.com/
Depression	Patient Health Questionnaire-2 (PHQ-2)	13+ yr	1 min	Patient	Brief screening tool for adolescents or parents (e.g., postpartum depression)	http://www.cqaimh.org/pdf/tool_phq2.pdf
	Center for Epidemiological Studies Depression Scale for Children (CES-DC)	6–17 yr	5–10 min	Child/adolescent	Originally used in adult populations	http://www.brightfutures.org/mentalhealth/pdf/professionals/bridges/ces_dc.pdf

Modified from American Academy of Pediatrics. Identifying infants and young children with developmental disorders in the medical home: an algorithm for developmental surveillance and screening. Pediatrics. 2006;118:405-420; American Academy of Pediatrics. Identification and evaluation of children with autism spectrum disorders. Pediatrics. 2007;120: 1183-1215; American Academy of Pediatrics. Mental health screening and assessment tools for primary care. From Addressing Mental Health Concerns in Primary Care: A Clinician's Toolkit. 2010; Robins DL, Casagrande K, Barton M, et al. Validation of the Modified Checklist for Autism in Toddlers, Revised with Follow-up (M-CHAT-R/F). Pediatrics. 2014;133:37-45.

Chapter 9 Development, Behavior, and Mental Health

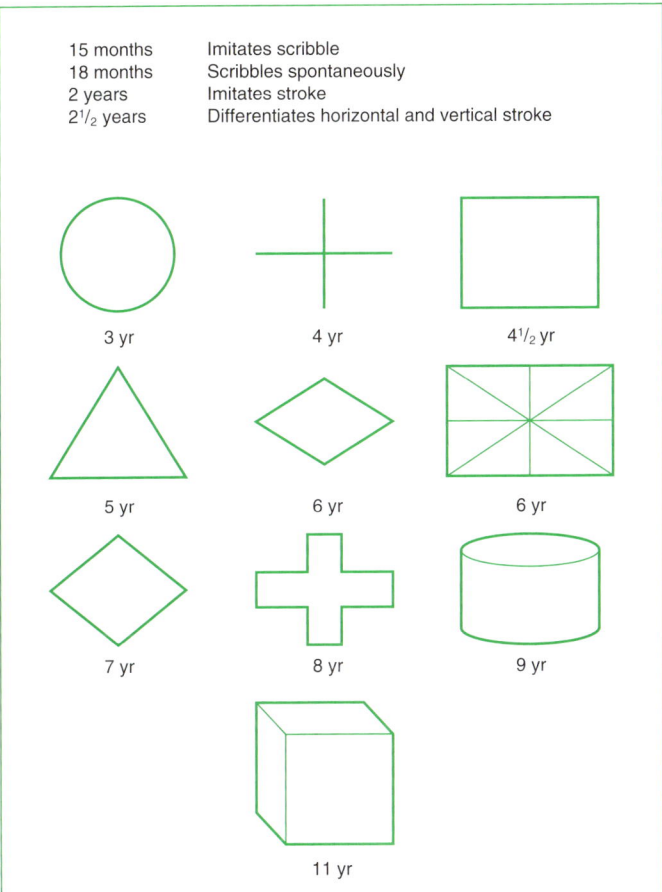

FIGURE 9.1
Gesell figures. *(From Illingsworth RS. The Development of the Infant and Young Child, Normal and Abnormal. 5th ed. Baltimore: Williams & Wilkins; 1972:229-232; and Cattel P. The Measurement of Intelligence of Infants and Young Children. New York: Psychological Corporation; 1960:97-261.)*

C. Laboratory Investigations, Imaging Studies, Other Tests

1. **Hearing and vision screening:** Hearing or vision loss may be part of a broader syndrome. Formal audiologic testing is indicated for all children with global developmental delay or any delay in communication or language.

TABLE 9.5
DEVELOPMENTAL RED FLAGS

Positive Indicators (Presence of Any of the Following)	Negative Indicators (Activities That the Child Cannot Do)
Loss of developmental skills at any age	Sit unsupported by 12 mo
Parental or professional concerns about vision, fixing, or following an object or a confirmed visual impairment at any age (simultaneous referral to pediatric ophthalmology)	Walk by 18 mo (boys) or 2 yr (girls) (check creatine kinase urgently)
Hearing loss at any age (simultaneous referral for expert audiologic or ear, nose, and throat assessment)	Walk other than on tiptoes
Persistently low muscle tone or floppiness	Run by 2.5 yr
No speech by 18 mo, especially if the child does not try to communicate by other means such as gestures (simultaneous referral for urgent hearing test)	Hold object placed in hand by 5 mo (corrected for gestation)
Asymmetry of movements or other features suggestive of cerebral palsy, such as increased muscle tone	Reach for objects by 6 mo (corrected for gestation)
Persistent toe walking	Point at objects to share interest with others by 16–18 mo
Complex disabilities	
Head circumference above the 99.6th percentile or below 0.4th percentile. Also, if circumference has crossed two percentiles (up or down) on the appropriate chart or is disproportionate to parental head circumference	
An assessing clinician who is uncertain about any aspect of assessment but thinks that development may be disordered	

Adapted from Bellman M, Byrne O, Sege R. Developmental assessment of children. BMJ. 2013;346:31-36.

2. **Neuroimaging:** If abnormal neurologic examination, concern about head circumference growth velocity, or global developmental delay. Discussion with neuroradiologist is of benefit in determining optimal imaging study.
3. **Electroencephalogram (EEG):** If history of seizure or concern about epilepsy syndrome
4. **Laboratory studies:** Consider CBC, CMP, lead level, CK, TSH based on history and exam
5. **Genetic studies:**
a. **Microarray** is the genetic test with the highest diagnostic yield, and is considered the first-line cytogenetic test for all patients with unexplained global developmental delay, intellectual disability, autism, and/or congenital anomalies.
b. **Whole exome sequencing** is clinically available to perform comprehensive assessment of the coding portion of the genome in

patients with unexplained global developmental delay. This test should only be ordered by a geneticist/genetic counselor after extensive pretest counseling.
c. Fragile X testing should be performed in all boys and girls with global developmental delay or intellectual disability of unknown cause.[3]
d. Karyotyping should be reserved for patients with signs of specific chromosomal syndromes (e.g., trisomy 13, 18, or 21).
e. Screening for *MECP2* mutations may be done in females with severe impairment to evaluate for Rett syndrome and related disorders.
f. Any abnormal result should be referred for comprehensive genetic counseling. See Chapter 13 for more details regarding these tests and diagnoses.

6. **Metabolic studies:**
a. Have a higher suspicion in children whose parents are consanguineous or have had children with similar problems, unexplained death, or fetal demise.
b. These children may have multiple organ system dysfunction, failure to thrive, dietary selectivity, unusual odors, hearing loss, or episodic symptoms (seizures or encephalopathy).[4]
c. Screening tests include plasma amino acids, homocysteine, acylcarnitine profile, and urine organic acids.[3] See Chapter 13 for more details.

VI. DISORDERS OF DEVELOPMENT

A. Overview
1. Mental and/or physical impairment(s) that cause significant limitations in functioning.
2. **Developmental diagnosis** is a functional description; identification of an etiology is important to further inform treatment, prognosis, comorbidities, and future risk.
3. School- and home-based programs are helpful interventions for all developmental disorders (see Section 9-VII, Developmental Referral and Intervention).

B. Intellectual Disability (ID)
1. **Definition and epidemiology**
a. Deficits in general mental abilities, previously known as mental retardation
b. Affects approximately 1% of the population[5]
c. Males more likely to be diagnosed with mild and severe ID[5]
2. **Clinical presentation**
a. Delay in milestones (motor, language, social)
b. Academic difficulty

c. Identifiable features of known associated genetic syndrome (e.g., Trisomy 21, Fragile X, Rett syndrome)

3. **Diagnosis**
a. Diagnostic criteria: 1) deficits in intellectual functioning, 2) deficits in adaptive functioning, 3) onset of these deficits during the developmental period
b. Deficits in adaptive functioning must be in one or more domains of activities of daily living
   i. ID is further categorized as mild, moderate, severe, or profound in the DSM-5 based on the degree of functional deficit (Table EC 9.C)

4. **Interventions/treatment**
a. Support, employment, and recreational programs through resources such as The Arc (www.thearc.org)

C. Communication Disorders

1. **Definition**
a. Deficits in communication, language, or speech
b. Can be subdivided into **receptive/expressive language disorder [includes social (pragmatic) communication disorder], speech sound disorders, childhood-onset fluency disorder (stuttering), and voice disorders**
c. Differential diagnosis includes ID, hearing loss, significant motor impairment, or severe mental health difficulties

2. **Interventions/treatment**
a. Referrals to speech-language pathology (SLP), audiology

D. Learning Disabilities (LDs)

1. **Definition**
a. A heterogeneous group of deficits in an individual's ability to perceive or process information efficiently and accurately

2. **Diagnosis**
a. Achievement on standardized tests that is substantially below expected for age, schooling, and level of intelligence in one or more of the following areas: basic reading skills, reading comprehension, reading fluency skills, oral expression, listening comprehension, written expression, mathematic calculation, and mathematic problem solving
b. There is no alternative diagnosis such as sensory impairment or ID[6,7]

E. Cerebral Palsy (CP)

1. **Definition and epidemiology**
a. **A group of disorders of the development of movement and posture** causing activity limitation that are attributed to **nonprogressive** disturbances that occurred in the developing fetal or infant brain[8]

TABLE 9.6
CLINICAL CLASSIFICATION OF CEREBRAL PALSY[10]

Type	Pattern of Involvement
I. SPASTIC (INCREASED TONE, CLASPED KNIFE, CLONUS, FURTHER CLASSIFIED BY DISTRIBUTION)	
Bilateral spasticity	Diplegia (legs primarily affected)
	Quadriplegia (all four extremities impaired; legs worse than arms)
Unilateral spasticity	Hemiplegia (ipsilateral arm and leg; arm worse than leg)
	Monoplegia (one extremity, usually upper; probably reflects a mild hemiplegia)
II. DYSKINETIC (LEAD-PIPE OR CANDLE-WAX RIGIDITY, VARIABLE TONE, ± CLONUS)	
Dystonic	Complex disorders often reflecting basal ganglia pathology, resulting in involuntary and uncontrolled movements. May be focal or generalized
Choreoathetoid	
III. OTHER	
Ataxic	Movement and tone disorders often reflecting cerebellar origin
Hypotonic	Usually related to diffuse, often severe cerebral and/or cerebellar cortical dysfunction. May be axial, appendicular, or generalized
Rigid	Muscle cocontraction, seen in rare neurogenetic diseases

Adapted from Caputo AJ, Accardo PJ, eds. Cerebral Palsy: Developmental Disabilities in Infancy and Childhood. 3rd ed. vol 2. Baltimore: Paul H. Brookes; 2008:83-86; and Rosenbaum P, Paneth N, Leviton A, et al. A report: the definition and classification of cerebral palsy April 2006. Dev Med Child Neurol Suppl. 2007;109:8-14.

b. Prevalence is 2–3/1000 live births and has remained stable over the past 40 years[9]
c. Manifestations may change with brain maturation and development

2. **Clinical presentation**
a. Delayed motor development, abnormal tone, atypical postures, persistent primitive reflexes past 6 months
b. History of known or suspected brain injury

3. **Diagnosis**
a. **Classification is based on physiologic and topographic characteristics as well as severity** (Table 9.6).[10] Different classifications often have very different etiologies and associated impairments
b. Brain imaging should be obtained with magnetic resonance imaging (MRI) (abnormal in 70%–90%)

4. **Interventions/treatment**
a. Ongoing care in a CP program as available
b. Baseline and ongoing medical subspecialty care, including developmental pediatrics, neurology, orthopedics, neurosurgery, and others as applicable
c. Multidisciplinary involvement by physical therapy (PT), occupational therapy (OT), SLP, social work, behavioral psychology, education, nutrition, audiology
d. Equipment to promote mobility and communication

e. Pharmacotherapy for spasticity (botulinum toxin injections, baclofen), dyskinesia, hypersalivation (glycopyrrolate, scopolamine patch)[11]
f. In carefully selected patients: intrathecal baclofen, selective dorsal rhizotomy, deep brain stimulation

F. Autism Spectrum Disorders (ASDs)

1. **Definition and epidemiology**
a. Encompasses previously named disorders of autistic disorder (autism), Asperger's disorder, childhood disintegrative disorder, and pervasive developmental disorder not otherwise specified (PDD-NOS)
b. Prevalence continues to increase, with **1 in 68** children in the United States diagnosed in 2010[12]
c. Almost five times more common in males than females[12]
2. **Screening**
a. **Formal screening for ASD recommended at the 18- and 24-month visits** (see the AAP practice guidelines for more detailed recommendations)[13]
b. Recommendation upheld by the AAP despite a U.S. Preventive Services Task Force (USPSTF) draft recommendation statement citing insufficient evidence for screening[14,15]
c. Evaluate using screening tools such as the **Modified Checklist for Autism in Toddlers (M-CHAT-R/F)** and **Childhood Autism Screening Test (CAST)** (see Table 9.4)
3. **Diagnosis**
a. Symptoms vary by age, developmental level, language ability, and supports in place
b. Diagnostic criteria include:
    i. **Impaired social communication and interaction**
    Examples: Lack of joint attention behaviors (e.g., showing toys, pointing for showing), diminished eye contact, no sharing of emotions, lack of imitation
    ii. **Restricted repetitive patterns of behavior, interests, or activities**
    Examples: Simple motor stereotypies (hand flapping, finger flicking), repetitive use of objects (spinning coins, lining up toys), repetitive speech (echolalia), resistance to change, unusual sensory responses
    iii. Presentation in early childhood and significant limitation of functioning[5]
4. **Interventions/treatment**
a. Educational interventions, visual supports, naturalistic developmental behavioral interventions (integrating behavioral and child-responsive strategies to teach developmentally appropriate skills in a more natural and interactive setting)[16]
b. Referral to SLP, OT/sensory-based interventions
c. Pharmacotherapy for coexisting mental health symptoms (Table 9.7)[17]

TABLE 9.7
COMMONLY USED PSYCHIATRIC DRUGS AND CORRESPONDING AGES OF FDA APPROVAL (YEARS)

Antidepressants/Anxiolytics*		Stimulants (ADHD)*		Antipsychotics*	
Fluoxetine (Prozac)	7–17 yr (OCD) 8–18 yr (MDD)	Dextroamphetamine + amphetamine (Adderall)	3–12 yr	Aripiprazole (Abilify)	6+ yr (irritability with ASD) 10+ yr (BPD) 13+ yr (schizophrenia)
Sertraline (Zoloft)	6–17 yr (OCD)	Methylphenidate (Concerta, Ritalin)	6–12 yr (Ritalin)	Haloperidol (Haldol)	Not established
Escitalopram (Lexapro)	12–17 yr (MDD)	Dexmethylphenidate (Focalin)	6–17 yr	Risperidone (Risperdal)	5–16 yr (irritability with ASD) 10+ yr (BPD) 13+ yr (schizophrenia)
		Lisdexamfetamine (Vyvanse)	6 yr–adult	Quetiapine (Seroquel)	10+ yr (BPD) 12+ yr (schizophrenia)

*For more detailed drug information, indications, and dosing, please refer to the Formulary (Chapter 29).

ASD, Autism spectrum disorder; BPD, bipolar disorder; GAD, generalized anxiety disorder; MDD, major depressive disorder; OCD, obsessive-compulsive disorder.

Adapted from the Centers for Medicare and Medicaid Services factsheets (www.CMS.gov) and the Food and Drug Administration (FDA).

VII. DEVELOPMENTAL REFERRAL AND INTERVENTION

A. State Support

1. **The Individuals with Disabilities Education Act (IDEA)** sets forth regulations in the following areas for states that receive federal funding:[7,18]
   a. Entitles all children with qualifying disabilities to a **free and appropriate public education** in the **least restrictive environment.**
   b. **Early intervention services:** Infants and toddlers younger than 3 years may be referred for evaluation to receive developmental services. Eligibility criteria vary by state; see The National Early Childhood Technical Assistance Center (www.ectacenter.org) for details.
   c. **Qualifying disabilities:** Children aged 3–21 years with autism, ID, specific LD, hearing or visual impairment, speech or language impairment, orthopedic impairment, traumatic brain injury, emotional disturbance, or other health impairment are eligible.
   d. **Individualized Education Program (IEP):** Written statement that includes a child's current capabilities, goals and how they will be measured, and services required. A comprehensive team is needed to develop and implement the IEP.
2. **Head Start and Early Head Start** are programs instituted by the federal government to promote school readiness of low-income children aged 3–5 years and younger than 3 years, respectively, within their communities.[19]
3. **Section 504 of the Rehabilitation Act of 1973** and the **Americans with Disabilities Act (ADA)** prohibit discrimination against individuals with any disability, more broadly defined as an impairment that limits function.

B. Multidisciplinary involvement

1. Neurodevelopmental pediatrician, child neurologist, developmental/behavioral pediatrician, other medical subspecialties as indicated
2. Genetic counseling for families of children with a genetic condition
3. Psychologists for formal testing, counseling
4. Rehabilitation and therapists
5. Educators

VIII. DISORDERS OF MENTAL HEALTH

A. Overview

1. Very common in the pediatric population, with an estimated **15%–20%** of children in primary care practices requiring ongoing intervention for mental health or psychological problems.[20]
2. **Surveillance for mental health issues should occur at all routine well-child visits from early childhood through adolescence,** including history of mood symptoms and any behavioral issues.

3. **The Pediatric Symptom Checklist (PSC) is a general mental health checklist that screens for a broad array of disorders** (see Table 9.4).
4. See the DSM-5 for a complete list of psychiatric diagnoses and full diagnostic criteria for the disorders mentioned.[5]
5. Pharmacotherapy for many disorders may be managed or monitored by the pediatrician. See Pediatric Psychopharmacology for Primary Care.[21]

B. Attention Deficit/Hyperactivity Disorder

1. **Definition and epidemiology**
   a. Persistent pattern of inattention and/or hyperactivity–impulsivity that interferes with functioning or development.
   b. Prevalence continues to rise. Affected 11.0% (6.4 million) of children in the United States in 2011, increased from 9.5% (5.4 million) of children in 2007.[22,23]
   c. Majority of children continue to meet diagnostic criteria through adolescence, and ADHD does not typically remit after onset of puberty. Symptoms may last through adulthood, with significant impairment noted.
2. **Screening**
   a. Evaluate all children aged 4–18 years who have academic and/or behavioral issues for ADHD and common comorbid conditions (depression, anxiety, oppositional defiant disorder, conduct disorder)[24]
3. **Diagnosis**
   a. Diagnostic criteria: Inattention, impulsivity/hyperactivity that are more frequent and severe than typically observed in children of the same developmental age
   b. Symptoms must persist for at least 6 months, occur before the age of 12 years, and be evident in two or more settings[5,25]
   c. Subtypes include **combined** (inattention, hyperactivity, and impulsivity), **predominantly inattentive**, or **predominantly hyperactive/impulsive**
   d. Diagnosis is made using history, observation, and behavioral checklists such as the **Vanderbilt Assessment Scale** (see Table 9.4)
   e. If the medical history is unremarkable, no further laboratory or neurologic testing is required
   f. Psychological and neuropsychological testing are not required for diagnosis but are recommended if other academic or developmental concerns are present[25]
4. **Treatment**
   a. Studies show pharmacologic treatment works best with behavioral therapy as an adjunct.
   b. Before starting a stimulant medication, history should be taken to exclude cardiac symptoms, Wolff–Parkinson–White syndrome, sudden

death in the family, hypertrophic cardiomyopathy, and long QT syndrome.
  c. See Table 9.7 for recommended pharmacologic treatments. The ADHD Medication Guide (www.adhdmedicationguide.com) provides visual information.
  d. Titrate medications to maximal symptom control with minimal side effects.
  e. Common side effects of stimulants to monitor include appetite suppression, abdominal pain, headaches, and sleep disturbance.[24]

C. Anxiety Disorders

1. **Definition and epidemiology**
  a. A group of disorders characterized by excessive fear, anxiety, and related behavioral disturbances and impairment of optimal developmental functioning.
  b. One of the most common mental health issues that presents in the general pediatric setting.
  c. An estimated 4.7% of all children aged 3–17 years are affected, with onset most often before the age of 25 and increased prevalence (15%–20%) among adolescents aged 13–17 years.[26-28]
  d. Children may develop new anxiety disorders over time, and are at higher risk for anxiety and depressive disorders than adults. They are also at risk for social, family, and academic impairments.

2. **Clinical presentation**
  a. May present with fear or worry and not recognize their fear as unreasonable
  b. Commonly have somatic complaints of headache and stomach ache
  c. May affect school performance or manifest as school avoidance
  d. Crying, irritability, angry outbursts, and disruptive behavior are expressions of fear and effort to avoid anxiety-provoking stimuli

3. **Screening**
  a. Multiple tools available such as the **SCARED** and **Spence Children's Anxiety Scale** (see Table 9.4)

4. **Diagnosis**
  a. Diagnostic criteria vary based on the specific disorder[5]:
     i. Generalized anxiety disorder
     ii. Separation anxiety disorder
     iii. Social anxiety disorder
     iv. Selective mutism
     v. Specific phobia
     vi. Panic disorder
     vii. Agoraphobia
  b. Differential diagnosis in addition to those listed above includes obsessive–compulsive disorder, post-traumatic stress disorder, and acute stress disorder

Chapter 9 Development, Behavior, and Mental Health

5. **Treatment**
   a. Psychotherapy with cognitive behavioral therapy (CBT), with or without pharmacotherapy (see Table 9.7), based on the disorder and severity[29]

D. Depressive Disorders

1. **Definition and epidemiology**
   a. A group of disorders characterized by mood changes as well as somatic and cognitive symptoms that disrupt functioning
   b. Major depressive disorder: 2% of children, 4%–8% of adolescents[27]
   c. Subclinical symptoms: 5%–10% of children
   d. Common comorbid conditions: Anxiety disorders, disruptive behavior disorders, ADHD, and substance use (adolescents)

2. **Screening**
   a. Routine screening is recommended for patients ≥ 11 years; the **Patient Health Questionnaire (PHQ-2)** is a brief but effective tool to use in adolescents.[30] Other screening tools include the **Center for Epidemiological Studies Depression Scale for Children (CES-DC)** (see Table 9.4)
   b. All patients with suspected depressive symptoms should be screened for suicidal ideation (SI) and referred for emergency evaluation if serious thoughts and/or action plans are endorsed

3. **Diagnosis**
   a. Major depressive disorder diagnostic criteria:
      i. Five or more of the following symptoms for ≥2 weeks:
         (1) Must include either depressed mood/irritability OR anhedonia
         (2) Changes in appetite/weight, sleep, or activity; fatigue or loss of energy; guilt/worthlessness; decreased concentration; suicidality
      ii. Symptoms cause significant impairment in functioning
      iii. Not due to substance use or a medical condition
      iv. No history of manic episodes[31]
   b. Other depressive disorders are defined by their own diagnostic criteria:[5]
      i. Disruptive mood dysregulation disorder
      ii. Persistent depressive disorder (dysthymia)
      iii. Premenstrual dysphoric disorder
   c. Differential diagnosis includes bipolar disorder, adjustment disorder

4. **Treatment**
   a. Selective serotonin reuptake inhibitors (SSRIs) may be initiated in the primary care setting. Referral to subspecialist may be required depending on severity or in the case of treatment failure.
   b. Literature shows that antidepressant medications (see Table 9.7) and CBT combined are the most effective treatment, followed by medication alone, then CBT alone.[32]
   c. SSRIs have a black box warning concerning a possible increase in suicidal thoughts or behaviors in children and adolescents after

initiation of medication. Patients should be followed closely for the first 2–4 weeks, then every other week thereafter.
d. Refer to the Physicians Med Guide prepared by the American Psychological Association (APA) and American Academy of Child and Adolescent Psychiatry (AACAP) for guidelines regarding medication use for depression in adolescent patients (parentsmedguide.org/physiciansmedguide.htm).[33]

E. Feeding and Eating Disorders
1. **Definition and epidemiology**
   a. Includes not only anorexia nervosa and bulimia nervosa, but also pica, rumination disorder (repeated regurgitation), avoidant/restrictive food intake disorder, and binge eating disorder
   b. 12-month prevalence of 0.4% (anorexia nervosa) and 1%–1.5% (bulimia nervosa); 10:1 female-to-male ratio[5]
   c. Common comorbidities include depressive, bipolar, and anxiety disorders
2. **Diagnosis**
   a. Anorexia nervosa
      i. Energy intake restriction and low weight (BMI < 18.5 kg/m^2; severity of the disorder is stratified by BMI)
      ii. Fear of gaining weight
      iii. Disturbance in perception of body weight or shape
   b. Bulimia nervosa
      i. Recurrent episodes of binge eating that occur at least once per week for 3 months
      ii. Recurrent inappropriate compensatory mechanisms to prevent weight gain, or purging (self-induced vomiting, medication use such as diuretics or laxatives, exercise)
      iii. Self-evaluation excessively influenced by body shape or weight[5]
3. **Treatment**
   a. Aimed at nutritional rehabilitation and therapy (family-based or as a component of day treatment programs). Hospitalization may be needed in the case of medical instability.
   b. SSRIs indicated in the treatment of bulimia nervosa (see Table 9.7; no medications have been approved for use in anorexia nervosa[34]).

F. Substance Use Disorders
1. **Definition and epidemiology**
   a. Lifetime diagnosis of alcohol abuse: 0.4%–9%, and dependence: 0.6%–4.3%[35]
   b. Lifetime diagnosis of drug abuse or dependence: 3.3%–9.8%[35]
   c. Common comorbid conditions: Disruptive behavior disorders, mood disorders, anxiety disorders

Chapter 9 Development, Behavior, and Mental Health

2. **Clinical presentation**
a. Acute change in mood, behavior, and cognition
   i. Mood: Low mood to elevated mood
   ii. Behavior: Disinhibition, lethargy, hyperactivity, agitation, somnolence, and hypervigilance
   iii. Cognition: Impaired concentration, changes in attention span, perceptual and overt disturbances in thinking (e.g., delusions)
b. Impairment in psychosocial and academic functioning (family conflict/dysfunction, interpersonal conflict, academic failure)
c. Deviant or risk-taking behavior[35]

3. **Diagnosis**
a. Establish standards of confidentiality
b. Administer CRAFFT Questionnaire (see Box 5.2 in Chapter 5)
c. Evaluate for age of onset of use; progression of use for specific substances; circumstances, frequency, and variability of use; and types of agents used
d. Urine/serum toxicology workup should be part of any routine evaluation if any concern for substance use

4. **Treatment**
a. Determine goals and readiness for change, and promote behavioral change through motivational interviewing[36]
b. Families should be involved with treatment
c. Medications can be used to manage withdrawal symptoms and/or cravings
d. Treatment of comorbid conditions should occur at the same time[35]
e. Find a treatment center at: www.SAMSHA.org

IX. MENTAL HEALTH REFERRAL AND INTERVENTION

A. Referral to outside mental health services may be necessary if patient care needs exceed scope of the provider's practice, or if incorporated liaisons such as social workers or counselors are not available
B. Varying levels of care depending on level of severity or concern
   1. Outpatient treatment and therapy
   a. Cognitive-behavioral therapy (CBT): Recognition and replacement of harmful or maladaptive behaviors and the thinking patterns that may accompany them
   2. Day treatment: Provides services such as counseling and skill building for at least 4 hours per day
   3. Inpatient hospitalization: Indicated for patients with active SI, concern for self-harm, severe eating disorders, or any other unsafe situation
   4. Emergency and crisis services: Resources available for crisis or emergency scenarios at all times, such as the National Suicide Prevention Lifeline (1-800-273-8255) or outreach teams[37]

REFERENCES

1. Caputé AJ, Shapiro BK, Palmer FB. Spectrum of developmental disabilities: continuum of motor dysfunction. *Orthop Clin North Am.* 1981;12:3-22.
2. American Academy of Pediatrics. Identifying infants and young children with developmental disorders in the medical home: an algorithm for developmental surveillance and screening. *Pediatrics.* 2006;118:405-420.
3. Moeschler JB, Shevell M, Committee on Genetics. Comprehensive evaluation of the child with intellectual disability or global developmental delays. *Pediatrics.* 2014;134:e903-e918.
4. Michelson DJ, Shevell MI, Sherr EH, et al. Evidence report: genetic and metabolic testing on children with global developmental delay: report of the Quality Standards Subcommittee of the American Academy of Neurology and the Practice Committee of the Child Neurology Society. *Neurology.* 2011;77:1629-1635.
5. American Psychiatric Association. *Diagnostic and Statistical Manual of Mental Disorders: Text Revision.* 5th ed. Arlington: APA; 2013.
6. Shapiro BK, Gallico RP. Learning disabilities. *Pediatr Clin North Am.* 1993;40:491-505.
7. Individuals with Disability Education Improvement Act of 2004, Pub. L. No. 108-445.
8. Rosenbaum P, Paneth N, Leviton A, et al. A report: the definition and classification of cerebral palsy April 2006. *Dev Med Child Neurol Suppl.* 2007;109:8-14.
9. Colver A, Fairhurst C, Pharoah PO. Cerebral palsy. *Lancet.* 2014;383(9924):1240-1249.
10. Caputé AJ, Accardo PJ, eds. *Cerebral Palsy: Developmental Disabilities in Infancy and Childhood.* Vol 2. 2nd ed. Baltimore: Paul H. Brookes; 1996.
11. Liptak GS, Murphy NA, Council on Children with Disabilities. Providing a primary care medical home for children and youth with cerebral palsy. *Pediatrics.* 2011;128:e1321-e1329.
12. Developmental Disabilities Monitoring Network Surveillance Year 2010 Principal Investigators; Centers for Disease Control and Prevention (CDC). Prevalence of autism spectrum disorder among children aged 8 years - autism and developmental disabilities monitoring network, 11 sites, United States, 2010. *MMWR Morb Mortal Wkly Rep.* 2014;63:1-21.
13. Johnson CP, Myers SM, American Academy of Pediatrics. Identification and evaluation of children with autism spectrum disorders. *Pediatrics.* 2007;120:1183-1215. Reaffirmed in AAP publications reaffirmed or retired. *Pediatrics.* 2014;134:e1520.
14. Hassink G. AAP Statement on U.S. Preventive Services Task Force Draft Recommendation on Autism Screening. August 3, 2015. <https://www.aap.org/en-us/about-the-aap/aap-press-room/pages/AAP-Statement-on-U-S-Preventive-Services-Task-Force-Draft-Recommendation-Statement-on-Autism-Screening.aspx>. Accessed September 10, 2015.
15. Draft Recommendation Statement: Autism Spectrum Disorder in Young Children: Screening. U.S. Preventive Services Task Force. August 2015. <http://www.uspreventiveservicestaskforce.org/Page/Document/draft-recommendation-statement15/autism-spectrum-disorder-in-young-children-screening>. Accessed September 10, 2015.

16. Schreibman L, Dawson G, Stahmer AC, et al. Naturalistic developmental behavioral interventions: empirically validated treatments for autism spectrum disorder. *J Autism Dev Disord*. 2015;45(8):2411-2428.
17. Myers SM, Johnson CP, American Academy of Pediatrics Council on Children with Disabilities. Management of children with autism spectrum disorders. *Pediatrics*. 2007;120:1162-1182.
18. Lipkin PH, Okamoto J, Council on Children with Disabilities and Council on School Health. The Individuals With Disabilities Education Act (IDEA) for Children With Special Educational Needs. *Pediatrics*. 2015;136(6):e1650-e1662.
19. Improving Head Start for School Readiness Act of 2007, Pub. L. No. 110-134.
20. Kelleher KJ, McInerny TK, Gardner WP, et al. Increasing identification of psychosocial problems: 1979-1996. *Pediatrics*. 2000;105:1313-1321.
21. Riddle MA, Foy JM, Baum RA, et al. Pediatric psychopharmacology for primary care. Illinois: American Academy of Pediatrics; 2016. <http://ebooks.aappublications.org/content/pediatric-psychopharmacology-for-primary-care>. Accessed January 27, 2016.
22. Centers for Disease Control and Prevention (CDC). Increasing prevalence of parent-reported attention-deficit/hyperactivity disorder among children—United States, 2003 and 2007. *MMWR Morb Mortal Wkly Rep*. 2010;59:1439-1443.
23. Visser SN, Danielson ML, Bitsko RH, et al. Trends in the parent-report of health care provider-diagnosed and medicated attention-deficit/hyperactivity disorder: United States, 2003-2011. *J Am Acad Child Adolesc Psychiatry*. 2014;53:34-46.e2.
24. Subcommittee on Attention-Deficit/Hyperactivity Disorder, Steering Committee on Quality Improvement and Management, Wolraich M, Brown L, et al. ADHD: clinical practice guideline for the diagnosis, evaluation, and treatment of attention-deficit/hyperactivity disorder in children and adolescents. *Pediatrics*. 2011;128:1007-1022.
25. Pliszka S, AACAP Work Group on Quality Issues. Practice parameter for the assessment and treatment of children and adolescents with attention-deficit/hyperactivity disorder. *J Am Acad Child Adolesc Psychiatry*. 2007;46:894-921.
26. Beesdo K, Knappe S, Pine DS. Anxiety and anxiety disorders in children and adolescents: developmental issues and implications for DSM-5. *Psychiatr Clin North Am*. 2009;32:483-524.
27. Perou R, Bitsko RH, Blumberg SJ, et al.; Centers for Disease Control and Prevention (CDC). Mental health surveillance among children—United States, 2005-2011. *MMWR Surveill Summ*. 2013;62(suppl 2):1-35.
28. Merikangas KR, He J, Burstein M, et al. Lifetime prevalence of mental disorders in U.S. adolescents: results from the National Comorbidity Survey Replication-Adolescent Supplement (NCS-A). *J Am Acad Child Adolesc Psychiatry*. 2010;40:980-989.
29. Connolly SD, Bernstein GA, Work Group on Quality Issues. Practice parameter for the assessment and treatment of children and adolescents with anxiety disorders. *J Am Acad Child Adolesc Psychiatry*. 2007;46:267-283.
30. Richardson LP, Rockhill C, Russo JE, et al. Evaluation of the PHQ-2 as a brief screen for detecting major depression among adolescents. *Pediatrics*. 2010;125(5):e1097-e1103.

31. Birmaher B, Brent D, AACAP Work Group on Quality Issues. Practice parameter for the assessment and treatment of children and adolescents with depressive disorders. *J Am Acad Child Adolesc Psychiatry*. 2007;46:1503-1526.
32. March J, Silva S, Petrycki S, et al. Fluoxetine, cognitive-behavioral therapy, and their combination for adolescents with depression: Treatment for Adolescents with Depression Study (TADS) randomized controlled trial. *JAMA*. 2004;292:807-820.
33. Physicians Med Guide. The use of medication in treating childhood and adolescent depression: information for physicians. Available at <http://www.parentsmedguide.org/physiciansmedguide.htm>. Prepared by the American Psychiatric Association and the American Academy of Child and Adolescent Psychiatry. October 7, 2009.
34. Rosen DS, the Committee on Adolescence. Clinical report—identification and management of eating disorders in children and adolescents. *Pediatrics*. 2010;126:1240-1253.
35. Bukstein OG, Bernet W, Arnold V, et al. Practice parameter for the assessment and treatment of children and adolescents with substance use disorders. *J Am Acad Child Adolesc Psychiatry*. 2005;44:609-621.
36. Jensen CD, Cushing CC, Aylward BS, et al. Effectiveness of motivational interviewing interventions for adolescent substance use behavior change: a meta-analytic review. *J Consult Clin Psychol*. 2011;79:433-440.
37. American Academy of Pediatrics. Supplemental appendix S9: Glossary of mental health and substance abuse terms. *Pediatrics*. 2010;125:S161-S170.

Chapter 10
Endocrinology

*Jessica Jack, MD, and
Sarah Brunelli Young, MD, MS*

See additional content on Expert Consult

I. WEB RESOURCES

- Children with Diabetes (www.childrenwithdiabetes.com)
- American Diabetes Association (www.diabetes.org)
- International Society for Pediatric and Adolescent Diabetes (www.ispad.org)
- Pediatric Endocrine Society (www.lwpes.org)
- UCSF Center of Excellence for Transgender Health (www.transhealth.ucsf.edu/)

II. DIABETES

A. Evaluation and Diagnosis[1-3]

1. Diagnostic criteria (must meet one of four):
a. Symptoms for diabetes (polyuria, polydipsia, or weight loss) and random blood glucose ≥ 200 mg/dL
b. Fasting plasma glucose (FPG = no caloric intake for at least 8 hours) ≥ 126 mg/dL*
c. Oral glucose tolerance test (OGTT) with a 2-hour post-load plasma glucose of ≥200 mg/dL*
d. Hemoglobin A_{1c} (HbA_{1c}) ≥ 6.5%
2. **Defining increased risk:** FPG 100–125 mg/dL, 2-hour post-OGTT 140–199 mg/dL, HbA_{1c} 5.7%–6.4%[†]
3. **Interpreting HbA_{1c}:** Estimates average blood glucose for the past 3 months; 6% approximately equals an average of 130 mg/dL, each additional 1% ≈ 30 mg/dL more. Unreliable in patients with hemoglobinopathies.
4. **Oral glucose tolerance test (OGTT):**
a. Pretest preparation:
   (1) Calorically adequate diet required for 3 days before the test, with 50% of total calories taken as carbohydrate.
   (2) The test should be delayed for 2 weeks after an illness.

---

*In the absence of symptoms of hyperglycemia, these values should be repeated on another day.
[†]These values are for adults; equivalent values not yet determined in children.

(3) All hyperglycemic and hypoglycemic agents (e.g., salicylates, diuretics, oral contraceptives, or phenytoin) should be discontinued.
b. Procedure: Give 1.75 g/kg (maximum 75 g) oral (PO) glucose after a 12-hour fast, allowing up to 5 minutes for ingestion. Mix glucose with water and lemon juice as a 20% dilution. Quiet activity is permissible during the OGTT. Draw blood samples at 0 and 120 minutes after ingestion.
c. Interpretation: 2-hour blood glucose < 140 mg/dL = normal, 140–199 mg/dL = impaired glucose tolerance; ≥200 mg/dL = diabetes mellitus (DM).

B. Diabetes Classification[1,2]

1. **Type 1 or type 2 (most common types, polygenic)**
a. Patient characteristics (Table 10.1)
b. Laboratory characteristics:
    (1) Diabetes autoantibodies: (GAD-65, insulin, islet cell antibodies (ICA), IA2 (ICA 512), and ZnT8) are suggestive of type 1 DM. However, ≈15% of children with type 1 DM will not have autoantibodies to a specific islet cell antigen, and ≈5% will not have any detectable ICAs.
    NOTE: Some children with type 2 DM will have measurable ICAs.
    (2) Ketoacidosis: Usually associated with type 1 DM but does not exclude type 2 DM (see Sections C and D). Recurrent ketosis, especially diabetic ketoacidosis (DKA), in a type 2 DM patient should prompt a reevaluation of the classification.
    (3) C-peptide: In a type 1 DM patient, a measurable level of C-peptide > 2 years after diagnosis should prompt a reevaluation of the classification.
    (4) Insulin and C-peptide: Often unhelpful in the initial classification. At presentation, insulin and C-peptide levels are usually low in type 1 DM but there is significant overlap with type 2 DM.
2. **Other forms of diabetes**[4,5]
a. Monogenic diabetes: 1%–2% of DM cases. Due to single-gene mutations, typically relating to insulin production or release. Identifying the gene can have clinical significance.

TABLE 10.1
CHARACTERISTICS SUGGESTIVE OF TYPE 1 VS. TYPE 2 DIABETES AT PRESENTATION

Characteristic	Type 1	Type 2
Onset	Usually prepubertal	Usually postpubertal
Polydipsia and polyuria	Present for days to weeks	Absent or present for weeks to months
Ethnicity	Caucasian	African American, Hispanic, Asian, Native American
Weight	Weight loss	Obese
Other physical findings		Acanthosis nigricans
Family history	Autoimmune diseases	Type 2 diabetes
Ketoacidosis	More common	Less common

b. Maturity-onset diabetes of youth (MODY):
   (1) Suspect if autosomal dominant inheritance pattern of early-onset (<25 years) DM, insulin independence, an absent type 2 DM phenotype (nonobese), or preservation of C-peptide.
   (2) Well-described subtypes: MODY1 and MODY3, which are due to mutations in transcription factors for insulin production, are responsive to sulfonylureas.
c. Neonatal diabetes (NDM):
   (1) Defined as DM onset <6 months of age
   (2) Rare: 1:160,000–260,000 live births, typically a *de novo* mutation
   (3) May be transient (50% recur) or permanent
   (4) Subset respond to sulfonylureas
d. Other causes of DM: Diseases of exocrine pancreas due to pancreatitis, trauma, infection, invasive disease (cystic fibrosis, hemochromatosis). Can also be drug– or chemically–induced DM.

C. Diabetic Ketoacidosis (DKA)[6,7]

1. **Definition:** Hyperglycemia, ketonemia, ketonuria, and metabolic acidosis (pH < 7.30, bicarbonate < 15 mEq/L)
2. **Assessment:**
a. History: In a *suspected* diabetic, a history of polydipsia, polyuria, polyphagia, weight loss, vomiting, abdominal pain, infection, or an inciting event should be determined. In a *known* diabetic, the usual insulin regimen, and the timing and amount of the last dose should also be determined.
b. Examination: Assessment should be performed for dehydration, Kussmaul respiration, fruity breath, change in mental status, and current weight.
c. Laboratory tests: See Fig. 10.1. HbA_{1c} should be assessed for chronic hyperglycemia. In a new-onset diabetic, autoantibodies, thyroid antibodies, thyroid function tests (TSH), and a celiac screen (endomesial IgA antibody or tissue transglutaminase IgA antibody, and total IgA) should be considered.
3. **Management:** See Fig. 10.1. Because the fluid and electrolyte requirements of DKA patients vary greatly, the following guidelines are only a starting point and therapy must be individualized based on patient dynamics.
a. Acidosis: pH is an indicator of insulin deficiency. If the acidosis is not resolving, the patient may need more insulin. **NOTE:** Initial insulin administration may cause transient worsening of the acidosis as potassium is driven into cells in exchange for hydrogen ions.
b. Hyperglycemia: Blood glucose, in part, is an indicator of hydration status.
4. **Cerebral edema:** Most severe complication of DKA. Overly aggressive hydration and rapid correction of hyperglycemia may play a role in its development.

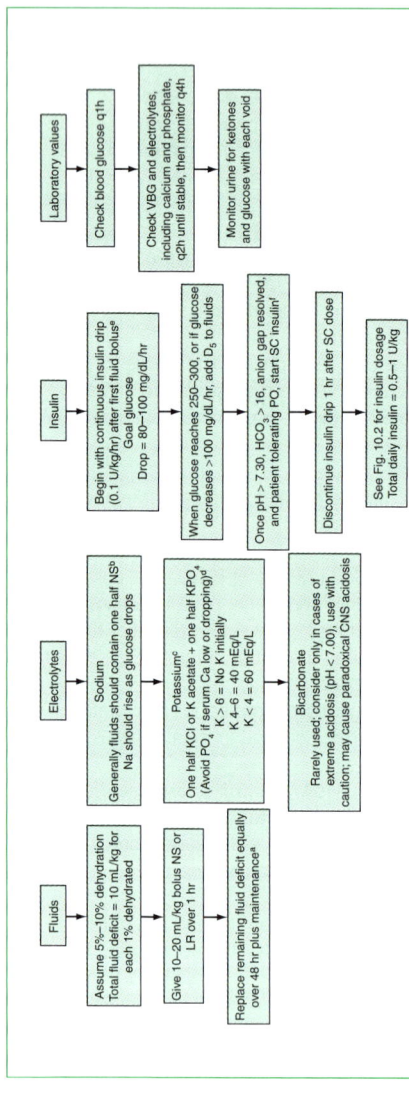

FIGURE 10.1

Management of diabetic ketoacidosis. (Modified from Cooke DW, Plotnick L. Management of diabetic ketoacidosis in children and adolescents. Pediatr Rev. 2008;29:431-436.)

TABLE 10.2
SUBCUTANEOUS INSULIN DOSING

	Insulin	Dose Calculation	Sample Calculation for 24-kg Child	Dose
Total daily dose		0.5–1 unit/kg/day	$0.75 \times 24 = 18$ units/day	18 units
Basal	Glargine	1/2 daily total	$\frac{1}{2} \times 18$ units $= 9$	9 units daily
	OR			
	Detemir	1/2 daily total ÷ BID	$\frac{1}{2} \times 18$ units $= 9$	4.5 units BID
Carbohydrate coverage ratio	Lispro, aspart	450 ÷ daily total	$450 \div 18 = 25$	1 unit: 25 g carbohydrate
	OR			
	Regular	500 ÷ daily total		
Correction factor	Lispro, aspart	1800 ÷ daily total	$1800 \div 18 = 100$	1 unit: 100 mg/dL >200 mg/dL
	OR			
	Regular	1500 ÷ daily total		

5. **Insulin requirements:** Once DKA is resolved, patient will need to be started on a regimen of subcutaneous (SQ) insulin. See Tables 10.2 and 10.3 for calculations. Insulin doses are subsequently adjusted based on actual blood sugars. Blood sugar should be checked before meals (QAC), at bedtime (QHS), and at 2 AM.

D. Type 2 Diabetes Mellitus[8-10]

1. **Prevalence:** Increasing among children, especially among African Americans, Hispanics, and Native Americans. Increase is related to increased prevalence of childhood obesity.
2. **Etiology:** Abnormality in glucose levels caused by insulin resistance and insulin secretory defect.
3. **Presentation:** Although not typical, can present in ketoacidosis (chronic high glucose impairs β-cell function and increases peripheral insulin resistance).
4. **Screening:**
a. Consider screening by measuring fasting blood glucose levels in children who are overweight (body mass index > 85th percentile for age and gender) *and* have two of the following risk factors:
   (1) Family history of type 2 DM in a first- or second-degree relative
   (2) Race/ethnicity: African American, Native American, Hispanic, Asian, or Pacific Islander
   (3) Signs associated with insulin resistance (acanthosis nigricans, hypertension, dyslipidemia, polycystic ovarian disease)

TABLE 10.3
CURRENTLY AVAILABLE INSULIN PRODUCTS

Insulin*	Onset	Peak	Effective Duration
Rapid acting	5–15 min	30–90 min	5 hr
Lispro (Humalog)			
Aspart (Novo Log)			
Glulisine (Apidra)			
Short acting	30–60 min	2–3 hr	5–8 hr
Regular U100			
Regular U500 (concentrated)			
Intermediate acting	2–4 hr	4–10 hr	10–16 hr
Isophane insulin (NPH, Humulin N/Novolin N)			
Long acting			
Glargine (Lantus)	2–4 hr†	No peak	20–24 hr
Detemir (Levemir)	Slow	6–8 hr	6–24 hr (dose related)
Premixed		Dual	10–16 hr
70% NPH/30% regular (Humulin 70/30)	30–60 min		
75% NPL/25% lispro (Humalog Mix 75/25)	5–15 min		
50% NPL/50% lispro (Humalog Mix 50/50)	5–15 min		
70% NPA/30% aspart (NovoLog Mix 70/30)	5–15 min		

*Assuming 0.1–0.2 U/kg per injection. Onset and duration vary significantly by injection site.
†Time to steady state
NPA, insulin aspart protamine (neutral protamine aspart); NPH, neutral protamine Hagedorn; NPL, insulin
(Modified from The American Diabetes Association. Practical Insulin: A Handbook for Prescribing Providers, 2nd ed. Alexandria, Va: American Diabetes Association; 2007)

    b. Screening should begin at the age of 10 years or at the onset of puberty (whichever occurs first), and should be repeated every 2 years.
    c. Based on adult data, HbA_{1c} may be used as a screening tool:
        HbA_{1c} = 5.7%–6.4% may indicate an increased risk for future diabetes
        HbA_{1c} = 6.0%–6.5% is abnormal and indicates the need for further testing (OGTT, fasting plasma glucose)
        $HbA_{1c} \geq 6.5\%$ is diagnostic of DM
5. **Treatment:** See Fig. 10.2

E. Monitoring

1. **Glucose control:** Daily blood glucose levels; HbA_{1c} level every 3 months
2. **Other involved organ systems:** Annual eye examinations (after age 10 years and 3 to 5 years of diabetes); annual screen for microalbuminuria (after 5 years of diabetes); screen for hyperlipidemia at diagnosis, then every 5 years if low-density lipoprotein [LDL] is <100 mg/dL; monitor for hypertension at each visit.

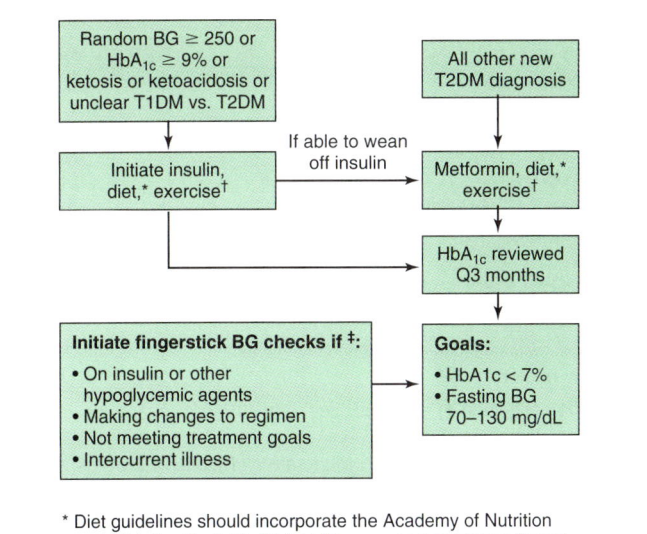

FIGURE 10.2

Treatment decision tree for management of type 2 diabetes (T2DM) in children and adolescents. *(Modified from Copeland KC, Silverstein J, Moore KR, et al. Clinical practice guidelines: management of newly diagnosed type 2 diabetes mellitus (T2DM) in children and adolescents. Pediatrics. 2013;131:364-382.)*

III. THYROID FUNCTION[11-13]

A. Thyroid Tests[12,14,15]

1. **Interpretation of thyroid function tests** (Table 10.4): See reference values for age (Table 10.5). Remember that preterm infants have different ranges (Table 10.6).
2. **Thyroid scan:** Used to study thyroid structure and function. Localizes ectopic thyroid tissue, and hyperfunctioning and nonfunctioning thyroid nodules.
3. **Technetium uptake:** Measures uptake of technetium by thyroid gland. Levels are increased in Graves disease and decreased in hashitoxicosis and hypothyroidism (except dyshormonogenesis, when levels may be increased).

TABLE 10.4
THYROID FUNCTION TESTS: INTERPRETATION

Disorder	TSH	T_4	Free T_4
Primary hyperthyroidism	L	H	High N to H
Primary hypothyroidism	H	L	L
Hypothalamic/pituitary hypothyroidism	L, N, H*	L	L
TBG deficiency	N	L	N
Euthyroid sick syndrome	L, N, H*	L	L to low N
TSH adenoma or pituitary resistance	N to H	H	H
Compensated hypothyroidism†	H	N	N

*Can be normal, low, or slightly high
†Treatment may not be necessary
H, high; L, low; N, normal; T_4, thyroxine; TBG, thyroxine-binding globulin; TSH, thyroid-stimulating hormone

B. Hypothyroidism (Table 10.7)

1. **Can be congenital or acquired.** See Table 10.7 for characteristics and types of hypothyroidism.
2. **Hypothyroidism and obesity**[16]: Moderate elevations in thyroid-stimulating hormone (TSH [4–10 mIU/L]), with normal or slightly elevated triiodothyronine (T_3) and thyroxine (T_4) are seen in 10%–23% of obese children and adolescents. In these individuals, there does not appear to be a benefit to treating with thyroxine. Values tend to normalize with weight loss, suggesting they are the result, rather than the cause, of obesity in these individuals. Could consider testing for thyroid antibodies to further clarify whether there is true thyroid dysfunction.
3. **Newborn screening for hypothyroidism**[13,17]: Mandated in all 50 states. Measures a combination of TSH and T_4, based on the particular state's algorithm; 1:25 abnormal tests are confirmed. Congenital hypothyroidism has prevalence of 1:3000–1:4000 U.S. infants. If abnormal results are found, clinicians should follow recommendations of the American College of Medical Genetics, ACT sheets and Algorithm for confirmation testing. See Chapter 13 for further resources on newborn screening.
NOTE: Because of the risk of inducing adrenal crisis if adrenocorticotropic hormone (ACTH) deficiency is present, the treatment of central hypothyroidism *should not be* started until normal ACTH/cortisol function is documented.

C. Hyperthyroidism

1. **General:**
a. Symptoms: Hyperactivity, irritability, altered mood, insomnia, heat intolerance, increased sweating, pruritus, tachycardia, palpitations, fatigue, weakness, weight loss despite increased appetite (or weight gain), increased stool frequency, oligomenorrhea or amenorrhea, fine tremor, hyperreflexia, and hair loss.

TABLE 10.5
AGE-BASED NORMAL VALUES FOR ROUTINE THYROID FUNCTION TESTS[14]

Age	Free T$_4$ (ng/dL)	TSH (mIU/L)	T$_4$ (mcg/dL)	T$_3$ (ng/dL)	Reverse T$_3$ (ng/dL)	TBG (mcg/mL)
Day of birth	0.94–4.39	2.43–24.3	5.85–18.68	19.53–266.26	19.53–358.70	19.17–44.7
1 wk	0.96–4.08	0.58–5.58*	5.90–18.58	20.83–265.61	19.53–338.52	19.16–44.68
1 mo	1.00–3.44	0.58–5.57*	6.06–18.27	25.39–264.31	19.53–283.84	19.12–44.59
3 mo	1.04–2.86	0.58–5.57*	6.39–17.66	36.46–259.75	19.53–197.90	19.02–44.35
6 mo	1.07–2.44	0.58–5.56*	6.75–17.04	51.43–252.59	19.53–137.36	18.87–44
1 yr	1.10–2.19	0.57–5.54	7.10–16.16	74.87–240.87	18.23–85.93	18.56–43.28
2 yr	1.11–2.05	0.57–5.51	7.16–14.98	103.51–228.50	16.93–55.99	17.94–41.82
5 yr	1.08–1.93	0.56–5.41	6.39–12.94	131.50–212.23	13.02–35.81	16–37.3
8 yr	1.04–1.87	0.55–5.31	5.72–11.71	130.85–202.46	11.72–30.60	14.2–33.09
12 yr	0.99–1.81	0.53–5.16	5.08–10.58	119.78–192.70	11.07–27.99	12.54–29.24
15 yr	1.03–1.77	0.52–5.05	4.84–10.13	110.02–184.88	10.42–27.34	11.96–27.89
18 yr	0.93–1.73	0.51–4.93		101.56–179.03	10.42–26.04	

*Some laboratories report that the reference range upper limit for TSH in children up to 12 months of age is 8.35 mU/L.
T$_3$, triiodothyronine; T$_4$, thyroxine; TBG, thyroxine-binding globulin; TSH, thyroid-stimulating hormone
NOTE: If age-specific reference ranges are provided by the laboratory that is running the assay, please refer to those ranges.
(Data modified from Lem AJ, de Rijke YB, van Toor H, et al. Serum thyroid hormone levels in healthy children from birth to adulthood and in short children born small for gestational age. J Clin Endocrinol Metab. *2012;97:3170-3178)*

TABLE 10.6
MEAN TSH AND T$_4$ OF PRETERM AND TERM INFANTS 0–28 DAYS[15]

Age ± SD	Cord (Day 0)	Day 7	Day 14	Day 28
T$_4$ (mcg/dL)				
23–27*	5.44 ± 2.02	4.04 ± 1.79	4.74 ± 2.56	6.14 ± 2.33
28–30	6.29 ± 2.02	6.29 ± 2.10	6.60 ± 2.25	7.46 ± 2.33
31–34	7.61 ± 2.25	9.40 ± 3.42	9.09 ± 3.57	8.94 ± 2.95
>37	9.17 ± 1.94	12.67 ± 2.87	10.72 ± 1.40	9.71 ± 2.18
FT$_4$ (ng/dL)				
23–27	1.28 ± 0.41	1.47 ± 0.56	1.45 ± 0.51	1.50 ± 0.43
28–30	1.45 ± 0.43	1.82 ± 0.66	1.65 ± 0.44	1.71 ± 0.43
31–34	1.49 ± 0.33	2.14 ± 0.57	1.96 ± 0.43	1.88 ± 0.46
>37	1.41 ± 0.39	2.70 ± 0.57	2.03 ± 0.28	1.65 ± 0.34
TSH (mIU/L)				
23–27	6.80 ± 2.90	3.50 ± 2.60	3.90 ± 2.70	3.80 ± 4.70
28–30	7.00 ± 3.70	3.60 ± 2.50	4.90 ± 11.2	3.60 ± 2.50
31–34	7.90 ± 5.20	3.60 ± 4.80	3.80 ± 9.30	3.50 ± 3.40
>37	6.70 ± 4.80	2.60 ± 1.80	2.50 ± 2.00	1.80 ± 0.90

*Weeks gestational age
FT$_4$, free thyroxine; T$_4$, thyroxine; TSH, thyroid-stimulating hormone
(Data modified from Williams FL, Simpson J, Delahunty C, et al. Collaboration from The Scottish Preterm Thyroid Group: Developmental trends in cord and postpartum serum thyroid hormones in preterm infants. J Clin Endocrinol Metab. *2004;89:5314-5320)*

TABLE 10.7
HYPOTHYROIDISM

Disease and Clinical Symptoms	Onset	Etiology	Management	Follow-up
PRIMARY/CONGENITAL				
Large fontanelles, lethargy, constipation, hoarse cry, hypotonia, hypothermia, jaundice	Symptoms usually develop within first 2 weeks of life; almost always present by 6 weeks. Some infants may be relatively asymptomatic if the cause is other than absence of the thyroid gland. Treated patients are still at risk for developmental delay.	Primary hypothyroidism: Most common cause is defect of fetal thyroid development. Other causes include TSH receptor mutation or thyroid dyshormonogenesis. *OR* Central hypothyroidism: Deficiency of thyrotropin-releasing hormone (TRH) or thyrotropin (TSH).	Goal is to achieve T_4 in the upper half of normal range. In primary hypothyroidism, TSH should be kept <5. A minority of infants maintain persistently high TSH despite correction of T_4. Replacement with L-thyroxine as soon as diagnosis is confirmed.	Monitor T_4 and TSH at the end of weeks 1 and 2 of therapy and 3–4 weeks after any dose change. If levels are adequate, follow every 1–3 months during the first 12 months.
ACQUIRED				
Growth deceleration; other signs may include coarse brittle hair, dry scaly skin, delayed tooth eruption, cold intolerance	Can occur as early as the first 2 years of life.	Hashimoto thyroiditis (diagnosis supported by presence of antithyroglobulin or antimicrosomal antibodies). Head/neck radiation. Central hypothyroidism (pituitary/hypothalamic insult).	Replacement with L-thyroxine.	As for primary/congenital. After 2 years, monitor levels every 6–12 months as dose changes become less frequent.

NOTE: Thyroid hormone levels in premature infants are lower than those seen in full-term infants. Furthermore, the TSH surge seen at approximately 24 hours of age in full-term babies does not appear in preterm infants. In this population, lower levels are associated with increased illness; however, the effect of replacement therapy remains controversial.
L-thyroxine, levothyroxine; TSH, thyroid-stimulating hormone

b. Epidemiology: Prevalence increases with age, beginning in adolescence; 4:1 female-to-male predominance.
  c. Etiology: Most common cause in childhood is Graves disease (see Section C.2). Other causes: Subacute thyroiditis, factitious hyperthyroidism (intake of exogenous hormone), TSH-secreting pituitary tumor (rare), and pituitary resistance to thyroid hormone (compensatory rise in T_4, but TSH remains within normal range).
  d. Laboratory findings: ↑ T_4, ↑ T_3, ↓ TSH. Further tests include TSH receptor–stimulating antibody, thyroid-stimulating immunoglobulin (TSI), antithyroglobulin and antimicrosomal antibodies, free T_4, and free T_3.

2. **Graves disease:**
  a. Physical examination: Diffuse goiter, a feeling of grittiness and discomfort in the eye, retrobulbar pressure or pain, eyelid lag or retraction, periorbital edema, chemosis, scleral injection, exophthalmos, extraocular muscle dysfunction, localized dermopathy, and lymphoid hyperplasia.
  b. Epidemiology: Peak incidence, age 11–15 years; 4:1 female-to-male ratio. Family history of autoimmune thyroid disease.
  c. Etiology: Autoimmune (positive TSI; may also have low titers of thyroglobulin ± microsomal antibodies).
  d. Laboratory findings: ↑ T_4, ↑ T_3, ↓ TSH [↑ iodine 123 (^{123}I) uptake distinguishes it from Hashimoto thyroiditis].
  e. Treatment and monitoring: Methimazole is the first-line treatment. Propylthiouracil (PTU) should not be used as the first-line treatment in children because of the higher risk of liver dysfunction compared to methimazole. PTU can be considered for patients with mild reactions to methimazole. Radioactive iodine (^{131}I) or surgical thyroidectomy are options for initial treatment or refractory cases. Symptoms, T_4, and TSH levels should be followed.

3. **Hashimoto thyroiditis:**
  a. Presentation: ± Initial hyperthyroidism, followed by eventual thyroid burnout and hypothyroidism.
  b. Etiology: Autoimmune (significantly elevated thyroglobulin and/or microsomal antibody).
  c. Laboratory findings: Mild to moderate ↑ T_4, ↓ TSH (↓^{123}I uptake distinguishes from Graves disease).
  d. Treatment: Hyperthyroid phase is usually self-limited; patient may eventually need thyroid replacement therapy. Propranolol if symptomatic during hyperthyroid phase.

4. **Thyroid storm:**
  a. Presentation: Acute onset of hyperthermia, tachycardia, and restlessness. May progress to delirium, coma, and death.
  b. Treatment: Propranolol is used to relieve signs and symptoms of thyrotoxicosis. Potassium iodide may also be used for acute

hyperthyroid management. Same long-term management as for Graves disease.

5. **Neonatal thyrotoxicosis:**
a. Presentation: Microcephaly, frontal bossing, intrauterine growth retardation (IUGR), tachycardia, systolic hypertension leading to widened pulse pressure, irritability, failure to thrive, exophthalmos, goiter, flushing, vomiting, diarrhea, jaundice, thrombocytopenia, and cardiac failure or arrhythmias. Onset from immediately after birth to weeks.
b. Etiology: Occurs exclusively in infants born to mothers with Graves disease. Caused by transplacental passage of maternal TSI. Occasionally, mothers are unaware they have Graves. Even if a mother has received definitive treatment (thyroidectomy or radiation therapy), passage of TSI remains possible.
c. Treatment and monitoring: Propranolol for symptom control. Methimazole to lower thyroxine levels. Digoxin may be indicated for heart failure. Disease usually resolves by 6 months of age.

IV. PARATHYROID GLAND FUNCTION AND VITAMIN D

A. Parathyroid Gland

1. **Parathyroid hormone (PTH) function:** Increases serum calcium by increasing bone resorption, increasing calcium and magnesium reuptake in the kidney, increasing phosphorus excretion in the kidney, and increasing 25-hydroxy vitamin D conversion to 1,25-dihydroxy vitamin D in order to increase calcium absorption in the intestine.
2. **Hypoparathyroidism:**
a. Presentation: Asymptomatic or mild muscle cramps to hypocalcemic tetany, prolonged QTc, and convulsions.
b. Etiology: Results from a decrease in PTH due to decreased function or absence of the parathyroid gland. This can be due to transient hypoparathyroidism in infants, autoimmune disease, DiGeorge syndrome, iatrogenic removal of the parathyroid gland during other surgical procedures. Pseudohypoparathyroidism results from PTH resistance and is distinguished by normal or elevated PTH.
c. Laboratory findings: ↓ PTH; ↓ serum Ca^{2+}, ↑ serum phosphorus, normal/↓ alkaline phosphatase, ↓ 1,25-OH–vitamin D.
d. Treatment and monitoring: Calcium supplementation for documented hypocalcemia, treatment with calcitriol. Carefully monitor serum calcium and phosphorus during therapy. Monitor urine calcium levels to avoid hypercalciuria.
3. **Hyperparathyroidism:**
a. Presentation: Hypercalcemia leads to vomiting, constipation, abdominal pain, weakness, paresthesias, malaise, and bone pain. Uncommon in childhood.

b. Etiology: Primary hyperparathyroidism is uncommon in children and is usually due to overproduction secondary to adenoma or hyperplasia. Adenomas can be associated with multiple endocrine neoplasia (MEN) syndromes (see Expert Consult, Box EC 10.A). Secondary hyperparathyroidism is more common; develops in response to hypocalcemic states like renal failure or rickets.
c. Laboratory findings, primary: ↑ PTH, ↑ serum Ca^{2+}, ↓ serum phosphorus, normal/↑ alkaline phosphatase. In secondary hyperparathyroidism, Ca^{2+} normal/↓.
d. Treatment for hypercalcemia associated with primary hyperparathyroidism: Hydration with intravenous (IV) normal saline is mainstay of treatment, as both the hydration and the natriuresis enhance calciuria. Furosemide may be used with caution with adequate hydration. Hydrocortisone (1 mg/kg Q6 hr) reduces intestinal absorption of calcium. Calcitonin transiently opposes bone resorption. In severe hypercalcemia, bisphosphates may be considered. Surgical removal of parathyroid glands (may result in hypoparathyroidism).

B. Vitamin D Deficiency (Table 10.8)[18-20]

1. **Current recommendations suggest 600 IU/day in children >12 months of age to meet daily requirements. Breastfed infants require 400 IU/day of supplementation.**
2. **The definition and consequences of vitamin D deficiency and insufficiency is an evolving field.** See Table 10.9 for suggested ranges of 25-hydroxyvitamin D.

V. ADRENAL FUNCTION[21-23]

A. Adrenal Insufficiency

1. **Etiology**
a. Common causes: Congenital adrenal hyperplasia (CAH) and chronic glucocorticoid treatment (suppresses ACTH secretion)

TABLE 10.8
VITAMIN D DEFICIENCY

Disease, Clinical Symptoms, and Onset	Etiology	Evaluation	Management
RICKETS (infancy/childhood): Failure of adequate bone mineralization, leading to soft bones/skeletal deformities **OSTEOMALACIA** (adults): Bone pain and muscle weakness	Decreased dietary intake Inadequate exposure to sunlight Increased melanin Impaired renal function Fat malabsorption (celiac disease, cystic fibrosis, Crohn's disease)	↓ 25-OH vitamin D	Supplementation for: • Breast-fed infants • Those with celiac disease, cystic fibrosis, Crohn's disease, pancreatic deficiency Repletion per Formulary

TABLE 10.9
VITAMIN D, 25-HYDROXY VITAMIN D[18-20]

25-Hydroxy Vitamin D	Value (ng/mL)
Deficiency	<10–15*
Insufficiency	15–20
Optimal level	>20–30†

NOTE: 1,25-dihydroxy vitamin D is the physiologically active form, but 25-hydroxy vitamin D is the value to monitor for vitamin D deficiency because it approximates body stores of vitamin D. Cut-off values are not yet well defined.
*Values of <10–15 ng/mL have been associated with the bone changes found in rickets.
†Controversy exists regarding the optimal 25-hydroxy vitamin D level. Some experts recommend a level of >30 ng/mL as being optimal.

TABLE 10.10
CORTISOL, 8 AM

Interpretation	Cortisol (mcg/dL)
Suggestive of adrenal insufficiency	<5 mcg/dL
Indeterminate	5–14 mcg/dL
Adrenal insufficiency unlikely	>14 mcg/dL

  b. Other causes: Addison disease, hypothalamic or pituitary disease secondary to tumors, surgery, radiation therapy, or congenital defects
2. **Evaluation**
  a. AM cortisol level (see Table 10.10 for interpretation)
  b. ACTH stimulation test: Most useful in diagnosis of adrenal insufficiency
    (1) Purpose: Measures ability of the adrenal gland to produce cortisol in response to ACTH.
    (2) Interpretation: Normally, a rise in serum cortisol follows ACTH administration. With ACTH deficiency or prolonged adrenal suppression, there is an inadequate rise in cortisol after a single ACTH dose. Blunted cortisol response can be indicative of CAH.
    (3) Standard-dose ACTH stimulation test: 250 mcg IV cortisol measured at 30 minutes and/or 60 minutes.
      (a) For evaluation of primary adrenal insufficiency:
        < 18 mcg/dL: Highly suggestive of adrenal insufficiency,
        > 18 mcg/dL: Normal (rules out adrenal insufficiency)
      (b) For evaluation of central adrenal insufficiency:
        < 16 mcg/dL: Highly suggestive of adrenal insufficiency,
        16–30 mcg/dL: Adrenal insufficiency less likely but not excluded
        > 30 mcg/dL: Normal (rules out adrenal insufficiency)
    (4) Low-dose ACTH stimulation test (1 mcg/1.73 m^2); cortisol measured at 30 minutes. May have higher sensitivity to detect central adrenal insufficiency than the standard dose test.

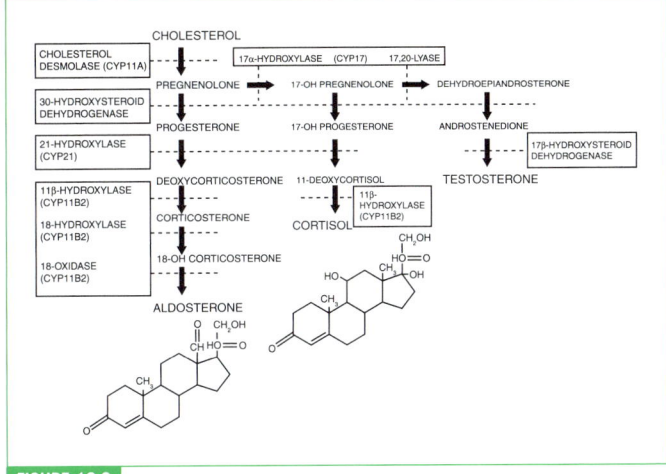

FIGURE 10.3
Biosynthetic pathway for steroid hormones.

Level <16 mcg/dL: Suggestive of adrenal insufficiency
Level 16–22 mcg/dL: Adrenal insufficiency less likely but not excluded
Level >22 mcg/dL: Adrenal insufficiency unlikely
NOTE: No test for adrenal insufficiency has perfect sensitivity or specificity, so results must be interpreted in the individual clinical context.
c. Mineralocorticoid deficiency confirmed with ↑ renin and ↓ aldosterone.
3. **Congenital adrenal hyperplasia**[22,23]
a. Group of autosomal recessive disorders characterized by a defect in one of the enzymes required in the synthesis of cortisol (Fig. 10.3). Cortisol deficiency results in oversecretion of ACTH and hyperplasia of the adrenal cortex.
b. Most common cause of ambiguous genitalia in females.
c. 21-Hydroxylase deficiency accounts for 90% of cases.
d. The enzymatic defect results in impaired synthesis of adrenal steroids beyond the enzymatic block and overproduction of the precursors before the block. Two major classifications:
   (1) Classic (complete enzyme deficiency):
      (a) Occurs with or without salt loss
      (b) Symptoms occur in the absence of stress
      (c) Adrenal crisis in untreated patients occurs at 1–2 weeks of life, with signs and symptoms of adrenal insufficiency rarely occurring before 3–4 days of life. (Non-salt-losing forms have

TABLE 10.11
17-HYDROXYPROGESTERONE, SERUM

Age	Baseline (ng/dL)
Premature (31–35 weeks)	≤360
Term infants (3 days)	≤420
1–12 mo	11–170
1–4 yr	4–115
5–9 yr	≤90
10–13 yr	≤169
14–17 yr	16–283
Males, Tanner II–III	12–130
Females, Tanner II–III	18–220
Male, Tanner IV–V	51–190
Females, Tanner IV–V	36–200
Male (18–30 yr)	32–307
Adult female	
Follicular phase	≤185
Midcycle phase	≤225
Luteal phase	≤285

Reference ranges from Quest Diagnostics LC/MS assay (liquid chromatography/tandem mass spectroscopy).
For preterm infants or infants born small for gestational age, see Olgemöller B, Roscher AA, Liebl B, et al. Screening for congenital adrenal hyperplasia: adjustment of 17-hydroxyprogesterone cut-off values to both age and birth weight markedly improves the predictive value. J Clin Endocrinol Metab. 2003;88:5790-5794.

       a less severe risk for adrenal crisis, owing to preservation of mineralocorticoid synthesis.)
    (d) Diagnosis: Elevated 17-hydroxyprogesterone (17-OHP) levels (often on newborn screening) (Table 10.11).
    (e) Elevated testosterone in girls and elevated androstenedione in girls and boys.
    (f) For apparent male infants who present with classic CAH, the karyotype should be evaluated to rule out the possibility of a severely masculinized female infant.
  (2) Nonclassic or simple virilizing form (partial enzyme deficiency):
    (a) Adrenal insufficiency tends to occur only under stress; manifests as androgen excess after infancy (i.e., precocious pubarche, irregular menses, hirsutism, acne, advanced bone age).
    (b) Morning 17-OHP levels may be elevated; however, the diagnosis may require an ACTH stimulation test. A significant rise in the 17-OHP level 60 minutes after ACTH injection is diagnostic. Cortisol response will be decreased.
  (3) Newborn screen:
    (a) Measures 17-OHP on filter paper; can be artificially elevated due to prematurity, sickness, stress; 2% specific, resulting in 98% false-positive rate.

(b) Results: If 17-OHP 40–100 ng/mL, repeat. If higher, check electrolytes and serum 17-OHP. If K ↑ and Na ↓, initiate treatment with hydrocortisone.

4. **Primary adrenal insufficiency (Addison disease)**[24]
  a. Syndrome of weakness, fatigue, and hyperpigmentation due to insufficient mineralocorticoid and glucocorticoid production, with compensatory ACTH overproduction.
  b. Autoimmune destruction of adrenal glands is the most common cause outside of infancy. In children, it may be part of autoimmune polyendocrine syndrome type 1 (APS-1), which also includes hypoparathyroidism and chronic mucocutaneous candidiasis. Individuals with autoimmune Addison disease should also be screened for other endocrinopathies.

5. **Management of adrenal insufficiency** (for relative potency of steroids see Table 10.12)
  a. Glucocorticoid maintenance: replacement of physiologic glucocorticoid production: 6–18 mg/m^2/day ÷ TID hydrocortisone PO or 1.5–3.5 mg/m^2/day prednisone ÷ BID (or equivalent glucocorticoid dose of another steroid). Typically, lower doses are required for central adrenal insufficiency, intermediate doses for primary adrenal insufficiency, and higher doses for CAH. Consultation with an endocrinologist is recommended.

TABLE 10.12
POTENCY OF VARIOUS THERAPEUTIC STEROIDS[‡]

Steroid	Glucocorticoid Effect* (in mg of Cortisol per mg of Steroid)	Mineralocorticoid Effect[†] (in mg of Cortisol per mg of Steroid)
Cortisol (hydrocortisone)	1	1
Cortisone acetate (oral)	0.8	0.8
Cortisone acetate (intramuscular)	0.8	0.8
Prednisone	4	0.25
Prednisolone	4	0.25
Methylprednisolone	5	0.4
Betamethasone	25	0
Triamcinolone	5	0
Dexamethasone	30	0
9α–fluorocortisone (fludrocortisone)	15	200
Deoxycorticosterone (DOC) acetate	0	20
Aldosterone	0.3	200–1,000

*To determine cortisol equivalent of a given steroid dose, multiply dose of steroid by corresponding number in column for glucocorticoid or mineralocorticoid effect. To determine dose of a given steroid based on desired cortisol dose, divide desired hydrocortisone dose by corresponding number in the column.
[†]Total physiologic replacement for salt retention is usually 0.1 mg Florinef, regardless of patient size.
[‡]Set relative to potency of cortisol.
(Modified from Sperling MA. Pediatric Endocrinology, 3rd ed. Philadelphia: Elsevier, 2008:476)

b. Mineralocorticoid maintenance:
   (1) For salt-losing forms of adrenal insufficiency (e.g., CAH, Addison disease): 0.1 mg/m^2/day (typical range: 0.05–0.15 mg) oral (PO) fludrocortisone acetate once daily is recommended. (**NOTE:** Synthetic steroids such as prednisone and dexamethasone do not supply appropriate mineralocorticoid effects.)
   (2) In a patient requiring mineralocorticoid replacement but unable to take oral medications, IV hydrocortisone at a dose of 50 mg/m^2/day or more will provide sufficient mineralocorticoid effect. Prednisone and dexamethasone, even at stress doses, will not provide adequate mineralocorticoid effect.
   (3) Infants also require 1–2 g (17–34 mEq) of sodium supplementation per day.
   (4) Always monitor blood pressure and electrolytes when supplementing mineralocorticoids.
c. Stress-dose glucocorticoids:
   (1) Glucocorticoid dosage should increase in patients with fever or other illness to mimic normal physiologic cortisol response to stress.
   (2) Minor ambulatory illness stress dose: 30–50 mg/m^2/day of hydrocortisone PO ÷ TID or 6–10 mg/m^2/day prednisone PO ÷ BID
   (3) Major stress (surgery/severe illness/adrenal crisis): Hydrocortisone 50 mg/m^2 IV bolus, then 25–100 mg/m^2/day IV (as a continuous infusion) or intramuscular (IM) injection of 25 mg/m^2/dose Q6 hr.

6. **Acute adrenal crisis**
   a. Often precipitated by acute illness, trauma, surgery, or exposure to excess heat.
   b. Presentation: Emesis, diarrhea, dehydration, hypotension, metabolic acidosis, shock.
   c. Laboratory values: Hypoglycemia, hyponatremia, and hyperkalemia. In addition, serum cortisol and aldosterone are decreased, and ACTH and renin are elevated. In infants with CAH, 17-OHP is increased.
   NOTE: Performing these studies before steroid administration is useful to confirm the diagnosis, but treatment should not be delayed.
   d. Management includes rapid volume expansion to support blood pressure, sufficient dextrose to maintain blood glucose, close monitoring of electrolytes, and corticosteroid administration.
      (1) Give 50 mg/m^2 of hydrocortisone by IV bolus (rapid estimate: infants = 25 mg; children = 50–100 mg), followed by 50 mg/m^2/24 hr by continuous drip (preferable) or divided Q3–4 hr.
      (2) Hydrocortisone and cortisone are the only glucocorticoids that provide the necessary mineralocorticoid effects; prednisone and dexamethasone do not.

7. **Cushing syndrome**[25]
   a. Signs and symptoms (including rapid weight gain with central obesity, buffalo hump, moon face, striae, thinning of skin and other

membranes, hypertension) associated with elevated cortisol levels and overexposure to glucocorticoids (either endogenous or exogenous). Relatively rare in children, with most cases resulting from iatrogenic causes.
b. Cushing evaluation:
   (1) 24-hour urine collection for excess cortisol (normal value range by mass spectrometry: ≤27–30 ng/mL).
   (2) Salivary cortisol level: Measured at 11 PM (*spit in a tube*); levels are akin to free serum cortisol. Normal range is <0.2 mcg/dL.
   (3) Dexamethasone suppression test:
      (a) Dexamethasone suppresses secretion of ACTH by the normal pituitary, decreasing endogenous production of cortisol. Useful in determining the etiology of glucocorticoid or androgen overproduction.
      (b) Overnight dexamethasone suppression test: Measure serum cortisol at 8 AM; preceded by 1 mg of dexamethasone PO given at 11 PM the night before. Level <1.8 mcg/dL (50 nmol/L) is within normal range of suppression.
      NOTE: Random cortisol is not useful in evaluation for Cushing syndrome.

B. Adrenal Medulla: Pheochromocytoma[26-28]

1. **Pheochromocytoma only accounts for ≈1% of pediatric hypertension.** Often associated with syndromes: MEN IIa and IIb, von Hippel-Lindau, neurofibromatosis (NF) 1, familial paraganglioma syndrome.
2. **Evaluation for pheochromocytoma should involve imaging and laboratory workup**.
3. **Measurement of free, fractionated metanephrines in plasma:**
a. Use: Detection of pheochromocytoma
b. Upper limits of normal: Somewhat assay–dependent
   (1) One study suggests upper normal limits to be metanephrines, 0.3 nmol/L; normetanephrines, 0.6 nmol/L.[27]
   (2) A pediatric study suggests metanephrines for boys, 0.52 nmol/L; girls, 0.37 nmol/L; normetanephrines for boys, 0.53 nmol/L; girls, 0.42 nmol/L.[28]

VI. POSTERIOR PITUITARY FUNCTION[29]

A. Posterior Pituitary Hormones: Targets and Actions

1. Oxytocin
a. Targets: Breast and uterus
b. Actions: Breast milk let down and uterine contractions
2. Vasopressin
a. Target: Nephron distal collecting duct
b. Actions: Reabsorption of water

B. Posterior Pituitary Disorders: Vasopressin

1. **Syndrome of Inappropriate Antidiuretic Hormone Secretion (SIADH)**
   a. **Presentation:** Serum hyponatremia (Na^+ < 135 mEq/L) with inappropriately concentrated urine (>100 mOsm/kg) in the setting of euvolemia or mild hypervolemia
   b. **Etiology:** Central nervous system trauma, infection, tumor, surgery (up to 1 week postoperatively, particularly tonsillectomy and adenoidectomy), pneumonia, and medications (e.g., anti-epileptics, chemotherapeutic agents, and antidepressants).
   c. **Laboratory findings:** ↓ serum Na^+ and Cl with inappropriately concentrated urine
   d. **Treatment:** Correct hyponatremia slowly with fluid restriction (≈10% rise in Na^+ per 24 hours). Chronic treatment can be with orally active osmotic agents (including urea or sodium). In addition, the key to treating SIADH with hypertonic saline is to be sure the osmolarity of hypertonic saline is greater than the osmolarity of the urine. This can be used to treat SIADH even if the patient is not comatose or seizing. *In the setting of coma or seizures,* use hypertonic saline to rapidly correct Na^+ to ≈ 120–125 mEq/L. Definitive therapy: identify and treat the underlying cause.

2. **Diabetes Insipidus (DI)**
   a. **Presentation:** Hypernatremia with inappropriately dilute urine in the setting of mild hypovolemia. Coexisting polyuria and polydipsia (>2 L/m^2/24 hr) may also be present. Infants may present with failure to thrive or obesity, vomiting, constipation, unexplained fevers. In more severe cases, severe dehydration, hypovolemic shock, and seizures may occur.
   b. **Etiology:**
      (1) Central: ↓ADH secretion from posterior pituitary
      (2) Nephrogenic: ADH resistance at the nephron–collecting duct
   c. **Work-up:**
      (1) Serum osmolality, Na, K, blood urea nitrogen (BUN), creatinine, glucose, calcium
      (2) Urine osmolality, specific gravity
   d. **Diagnosis:**
      (1) Serum osmolality > 300 mOsm/kg and urine osmolality <300 mOsm/kg. If the serum osmolality is >270 mOsm but <300 mOsm with polyuria and polydipsia, a water deprivation test followed by a vasopressin test is necessary to further evaluate for DI.
      (2) **Water deprivation test:**
         (a) **Purpose:** Determines ability to concentrate urine. Useful in diagnosing DI in general, but need vasopressin test (see below) to differentiate central and nephrogenic DI. Risk of dehydration and hypernatremia, so careful supervision is required.

(b) **Method**:
  i. Begin test after a 24-hour period of adequate hydration and stable weight.
  ii. Obtain a baseline weight after bladder emptying.
  iii. Restrict fluids. Measure body weight and urine–specific gravity and volume hourly.
  iv. Check serum Na and urine and serum osmolality Q2 hr. (Hematocrit and blood urea nitrogen [BUN] levels may also be obtained but are not critical.) Monitor carefully to ensure fluids are not ingested during the test.
  v. Terminate test if weight loss approaches 5%.
(c) **Interpretation:** See Table 10.13
(3) Vasopressin test:
  (a) **Purpose:** Differentiate central versus nephrogenic DI
  (b) **Method:** Administer vasopressin 1 U/m^2 subcutaneously at end of water deprivation test. Assess urine output, urine specific gravity, and water intake.
  (c) **Interpretation:** See Table 10.14
e. **Central DI**
  (1) **Etiology**: Trauma or surgical injury to vasopressin neurons, gene mutations, congenital malformations, infection, autoimmune diseases, and drugs

TABLE 10.13
RESULTS OF WATER DEPRIVATION TEST IN NORMAL VS. CENTRAL/NEPHROGENIC DI

	Normal (Psychogenic DI)	Central Nephrogenic
Urine Volume	↓	No change
Weight Loss	No change	≤5%
Urine Osmolality	500–1400 mOsm/L	<150
Plasma Osmolality	288–291 mOsm/L	>290 mOsm/L
Urine Specific Gravity	≥1.010	<1.005
Urine:Plasma Osmolality Ratio	>2	<2
Key	Urine Osmolality >1000 mOsm/L generally excludes diagnosis of DI	

DI, diabetes insipidus

TABLE 10.14
RESULTS OF VASOPRESSIN ADMINISTRATION IN EVALUATION OF DI

	Psychogenic	Central*	Nephrogenic
Urine Volume	↓	↓	No change
Urine Specific Gravity	≥1.010	≥1.010	No change
Oral Fluid Intake	No change	↓	No change

*In central DI, urine osmolality increases by 200% or more in response to vasopressin administration.
DI, diabetes insipidus

(a) Trauma or surgical injury (often a triphasic response)
  i. 1–5 days: Transient DI due to initial edema
  ii. Up to 10 days: SIADH due to dying neurons releasing ADH
  iii. May be permanent if sufficient neuronal damage has occurred
(b) Genetic
  i. Autosomal recessive (present at birth) or autosomal dominant (occurs within 5 years of life)
  ii. Septo-optic dysplasia (agenesis of corpus callosum)
  iii. Holoprosencephaly
(2) **Laboratory findings**: Low vasopressin (<0.5 pg/mL). See Table 10.14.
(3) **Treatment:** IV, PO, SQ, or nasal desmopressin acetate (DDAVP) titrate dosage to urine output. Goal is ≥1-hour period of diuresis per day that stimulates thirst. Monitor electrolytes. Infants are often not treated with DDAVP because of difficulty monitoring input and output. Rather, they can be treated with increased free water and salt restriction.

f. **Nephrogenic DI**
(1) **Etiology:**
  (a) Genetic: X-linked (V2 receptor), autosomal dominant, and recessive (Aquaporin-2)
  (b) Acquired: Drugs, anatomical kidney disease
(2) **Laboratory findings:** Increased serum vasopressin level.
(3) **Treatment:** Ensure free water consumption, caloric intake, and a low-salt diet. Consider thiazide diuretics to increase proximal Na reabsorption. Indomethacin may increase ADH- and V2-binding affinity.

VII. GROWTH[29-31]

A. Height
1. **Target height range:** Mid-parental height ± 2 SD (1 SD = 4 inches).
a. Mid-parental height for boys: (Paternal height + maternal height + 5 inches)/2
b. Mid-parental height for girls: (Paternal height + maternal height − 5 inches)/2
c. Estimated average growth velocity per year: See Table 10.15.
2. **Short stature** (Fig. 10.4)
a. **Definition**: Height less than 3rd percentile, height percentile below target height range
b. **Differential diagnosis**:
  (1) **Familial short stature:** Characterized by slow growth rate during the first 2–3 years of life, followed by a low-normal growth velocity. Bone-age X-rays (left wrist and hand) may be within normal limits for age.

TABLE 10.15
ESTIMATED GROWTH VELOCITY IN CHILDREN BASED ON AGE

Age	Growth (cm/yr)
Birth to 1 year old	25 cm/yr
1 year old to 4 years old	10 cm/yr
4 years old to 8 years old	5 cm/yr
8 years old to 12 years old	5 cm/yr*

*Rates may be considerably higher at later end of this age range when individuals have entered their pubertal growth spurt.

   (2) **Constitutional growth delay:** Characterized by slow growth rate during the first 2–3 years of life. Bone-age X-rays may be delayed for age. This delay in bone-age X-rays corresponds with a delay in pubertal onset and skeletal maturation, leading to a period of catch-up growth. A family history of delayed puberty is often present.
   (3) **Pathologic short stature** (see Fig. 10.4). Differentiate from benign causes of short stature by the following workup:
      (a) Detailed history/physical examination, evaluation of growth curves and pubertal stage.
      (b) Labs: Electrolytes, LFTs, CBC, ESR, urinalysis, TFTs, serum insulin-like growth factor (IGF)-1 (see Table 10.16) and IGF-binding protein-3 (IGFBP-3), and tissue transglutaminase (TTG) for celiac disease. Consider karyotype in girls.
      (c) Imaging: Bone age x-ray. Consider a skeletal survey in patients with disproportionate features.
3. **Tall stature:** Most common cause is familial tall stature or precocious puberty. Differential also includes growth hormone excess. Bone age may be helpful.

VIII. SEXUAL DEVELOPMENT [32-38]

1. **Definitions:** For normal pubertal stages, please see Chapter 5.
2. **Delayed puberty**
a. **Definition:**
   (1) Girls: No pubertal development by 13 years or >5 years between thelarche and menarche. Primary amenorrhea: no menarche by age 16 years in the presence of secondary sexual characteristics, or no menarche and no secondary sexual characteristics by age 14 years.
   (2) Boys: No testicular enlargement by 14 years.
b. **Initial evaluation** (Fig. 10.5)
   (1) Physical exam for Tanner staging. Pubertal milestones and growth chart.
   (2) Labs: LH, FSH, and thyroid studies. See Tables 10.17 and 10.18.
   (3) Imaging: Bone age x-ray

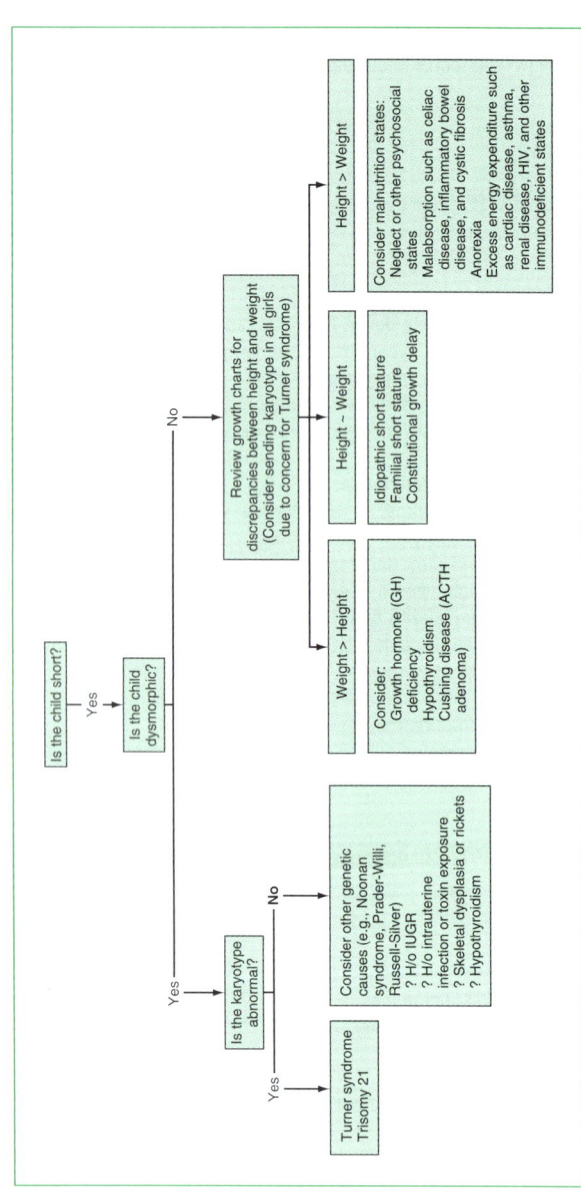

FIGURE 10.4 Differential diagnosis of short stature.

TABLE 10.16
INSULIN-LIKE GROWTH FACTOR 1 (IGF-1)*

Age (years)	Male (ng/mL)	Females (ng/mL)
<1	≤142	≤185
1–1.9	≤134	≤175
2–2.9	≤135	≤178
3–3.9	30–155	38–214
4–4.9	28–181	34–238
5–5.9	31–214	37–272
6–6.9	38–253	45–316
7–7.9	48–298	58–367
8–8.9	62–347	76–424
9–9.9	80–398	99–483
10–10.9	100–449	125–541
11–11.9	123–497	152–593
12–12.9	146–541	178–636
13–13.9	168–576	200–664
14–14.9	187–599	214–673
15–15.9	201–609	218–659
16–16.9	209–602	208–619
17–17.9	207–576	185–551

*A clearly normal IGF-1 level argues against growth hormone (GH) deficiency, except in young children in whom there is considerable overlap between normals and those with GH deficiency.
Reference ranges from Quest Diagnostics LC/MS (liquid chromatography/tandem mass spectrometry) assay.

TABLE 10.17
LUTEINIZING HORMONE

Age	Males (mIU/mL)	Females (mIU/mL)
0–2 yr	Not established	Not established
3–7 yr	≤0.26	≤0.26
8–9 yr	≤0.46	≤0.69
10–11 yr	≤3.13	≤4.38
12–14 yr	0.23–4.41	0.04–10.80
15–17 yr	0.29–4.77	0.97–14.70
Tanner Stages	**Males (mIU/mL)**	**Females (mIU/mL)**
I	≤0.52	≤0.15
II	≤1.76	≤2.91
III	≤4.06	≤7.01
IV–V	0.06–4.77	0.10–14.70

Data from Quest Diagnostics immunoassay. For more information, see www.questdiagnostics.com.

TABLE 10.18
FOLLICLE-STIMULATING HORMONE

Age	Male (mIU/mL)	Female (mIU/mL)
0–4 yr	Not established	Not established
5–9 yr	0.21–4.33	0.72–5.33
10–13 yr	0.53–4.92	0.87–9.16
14–17 yr	0.85–8.74	0.64–10.98

Data from Quest Diagnostics immunoassay. For more information, see www.questdiagnostics.com.

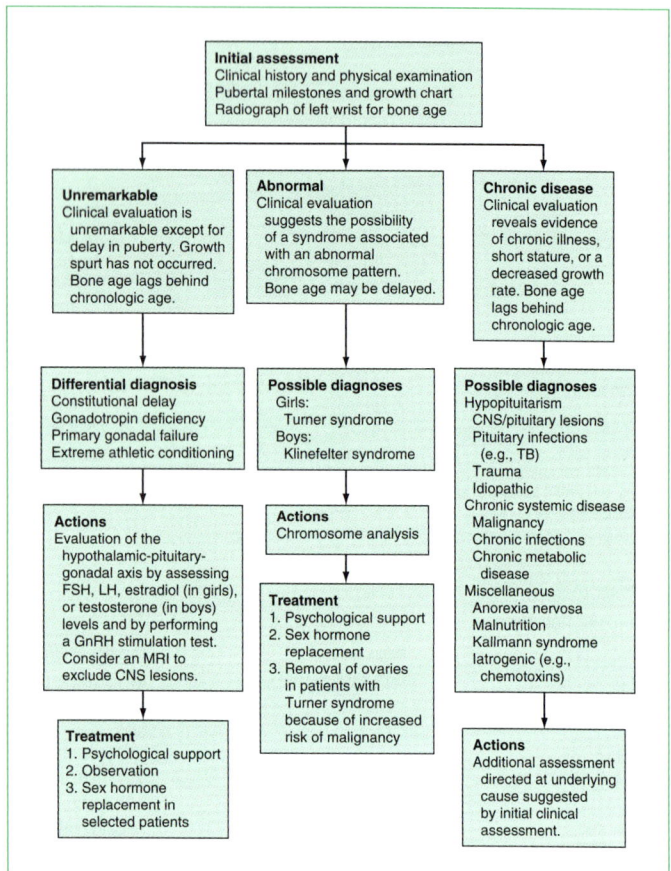

FIGURE 10.5

An approach to the child presenting with delayed puberty. CNS, central nervous system; FSH, follicle-stimulating hormone; GnRH, gonadotropin-releasing hormone; LH, luteinizing hormone; MRI, magnetic resonance imaging; TB, tuberculosis *(From Blondell R, Foster MB, Dave KC. Disorders of puberty. Am Fam Physician. 1999;60: 209-218.)*

  c. **Further work-up**
    (1) Hypergonadotropic hypogonadism (high LH and FSH):
      (a) Primary gonadal failure
      (b) Differential diagnosis: Turner or Klinefelter syndromes, androgen insensitivity, tumor, chemotherapy.
    (2) Hypogonadotropic hypogonadism (low or normal LH/FSH):

(a) May be due to constitutional delay or central gonadotropin deficiency.
(b) Of the latter cause, etiologies include Kallmann syndrome (most common cause of isolated gonadotropin deficiency), CNS tumors, hypopituitarism.

(3) GnRH stimulation test[39]
(a) Measures pituitary LH and FSH reserve: Helpful in the differential diagnosis of precocious or delayed sexual development.
(b) Method: Give 20 mcg/kg GnRH analog (Leuprolide) SQ, and measure LH and FSH levels at 0 and 60 minutes.
(c) Interpretation: Prepubertal children should show no or minimal increase in LH and FSH in response to GnRH. A rise of LH to >3.3–5.0 IU/L is evidence of central puberty.

3. **Precocious puberty**
a. **Definition:** Secondary sexual maturation before age 8 years in girls and 9 years in boys.
b. **Classification**
   (1) **Central (Gonadotropin Dependent):** Premature activation of hypothalamic-pituitary-gonadal axis, resulting in increased GnRH secretion and subsequently increased LH/FSH.
      (a) Male to female ratio 1:5.
      (b) Presentation: Pubertal progression and osseous maturation.
   (2) **Peripheral (Gonadotropin Independent):** No activation of hypothalamic-pituitary-gonadal axis. Sources of hormone production include the adrenals, gonads, ectopic, or exogenous. Most common causes are CAH, adrenal tumors, McCune-Albright syndrome, gonadal tumors, human chorionic gonadotropin (hCG)-producing tumors, and exogenous sex hormones. Hypothyroidism can also cause GnRH-independent precocity. Penile length is disproportionately greater than testicular size in peripheral precocious puberty, whereas testicular volume is disproportionately greater than penile size in normal puberty and central precocious puberty.
c. **Evaluation:** History of premature thelarche/adrenarche with detailed physical examination and assessment of growth curves.
   (1) Laboratory studies: Dependent upon male or female patient in addition to whether androgen effect, estrogen effect, or both are present.
   (2) Most often, 17-hydroxyprogesterone (17 OHP; see Table 10.11) should be measured to rule out CAH.
   (3) Other tests to consider include estradiol in females (Table 10.19), testosterone in males (Tables 10.20 and 10.21), dehydroepiandrosterone (DHEA) (Table 10.22), dehydroepiandrosterone sulfate (DHEA-S) (Table 10.23), thyroid studies, and LH (see Table 10.17).

TABLE 10.19
ESTRADIOL*

Age	Level (pg/mL)
Prepubertal children	<25
Men	6–44
Women	
Luteal phase	26–165
Follicular phase	None detected–266
Midcycle	118–355
Adult women on OCP	None detected–102

*Normal infants have elevated estradiol at birth, which decreases to prepubertal values during the first week of life. Estradiol levels increase again between age 1 and 2 months and return to prepubertal values by age 6–12 months.
OCP, oral contraceptive pill
Data from JHH Laboratories.

d. **Imaging:**
   (1) Initial evaluation may include bone age. In general, bone age is >2 years in advance of chronologic age in long-standing precocious puberty due to the action of sex hormones.
   (2) Depending on the differential diagnosis, imaging may also include brain magnetic resonance imaging (MRI), pelvic ultrasound, or testicular ultrasound. Testicular ultrasound should be considered with asymmetrical testicular volume (see Table 10.24 for normal testicular size and volume).
4. **Polycystic ovarian syndrome (PCOS)**[32]
a. **Definition**: Syndrome of hyperandrogenism and menstrual dysfunction
b. **Diagnostic criteria**:
   (1) **Hyperandrogenism**: Clinical characteristics are hirsutism, acne, and male pattern alopecia. Biochemical characteristics include elevated free testosterone, measured from total serum testosterone and sex hormone-binding protein (SHBG).
   (2) **Menstrual dysfunction**: Amenorrhea or oligomenorrhea.
   (3) **Polycystic ovaries:** Ultrasound (US) characteristics are increased ovarian volume (reliable in adolescents via transabdominal US) or follicular phase with ≥12 follicles measuring 2–9 mm (reliable via transvaginal US only).
c. **Management:**
   (1) Weight reduction and other lifestyle changes increase SHBG (thus decreasing free testosterone) can restore ovulation and increase insulin sensitivity.
   (2) Treatment of hirsutism/acne: Hormonal contraceptives
   (3) Insulin-sensitizing agents (e.g., metformin) may help mitigate metabolic consequences, but are off-label and are of uncertain benefit unless interested in becoming pregnant.

TABLE 10.20
TESTOSTERONE, TOTAL SERUM*

Age	Male (ng/dL)	Female (ng/dL)
Cord blood	17–61	16–44
1–10 days	≤187	≤24
1–3 mo	72–344	≤17
3–5 mo	≤201	≤12
5–7 mo	≤59	≤13
7–12 mo	≤16	≤11
1–5.9 yr	≤5	≤8
6–7.9 yr	≤25	≤20
8–10.9 yr	≤42	≤35
11–11.9 yr	≤260	≤40
12–13.9 yr	≤420	≤40
14–17.9 yr	≤1000	≤40
≥18 (adult)	250–1100	2–45
TANNER STAGE		
Stage I	≤5	≤8
Stage II	≤167	≤24
Stage III	21–719	≤28
Stage IV	25–912	≤31
Stage V	110–975	≤33

*Normal testosterone/dihydrotestosterone (T/DHT) ratio is <18 in adults and older children, and <10 in neonates. A T/DHT ratio >20 suggests 5-alpha-reductase deficiency or androgen insensitivity syndrome.
Data from Quest Diagnostics LC/MS (liquid chromatography/tandem mass spectrometry) assay.

TABLE 10.21
TESTOSTERONE, FREE

Age	Male (pg/mL)	Female (pg/mL)
5.9–9 yr	≤5.3	0.2–5.0
10–13.9 yr	0.7–52	0.1–7.4
14–17.9 yr	18–111	0.5–3.9
18–69 yr	35–155	0.1–6.4

Data from Quest Diagnostics LC/MS (liquid chromatography/tandem mass spectrometry) assay.

TABLE 10.22
DEHYDROEPIANDROSTERONE (DHEA), UNCONJUGATED

Age	ng/dL
1–5 yr	≤377
6–9 yr	19–592
10–13 yr	42–1067
14–17 yr	137–1489
Adult male	61–1636
Adult female	102–1185

Data from Quest Diagnostics LC/MS (liquid chromatography/tandem mass spectrometry) assay.

TABLE 10.23
DEHYDROEPIANDROSTERONE SULFATE (DHEA-S)

Age	Male (mcg/dL)	Female (mcg/dL)
<1 mo	≤316	15–261
1–6 mo	≤58	≤74
7–11 mo	≤26	≤26
1–3 yr	≤15	≤22
4–6 yr	≤27	≤34
7–9 yr	≤91	≤92
10–13 yr	≤138	≤148
14–17 yr	38–340	37–307
TANNER STAGES (AGES 7–17)		
I	≤49	≤46
II	≤81	15–133
III	22–126	42–126
IV	33–177	42–241
V	110–370	45–320

Data from Quest Diagnostics assay. For more information see www.questdiagnostics.com.

TABLE 10.24
TESTICULAR SIZE

Tanner Stage (Genital)	Length (cm) (Mean ± SD)	Volume (mL)*
I	2.0 ± 0.5	2
II	2.7 ± 0.7	5
III	3.4 ± 0.8	10
IV	4.1 ± 1.0	20
V	5.0 ± 0.5	29

*Testicular volume of >4 mL or a long axis of >2.5 cm is evidence that pubertal testicular growth has begun.
SD, standard deviation

(4) Prevention of endometrial hyperplasia (increased risk of endometrial cancer) by intermittent induction of menstruation with progesterone or prevention of endometrial proliferation by hormonal contraception.
5. **Ambiguous genitalia**[36]
   a. **Clinical findings in a neonate suspicious for ambiguous genitalia:**
      (1) Anogenital ratio (distance between anus and posterior fourchette divided by distance between anus and base of phallus) > 0.5 cm
      (2) Phallus length < 1.9 cm
      (3) Clitoromegaly (length > 1 cm)
      (4) Non-palpable gonads in an apparent male
      (5) Hypospadias associated with separation of scrotal sacs or undescended testis

b. **Etiology:**
   (1) Most common cause is CAH (see Section V.A.3).
   (2) Other causes: Testicular regression syndrome, androgen insensitivity, testosterone biosynthesis disorders, and chromosomal abnormalities.
c. **Evaluation:**
   (1) Labs: Timing of collection is important.
      (a) Day 0-1: LH, testosterone, dihydrotestosterone (DHT), and karyotype.
      (b) Day 3-4: Cortisol, 17-OHP, DHEA, androstenedione, and karyotype.
   (2) Imaging: Voiding cysto-urethrogram (VCUG), pelvic and renal US, pelvic computerized tomography (CT)
6. **Cryptorchidism:**
a. **Prevalence:** 3% of term male infants. About 50% of cryptorchid testicles descend by age 3 months and 80% by age 12 months. Neoplasm occurs in 48.9% of individuals with untreated cryptorchidism, and 25% of those tumors occur in the contralateral testis.
b. **Evaluation:** Consider karyotyping to rule out a virilized female. A hCG stimulation test measures the capacity for testosterone biosynthesis and can be used to differentiate cryptorchidism from anorchia (absent testes).
   (1) Method: Give 1000 units of intravenous (IV) or intramuscular (IM) hCG for 3 days, and measure serum testosterone and dihydrotestosterone on day 0 and day 4.
   (2) Interpretation: Testosterone level >100 ng/dL in response to hCG stimulation is evidence for adequate testosterone biosynthesis. In cryptorchidism, testosterone rises to adult levels; in anorchia, there is no rise.
c. **Treatment:** Observe until age 12 months, at which time if testis remains undescended, surgical removal is indicated.
7. **Gender dysphoria**[40]
   See Chapter 5. Gender dysphoria is diagnosed when there is a marked difference between the individual's expressed/experienced gender and the gender others would assign him or her characterized by significant distress or impairment.[40] The DSM-V criteria recommends a diagnosis occur after 6 months of continuous incongruence, and for pre-pubescent children, must be present and verbalized. The primary focus in caring for pre-pubescent children is parental support and education to create a safe environment for the child.[41] Familial support of social transition for transgender children has been associated with better mental health outcomes.[42]
   Transgender children and adolescents for whom medical interventions are appropriate may initially undergo treatment to suppress pubertal development. Patient must be Tanner Stage 2–3 confirmed by

pubertal levels of estradiol and testosterone. Suppression of endogenous hormones can be achieved with GnRH analogue (Lupron, Supprelin). In adolescence, initiation of opposite sex pubertal development may occur with exogenous hormones. Oral estradiol induces female puberty. Intramuscular testosterone induces male puberty.[43] Generally, gender confirming surgery is deferred until the patient reaches the age of majority. A valuable online reference for transgender medicine can be found at UCSF's Center of Excellence for Transgender Health (http://www.transhealth.ucsf.edu/).

IX. NEONATAL HYPOGLYCEMIA EVALUATION[44]

A. Definition of Hypoglycemia:

Serum glucose level insufficient to meet metabolic requirements; can vary with perinatal stress, birth weight, and maternal factors. For practical purposes, value is defined as a point-of-care glucose (POCG) <45 mg/dL. **NOTE:** Bedside glucometer is inaccurate at levels < 40 mg/dL; stat serum glucose must be sent if POCG ≤40.

B. Symptoms:

Abnormal cry, seizures, apnea, hypotonia, bradycardia, hypothermia.

C. Treatment:

Do not delay while awaiting serum glucose results:
1. Plasma glucose 25–45 mg/dL (1.4–2.5 mM), asymptomatic: breastfeed or nipple/gavage with formula.
2. Plasma glucose level < 25 mg/dL (<1.4 mM) ± symptoms, asymptomatic infants who do not tolerate enteral feeding, or symptomatic infants:
a. Give IV bolus of glucose 0.25 g/kg (2.5 mL/kg of 10% glucose, or 1 mL/kg of 25% glucose) over 1–2 minutes.
b. Continue IV glucose at a rate of 6–8 mg/kg/min (3.6–4.8 mL/kg/hr of 10% glucose).
c. Monitor blood glucose Q30–60 min, and increase glucose delivery by 1–2 mg/kg/min if blood glucose is consistently < 50 mg/dL.
3. If serum glucose is consistently < 45 mg/dL: Further endocrine workup warranted. At the time of hypoglycemia (serum glucose < 45 mg/dL):
a. Obtain serum glucose, insulin, growth hormone, cortisol, free fatty acids, and β-hydroxybutyrate.
b. Glucagon Stimulation Test: Administer glucagon and obtain serum glucose levels Q10 min ×4. Repeat growth hormone and cortisol levels 30 minutes after documented hypoglycemia.
   (1) A rise in glucose ≥ 30 mg/dL along with elevated insulin levels, low serum levels of free fatty acids and β-hydroxybutyrate, and a glucose requirement >8 mg/kg/min suggests a diagnosis of **hyperinsulinemia**.

(2) Hypoglycemia with midline defects and micropenis in a male suggest hypopituitarism, supported by low serum levels of growth hormone and cortisol at the time of hypoglycemia.

X. ADDITIONAL NORMAL VALUES

NOTE: Normal values may differ among laboratories because of variation in technique and type of assay used.

See Expert Consult, Chapter 10, for normal values of:
Table EC 10.A, Dihydrotestosterone (DHT)
Table EC 10.B, Catecholamines, urine
Table EC 10.C, Catecholamines, plasma
Table EC 10.D, Insulin-like growth factor binding protein
Table EC 10.E, Mean stretched penile length
Table EC 10.F, Androstenedione, serum

REFERENCES

1. American Diabetes Association. Diagnosis and classification of diabetes mellitus. *Diabetes Care*. 2012;35(Suppl 1):S64-S71.
2. Craig ME, Hattersley A, Donaghue KC. ISPAD Clinical Practice Consensus Guidelines 2009 Compendium: definition, epidemiology, and classification of diabetes in children and adolescents. *Pediatr Diabetes*. 2009;10(Suppl 12): 3-12.
3. International Expert Committee report on the role of the A1c assay in the diagnosis of diabetes. *Diabetes Care*. 2009;32:1327-1334.
4. Hattersley A, Bruining J, Shield J, et al. ISPAD Clinical Practice Consensus Guidelines 2009. The diagnosis and management of monogenic diabetes in children. *Pediatr Diabetes*. 2009;10(Suppl 12):33-42.
5. Steck AK, Winter WE. Review on monogenic diabetes. *Curr Opin Endocrinol Diabetes Obes*. 2011;18:252-258.
6. Cooke DW, Plotnick L. Management of diabetic ketoacidosis in children and adolescents. *Pediatr Rev*. 2008;29:431-436.
7. Dunger DB, Sperling MA, Acerini CL, et al. European Society for Pediatric Endocrinology/Lawson Wilkins Pediatric Endocrine Society consensus statement on diabetic ketoacidosis in children and adolescents. *Pediatrics*. 2004;113:e133-e140.
8. Alberti G, Zimmet P, Shaw J, et al. Type 2 diabetes in the young: the evolving epidemic. The International Diabetes Federation consensus workshop. *Diabetes Care*. 2004;27:1798-1811.
9. Rosenbloom AL, Silverstein JH, Amemiya S. ISPAD Consensus Practice Guidelines 2009 Compendium: type 2 diabetes in children and adolescents. *Pediatr Diabetes*. 2009;10(suppl 12):17-22.
10. Copeland KC, Silverstein J, Moore KR et al. Management of newly diagnosed type 2 diabetes mellitus (T2DM) in children and adolescents. *Pediatrics*. 2013;131:364-382.
11. Fisher DA. The thyroid. In: Rudolph CD, Rudolph AM, Lister GE, et al., eds. *Rudolph's Pediatrics*. New York: McGraw-Hill; 2011.
12. Fisher DA. Thyroid function and dysfunction in premature infants. *Pediatr Endocrinol Rev*. 2007;4:317-328.

13. Büyükgebiz A. Newborn screening for congenital hypothyroidism. *J Pediatr Endocrinol Metab*. 2006;19:1291-1298.
14. Lem AJ, de Rijke YB, van Toor H, et al. Serum thyroid hormone levels in healthy children from birth to adulthood and in short children born small for gestational age. *J Clin Endocrinol Metab*. 2012;97:3170-3178.
15. Williams FL, Simpson J, Delahunty C, et al. Developmental trends in cord and postpartum serum thyroid hormones in preterm infants. *J Clin Endocrinol Metab*. 2004;89:5314-5320.
16. Reinehr T. Thyroid function in the nutritionally obese child and adolescent. *Curr Opin Pediatr*. 2011;23:415-420.
17. Screening for congenital hypothyroidism: US Preventative Services Task Force reaffirmation recommendation. *Ann Fam Med*. 2008;6:166.
18. Ross AC, Manson JE, Abrams SA, et al. The 2011 report on dietary reference intakes for calcium and vitamin D from the Institute of Medicine: what clinicians need to know. *J Clin Endocrinol Metab*. 2010;96:53-58.
19. Greer FR. Defining vitamin D deficiency in children: beyond 25-OH vitamin D serum concentrations. *Pediatrics*. 2009;124:1471-1473.
20. Misra M, Pacaud D, Petryk A, et al. Vitamin D deficiency in children and its management: review of current knowledge and recommendations. *Pediatrics*. 2008;122:398-417.
21. Stewart PM. The adrenal cortex. In: Melmed S, Polonsky KS, Reed Larsen P, et al., eds. *Williams Textbook of Endocrinology*. Philadelphia: Saunders; 2011.
22. American Academy of Pediatrics, Section on Endocrinology and Committee on Genetics. Technical report: congenital adrenal hyperplasia. *Pediatrics*. 2000;106:1511-1518.
23. Autal Z, Zhou P. Congenital adrenal hyperplasia: diagnosis, evaluation, and management. *Pediatr Rev*. 2009;30:e49-e57.
24. Autal Z, Zhou P. Addison disease. *Pediatr Rev*. 2009;30:491-493.
25. Stratakis CA. Cushing syndrome in pediatrics. *Endocrinol Metab Clin North Am*. 2012;41:793-803.
26. Edmonds S, Fein DM, Gurtman A. Pheochromocytoma. *Pediatr Rev*. 2011;32:308-310.
27. Lenders JW, Pacak K, Walther MM, et al. Biomedical diagnosis of pheochromocytoma: which test is best? *JAMA*. 2002;287:1427-1434.
28. Weise M, Merke DP, Pacak K, et al. Utility of plasma free metanephrines for detecting childhood pheochromocytoma. *J Clin Endocrinol Metab*. 2002;87:1955-1960.
29. Robinson AG, Verbalis JG. Posterior pituitary. In: Melmed S, Polonsky KS, Reed Larsen P, et al., eds. *Williams Textbook of Endocrinology*. Philadelphia: Saunders; 2011.
30. Plotnick L, Miller R. Growth, growth hormone, and pituitary disorders. In: McMillan J, ed. *Oski's Pediatrics: Principles and Practice*. Philadelphia: Lippincott Williams & Wilkins; 2006:2084-2092.
31. MacGillivray MH. The basics for the diagnosis and management of short stature: a pediatric endocrinologist's approach. *Pediatr Ann*. 2000;29:570-575.
32. Norman RJ, Dewailly D, Legro RS, et al. Polycystic ovary syndrome. *Lancet*. 2007;370:685-697.
33. Styne DM. New aspects in the diagnosis and treatment of pubertal disorders. *Pediatr Clin North Am*. 1997;44:505-529.
34. Kaplowitz PB. Delayed puberty. *Pediatr Rev*. 2010;31:189-195.

35. Carel JC, Leger J. Clinical practice. Precocious puberty. *N Engl J Med*. 2008;358:2366-2377.
36. American Academy of Pediatrics, Committee on Genetics, Sections on Endocrinology and Urology. Evaluation of newborn with developmental anomalies of the external genitalia. *Pediatrics*. 2000;106:138-142.
37. Blondell R, Foster MB, Dave KC. Disorders of puberty. *Am Fam Physician*. 1999;60:209-218.
38. Master-Hunter T, Heiman DL. Amenorrhea: evaluation and treatment. *Am Fam Physician*. 2006;73:1374-1382.
39. Carel JC, Eugster EA, Rogol A, et al. Consensus statement on the use of gonadotropin-releasing hormone analogs in children. *Pediatrics*. 2009;123:e752-e762.
40. World Professional Association for Transgender Health. Standard of care or the health of transsexual, transgender, and gender- nonconforming people [Version 7]. Retrieved from <http://www.wpath.org/site_page.cfm?pk_association_webpage_menu=1351&pk_association_webpage=3926> 2012.
41. University of California—San Francisco. Youth: Special considerations. Retrieved from <http://www.transhealth.ucsf.edu/trans?page=protocol-youth> 2016.
42. Olsen KR, Durwood L, DeMueles M, McLaughlin KA. Mental health of transgender children who are supported in their identities. *Pediatrics*. 2016;137(3):e20153223. doi:10.1542/peds.2015-3223.
43. Hembree WC, et al. Endocrine Treatment of Transsexual Persons: An Endocrine Society Clinical Practice Guideline. *J Clin Endocrinol Metab*. 2009;94(9):3132-3154.
44. Cooke DW. Metabolism and endocrinology. In: Seidel HM, Rosenstein BJ, Pathak A, eds. *Primary Care of the Newborn*. 4th ed. Philadelphia: Mosby; 2006.

Chapter 11
Fluids and Electrolytes
Candice M. Nalley, MD

In memory of Idoreyin P. Montague, MD

See additional content on Expert Consult

I. OVERALL GUIDANCE IN FLUID AND ELECTROLYTE MANAGEMENT

Fluid therapy is an essential component of the care of hospitalized children. Some basic principles should be followed whether providing enteral or parenteral fluids. Appropriate fluid management involves the calculation and administration of water volume and electrolyte concentration of:
A. **Maintenance requirements**
B. **Deficit repletion**
C. **Ongoing losses**

Clinical context is paramount. One should always strive to treat the underlying etiology of a fluid or electrolyte abnormality, rather than responding to scenarios or laboratory values in a rote manner. For example, patients in cardiac, hepatic, or renal failure may experience hypervolemic hyponatremia, and attempted correction of their hyponatremia via administration of intravenous (IV) fluids would be inappropriate. Similarly, clinical context should inform the decision to start or hold maintenance IV fluids (the healthy adolescent may not need maintenance fluids overnight prior to a procedure) and whether to administer isotonic or hypotonic fluids (see Section II. B. for more on this issue).

II. MAINTENANCE REQUIREMENTS

Maintenance requirements constitute the amount of water and electrolytes lost during basal metabolism. Metabolism creates two byproducts, heat and solute, that must be eliminated to maintain homeostasis. The amount of heat dissipated through insensible fluid losses and the amount of solute excreted in bodily fluids are directly related to caloric expenditure (Fig. 11.1).[1]

Metabolic demands do not increase in direct proportion to body mass (weight) across the continuum. The metabolic rate per kg body weight declines with age; an infant generates significantly more solute and heat per kg than a child or an adolescent. To accurately calculate maintenance needs, it is necessary to determine caloric expenditure.

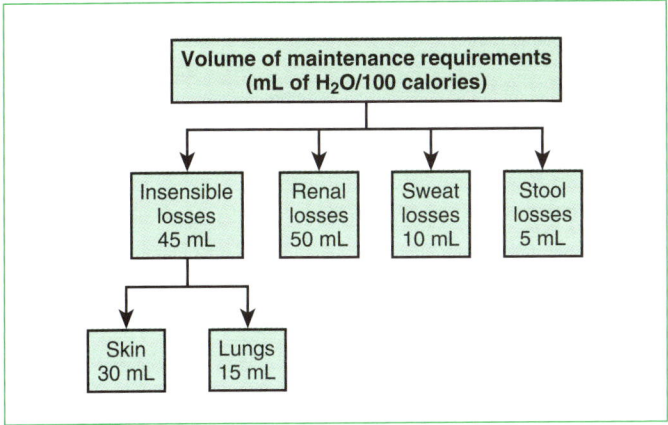

FIGURE 11.1

For every 100 calories metabolized in 24 hours, approximately 55–60 mL of fluid is required to provide for insensible losses as well as basal stool and sweat losses, and 50 mL of fluid is required for the kidneys to excrete an ultrafiltrate of plasma at 300 mOsm/L, without having to concentrate the urine. *(Modified from Roberts KB. Fluids and electrolytes: parenteral fluid therapy. Pediatr Rev. 2001;22:380-387.)*

A. Maintenance Volume: Caloric Calculations

There are three basic methods to calculate maintenance fluid volume needs:

1. **Basal calorie method:** Useful for all ages, types of body habitus, and clinical states
   a. Determine the child's estimated energy requirements based on age and activity level (see Table 21.1).
   b. For each 100 calories metabolized in 24 hours, the average patient will need 100–120 mL H_2O, 2–4 mEq Na^+, and 2–3 mEq K^+.
2. **Holliday-Segar method** (Table 11.1 and Box 11.1)[2]: Estimates caloric expenditure in fixed-weight categories and makes the same assumption for water and electrolyte needs based on 100 kcal burned as in A.1.b above. This is the most commonly used method of determining maintenance fluid volume and is often referred to as the "4-2-1 Rule" for its ease in approximating IV fluid rates in mL/kg/hr.
   NOTE: The Holliday-Segar method is not suitable for neonates <14 days old. In general, it overestimates fluid needs in neonates compared with the basal calorie method. (See Chapter 18 for neonatal fluid management.)
3. **Body surface area (BSA) method:** See Table EC 11.A on Expert Consult for information on this method, which is not commonly used.[3]

TABLE 11.1
HOLLIDAY-SEGAR METHOD

Body Weight	Water	
	mL/kg/day	mL/kg/hr
First 10 kg	100	≈4
Second 10 kg	50	≈2
Each additional kg	20	≈1

To calculate needed electrolytes: Na^+ 3 mEq/100 mL H_2O; Cl^- 2 mEq/100 mL H_2O; K^+ 2 mEq/100 mL H_2O.

BOX 11.1
HOLLIDAY-SEGAR METHOD

Example: Determine the correct fluid rate for an 8-year-old child weighing 25 kg:

First 10 kg:	4 mL/kg/hr × 10 kg = 40 mL/hr	100 mL/kg/day × 10 kg = 1000 mL/day
Second 10 kg:	2 mL/kg/hr × 10 kg = 20 mL/hr	50 mL/kg/day × 10 kg = 500 mL/day
Each additional 1 kg:	1 mL/kg/hr × 5 kg = 5 mL/hr	20 mL/kg/day × 5 kg = 100 mL/day
	Answer: 65 mL/hr	Answer: 1600 mL/day

B. Maintenance Solute

1. **For the purposes of fluid calculation,** fluid lost via insensible losses through the skin and respiratory tract can be considered electrolyte-free. Urine represents the primary source of electrolyte loss, with variability based on renal ability to dilute and concentrate. Average electrolyte requirements per 100 mL H_2O are seen in Table 11.1 and are based on the electrolyte composition of human milk.[2] With the addition of 5%–10% dextrose (depending on need) to prevent ketosis, basic solute needs can be met by administering D5 ¼ normal saline (NS) with 20 mEq/L potassium chloride (KCl). However, outside of the neonatal period, ¼ NS is generally not used as a maintenance fluid.

2. **Cautions regarding hypotonic fluid administration:** Although 3 mEq of Na^+ per 100 mL of water should be sufficient to maintain basic sodium needs, there is overwhelming evidence that administration of hypotonic fluids to hospitalized children can lead to hyponatremia.[4-10] Children who are hospitalized are ill, and various disease states and processes including pulmonary disease (e.g., asthma, bronchiolitis, or pneumonia), central nervous system (CNS) processes, nausea, pain, and even stress can lead to an increased secretion of antidiuretic

BOX 11.2
CLINICAL SETTING OF INCREASED ADH RELEASE IN CHILDREN

Hemodynamic Stimuli for ADH Release (Decreased Effective Volume)	Non-hemodynamic Stimuli for ADH Release
Hypovolemia	CNS disturbances (meningitis, encephalitis, brain tumors, head injury)
Nephrosis	Pulmonary disease (pneumonia, asthma, bronchiolitis)
Cirrhosis	
Congestive heart failure	Cancer
Hypoaldosteronism	Medications (cytoxan, vincristine, morphine)
Hypotension	
Hypoalbuminemia	GI disturbances (nausea, emesis)
	Pain or stress
	Postoperative state

Modified from Moritz ML, Ayus JC. Prevention of hospital-acquired hyponatremia: a case for using isotonic saline. Pediatrics. 2003;111:227-230.
ADH, antidiuretic hormone; CNS, central nervous system; GI, gastrointestinal.

hormone (ADH) and hence, retention of free water[10] (Box 11.2). These children may also have prior or ongoing losses of water and electrolytes that make them unsuitable candidates for mere "maintenance" fluid replacement. Their clinical context requires further volume and electrolyte deficit calculations, and appropriate adjustment of replacement fluids in their management (Tables 11.3 and 11.4 show fluid composition).

III. DEFICIT REPLETION[1,11,12]

A. Water Deficit Volume

1. **Calculated assessment:** The most precise method of assessing fluid deficit uses weight loss:
   Water deficit (L) = pre-illness weight (kg) − illness weight (kg)
   % Dehydration = (pre-illness weight − illness weight)/pre-illness weight × 100%
2. **Clinical assessment:** If weight loss is not known, clinical observation may be used (Table 11.2).[13,14] Each 1% dehydration corresponds to 10 mL/kg fluid deficit.

B. Solute Deficit: Isonatremic Dehydration

Fluid losses and electrolyte deficits come from the body's intracellular and extracellular compartments. One can use sophisticated calculations, factoring in number of days of illness and percentage deficit from each compartment, to arrive at a precise composition for electrolyte replacement (see Section III. B. 1-5 on Expert Consult for such equations). However, in clinical practice, for isonatremic dehydration, one can estimate a sodium repletion requirement of 8–10 mEq/100 mL fluid deficit (in addition to 3 mEq/100 mL of maintenance fluid).[11] Unless

TABLE 11.2
CLINICAL OBSERVATIONS IN DEHYDRATION*

	Older Child		
	3% (30 mL/kg)	6% (60 mL/kg)	9% (90 mL/kg)
	Infant		
	5% (50 mL/kg)	10% (100 mL/kg)	15% (150 mL/kg)
EXAMINATION			
Dehydration	Mild	Moderate	Severe
Skin turgor	Normal	Tenting	None
Skin (touch)	Normal	Dry	Clammy
Buccal mucosa/lips	Dry	Dry	Parched/cracked
Eyes	Normal	Deep set	Sunken
Tears	Present	Reduced	None
Fontanelle	Flat	Soft	Sunken
Mental status	Alert		Lethargic/obtunded
Pulse rate	Normal	Slightly increased	Increased
Pulse quality	Normal	Weak	Feeble/impalpable
Capillary refill	Normal	≈2–3 seconds	>3 seconds
Urine output	Normal/mild oliguria	Mild oliguria	Severe oliguria

*Serum sodium concentration affects the clinical manifestations of dehydration, such as skin turgor and mucous membranes. For example, hyponatremia exaggerates instability, and hypernatremia maintains intravascular volume at the expense of intracellular volume.
Data from Kliegman RM, Behrman RE, Jenson HB, et al: Nelson textbook of pediatrics, 18th ed. Philadelphia, WB Saunders, 2007; and Oski FA: Principles and practice of pediatrics, 4th ed. Philadelphia, JB Lippincott, 2007.

hypokalemia is present (see section V.B.1.), maintenance potassium requirements (20 mEq/L of fluid) should be given, as long as the child is not in renal failure.[11] See Box 11.3 for sample calculations of solute deficit in isonatremic dehydration.

C. Solute Deficit: Hyponatremic Dehydration (Hyponatremic Hypovolemia)

Although there is a vast differential for hyponatremia (see Section V.A.1.), the calculations and fluid replacement discussed here should only be used to manage hypovolemic hyponatremia, most commonly due to gastrointestinal losses.

The general equation used to calculate the excess sodium deficit in hypovolemic hyponatremia is:

$$Na^+ \text{ deficit (mEq required)} = [\text{Desired } Na^+ \text{ (mEq/L)} - \text{Serum } Na^+ \text{ (mEq/L)}] \times 0.6 \times \text{weight (in kg)}*$$

Where 0.6 represents the percentage of body water for a child or infant (and hence 0.6 × weight = total body water or TBW)
See Box 11.4 for sample calculations.

---

*This represents the *excess* sodium deficit in hyponatremic dehydration. It must be added to the isotonic sodium deficit of 8–10 mEq/100 mL of fluid (see Section B, above).

BOX 11.3
SAMPLE CALCULATIONS: ISONATREMIC DEHYDRATION
Isonatremic Dehydration

Example: A 15-kg (pre-illness weight) child with 10% dehydration and normal serum sodium

Requirement	Formula	Sample Calculation
Maintenance fluid requirements	Holliday–Segar formula	(100 mL/kg/day × 10 kg) + (50 mL/kg/day × 5 kg) = 1250 mL/24 hr = 52 mL/hr
Fluid deficit	10 mL per kg for each percent dehydration	10 mL × 15 kg × 10% = 1500 mL

Fluid Replacement Rate Over 24 hrs

½ fluid deficit replaced in first 8 hrs	750 mL/8 hr = 94 mL/hr + 52 mL/hr maintenance = 146 mL/hr	
½ fluid deficit replaced over 16 hrs	750 mL/16 hr = 47 mL/hr + 52 mL/hr maintenance = 99 mL/hr	

Note: if patient received an initial 20 mL/kg bolus (300 mL): 1500 mL − 300 mL = 1200 mL

½ fluid deficit in first 8 hrs: 600 cc/8 hr = 75 mL + 52 mL/hr maintenance = 127 mL/hr

½ fluid deficit over next 16 hrs: 600 cc/16 hr = 38 mL/hr + 52 mL/hr maintenance = 90 mL/hr

Calculations for Fluid Selection

Maintenance sodium requirements	3 mEq per 100 mL of maintenance fluid	3 mEq × (1250 mL/100 mL) = 38 mEq Na+
Isotonic sodium deficit	8–10 mEq Na+ per each 100 mL of fluid deficit	10 mEq × (1500 mL/100 mL) = 150 mEq Na+
Total sodium required	Add maintenance sodium and isotonic sodium deficit	38 mEq + 150 mEq = 188 mEq
Sodium required per L	Divide total sodium by fluid deficit	188 mEq/1.5 L = 125 mEq
Fluid that best approximates sodium required per L	Compare sodium needed to fluid composition (Table 11.3); add dextrose and potassium per needs	D5 normal saline (154 mEq/L) + 20 mEq KCl or KAcetate

In the absence of hypokalemia, 20–30 mEq/L of potassium is commonly used and is typically sufficient. Monitor carefully for hyperkalemia (via lab draws and cardiorespiratory monitoring) and for adequate urine output if high concentrations (>0.5 mEq/kg/hr) are used. Potassium infusion rate should not exceed 1 mEq/kg/hr.

BOX 11.4
SAMPLE CALCULATIONS: HYPONATREMIC DEHYDRATION
Hyponatremic Dehydration

Example: A 15-kg (pre-illness weight) child with 10% dehydration and serum sodium 125 mEq/L without CNS symptoms

Requirement	Formula	Sample Calculation
Maintenance fluid requirements	Holliday–Segar formula	(100 mL/kg/d × 10 kg) + (50 mL/kg/d × 5 kg) = 1250 mL/24 hr = 52 mL/hr
Fluid deficit	10 mL/kg for each percent dehydration	10 mL × 15 kg × 10% = 1500 mL

Fluid Replacement Rate Over 24 hrs

1500 mL/24 hr = 63 mL/hr + 52 mL/hr maintenance = 115 mL/hr

Calculations for Fluid Selection

Maintenance sodium requirements	3 mEq per 100 mL of maintenance fluid	3 mEq × (1250 mL/100 mL) = 38 mEq Na^+
Isotonic sodium deficit	8–10 mEq Na^+ per each 100 mL of fluid deficit	10 mEq × (1500 mL/100 mL) = 150 mEq Na^+
Excess sodium deficit	[Desired Na^+ (in mEq) − Serum Na^+ in mEq)]* × 0.6 × wt (in kg)	(135 mEq − 125 mEq) × 0.6 × 15 kg = 90 mEq Na^+
Total sodium deficit	Add isotonic sodium deficit + excess sodium deficit	150 mEq + 90 mEq = 240 mEq
Total sodium required	Add maintenance sodium requirement and total sodium deficit	38 mEq + 240 mEq = 278 mEq
Sodium required per L	Divide total sodium by fluid deficit in L	278 mEq/1.5 L = 185 mEq
Fluid that best approximates sodium required per L	Compare sodium needed to fluid composition (Table 11.3); add dextrose and potassium per needs	D5 normal saline (154 mEq/L) + 20 mEq KCl or KAcetate

*The difference between desired Na^+ and serum Na^+ should be no greater than 10 mEq per 24 hr to avoid rapid correction of Na^+. In this case, if the serum Na^+ was 115 mEq/L with 10% dehydration and no CNS symptoms, the excess sodium deficit would still be calculated as 90 mEq for a 24-hr period (using 125 mEq − 115 mEq in the calculation), and one would plan to use D5 NS + 20 mEq KCl to replace half the fluid deficit (750 mL) over 24 hrs (at 31 mL/hr + 52 mL/hr maintenance = 83 mL/hr) and the other half over the following 24 hrs to restore to isonatremia and isovolemia in 48 hrs.

In the absence of hypokalemia, 20–30 mEq/L of potassium is commonly used and is typically sufficient. Monitor carefully for hyperkalemia (via lab draws and cardiorespiratory monitoring) and for adequate urine output if high concentrations (>0.5 mEq/kg/hr) are used. Potassium infusion rate should not exceed 1 mEq/kg/hr.

D. Water and Solute Deficits: Hypernatremic Dehydration

Hypernatremic dehydration occurs in scenarios where free water is either unavailable/restricted (as in a poorly breastfeeding infant) or there is excessive loss of solute-free water (as in diabetes insipidus or a diarrheal illness with very watery stools). The free water deficit (FWD) can be calculated based on the estimate that it requires 4 mL/kg to decrease serum Na^+ by 1 mEq/L. **NOTE:** If serum Na^+ is >170, the estimate decreases to 3 mL/kg.

$$FWD \text{ (mL)} = 4 \text{ mL/kg} \times \text{pre-illness weight (in kg)} \\ \times [\text{Serum } Na^+ \text{ (mEq/L)} - \text{Desired } Na^+ \text{ (mEq/L)}]$$

The amount of additional fluid volume loss beyond free water loss in a patient with hypernatremic dehydration is referred to as the solute fluid deficit (SFD) and is used to calculate Na^+ and K^+ deficits in these patients.

$$SFD = \text{total fluid deficit} - FWD$$

See Box 11.5 for sample calculations.

E. Deficit Replacement Strategy

1. **Phase I: Initial Stabilization**
a. Rapid fluid resuscitation with isotonic fluid [NS or Lactated Ringers (LR)] should be reserved for patients with need for rapid volume expansion (see Chapter 1). In general, administration of isotonic fluid expands the intravascular volume without causing significant fluid shifts; however, excessive administration of isotonic fluids can be dangerous in patients with hyperosmolarity [e.g., diabetic ketoacidosis (DKA) with hyperglycemia].
b. For severe, symptomatic hyponatremic dehydration in which CNS symptoms, such as seizure or altered mental status, are present, hypertonic saline (HTS) should be administered over 3–4 hours to correct the hyponatremia by ~5 mEq/L, which is generally sufficient to control seizures and improve mental status.[11,15] (see Box 11.6 for sample calculations.) If severe CNS symptoms persist, the HTS administration may be repeated. Once CNS symptoms have improved, one can proceed to correct the remaining sodium deficit as per (2.b.) below.
c. In severe hypernatremic dehydration (serum Na^+ > 175 mEq/L), most commonly seen in poorly breastfeeding neonates, initial resuscitation with NS may decrease the serum sodium too rapidly, leading to cerebral edema, as the concentration of NS (154 mEq/L) is significantly lower than the child's serum Na^+.[16] In this case, one can resuscitate by simultaneously running NS and HTS to avoid giving a fluid whose concentration is more than 15 mEq/L below that of the serum Na^+ (see Box 11.7 for calculations).

BOX 11.5

SAMPLE CALCULATIONS: HYPERNATREMIC DEHYDRATION

Hypernatremic Dehydration

Example: A 15-kg (pre-illness weight) child with 10% dehydration and serum sodium 155 mEq/L

Requirement	Formula	Sample Calculation
Maintenance fluid requirements	Holliday–Segar formula	(100 mL/kg/d × 10 kg) + (50 mL/kg/d × 5 kg) = 1250 mL/24 hr = 52 mL/hr
Total fluid deficit	10 mL/kg for each percent dehydration	10 mL × 15 kg × 10% = 1500 mL

Fluid Replacement Rate Over 24 hrs

1500 mL/24 hr = 63 mL/hr + 52 mL/hr maintenance = 115 mL/hr

Calculations for Fluid Selection

Free water deficit	4 mL/kg × wt (in kg) × [Serum Na$^+$ (mEq/L) − Desired Na$^+$ (mEq/L)]*	4 mL/kg × 15 kg × (155 mEq/L − 145 mEq/L) = 600 mL
Solute fluid deficit	Total fluid deficit − free water deficit	1500 mL − 600 mL = 900 mL
Maintenance sodium requirements	3 mEq per 100 mL of maintenance fluid	3 mEq × (1250 mL/100 mL) = 38 mEq Na$^+$
Sodium deficit	8–10 mEq Na$^+$ per each 100 mL of solute fluid deficit	10 mEq × (900 mL/100 mL) = 90 mEq Na$^+$
Total sodium required	Add maintenance sodium requirement and sodium deficit	38 mEq + 90 mEq = 128 mEq
Sodium required per L	Divide total sodium by fluid deficit in L	128 mEq/1.5 L = 85 mEq
Fluid that best approximates sodium required per L	Compare sodium needed to fluid composition (Table 11.3); add dextrose and potassium per needs	D5 ½ normal saline† (77 mEq/L) + 20 mEq KCl or KAcetate

*The difference between serum Na$^+$ and desired Na$^+$ should be no greater than 10 mEq per 24 hr to avoid rapid correction of Na$^+$. In this case, if the serum Na$^+$ was 165 mEq/L with 10% dehydration, the free water deficit would still be calculated as 600 mL for a 24-hr period (using 165 mEq−155 mEq in the calculation), and one would plan to use D5 ½ NS + 20 mEq KCl to replace half the fluid deficit (750 mL) over 24 hrs (at 31 mL/hr + 52 mL/hr maintenance = 83 mL/hr) and the other half over the following 24 hrs to restore to isonatremia and isovolemia in 48 hrs.

†There is some controversy regarding whether NS or ½ NS should be used in this circumstance. Although the tonicity of ½ NS is significantly below that of the patient's serum sodium, most experts[3,11,12,17] recommend use of hypotonic fluids, administered slowly over a minimum of 24 hours to slowly correct hypernatremia. Refer to Section III. E.2.c for use of an equation to calculate the expected change in serum sodium per L of fluid administered.

In the absence of hypokalemia, 20–30 mEq/L of potassium is commonly used and is typically sufficient. Monitor carefully for hyperkalemia (via lab draws and cardiorespiratory monitoring) and for adequate urine output if high concentrations (>0.5 mEq/kg/hr) are used. Potassium infusion rate should not exceed 1 mEq/kg/hr.

BOX 11.6
SAMPLE CALCULATIONS: SEVERE SYMPTOMATIC HYPONATREMIC DEHYDRATION
Initial Fluid Replacement for Neurologic Stabilization

Example: A 15-kg (pre-illness weight) child with altered mental status and serum sodium 110 mEq/L
Fluid to be used: 3% hypertonic saline (HTS)

Requirement	Formula	Sample Calculation
Sodium deficit	Desired change in plasma sodium (5 mEq/L) × 0.6 × wt (kg)	5 mEq/L × 0.6 × 15 kg = 45 mEq Na$^+$
mEq Na$^+$ per mL 3% HTS	Divide total mEq Na$^+$ in 1 L of 3% HTS (from Table 11.3) by 1000 mL	513 mEq / 1000 mL = 0.513 mEq/mL*
mL 3% HTS required	Divide sodium deficit by mEq/mL 3% Na$^+$	45 mEq Na$^+$/0.513 mEq/mL = 88 mL of 3% HTS
Rate of administration	Divide mL required by 4 hrs (optimal time over which to correct deficit by 5 mEq/L)[8]	88 mL/4 hr = 22 mL/hr of 3% HTS

*Note: if using 2% HTS, this calculation is 342 mEq/1000 mL = 0.342 mEq/mL.
Note: This sequence of calculations can be simplified as: [Sodium deficit (in mEq) × 1000 mL]/[infusate Na$^+$ (in mEq) × time (in hours)] = rate of administration in mL/hr.
Example: 45 mEq × 1000 mL/513 mEq × 4 hr = 22 mL/hr.

d. Recognize that a bolus of 20 mL/kg represents only a 2% body weight replacement. A child calculated to be above 2% dehydrated will not be sufficiently repleted after a single bolus.
e. Consider subtracting fluid and electrolytes given during resuscitation from the total deficits when calculating replacement of fluid and electrolytes.

2. **Phase II:** Deficit repletion, maintenance, and ongoing losses
After initial stabilization, the remaining deficit is replaced over the next 24–48 hours.

a. **Isonatremic dehydration**: Proportional loss of sodium and water (serum Na$^+$ 130–149 mEq/L).
Replace half of the remaining deficit after stabilization over the first 8 hours and the second half over the following 16 hours, making sure to also administer maintenance fluids (see Box 11.3 for sample calculations).

b. **Hyponatremic dehydration:** Excess Na$^+$ loss (Na$^+$ <130 mEq/L).
For hyponatremia without CNS symptoms, hypertonic saline is not needed, and one should plan to correct the sodium deficit by ~10 mEq per 24 hours until isonatremia is achieved (see Box 11.4 for

> **BOX 11.7**
>
> **SAMPLE CALCULATIONS: SEVERE HYPERNATREMIC DEHYDRATION**
>
> **Initial Fluid Resuscitation Strategy to Avoid Rapid Sodium Correction when Serum Na⁺ >175 mEq/L[16]**
>
> Example: A 3-kg (pre-illness-weight) breastfed neonate appearing severely dehydrated with serum sodium 185 mEq/L and hemodynamic instability
> Resuscitation with NS may drop the serum Na⁺ too quickly. Plan to simultaneously run NS and 3% hypertonic saline (HTS), given rapidly together (i.e. over 5 minutes), to effectively give resuscitation fluid with a concentration no more than 15 mEq/L below the child's serum Na⁺. Repeat the boluses as needed to achieve hemodynamic stability.
>
> | Requirement | Formula | Sample Calculation |
> | --- | --- | --- |
> | Ideal bolus fluid concentration | Serum sodium (in mEq/L) – 15 mEq/L | 185 mEq/L – 15 mEq/L = 170 mEq/L |
> | mL of HTS required per L of NS | [1000 mL × (Ideal bolus fluid concentration – Concentration of NS)]/(Concentration of HTS – Desired fluid concentration) | 1000 mL × (170 mEq/L – 154 mEq/L)/ (513 mEq/L – 170 mEq/L) = 47 mL |
> | Bolus NS amount in mL | 20 mL/kg × wt (in kg) | 20 mL/kg × 3 kg = 60 mL |
> | Bolus amount HTS in mL | mL HTS required per L of NS × NS bolus amount (in mL)/1000 mL | 47 mL × 60 mL /1000 mL = 2.8 mL |

Note: In clinical practice, one will often not have laboratory data available quickly enough to employ this strategy. However, severe hypernatremia should be suspected in the clinical scenario of a solely breastfed neonate who appears severely dehydrated.[16] STAT labs should be sent, and the strategy may be employed as soon as laboratory values are available.

sample calculations). Rapid correction of serum Na⁺ can result in central pontine myelinolysis and should be reserved for symptomatic patients.[15] In asymptomatic patients, the rate of rise should not exceed 0.5–1 mEq/L per hour or 10–12 mEq/L in 24 hours.[11]

c. **Hypernatremic dehydration:** Excess free water loss (Na⁺ >150 mEq/L). Plan to correct the free water deficit and solute fluid deficits while lowering the serum sodium no more than 10 mEq/L per 24 hours to minimize the risk of cerebral edema[11] (see Box 11.5 for sample calculations).

Note: The calculations above provide a starting rate for fluid administration and cannot account for other factors that may affect a patient's rate of rise or fall of serum sodium. One should obtain frequent lab draws (every 2–4 hrs) when correcting solute or free water deficits to ensure an appropriate rate of correction and recalculation of fluid rates based on the results. As a "check" on the rate of rise or fall you should expect from your calculated fluid rate, the following equation gives the expected change in sodium per 1 L of parenteral fluid:[17]

Change in Serum Na^+ = [(Infusate Na^+ + Infusate K^+) − Serum Na^+]/TBW + 1

Where TBW = 0.6 × pre-illness weight for infants, children, and adult men, and 0.5 × pre-illness weight in adult women

F. Calculation of Appropriate Fluids

After completing the previous calculations for the patient, divide the desired amount of each solute by the total volume of fluid required to calculate the concentration of fluid and additives. Choose the appropriate corresponding fluid from Table 11.3, and add any other necessary solute components.

1. **Parenteral fluid composition** (see Table 11.3)
2. **Oral fluid composition** (see Table 11.3)
   Oral rehydration therapy should be used in patients with mild to moderate dehydration without signs of shock, coma, acute abdomen, gastric distension, intractable vomiting, sodium derangements, or excess stool losses.
  a. Method: Give 5–10 mL of oral rehydration solution (ORS) every 5–10 minutes, gradually increasing the volume as tolerated.[12]
  b. Deficit replacement:
     (1) Mild dehydration = 50 mL/kg pre-illness weight over 4 hours
     (2) Moderate dehydration = 100 mL/kg pre-illness weight over 4 hours
  c. Maintenance: Infants should resume formula/breast milk by mouth (PO) ad lib. Children should continue with a regular, bland diet.
  d. Ongoing losses: Regardless of the degree of dehydration, give additional 10 mL/kg body weight of ORS for each additional diarrheal stool and 2 mL/kg body weight ORS for each additional episode of emesis.[12]

IV. ONGOING LOSSES

Ongoing losses represent continued losses of fluid and solute after initial presentation, as in persistent vomiting and/or diarrhea, high fever with diuresis, or nasogastric suction. If the losses can be measured directly, they should be replaced 1:1 concurrently ("piggybacked" or "Y'ed in") with an appropriate fluid based on known bodily fluid electrolyte composition (Table 11.4).[13] If the losses cannot be measured, an estimate of 10 mL/kg body weight for each watery stool and 2 mL/kg body weight for each episode of emesis should be administered.[12]

TABLE 11.3
COMPOSITION OF FREQUENTLY USED PARENTERAL AND ORAL REHYDRATION FLUIDS

	D% CHO (g/100 mL)	Protein* (g/100 mL)	Cal/L	Na+ (mEq/L)	K+ (mEq/L)	Cl− (mEq/L)	HCO3−† (mEq/L)	Ca2+ (mEq/L)	mOsm/L
PARENTERAL FLUID									
D5W	5	—	170	—	—	—	—	—	252
D10W	10	—	340	—	—	—	—	—	505
NS (0.9% NaCl)	—	—	—	154	—	154	—	—	308
½ NS (0.45% NaCl)	—	—	—	77	—	77	—	—	154
D5 ¼ NS (0.225% NaCl)	5	—	170	38.5	—	34	—	—	329
2% NaCl	—	—	—	342	—	342	—	—	684
3% NaCl	—	—	—	513	—	513	—	—	1027
8.4% sodium bicarbonate (1 mEq/mL)	—	—	—	1000	—	—	1000	—	2000
Ringer's solution	0–10	—	0–340	147	4	155.5	—	≈4	—
Lactated Ringer's	0–10	—	0–340	130	4	109	28	3	273
Amino acid 8.5% (Travasol)	—	8.5	340	3	—	34	52	—	880
Plasmanate	—	5	200	110	2	50	29	—	—
Albumin 25% (salt poor)	—	25	1000	100–160	—	<120	—	—	300
Intralipid‡	2.25	—	1100	2.5	0.5	4.0	—	—	258–284
ORAL FLUID									
Pedialyte	2.5	—	—	45	20	35	30	—	250
WHO solution	2	—	—	90	20	80	30	—	310
Rehydralyte	2.5	—	—	75	20	65	30	—	310

Continued

APPROXIMATE ELECTROLYTE COMPOSITION OF COMMONLY CONSUMED FLUIDS (NOT RECOMMENDED FOR ORAL REHYDRATION THERAPY)**							
Apple juice	11.9	—	0.4	26	—	—	700
Coca-Cola	10.9	—	4.3	0.1	—	13.4	656
Gatorade	5.9	—	21	2.5	17	—	377
G2	4.7	—	20	3.2	—	—	—
Ginger ale	9	—	3.5	0.1	—	3.6	565
Milk	4.9	—	22	36	28	30	260
Orange juice	10.4	—	0.2	49	—	50	654
Powerade	5.8	—	18	2.7	—	—	264

CHO, carbohydrate; HCO_3^-, bicarbonate; NS, normal saline; WHO, World Health Organization

*Protein or amino acid equivalent.

†Bicarbonate or equivalent (citrate, acetate, lactate).

‡Values are approximate; may vary from lot to lot. Also contains < 1.2% egg phosphatides.

**Values vary slightly depending on source.

TABLE 11.4
ELECTROLYTE COMPOSITION OF VARIOUS BODY FLUIDS

Fluid	Na⁺ (mEq/L)	K⁺ (mEq/L)	Cl⁻ (mEq/L)	Replacement Fluid
Gastric	20–80	5–20	100–150	½ NS
Pancreatic	120–140	5–15	90–120	NS
Small bowel	100–140	5–15	90–130	NS
Bile	120–140	5–15	80–120	NS
Ileostomy	45–135	3–15	20–115	½ NS or NS
Diarrhea	10–90	10–80	10–110	½ NS
Burns*	140	5	110	NS or LR
Sweat				
Normal	10–30	3–10	10–35	½ NS
Cystic fibrosis†	50–130	5–25	50–110	

LR, lactated Ringer solution; NS, normal saline
*3–5 g/dL of protein may be lost in fluid from burn wounds.
†Replacement fluid dependent on sodium content.
Modified from Kliegman RM, Stanton B, St. Gene J, et al. Nelson Textbook of Pediatrics. *19th ed. Philadelphia: Saunders; 2011.*

V. SERUM ELECTROLYTE DISTURBANCES

A. Sodium

1. **Hyponatremia:**
a. Etiologies, diagnostic studies, and management (Table 11.5)
b. Factitious etiologies:
   (1) Hyperglycemia: Na⁺ decreased 1.6 mEq/L for each 100-mg/dL rise in glucose
   (2) Hyperlipidemia: Na⁺ decreased by 0.002 × lipid (mg/dL)
   (3) Hyperproteinemia: Na⁺ decreased by 0.25 × [protein (g/dL) − 8]
c. Clinical manifestations: Nausea, headache, lethargy, seizure, coma
2. **Hypernatremia:** Etiologies, diagnostic studies, and management (Table 11.6)

B. Potassium

1. **Hypokalemia:**
a. Etiologies and laboratory data (Table 11.7)
b. Clinical manifestations: Skeletal muscle weakness or paralysis, ileus, cardiac arrhythmias.[18,19] Electrocardiogram (ECG) changes include delayed depolarization, with flat or absent T waves, and, in extreme cases, U waves.
c. Diagnostic studies:
   (1) Blood: Electrolytes, blood urea nitrogen/creatinine (BUN/Cr), creatine kinase (CK), glucose, renin, arterial blood gas (ABG)
   (2) Urine: Urinalysis, K⁺, Na⁺, Cl⁻, osmolality, 17-ketosteroids
   (3) Other: ECG, consider evaluation for Cushing's syndrome (Chapter 10)

TABLE 11.5
HYPONATREMIA*

Decreased Weight		Increased or Normal Weight
Renal Losses	**Extrarenal Losses**	
Na+-losing nephropathy	GI losses	Nephrotic syndrome
Diuretics	Skin losses	Congestive heart failure
Adrenal insufficiency	Third spacing	SIADH (see Chapter 10)
Cerebral salt-wasting syndrome	Cystic fibrosis	Acute/chronic renal failure
		Water intoxication
		Cirrhosis
		Excess salt-free infusions
LABORATORY DATA		
↑ Urine Na+	↓ Urine Na+	↓ Urine Na+†
↑ Urine volume	↓ Urine volume	↓ Urine volume
↓ Specific gravity	↑ Specific gravity	↑ Specific gravity
↓ Urine osmolality	↑ Urine osmolality	↑ Urine osmolality
MANAGEMENT (IN ADDITION TO TREATING UNDERLYING CAUSE)		
Replace losses	Replace losses	Restrict fluids

GI, gastrointestinal; SIADH, syndrome of inappropriate antidiuretic hormone secretion
*Hyperglycemia and hyperlipidemia cause spurious hyponatremia.
†Urine Na+ may be appropriate for the level of Na+ intake in patients with SIADH and water intoxication.

TABLE 11.6
HYPERNATREMIA

Decreased Weight		Increased Weight
Renal Losses	**Extrarenal Losses**	
Nephropathy	GI losses	Exogenous Na+
Diuretic use	Skin losses	Mineralocorticoid excess
Diabetes insipidus	Respiratory*	Hyperaldosteronism
Postobstructive diuresis		
Diuretic phase of ATN		
LABORATORY DATA		
↑ Urine Na+	↓ Urine Na+	Relative ↓ urine Na+†
↑ Urine volume	↓ Urine volume	Relative ↓ urine volume
↓ Specific gravity	↑ Specific gravity	Relative ↑ specific gravity
CLINICAL MANIFESTATIONS		
Predominantly neurologic symptoms: lethargy, weakness, altered mental status, irritability, and seizures.[18,19] Additional symptoms may include muscle cramps, depressed deep tendon reflexes, and respiratory failure.		
MANAGEMENT		
Replace free water losses based on the calculations in the text, and treat cause. Consider a natriuretic agent if there is increased weight.		

ATN, acute tubular necrosis; GI, gastrointestinal
*This cause of hypernatremia is usually secondary to free water loss; therefore, the fractional excretion of sodium may be decreased or normal.
†Exogenous Na+ administration will cause an increase in the fractional excretion of sodium.

TABLE 11.7
CAUSES OF HYPOKALEMIA

	Decreased Stores		Normal Stores*
	Normal Blood Pressure		
Hypertension	**Renal**	**Extrarenal**	
Renovascular disease	RTA	Skin losses	Metabolic alkalosis
Excess renin	Fanconi syndrome	GI losses	Hyperinsulinemia
Excess mineralocorticoid	Bartter syndrome	High CHO diet	Leukemia
Cushing's syndrome	DKA	Enema abuse	β_2-Catecholamines
	Antibiotics	Laxative abuse	Familial hypokalemic
	Diuretics	Anorexia nervosa	periodic paralysis
	Amphotericin B	Malnutrition	Familial
LABORATORY DATA			
↑ Urine K$^+$	↑ Urine K$^+$	↓ Urine K$^+$	↑ Urine K$^+$

CHO, carbohydrate; DKA, diabetic ketoacidosis; GI, gastrointestinal; RTA, renal tubular acidosis
*Blood pressure may vary.

TABLE 11.8
CAUSES OF HYPERKALEMIA

Increased Stores		Normal Stores
Increased Urine K$^+$	**Decreased Urine K$^+$**	
Transfusion with aged blood	Renal failure	Tumor lysis syndrome
Exogenous K$^+$ (e.g., salt substitutes)	Hypoaldosteronism	Leukocytosis (>100 K/µL)
Spitzer syndrome	Aldosterone insensitivity	Thrombocytosis (>750 K/µL)
	↓ Insulin	Metabolic acidosis*
	K$^+$-sparing diuretics	Type IV RTA
	Congenital adrenal hyperplasia	Blood drawing (hemolyzed sample)
		Rhabdomyolysis/crush injury
		Malignant hyperthermia
		Theophylline intoxication

RTA, renal tubular acidosis
*For every 0.1-unit reduction in arterial pH, there is approximately a 0.2–0.4 mEq/L increase in plasma K$^+$.

d. Management: The rapidity of treatment should depend on the symptom severity. See Formulary for dosage information:
   (1) Acute: Calculate deficit, and replace with potassium acetate or potassium chloride. Enteral replacement is safer when feasible, with less risk for iatrogenic hyperkalemia. Closely follow serum K$^+$.
   (2) Chronic: Determine daily requirement and replace with potassium chloride or potassium gluconate.
2. **Hyperkalemia:**
a. Etiologies (Table 11.8)

b. Clinical manifestations: Skeletal muscle weakness, paresthesias, and ECG changes. The typical ECG changes of hyperkalemia progress with increasing serum K$^+$ values:
   (1) Peaked T waves
   (2) Loss of P waves with widening of QRS
   (3) ST-segment depression with further widening of QRS
   (4) Bradycardia, atrioventricular (AV) block, ventricular arrhythmias, torsades de pointes, and cardiac arrest
c. Management: Stop all IV infusions containing potassium; see algorithm in Fig. 11.2.

C. Calcium
1. **Hypocalcemia:**
a. Etiologies (Box 11.8)
b. Clinical manifestations: Tetany, neuromuscular irritability with weakness, paresthesias, fatigue, cramping, altered mental status, seizures, laryngospasm, cardiac arrhythmias[18,19]:
   (1) ECG changes (prolonged QT interval)
   (2) Trousseau's sign (carpopedal spasm after arterial occlusion of an extremity for 3 minutes)
   (3) Chvostek's sign (muscle twitching on percussion of the facial nerve)
c. Diagnostic studies:
   (1) Blood: Total and ionized Ca^{2+}, phosphate, alkaline phosphatase, Mg^{2+}, total protein, BUN, creatinine, 25-hydroxy (25-OH) vitamin D, parathyroid hormone (PTH):
      (a) Albumin: Δ of 1 g/dL changes the total serum Ca^{2+} in the same direction by 0.8 mg/dL.
      (b) pH: Acidosis increases ionized calcium.
   (2) Urine: Ca^{2+}, phosphate, creatinine
   (3) Other: Chest x-ray (visualize the thymus), ankle, and wrist films (assessment for rickets), ECG (QT interval)
d. Management: See Formulary for dosing information:
   (1) Acute: Consider IV replacement [calcium gluconate, calcium gluceptate, or calcium chloride (cardiac arrest dose)].
   (2) Chronic: Consider use of oral supplements of calcium carbonate, calcium gluconate, calcium glubionate, or calcium lactate.
e. Special considerations:
   (1) Symptoms of hypocalcemia refractory to Ca^{2+} supplementation may be caused by hypomagnesemia.
   (2) Significant hyperphosphatemia should be corrected before the correction of hypocalcemia because renal calculi or soft-tissue calcification may occur if total [Ca^{2+}] × [PO$_4^{3-}$] ≥ 55.

2. **Hypercalcemia:**
a. Etiologies (see Box 11.8)
b. Clinical manifestations: Weakness, irritability, lethargy, seizures, coma, abdominal cramping, anorexia, nausea, vomiting, polyuria,

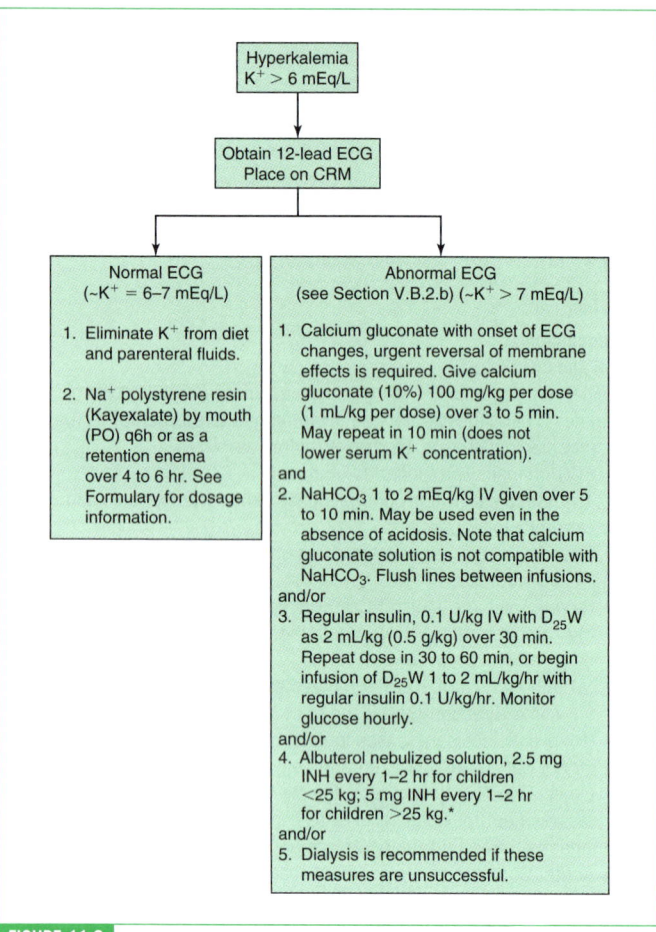

FIGURE 11.2

Algorithm for hyperkalemia. CRM, cardiorespiratory monitor; D25W, 25% dextrose in water; ECG, electrocardiogram; INH, inhaled; IV, intravenous. *Dosing for Albuterol. *(Data from DRUGDEX System (Internet database). Greenwood Village, Colo: Thomson Reuters (Healthcare). Updated periodically.)*

polydipsia, renal calculi, pancreatitis, ECG changes (shortened QT interval)
c. Diagnostic studies:
 (1) Blood: Total and ionized Ca^{2+}, phosphate, alkaline phosphatase, total protein, albumin, BUN, creatinine, PTH, 25-OH vitamin D

BOX 11.8
ETIOLOGIES OF HYPOCALCEMIA AND HYPERCALCEMIA

Hypocalcemia	Hypercalcemia
Hypoparathyroidism	Hyperparathyroidism
Vitamin D deficiency	Vitamin D intoxication
Hyperphosphatemia	Excessive exogenous calcium administration
Pancreatitis	Malignancy
Malabsorption states (malnutrition)	Prolonged immobilization
Drugs (anticonvulsants, cimetidine, aminoglycosides, calcium channel blockers)	Thiazide diuretics
Hypomagnesemia/hypermagnesemia	Subcutaneous fat necrosis
Maternal hyperparathyroidism (in neonates)	Williams syndrome
Ethylene glycol ingestion	Granulomatous disease (e.g., sarcoidosis)
Calcitriol (activated vitamin D) insufficiency	Hyperthyroidism
Tumor lysis syndrome	Milk-alkali syndrome

    (2) Urine: Ca^{2+}, phosphate, creatinine
    (3) Other: ECG (calculate QT interval), kidney, ureter, bladder (KUB) radiograph or renal ultrasound (assess for renal calculi)[19]
  d. Management:
    (1) Treat the underlying disease.
    (2) Hydration: Increase urine output and Ca^{2+} excretion. If the glomerular filtration rate and blood pressure are stable, give NS with maintenance K^+ at two to three times the maintenance rate until Ca^{2+} is normalized.
    (3) Diuresis with furosemide.
    (4) Consider hemodialysis for severe or refractory cases.
    (5) Consider steroids in malignancy, granulomatous disease, and vitamin D toxicity to decrease vitamin D and Ca^{2+} absorption (in consultation with appropriate specialists).
    (6) Severe or persistently elevated Ca^{2+}: Consider calcitonin or bisphosphonate in consultation with endocrinologist.

D. Magnesium
1. **Hypomagnesemia:**
  a. Etiologies (Box 11.9)
  b. Clinical manifestations: Anorexia, nausea, weakness, malaise, depression, nonspecific psychiatric symptoms, hyperreflexia, carpopedal spasm, clonus, tetany, ECG changes (atrial and ventricular ectopy; torsades de pointes)

> **BOX 11.9**
> **ETIOLOGIES OF HYPOMAGNESEMIA AND HYPERMAGNESEMIA**
>
> | Hypomagnesemia | Hypermagnesemia |
> |---|---|
> | **Increased Urinary Losses:** Diuretic use, renal tubular acidosis, hypercalcemia, chronic adrenergic stimulants, chemotherapy
Increased Gastrointestinal Losses: Malabsorption syndromes, severe malnutrition, diarrhea, vomiting, short bowel syndromes, enteric fistulas
Endocrine Etiologies: Diabetes mellitus, parathyroid hormone disorders, hyperaldosterone states
Decreased Intake: Prolonged parenteral fluid therapy with Mg^{2+}-free solutions | **Renal Failure**
Excessive Administration: Status asthmaticus, eclampsia/preeclampsia, cathartics, enemas, phosphate binders |

    c. Diagnostic studies:
       (1) Blood: Mg^{2+}, total and ionized Ca^{2+}
       (2) Other: Consider evaluation for renal/gastrointestinal losses or endocrine etiologies
    d. Management: (see Formulary for dosing and side effects):
       (1) Acute: Magnesium sulfate
       (2) Chronic: Magnesium oxide or magnesium sulfate
  2. **Hypermagnesemia:**
    a. Etiologies (see Box 11.9)
    b. Clinical manifestations: Depressed deep tendon reflexes, lethargy, confusion, respiratory failure (in extreme cases)
       NOTE: Neonates born prematurely after tocolysis with magnesium sulfate are at high risk for respiratory sequelae; however, serum magnesium levels tend to normalize within 72 hours.
    c. Diagnostic studies: Mg^{2+}, total and ionized Ca^{2+}, BUN, creatinine
    d. Management:
       (1) Stop supplemental Mg^{2+}
       (2) Diuresis
       (3) Ca^{2+} supplements, such as calcium chloride (cardiac arrest doses), or calcium gluconate (see Formulary for dosing)
       (4) Dialysis if life-threatening levels are present

E. Phosphate

1. **Hypophosphatemia:**
a. Etiologies (Box 11.10)
b. Clinical manifestations: Symptomatic only at very low levels (<1 mg/dL) with irritability, paresthesias, confusion, seizures, myocardial depression, apnea in very low-birth-weight infants, and coma

BOX 11.10	
ETIOLOGIES OF HYPOPHOSPHATEMIA AND HYPERPHOSPHATEMIA	
Hypophosphatemia	**Hyperphosphatemia**
Starvation	Hypoparathyroidism (rarely in the absence of renal insufficiency)
Protein-energy malnutrition	
Malabsorption syndromes	Excessive administration of phosphate (oral, intravenous, or enemas)
Intracellular shifts associated with respiratory or metabolic alkalosis	
Treatment of diabetic ketoacidosis	Tumor lysis syndrome
Corticosteroid administration	Reduction of glomerular filtration rate to <25% (may occur at smaller reductions in neonates)
Increased renal losses (e.g., renal tubular defects, diuretic use)	
Vitamin D-deficient and vitamin D-resistant rickets	
Very low-birth-weight infants when intake does not meet demand	

    c. Diagnostic studies
       (1) Blood: Phosphate, total and ionized Ca^{2+}, BUN, creatinine, Na^+, K^+, Mg^{2+}; consider PTH and vitamin D
       (2) Urine: Ca^{2+}, phosphate, creatinine, pH
    d. Management:
       (1) Insidious onset of symptoms: PO potassium phosphate or sodium phosphate (see Formulary for dosing)
       (2) Acute onset of symptoms: IV potassium phosphate or sodium phosphate (see Formulary for dosing)
2. **Hyperphosphatemia:**
a. Etiologies (see Box 11.10)
b. Clinical manifestations: Symptoms of resulting hypocalcemia (see section V.C.1)
c. Diagnostic studies:
    (1) Blood: Phosphate, total, and ionized Ca^{2+}, BUN, creatinine, Na^+, K^+, Mg^{2+}; consider PTH, vitamin D, complete blood cell count (CBC), arterial blood gas
    (2) Urine: Ca^{2+}, phosphate, creatinine, urinalysis
d. Management:
    (1) Restrict dietary phosphate.
    (2) Phosphate binders (calcium carbonate, aluminum hydroxide; use with caution in renal failure). See Formulary for dosing.
    (3) For cell lysis (with normal renal function), give an NS bolus and IV mannitol. See Chapter 22 for management of tumor lysis syndrome.
    (4) If the patient has poor renal function, consider dialysis.

VI. ACID–BASE/OSMOLAR GAP DISTURBANCES

A. Definitions

1. **Serum osmolality:** Number of dissolved particles per kg. Can be calculated as follows:

    $$2[\text{serum Na}^+] + \text{glucose(mg/dL)}/18 + \text{BUN(mg/dL)}/2.8$$

    a. Normal range: 275–295 mOsm/kg
    b. Serum osmolar gap = calculated serum osmolality − laboratory measured osmolality
    NOTE: The serum osmolar gap may be elevated in some anion gap acidosis; however, a markedly elevated osmolar gap in the setting of an anion gap acidosis is highly suggestive of acute methanol or ethylene glycol intoxication.

2. **Anion gap (AG):** Represents anions other than bicarbonate and chloride required to balance the positive charge of Na^+. (K^+ is considered negligible in AG calculations.)

    $$AG = Na^+ - (Cl^- + HCO_3^-) \text{ (Normal: 12 mEq/L} \pm 2 \text{ mEq/L)}$$

    a. The majority of unmeasured anions contributing to the anion gap in normal individuals are albumin and phosphate. A decrease in either of these components will decrease the anion gap and could mask an increase in organic acids such as lactate. Correcting the anion gap for albumin concentration increases the utility of the traditional method. The following equation can be used; AG is measured in mEq/L and albumin is measured in g/dL[20]:
    b. Corrected AG = Observed AG + 2.5 × (Normal albumin − Measured albumin)

3. **Acidosis (pH < 7.35):**
    a. Respiratory acidosis: PCO_2 > 45 mm Hg
    b. Metabolic acidosis: Arterial bicarbonate < 22 mmol/L

4. **Alkalosis (pH > 7.45):**
    a. Respiratory alkalosis: PCO_2 < 35 mm Hg
    b. Metabolic alkalosis: Arterial bicarbonate > 26 mmol/L

B. Rules for Determining Primary Acid–Base Disorders (See Table 24.3; Calculation of Expected Compensatory Response)[21,22]

1. **Determine the pH:** The body does not fully compensate for primary acid–base disorders; therefore, the primary disturbance will shift the pH away from 7.40. Examine the PCO_2 and HCO_3^- to determine whether the primary disturbance is a metabolic acidosis/alkalosis or respiratory acidosis/alkalosis.

2. **Calculate the anion gap:** If the anion gap is elevated (>15), an elevated anion gap metabolic acidosis (AGMA) is diagnosed. If the anion gap is <12, there is a nonelevated anion gap metabolic acidosis (NAGMA). If the anion gap is >20 mmol/L, there is a primary metabolic acidosis regardless of the pH or serum bicarbonate concentration. (The body

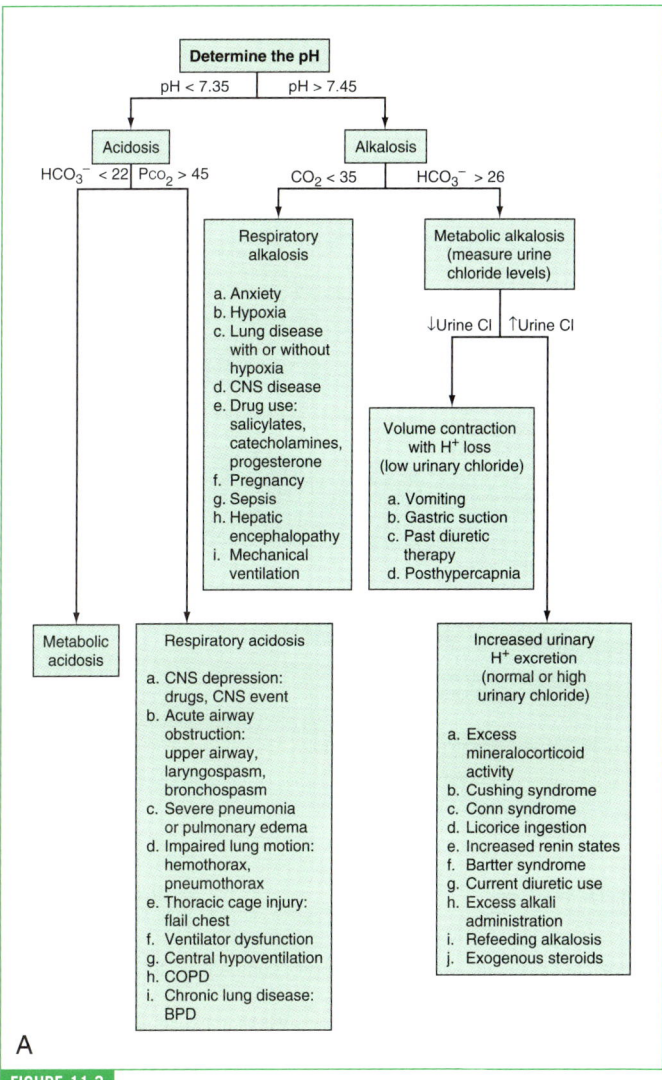

FIGURE 11.3

A and B, Etiology of acid-base disturbances. BPD, bronchopulmonary dysplasia; CNS, central nervous system; COPD, chronic obstructive pulmonary disease; NSAID, non-steroidal anti-inflammatory drug.

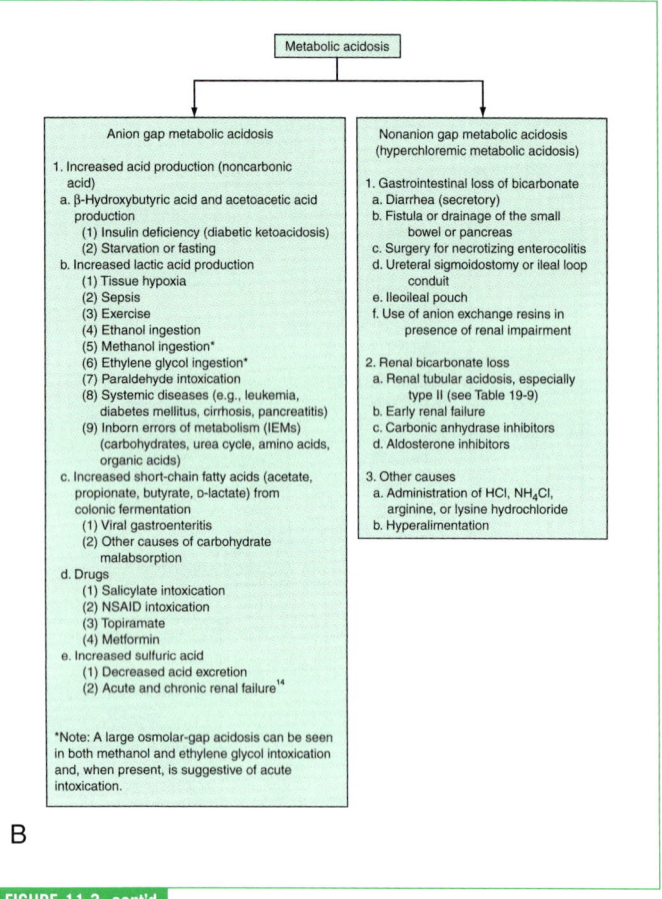

FIGURE 11.3, cont'd

does not generate a large anion gap to compensate for a primary disorder.)

3. **Calculate the delta gap:** If there is an AGMA, calculating the delta gap will help to determine if there is another, concurrent metabolic abnormality:

Delta gap = (AG − 12) − (24 − HCO_3^-)

If the delta gap is greater than 6, there is a combined AGMA and metabolic alkalosis.

If the delta gap is less than −6, there is a combined AGMA and NAGMA.

C. Etiology of Acid–Base Disturbances (Fig. 11.3)

REFERENCES

1. Roberts KB. Fluids and electrolytes: parenteral fluid therapy. *Pediatr Rev*. 2001;22:380-387.
2. Holliday MA, Segar WE. The maintenance need for water in parenteral fluid therapy. *Pediatrics*. 1957;19(5):823-832.
3. Finberg L, Kravath RE, Hellerstein S. *Water and Electrolytes in Pediatrics: Physiology, Pathology, and Treatment*. 2nd ed. Philadelphia: Saunders; 1993.
4. Choong K, Kho ME, Menon K, et al. Hypotonic versus isotonic saline in hospitalized children: a systematic review. *Arch Dis Child*. 2006;91:828-835.
5. Neville KA, Sandeman DJ, Rubinstein A. Prevention of hyponatremia during maintenance intravenous fluid administration: a prospective randomized study of fluid type versus fluid rate. *J Pediatr*. 2010;156:313-319.
6. Moritz ML, Ayus JC. Intravenous fluid management for the acutely ill child. *Curr Opin Pediatr*. 2011;23:186-193.
7. Beck CE. Hypotonic versus isotonic maintenance intravenous fluid therapy in hospitalized children: a systematic review. *Clin Pediatr (Phila)*. 2007;46(9):764-770.
8. Foster BA, Tom D, Hill V. Hypotonic versus isotonic fluids in hospitalized children: a systematic review and meta-analysis. *J Pediatr*. 2014;165(1):163-169.
9. Wang J, Xu E, Xiao Y. Isotonic versus hypotonic maintenance IV fluids in hospitalized children: a meta-analysis. *Pediatrics*. 2014;133(1):105-113.
10. Moritz ML, Ayus JC. Prevention of hospital-acquired hyponatremia: a case for using isotonic saline. *Pediatrics*. 2003;111(2):227-230.
11. Jospe N, Forbes G. Fluids and electrolytes: clinical aspects. *Pediatr Rev*. 1996;17(11):395-403.
12. Powers KS. Dehydration: isonatremic, hyponatremic, and hypernatremic recognition and management. *Pediatr Rev*. 2015;36(7):274-283.
13. Kliegman RM, Stanton B, St. Gene J, et al. *Nelson Textbook of Pediatrics*. 19th ed. Philadelphia: Saunders; 2011.
14. Oski FA. *Principles and Practice of Pediatrics*. 4th ed. Philadelphia: Saunders; 2006.
15. Adrogue HJ, Madias NE. Hyponatremia. *N Engl J Med*. 2000;342(21):1581-1589.
16. Schwaederer AL, Schwartz GJ. Treating hypernatremic dehydration. *Pediatr Rev*. 2005;26(4):148-150.
17. Adrogue HJ, Madias NE. Hypernatremia. *N Engl J Med*. 2000;342(20):1493-1499.
18. Feld LG, Kaskel FJ, Schoeneman MJ. The approach to fluid and electrolyte therapy in pediatrics. *Adv Pediatr*. 1988;35:497-535.
19. Fleisher G, Ludwig S, Henretig F. *Textbook of Pediatric Emergency Medicine*. Baltimore: Williams & Wilkins; 2010.
20. Figge J, Jabor A, Kazda A, Fencl V. Anion gap and hypoalbuminemia. *Crit Care Med*. 1998;26:1807-1810.
21. Haber RJ. A practical approach to acid-base disorders. *West J Med*. 1991;155:146-151.
22. Carmody JB, Norwood VF. A clinical approach to pediatric acid-base disorders. *Postgrad Med J*. 2012;88(1037):143-151.

Chapter 12
Gastroenterology
Nina Guo, MD, and Ammarah Iqbal, MD, MPH

See additional content on Expert Consult

I. WEB RESOURCES
- American College of Gastroenterology: www.acg.gi.org
- North American Society for Pediatric Gastroenterology, Hepatology, and Nutrition: www.naspghan.org

II. GASTROINTESTINAL EMERGENCIES

A. Gastrointestinal Bleeding
1. **Presentation**: Blood loss from the gastrointestinal (GI) tract occurs in four ways: hematemesis, hematochezia, melena, and occult bleeding.
2. **Differential diagnosis of GI bleeding:** Table 12.1
3. **Diagnosis/Management**
    a. Assess airway, breathing, circulation, and hemodynamic stability.
    b. Perform physical examination, looking for evidence of bleeding.
    c. Verify bleeding with rectal examination, testing of stool or emesis for occult blood, and/or gastric lavage.
    d. Obtain baseline laboratory tests. Complete blood cell count (CBC), prothrombin time/partial thromboplastin time (PT/PTT), blood type and cross-match, reticulocyte count, blood smear, blood urea nitrogen (BUN)/creatinine, electrolytes, and a panel to assess for disseminated intravascular coagulation (D-dimer, fibrinogen).
    e. Begin initial fluid resuscitation with normal saline or lactated Ringer solution. Consider transfusion if there is continued bleeding, symptomatic anemia, and/or a hematocrit level <20%. Initiate intravenous acid suppression therapy, preferably with a proton pump inhibitor (PPI).
    f. Further evaluation and therapy based on the assessment and site of bleeding:
       (1) Positive Gastric lavage: Consider esophagogastroduodenoscopy (EGD) and testing for *H. Pylori*. Treatment may include a histamine-2 (H2) blocker or a PPI. (Use nasogastric tube with caution if esophageal varices are suspected.[1])
       (2) Positive Stool hemoccult: Abdominal film, upper GI study (± small bowel follow-through), air-contrast barium enema, colonoscopy, Meckel scan, and tagged red cell scan. Consider computed tomography (CT) and magnetic resonance enterography. If signs/

TABLE 12.1
DIFFERENTIAL DIAGNOSIS OF GI BLEEDING

Age	Upper GI Tract	Lower GI Tract
Newborns (0–30 days)	Swallowed maternal blood Gastritis	Necrotizing enterocolitis Malrotation with midgut volvulus Anal fissure Hirschsprung disease
Infant (30 days–1 year)	Gastritis Esophagitis Peptic ulcer disease	Anal fissure Allergic proctocolitis Intussusception Meckel diverticulum Lymphonodular hyperplasia Intestinal duplication Infectious colitis
Preschool (1–5 years)	Gastritis Esophagitis Peptic ulcer disease Esophageal varices Epistaxis	Juvenile polyps Lymphonodular hyperplasia Meckel diverticulum Hemolytic-uremic syndrome Henoch-Schönlein purpura Infectious colitis Anal fissure
School age and adolescence	Esophageal varices Peptic ulcer disease Epistaxis Gastritis	Inflammatory bowel disease Infectious colitis Juvenile polyps Anal fissure Hemorrhoids

Modified from Pearl R. The approach to common abdominal diagnoses in infants and children. Part II. Pediatr Clin North Am. 1998;45:1287-1326.

symptoms of infection exist, consider stool culture, stool ova and parasites, and *Clostridium difficile* toxin.

B. Acute Abdominal Pain[2]

1. **Definition:** Severe abdominal pain (localized or generalized). May require emergency surgical evaluation/intervention.
2. **Differential diagnosis:** Table 12.2
3. **Diagnosis:**
a. History: Course and characterization of the pain (e.g., visceral vs. parietal vs. referred); GI history such as emesis, melena, hematochezia, diet, and stool history; fever; travel history; menstrual history; vaginal symptoms; urinary symptoms; and respiratory symptoms.
b. Physical examination: Vital signs, general appearance, rashes, arthritis, and jaundice. A thorough abdominal examination including abdominal tenderness on palpation, rebound/guarding, rigidity, masses, distention, or abnormal bowel sounds, rectal examination with stool hemoccult testing, pelvic examination (discharge, masses, adnexal/cervical motion tenderness), and genital examinations.

TABLE 12.2
ACUTE ABDOMINAL PAIN

GI source	Appendicitis, pancreatitis, intussusception, malrotation with volvulus, inflammatory bowel disease, gastritis, bowel obstruction, mesenteric lymphadenitis, irritable bowel syndrome, abscess, hepatitis, perforated ulcer, Meckel diverticulitis, cholecystitis, choledocholithiasis, constipation, gastroenteritis, abdominal trauma
Renal source	Urinary tract infection, pyelonephritis, nephrolithiasis
Genitourinary source	Ectopic pregnancy, ovarian cyst/torsion, pelvic inflammatory disease, testicular torsion
Oncological source	Wilm tumor, neuroblastoma, rhabdomyosarcoma, lymphoma
Other sources	Henoch-Schönlein purpura, pneumonia, sickle cell anemia, diabetic ketoacidosis, juvenile rheumatoid arthritis, incarcerated hernia

c. Radiologic studies: Obtain plain abdominal radiographs to assess for obstruction, constipation, free air, gallstones, and kidney stones. Consider chest radiograph to evaluate for pneumonia, abdominal/pelvic ultrasonography, and abdominal CT with contrast.
d. Laboratory studies to consider: Electrolytes, chemistry panel, CBC, liver and kidney function tests, coagulation studies, blood type and screen/cross-match, urinalysis, amylase, lipase, gonorrhea/chlamydia cultures (or polymerase chain reaction probes), beta-human chorionic gonadotropin (β-hCG), erythrocyte sedimentation rate (ESR), and C-reactive protein (CRP).
4. **Management:**
a. Immediate: Ensure that the patient has nothing by mouth. Begin rehydration. Consider nasogastric decompression, serial abdominal examinations, surgical/gynecologic/GI evaluation, pain control, and antibiotics as indicated.

III. CONDITIONS OF THE GI TRACT (ESOPHAGUS/STOMACH/BOWEL)

A. Vomiting
1. **Definition:** Forceful oral expulsion of gastric contents, can be bilious (green or yellow) or nonbilious.
2. **Differential Diagnosis:** Table 12.3
3. **Diagnosis:** Review diet and medication history. Assess: bilious, hematemesis, acute vs. chronic. Consider: Electrolytes, CBC, UA, β-hCG, pancreatic enzymes, abdominal and neurologic exam. Imaging: Plain abdominal film with upright view (to rule out obstruction or free air), abdominal ultrasound, upper GI, neurologic evaluation imaging if history and physical suggest neurologic cause of emesis. Nasogastric/orogastric tube decompression if GI obstruction suspected. Consider surgical consultation if the vomiting is bilious or if there is hematemesis.
4. **Management:** Hydration. Avoid antiemetic unless a specific benign etiology is identified.

TABLE 12.3
DIFFERENTIAL DIAGNOSIS OF VOMITING

Age	Typically Nonbilious	Typically Bilious
Newborn & infant (0 days–1 year)	Overfeeding, physiologic reflux, milk protein sensitivity, pyloric stenosis, necrotizing enterocolitis, metabolic disorder, infection (GU, respiratory, GI), esophageal/intestinal atresia/stenosis, Hirschsprung disease	Malrotation ± volvulus, intestinal atresia/stenosis, intussusception, pancreatitis
Preschool (1–5 years)	Cyclic vomiting, infectious (GI, GU), toxin ingestion, diabetic ketoacidosis (DKA), central nervous system (CNS) mass effect, eosinophilic esophagitis, post-tussive, peptic disease, appendicitis	Malrotation, intussusception, incarcerated hernia, pancreatitis, intestinal dysmotility
School age & adolescence	Eating disorders, pregnancy, CNS mass effect, eosinophilic esophagitis, DKA, peptic disease, cyclic vomiting, toxins/drugs of abuse, infectious (GU, GI), appendicitis	Peritoneal adhesions, malrotation, incarcerated hernia, pancreatitis, intestinal dysmotility

B. Diarrhea[3]

1. **Definition:** Usual stool output is 10 g/kg/day in children and 100 g/day in adults. Stool loss of >10 g/kg/day in infants and young children or >200 g/day in older children or adults is considered as diarrhea. Acute diarrhea is >3 loose or watery stools per day. Chronic diarrhea is diarrhea lasting more than 2–4 weeks.
2. **Pathogenesis:** It can be infectious or malabsorptive with an osmotic or secretory mechanism.
a. Osmotic diarrhea: Water is drawn into intestinal lumen by maldigested nutrients (e.g., celiac or pancreatic disease, lactose) or other osmotic compounds. Stool volume depends on diet and decreases with fasting (stool osmolar gap ≥100 mOsm/kg).
b. Secretory diarrhea: Water accompanies secreted or unabsorbed electrolytes into the intestinal lumen (e.g., excessive secretion of chloride ions caused by cholera toxin). Stool volume is increased and does not vary with diet (stool osmolar gap <50 mOsm/kg).
c. Stool osmolar gap = Stool Osm − {2 × [stool (Na) m Eq/L + stool (K) m Eq/L]}. Stool Osm is not frequently measured. The standard value is 290 mOsm/kg.[4]
4. **Differential Diagnosis:** Table 12.4
5. **Diagnosis:** History to assess acute vs. chronic, travel, recent antibiotic use, and immune status. Consider laboratory evaluation: Electrolytes, CBC, stool hemoccult testing, urine culture, stool culture, *C. difficile*

TABLE 12.4
DIFFERENTIAL DIAGNOSIS OF COMMON CAUSES OF DIARRHEA

Diagnosis	Major Clinical Features
Infectious colitis (viral, bacterial, protozoal)	+ve stool culture, +ve lactoferrin/calprotectin, possible blood or mucous in stool, possible exposure history
Lactose malabsorption	Bloating, flatulence, abdominal pain, elevated breath hydrogen concentration post-lactose ingestion
Small bowel bacterial overgrowth	Abdominal discomfort, increased risk if ileocecal valve removed
Irritable bowel syndrome	Constipation and/or diarrhea, absence of laboratory or imaging findings
Allergic enteropathy	Growth failure, hypoalbuminemia, anemia, may have elevated serum IgE
Hirschsprung disease	Distended abdomen, abnormal barium enema, absent ganglion cells on rectal biopsy
Cystic fibrosis	Decreased fecal elastase, steatorrhea, poor growth
IBD and celiac disease	See sections XII.III.D and XII.III.G
Other: hyperthyroidism, UTI, encopresis	Dependent on etiology

Modified from Zella GC, Israel EJ. Chronic Diarrhea in Children. Pediatrics in Review. 2012;33(5):207-218.

toxin, ova and parasites, and viral antigens (see Chapter 17 for a list of common bacterial and viral pathogens).

6. **Management**
   a. Oral rehydration therapy (ORT)[5]: Mainstay of initial management regardless of etiology. Enteral hydration has proven superior in reducing the length of hospital stay and adverse events.[6] Parenteral hydration is indicated in severe dehydration, hemodynamic instability, or failure of ORT. See Chapter 11 for oral rehydration solutions and calculation of deficit and maintenance fluid requirements.
   b. Diet: Restart regular diet once patient is rehydrated, unless food has been found to be the source of the diarrhea [e.g., gluten in celiac disease (CD)].
   c. Other: Nonspecific antidiarrheal agents (e.g., adsorbents such as kaolin-pectin), antimotility agents (e.g., loperamide), antisecretory drugs, and toxin binders (e.g., cholestyramine); however, limited data exist regarding their efficacy, and they may adversely affect motility. If diarrhea is infectious, antimicrobial therapy may be indicated. If malabsorptive (e.g., CD or inflammatory bowel disease), therapy should be tailored to disease process.
   d. Probiotics[7]: Evidence supporting use of probiotics (live microorganisms in fermented foods that promote optimal health by establishing improved balance in intestinal microflora) is limited. However, their efficacy has been demonstrated in the following circumstances: antibiotic-associated diarrhea, mild to moderate acute diarrhea, *C. difficile* diarrhea (severe recurrent disease only), hepatic

encephalopathy, the prevention of atopic dermatitis, and possibly preventing necrotizing enterocolitis in premature infants.[8] Probiotics are not regulated by the U.S. Food and Drug Administration; therefore, there is no oversight of quality control (including potency).

C. Constipation and Encopresis[9]

Normal stooling patterns by age: Infants 0–3 months, 2–3 bowel movements/day; 6–12 months, 1.8/day; 1–3 years, 1.4/day; >3 years, 1/day

1. **Definitions:**
a. Constipation: Delay or difficulty in defecation for 2 or more weeks. Functional causes of constipation are the most common.
   (1) Functional: Consider Rome III Criteria (Table EC 12.A)
   (2) Nonfunctional: See Table 12.5 for differential diagnosis.
2. **Diagnosis:**
a. History: Timing of first meconium stool, family's definition of constipation, duration of condition and age of onset, toilet training experience, frequency/consistency/size of stools, pain or bleeding with defecation, presence of abdominal pain, soiling of underwear, stool-withholding behavior, change in appetite, abdominal distention, anorexia, nausea, vomiting, weight loss or poor weight gain, allergies, dietary history, medications, developmental history, psychosocial history, and family history (e.g., constipation, thyroid disorders, or cystic fibrosis).

TABLE 12.5
DIFFERENTIAL DIAGNOSIS OF NONFUNCTIONAL CONSTIPATION*

Anatomic malformations	Anal stenosis, anterior displaced anus, imperforate anus, pelvic mass (e.g., sacral teratoma)
Metabolic and GI	Cystic fibrosis, diabetes mellitus, gluten enteropathy, hypercalcemia, hypokalemia, hypothyroidism, multiple endocrine neoplasia type 2B
Neuropathic conditions	Neurofibromatosis, spinal cord abnormalities, spinal cord trauma, static encephalopathy, tethered cord
Intestinal nerve or muscle disorders	Hirschsprung disease, intestinal neuronal dysplasia, visceral myopathies, visceral neuropathies
Abnormal abdominal musculature	Down syndrome, gastroschisis, prune belly
Connective tissue disorders	Ehlers-Danlos syndrome, scleroderma, systemic lupus erythematosus
Drugs	Antacids, anticholinergics, antidepressants, antihypertensives, opiates, phenobarbital, sucralfate, sympathomimetics
Other	Botulism, cow's milk protein intolerance, heavy metal ingestion (lead), vitamin D intoxication

*Remember that functional constipation remains the most common cause.
Constipation Guideline Committee of the North American Society for Pediatric Gastroenterology, Hepatology, and Nutrition. Evaluation and treatment of constipation in infants and children: Evidence-Based Recommendations from ESPGHAN and NASPGHAN. J Pediatr Gastroenterol Nutr. 2014;58(2):258-274.

b. Physical examination: External perineum, perianal examination, and digital anorectal examination. Stool occult blood test for all infants with constipation and for any child with abdominal pain, failure to thrive, intermittent diarrhea, or a family history of colon cancer or colonic polyps. Fecal impaction may be diagnosed on physical examination (hard mass within the abdomen) or digital examination (dilated rectal vault filled with stool). Evidence does not support using digital rectal examination or abdominal radiography to diagnose functional constipation.
2. **Treatment of functional constipation:**
a. Disimpaction (2–5 days)
   (1) Oral/nasogastric approach: Polyethylene glycol (PEG) electrolyte solutions are effective for initial disimpaction. May also use magnesium hydroxide, magnesium citrate, sorbitol, senna, or bisacodyl laxatives (avoid magnesium-containing products in infants owing to potential toxicity; beware of overdose in children).
   (2) Rectal approach: Saline or mineral oil enemas. Avoid soapsuds, tap water, and magnesium enemas because of potential toxicity. Avoid enemas in infants; may use glycerin suppositories. Avoid phosphate-containing products owing to risk of acute phosphate nephropathy (reported with use of oral sodium phosphate products).
b. Maintenance therapy (usually 3–12 months): Goal is to prevent recurrence.
   (1) Dietary changes: Increase intake of absorbable and nonabsorbable carbohydrates to soften stools. Current evidence is limited regarding increasing fluid intake for functional constipation. A balanced diet that includes whole grains, fruits, and vegetables is recommended. Evidence does not support the use of fiber supplementation in the treatment of functional constipation in children.
   (2) Behavioral modifications: Regular toilet habits with positive reinforcement. Referral to a mental health specialist for help with motivational or behavioral concerns.
   (3) Medications: Polyethylene glycol (PEG; osmotic laxatives), lactulose (if PEG solution is not available, lactulose is the best and safest alternative), magnesium hydroxide, or sorbitol recommended. Avoid prolonged use of stimulant laxatives. Discontinue therapy gradually only after return of regular bowel movements with good evacuation. Evidence does not support use of probiotics.
c. **Special considerations in infants aged <1 year:** 2–4 oz of 100% fruit juice (e.g., prune, pear, or apple) recommended in younger infants. Barley cereal, sorbitol-containing fruit purees, or lactulose can be used in infants taking solid foods. Glycerin suppositories may be useful. Avoid mineral oil, stimulant laxatives, and phosphate enemas.

D. Inflammatory Bowel Disease (IBD)[10,11]

1. **Classification:**
a. **Crohn's disease:** Transmural inflammatory process affecting any segment of the GI tract. Abdominal pain in majority of cases. Other common symptoms include weight loss, diarrhea, lethargy, anorexia, fever, nausea, vomiting, growth retardation, malnutrition, delayed puberty, psychiatric symptoms, arthropathy, and erythema nodosum.
b. **Ulcerative colitis (UC):** Chronic, relapsing, inflammatory disease of the colon and rectum. Symptoms (present for at least 2 weeks) include gross or occult rectal bleeding, diarrhea, and abdominal pain with or around the time of defecation. Exclusion of enteric pathogens (e.g., *Salmonella, Shigella, Yersinia, Campylobacter, Escherichia coli* 0157:H7, *C. difficile*) is necessary.[12]
2. **Diagnosis:**
a. Complete medical history and physical examination, including family history, exposure to infectious agents or antibiotic treatment, assessment of hydration and nutritional status, signs of peritoneal inflammation, and signs of systemic chronic disease. Stomatitis, perianal skin tags, fissures, and fistulas are suggestive of Crohn's disease. Presence of fever, orthostasis, tachycardia, abdominal tenderness, distention, or masses suggests moderate to severe disease and need for hospitalization.
b. Laboratory assessment: CBC, ESR, CRP, serum urea and creatinine, serum albumin, and liver function tests. IBD is typically associated with decreased hemoglobin and albumin, rise in platelet count, ESR, and CRP. Fecal lactoferrin and fecal calprotectin have been shown to be elevated in IBD and may serve as sensitive, noninvasive markers of IBD when used individually and with greater specificity when used together[13]. Diagnostic endoscopy is typically used to make diagnosis.
3. **Treatment/Management[14]:**
a. Induction of remission: Corticosteroids, exclusive enteral nutrition (100% caloric need by liquid formula), 5-aminosalicylates, anti-tumor necrosis factor (TNF) agents, and if indicated, antibiotics or surgery.
b. Maintenance of remission: Immunosuppression includes thiopurines, methotrexate, cyclosporine, tacrolimus, and anti-TNF monoclonal antibodies.
c. Surgical intervention is indicated only after medical management has failed in both Crohn's disease and UC. In Crohn's disease, surgery is indicated for localized disease (strictures), abscess, or disease refractory to medical management.

E. Gastrointestinal Reflux Disease[15]

1. **Definitions:** Gastroesophageal reflux (GER) is passage of gastric contents into the esophagus, and gastroesophageal reflux disease (GERD) is defined as symptoms or complications of GER.

2. **Diagnosis:**
   a. History and physical examination: Usually sufficient to reliably diagnose GER, identify complications and initiate management. Signs and symptoms include recurrent regurgitation, vomiting, heartburn, chest pain, dysphagia, stridor or wheezing, cough, recurrent aspiration pneumonia, and dental erosions. In infants, GER may present as irritability, feeding refusal, or Sandifer syndrome.
   b. Esophageal pH monitoring: Valid and reliable method of measuring acid reflux.
   c. Esophageal impedance monitoring: Combine with esophageal pH monitoring to detect both acid and nonacid reflux with greater sensitivity than pH monitoring alone.[16]
3. **Management:**
   a. Diet: Consider a 2- to 4-week trial of extensively hydrolyzed protein formula in infants to eliminate milk protein sensitivity as a cause of unexplained vomiting in formula-fed infants. Milk-thickening agents decrease overt regurgitation but do not decrease reflux. No evidence to support routine elimination of specific foods to treat GERD in older children.
   b. Lifestyle: A prone or left-sided sleeping position and elevation of head of bed may improve GER symptoms in adolescents. Infants up to 12 months should continue to sleep supine—sudden infant death syndrome risk far outweighs benefit of prone or lateral sleeping in GERD. (May consider prone positioning for infants while awake and monitored.) Obesity and large meal volumes are associated with increased GER in adults.
   c. Acid-suppressant therapy: Both PPIs and H_2 receptor antagonists (H_2RAs) are effective in relieving symptoms and promoting mucosal healing. PPIs are superior to H_2RAs; however, they may have more side effects. Smallest effective dose should be used for acid suppression.
   d. Prokinetic therapy: Potential side effects of each currently available prokinetic agent outweigh potential benefits. There is insufficient evidence to support routine use of metoclopramide, erythromycin, bethanechol, or domperidone for GERD.

F. Eosinophilic Esophagitis (EE)[17]

1. **Definition:** Symptoms of esophageal dysfunction with ≥15 eosinophils/high-power field (hpf) on peripheral blood smear and absence of pathologic GERD as evidenced by lack of responsiveness to high-dose PPI or normal pH monitoring of the distal esophagus.
2. **Differential diagnosis**: GERD, eosinophilic gastroenteritis, Crohn's disease, connective tissue disease, hypereosinophilic syndrome, infection, and drug hypersensitivity.

3. **Clinical Presentation:** Dysphagia, food impaction, chest pain, food refusal or intolerance, GER symptoms, emesis, abdominal pain, and failure to thrive. High rate of atopy in children with EE.
4. **Diagnosis:** Endoscopy and esophageal biopsy, and an allergy evaluation for other atopic conditions.
5. **Treatment:** Dietary therapy (elemental formula or removal of specific foods identified by skin prick or atopy patch testing), PPI therapy (as cotreatment), may consider systemic steroids for short-term use (e.g., dysphagia leading to dehydration or weight loss), and topical steroids for less severe symptoms [e.g., 6- to 8-week course of fluticasone or budesonide metered-dose inhaler administered orally *without* a spacer].

G. Celiac Disease[18]

1. **Definition:** An immune-mediated enteropathy caused by permanent GI tract sensitivity to gluten in genetically susceptible individuals. Increased occurrence in children with type 1 diabetes mellitus, autoimmune thyroiditis, Down syndrome, Turner syndrome, William syndrome, selective immunoglobulin (Ig) A deficiency, and in first-degree relatives of those with celiac disease (CD).
2. **Clinical presentation:** Diarrhea, vomiting, abdominal pain, constipation, abdominal distention, and failure to thrive. Non-GI symptoms include dermatitis herpetiformis, dental enamel hypoplasia of the permanent teeth, osteoporosis, short stature, delayed puberty, and iron deficiency anemia that is resistant to oral iron.
3. **Diagnosis:** Measure IgA antibody to human recombinant tissue transglutaminase (TTG) and serum IgA (high prevalence of IgA deficiency in CD). If there is known selective IgA deficiency and symptoms are suggestive of CD, testing with TTG IgG is recommended. Confirmation requires intestinal biopsy in all cases with findings of villous atrophy as a characteristic histopathologic feature.
4. **Management:** Lifetime, gluten-free diet.

IV. CONDITIONS OF THE LIVER

A. Liver Function Studies: Table 12.6

1. **Synthetic function:** Albumin, prealbumin, PT, activated PTT, and cholesterol levels. Elevated NH_3 is evidence of decreased ability to detoxify ammonia.
2. **Liver cell injury:** Elevation of aspartate aminotransferase, alanine aminotransferase, and lactate dehydrogenase.
3. **Cholestasis:** Increased bilirubin, urobilinogen, γ-glutamyltransferase, alkaline phosphatase, 5′-nucleotidase, and serum bile acids.

B. Acute Liver Failure (ALF)[19,20]

1. **Definition:** Biochemical evidence of liver injury with no known history of chronic liver disease, the presence of coagulopathy not corrected by vitamin K administration, and an international normalized ratio

TABLE 12.6
EVALUATION OF LIVER FUNCTION TESTS

Enzyme	Source	Increased	Decreased	Comments
AST/ALT	Liver, heart, skeletal muscle, pancreas, RBCs, kidney	Hepatocellular injury, rhabdomyolysis, muscular dystrophy, hemolysis, liver cancer	Vitamin B_6 deficiency, uremia	ALT more specific than AST for liver, AST > ALT in hemolysis, AST/ALT >2 in 90% of alcohol disorders in adults
Alkaline phosphatase	Osteoblasts, liver, small intestine, kidney, placenta	Hepatocellular injury, bone growth, disease, trauma, pregnancy, familial	Low phosphate, Wilson disease, zinc deficiency, hypothyroidism, pernicious anemia	Highest in cholestatic conditions; must be differentiated from bone source
GGT	Renal tubules, bile ducts, pancreas, small intestine, brain	Cholestasis, newborn period, induced by drugs	Estrogen therapy, artificially low in hyperbilirubinemia	Not found in bone, increased in 90% of primary liver disease, specific for hepatobiliary disease in nonpregnant patient
5′-NT	Intestine, liver cell membrane, brain, heart, pancreas	Cholestasis		Specific for hepatobiliary disease in nonpregnant patient
NH_3	Bowel flora, protein metabolism	Hepatic disease secondary to urea cycle dysfunction, hemodialysis, valproic acid therapy, urea cycle enzyme deficiency, organic acidemia and carnitine deficiency		Converted to urea in liver

AST/ALT, Aspartate aminotransferase/alanine aminotransferase; 5′-NT, 5′-nucleotidase; GGT, γ-glutamyl transpeptidase; RBCs, red blood cells

(INR) >1.5 if patient has encephalopathy or >2.0 if patient does not have encephalopathy. Causes of ALF and its reversibility vary with age (with treatment or withdrawal of offending agent).

2. **Pathogenesis** (incidence varies by age):
a. Infection: Herpes virus, hepatitis A, hepatitis B, adenovirus, cytomegalovirus, Epstein-Barr virus, enterovirus, human herpes

virus 6, parvovirus B19, Dengue fever, and indeterminate causes.
b. Vascular: Budd-Chiari syndrome, portal vein thrombosis, veno-occlusive disease, and ischemic hepatitis.
c. Immune dysregulation: Natural killer cell dysfunction (hemophagocytic lymphohistiocytosis), autoimmune, and macrophage activation syndrome.
d. Inherited/metabolic: Wilson disease, mitochondrial, tyrosinemia, galactosemia, hemochromatosis, fatty acid oxidation defect, and iron storage disease.
e. Drugs/toxins: Acetaminophen, anticonvulsants, and chemotherapy.
f. Other: Unknown, cancer/leukemia.
3. **Diagnosis:**
a. Clinical: Neurologic status, signs of chronic liver disease, and signs of other chronic disease. Jaundice and encephalopathy (hyperammonemia, cerebral edema) may be delayed by hours to weeks. Glucose instability with hypoglycemia and/or coagulopathy are common.
b. Laboratory: Electrolytes, BUN, creatinine, blood glucose, calcium, magnesium, phosphorous, blood gas, CBC with peripheral smear, reticulocyte count, liver function/production [albumin, aspartate aminotransferase, alanine aminotransferase, alkaline phosphatase], INR, PT, PTT, ammonia, factors V, VII (depleted first in ALF), VIII, and fibrinogen. A urine toxicology screen should be performed and a serum acetaminophen level should be taken. Consider viral studies, immune function studies, and metabolic studies.
NOTE: See Table 12.7 for interpretation of serologic markers of hepatitis B.
c. Imaging: Abdominal ultrasound with Doppler flow, head CT scan to exclude hemorrhage/edema, and chest radiography.
d. Other: Consider tissue biopsies.

C. Hyperbilirubinemia[21,22]

1. **Definition**: Bilirubin is the product of hemoglobin metabolism. There are two forms: direct (conjugated) and indirect (unconjugated). Hyperbilirubinemia is usually the result of increased hemoglobin load, reduced hepatic uptake, reduced hepatic conjugation, or decreased excretion. Direct hyperbilirubinemia is defined as a direct bilirubin >20% of the total bilirubin or a direct bilirubin of >2 mg/dL.
2. **Differential Diagnosis**: Table 12.8
3. **Treatment**: Highly dependent upon etiology in older children. Evaluation and diagnosis should be guided by history; however, liver function tests and ultrasounds are warranted in most patients. Refer to Chapter 18 for evaluation and treatment of neonatal hyperbilirubinemia.

TABLE 12.7
INTERPRETATION OF THE SEROLOGIC MARKERS OF HEPATITIS B IN COMMON SITUATIONS

Serologic Marker				
HBsAg	Total HBcAb	IgM HBcAb	HBsAb	Interpretation
−	−	−	−	No prior infection, not immune
−	−	−	+	Immune after hepatitis B vaccination (if concentration ≥ 10 IU/mL or passive immunization from HBIG administration)
−	+	−	+	Immune after recovery from HBV infection
+	+	+	−	Acute HBV infection
+	+	−	−	Chronic HBV infection

HBsAg, Hepatitis B surface antigen; HBcAb, antibody to hepatitis B core antigen; HBsAb, antibody to hepatitis B surface antigen; HBIG, hepatitis B immune globulin; HBV, hepatitis B virus; IgM, immunoglobulin M
From Davis AR, Rosenthal P. Hepatitis B in Children. Pediatr Rev. 2008;29(4):111-120.

V. PANCREATITIS[23-25]

Definition: Inflammatory disease of the pancreas; falls into two major categories: acute and chronic.

A. Acute Pancreatitis

1. **Clinical Presentation:** Sudden onset of abdominal pain associated with rise in pancreatic digestive enzymes in the serum or urine, with or without radiographic changes in the pancreas. Reversible process. Most common etiologies: Trauma, multisystem disease, drugs, infections, idiopathic, and congenital anomalies. See Table 12.9 for conditions associated with acute pancreatitis.
2. **Diagnosis:**
  a. Clinical signs/symptoms: History of abdominal pain (sudden or gradual, most commonly epigastric), anorexia, nausea, and vomiting. On physical examination, clinical signs include tachycardia, fever, hypotension, guarding/rebound tenderness, and decreased bowel sounds. Imaging with sonographic or radiologic evidence of pancreatic inflammation.
  b. Laboratory findings:
    (1) Elevated lipase and amylase; ≥3 times above normal limit (but no correlation with disease severity). Lipase is more sensitive and specific for acute pancreatitis but normalizes more slowly.
    (2) Additional findings: leukocytosis, hyperglycemia, glucosuria, hypocalcemia, and hyperbilirubinemia.
3. **Management:**
  a. Pancreatic rest: Nasogastric decompression, analgesia, aggressive intravenous fluid hydration, and initial oral intake restriction. Early enteral feeding is now recommended for nutrition over parenteral

TABLE 12.8
DIFFERENTIAL DIAGNOSIS OF HYPERBILIRUBINEMIA

INDIRECT HYPERBILIRUBINEMIA

Transient neonatal jaundice	Breast milk jaundice, physiological jaundice, Polycythemia, reabsorption of extravascular blood
Hemolytic disorders	Autoimmune disease, blood group incompatibility, hemoglobinopathies, microangiopathies, red cell enzyme deficiencies, red cell membrane disorders
Enterohepatic recirculation	Cystic fibrosis, Hirschsprung disease, ileal atresia, pyloric stenosis
Disorders of bilirubin metabolism	Acidosis, Crigler-Najjar syndrome, Gilbert syndrome, hypothyroidism, hypoxia
Miscellaneous	Dehydration, drugs, hypoalbuminemia, sepsis

DIRECT HYPERBILIRUBINEMIA

Biliary obstruction	Biliary atresia, choledochal cyst, fibrosing pancreatitis, gallstones or biliary sludge, inspissated bile syndrome, neoplasm, primary sclerosing cholangitis
Infection	Cholangitis, cytomegalovirus, Epstein-Barr virus, herpes simplex virus, histoplasmosis, HIV, leptospirosis, liver abscess, sepsis, syphilis, rubella, toxocariasis, toxoplasmosis, tuberculosis, urinary tract infection, varicella-zoster virus, viral hepatitis
Genetic/metabolic disorders	α_1-Antitrypsin deficiency, Alagille syndrome, Caroli disease, cystic fibrosis, Dubin-Johnson syndrome, galactokinase deficiency, galactosemia, glycogen storage disease, hereditary fructose intolerance, hypothyroidism, Niemann-Pick disease, rotor syndrome, tyrosinemia, Wilson disease
Chromosomal abnormalities	Trisomy 18, Trisomy 21, Turner syndrome
Drugs	Acetaminophen, aspirin, erythromycin, ethanol, iron, isoniazid, methotrexate, oxacillin, rifampin, steroids, sulfonamides, tetracycline, vitamin A
Miscellaneous	Neonatal hepatitis syndrome, parenteral alimentation, Reye syndrome

nutrition. The method of enteral feeding (prepyloric vs. postpyloric) remains controversial. In adults, enteral nutrition is associated with a lower incidence of infection, surgical intervention, and shorter hospital stay. Minimal pediatric evidence available.

b. Antibiotics are reserved only for the most severe cases.

B. Chronic Pancreatitis

1. **Definition:** Progressive inflammatory process causing irreversible changes in the architecture and function of the pancreas. Common complications include chronic abdominal pain and loss of exocrine function (malabsorption, malnutrition) and/or endocrine function (diabetes mellitus). Two major morphologic forms: calcific and obstructive (Table EC 12.B).

TABLE 12.9
CONDITIONS ASSOCIATED WITH ACUTE PANCREATITIS

SYSTEMIC DISEASES

Infections	Coxsackie, CMV, cryptosporidium, EBV, hepatitis, influenza A or B, leptospirosis, mycoplasma, mumps, rubella, typhoid fever, varicella
Inflammatory and vasculitic disorders	Collagen vascular diseases, hemolytic uremic syndrome, Henoch-Schönlein purpura, IBD, Kawasaki disease
Sepsis/peritonitis/shock	
Transplantation	

IDIOPATHIC (UP TO 25% OF CASES)

MECHANICAL/ STRUCTURAL

Trauma	Blunt trauma, child abuse, ERCP
Perforation	
Anomalies	Annular pancreas, choledochal cyst, pancreatic divisum, stenosis, other
Obstruction	Parasites, stones, tumors

METABOLIC AND TOXIC FACTORS

Cystic fibrosis	
Diabetes mellitus	
Drugs/toxins	Salicylates, cytotoxic drugs (L-asparaginase), corticosteroids, chlorothiazides, furosemide, oral contraceptives (estrogen), tetracyclines, sulfonamides, valproic acid, azathioprine, 6-mercaptopurine
Hypercalcemia	
Hyperlipidemia	
Hypothermia	
Malnutrition	
Organic acidemia	
Renal disease	

CMV, Cytomegalovirus; EBV, Epstein-Barr virus; ERCP, endoscopic retrograde cholangiopancreatography; IBD, inflammatory bowel disease

Modified from Robertson MA. Pancreatitis. In: Walker WA et al, eds. Pediatric Gastrointestinal Disease. 3rd ed. New York: BC Decker; 2000:1321-1344; Werlin SL. Pancreatitis. In: McMillan JA et al, eds. Oski's Pediatrics. Philadelphia: Lippincott Williams & Wilkins; 2006:2010-2012.

2. **Management:** (For acute exacerbations) same as management of acute pancreatitis. See Section V.A.3.

VI. MISCELLANEOUS TESTS

For descriptions, see Expert Consult.

A. Occult Blood

B. Quantitative Fecal Fat

REFERENCES

1. Koletzko S, Jones N, Goodman K, et al. Evidence-based guidelines from ESPGHAN and NASPGHAN for Helicobacter pylori infection in children.

Pediatric Gastroenterology, Hepatology and Nutrition. *J Pediatr Gastroenterol Nutr*. 2011;53:230-243.
2. Leung A, Sigalet DL. Acute abdominal pain in children. *Am Fam Physician*. 2003;67(11):2321-2326.
3. Zella GC, Israel EJ. Chronic Diarrhea in Children. *Pediatr Rev*. 2012;33(5):207-218.
4. Thomas PD, Forbes A, Green J, et al. Guidelines for the investigation of chronic diarrhoea, 2nd ed. *Gut*. 2003;52(suppl 5):v1-v15.
5. King CK, Glass R, Bresee JS, et al. Managing acute gastroenteritis among children: oral rehydration, maintenance, and nutritional therapy. *MMWR Recomm Rep*. 2003;52:1-16.
6. Fonseca BK, Holdgate A, Craig JC. Enteral vs. intravenous rehydration therapy for children with gastroenteritis. A meta-analysis of randomized controlled trials. *Arch Pediatr Adolesc Med*. 2004;158:483-490.
7. Clinical Practice Guidelines. Clinical efficacy of probiotics: review of the evidence with focus on children. NASPGHAN Nutrition Committee Report. *J Pediatr Gastroenterol Nutr*. 2006;43:550-557.
8. Shane AL. Improved Neonatal Outcomes with Probiotics. *JAMA Pediatr*. 2013;167(10):885-886.
9. Constipation Guideline Committee of the North American Society for Pediatric Gastroenterology, Hepatology, and Nutrition. Evaluation and treatment of constipation in infants and children: Evidence-based recommendations from ESPGHAN and NASPGHAN. *J Pediatr Gastroenterol Nutr*. 2014;58(2):258-274.
10. McMillan JA, Feigin RD, DeAngelis CD. *Oski's Pediatrics*. 4th ed. Philadelphia: Lippincott Williams & Wilkins; 2011.
11. Beattie RM, Croft NM, Fell JM, et al. Inflammatory bowel disease. *Arch Dis Child*. 2006;91:426-432.
12. Clinical Report: Differentiating ulcerative colitis from Crohn disease in children and young adults: report of a working group of the North American Society for Pediatric Gastroenterology, Hepatology, and Nutrition and the Crohn's and Colitis Foundation of America. *J Pediatr Gastroenterol Nutr*. 2007;44:653-674.
13. Joishy M, Davies I, Ahmed M, et al. Fecal calprotectin and lactoferrin as noninvasive markers of pediatric inflammatory bowel disease. *J Pediatr Gastroenterol Nutr*. 2008;48(10):48-54.
14. Rosen MJ, Dhawan A, Saeed SA. Inflammatory Bowel Disease in Children and Adolescents. *JAMA Pediatr*. 2015;169(11):1053-1060.
15. Vandenplas Y, Rudolph CD, DiLorenzo C, et al. Pediatric gastroesophageal reflux clinical practice guidelines: joint recommendations of the North American Society of Pediatric Gastroenterology, Hepatology, and Nutrition and the European Society of Pediatric Gastroenterology, Hepatology, and Nutrition. *J Pediatr Gastroenterol Nutr*. 2009;49:498-547.
16. Hirano I, Richter JE. Practice Parameters Committee of the American College of Gastroenterology. ACG practice guidelines: esophageal reflux testing. *Am J Gastroenterol*. 2007;102:668-685.
17. Furuta GT, Liacouras CA, Collins MH, et al. Eosinophilic esophagitis in children and adults: a systematic review and consensus recommendations for diagnosis and treatment. *Gastroenterology*. 2007;133:1342-1363.
18. Hill ID, Dirks MH, Liptak GS, et al. Guideline for the diagnosis and treatment of celiac disease in children: recommendations of the North American Society

for Pediatric Gastroenterology, Hepatology and Nutrition. *J Pediatr Gastroenterol Nutr.* 2005;40:1-19.
19. Bucuvalas J, Yazigi N, Squires Jr RH. Acute liver failure in children. *Clin Liver Dis.* 2006;10:149-168.
20. Devictor D, Tissieres P, Afanetti M, et al. Acute liver failure in children. *Clin Res Hepatol Gastroenterol.* 2011;35:430-437.
21. Brumbaugh D, Mack C. Conjugated hyperbilirubinemia in children. *Pediatr Rev.* 2012;13(7):291-302.
22. Moyer V, Freese DK, Whitington PF, et al. Guideline for the evaluation of cholestatic jaundice in infants: recommendations of the North American Society for Pediatric Gastroenterology, Hepatology and Nutrition. *J Pediatr Gastroenterol Nutr.* 2004;39:115-128.
23. Lowe ME. Pancreatitis in childhood. *Curr Gastroenterol Rep.* 2004;6:240-246.
24. Nydegger A, Couper RT, Oliver MR. Childhood pancreatitis. *J Gastroenterol Hepatol.* 2006;21(3):499-509.
25. Srinath AI, Lowe ME. Pediatric pancreatitis. *Pediatr Rev.* 2013;34(2):79-90.

Chapter 13
Genetics: Metabolism and Dysmorphology
Christina Peroutka, MD

See additional content on Expert Consult

Genetics is the frontier of medicine. Continuous technologic advances have brought a constantly evolving field to the forefront of medical research and to the bedside of the everyday pediatric patient. Genetics is best considered in two broad categories: metabolism and dysmorphology. When considering a particular diagnosis, a complete patient history, including details of conception, pregnancy, prenatal screening and diagnostic studies, delivery, postnatal growth, development, and a three-generation family history in the form of a pedigree should accompany a comprehensive physical examination.

I. WEB RESOURCES

- American College of Medical Genetics: www.acmg.net (Search for ACT sheets and algorithms to help guide physicians after a positive newborn metabolic screen.)
- Genetics Home Reference: http://ghr.nlm.nih.gov/. (Patient–friendly information about genetic conditions.)
- GeneReviews: www.genereviews.org. (Expert-authored and peer-reviewed descriptions of inherited disorders.)
- GeneTests: www.genetests.org. (Information on genetic diagnostic tests, genetic clinics in the United States and laboratories that perform genetic testing.)
- LactMed: A Toxnet Database: toxnet.nlm.nih.gov. (Drugs and lactation database available through the U.S. National Library of Medicine.)
- National Newborn Screening and Genetics Resource Center: genes-r-us.uthscsa.edu/resources.htm.
- National Organization for Rare Disorders: www.rarediseases.org.
- Online Mendelian Inheritance in Man (OMIM): http://omim.org. (Search engine for identifying genetic diseases based on clinical phenotype, gene, and OMIM number; the "Clinical Synopsis" is particularly helpful.)
- Reprotox through Micromedex. (Subscription database of drug teratogenicity and toxicology.)

II. THE PEDIGREE

A. Pedigree Construction (Fig. 13.1)

B. Patterns of Inheritance

See Expert Consult

C. U.S. Department of Health and Human Services My Family Health Portrait Tool

1. This tool can be used to create a pedigree; it may be saved and updated: http://www.hhs.gov/familyhistory/portrait/index.html

III. METABOLISM

A. Clinical Presentation of Metabolic Disease[1-4] (Box 13.1)

1. Most metabolic diseases are inherited in an autosomal recessive pattern. Some, like ornithine transcarbamylase deficiency and mucopolysaccharidosis type 2 (Hunter syndrome), are X-linked. The presentation of small molecule (metabolic) diseases in neonates tends to be nonspecific, and may include lethargy, irritability, seizures, hypotonia, poor feeding, hypoglycemia, vomiting, and temperature instability. The family history may be remarkable for siblings who died of similar presentations (often mistaken for "sepsis" or "SIDS"). After the neonatal period, the presentation may include recurrent vomiting, lethargy progressing to coma, or organ dysfunction. Symptoms may wax and wane with intercurrent illness. A high index of suspicion is required, as routine investigations may be unrevealing. For the diseases included in this handbook, please see the sections on "Evaluation" and "Treatment of Metabolic Crisis" for empiric management; special considerations are listed under each disease.

B. Evaluation[1,4]

1. **Initial laboratory tests:** Comprehensive metabolic panel (CMP), blood glucose, venous blood gas (VBG), ammonia, lactate, creatine kinase (CK), complete blood cell count (CBC) with differential, urine ketones.
2. **Subsequent evaluation for metabolic disease:** Consult a geneticist. General metabolic workup includes plasma amino acids (PAA), urine organic acids (UOA), acylcarnitine profile, quantitative (free and total) plasma carnitine, lactate/pyruvate ratio (see Table 13.1 for collection information).
3. **Special considerations**[4,6,7]
   a. Hyperammonemia: VBG, UOA, PAA, acylcarnitine profile, urine orotic acid (Fig. 13.2)
   b. Hypoglycemia: During acute illness consider urine ketones, acylcarnitine profile, PAA, UOA, insulin, growth hormone, cortisol, C-peptide (Fig. 13.3)[8]
   c. Metabolic acidosis: Ammonia, lactic acid, UOA, UA with urine pH, CMP (Fig. 13.4)

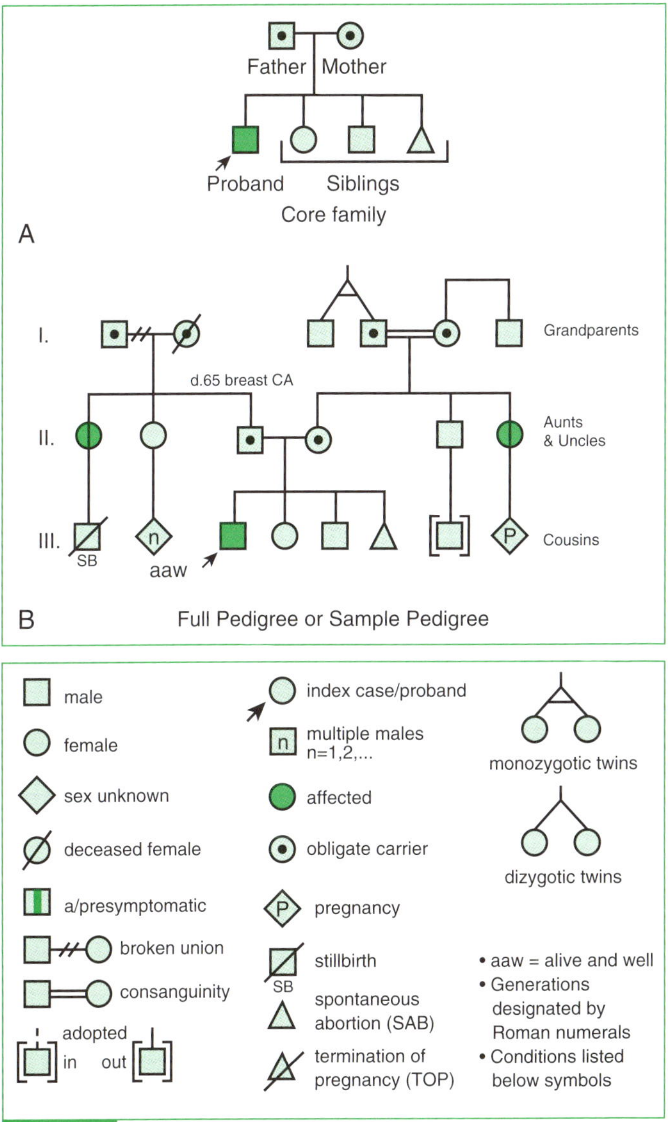

Chapter 13 Genetics: Metabolism and Dysmorphology

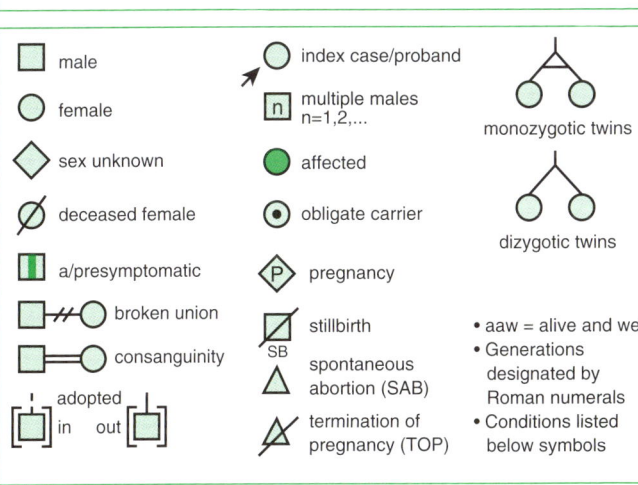

FIGURE 13.1
Pedigree construction.

BOX 13.1
WHEN TO SUSPECT METABOLIC DISEASE[1,4]

Overwhelming illness in the neonatal period
Vomiting
Acute acidosis, anion gap
Massive ketosis
Hypoglycemia
Coagulopathy
Deep coma
Seizures, especially myoclonic
Hypotonia
Unusual odor of urine
Extensive dermatosis, especially monilial
Neutropenia, thrombocytopenia, or pancytopenia
Family history of siblings dying early

TABLE 13.1
SAMPLE COLLECTION

Specimen Name	Volume (mL)	Tube	Handling Instructions
Chromosome microarray (SNP array)	2–5	Purple top	Do not freeze, may refrigerate.
Karyotype	2–5	Green top	Room temperature.
DNA-based testing (see Table 13.2)	5–10	Purple top	Room temperature; ship in insulated container overnight. Refrigerate for long term storage.
Plasma ammonia	1–3	Purple top	Place on ice and transport immediately to laboratory.
Plasma amino acids	1–3	Green top	Take to laboratory immediately on ice water; if must store, spin down and separate plasma and store at −20°C.
Quantitative carnitine (free and total carnitine)	1–3	Green top	Transport on ice.
Acylcarnitine profile	0.5–2.0	Green top	Transport on ice.
Lactate	2–3	Gray top	Immediately transport on ice.
Urine organic acids	3–5	Urine specimen container	Take immediately to laboratory on ice; if must store, store at −20°C.
Urine amino acids	1–5	Urine specimen container	Take immediately to laboratory on ice; if must store, store at −20°C.

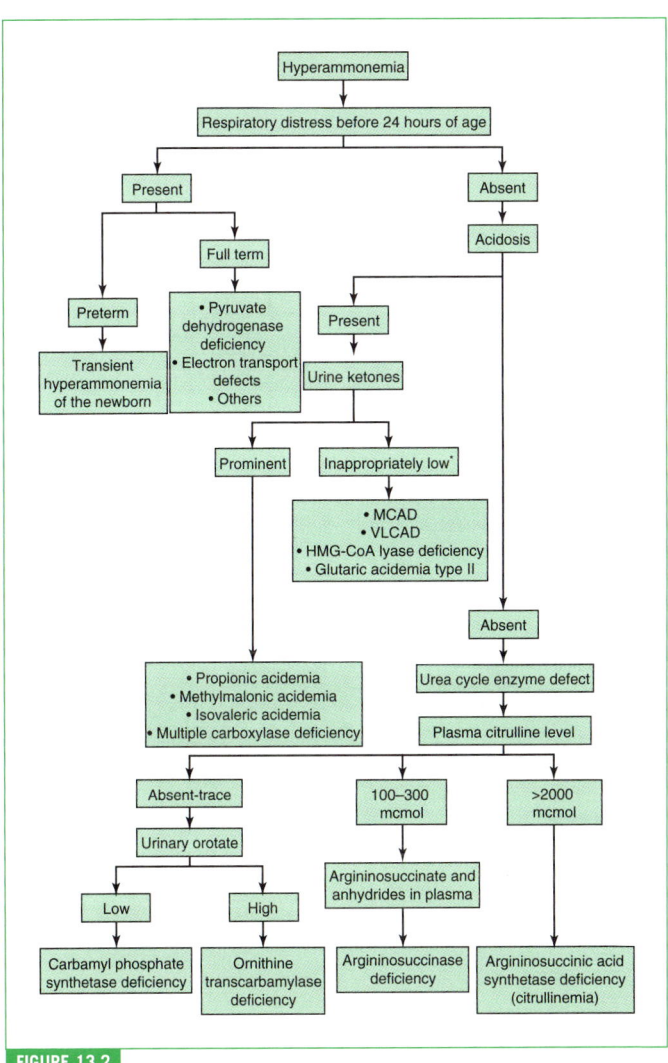

FIGURE 13.2

Differential diagnosis of hyperammonemia. *Indicates inappropriately low urinary ketones in the setting of symptomatic hypoglycemia. HMG-CoA, Hydroxymethylglutaryl-CoA; MCAD, medium-chain acyl-CoA dehydrogenase; VLCAD, very long-chain acyl-CoA dehydrogenase.

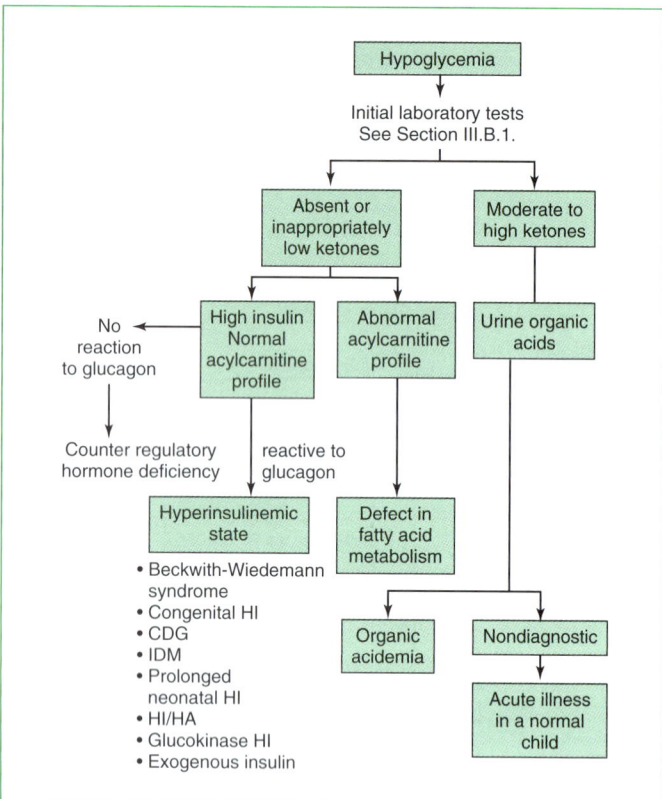

FIGURE 13.3

Evaluation of hypoglycemia. B-W, Beckwith-Wiedemann syndrome; CDG, congenital disorder of glycolization; HI, hyperinsulinism; HI/HA, hyperinsulinism/hyperammonemia; IDM, infant of a diabetic mother. *(Modified from Burton BK. Inborn errors of metabolism in infancy: a guide to diagnosis. Pediatrics. 1998;102:E69 and Cox GF. Diagnostic approaches to pediatric cardiomyopathy of metabolic genetic etiologies and their relation to therapy. Prog Pediatr Cardiol. 2007;24:15-25.)*

d. Neonatal seizures: CSF and plasma amino acids (done simultaneously to determine the glycine ratio to evaluate for nonketotic hyperglycinemia), CSF/serum glucose ratio, serum neurotransmitters, serum very long-chain fatty acids, urine organic acids, serum uric acid, urine sulfites. Consider trial of pyridoxine (100 mg intravenously [IV] once; see Formulary for specific dosing instructions).
e. Urine reducing substances (finding with differential):
   i. Galactose: Galactosemia
   ii. Fructose: Hereditary fructose intolerance, fructosuria

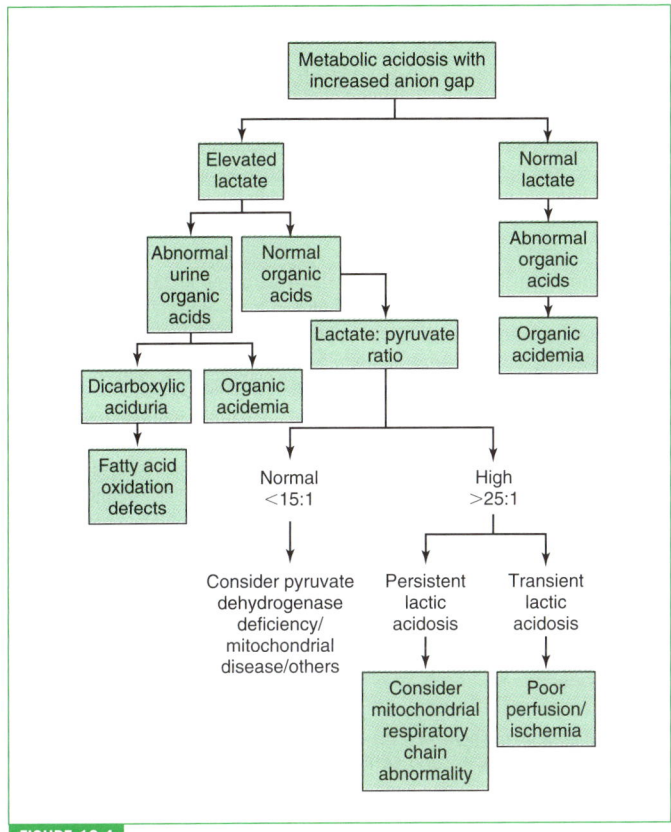

FIGURE 13.4

Metabolic acidosis with increased anion gap. *(From Burton B. Inborn errors of metabolism in infancy: a guide to diagnosis.* Pediatrics. *1998;102:E69.)*

    iii. Glucose: Diabetes mellitus, renal tubular defect
    iv. Xylose: Pentosuria
    v. P-hydroxyphenylpyruvic acid: Tyrosinemia
    vi. False positive: Cephalosporins, nalidixic acid

C. Treatment of Metabolic Crisis[4,6,7]

1. **Initial intervention**
a. Normal saline (NS) bolus, 10–20 mL/kg
b. Start 10% dextrose (D_{10}) + 1/4 to 1/2 NS + KCl (10–20 mEq/L) at 1.5–2 times maintenance rate.
c. Patient should have nothing by mouth except in the diagnosis of Maple Syrup Urine Disease (MSUD). In MSUD it is essential to continue leucine-free synthetic protein formula to give amino acids

that can compete with elevated leucine for the blood brain barrier to prevent cerebral edema.
   d. Bicarbonate should be included in the fluids, equivalent to the patient's home dose or if pH is <7.1.
2. **Hemodialysis:** Should be initiated as soon as possible in infants with hyperammonemia > 250, and in patients with any small-molecule disease that is unresponsive to initial management.
3. **Commonly used medications**
   a. Carnitine 50 mg/kg/dose IV Q6 hr when ill, or 100 mg/kg/day orally (PO) divided Q8 hr when well.
   b. Sodium phenylacetate (10%) + sodium benzoate (10%) (Ammonul) should be combined with arginine HCl in a 25–35 mL/kg 10% dextrose solution to treat acute hyperammonemia in a urea cycle patient. The dose of Ammonul is 250 mg/kg for a child < 20 kg, and 5.5 g/m^2 for a child > 20 kg. The dose of arginine HCl is 2–6 g/m^2, depending on the diagnosis (2 g/m^2 for carbamylphosphate synthase deficiency (CPS) and ornithine transcarbamylase deficiency (OTC); 4–6 g/m^2 for citrullinemia; 6 g/m^2 alone for argininosuccinase deficiency). Administer as a loading dose over 90–120 minutes, followed by an equivalent dose as a maintenance infusion over 24 hours. As all of these medications have significant side effects and narrow therapeutic windows, treatment should always be undertaken in consultation with a biochemical geneticist.
   c. Arginine HCl 0.15–0.4 g/kg/day IV for MELAS stroke-like episode. (MELAS: mitochondrial encephalomyopathy, lactic acidosis, stroke-like episodes)[9,10]
   d. Sodium benzoate for nonketotic hyperglycinemia (NKH): start with 500 mg/kg/day added to a 24 hour supply of formula or divided at least four times daily, and consult a biochemical geneticist.

D. Newborn Metabolic Screening[1,2,11,29]

1. **Overview by state:** http://genes-r-us.uthscsa.edu
2. **Timing**
   a. First screen should be performed within the first 48–72 hours of life (at least 24 hours after initiation of feeding).
   b. Second screen (requested in some states) should be performed between the age of 1 and 4 weeks (after 7 days).
   c. Preterm infants: Perform initial screen at birth (to collect DNA before transfusions), another at age 48–72 hours, a third at age 7 days, and a final at age 28 days or before discharge (whichever comes first).
3. **Abnormal results**
   a. Requires immediate follow-up and confirmatory testing; consult a geneticist.
   b. ACT Sheets and Confirmatory Algorithms are available for more information on how to proceed with specific abnormalities: www.acmg.net/ (search ACT sheets).

E. Categories of Metabolic Diseases[1,3,4,6,7]

1. **Fatty acid oxidation (FAO) and carnitine metabolism disorders**
a. Presentation:
   i. Hypoketotic hypoglycemia
   ii. Disorders of long chain fatty acid metabolism can present with rhabdomyolysis and/or cardiomyopathy.
b. Diagnostic evaluation: Initial laboratory tests (section III.B.1.) with acylcarnitine profile, quantitative (free and total) carnitine
c. Acute management: Treatment of metabolic crisis (section III.C.1.). Consider bolus of D_{10} 2 mL/kg in hypoglycemia.
   i. Treat fever aggressively with antipyretics and treat intercurrent infection.
d. Chronic management:
   i. Carnitine supplementation for primary carnitine deficiencies and medium-chain acyl-CoA dehydrogenase disorders (avoid in very long-chain acyl-CoA dehydrogenase and long-chain 3-hydroxyl-CoA dehydrogenase disorders).
   ii. In very long-chain fatty acid disorders, limit intake to low-fat foods and supplement with medium-chain triglyceride oil.
   iii. In all FAO patients with mild intercurrent illness or decreased daytime intake, nighttime feeds Q4 hr are necessary.

2. **Organic acidemias**
a. Epidemiology
   i. Includes glutaric acidemia type 1 (GA1), methylmalonic acidemia (MMA), propionic acidemia (PA), isovaleric acidemia, maple syrup urine disease (MSUD), and 3-methylcrotonyl-CoA carboxylase deficiency (3-MCC).
   ii. 3-MCC is detected on newborn screens, but most children are unaffected without problems during illness. Rarely, patients may have more severe presentation with acidosis.
b. Presentation
   i. Neonatal: nonspecific as described above
   ii. Older infant/child: global developmental delays, choreoathetoid or dystonic movements secondary to metabolic stroke in the basal ganglia, bone marrow suppression, frequent infections, pancreatitis, cardiomyopathy
c. Diagnostic evaluation: Initial laboratory tests (section III.B.1.) with UOA, acylcarnitine profile, PAA, quantitative (free and total) carnitine
d. Acute management
   i. Follow treatment of metabolic crisis (section III.C.1.)
   ii. May need bicarbonate, essential if on it daily at baseline
   iii. Stop all protein feeds (except in MSUD, where leucine-free synthetic formula should be used at all times to help decrease cerebral edema)
   iv. Carnitine 50 mg/kg IV Q6 hr in MMA, PA
   v. 10% glycine 500 mg/kg/day in isovaleric acidemia

e. Chronic management: Formula that appropriately restricts amino acids; treatment with carnitine; anticipatory management of complications including renal insufficiency in MMA and cardiomyopathy in PA

3. **Urea cycle defects**
a. Epidemiology:
    i. Most common is OTC deficiency, which is X linked.
    ii. OTC deficiency and CPS deficiency are not picked up on newborn screening because it is difficult to distinguish between low and normal citrulline levels.
b. Presentation: Episodes of acute decompensation characterized by headache, vomiting, lethargy, and altered mental status due to hyperammonemia that causes respiratory alkalosis. Seizures are very rare. Failure to thrive and poor appetite are chronic symptoms in undiagnosed patients with mild urea cycle defects.
c. Diagnostic evaluation: Initial laboratory tests (section III.B.1.) with PAA, urine orotic acid.
d. Acute management:
    i. Treatment of metabolic crisis (section III.C.1.), stop all protein intake, dialysis as indicated for ammonia >250 μmol/L.
    ii. Sodium benzoate + sodium phenylacetate (Ammonul) and arginine IV (section III.C.3.b.)
e. Chronic management: Sodium phenylbutyrate or glycerol phenylbutyrate, citrulline (for OTC deficiency and CPS deficiency), arginine (for citrullinemia and argininosuccinate lyase deficiency), protein-restricted diet.

4. **Aminoacidopathies**
a. **Phenylketonuria (PKU)**
    i. Presentation: Intellectual disability if untreated
    ii. Diagnostic evaluation: Most infants diagnosed by newborn screening before clinical appearance; PAA to look at phenylalanine and tyrosine.
    iii. Acute management: Phenylalanine-restricted diet
    iv. Chronic management: Phenylalanine-restricted diet; sapropterin effective in a subset of patients at a dose of 10–20 mg/kg/day
b. **Hereditary tyrosinemia (HT1)**
    i. Presentation: Severe liver failure, vomiting, porphyria-like crisis, bleeding, sepsis, hypoglycemia, hyponatremia, renal tubulopathy (Fanconi syndrome). Chronic untreated HT1 leads to cirrhosis and liver cancer, failure to thrive, rickets, neuropathy, tubulopathy, neurologic crises.
    ii. Diagnostic evaluation: Initial laboratory tests (section III.B.1.) with coagulation studies, UOA to quantitate succinylacetone, PAA
    iii. Acute management: Manage bleeding complications and provide replacement factors; nitisinone (NTBC) 1–2 mg/kg divided twice daily
    iv. Chronic management: Tyrosine- and phenylalanine-restricted diet, NTBC 1–2 mg/kg divided twice daily

5. **Lactic acidemias and mitochondrial diseases**[6,12]
   a. Presentation: Can involve any organ system; symptoms usually neurologic and myopathic. For in-depth discussion, access GeneReviews at www.ncbi.nlm.nih.gov/books/NBK1224/.
   b. Diagnostic Evaluation: Initial laboratory tests (section III.B.1.) with lactate/pyruvate ratio, CSF levels of lactate and pyruvate, plasma and CSF amino acids, UOA, urine amino acids, brain imaging, mitochondrial DNA testing. Of note, mitochondrial disease can be caused by mutations in nuclear or mitochondrial DNA. Muscle biopsy is no longer indicated except in the case of severe myopathy, as diagnosis can be made by molecular testing of blood.
   c. Acute management: ABCs, supportive therapy, encourage anaerobic metabolism. For MELAS syndrome, IV arginine may abort a crisis (section III.C.3.).
   d. Chronic management: Cocktail of antioxidants, vitamins, and cofactors.
6. **Disorders of carbohydrate metabolism**
   a. **Galactosemia**[13,14]
      i. Epidemiology: classical variant, clinical variant (may be missed on newborn screen unless both Gal-1P and GALT enzyme activity are measured), biochemical variant (Duarte variant; most often no clinical significance).
      ii. Presentation:
         (1) Presents at 3–4 days of life (before the newborn screen returns) with nonspecific findings as described above. Other presenting symptoms include failure to thrive, lethargy, hemolytic anemia, hyperbilirubinemia, cataracts, hepatic dysfunction, and renal dysfunction.
         (2) Galactosemia should be considered in an infant with overwhelming *Escherichia coli* sepsis.
      iii. Diagnostic evaluation: Diagnosis often made on newborn screening. Obtain initial laboratory tests (section III.B.1) with coagulation studies, urine for reducing substances, erythrocyte galactose-1-phosphate, galactose-1-phosphate uridyltransferase (GALT) activity.
      iv. Acute management: ABCs, discontinue feeds, dextrose containing fluids. If infant is not critically ill, simply initiate soy-based formula.
      v. Chronic management: Lactose-free and galactose-restricted diet for life.
   b. **Glycogen storage disease (GSD)**[15,16,63]
      i. Presentation
         (1) GSD type I (von Gierke): Glycogen accumulation leads to hepatomegaly, renomegaly, and short stature. Most commonly presents by 3–4 months with hepatomegaly, hyperuricemia, hyperlipidemia and hypoglycemia with lactic acidosis that develop within 2–4 hours of fasting. Other features include doll-like facies, xanthomas, hepatic adenomas, polycystic ovaries, and pancreatitis. Recurrent bacterial infections and mucosal ulcers occur in type Ib.

    (2) GSD type II (Pompe): Classic infantile disease presents by 2 months with hypotonia, generalized muscle weakness, cardiomegaly with short PR interval, and failure to thrive (FTT). Without treatment with enzyme replacement, death occurs by one year from hypertrophic cardiomyopathy causing LV outflow obstruction.
    (3) GSD type III (Cori): Liver disease in infancy and early childhood is marked by ketotic hypoglycemia, hepatomegaly, hyperlipidemia, and elevated hepatic transaminases, but tends to become less prominent with time. Hypertrophic cardiomyopathy develops in childhood, followed by skeletal myopathy in the third to fourth decade.
  ii. Diagnostic evaluation: Ketotic hypoglycemia with fasting lactic acid, uric acid, lipid panel, transaminases, CK, electrocardiogram (ECG), echocardiogram (ECHO), molecular testing.
  iii. Acute management: Prevent hypoglycemia, treat with dextrose-containing fluids.
  iv. Chronic management
    (1) GSD type I: Prevent hypoglycemia; patients < 18 months require continuous feeds overnight. After age 18 months, consider cornstarch or newly available Glycosade (modified slow release starch) after consulting a geneticist. Allopurinol to prevent gout. Lipid-lowering medications. Supplement citrate to help prevent nephrolithiasis, nephrocalcinosis. Angiotensin-converting enzyme (ACE) inhibitors to treat microalbuminuria. Kidney transplant for end-stage renal disease. Granulocyte-colony stimulating factor (G-CSF) for recurrent infections in glycogen storage disease type 1b (GSD1b).
    (2) GSD type II: Enzyme replacement (alglucosidase alfa) as soon as diagnosis is made, must be initiated before age 6 months to be effective.
    (3) GSD type III: High-protein diet and frequent feedings (Q3–4 hr) in infancy. Corn starch or Glycosade to prevent hypoglycemia overnight after age 18 months.
7. **Lysosomal storage diseases**
a. **Mucopolysaccharidoses**[6,17]
  i. Epidemiology: Includes Hurler (MPS I), Hunter (MPS II), Sanfilippo (MPS III), Morquio (MPS IV), Maroteaux-Lamy (MPS VI), and Sly (MPS VII) syndromes.
  ii. Presentation
    (1) Infants normal at birth, except in Sly syndrome (MPS VII), where infants usually die from hydrops. Coarsening of facial features noted by age 1 year in most. Progressive dysostosis multiplex, growth failure, hepatomegaly, psychomotor retardation, intellectual disability, hearing loss.

(2) Hurler syndrome (MPS I): Lethal by age 10 years if not treated with bone marrow transplantation by age 2 years.
(3) Sanfilippo syndrome (MPS III): Extremely hyperkinetic behavior, challenging behavior and sleep disturbance. Somatic abnormalities relatively mild.
(4) Morquio syndrome (MPS IV): Small stature with severe skeletal abnormalities
(5) Maroteaux-Lamy syndrome (MPS VI): Visceral involvement, normal intelligence

iii. Diagnostic evaluation: CBC with differential, skeletal survey for dysostosis, specific enzyme activity and/or molecular testing.
iv. Acute management: Supportive therapy
v. Chronic management
(1) Hurler syndrome (MPS I): Stem cell transplantation before 2 years of age arrests progression of cognitive decline, and slows but does not prevent skeletal manifestations or corneal clouding.
(2) Enzyme replacement is available for Hurler-Scheie syndrome type MPS I, nonneuronopathic manifestations of Hunter syndrome (MPS II), Morquio syndrome (MPS IV), and Maroteaux-Lamy syndrome (MPS VI).

b. **Sphingolipidoses**[2,6,18-21]
   i. Epidemiology: includes Tay-Sachs, Niemann-Pick, Gaucher and Krabbe diseases.
   ii. Presentation:
   (1) Sphingolipids are major components of the cell membrane, especially in the nervous system. Clinical features therefore include progressive psychomotor retardation and neurologic problems, such as epilepsy, ataxia, and spasticity. Hepatosplenomegaly is not uncommon. Skeletal dysplasias or dysmorphic features are rare. Ophthalmologic evaluation may show a cherry red spot on the macula.
   (2) Tay-Sachs: Infantile form presents at age 4–6 months with hypotonia, loss of motor skills, increased startle reaction and a cherry-red spot. Eventual blindness, spastic tetraparesis, decerebration and macrocephaly (by age 18 months) lead to death by age 4 years.
   (3) Niemann-Pick: Neuropathic (type A), non-neuropathic (type B), and type C forms exist. Type A presents with hypotonia, FTT, massive hepatosplenomegaly and a cherry red spot progressing to blindness, deafness and neurologic deterioration with death by age 1.5–3 years. Type B involves hepatosplenomegaly, interstitial lung disease and growth restriction, but individuals have normal intellectual function and may survive to adulthood. Type C has an extremely heterogeneous presentation and is beyond the scope of this chapter.

(4) Gaucher: Neuropathic (types II and III) and non-neuropathic (type I) forms exist. Types II and III are distinguished by age of onset of primary neurologic disease, with type II having rapid progression of brainstem dysfunction and spasticity in infancy, with death by age 2 years. Type I is more characterized by hematological and skeletal findings including severe hepatosplenomegaly, anemia, thrombocytopenia, bleeding dyscrasias, splenic and medullary infarctions, osteopenia, and fractures. Intellectual function is normal.

(5) Krabbe: Infantile and late-onset forms, with infantile-onset presenting by age 3–6 months, followed by progressive neurologic deterioration (irritability, increased startle, neuropathy, decerebration, blindness, and deafness); death by age 2. Late onset forms include progressive ataxia, spastic paresis, and visual failure. Onset can be between ages 1 and 50 years; progression is variable.

iii. Diagnostic evaluation: Specific enzyme activity in fibroblasts or leukocytes; some conditions show elevated urine oligosaccharides

iv. Acute management: Supportive therapy

v. Chronic management: Mostly supportive

(1) Tay-Sachs: Manage seizures with conventional antiepileptic drugs; avoid severe constipation.

(2) Niemann-Pick: Transfuse blood products for life-threatening bleeding; provide supplemental oxygen for symptomatic pulmonary disease. Enzyme replacement is being developed.

(3) Gaucher: Manage at a Comprehensive Gaucher Center including enzyme replacement (ERT) or substrate reduction therapy (SRT); transfusion of blood products; joint replacements and osteoporosis management. Initiation of ERT or SRT prevents occurrence of progressive manifestations, such as bone disease.

(4) Krabbe: Manage severe pain and spasticity in advanced disease. Hematopoietic stem cell transplantation only in presymptomatic infants prior to age 3 weeks and older individuals with late-onset disease.

8. **Cholesterol synthesis disorders**[2,22]

a. **Smith-Lemli-Opitz**

i. Presentation: Growth retardation, craniofacial dysmorphism (microcephaly, micrognathia, anteverted nostrils, ptosis), 2–3-toe syndactyly (almost obligatory), relative adrenal insufficiency, midline defects (holoprosencephaly, genital malformations in boys, cardiac defects). The clinical spectrum is wide and ranges from intrauterine demise to mild malformations and normal lifespan.

ii. Diagnostic Evaluation: Elevated serum concentrations of 7-dehydrocholesterol (7-DHC); serum cholesterol concentrations low in 90% of cases. Sequence analysis of DHCR7.

Chapter 13 Genetics: Metabolism and Dysmorphology

iii. Acute management: Supportive; treat with stress-related doses of steroids during illness or other stress; fresh frozen plasma can be given as an emergency source of LDL cholesterol.
iv. Chronic management: Cholesterol supplementation 50–100 mg/kg/day may lead to clinical improvement; simvastatin 0.5–1 mg/kg divided BID may be useful for mildly affected patients (simvastatin specifically crosses the blood brain barrier; decreases accumulation of 7-DHC and 8-DHC).

IV. DYSMORPHOLOGY[1,26-30]

A. History
Past medical history including pregnancy history, prenatal drug/other exposures, type of conception (natural or assisted), perinatal history, developmental milestones, three-generation pedigree.

B. Physical Examination[26,30]
1. **Major anomalies:** Structural anomalies that are found in < 5% of the population and cause significant cosmetic or functional impairment, often requiring medical or surgical management. Examples include structural brain abnormalities, growth < 3%, cleft lip and/or palate, congenital heart defects, or skeletal dysplasia.
2. **Minor anomalies:** Structural anomalies that are found in < 5% of the population with little or no cosmetic or functional significance to the patient. Three or more minor anomalies may be a nonspecific indicator of occult or major anomaly (~20%–25% risk). Examples include atypically shaped ears or eyes, inverted nipples, birthmarks, atypical skin folds or creases (e.g., single palmar crease). Seventy-one percent of minor anomalies are present in the craniofacies and hands.[31]

C. Workup
1. **Imaging**
a. Abdominal ultrasound, echocardiogram, brain imaging (head ultrasound, or magnetic resonance imaging [MRI]).
b. Genetic skeletal survey for patients with apparent short bones, short stature, visible external anomalies (e.g., asymmetry, proximal thumbs, skin dimpling).
2. **Ophthalmology evaluation**
3. **Hearing evaluation**
4. **Genetic testing:** See Table 13.2. The patient should be referred to genetics for a dysmorphology evaluation and appropriate testing.

D. Specific Dysmorphology Conditions
This section is not comprehensive; it covers some common genetic syndromes. More complete information can be found in the following references: Jones,[27] Hall and colleagues,[26] http://www.omim.org, and http://www.genereviews.org.
1. **Aneuploidy syndromes:** All aneuploidy syndromes are most commonly due to maternal nondisjunction. Therefore, the risk increases with

maternal age. In trisomy 21 specifically, maternal nondisjunction causes around 95% of cases, but in 3%–4% of cases, the condition is a result of a chromosomal translocation. The diagnostic evaluation for aneuploidy often begins prenatally with an abnormal first trimester screen (nuchal translucency, nasal bone, free β-hcG, PAPP-A), followed by further screening options including noninvasive circulating cell free fetal DNA analysis and a second trimester anatomy screen, diagnostic testing via chorionic villus sampling in the first trimester, or amniocentesis during or after the second trimester. Fluorescence *in situ* hybridization (FISH) may be performed in the first 24–48 hours of life to indicate number of chromosomes, but will not determine the morphology of the chromosomes (i.e., if a translocation is present). Therefore, karyotype analysis is still indicated in aneuploidy syndromes, both to provide a diagnosis, and to provide accurate genetic counseling.

a. **Trisomy 21**[32]
   i. Presentation: Hypotonia, brachycephaly, epicanthal folds, flat nasal bridge, upward-slanting palpebral fissures, Brushfield spots, small mouth and ears, excessive skin at the nape of the neck, single transverse palmar crease, short fifth finger with clinodactyly, wide gap between the first and second toes, intellectual disability with a range from mild to severe, increased risk of congenital heart defects (50%), hearing loss (75%), otitis media (50%–70%), Hirschsprung disease (<1%), gastrointestinal atresias (12%), eye disease (60%) including cataracts (15%) and severe refractive errors (50%), acquired hip dislocation (6%), obstructive sleep apnea (50%–75%), and thyroid disease (15%). Of note, transient myeloproliferative disease (TMD) occurs almost exclusively in infants with Down syndrome (10%) and usually regresses by age 3 months. However, infants with TMD are at increased risk of developing leukemia later on (10%–30%).
   ii. Health supervision: AAP guideline available at http://pediatrics.aappublications.org/content/107/2/442
      (1) Neonatal: Ophthalmologic evaluation for cataracts, hearing screen, echocardiogram, CBC, consider ear-nose-throat (ENT) evaluation for any airway concerns, check thyroid studies or confirm normal on newborn screen (1% congenital hypothyroidism), early intervention services.
      (2) Infancy: Risk of serous otitis media 50%–70% (may need referral to ENT), behavioral audiogram in all children at 1 year, ophthalmology referral at 6 months, thyroid studies at 6 and 12 months and then annually, early intervention services.
      (3) Early childhood and on: Annual thyroid studies, CBC (add ferritin and CRP for any child at risk of iron deficiency), hearing and vision assessments; ophthalmology assessments may be spaced to every 3 years after age 13 years; cervical spine roentgenogram at age 3 years if asymptomatic (sooner

imaging with immediate neurosurgical referral if symptomatic); monitor for signs of obstructive sleep apnea.
b. **Trisomy 18**[27]
  i. Features: Intrauterine growth restriction and polyhydramnios, small for gestational age at birth, clenched hands with overlapping fingers, hypoplastic nails, short sternum, prominent occiput, low-set and structurally abnormal ears, micrognathia, rocker-bottom feet, congenital heart disease, cystic and horseshoe kidneys, seizures, hypertonia, significant developmental and cognitive impairments.
  ii. Previously thought to be invariably lethal in the neonatal period, now approximately 5%–10% survive to their first birthday.
c. **Trisomy 13**[27]
  i. Features: Defects of forebrain development (holoprosencephaly), severe developmental disability, low-set malformed ears, cleft lip and palate, microphthalmia, aplasia cutis congenita, polydactyly (most frequently of the postaxial type), narrow hyperconvex nails, apneic spells, cryptorchidism, congenital heart defects.
  ii. Roughly 5% of pregnancies with trisomy 13 survive to birth, and only 5% of those survive the first 6 months of life.
d. **Turner syndrome (45, X)**[27,33,34]
  i. Features: Characterized by partial or complete absence of one X chromosome. The diagnosis should be considered in a female fetus with hydrops, increased nuchal translucency, cystic hygroma, or lymphedema. Other features may include short stature, gonadal dysgenesis with amenorrhea and lack of a pubertal growth spurt, broad chest with hypoplastic or inverted nipples, renal abnormalities, webbed neck, hypertension, congenital heart disease (most commonly bicuspid aortic valve and coarctation of the aorta), and hypothyroidism. Intelligence is usually normal, but patients are at risk for cognitive, behavioral, and social disabilities.
  ii. Health supervision: Guidelines available at http://www.aafp.org/afp/2007/0801/p405.html
    (1) Endocrine: Growth hormone usually initiated when height < fifth percentile (refer early to pediatric endocrinology), monitor for obesity and glucose intolerance, thyroid dysfunction, and dyslipidemia. Estrogen therapy for sexual development and preservation of bone mineral density. TTG and IgA every 2–4 years starting at age 4 for celiac disease.
    (2) Cardiology: Baseline echocardiogram, close cardiac follow-up to monitor for aortic dilatation, monitor for hypertension and manage aggressively.
    (3) HEENT: Audiology assessment at diagnosis and periodically thereafter; monitor for strabismus.
    (4) Renal: Ultrasound for renal abnormalities (most commonly a horseshoe kidney).

(5) Orthopedic: Hip examinations in infancy because of increased risk of congenital developmental hip dysplasia; monitor for scoliosis.
(6) Provide psychosocial support.

e. **Klinefelter syndrome (47, XXY; 48, XXYY; 48, XXXY; and 49, XXXXY)**[35,36]
  i. Features: Klinefelter syndrome is a spectrum of diseases characterized by the presence of at least one extra X added to a normal male karyotype. It is the most common congenital cause of primary hypogonadism. Infants may present with hypospadias or cryptorchidism. Children may present with expressive language delay or learning disabilities. Adolescent and adult males may present with infertility and hypoandrogenism with eunuchoid body habitus, gynecomastia and small testes. There is an increased risk of breast carcinoma in 47, XXY.
  ii. Health supervision: Androgen replacement should begin at puberty (as early as age 10 years) and be titrated to keep age-appropriate levels of follicle-stimulating hormone, luteinizing hormone, estradiol, and testosterone. Testicular sperm extraction in early puberty and intracytoplasmic sperm injection may be considered if fatherhood is desired.

2. **Connective tissue diseases**[27,37,38]
Examples include Marfan syndrome, Loeys-Dietz syndrome, familial thoracic aortic aneurysm disease, bicuspid aortic valve and aneurysm syndromes, Ehlers-Danlos syndrome, Shprintzen-Goldberg syndrome, cutis laxa syndromes, arterial tortuosity syndrome, Stickler syndrome (description of all of these is beyond the scope of this chapter).

a. **Marfan syndrome**[38]
  i. Presentation: Myopia, ectopia lentis (60%), dilatation of the aorta at level of sinuses of Valsalva, predisposition to aortic tear and rupture, mitral valve prolapse, enlargement of proximal pulmonary artery, pneumothorax, bone overgrowth and joint laxity, extremities disproportionately long for size of trunk, pectus carinatum or excavatum, scoliosis, pes planus.
  ii. Physical examination: Scoring of systemic features based on evaluation of the literature available at http://www.marfan.org/dx/score.
  iii. Diagnostic evaluation: Clinical diagnosis based on the revised Ghent criteria; may be confirmed by molecular genetic testing of FBN1.
  iv. Health supervision: Annual ophthalmologic examination; annual echocardiography unless aortic root diameter exceeds ≈ 4.5 cm in adults (or if rates of aortic dilation exceed ≈ 0.5 cm/year) and significant aortic regurgitation is present, then valve-sparing surgery to replace the aortic root; intermittent surveillance of the entire aorta with computed tomography (CT) or magnetic resonance

angiography (MRA) scans beginning in young adulthood. Avoid contact sports, competitive sports, isometric exercise.
v. Guidelines are available at http://pediatrics.aappublications.org/content/132/4/e1059.short.
vi. Treatment with β-blocker (atenolol) and an angiotensin-II type 1 receptor blocker (losartan) is current standard of care. A large-scale trial published in 2014 did not show a significant difference in the rate of aortic-root dilation with angiotensin-II type 1 receptor blocker (losartan) versus atenolol. However, other studies suggest a benefit with combination therapy.[39] Treatment by a geneticist and/or cardiologist is recommended.

b. **Ehlers-Danlos syndrome (EDS)**[40,41]
  i. Presentation: At least six types were recognized in the revised Beighton criteria used to make a clinical diagnosis. Most are inherited in an autosomal dominant pattern. The most common forms are the classical and hypermobility types, while the vascular type involves the highest risk. Features of Ehlers-Danlos syndrome may include smooth, velvety, hyperextensible skin, widened scars, easy bruising, joint hypermobility with recurrent dislocations, chronic joint or limb pain and a positive family history. The vascular type EDS involves translucent skin, characteristic facies (pinched nose), as well as risk for arterial, intestinal and uterine fragility or rupture.
  ii. Diagnostic evaluation: Clinical evaluation (≥5 of 9 Beighton criteria) and family history.
  iii. Chronic management: Physical therapy to improve joint stability, low-resistance exercise, and pain medications as needed; treat gastroesophageal reflux. Vascular EDS requires management in a clinic specializing in connective tissue disorders.

3. **Neurocutaneous syndromes**
a. **Neurofibromatosis type I (NF1)**[27,42]
  i. Epidemiology: Autosomal dominant condition; 1/2 cases spontaneous or *de novo* genetic mutations.
  ii. Presentation and diagnosis
     (1) Two or more of the following: ≥6 café au lait macules over 5 mm in greatest diameter in prepubertal individuals and over 15 mm in greatest diameter in postpubertal individuals, ≥2 neurofibromas of any type or one plexiform neurofibroma, freckling in the axilla or inguinal area, optic glioma, ≥2 Lisch nodules, a distinctive osseous lesion (e.g., sphenoid dysplasia, tibial pseudarthrosis), a first-degree relative (parent, sibling, offspring) with NF1 as defined by the above criteria.
     (2) Other features: Short stature, macrocephaly, progressive scoliosis
     (3) Genetic testing: Molecular confirmation by NF1 gene testing
  iii. Surveillance: Annual genetics examination, annual ophthalmologic examination, developmental assessment of children, regular blood

pressure monitoring, MRI for follow-up of clinically symptomatic tumors

b. **Tuberous Sclerosis**[43,44]
  i. Epidemiology: Autosomal dominant condition; 2/3 cases spontaneous or *de novo* genetic mutations. Variable expression leads to a heterogeneous presentation, even within families.
  ii. Presentation: Benign tumors form in the brain, kidneys, heart, eyes, lungs and skin.
  iii. Diagnostic evaluation: At least two major or one major plus two minor features are required.
      (1) Major features: **Cortical tuber (characteristic lesion)**, subependymal nodule or giant cell astrocytoma, **facial angiofibroma** or forehead plaque (age 4–6 years; may be confused with acne), ungual or periungual fibroma (nontraumatic), **>3 hypomelanotic "ash leaf" macules** (present in more than 90%), **shagreen patch** (lumbosacral region), retinal hamartomas, **cardiac rhabdomyoma** (50% of children), **renal angiomyolipoma** (75%–80% of children age > 10 years), pulmonary lymphangioleiomyomatosis.
      (2) Minor features: Cerebral white matter migration lines, dental pits, gingival fibromas, bone cysts, retinal chromatic patch, confetti skin lesions, nonrenal hamartomas, multiple renal cysts, hamartomatous rectal polyps.
  iv. Health supervision
      (1) Brain MRI best to detect cortical tubers; repeat every 1–3 years. Monitor for signs of hydrocephalus, seizures, cognitive impairment and autism spectrum disorders.
      (2) Visualize ash leaf spots with a Wood ultraviolet lamp.
      (3) Renal angiomyolipomas: Monitor for hematuria; follow with yearly imaging and embolize if > 4 cm.
  v. Treatment: Manage complications of disease as they arise.

4. **Skeletal conditions**
a. **Achondroplasia**[44-46]
  i. Epidemiology: Most common condition characterized by disproportionate short stature. Autosomal dominant, with 80% of cases being *de novo*. Associated with advanced paternal age (>35 years).
  ii. Features: Short arms and legs (especially involving proximal segment); bowing of the lower legs; large head with characteristic facial features including frontal bossing (prominent forehead) and midface retrusion. Infantile hypotonia is typical, followed by delayed motor development. Gibbus deformity of the thoracolumbar spine leads to exaggerated lumbar lordosis. Rarely, children have hydrocephalus and restrictive pulmonary disease. Stenosis at the foramen magnum in infancy increases the risk of death; lumbar spinal stenosis may present in childhood, but is

more common in adulthood. Intelligence and lifespan are usually normal. Average adult height for males and females is around 4 feet.
   iii. Diagnostic evaluation: Clinical diagnosis based on characteristic physical exam described above and radiographic findings including a contracted skull base, square shaped pelvis with small sacrosciatic notch, short vertebral pedicles, rhizomelic shortening of long bones, trident hands, proximal femoral radiolucency and chevron shape of distal femoral epiphysis. *FGFR3* mutation testing available if diagnostic uncertainty.
   iv. Health supervision: Use standard growth charts for achondroplasia. Monitor orthopedic growth and development closely. Baseline head CT in infancy. Monitor for signs of obstructive sleep apnea (OSA) and middle ear complications (i.e. otitis media). In adults, screen for spinal stenosis every 3–5 years with neurologic exam.
   v. Treatment: Manage complications of disease: VP shunt placement for increased ICP, suboccipital or lumbar decompression for spinal stenosis, orthopedic management of leg bowing, management of OSA and otitis media. Growth hormone treatment and surgical limb lengthening are controversial.
b. **Craniosynostosis**[44,47,48]
   i. See Fig. EC13.A.
   ii. Features: Primary craniosynostosis results from premature fusion of the cranial sutures, an event which usually occurs prenatally. Both syndromic and nonsyndromic forms exist. Most cases are of unknown etiology; genetic syndromes account for 10%–20% of cases, of which Apert, Crouzon and Pfeiffer syndromes are the most common. Scaphocephaly occurs from premature closer of the sagittal suture and is the most common form of craniosynostosis. Frontal plagiocephaly is the next most common form and results from premature fusion of a coronal and sphenofrontal suture.
   iii. Diagnostic evaluation: Palpation of the suture at birth often reveals a bony ridge. Skull radiograph or head CT may be considered. Certain genetic forms of craniosynostosis are caused by mutations in *TWIST*, *FGFR1*, *FGFR2*, or *FGFR3*.
   iv. Treatment: Management by a multidisciplinary craniofacial clinic is recommended, as staged surgical procedures are often required beginning at age 3–6 months. Early treatment and management may decrease the risk of associated complications such as hydrocephalus and cognitive impairment.
5. **Disorders of methylation/epigenetics**
a. **Prader-Willi syndrome**[30,49]
   i. Features: Characterized by severe hypotonia and feeding difficulties in infancy, followed by an insatiable appetite in later

infancy or early childhood. Developmental delays in motor and language abilities are present, and all affected individuals have some degree of intellectual disability. Short stature is common; males and females have hypogonadism, and in most, infertility.

ii. Diagnostic evaluation: Results from missing *paternally* contributed region. The patient has abnormal paternal-specific imprinting, a paternal deletion, or maternal uniparental disomy within the Prader-Willi/Angelman critical region of 15q.

iii. Health Supervision: Special attention to feeding in infancy; manage cryptorchidism in males; also screen for strabismus. Strict supervision in childhood is required to maintain a healthy BMI and avoid development of noninsulin dependent diabetes mellitus. Annual testing for hypothyroidism. Evaluate and treat sleep disturbance.

iv. Treatment: Growth hormone may normalize height. Replace sex hormones in puberty for secondary sexual characteristics and bone health. SSRIs may help with behavioral problems. Topiramate may help with skin picking. Modafinil treats daytime sleepiness. No medication available to treat hyperphagia.

b. **Angelman syndrome**[30,50]
   i. Features: Happy demeanor, hand-flapping and fascination with water. Severe developmental delay or intellectual disability beginning at age 6 months, severe speech impairment, gait ataxia with tremulous limbs, hypotonia, microcephaly and seizures.
   ii. Diagnostic evaluation: Results from missing *maternally* contributed region. The patient has abnormal maternal-specific imprinting, a maternal deletion, paternal uniparental disomy, or a mutation of *UBE3A* on the maternal allele within the Prader-Willi/Angelman critical region of 15q.
   iii. Health supervision: Monitor for behavior problems, feeding issues, sleep disturbance, scoliosis, strabismus, constipation, and gastroesophageal reflux disease.
   iv. Treatment: Antiepileptic drugs for seizures; be careful not to overtreat, since Angelman syndrome also associated with movement abnormalities (*avoid* carbamazepine, vigabatrin, and tigabine). Speech therapy with a focus on nonverbal communication. Sedatives for nighttime wakefulness.

c. **Rett syndrome**[44,51]
   i. Epidemiology: Most common in females, since pathogenic *MECP2* variants are most often lethal in males. *MECP2* variants are on the differential diagnosis for Angelman syndrome, intellectual disability with spasticity or tremor, learning disabilities or autism.
   ii. Features: Classic Rett syndrome is a neurodevelopmental syndrome that presents after 6-18 months of typical development with acquired microcephaly, then developmental stagnation,

followed by rapid regression in language and motor skills, and finally long-term stability with autistic features. Repetitive, sterotypical hand-wringing, fits of screaming or inconsolable crying, autistic features, episodic breathing abnormalities (sighing, apnea or hyperpnea), gait ataxia, tremors, and generalized tonic-clonic seizures are observed.

  iii. Diagnostic evaluation: Molecular testing of *MECP2* is indicated for classic Rett syndrome and for all related disorders.
  iv. Health supervision: Regular ECG to evaluate QT interval; regular assessment of feeding and monitor for scoliosis.
  v. Treatment: Supportive. Avoid drugs that prolong the QT interval.

6. **Cleft Lip and Palate (CLP)**[30,52]
  a. See Fig. EC13.B.[40]
  b. Epidemiology: Cleft lip and palate are still considered to be multifactorial conditions due to interaction of genetic and environmental factors. Multiple genes are being discovered, which may be causative in syndromic forms of cleft lip and palate, and may also play a role in nonsyndromic forms. The most common syndromic form is autosomal dominant Van der Woude syndrome (VDWS); other syndromes include 22q11.2, Apert, Crouzon, hemifacial microsomia, Pierre Robin and Treacher Collins. Maternal smoking, heavy alcohol use (more than five drinks per occasion), systemic corticosteroid use, folic acid and cobalamin deficiency increase the risk of cleft palate. The evidence is not as clear for maternal epilepsy syndromes and/or antiepileptic medications.
  c. Features: Spectrum of malformation (see Fig. EC13.B). Submucosal clefts may be indicated by a bifid uvula. Infants present with facial malformation, feeding problems and recurrent middle ear infections.
  d. Diagnostic evaluation: If the patient has cleft lip and/or palate, assess for additional major malformation(s), cognitive impairment, failure to thrive/unmet genetic potential, family history of Mendelian condition, or characteristic dysmorphism(s) of a specific condition. If any of these are present, pursue a full workup for occult anomalies including ophthalmology, audiology, abdominal ultrasound, ECHO and SNP array. Full workup recommended for cleft palate alone without additional features. For cleft palate with microretrognathia and/or severe midface hypoplasia, consider sending a Stickler panel (includes *COL2A1*, *COL11A1*, and *COL11A2*). If the patient has cleft lip, or cleft lip and palate without additional features, follow patient's growth and development without further tests.[53]
  e. Health supervision: Monitor for difficulty with speech, orthodontic concerns, and hearing loss.
  f. Treatment: A multidisciplinary approach including general pediatrics, genetics, plastic surgery, otolaryngology, lactation (early), speech therapy (later), and dentistry is recommended.

7. **Hypotonia**[54,55]

a. **Definition:** Reduced resistance to passive range of motion in joints, characterized by an impaired ability to sustain postural control and movement against gravity.
b. There can be central, peripheral, or combined forms of hypotonia. The workup is extensive and often involves a genetic metabolic workup as well as SNP array. These patients should be referred to genetics or neurology.
    i. **Central:** Depressed level of consciousness, predominantly axial weakness, normal strength with hypotonia, abnormalities of brain function, dysmorphic features, and other congenital malformations.
    ii. **Peripheral:** Alert, responds appropriately to surroundings, normal sleep/wake cycles, profound weakness, absent reflexes, feeding difficulties, decreased and/or lack of antigravity movement.
8. **Other**
    a. **Noonan syndrome**[56,57]
        i. Epidemiology: Autosomal dominant syndrome that may affect males or females, though a frequent misnomer is "male Turners" (historically due to some similar physical features).
        ii. Features: Short stature, congenital heart defects (specifically pulmonary valve stenosis and/or hypertrophic cardiomyopathy), broad or webbed neck, chest with superior pectus carinatum and inferior pectus excavatum, cryptorchidism in males, lymphatic dysplasias, mild intellectual disability (~33%), coagulation defects, and characteristic facies (inverted triangular shaped face, low-set, posteriorly rotated ears with fleshy helices, telecanthus and/or hypertelorism, epicanthal folds, thick or droopy eyelids). Adult height at the lower limit of normal.
        iii. Diagnostic Evaluation: Fifty percent have *PTPN11* mutations; various molecular panels are available including other genes, which explain up to 61% of cases. Thus, NS remains a clinical diagnosis. Infants with pulmonic stenosis and small size may have another rasopathy with a more severe prognosis than Noonan syndrome. Therefore molecular testing is indicated.
        iv. Health supervision: Guidelines available at http://pediatrics.aappublications.org/content/126/4/746. Specifically, obtain ECG and ECHO; renal ultrasound, PT, aPTT, platelet count, and bleeding time in all patients. Thyroid function studies if symptomatic. Monitor for feeding difficulties including recurrent emesis.
        v. Treatment: Involves management of specific features (i.e., cardiology management, early intervention for developmental delays). Treatment for serious bleeding may be required (must know specific factor deficiency or platelet aggregation anomaly). Growth hormone will increase growth velocity.
    b. **22q11 Deletion Syndrome (velocardiofacial syndrome, DiGeorge syndrome)**[28]

i. Features: Congenital heart disease (tetralogy of Fallot, interrupted aortic arch, ventricular septal defect, and truncus arteriosus most common), palatal abnormalities (velopharyngeal incompetence [VPI], cleft palate), characteristic facial features, learning difficulties, immune deficiency (70%), hypocalcemia (50%), significant feeding problems (30%), renal anomalies (37%), hearing loss (both conductive and sensorineural), laryngotracheoesophageal anomalies, growth hormone deficiency, autoimmune disorders, seizures (with or without hypocalcemia), and skeletal abnormalities.
ii. Diagnostic Evaluation: SNP array is the gold standard; FISH is no longer recommended. Assessments should include serum calcium, absolute lymphocyte count, B- and T-cell subsets, renal ultrasound, chest x-ray, cardiac examination, and echocardiogram.
iii. Hold live vaccines until immune function is assessed.

c. **Fragile X syndrome**[58]
   i. Epidemiology: Twice as common in males as in females; X-linked (Xq27.3); most common cause of inherited intellectual disability.
   ii. Features
      (1) Males: Mild to moderate intellectual disability, cluttered speech, autism, macrocephaly, large ears, prominent forehead, prognathism, postpubertal macro-orchidism, tall stature in childhood that slows in adolescence, seizures, and connective tissue dysplasia. Early physical recognition is difficult, so the diagnosis should be considered in males with developmental delay.
      (2) Females: Intellectual abilities range from normal to significant intellectual disability due to the degree of X inactivation of the affected chromosome. A condition unique to female premutation carriers (55–200 repeats) is primary ovarian insufficiency.
   iii. Diagnostic Evaluation: Molecular genetic testing of the *FMR1* gene to detect expansion (≥200 repeats) of the CGG trinucleotide.
   iv. Health supervision: Guidelines available at http://pediatrics.aappublications.org/content/127/5/994.short.

V. DIAGNOSTIC GENETIC TESTING AND CLINICAL CONSIDERATIONS

A. Ethics of Genetic Testing in Pediatrics[59]

Genetic testing in pediatric patients poses unique challenges given that children require proxies (most often parents) to give consent for testing. With advances in the scope and availability of genetic technology, as well as the familial implications of genetic testing, it is especially important to consider how genetic testing may influence the care and future of the pediatric patient. Several publications and statements have been made with regard to genetic testing in children, including the "Ethical Issues with Genetic Testing in Pediatrics" statement made by the AAP. Please see Expert Consult for important considerations and information on informed consent.

TABLE 13.2
DIAGNOSTIC GENETIC TESTING AND CLINICAL CONSIDERATIONS

Genetic Testing Technology	Description of Technology	Turnaround Time	Able to Detect	Specific Indications
Karyotype	Systematically arranged photomicrograph of chromosomes	1–2 weeks	Aneuploidy, larger deletions/duplications, translocation or balanced rearrangements	Patient confirmation and family studies in aneuploidy, recurrent miscarriages to detect a balanced translocation in parents, family studies in the setting of an unbalanced translocation
Fluorescence *in situ* hybridization (FISH)	Mapping a segment of DNA by molecular hybridization of a fluorescent probe	<1 week	Presence or absence of a specific site or chromosome	Not indicated, except in family studies and for rapid diagnosis of a suspected trisomy
Array CGH (i.e., SNP or oligo chromosomal microarray)	Comparative genome hybridization using a high-density SNP profile or oligos (short segments of DNA) across the genome	2–4 weeks	Genomic gains or losses (CNVs), regions of homozygosity. Incidental findings unrelated to phenotype. SNP arrays will reveal consanguinity.	First-line cytogenetic test for all patients with unexplained global developmental delay, intellectual disability, autism, and/or at least 1 major + 2 minor congenital anomalies.
Single gene testing, Sanger sequencing	Nucleotide-by-nucleotide sequencing using DNA base pairing	<1 month	Mutations in specific gene of interest	Indicated only when there is a strong clinical suspicion of a single gene disorder
Targeted mutation analysis, Sanger sequencing	Detection of previously identified familial mutation or common population mutation	<1 month	Confirmation of clinical diagnosis, presymptomatic genetic diagnosis, identification of carrier status, preimplantation genetic diagnosis, prenatal testing	Confirmation testing in single gene disorders or in family studies

Test	Method	Turnaround	Detects	Indications/Notes
Repeat expansion testing	Southern blot or triplet-repeat primed PCR	<1 month	Pathogenic expansion of repeats	Indicated only when there is a strong clinical suspicion of a triplet repeat disorder, which cannot be detected on SNP array or WES.
Methylation analysis	Methylation multiplex ligation-dependent probe amplification	<1 month	Identification of imprinting defect (e.g., Prader-Willi)	Indicated only when there is a strong clinical suspicion of a methylation defect
Next-generation sequencing (multiple gene panels)	Massively-parallel sequencing of specific genes	1–2 months	Mutations in more than one gene of interest	Used for syndromes with genetic heterogeneity where mutations in different genes can cause the same phenotype
Whole exome sequencing	Massively-parallel sequencing of ~80% of exons	2–6 months	Variants in the coding portions of the genes that are captured. Incidental findings unrelated to phenotype.	More comprehensive genomic test indicated in an otherwise negative workup, or when cost-benefit ratio of more targeted testing is in favor of WES
Whole genome sequencing	Massively parallel sequencing of entire genome	Variable depending on laboratory	More uniform coverage of exonic, intronic, and splice site mutations. Incidental findings unrelated to phenotype.	Not widely clinically available. Used mostly in research studies.

NOTE: It is recommended that genetic testing be sent in consultation with a geneticist, genetic counselor, or other provider who can guide appropriate testing, provide pretest counseling, interpretation of results, and posttest follow-up.

Courtesy Weiyi Mu, ScM, CGC, and Christina Peroutka, MD, McKusick Nathans Institute of Genetic Medicine, Johns Hopkins Hospital; Zachary Cordner, PhD, Department of Psychiatry and Behavioral Sciences, Johns Hopkins University.

B. Informed Consent[60]

As genetic testing has become more available, patients may have genetic testing sent without direct consultation of a geneticist or genetics counselor. Specifically, the chromosome microarray (SNP array) has become the most common test sent in the initial workup of developmental delay or disability. Pretest counseling and informed consent are important prior to sending any genome-wide testing, given that incidental findings or variants of unknown significance may be found. With this in mind, it is recommended that pretest counseling be provided including the following possibilities:
1. Positive—a causative/related variant is found
2. Negative—either no causative/related variant is present, *or* the available technology or scope of the test methodology was unable to detect the causative/ related variant. This does not mean that the condition of the patient is not genetic.
3. Variant(s) of uncertain significance—variants for which the meaning is uncertain (could be variants without clinical significance or related to the patient's presentation but not previously reported).
4. Incidental finding(s)—variants anticipated to affect the patient's health that are unrelated to the indication for sending the test.
5. Discovery that parents are blood relatives.
   Documentation of informed consent for genetic testing is also recommended.

C. Professional Disclosure of Familial Genetic Information[61]
See Expert Consult.

D. Disclosure of Incidental Findings[62]
See Expert Consult.

E. Diagnostic Genetic Testing and Clinical Considerations
(see Table 13.2)

REFERENCES

1. McMillan JA, Feigin RD, DeAngelis C. *Oski's Pediatrics: Principles and Practice.* 4th ed. Philadelphia: Lippincott Williams & Wilkins; 2006.
2. Zschocke J, Hoffman GF. *Vademecum Metabolicum.* 3rd ed. Friedrichsdorf, Germany: Milupa Metabolics; 2011.
3. Burton BK. Inborn errors of metabolism in infancy: a guide to diagnosis. *Pediatrics.* 1998;102:E69.
4. Hoffman GF, Zschocke J, Nyhan W. *Inherited Metabolic Diseases: A Clinical Approach.* Heidelberg: Springer; 2010.
5. Deleted in page proofs.
6. Saudubray JM, van den Berghe G, Walter JH. *Inborn Metabolic Diseases: Diagnosis and Treatment.* 5th ed. Heidelberg: Springer; 2012.
7. Scriver CR, Sly WS, Childs B, et al. *The Metabolic and Molecular Bases of Inherited Disease.* 8th ed. New York: McGraw-Hill Professional; 2001.
8. Hoe FM. Hypoglycemia in infants and children. *Adv Pediatr.* 2008;55:367-384.

9. Koga Y, Akita Y, Nishioka J, et al. L-arginine improves the symptoms of strokelike episodes in MELAS. *Neurology*. 2005;64(4):710-712.
10. Moutaouakil F, El Otmani H, Fadel H, et al. l-arginine efficiency in MELAS syndrome: A case report. [Article in French] *Rev Neurol (Paris)*. 2009;165(5):482-485.
11. Kaye CI. Committee on Genetics. Introduction to the newborn screening fact sheets. *Pediatrics*. 2006;118:1304-1312.
12. Chinnery PF. Mitochondrial Disease Overview; 2000. Last update 2010. GeneReviews. Available at <http://www.ncbi.nlm.nih.gov/books/NBK1224/>.
13. Berry GT. Classic Galactosemia and Clinical Variant Galactosemia; 2000. Last update 2014. GeneReviews. Available at <http://www.ncbi.nlm.nih.gov/books/NBK1518/>.
14. Fridovich-Keil JL, et al. Duarte Variant Galactosemia; 2014. GeneReviews. Available at <http://www.ncbi.nlm.nih.gov/books/NBK258640/>.
15. Bali DS, et al. Glycogen Storage Disease Type 1; 2006. Last update 2013. GeneReviews. Available at <http://www.ncbi.nlm.nih.gov/books/NBK1312/>.
16. Dagli A, et al. Glycogen Storage Disease Type III; 2010. Last update 2012. GeneReviews. Available at <http://www.ncbi.nlm.nih.gov/books/NBK26372/>.
17. Staretz-Chacham O, Lang TC. Lysosomal storage diseases in the newborn. *Pediatrics*. 2009;123:1191-1207.
18. Kaback MM, Desnick RJ. Hexosaminidase A Deficiency; 1999. Last update 2011. GeneReviews. Available at <http://www.ncbi.nlm.nih.gov/books/NBK1218/?report=printable>.
19. Wasserstein MP, Schuchman EH. Acid Sphingomyelinase Deficiency; 2006. Last update 2015. GeneReviews. Available at <http://www.ncbi.nlm.nih.gov/books/NBK1370/>.
20. Pastores GM, Hughes DA. Gaucher Disease; 2000. Last update 2015. GeneReviews. Available at <http://www.ncbi.nlm.nih.gov/books/NBK1269/>.
21. Wenger DA. Krabbe Disease; 2000. Last update 2011. GeneReviews. Available at <http://www.ncbi.nlm.nih.gov/books/NBK1238/>.
22. Nowaczyk MJM. Smith-Lemli-Opitz Syndrome; 1998. Last update 2013. GeneReviews. Available at <http://www.ncbi.nlm.nih.gov/books/NBK1143/>.
23. Steinberg SJ, et al. Peroxisome Biogenesis Disorders, Zellweger Syndrome Spectrum; 2003. Last update 2012. GeneReviews. Available at <http://www.ncbi.nlm.nih.gov/books/NBK1448/>.
24. Steinberg SJ, et al. X-linked Adrenoleukodystrophy; 1999. Last update 2015. GeneReviews. Available at <http://www.ncbi.nlm.nih.gov/books/NBK1315/>.
25. Weiss KH. Wilson Disease; 1999. Last update 2013. GeneReviews. Available at <http://www.ncbi.nlm.nih.gov/books/NBK1512/>.
26. Hall JG, Allanson J, Gripp K, et al. *Handbook of Physical Measurements*. 2nd ed. Oxford, UK: Oxford University Press; 2007.
27. Jones KL. *Smith's Recognizable Patterns of Human Malformation*. 6th ed. Philadelphia: Saunders; 2006.
28. Hennekam R, Allanson J, Krantz I. *Gorlin's Syndromes of the Head and Neck*. 5th ed. New York: Oxford University Press; 2010.
29. Seidel HM, Rosenstein B, Pathak A, et al. *Primary Care of the Newborn*. 4th ed. St Louis: Mosby; 2006.
30. Saul RA. *Medical Genetics in Pediatric Practice: Policy of the American Academy of Pediatrics*. United States of America: American Academy of Pediatrics; 2013.
31. Hoyme HE. Minor anomalies: diagnostic clues to aberrant human morphogenesis. *Genetica*. 1993;89:307-315.

32. Bull MJ. Committee on Genetics. Health supervision for children with Down syndrome. *Pediatrics*. 2011;128:393-406.
33. Frias JL, Davenport ML. Committee on Genetics and Section on Endocrinology. Health supervision for children with Turner syndrome. *Pediatrics*. 2003;111:692-702, reaffirmed 2009.
34. Morgan T. Turner syndrome: diagnosis and management. *Am Fam Physician*. 2007;76(3):405-410.
35. Visootsak J, Graham JM Jr. Klinefelter syndrome and other sex chromosomal aneuploidies. *Orphanet J Rare Dis*. 2006;1:42.
36. Mehta A, Clearman T, Paduch DA. Safety and efficacy of testosterone replacement therapy in adolescents with Klinefelter syndrome. *J Urol*. 2014;191:1527-1531.
37. Loeys BL, Dietz HC, Braverman AC, et al. The revised Ghent nosology for the Marfan; syndrome. *J Med Genet*. 2010;47:476-485. doi:10.1136/jmg.2009.072785.
38. Tinkle BT, Saal HM, the American Academy of Pediatrics, Committee on Genetics. Health supervision for children with Marfan syndrome. *Pediatrics*. 2003;132:e1059-e1072.
39. Lacro RV, Dietz HC, Sleeper LA, et al. Atenolol versus losartan in children and young adults with Marfan's syndrome. *N Engl J Med*. 2014;371(22):2061-2071.
40. Beighton P, De Paepe A, Steinmann B, et al. Ehlers-Danlos syndromes: revised nosology, Villefranche, 1997. *Am J Med Genet*. 1998;77:31-37.
41. Levy HP. Ehlers-Danlos Syndrome, Hypermobility Type; 2004. Last update 2012. GeneReviews. Available at <http://www.ncbi.nlm.nih.gov/books/NBK1279/>.
42. Hersh JH. Health supervision for children with neurofibromatosis. *Pediatrics*. 2008;121:633-642.
43. National Institute of Neurological Disorders and Stroke (NINDS) Tuberous Sclerosis Information Page. Last update 2015. NINDS. Available at <http://www.ninds.nih.gov/disorders/tuberous_sclerosis/tuberous_sclerosis.htm>.
44. Kliegman RM. *Nelson Textbook of Pediatrics*. 20th ed. Philadelphia: Elsevier; 2016.
45. Pauli RM. Achondroplasia; 1998. Last update 2012. GeneReviews. Available at <http://www.ncbi.nlm.nih.gov/books/NBK1152/>.
46. Trotter TL, Hall JG, the American Academy of Pediatrics, Committee on Genetics. Health supervision for children with Achondroplasia. *Pediatrics*. 2005;116(3):771-783.
47. Robin NH, et al. FGFR-Related Craniosynostosis Syndromes; 1998. Last update 2011. GeneReviews. Available at <http://www.ncbi.nlm.nih.gov/books/NBK1455/>.
48. Gallagher ER, Hing AV, Cunningham ML. Evaluating fontanels in the newborn skull. *Contemp Pediatr*. 2013;20:12-20.
49. Driscoll DJ, et al. Prader-Willi Syndrome; 1998. Last update 2014. GeneReviews. Available at <http://www.ncbi.nlm.nih.gov/books/NBK1330/>.
50. Dagli AI, et al. Angelman Syndrome; 1998. Last update 2015. GeneReviews. Available at <http://www.ncbi.nlm.nih.gov/books/NBK1144/>.
51. Christodoulou J, Gladys H. MECP2-Related Disorders; 2001. Last update 2012. GeneReviews. Available at <http://www.ncbi.nlm.nih.gov/books/NBK1497/>.
52. Kohli SS, Kohli VS. A comprehensive review of the genetic basis of cleft lip and palate. *J Oral Maxillofac Pathol*. 2012;16(1):64-72.

53. Unpublished recommendations courtesy of Julie Hoover-Fong, M.D., Ph.D., Director, Greenberg Center for Skeletal Dysplasias, McKusick-Nathans Institute of Genetic Medicine, Johns Hopkins, Baltimore, MD.
54. Peredo DE, Hannibal MC. The floppy infant: evaluation of hypotonia. *Pediatr Rev*. 2009;30:e66-e76.
55. Lisi EC, Cohn RD. Genetic evaluation of the pediatric patient with hypotonia: perspective from a hypotonia specialty clinic and review of the literature. *Dev Med Child Neurol*. 2011;53:586-599.
56. Allanson JE, Roberts AE. Noonan Syndrome; 2001. Last update 2011. GeneReviews. Available at <http://www.ncbi.nlm.nih.gov/books/NBK1124/>.
57. Romano AA, et al. Noonan Syndrome: Clinical Features, Diagnosis, and Management Guidelines. *Pediatrics*. 2010;126(4):746-759.
58. Hersh JH, Saul RA; Committee on Genetics. Health supervision for children with Fragile X syndrome. *Pediatrics*. 2011;127:994-1006.
59. American Academy of Pediatrics, Committee on Bioethics. Ethical issues with genetic testing in pediatrics. *Pediatrics*. 2001:107(6):1451-1455.
60. Cohen J, Hoon A, Wilms Floet AM. Providing family guidance in rapidly shifting sand: informed consent for genetic testing. *Dev Med Child Neurol*. 2013:55:766-769.
61. The American Society of Human Genetics Social Issues Subcommittee on Familial Disclosure. Professional Disclosure of Familial Genetic Information. *Am J Hum Genet*. 1998; 62:474-483.
62. Green RC, Berg JS, Grody WW, et al. American College of Medical Genetics and Genomics (ACMG) recommendations for reporting of incidental findings in clinical exome and genome sequencing. *Genet Med*. 2013;15(7):565-574.
63. Leslie N, et al. Glycogen Storage Disease Type II (Pompe Disease); 2007. Lasted update 2013. GeneReviews. Available at <https://www.ncbu.nlm.nih.gov/books/NBK12V1>.

Chapter 14
Hematology
Katherine Costa, MD

I. WEB RESOURCES
- http://g6pddeficiency.org/index.php?cmd=contraindicated
- www.redcrossblood.org

II. ANEMIA

A. General Evaluation
Anemia is defined as a reduction in hemoglobin (Hb) two standard deviations below the mean, based on age-specific norms (Table 14.1). Evaluation should include:
1. **Complete history,** including nutrition, menstruation, ethnicity, fatigue, pica, medication exposure, growth and development, blood loss, hyperbilirubinemia and family history of anemia, splenectomy, or cholecystectomy
2. **Physical examination,** including evaluation of pallor, tachycardia, cardiac murmur, jaundice, hepatosplenomegaly, glossitis, tachypnea, koilonychia, angular cheilitis, or signs of systemic illness
3. **Initial laboratory tests** including complete blood cell count (CBC) with red blood cell (RBC) indices [mean corpuscular volume (MCV), mean corpuscular hemoglobin (MCH), red cell distribution width (RDW)], reticulocyte count, stool for occult blood, urinalysis, and serum bilirubin. Complete evaluation always includes a peripheral blood smear

B. Diagnosis
Anemias may be categorized as macrocytic, microcytic, or normocytic. Table 14.2 gives an approach to diagnosis based on RBC production as measured by reticulocyte count and cell size. Note that normal ranges for Hb and MCV are age dependent.

C. Evaluation of Specific Causes of Anemia (Decreased Production, Hemorrhage, or Increased Destruction)
1. **Iron-deficiency anemia:** Hypochromic/microcytic anemia with a low reticulocyte count and an elevated RDW.
   a. Serum ferritin reflects total body iron stores after age 6 months, and is the first value to fall in iron deficiency; may be falsely elevated with inflammation or infection.
   b. Other indicators: Low serum iron, elevated total iron-binding capacity (TIBC), low mean corpuscular hemoglobin concentration (MCHC), elevated transferrin receptor level, and low reticulocyte Hb content.

TABLE 14.1
AGE-SPECIFIC BLOOD CELL INDICES

Age	Hb (g/dL)*	HCT (%)*	MCV (fL)*	MCHC (g/dL RBC)*	Reticulocytes	WBCs (×10³/mL)†	Platelets (10³/mL)†
26-30 wk gestation[‡]	13.4 (11)	41.5 (34.9)	118.2 (106.7)	37.9 (30.6)	—	4.4 (2.7)	254 (180-327)
28 wk	14.5	45	120	31.0	(5-10)	—	275
32 wk	15.0	47	118	32.0	(3-10)	—	290
Term[§] (cord)	16.5 (13.5)	51 (42)	108 (98)	33.0 (30.0)	(3-7)	18.1 (9-30)[∥]	290
1-3 days	18.5 (14.5)	56 (45)	108 (95)	33.0 (29.0)	(1.8-4.6)	18.9 (9.4-34)	192
2 wk	16.6 (13.4)	53 (41)	105 (88)	31.4 (28.1)	—	11.4 (5-20)	252
1 mo	13.9 (10.7)	44 (33)	101 (91)	31.8 (28.1)	(0.1-1.7)	10.8 (4-19.5)	—
2 mo	11.2 (9.4)	35 (28)	95 (84)	31.8 (28.3)	—	—	—
6 mo	12.6 (11.1)	36 (31)	76 (68)	35.0 (32.7)	(0.7-2.3)	11.9 (6-17.5)	—
6 mo-2 yr	12.0 (10.5)	36 (33)	78 (70)	33.0 (30.0)	—	10.6 (6-17)	(150-350)
2-6 yr	12.5 (11.5)	37 (34)	81 (75)	34.0 (31.0)	(0.5-1.0)	8.5 (5-15.5)	(150-350)
6-12 yr	13.5 (11.5)	40 (35)	86 (77)	34.0 (31.0)	(0.5-1.0)	8.1 (4.5-13.5)	(150-350)
12-18 YR							
Male	14.5 (13)	43 (36)	88 (78)	34.0 (31.0)	(0.5-1.0)	7.8 (4.5-13.5)	(150-350)
Female	14.0 (12)	41 (37)	90 (78)	34.0 (31.0)	(0.5-1.0)	7.8 (4.5-13.5)	(150-350)
ADULT							
Male	15.5 (13.5)	47 (41)	90 (80)	34.0 (31.0)	(0.8-2.5)	7.4 (4.5-11)	(150-350)
Female	14.0 (12)	41 (36)	90 (80)	34.0 (31.0)	(0.8-4.1)	7.4 (4.5-11)	(150-350)

Hb, Hemoglobin; HCT, hematocrit; MCHC, mean cell hemoglobin concentration; MCV, mean corpuscular volume; RBC, red blood cell; WBC, white blood cell
*Data are mean (−2 SD)
†Data are mean (±2 SD)
‡Values are from fetal samplings.
§1 mo, capillary hemoglobin exceeds venous: 1 hr: 3.6-g difference; 5 day: 2.2-g difference; 3 wk: 1.1-g difference
∥Mean (95% confidence limits)

Data from Forestier F, Dattos F, Galacteros F, et al. Hematologic values of 163 normal fetuses between 18 and 30 weeks of gestation. Pediat Res. 1986;20:342; Oski FA, Naiman JL. Hematological Problems in the Newborn Infant. Philadelphia: WB Saunders; 1982; Nathan D, Oski FA. Hematology of Infancy and Childhood. Philadelphia: WB Saunders; 1998; Matoth Y, Zaizor K, Varsano I, et al. Postnatal changes in some red cell parameters. Acta Paediatr Scand. 1971;60:317; and Wintrobe MM. Clinical Hematology. Baltimore: Williams & Wilkins; 1999.

TABLE 14.2
CLASSIFICATION OF ANEMIA

Reticulocyte Count	Microcytic Anemia	Normocytic Anemia	Macrocytic Anemia
Low	Iron deficiency Lead poisoning Chronic disease Aluminum toxicity Copper deficiency Protein malnutrition	Chronic disease RBC aplasia (TEC, infection, drug–induced) Malignancy Juvenile rheumatoid arthritis Endocrinopathies Renal failure	Folate deficiency Vitamin B_{12} deficiency Aplastic anemia Congenital bone marrow dysfunction (Diamond–Blackfan or Fanconi syndromes) Drug–induced Trisomy 21 Hypothyroidism
Normal	Thalassemia trait Sideroblastic anemia	Acute bleeding Hypersplenism Dyserythropoietic anemia II	—
High	Thalassemia syndromes Hemoglobin C disorders	Antibody-mediated hemolysis Hypersplenism Microangiopathy (HUS, TTP, DIC, Kasabach–Merritt) Membranopathies (spherocytosis, elliptocytosis) Enzyme disorders (G6PD, pyruvate kinase) Hemoglobinopathies	Dyserythropoietic anemia I, III Active hemolysis

DIC, Disseminated intravascular coagulation; G6PD, glucose-6-phosphate dehydrogenase; HUS, hemolytic-uremic syndrome; RBC, red blood cell; TEC, transient erythroblastopenia of childhood; TTP, thrombotic thrombocytopenic purpura
Data from Nathan D, Oski FA. Hematology of Infancy and Childhood. 6th ed. Philadelphia: WB Saunders; 2003.

    c. Iron therapy should result in an increased reticulocyte count in 2–3 days and an increase in hematocrit (HCT) after 1–4 weeks of therapy. Iron stores are generally repleted after 3 months of therapy.
    d. Mentzer index (MCV/RBC): Index > 13.5 suggests iron deficiency; expect elevated RDW. Mentzer index < 11.5 suggests thalassemia minor; expect low/normal RDW.
2. **Physiologic anemia of infancy (physiologic nadir):** Decrease in Hb until oxygen needs exceed oxygen delivery, usually at Hb of 9–11 mg/dL. Normally occurs at age 8–12 weeks for full-term infants and age 3–6 weeks for preterm infants.

3. **Anemia of chronic inflammation:** Usually normocytic with normal-to-low reticulocyte count. Iron studies reveal low iron, TIBC, and transferrin and elevated ferritin.
4. **Red cell aplasia:** Variable cell size, low reticulocyte count, variable platelet and white blood cell (WBC) counts. Bone marrow aspiration for evaluation of RBC precursors in the marrow may detect marrow dysfunction, neoplasm, or specific signs of infection.
a. Acquired aplasias:
   (1) Infectious causes: Parvovirus in children with rapid RBC turnover (infects RBC precursors), Epstein–Barr virus, cytomegalovirus (CMV), human herpesvirus type 6, or human immunodeficiency virus (HIV).
   (2) Transient erythroblastopenia of childhood (TEC): Occurs from age 6 months to 4 years, with > 80% of cases presenting after age 1 year with a normal or slightly low MCV and low reticulocyte count. Spontaneous recovery usually occurs within 4–8 weeks.
   (3) Exposures include radiation and various drugs and chemicals (including lead).
b. Congenital aplasias: Typically macrocytic anemias
   (1) Fanconi anemia: Autosomal recessive disorder, usually presents before 10 years of age; may present with pancytopenia. Patients may have thumb abnormalities, renal anomalies, microcephaly, or short stature. Chromosomal fragility studies can be diagnostic.
   (2) Diamond–Blackfan anemia: Autosomal recessive pure RBC aplasia; presents in the first year of life. Associated with congenital anomalies in 30%–47%[13] of cases, including triphalangeal thumb, short stature, and cleft lip.
c. Aplastic anemia: Idiopathic bone marrow failure, usually macrocytic.
5. **Hemolytic anemia:** Rapid RBC turnover. Etiologies: Congenital membranopathies, hemoglobinopathies, enzymopathies, metabolic defects, thrombotic microangiopathies (see Thrombocytopenia, below), and immune-mediated destruction. Useful studies include:
a. Reticulocyte count: Usually elevated; indicates increased production of RBCs to compensate for increased destruction.
b. Corrected reticulocyte count (CRC) accounts for differences in HCT, and is an indicator of erythropoietic activity. CRC > 1.5 suggests increased RBC production secondary to hemolysis or blood loss.

$$CRC = \%Reticulocytes \times Patient\ HCT/Normal\ HCT$$

c. Plasma aspartate aminotransferase (AST) and lactate dehydrogenase (LDH): Increased from release of intracellular enzymes. Serum LDH levels are significantly elevated in intravascular hemolysis and mildly elevated in extravascular hemolysis.
d. Haptoglobin: Binds free Hb; decreased with intravascular and extravascular hemolysis. Can also be decreased in patients with liver

dysfunction secondary to decreased hepatic synthesis and in neonates.
e. Direct Coombs test: Tests for presence of antibody or complement on patient RBCs. May be falsely negative if affected cells have already been destroyed or antibody titer is low.
f. Indirect Coombs test: Tests for free autoantibody in patient's serum after RBC antibody binding sites are saturated. Positive indirect test with negative direct test is typical of alloimmune sensitization (e.g., transfusion reaction).
g. Osmotic fragility test: Useful in diagnosis of hereditary spherocytosis. Can also be positive in ABO incompatibility, autoimmune hemolytic anemia, or anytime spherocytes are present.
h. Glucose-6-phosphate dehydrogenase (G6PD) assay: Quantitative test to diagnose G6PD deficiency, an X-linked disorder affecting 10%–14% of African-American males. May be normal immediately after a hemolytic episode because older, more enzyme-deficient cells have been lysed. For a comprehensive list of oxidizing drugs, go to http://g6pddeficiency.org/index.php?cmd=contraindicated.
i. Heinz body preparation: Detects precipitated Hb within RBCs; present in unstable hemoglobinopathies and enzymopathies during oxidative stress (e.g., G6PD deficiency).

III. HEMOGLOBINOPATHIES

A. Hemoglobin Electrophoresis
Involves separation of Hb variants based on molecular charge and size. All positive sickle preparations and solubility tests for sickle Hb (e.g., Sickledex) should be confirmed with electrophoresis or isoelectric focusing (component of mandatory newborn screening in many states). Table 14.3 outlines neonatal Hb electrophoresis patterns.

B. Sickle Cell Anemia
Caused by a genetic defect in β-globin; 8% of African Americans are carriers; 1 in 500 African Americans have sickle cell anemia.
1. **Diagnosis:** Often made on newborn screen with Hb electrophoresis. The sickle preparation and Sickledex are rapid tests that are positive in all sickle hemoglobinopathies. False-negative test results may be seen in neonates and other patients with a high percentage of fetal Hb.
2. **Complications (Table 14.4):** A hematologist should be consulted.
3. **Health maintenance**[1,2]**:** Ongoing consultation and clinical involvement with a pediatric hematologist and/or sickle cell program are essential (Table 14.5).
4. **Hb electrophoresis (outside neonatal period):** Hb SF, SCF, SAF—other Hb combinations may sickle (see Table 14.3).

TABLE 14.3
NEONATAL HEMOGLOBIN (HB) ELECTROPHORESIS PATTERNS*

FA	Fetal Hb and adult normal Hb; the normal newborn pattern.
FAV	Indicates presence of both HbF and HbA, but an anomalous band (V) is present that does not appear to be any of the common Hb variants.
FAS	Indicates fetal Hb, adult normal HbA, and HbS, consistent with benign sickle cell trait.
FS	Fetal and sickle HbS without detectable adult normal HbA. Consistent with clinically significant homozygous sickle Hb genotype (S/S) or sickle β-thalassemia, with manifestations of sickle cell anemia during childhood.
FC[†]	Designates presence of HbC without adult normal HbA. Consistent with clinically significant homozygous HbC genotype (C/C), resulting in a mild hematologic disorder presenting during childhood.
FSC	HbS and HbC present. This heterozygous condition could lead to manifestations of sickle cell disease during childhood.
FAC	HbC and adult normal HbA present, consistent with benign HbC trait.
FSA	Heterozygous HbS/β-thalassemia, a clinically significant sickling disorder.
F[†]	Fetal HbF is present without adult normal HbA. May indicate delayed appearance of HbA, but is also consistent with homozygous β-thalassemia major or homozygous hereditary persistence of fetal HbF.
FV[†]	Fetal HbF and an anomalous Hb variant (V) are present.
AF	May indicate prior blood transfusion. Submit another filter paper blood specimen when infant is 4 mo of age, at which time the transfused blood cells should have been cleared.

NOTE: HbA: $\alpha_2\beta_2$; HbF: $\alpha_2\gamma_2$; HbA$_2$: $\alpha_2\delta_2$
*Hemoglobin variants are reported in order of decreasing abundance; for example, FA indicates more fetal than adult hemoglobin.
[†]Repeat blood specimen should be submitted to confirm original interpretation.

C. Thalassemias

Defects in α- or β-globin production. The predominant adult hemoglobin is HbA ($\alpha_2\beta_2$), a tetramer composed of two α- and two β-chains. α-globin production is dependent on four genes, and β-globin production is dependent on two genes. Imbalance in production of globin chains leads to precipitation of excess chains, causing ineffective erythropoiesis and shortened survival of mature RBCs.

1. **α-Thalassemias:**
a. Silent carriers (α–/αα): not anemic, childhood and adult Hb electrophoresis usually normal.
b. α-Thalassemia trait (α–/α–) or (αα/––): Causes mild microcytic anemia from birth; childhood and adult Hb electrophoresis usually normal. Hb Barts can be seen in infancy (e.g., on state newborn screens) in patients with α-thalassemia trait.
c. HbH disease (β$_4$) (α–/––): Causes moderately severe anemia from birth; HbH (β-tetramer) may be seen on newborn screen and subsequent electrophoresis.
d. Hb Bart/hydrops fetalis (––/––): Hb Barts (γ$_4$) cannot deliver oxygen; usually fatal *in utero* or in neonatal period.

TABLE 14.4
SICKLE CELL DISEASE COMPLICATIONS

Complication	Evaluation	Treatment
Fever (T ≥ 38.5°C)	History and physical CBC with differential Reticulocyte count Blood cultures Chest X-ray Other cultures as indicated	IV antibiotics (third-generation cephalosporin, other antibiotics as indicated, especially if penicillin-resistant pneumococcus suspected) Admit if ill appearing, aged <3 yr, concerning lab results, or complications Some centers use antibiotics with a long half-life and reevaluate in 24 h as an outpatient
Vaso-occlusive crisis Children < 2 yr, dactylitis Children > 2 yr, unifocal or multifocal pain	History and physical CBC with differential Reticulocyte count Type and screen	Oral analgesics as an outpatient, as tolerated IV analgesics and IV fluids if outpatient therapy fails (parenteral narcotics in form of PCA and parenteral NSAIDs, usually in combination) Aggressive early treatment of pain is essential
Acute chest syndrome (new pulmonary infiltrate with fever, cough, chest pain, tachypnea, dyspnea, or hypoxia)	History and physical CBC with differential Reticulocyte count Blood cultures Chest X-ray Type and screen	Admit O_2, incentive spirometry, bronchodilators IV antibiotics (third-generation cephalosporin and macrolide) Analgesia, IV fluids Simple transfusion or partial exchange for moderately severe illness; double the packed cell volume exchange transfusion for severe or rapidly progressing illness High-dose dexamethasone controversial (risk of readmission for pain or other SCD-related issues)[9]

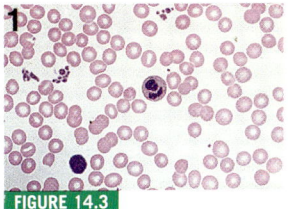

FIGURE 14.3

Normal smear. Round RBCs with central pallor about one-third of the cell's diameter, scattered platelets, occasional white blood cells.

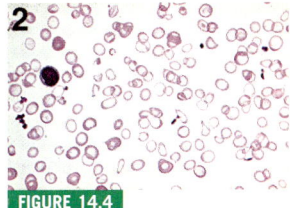

FIGURE 14.4

Iron deficiency. Hypochromic/microcytic RBCs, poikilocytosis, plentiful platelets, occasional ovalocytes and target cells.

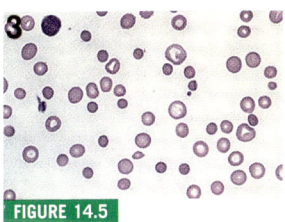

FIGURE 14.5

Spherocytosis. Microspherocytes a hallmark (densely stained RBCs with no central pallor).

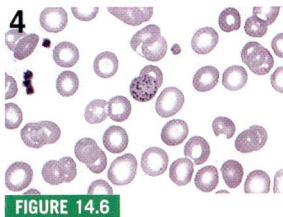

FIGURE 14.6

Basophilic stippling as a result of precipitated RNA throughout the cell; seen with heavy metal intoxication, thalassemia, iron deficiency, and other states of ineffective erythropoiesis.

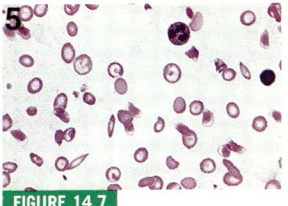

FIGURE 14.7

Hemoglobin SS disease. Sickled cells, target cells, hypochromia, poikilocytosis, Howell–Jolly bodies; nucleated RBCs common (not shown).

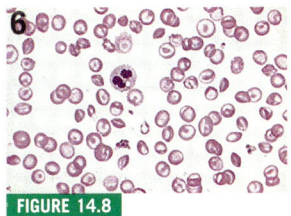

FIGURE 14.8

Hemoglobin SC disease. Target cells, oat cells, poikilocytosis; sickle forms rarely seen.

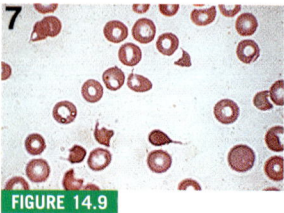

FIGURE 14.9
Microangiopathic hemolytic anemia. RBC fragments, anisocytosis, polychromasia, decreased platelets.

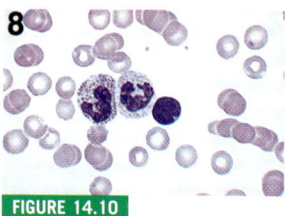

FIGURE 14.10
Toxic granulations. Prominent dark blue primary granules; commonly seen with infection and other toxic states (e.g., Kawasaki disease).

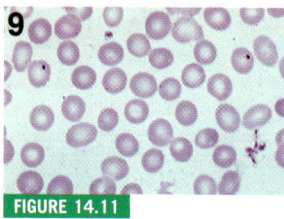

FIGURE 14.11
Howell–Jolly body. Small, dense nuclear remnant in an RBC; suggests splenic dysfunction or asplenia.

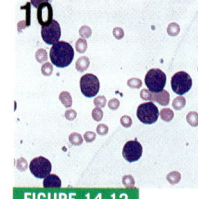

FIGURE 14.12
Leukemic blasts showing large nucleus-to-cytoplasm ratio.

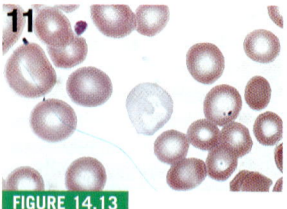

FIGURE 14.13
Polychromatophilia. Diffusely basophilic because of RNA staining; seen with early release of reticulocytes from the marrow.

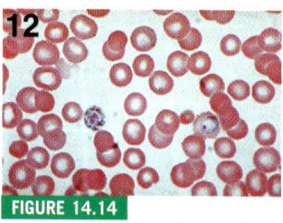

FIGURE 14.14
Malaria. Intraerythrocytic parasites.

TABLE 14.4
SICKLE CELL DISEASE COMPLICATIONS—cont'd

Complication	Evaluation	Treatment
Splenic sequestration (acutely enlarged spleen and Hb level ≥ 2 g/dL below patient's baseline)	History and physical CBC Reticulocyte count Type and screen	Serial abdominal exams IV fluids and fluid resuscitation as necessary RBC transfusion or, in severe cases, exchange transfusion for cardiovascular compromise and Hb < 4.5 g/dL. (Autotransfusion may occur with recovery, leading to increased Hb and CHF. Transfuse cautiously)
Aplastic crisis (acute illness with Hb below patient's baseline and low reticulocyte count; may follow viral illnesses, especially parvovirus B19)	History and physical CBC with differential Reticulocyte count Type and screen Parvovirus serology and polymerase chain reaction	Admit IV fluids PRBCs for symptomatic anemia Isolation to protect susceptible individuals and women of childbearing age until parvovirus excluded
Other complications: Priapism, CVA, TIA, gallbladder disease, avascular necrosis, hyphema*		

NOTE: CVA requires emergency transfusion guided by a hematologist and a neurologist experienced with sickle cell disease. Exchange transfusion preferable to simple transfusion if possible.[10]
*Hyphema in a patient with sickle cell trait is an ophthalmologic emergency.
CBC, Complete blood cell count; CHF, congestive heart failure; CVA, cerebrovascular accident; Hb, hemoglobin; IV, intravenous; NSAIDs, nonsteroidal antiinflammatory drugs; PCA, patient-controlled analgesia; PRBCs, packed red blood cells; RBC, red blood cells; SCD, sickle cell disease; T, temperature; TIA, transient ischemic attack.

2. **β-Thalassemia:** Found throughout the Mediterranean, Middle East, India, and Southeast Asia. Ineffective erythropoiesis is more severe in β-thalassemia than α-thalassemia because excess α-chain tetramers are more unstable than β-chain tetramers. Adult Hb electrophoresis with decreased Hb A, increased Hb A_2, and increased Hb F.
  a. Thalassemia trait/thalassemia minor (β/β+) or (β/β0): Mildly decreased β-globin production. Usually asymptomatic, with microcytosis out of proportion to anemia, sometimes with erythrocytosis.
  b. Thalassemia intermedia (β+/β+): Markedly decreased β-globin production. Presents at about age 2 years with moderate compensated anemia that may become symptomatic, leading to heart failure, pulmonary hypertension, splenomegaly, and bony expansion, usually in second or third decade of life.

TABLE 14.5
SICKLE CELL DISEASE HEALTH MAINTENANCE

Immunizations	Maintenance
Pneumococcal vaccine	Give 13-valent conjugate vaccine per routine childhood schedule; give 23-valent polysaccharide vaccine at age 2 years followed by booster 5 years after 1st dose (age 7 years).
Meningococcal vaccine (Menactra)	Give 2-dose primary series 8–12 weeks apart, starting at age 2 years. Give booster 3 years after primary series (age 5 years) and then every 5 years.
Influenza vaccine	Vaccinate yearly beginning at age 6 mo.
MEDICATIONS	
PCN	Begin as soon as SCD diagnosis made (125 mg BID; increase dose to 250 mg BID at age 3 years*).
Folic acid	Consider supplementation, start by age 1 year.
Hydroxyurea	Offer to all patients ≥ 9 months of age. Requires close monitoring.[†]
Contraceptives	Consider progestin-only or nonhormonal options to limit risk of stroke.
IMAGING	
Transcranial Doppler (TCD)	Perform annually from ages 2 to 16 years to evaluate for increased risk of cerebrovascular accident (CVA).
OTHER	
Ophthalmology	Refer annually from age 10 years to evaluate for sickle cell retinopathy.
Growth and development, school/social issues, counseling regarding fevers	Review closely at all visits.

*Prophylaxis may be discontinued by age 5 years if patient has no prior severe pneumococcal infections or splenectomy and has documented pneumococcal vaccinations, including second 23-valent vaccination. Practice patterns vary. Some continue penicillin indefinitely.
[†]Increases levels of fetal Hb and decreases HbS polymerization in cells. Has been shown to significantly decrease episodes of vaso-occlusive crises, dactylitis, acute chest syndrome, number of transfusions, and hospitalizations.[14] May decrease mortality in adults.
PCN, Penicillin; SCD, sickle cell disease
Data from Yawn BP, Buchanan GR, Afenyi-Annan AN, et al. Management of sickle cell disease: summary of the 2014 evidence-based report by expert panel members. JAMA. 2014;312(10):1033-1048.

c. Thalassemia major/Cooley anemia (β0/β0, β+/β0, or β+/β+): Minimal to no β-globin production. Presence of anemia within first 6 months of life, with hepatosplenomegaly and progressive bone marrow expansion that may lead to frontal bossing, maxillary hyperplasia, and other skeletal deformities. Regular transfusions required to avoid anemia.

IV. NEUTROPENIA

An absolute neutrophil count (ANC) < 1500/μL, although neutrophil counts vary with age (Table 14.6). Severe neutropenia is defined as an ANC < 500/μL. Children with significant neutropenia are at risk for

TABLE 14.6
AGE-SPECIFIC LEUKOCYTE DIFFERENTIAL

Age	Total Leukocytes* Mean (Range)	Neutrophils† Mean (Range)	%	Lymphocytes Mean (Range)	%	Monocytes Mean	%	Eosinophils Mean	%
Birth	18.1 (9–30)	11 (6–26)	61	5.5 (2–11)	31	1.1	6	0.4	2
12 hr	22.8 (13–38)	15.5 (6–28)	68	5.5 (2–11)	24	1.2	5	0.5	2
24 hr	18.9 (9.4–34)	11.5 (5–21)	61	5.8 (2–11.5)	31	1.1	6	0.5	2
1 wk	12.2 (5–21)	5.5 (1.5–10)	45	5.0 (2–17)	41	1.1	9	0.5	4
2 wk	11.4 (5–20)	4.5 (1–9.5)	40	5.5 (2–17)	48	1.0	9	0.4	3
1 mo	10.8 (5–19.5)	3.8 (1–8.5)	35	6.0 (2.5–16.5)	56	0.7	7	0.3	3
6 mo	11.9 (6–17.5)	3.8 (1–8.5)	32	7.3 (4–13.5)	61	0.6	5	0.3	3
1 yr	11.4 (6–17.5)	3.5 (1.5–8.5)	31	7.0 (4–10.5)	61	0.6	5	0.3	3
2 yr	10.6 (6–17)	3.5 (1.5–8.5)	33	6.3 (3–9.5)	59	0.5	5	0.3	3
4 yr	9.1 (5.5–15.5)	3.8 (1.5–8.5)	42	4.5 (2–8)	50	0.5	5	0.3	3
6 yr	8.5 (5–14.5)	4.3 (1.5–8)	51	3.5 (1.5–7)	42	0.4	5	0.2	3
8 yr	8.3 (4.5–13.5)	4.4 (1.5–8)	53	3.3 (1.5–6.8)	39	0.4	4	0.2	2
10 yr	8.1 (4.5–13.5)	4.4 (1.5–8.5)	54	3.1 (1.5–6.5)	38	0.4	4	0.2	2
16 yr	7.8 (4.5–13.0)	4.4 (1.8–8)	57	2.8 (1.2–5.2)	35	0.4	5	0.2	3
21 yr	7.4 (4.5–11.0)	4.4 (1.8–7.7)	59	2.5 (1–4.8)	34	0.3	4	0.2	3

*Numbers of leukocytes are ×10³/µL; ranges are estimates of 95% confidence limits; percentages refer to differential counts.
†Neutrophils include band cells at all ages and a small number of metamyelocytes and myelocytes in the first few days of life.
Adapted from Cairo MS, Brauho F. Blood and blood-forming tissues. In: Randolph AM, ed. Pediatrics. 21st ed. New York: McGraw-Hill; 2003.

bacterial and fungal infections. Granulocyte colony-stimulating factor may be indicated. Transient neutropenia secondary to viral illness rarely causes significant morbidity. Autoimmune neutropenia is a common cause of neutropenia in children 6 months to 6 years. Testing for antineutrophil antibodies is indicated in this age group, and may obviate the need for more extensive workup. For management of fever and neutropenia in oncology patients, see Chapter 22, Fig. 22.1. Box 14.1 lists causes.

V. THROMBOCYTOPENIA

A. Definition

Platelet count < 150,000/µL. Clinically significant bleeding is unlikely with platelet counts > 20,000/µL in the absence of other complicating factors.

B. Causes of Thrombocytopenia

1. **Idiopathic thrombocytopenic purpura (ITP):** A diagnosis of exclusion; can be acute or chronic. WBC count, Hb level, and peripheral blood smear are normal. Risk of intracranial hemorrhage (ICH) is 0.5%, associated with history of head trauma, mucosal bleeding, hematuria, and platelet count < 10,000. Treatment indicated for ICH, other

BOX 14.1
DIFFERENTIAL DIAGNOSIS OF CHILDHOOD NEUTROPENIA

Acquired	Congenital
Infection	Cyclic neutropenia
Immune-mediated	Severe congenital neutropenia (e.g., Kostmann syndrome)
Chronic benign neutropenia of childhood	Shwachman–Diamond syndrome
Hypersplenism	Fanconi anemia
Vitamin B_{12}, folate, copper deficiency	Metabolic disorders (e.g., aminoacidopathies, Barth syndrome, glycogen storage disorders)
Drugs or toxic substances	
Aplastic anemia	
Malignancies or preleukemic disorders	Osteopetrosis
Ionizing radiation	Neutropenia with pigmentation abnormalities (e.g., Chédiak–Higashi anomaly)

symptomatic bleeding, or at increased risk of ICH; otherwise, may monitor, as acute ITP is likely to self-resolve within 6 months.[3]

a. Treatment options:
   (1) Observation
   (2) Intravenous immune globulin (see Formulary for dosing).
   (3) Corticosteroids (consider bone marrow biopsy prior to administering steroids in case of leukemia or aplastic anemia)
   (4) Anti-Rh (D) immune globulin (WinRho). Useful only in Rh-positive, nonsplenectomized patients. Should not be used in patients with preexisting hemolysis or renal disease; monitor for signs of intravascular hemolysis after administration. Disseminated intravascular coagulation (DIC) has been reported. See package insert for black box warning and monitoring guidelines.
   (5) Platelet transfusions, only in life-threatening bleeding.
   (6) Consider rituximab, splenectomy, or chemotherapy in chronic ITP.[4]

2. **Neonatal thrombocytopenia.** May be caused by:
a. Decreased production: Results from aplastic disorders, congenital malignancy such as leukemia, and viral infections.
b. Increased consumption: Usually result of DIC due to infection or asphyxia.
c. Immune mediated: Immunoglobulin G (IgG) or complement attach to platelets and cause destruction. Specific causes include preeclampsia, sepsis, maternal ITP, and platelet alloimmunization.
   (1) Neonatal alloimmune thrombocytopenia (NAIT): Transplacental maternal antibodies (usually against paternally inherited PLA-1/HPA-1a) cause fetal platelet destruction. High risk of *in utero* or neonatal ICH. If severely thrombocytopenic, a transfusion of

maternal platelets will be more effective than random donor platelets in raising infant's platelet count.
   i. Evaluation/diagnosis:
      (a) Exclude maternal ITP: check maternal platelet count and platelet-associated IgG. Mother's platelet count should be normal and platelet-associated IgG negative.
      (b) Confirm NAIT: maternal and paternal platelet antigen typing, and mixing study of maternal or neonatal plasma against minor platelet antigen panel or paternal platelets and/or direct identification of maternal antibodies against paternal PLA-1a/HPA-1a.
3. **Microangiopathies**
a. Characterized by microangiopathic hemolytic anemia (MAHA), thrombocytopenia, and end-organ injury (renal failure, neurologic changes)
b. Causes: Intravascular prostheses, hypersplenism, drug-induced, malignant hypertension, DIC, systemic infection, SLE, malignancy, s/p BMT or solid organ transplant, HELLP syndrome, or primary thrombotic microangiopathy (TMA)
c. Primary TMAs include Shiga toxin–mediated hemolytic-uremic syndrome (ST-HUS); complement-mediated TMA, drug-mediated TMA (immune versus direct toxicity), metabolism-mediated TMA, coagulation-mediated TMA, and thrombotic thrombocytopenic purpura (TTP)[5]
   (1) ST-HUS: Triad of MAHA, thrombocytopenia, and acute renal failure. Associated with *Escherichia coli* O157:H7 and *Shigella*, although *S. pneumococcus* and HIV have also been linked to HUS. Supportive care includes packed red blood cells (PRBCs) and platelet transfusions as needed, careful fluid and electrolyte management, antihypertensives, and close monitoring for any neurologic complications. Avoid blood products in patients with HUS thought to be secondary to pneumococcal infection.
   (2) Complement-mediated TMA: May use eculizumab.
   (3) TTP: Caused by decreased activity of ADAMTS13 either by inherited mutation or by acquired inhibitor (more common in adults). Acquired TTP is lethal if not managed aggressively with plasma exchange and corticosteroids.
   (4) DIC (see Box 14.5)
4. **Other causes of thrombocytopenia:** Infection-induced marrow suppression, malignancy, myelodysplasia or marrow infiltration, HIV, drug-induced thrombocytopenia, cavernous hemangiomas (Kasabach–Merritt syndrome), thrombocytopenia with absent radii syndrome (TAR), thrombosis, hypersplenism, and other rare inherited disorders (e.g., Wiskott–Aldrich, Paris-Trousseau, Noonan, and DiGeorge syndromes; myosin 9–associated megaplatelet disorders; chromosomal abnormalities).

VI. COAGULATION

See Fig. 14.1.

A. Tests of Coagulation

An incorrect anticoagulant-to-blood ratio will give inaccurate results. Table 14.7 lists normal hematologic values for coagulation testing.

1. **Activated partial thromboplastin time (aPTT):** Measures intrinsic system; requires factors V, VIII, IX, X, XI, XII, fibrinogen, and prothrombin. May be prolonged in heparin administration, hemophilia, von Willebrand disease (vWD), DIC, and in the presence of circulating inhibitors (e.g., lupus anticoagulants).
2. **Prothrombin time (PT):** Measures extrinsic pathway; requires factors V, VII, X, fibrinogen, and prothrombin. May be prolonged in warfarin administration, deficiencies of vitamin K–associated factors, malabsorption, liver disease, DIC, and the presence of circulating inhibitors.
3. **Platelet function testing:** Platelet aggregation and the Platelet Function Analyzer-100 (PFA-100) system are *in vitro* methods for measuring platelet function. Bleeding time (BT) evaluates clot formation,

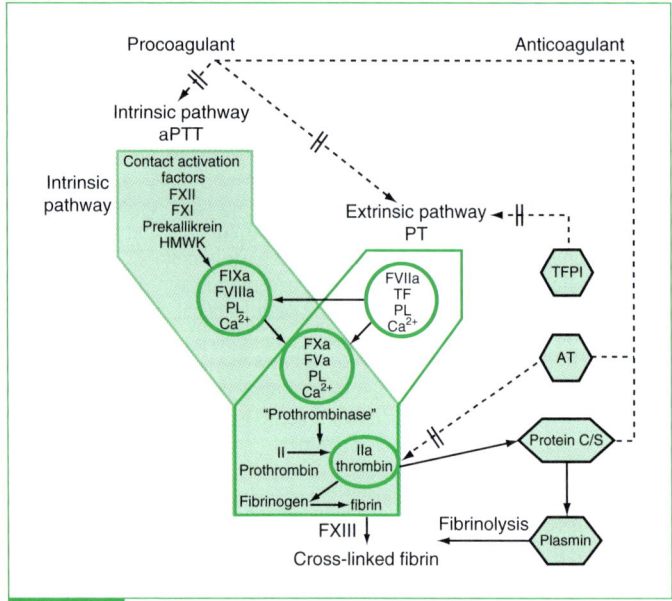

FIGURE 14.1

Coagulation cascade. AT, Antithrombin; F, factor; HMWK, high-molecular-weight kininogen; PL, phospholipid; TF, tissue factor; TFPI, tissue factor pathway inhibitor. *(Adaptation courtesy James Casella and Clifford Takemoto.)*

TABLE 14.7
AGE-SPECIFIC COAGULATION VALUES

Coagulation Test	Preterm Infant (30–36 wk), Day of Life 1*	Term Infant, Day of Life 1	Day of Life 3	1 mo–1 yr	1–5 yr	6–10 yr	11–16 yr	Adult
PT (s)	13.0 (10.6–16.2)	15.6 (14.4–16.4)	14.9 (13.5–16.4)	13.1 (11.5–15.3)	13.3 (12.1–14.5)	13.4 (11.7–15.1)	13.8 (12.7–16.1)	13.0 (11.5–14.5)
INR		1.26 (1.15–1.35)	1.20 (1.05–1.35)	1.00 (0.86–1.22)	1.03 (0.92–1.14)	1.04 (0.87–1.20)	1.08 (0.97–1.30)	1.00 (0.80–1.20)
aPTT (s)†	53.6 (27.5–79.4)	38.7 (34.3–44.8)	36.3 (29.5–42.2)	39.3 (35.1–46.3)	37.7 (33.6–43.8)	37.3 (31.8–43.7)	39.5 (33.9–46.1)	33.2 (28.6–38.2)
Fibrinogen (g/L)	2.43 (1.50–3.73)	2.80 (1.92–3.74)	3.30 (2.83–4.01)	2.42 (0.82–3.83)	2.82 (1.62–4.01)	3.04 (1.99–4.09)	3.15 (2.12–4.33)	3.1 (1.9–4.3)
Bleeding time (min)*					6 (2.5–10)	7 (2.5–13)	5 (3–8)	4 (1–7)
Thrombin time (s)	14 (11–17)	12 (10–16)*		17.1 (16.3–17.6)	17.5 (16.5–18.2)	17.1 (16.1–18.5)	16.9 (16.2–17.6)	16.6 (16.2–17.2)
Factor II (U/mL)	0.45 (0.20–0.77)	0.54 (0.41–0.69)	0.62 (0.50–0.73)	0.90 (0.62–1.03)	0.89 (0.70–1.09)	0.89 (0.67–1.10)	0.90 (0.61–1.07)	1.10 (0.78–1.38)
Factor V (U/mL)	0.88 (0.41–1.44)	0.81 (0.64–1.03)	1.22 (0.92–1.54)	1.13 (0.94–1.41)	0.97 (0.67–1.27)	0.99 (0.56–1.41)	0.89 (0.67–1.41)	1.18 (0.78–1.52)
Factor VII (U/mL)	0.67 (0.21–1.13)	0.70 (0.52–0.88)	0.86 (0.67–1.07)	1.28 (0.83–1.60)	1.11 (0.72–1.50)	1.13 (0.70–1.56)	1.18 (0.69–2.00)	1.29 (0.61–1.99)
Factor VIII (U/mL)	1.11 (0.50–2.13)	1.82 (1.05–3.29)	1.59 (0.83–2.74)	0.94 (0.54–1.45)	1.10 (0.36–1.85)	1.17 (0.52–1.82)	1.20 (0.59–2.00)	1.60 (0.52–2.90)
vWF (U/mL)*	1.36 (0.78–2.10)	1.53 (0.50–2.87)			0.82 (0.47–1.04)	0.95 (0.44–1.44)	1.00 (0.46–1.53)	0.92 (0.5–1.58)
Factor IX (U/mL)	0.35 (0.19–0.65)	0.48 (0.35–0.56)	0.72 (0.44–0.97)	0.71 (0.43–1.21)	0.85 (0.44–1.27)	0.96 (0.48–1.45)	1.11 (0.64–2.16)	1.30 (0.59–2.54)
Factor X (U/mL)	0.41 (0.11–0.71)	0.55 (0.46–0.67)	0.60 (0.46–0.75)	0.95 (0.77–1.22)	0.98 (0.72–1.25)	0.97 (0.68–1.25)	0.91 (0.53–1.22)	1.24 (0.96–1.71)
Factor XI (U/mL)	0.30 (0.08–0.52)	0.30 (0.07–0.41)	0.57 (0.24–0.79)	0.89 (0.62–1.25)	1.13 (0.65–1.62)	1.13 (0.65–1.62)	1.11 (0.65–1.39)	1.12 (0.67–1.96)
Factor XII (U/mL)	0.38 (0.10–0.66)	0.58 (0.43–0.80)	0.53 (0.14–0.80)	0.79 (0.20–1.35)	0.85 (0.36–1.35)	0.81 (0.26–1.37)	0.75 (0.14–1.17)	1.15 (0.35–2.07)
PK (U/mL)*	0.33 (0.09–0.57)	0.37 (0.18–0.69)			0.95 (0.65–1.30)	0.99 (0.66–1.31)	0.99 (0.53–1.45)	1.12 (0.62–1.62)
HMWK (U/mL)*	0.49 (0.09–0.89)	0.54 (0.06–1.02)			0.98 (0.64–1.32)	0.93 (0.60–1.30)	0.91 (0.63–1.19)	0.92 (0.50–1.36)
Factor XIIIa (U/mL)*	0.70 (0.32–1.08)	0.79 (0.27–1.31)			1.08 (0.72–1.43)	1.09 (0.65–1.51)	0.99 (0.57–1.40)	1.05 (0.55–1.55)
Factor XIIIs (U/mL)*	0.81 (0.35–1.27)	0.76 (0.30–1.22)			1.13 (0.69–1.56)	1.16 (0.77–1.54)	1.02 (0.60–1.43)	0.97 (0.57–1.37)

Continued

TABLE 14.7
AGE-SPECIFIC COAGULATION VALUES—cont'd

Coagulation Test	Preterm Infant (30–36 wk), Day of Life 1*	Term Infant, Day of Life 1	Day of Life 3	1 mo–1 yr	1–5 yr	6–10 yr	11–16 yr	Adult
D-dimer			1.34 (0.58–2.74)	0.22 (0.11–0.42)	0.25 (0.09–0.53)	0.26 (0.10–0.56)	0.27 (0.16–0.39)	0.18 (0.05–0.42)
FDPs*		1.47 (0.41–2.47)						Borderline titer = 1.25–1:50 Positive titer < 1:50
COAGULATION INHIBITORS								
ATIII (U/mL)*	0.38 (0.14–0.62)	0.63 (0.39–0.97)			1.11 (0.82–1.39)	1.11 (0.90–1.31)	1.05 (0.77–1.32)	1.0 (0.74–1.26)
α_2-M (U/mL)*	1.10 (0.56–1.82)	1.39 (0.95–1.83)			1.69 (1.14–2.23)	1.69 (1.28–2.09)	1.56 (0.98–2.12)	0.86 (0.52–1.20)
C1-Inh (U/mL)*	0.65 (0.31–0.99)	0.72 (0.36–1.08)			1.35 (0.85–1.83)	1.14 (0.88–1.54)	1.03 (0.68–1.50)	1.0 (0.71–1.31)
α_2-AT (U/mL)*	0.90 (0.36–1.44)	0.93 (0.49–1.37)			0.93 (0.39–1.47)	1.00 (0.69–1.30)	1.01 (0.65–1.37)	0.93 (0.55–1.30)
Protein C (U/mL)	0.28 (0.12–0.44)	0.32 (0.24–0.40)	0.33 (0.24–0.51)	0.77 (0.28–1.24)	0.94 (0.50–1.34)	0.94 (0.64–1.25)	0.88 (0.59–1.12)	1.03 (0.54–1.66)
Protein S (U/mL)	0.26 (0.14–0.38)	0.36 (0.28–0.47)	0.49 (0.33–0.67)	1.02 (0.29–1.62)	1.01 (0.67–1.36)	1.09 (0.64–1.54)	1.03 (0.65–1.40)	0.75 (0.54–1.03)
FIBRINOLYTIC SYSTEM*								
Plasminogen (U/mL)	1.70 (1.12–2.48)	1.95 (1.60–2.30)			0.98 (0.78–1.18)	0.92 (0.75–1.08)	0.86 (0.68–1.03)	0.99 (0.7–1.22)
TPA (ng/mL)					2.15 (1.0–4.5)	2.42 (1.0–5.0)	2.16 (1.0–4.0)	4.90 (1.40–8.40)
α_2-AP (U/mL)	0.78 (0.4–1.16)	0.85 (0.70–1.0)			1.05 (0.93–1.17)	0.99 (0.89–1.10)	0.98 (0.78–1.18)	1.02 (0.68–1.36)
PAI (U/mL)					5.42 (1.0–10.0)	6.79 (2.0–12.0)	6.07 (2.0–10.0)	3.60 (0–11.0)

*Data from Andrew M, Paes B, Milner R, et al. Development of the human anticoagulant system in the healthy premature infant. Blood. 1987;70:165-172; Andrew M, Paes B, Milner R, et al. Development of the human anticoagulant system in the healthy premature infant. Blood. 1988;72:1651-1657; and Andrew M, Vegh P, Johnston M, et al. Maturation of the hemostatic system during childhood. Blood. 1992;8:1998-2005.
†aPTT values may vary depending on reagent.

α_2-AP, Antiplasmin; α_2-AT, α_1-antitrypsin; α_2-M, α_2-macroglobulin; aPTT, activated partial thromboplastin time; ATIII, antithrombin III; FDPs, fibrin degradation products; HMWK, high-molecular-weight kininogen; INR, international normalized ratio; PAI, plasminogen activator inhibitor; PK, prekallikrein; PT, prothrombin time; TPA, tissue plasminogen activator; VIII, factor VIII procoagulant; vWF, von Willebrand factor
Adapted from Monagle P, Barnes C, Ignjatovic, V, et al. Developmental haemostasis. Impact for clinical haemostasis laboratories. Thromb Haemost. 2006;95:362-372.

> **BOX 14.2**
> **HYPERCOAGULABLE CONDITIONS**
>
> | Congenital | Acquired |
> |---|---|
> | Protein C and S deficiency: Hereditary autosomal dominant disorder. Heterozygotes have three- to six-fold increased risk for venous thrombosis.
Antithrombin III deficiency: Hereditary autosomal dominant disorder. Homozygotes die in infancy.
Factor V Leiden (activated protein C resistance): 2%–5% of European whites are heterozygotes with two- to four-fold increased risk for venous thrombosis; 1 in 1000 are homozygotes, with 80- to 100-fold increased risk for venous thrombosis.
Homocystinemia: Increased levels of homocysteine associated with arterial and venous thromboses, often due to MTHFR abnormalities.
Others: Prothrombin mutation (G20210A), plasminogen abnormalities, fibrinogen abnormalities. | Endothelial damage: Causes include vascular catheters, smoking, diabetes, hypertension, surgery, hyperlipidemia.
Hyperviscosity: Macroglobulinemia, polycythemia, sickle cell disease.
Antiphospholipid antibodies: Seen in patients with systemic lupus erythematosus or other autoimmune diseases; can occur with infections or idiopathically. Associated with venous and arterial thromboses and spontaneous abortions.
Platelet activation: Caused by essential thrombocytosis, oral contraceptives, heparin-induced thrombocytopenia.
Others: Drugs, malignancy, liver disease, inflammatory disease such as inflammatory bowel disease, paroxysmal nocturnal hemoglobinuria, lipoprotein A. |

MTHFR, Methyltetrahydrofolate reductase

including platelet number and function and von Willebrand factor (vWF). Always assess the platelet number and history of ingestion of platelet inhibitors (e.g., nonsteroidal antiinflammatory drugs [NSAIDs]) before any platelet function testing.

B. Hypercoagulable States

Present clinically as venous or arterial thrombosis (Box 14.2)

1. **Laboratory evaluation**[6,7]:
a. Initial laboratory screening includes PT and high-sensitivity aPTT; if PT or aPTT are prolonged, it may be useful to obtain a mixing study to evaluate for the presence of a circulating anticoagulants versus factor deficiency.
b. Extended workup for hypercoagulable states (Box 14.3): A hematologist should be consulted.
c. Identification of one risk factor (e.g., indwelling vascular catheter) does not preclude the search for others, especially when accompanied by a familial or personal history of thrombosis.

> **BOX 14.3**
>
> **EXTENDED WORKUP FOR HYPERCOAGULABLE STATES***
>
> Suggested tiered testing approach:
>
> **First Tier:**
>
> - Antithrombin III activity (antithrombin III deficiency and dysfunction)
> - Activated protein C resistance assay (screening test for factor V Leiden)
> - Factor V Leiden (DNA-based assay for factor V Leiden)
> - Factor II 20210A (prothrombin mutation)
> - Homocysteine
> - Methyltetrahydrofolate reductase (MTHFR) genetic testing if homocysteine elevated
> - Dilute Russell viper venom test (antiphospholipid antibody syndrome)
> - Anticardiolipin screening enzyme-linked immunosorbent assay (ELISA; anticardiolipin antibodies)
> - Protein C activity (protein C deficiency and dysfunction)
> - Protein S activity (protein S deficiency and dysfunction)
> - Factor VIII, IX, XI
>
> **Second Tier (Less Common Conditions):**
>
> - Platelet neutralization procedure (lupus anticoagulant)
> - Plasminogen activity
> - Tissue plasminogen activator (tPA) antigen
> - Plasminogen activator inhibitor-1 activity (PAI-1; measures activity of this tPA inhibitor)
> - α_2-Antiplasmin activity (measures activity of this plasmin inhibitor)
> - Lipoprotein(a) (Lp[a]) promotes decreased fibrinolysis

*Where necessary, abnormality tested for is listed in parentheses.

2. **Treatment of thromboses[12]:**
a. Unfractionated heparin (UFH): Used for treatment or prevention of deep venous thrombosis (DVT) or pulmonary embolism (PE), atrial fibrillation, mechanical heart valve, arterial thrombosis, cerebral sinovenous thrombosis, cardioembolic arterial ischemic stroke, homozygous purpura fulminans, and for bridge to warfarin therapy.
    (1) See Tables 14.8 and 14.9 for UFH bolus and drip adjustment guidelines for goal heparin anti-Xa level range of 0.3–0.7 U/mL or aPTT range 50–80 seconds.
    (2) UFH may be reversed with protamine.
    (3) UFH or low-molecular-weight-heparin (LMWH) therapy should continue for at least 5–7 days while initiating warfarin for treatment of venous thrombosis.
        i. Contraindications: Patients with known hypersensitivity to heparin, major active bleeding, known or suspected heparin-induced thrombocytopenia (HIT), or concurrent epidural therapy.

TABLE 14.8

UNFRACTIONATED HEPARIN DOSE INITIATION GUIDELINES FOR GOAL APTT RANGE OF 50–80 SECONDS* OR ANTI-XA ACTIVITY OF 0.3–0.7 UNITS/ML[†]

Age	Loading Dose (No Loading Dose for Stroke Patients)	Initial Infusion Rate	Monitoring Parameters
Neonates and infants < 1 yr	75 units/kg	28 units/kg/hr	Obtain aPTT or anti-Xa 4 hr after loading dose.
Children ≥1 yr–16 yr	75 units/kg IV (max dose = 7700 units)	20 units/kg/hr (initial max rate = 1650 units/hr)	Obtain aPTT or anti-Xa 4 hr after loading dose.
Patients >16 yr	70 units/kg (max dose = 7700 units)	15 units/kg/hr (initial max rate = 1650 units/hr)	Obtain aPTT or anti-Xa 4 hr after loading dose.

*Therapeutic aPTT range may vary with different aPTT reagents.
[†]Reflects anti factor Xa level of 0.3–0.7 IU/mL with current activated partial thromboplastin time (aPTT) reagents Johns Hopkins Hospital

TABLE 14.9

UNFRACTIONATED HEPARIN DOSE ADJUSTMENT ALGORITHM FOR GOAL APTT RANGE OF 50–80 SECONDS* OR GOAL ANTI-XA ACTIVITY OF 0.3–0.7 UNITS/ML[‡]

aPTT (seconds)	Anti-Xa level	Bolus (units/kg)	Hold (minutes)	Rate Change	Repeat aPTT (hours)
≤39	≤0.1	50	0	Increase 20%	4 hr
40–49	0.2	0	0	Increase 10%	4 hr
50–80	0.3–0.7	0	0	0	4 hr, then next day once two consecutive values are in range
81–100	0.8–0.9	0	0	Decrease 10%	6 hr
101–125	1.0–1.1	0	30–60 min	Decrease 20%	6 hr
≥125[†]	>1.2[†]	0	60–120 min until aPTT < 115 s or anti-Xa < 1.0	Decrease 30%; restart when aPTT <115 s or anti-Xa < 1.0	6 hr after infusion is restarted

*Therapeutic aPTT range may vary with different aPTT reagents.
[†]Confirm that specimen was not drawn from heparinized line or same extremity as site of heparin infusion.
[‡]Reflects anti factor Xa level of 0.3–0.7 IU/mL with current activated partial thromboplastin time (aPTT) reagents Johns Hopkins Hospital.

ii. Precautions: Patients at high risk for bleeding (general bleeding precaution protocols must be implemented) or with platelet count < 50,000/mm^3. Avoid intramuscular injections and avoid other drugs that affect platelet function (e.g., NSAIDs, aspirin, clopidogrel).
iii. Baseline labs prior to institution of UFH therapy (to assess baseline coagulation state): aPTT, PT, BMP, Heme-8.

b. LMWH[6,7]: Administered subcutaneously, has a longer half-life, more predictable pharmacokinetics, and requires less monitoring. Also associated with lower risk for HIT.
   (1) Dose depends on preparation. See Formulary for enoxaparin dosage information.
   (2) Monitor LMWH therapy by following anti-Xa activity. Therapeutic range is 0.5–1.0 U/mL for thrombosis treatment and 0.1–0.3 U/mL for prophylactic dosing. Blood for anti-Xa activity should be drawn 4 hours after dose.
   (3) LMWH-induced bleeding can be partially reversed with protamine. Consult hematologist for protamine reversal protocol.

c. Warfarin: Used for long-term anticoagulation. Patient should receive heparin (UFH or LMWH) while initiating warfarin therapy, owing to possibility of hypercoagulability from decreased protein C and S levels.
   (1) Usually administered orally at an initiation dose for 1–2 days, followed by a daily dose sufficient to maintain the PT/international normalized ratio (INR) in the desired range. Infants often require higher daily doses. Levels should be measured every 1–4 weeks. Table 14.10 lists dose adjustment guidelines, and Table 14.11 outlines management of excessive anticoagulation.
   (2) Efficacy is greatly affected by dietary intake of vitamin K. Patients should receive appropriate dietary education.
   (3) Box 14.4 lists medications that influence warfarin therapy.

d. Anticoagulant therapy alters many coagulation tests:
   (1) Heparin prolongs aPTT, thrombin time, dilute Russell viper venom test (dRVVT), and mixing studies.
   (2) Warfarin prolongs PT, aPTT, and dRVVT. Warfarin reduces the activity of vitamin K–dependent factors (II, VII, IX, X, protein C and S).

e. Thrombolytic therapy should be considered for life- or limb-threatening thrombosis. Consult a hematologist.

NOTE: Children receiving anticoagulation therapy should be protected from trauma. Subcutaneous injections should be used when possible, and caution should be used with intramuscular injections. The use of antiplatelet agents and arterial punctures should be avoided.

C. Bleeding Disorders (Fig. 14.2 and Box 14.5)

1. Differential diagnosis of bleeding disorders (Table 14.12 and Box 14.5)
2. Desired factor replacement goals in hemophilia (Table 14.13)

TABLE 14.10
ADJUSTMENT AND MONITORING OF WARFARIN TO MAINTAIN AN INTERNATIONAL NORMALIZED RATIO (INR) BETWEEN 2 AND 3[*,12]

I. DAY 1 INITIAL DOSING
Newborns age <3 months: there are limited data for safety and efficacy of warfarin.
Infants and children:
If baseline INR is ≤1.3, dose = 0.2 mg/kg/dose orally Q24 hr (max 7.5 mg/dose)[‡]
If baseline INR >1.3, liver dysfunction, NPO/poor nutrition, receiving broad-spectrum antibiotics, receiving medications causing significant drug/drug interactions, receiving medications with CYP2C9 enzyme inhibition (e.g., amiodarone, metronidazole, fluconazole, Bactrim), or slow metabolizer of warfarin, dose = 0.05–0.1 mg/kg/dose Q24 hr (max 5 mg/dose)
If immediate post-operative after Fontan = 0.05 mg/kg/dose orally Q24 hr (max 2.5 mg/dose)

II. DAYS 2–4*
DOSE ADJUSTMENT FOR GOAL INR OF 2–3

Day 2		Days 3 and 4	
INR Level	Action	INR Level	Action
1.1–1.3	Repeat initial dose	1.1–1.4	Increase dose by 20–50%
1.4–1.9	50% of initial dose	1.5–1.9	Continue current dose
≥2	Hold dose for 24 hr, then restart at 50% of initial dose on day 3	2–3	25–50% of initial dose
		3.1–3.5	25% of initial dose
		>3.5	Hold dose until INR <3.5, then restart at 25% of initial dose

III. DAY 5 AND MAINTENANCE*
MAINTENANCE DOSING[†]
≥5 Days

INR Level	Action
1.1–1.4	Increase weekly dose by 20%
1.5–1.9	Increase weekly dose by 10%
2–3	Continue current dose
3.1–3.5	Decrease weekly dose by 10%
>3.5	Hold dose, recheck INR daily until INR <3.5, then restart at 20% less than previous dose

*Effects of new warfarin dose will not be reflected in the INR until 2–3 days after a dose change; daily changes in dose are not typically recommended. For abrupt fluctuations in INR, deviation from guidelines is warranted and cautious dosing is recommended.
[†]Reported average daily dose to maintain INR of 2–3 for infants is 0.33 mg/kg; for adolescents, 0.09 mg/kg; and for adults, from 0.04–0.08 mg/kg
Adapted from The Johns Hopkins Hospital Children's Center pediatric policies, procedures, and protocols general care (Policy Number GEN069): Baltimore; 2016.

TABLE 14.11
MANAGEMENT OF EXCESSIVE WARFARIN ANTICOAGULATION

INR and Bleeding	Intervention
INR 4–4.5 without serious bleeding	Hold or lower next warfarin dose. Recheck INR daily. For patients with high bleeding risk, consider standard dose of oral vitamin K (0.03 mg/kg for patients <40 kg in weight; 1–2.5 mg for patients >40 kg). When INR approaches therapeutic range, resume warfarin therapy.*
INR ≥4.5 but <10 without serious bleeding	Hold warfarin. Recheck INR every 24 hr until <4. If high risk for bleeding, give standard dose of oral vitamin K (0.03 mg/kg for patients <40 kg in weight; 1–2.5 mg for patients >40 kg). When INR approaches therapeutic range, resume warfarin at a lower dose.*
INR ≥10 without serious bleeding	Hold warfarin. Recheck INR every 12–24 hr. Give high dose oral vitamin K every 12–24 hours as necessary (0.06 mg/kg for patients <40 kg in weight; 5–10 mg for patients >40 kg). When INR approaches therapeutic range, resume warfarin at a lower dose.*
Minor bleeding at any INR elevation	Hold warfarin. Monitor INR every 12–24 hr. Give standard dose vitamin K (oral: 0.03 mg/kg for patients <40 kg, 1–2.5 mg for patients ≥40 kg; IV: 0.5–2.5 mg); Vitamin K may be repeated as needed. Restart warfarin when INR approaches therapeutic range and when clinically appropriate at a lower dose.*
Significant or life-threatening bleeding at any INR	Hold warfarin. Monitor INR every 4–6 hr. Administer high dose vitamin K IV at 5–10 mg. Repeat vitamin K as needed. Transfuse FFP (10–15 mL/kg IV), consider prothrombinase complex concentrate; consult blood bank and/or hematology for dosing. Restart warfarin when INR approaches therapeutic range and when clinically appropriate at a lower dose.*

*Refer to Table 14.10.
NOTE: Always evaluate for bleeding risks and potential drug interactions.
FFP, Fresh frozen plasma; INR, international normalized ratio; IV, intravenous.
Adapted from The Johns Hopkins Hospital Children's Center pediatric policies, procedures, and protocols general care (Policy Number GEN069): Baltimore; 2016.

BOX 14.4
MEDICATIONS THAT INFLUENCE WARFARIN THERAPY*

Significant Increase in INR	Significant Decrease in INR
Amiodarone	Amobarbital
Anabolic steroids	Aprepitant
Bactrim (TMP/SMZ)	Butabarbital
Chloramphenicol	Carbamazepine
Disulfiram	Dicloxacillin
Fluconazole	Griseofulvin
Isoniazid	Methimazole
Metronidazole	Phenobarbital
Miconazole	Phenytoin
Phenylbutazone	Primidone
Quinidine	Propylthiouracil
Sulfinpyrazone	Rifabutin
Sulfisoxazole	Rifampin
Tamoxifen	Secobarbital

Moderate Increase in INR	Moderate Decrease in INR
Cimetidine	Atazanavir
Ciprofloxacin	Efavirenz
Clarithromycin	Nafcillin
Delavirdine	Ritonavir
Efavirenz	
Itraconazole	
Lovastatin	
Omeprazole	
Propafenone	
Ritonavir	

INR, International normalized ratio; TMP/SMZ, trimethoprim/sulfamethoxazole
*Numerous medications not listed in this table can affect warfarin administration.

VII. BLOOD COMPONENT REPLACEMENT

A. Blood Volume
Requirements are age specific (Table 14.14).

B. Complications of Transfusions

1. **Acute transfusion reactions**
   a. Acute hemolytic reaction: Most often the result of blood group incompatibility leading to intravascular hemolysis, acute renal failure, and DIC. Signs and symptoms include fever, chills, tachycardia, hypotension, shock, hematuria, and bleeding. Treatment includes immediate cessation of blood transfusion and institution of supportive measures. Laboratory findings include DIC, hemoglobinuria, and positive Coombs test.
   b. Febrile nonhemolytic reaction: Usually the result of inflammatory cytokines; common in previously transfused patients. Symptoms

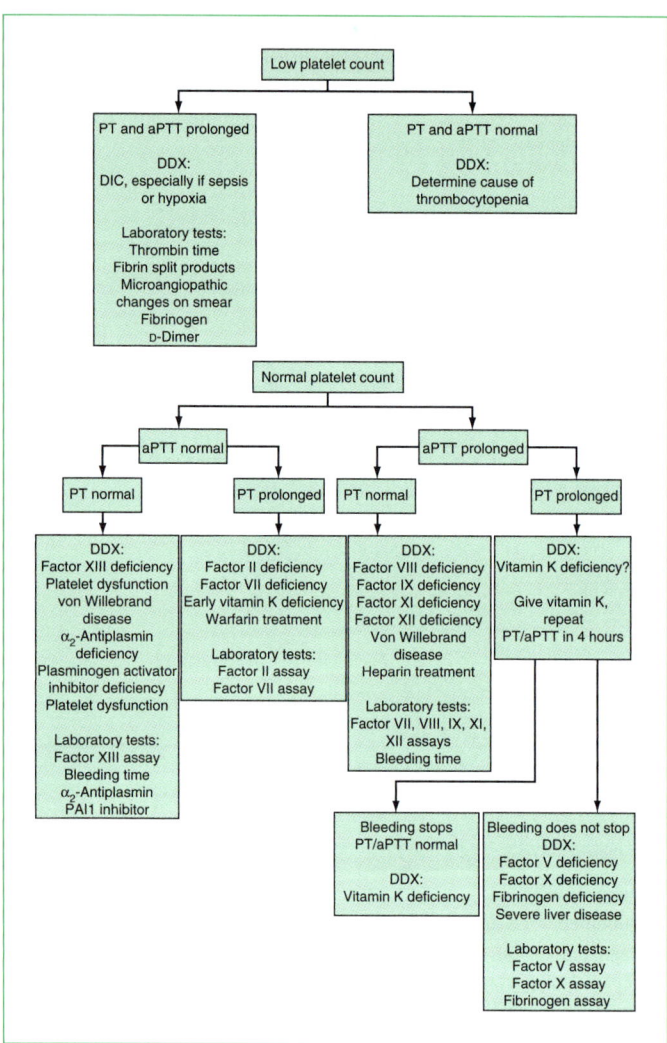

FIGURE 14.2

Differential diagnosis (DDX) of bleeding disorders.
aPTT, Activated partial thromboplastin time; DIC, disseminated intravascular coagulation; PT, prothrombin time.

BOX 14.5
ACQUIRED COAGULOPATHIES

Disseminated Intravascular Coagulation:

Characterized by prolonged PT and aPTT, decreased fibrinogen and platelets, increased fibrin degradation products, and elevated D-dimer. Treatment includes identifying and treating underlying disorder. Replacement of depleted coagulation factors with FFP may be necessary in severe cases, especially when bleeding is present; 10–15 mL/kg will raise clotting factors by 20%. Fibrinogen, if depleted, can be given as cryoprecipitate. Platelet transfusions may also be necessary.

Liver Disease:

Liver is the major site of synthesis of factors V, VII, IX, X, XI, XII, XIII, prothrombin, plasminogen, fibrinogen, proteins C and S, and ATIII. Treatment with FFP and platelets may be needed, but this will increase hepatic protein load. Vitamin K should be given to patients with liver disease and clotting abnormalities.

Vitamin K Deficiency:

Factors II, VII, IX, X, protein C, and protein S are vitamin K dependent. Early vitamin K deficiency may present with isolated prolonged PT because factor VII has the shortest half-life. Fibrinogen should be normal.

aPTT, Activated partial thromboplastin time; ATIII, antithrombin III; FFP, fresh frozen plasma; PT, prothrombin time

TABLE 14.12
COMMON COAGULATION DISORDERS

Factor VIII deficiency (hemophilia A)*	Characteristics: X-linked recessive, prolonged aPTT, normal PT and BT; reduced factor VIII activity.
	Classification: "Severe" if < 1% factor VIII activity; "moderate" if 1%–5% activity; "mild" if 5%–40% of activity.
	Severe hemophiliacs should be maintained on prophylactic factor therapy.
	Complications include development of factor 8 or 9 inhibitors. These patients may require recombinant factor VII; consult Hematology.
	Treatment for acute bleeds:
	  a. Treat with recombinant factor VIII.
	  b. Factor VIII level recovers by 2% per one unit of factor VIII per kg.
	  c. Dose calculation: Units of factor VIII needed = weight (kg) × desired % replacement (refer to Table 14.13) × 0.5. Replete 50 units/kg for 100% activity.
	  d. Dose q 12 hr.
	  e. Consider continuous infusion in surgical patients; 50 units/kg loading dose, then 3–5 units/kg/hr.
	  f. For suspected intracranial bleed, replete to 100% factor level before diagnostic procedure (e.g., computed tomography scan).
	  g. Other therapeutic options include DDAVP (desmopressin acetate) and aminocaproic acid.

Continued

TABLE 14.12
COMMON COAGULATION DISORDERS—cont'd

Factor IX deficiency (hemophilia B or Christmas disease)*	Characteristics: X-linked recessive, prolonged aPTT, normal PT and BT; reduced factor IX activity.
	Classification: "Severe" if < 1% factor IX activity; "moderate" if 1%–5% activity; "mild" if 5%–40% of activity.
	Severe hemophiliacs should be maintained on prophylactic factor therapy.
	Complications include development of factor IX inhibitors. These patients may require recombinant factor VII; consult Hematology.
	Treatment for acute bleeds:
	  a. Treat with recombinant factor IX.
	  b. Factor IX level recovers by 1% per 1–1.2 units of factor IX per kg.
	  c. Dose calculation: Units of factor IX needed = weight (kg) × desired % replacement (refer to Table 14.13) × 1.0 or 1.2. Replete 120 units/kg for 100% activity.
	  d. Dose q 18–24 hr.
	  e. For suspected intracranial bleed, replete to 100% factor level before diagnostic procedure (e.g., computed tomography scan).
	  f. Other therapeutic options include DDAVP and aminocaproic acid.

von Willebrand disease	Characteristics: vWF binds platelets to subendothelial surfaces and carries and stabilizes factor VIII.
	Type 1 (75%, AD): Partial quantitative deficiency of vWF. Mild-to-moderate bleeding. Prolonged BT, normal platelet count, platelet dysfunction on platelet function testing, aPTT normal in most cases but may be mildly prolonged.
	Type 2 (2A, 2B, 2M, 2N): Qualitative dysfunction of vWF. Mild-to-moderate bleeding, but in some cases can be severe.
	Type 3: Absence or near absence of vWF, with reduction of factor VIII and severe bleeding.
	Treatment:
	  a. Majority of patients with type 1 vWD respond to DDAVP with increases in vWF activity from two- to three-fold over baseline (DDAVP responsiveness should be established by prior testing). IV or intranasal DDAVP may be used for minor bleeding or surgical procedures.
	  b. DDAVP may be contraindicated in the rare vWD type 2B, because it may exacerbate thrombocytopenia.
	  c. For more severe disease or patients who do not respond to DDAVP, treatments of choice are purified plasma-derived products containing both vWF and factor VIII (Humate-P, Alphanate, or Wilate). These concentrates are preferred because they are virally inactivated.
	  d. Aminocaproic acid 100 mg/kg IV or PO every 4–6 hr (up to 30 g/day) may be useful for treatment of mucosal bleeding and as prophylaxis for dental extraction.

*All patients with hemophilia should be vaccinated with hepatitis A and B vaccines.
aPTT, Activated partial thromboplastin time; BT, bleeding time; IV, intravenous; PO, *per os*; PT, prothrombin time; vWF, von Willebrand factor

TABLE 14.13
DESIRED FACTOR REPLACEMENT IN HEMOPHILIA

Bleeding Site	Desired Level (%)	Factor VIII dose	Factor IX dose
Minor soft tissue bleeding	20–30	10–15 units/kg	20–35 units/kg
Joint	40–70	20–35 units/kg	40–85 units/kg
Simple dental extraction	50	25 units/kg	60 units/kg
Major soft tissue bleeding	80–100	40–50 units/kg	80–120 units/kg
Serious oral bleeding	80–100	40–50 units/kg	80–120 units/kg
Head injury	100+	50 units/kg	120 units/kg
Major surgery (dental, orthopedic, other)	100+	50 units/kg Consider continuous infusion	120 units/kg Consider continuous infusion

NOTE: A hematologist should be consulted for all major bleeding and before surgery.
Round to the nearest vial; do not exceed 200%.
Dosing adapted from Nathan D, Oski FA. Hematology of Infancy and Childhood. *Philadelphia: WB Saunders; 1998.*

TABLE 14.14
ESTIMATED BLOOD VOLUME (EBV)

Age	Total Blood Volume (mL/kg)
Preterm infants	90–105
Term newborns	78–86
1–12 mo	73–78
1–3 yr	74–82
4–6 yr	80–86
7–18 yr	83–90
Adults	68–88

Data from Nathan D, Oski FA. Hematology of Infancy and Childhood. *Philadelphia: WB Saunders; 1998.*

include fever, chills, and diaphoresis. Stop transfusion and evaluate. Prevention includes premedication with antipyretics, antihistamines, corticosteroids, and if necessary, use of leukocyte-poor PRBCs.

c. Urticarial reaction: Reaction to donor plasma proteins. Stop transfusion immediately; treat with antihistamines, and epinephrine and steroids if there is respiratory compromise (see also treatment of anaphylaxis in Chapter 1). Use leukocyte-poor RBCs with the next transfusion.

d. Evaluation of acute transfusion reaction:
   (1) Patient's urine: Test for Hb.
   (2) Patient's blood: Confirm blood type, screen for antibodies, and repeat direct Coombs test (DCT) on pretransfusion and posttransfusion sera.
   (3) Donor blood: Culture for bacteria.

2. **Delayed transfusion reaction:** Usually due to minor blood group antigen incompatibility, with low or absent titer of antibodies at time of transfusion. Occurs 3–10 days after transfusion. Symptoms include

fatigue, jaundice, and dark urine. Laboratory findings include anemia, positive Coombs test, new RBC antibodies, and hemoglobinuria. The need for acute intervention is much less likely than with acute reactions.

3. **Transmission of infectious diseases[8,11]:** Blood supply is tested for HIV types 1 and 2, human T-lymphotropic virus (HTLV) types I and II, hepatitis B, hepatitis C, syphilis, and West Nile virus. Data from *2009 Red Book* estimate the risk for transmitting infection (estimated per unit) as follows: HIV (1 in 2,000,000); HTLV (1 in 641,000); hepatitis B (1 in 63,000–500,000); hepatitis C (1 in 100,000); parvovirus (1 in 10,000). CMV, hepatitis A, parasitic, tickborne, and prion diseases may also be transmitted by blood products.
4. **Sepsis:** Occurs with products contaminated with bacteria, particularly platelets, because they are stored at room temperature. Risk for transmitting bacteria in PRBCs is 1 in 5 million units, and in platelets is 1 in 100,000.

C. Reasons Not to Consider a Directed Donor
1. **Donors less likely to be truthful about risk.**
2. **Increased risk of transfusion-related graft-versus-host disease (GVHD) if from a relative.**
3. **Can alloimmunize if potential bone marrow donor.**

D. Reasons to Consider a Directed Donor
1. **Chronic transfusion programs** (e.g., thalassemia or sickle cell disease), where donors provide antigen-matched red cells repetitively for the same patient.
2. **NAIT,** where maternal platelets lack causative antigens and represent optimal therapy.

E. Blood Product Components
1. **RBCs:** Decision to transfuse RBCs should be made with consideration of clinical symptoms and signs, degree of cardiorespiratory or central nervous system disease, cause and course of anemia, and options for alternative therapy, noting risks for transfusion-associated infections and reactions.
a. PRBC transfusion: Concentrated RBCs with HCT of 55%–70%. Typed and cross-matched blood products are preferred when possible; O-negative (or O-positive) blood may be used if transfusion cannot be delayed. O-negative is preferred for females of childbearing age to reduce risk for Rh sensitization.
   (1) Unless rapid replacement is required for acute blood loss or shock, infuse no faster than 2–3 mL/kg/hr (generally 10–15 mL/kg aliquots over 4 hr) to avoid congestive heart failure.[15]
   (2) Rule of thumb in severe compensated anemia: where X = patient Hb (g/dL), give an X mL/kg aliquot; for example, if Hb = 5 g/dL, transfuse 5 mL/kg over 4 hours.

(3) To calculate the volume of PRBC to achieve a desired HCT, use the following equation:

$$\text{Volume of PRBCs (mL)} = \text{EBV (mL)} \times (\text{desired HCT} - \text{actual HCT}) \div \text{HCT of PRBCs}$$

where EBV is the estimated blood volume (see Table 14.14 for age-specific EBV), and HCT of PRBCs is usually 55%–70%.

(4) A unit of blood is 500 mL, but approximately 300 mL after processing without significant loss of red cells. This may vary with type of diluents used and time of storage, owing to red cell compaction.

b. Leukocyte-poor PRBCs:
  (1) Filtered RBCs: 99.9% of WBCs removed from product; used for CMV-negative patients to reduce risk for CMV transmission. Also reduces likelihood of a nonhemolytic febrile transfusion reaction.
  (2) Washed RBCs: 92%–95% of WBCs removed from product. Although filtered leukocyte-poor blood is now more commonly used, washing may be helpful if a patient has preexisting antibodies to blood products (e.g., patients who have complete IgA deficiency or history of urticarial transfusion reactions).

c. CMV-negative blood: Obtained from donors who test negative for CMV. May be given to neonates or other immunocompromised patients, including those awaiting organ or marrow transplant who are CMV negative.

d. Irradiated blood products:
  (1) Many blood products [PRBCs, platelet preparations, leukocytes, fresh frozen plasma (FFP), and others] contain viable lymphocytes capable of proliferation and engraftment in the recipient, causing GVHD. Engraftment is most likely in young infants, immunocompromised patients, and patients receiving blood from first-degree relatives. Irradiation with 1500 cGy before transfusion may prevent GVHD but does not prevent antibody formation against donor white cells.
  (2) Indications: Intensive chemotherapy, leukemia, lymphoma, bone marrow transplantation, solid organ transplantation, known or suspected immune deficiencies, intrauterine transfusions, and transfusions in neonates.

2. **Platelets:** Indicated to treat severe or symptomatic thrombocytopenia. Not refrigerated (cold promotes premature platelet activation and clumping); this lack of refrigeration leads to a higher risk of bacteremia with platelet transfusions than with other blood products.

a. Hemorrhagic complications are rare with platelet counts > 20,000/µL. A transfusion *trigger* of 10,000/µL is recommended by many in the absence of serious bleeding complications. Platelet count >50,000/µL is advisable for minor procedures; >100,000/µL is advisable for major surgery or intracranial operation.

b. Single-donor product: Preferred over pooled concentrate for patients with antiplatelet antibodies.
c. Leukocyte-poor: Use if there is a history of significant acute febrile platelet transfusion reactions.
d. Give 5–10 mL/kg of normally concentrated platelet product.[15] For infants and children, 10 mL/kg will increase platelet count by about 50,000/μL.
e. Usually 1 unit = 50 mL after processing, $\geq 5.5 \times 10^{11}$ plt/unit.
3. **FFP:** Contains all clotting factors except platelets and fibrinogen. Also replaces anticoagulant factors (antithrombin III, protein C, protein S).
a. Used in severe clotting factor deficiencies with active bleeding or in combination with vitamin K to achieve rapid reversal of effects of warfarin. Used in treatment of DIC, vitamin K deficiency with active bleeding, or TTP (plasma exchange is treatment of choice for active TTP).
b. One milliliter of FFP expected to provide one unit of activity of all factors except labile factor V and VIII, but individual units may vary. One unit usually equals 250–300 mL after processing.
c. Dose 10–15 mL/kg; repeat doses as needed.[15]
4. **Cryoprecipitate:** Enriched for factor VIII (5–10 U/mL), vWF, factor XIII, fibrinogen, and fibronectin.
a. Use when hypofibrinogenemia or dysfibrinogenemia are expected.
b. One unit usually contains 80 units of factor VIII and 250 mg of fibrinogen, in a volume of 10–15 mL.
c. Dose 1–2 units per 10 kg; repeat as needed.[15]
5. **Monoclonal factor VIII:** Highly purified factor derived from pooled human blood using monoclonal antibodies.
6. **Recombinant factor VIII or IX:** Highly purified with less (theoretical) infectious risk than pooled human products. There is risk for inhibitor formation, as with other products.

F. PRBC Exchange Transfusion

1. **Partial PRBC exchange transfusion** may be indicated for sickle cell patients with acute chest syndrome, stroke, intractable pain crisis, or refractory priapism. Replace with Sickledex-negative cells. Follow HCT carefully during transfusion to avoid hyperviscosity, maintaining HCT < 35%.
2. **Indications for double packed volume PRBC exchange transfusion** include severe acute chest syndrome and cerebrovascular accident (CVA). This is based on twice the patient's calculated packed cell volume. Goal is to reduce percentage of HbS to <30%. The expected reduction in percentage of circulating sickle cells is 60%–80%.
3. **To calculate the volume of PRBC needed for a double packed volume PRBC exchange, use the following equation:**

$$\text{Desired volume of exchange} = \text{EBV (mL)} \times (\text{patient HCT} \times 2) \div \text{HCT of PRBCs}$$

where EBV is the age-dependent estimated blood volume (see Table 14.14), and HCT of PRBC is 55%–70%.

VIII. INTERPRETING BLOOD SMEARS

See Figs. 14.3 through 14.14 for examples of blood smears. Examine the blood smear in an area where the RBCs are nearly touching but do not overlap.

A. RBC
Examine size, shape, and color.

B. WBC
A rough estimate of the WBC count can be made by looking at the smear under high power (×100 magnification). Each one cell per high-power field correlates with approximately 500 WBC/mm³ (×20 magnification).

C. Platelets
A rough estimate of platelet count is one platelet per high-power field corresponds to 10,000–15,000/µL. Platelet clumps usually indicate > 100,000 platelets/µL.

REFERENCES

1. Yawn BP, Buchanan GR, Afenyi-Annan AN, et al. Management of sickle cell disease: summary of the 2014 evidence-based report by expert panel members. *JAMA*. 2014;312(10):1033-1048.
2. Kavanagh PL, Sprinz PG, Vinci SR, et al. Management of children with sickle cell disease: a comprehensive review of the literature. *Pediatrics*. 2011;128:e1552-1574.
3. Provan D, Stasi R, Newland AC, et al. International consensus report on the investigation and management of primary immune thrombocytopenia. *Blood*. 2010;115:168-186.
4. Bennett CM, Rogers ZR, Kinnamon DD, et al. Prospective phase 1/2 study of rituximab in childhood and adolescent chronic immune thrombocytopenic purpura. *Blood*. 2006;107(7):2630-2642.
5. George JN, Nester CM. Syndromes of thrombotic microangiopathy. *N Engl J Med*. 2014;371:654-656.
6. Streiff MB, Kickler TS. *The Johns Hopkins Hospital Hemostatic Testing and Antithrombotic Therapy Manual*. 3rd ed. Baltimore: Johns Hopkins Hospital; 2007.
7. The Johns Hopkins Hospital Children's Center pediatric policies, procedures, and protocols general care. Baltimore; 2012.
8. Red Book. *2009 Report of the Committee on Infectious Diseases*. 28th ed. Elk Grove Village, IL: American Academy of Pediatrics; 2009.
9. Strouse JJ, Takemoto CM, Keefer JR, et al. Corticosteroids and increased risk of readmission after acute chest syndrome in children with sickle cell disease. *Pediatr Blood Cancer*. 2008;50:1006-1012.
10. Hulbert ML, Scothorn DJ, Panepinto JA, et al. Exchange blood transfusion for first overt stroke is associated with a lower risk of subsequent stroke than simple transfusion: a retrospective cohort of 137 children with sickle cell anemia. *J Pediatr*. 2006;149:710-712.

11. Red Cross Blood Testing. <www.redcrossblood.org>. Accessed December 10, 2010.
12. Monagle P, Chan AC, Goldenberg NA. Antithrombotic therapy in neonates and children: antithrombotic therapy and prevention of thrombosis: American College of Chest Physicians evidence-based clinical practice guidelines. *Chest.* 2012;14(suppl 2):e737S-e801S.
13. Lipton JM, Ellis SR. Diamond-Blackfan anemia: diagnosis, treatment, and molecular pathogenesis. *Hematol Oncol Clin North Am.* 2009;23:261-282.
14. Wang WC, Ware RE, Miller ST. Hydroxycarbamide in very young children with sickle-cell anaemia: a multicentre, randomised, controlled trial (BABY-HUG). *Lancet.* 2011;377:1663-1672.
15. Behrman RE, et al. *Nelson Textbook of Pediatrics.* 17th ed. Philadelphia: Saunders; 2004.

Chapter 15
Immunology and Allergy
Jeremy Snyder, MD

I. ALLERGIC RHINITIS (AR) [1-6]

A. Epidemiology

1. **Most common chronic condition:** Prevalence in children up to 40%
2. **Significant impact on quality of life,** including mood, behavior, school performance and sleep patterns, as demonstrated in multiple studies
3. **Increases risk for** recurrent otitis media, asthma, acute and chronic sinusitis
4. **Risk factors:** Atopic family history, serum immunoglobulin (Ig) E > 100 IU/mL before age 6 years, higher socioeconomic status, maternal smoke exposure in first year of life

B. Diagnosis

1. **History**
   a. Allergen-driven mucosal inflammation leading to cyclical exacerbations or persistent symptoms
   b. Symptoms: Nasal (congestion, rhinorrhea, pruritus), ocular (pruritus, tearing), postnasal drip (sore throat, cough, pruritus)
   c. Patterns: Seasonal (depending on local allergens) vs. perennial (with seasonal peaks)
   d. Coexisting atopic diseases common (eczema, asthma, food allergy)
2. **Physical Examination**
   a. Allergic facies with shiners, mouth breathing, transverse nasal crease ("allergic salute"), accentuated lines below lower eyelids (Dennie-Morgan lines)
   b. Nasal mucosa may be normal to pink to pale gray, ± swollen turbinates
   c. Injected sclera with or without clear discharge, conjunctival cobblestoning
3. **Diagnostic Studies**
   a. Diagnosis can be made on clinical grounds, and allergy testing can identify specific allergic sensitivities.
   b. Allergy testing can be performed with skin tests or allergen-specific IgE testing.
   c. Total IgE: Nonspecific and of limited value.
   d. Peripheral blood eosinophil count: Not sensitive enough to be diagnostic.
   e. Imaging studies: Not useful.
   f. Consider sleep study to evaluate for obstructive sleep apnea and pulmonary function tests to evaluate for asthma.

C. Differential Diagnosis

1. **Vasomotor/nonallergic rhinitis:** Symptoms made worse by scents, alcohol, or changes in temperature or humidity
2. **Infectious rhinitis:** Viral vs. bacterial
3. **Adenoid hypertrophy**
4. **Rhinitis medicamentosa:** Rebound rhinitis from prolonged use of nasal vasoconstrictors
5. **Sinusitis:** Acute or chronic
6. **Nonallergic rhinitis with eosinophilia syndrome**
7. **Nasal polyps**

D. Treatment

1. **Allergen avoidance:**
   a. Relies on identification of triggers, most common of which are pollens, fungi, dust mites, insects, animals.
   b. Difficult to avoid ubiquitous airborne allergens.
   c. HEPA filter may be useful when animal allergens are a concern.
   d. Thorough housecleaning and allergy-proof bed coverings can be useful.
2. **Oral antihistamines** (e.g., diphenhydramine, cetirizine):
   a. First-line treatment
   b. Second– and third–generation preparations preferable (loratadine, desloratadine, fexofenadine, cetirizine, levocetirizine)
   c. Adverse effects: Sedation and anticholinergic side effects more prominent with first-generation agents
3. **Intranasal corticosteroids** (fluticasone, mometasone, budesonide, flunisolide, ciclesonide, and triamcinolone):
   a. Second-line treatment
   b. Most effective maintenance therapy for nasal congestion
   c. Potential benefit for ocular symptoms
   d. No proven adverse effect on long-term growth
   e. Adverse effects: nasal irritation, sneezing, bleeding
   f. Recognize potential risk of adrenal suppression at high doses of inhaled or intranasal steroids, especially for patients on multiple steroid preparations
4. **Leukotriene inhibitors** (montelukast): Alone or in combination with antihistamines
5. **Mast cell stabilizers** (intranasal cromolyn):
   a. Available over the counter
   b. Effective as prophylaxis
   c. Few adverse effects
6. **Intranasal antihistamines** (azelastine, olopatadine):
   a. Effective for acute symptoms and prophylaxis
   b. Not studied in children younger than 5 years
   c. Adverse effects: Bitter taste, systemic absorption with potential for sedation

7. **Intranasal combination agents** (azelastine/fluticasone): Useful for patients with moderate-to-severe allergic rhinitis
8. **Anticholinergics** (ipratropium):
a. Useful for rhinorrhea only, especially for nonallergic rhinitis
b. Adverse effects: Drying of nasal mucosa
9. **Immunotherapy**
a. Success rate is high when patients are chosen carefully and when performed by an allergy specialist.
b. Consider when symptoms are inadequately controlled with medications and allergen avoidance.
c. In addition to traditional subcutaneous immunotherapy, sublingual products have now been approved for several allergens.
d. Not recommended for patients with poor adherence to therapy or those with poorly-controlled asthma.
e. Not well studied in children younger than 5 years.
f. May reduce risk for future development of asthma, and treatment of allergic rhinitis may improve asthma control.
10. **Nasal rinsing with hypertonic saline:** Tolerable and inexpensive
11. **Ophthalmic agents:** Can be used to treat allergic conjunctivitis. Up to 60% of patients with allergic rhinitis have concomitant conjunctivitis
a. Mast cell stabilizers: Cromolyn sodium (Opticrom), lodoxamide-tromethamine (Alomide), nedocromil (Alocril), pemirolast (Alamast)
b. H_1-antagonists and mast cell stabilizers: Alcaftadine (Lastacaft), azelastine HCl (Optivar), bepotastine (Bepreve), emedastine (Emadine), epinastine (Elestat), ketotifen fumarate (Zaditor), olopatadine (Pantanol, Pataday)

II. FOOD ALLERGY[7-12]

A. Epidemiology
1. **Prevalence is 6%–8% in young children, 3% to 4% by adolescence**
2. **Most common allergens in children:** Milk, eggs, peanuts, tree nuts (e.g., cashew, walnut), soy, and wheat

B. Manifestations of Food Allergy
1. **Often a combination of several syndromes;** symptoms can occur within minutes to hours of ingesting food.
2. **Diagnosis** requires both sensitization (demonstration of allergen-specific IgE) and clinical symptoms after exposure to allergens.
3. **Rarely presents with isolated respiratory symptoms**
4. **Anaphylaxis:** see Chapter 1, Allergic Emergencies (Anaphylaxis)
5. **Skin syndromes:**
a. Urticaria/angioedema:
   (1) Chronic urticaria is rarely related to food allergy.
   (2) Acute urticaria due to food allergy may be a risk factor for future anaphylaxis.

b. Atopic dermatitis/eczema:
    (1) Food allergy is more common in patients with atopic dermatitis.
    (2) Even if not apparent by history, at least one-third of children with moderate to severe atopic dermatitis have IgE-mediated food allergies.
    (3) Acute and chronic skin changes often coexist.
6. **Gastrointestinal syndromes:**
a. Oral allergy syndrome:
    (1) Pollen-associated food allergy caused by cross-reactivity of antibodies to pollens (e.g., apple and tree pollen).
    (2) Pruritus of oral mucosa after ingestion of certain fresh fruits and vegetables in patients with pollen allergies
    (3) Rarely results in edema of oral mucosa
    (4) Symptoms rarely progress beyond mouth/throat
    (5) Inciting antigens are usually denatured by cooking
b. Allergic eosinophilic gastroenteritis, esophagitis:
    (1) May cause abdominal pain, diarrhea, vomiting, dysphagia, early satiety
    (2) May be confused with reflux
    (3) Characterized by eosinophilic infiltration of digestive tract; 50%–60% of patients with elevated serum IgE levels
    (4) Dietary therapy can be effective; often guided by allergy testing
    (5) In some cases, topical steroids, or a combination of dietary avoidance and topical steroids, may be needed for effective control
c. Food-induced enterocolitis:
    (1) Presents in infancy
    (2) Vomiting and diarrhea (may contain blood); when severe, may lead to lethargy, dehydration, hypotension, acidosis
    (3) Most commonly associated with milk and soy but may occur with a wide variety of foods (e.g., rice, oat, fruits, vegetables)
d. Infantile proctocolitis:
    (1) Confined to distal colon and can present with diarrhea or blood-streaked and mucous stools
    (2) Symptoms usually resolve within 72 hours of stopping offending agent; rarely leads to anemia

C. Diagnosis of Food Allergy (Fig. 15.1)
1. **History and physical examination:**
a. Identify specific foods and whether fresh vs. cooked
b. Establish timing and nature of reactions; patient should keep a food diary
c. Mainstays of diagnosis, but skin and/or IgE testing needed to identify trigger foods
2. **Skin testing:**
a. Skin prick test has poor positive predictive value but very good negative predictive value

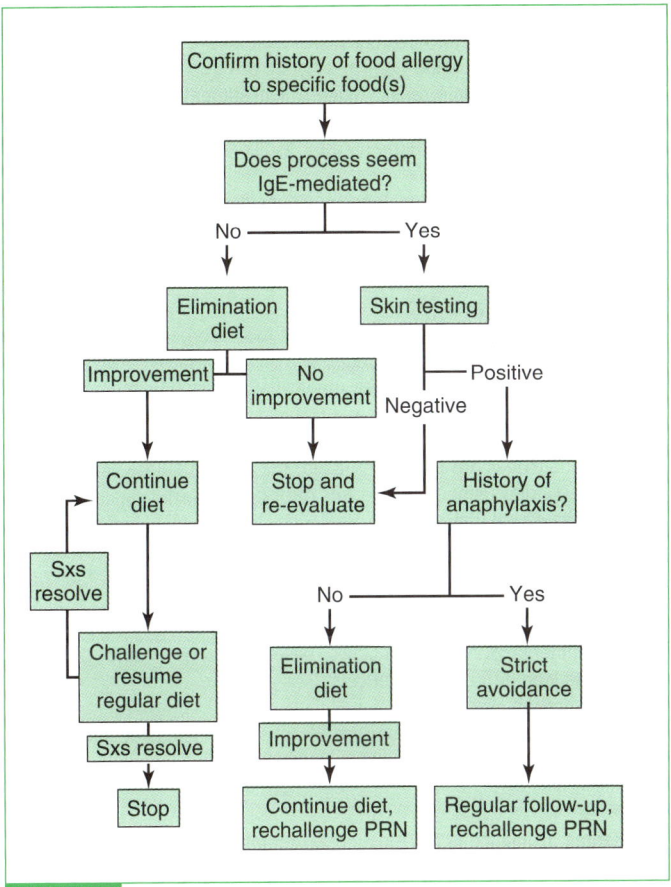

FIGURE 15.1

Evaluation and management of food allergy. IgE, immunoglobulin E; PRN, as needed; Sxs, Symptoms. (Data from Wood RA. The natural history of food allergy. Pediatrics. 2003;111:1631-1637; Wood RA. Up to Date 2009. http://www.uptodate.com.)

    b. Patient must not be taking antihistamines
    c. Widespread skin conditions (e.g., dermatographism, urticaria, severe eczema) may limit ability to perform skin tests
    d. Intradermal tests have high false-positive rates and higher risk
    e. Atopy patch testing (APT): Under investigation; no guidelines for use at present

3. **Measurement of allergen-specific IgE:**
a. Similar to skin tests, it has poor positive predictive value, excellent negative predictive value
b. Levels above a certain range (different for different antigens) have increasing positive predictive value
c. Useful in patients with dermatologic conditions that preclude skin testing
d. Component testing (measuring IgE to specific food proteins rather than crude extracts) may improve diagnostic accuracy for peanut, possibly, other foods
e. IgG testing not useful
4. **Oral food challenges:**
a. Can verify clinical reactivity to a specific food allergen or document that a food allergy has been outgrown
b. Must be performed under close medical supervision with emergency medications readily available
c. Patient must not be taking antihistamines
d. Open challenges are most often used, but most accurate when double-blinded using graded doses of disguised food
5. **Trial elimination diet:**
a. Helpful if improvement with removal of food from diet
b. Essential, especially in infants and for non-IgE–mediated food allergy

D. Differential Diagnosis
1. **Food intolerance:** Nonimmunologic, based on toxins or other properties of foods leading to adverse effects
2. **Malabsorption syndromes:**
a. Cystic fibrosis, celiac disease (see Chapter 12), lactase deficiency
b. Gastrointestinal (GI) malformations

E. Treatment
1. **Allergen avoidance** is the most important intervention for all types of food allergy.
a. Patients must pay close attention to food ingredients.
b. Infants with milk, soy allergies may be placed on elemental formula.
c. Nutritional counseling and regular growth monitoring are recommended.
2. **For angioedema, urticaria:**
a. Epinephrine is first-line treatment
b. Antihistamines, corticosteroids
c. Omalizumab used for chronic urticaria
3. **Atopic dermatitis:** Symptomatic control (see Chapter 8)
4. **Anaphylaxis:** Epinephrine, all at-risk patients should have an **epinephrine** auto-injector
5. **Food-specific immunotherapy** is under investigation. It is used to induce clinical desensitization to specific allergens.

F. Natural History

1. **About 50% of milk, egg, soy, and wheat allergies outgrown by school age.**
2. Peanut, tree nut, and shellfish allergies are outgrown only in 10% to 20%.
3. **Skin tests and allergen-specific IgE** may remain positive, even though symptoms resolve.

III. DRUG ALLERGY[13-14]

A. Epidemiology

1. **Drug allergy:** Immunologically mediated response to an agent in a sensitized person.
2. **Drug intolerance:** Undesirable pharmacologic effect.
3. **Although 10% of patients report penicillin allergy,** after evaluation, about 90% of these individuals can tolerate penicillin.

B. Diagnosis

1. **History:** Cutaneous manifestations are the most common presentation for drug allergic reactions.
2. **Diagnostic studies:**
a. Penicillin is the only agent for which optimal negative predictive values for IgE-mediated reactions have been established.
b. Skin testing with major and minor antigens of penicillin.

C. Management (Fig. 15.2)

1. **Desensitization:** Immunologic IgE induction of tolerance, progressive administration of an allergenic substance to render effector cells less reactive
2. **Graded challenge:** Administration of progressively increasing doses of a drug until full dose is reached; does not modify a patient's response to the drug

IV. EVALUATION OF SUSPECTED IMMUNODEFICIENCY

See Tables 15.1 and 15.2.[15-23]

V. IMMUNOGLOBULIN THERAPY[24-27]

A. Intravenous Immunoglobulin (IVIG)

1. **Indications:**
a. Replacement therapy for antibody-deficient disorders:
   (1) See Formulary for dosages.
   (2) Children with severe hypogammaglobulinemia (<100 mg/dL) may benefit from a higher total *loading* dose in two separate doses a few days apart, followed by standard dosing every 3–4 weeks.
   (3) Adjust dosing based on clinical response.

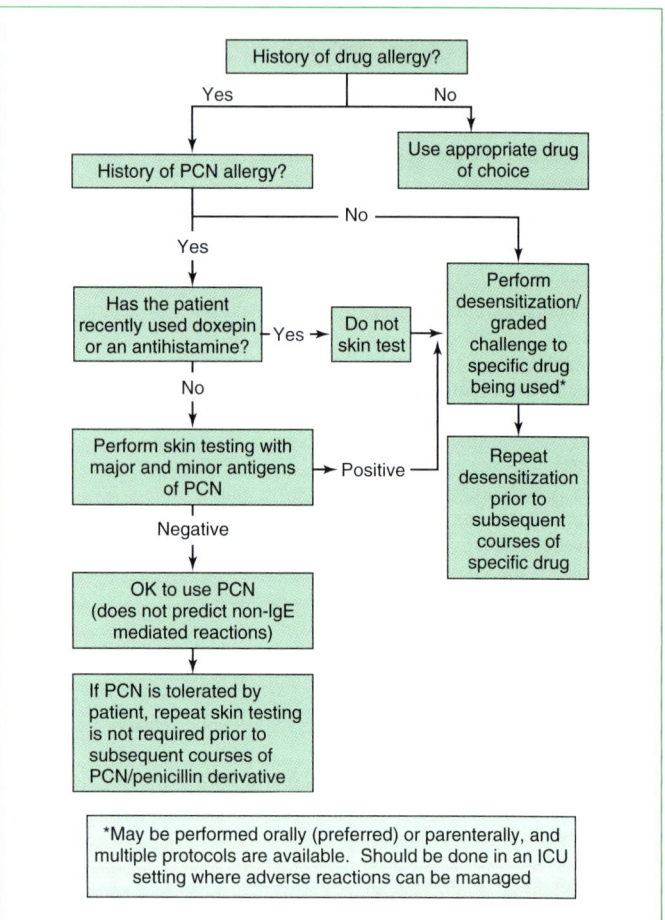

FIGURE 15.2

Evaluation and management of drug allergy. ICU, Intensive care unit; IgE, immunoglobulin E; PCN, penicillin. *(Adapted from Solensky R. Allergy to penicillins. Up to Date 2009. http://www.uptodate.com.)*

TABLE 15.1
WHEN TO SUSPECT IMMUNODEFICIENCY

Recurrent Infections	Opportunistic Infections	Severe Infections	Other Conditions
6 or more new infections in 1 yr Recurrent tissue or organ abscesses 2 or more serious sinus infections in 1 yr 2 or more pneumonias in 1 yr	*Pneumocystis jirovecii* pneumonia *Pseudomonas* sepsis Invasive infection with *Neisseria* spp.	2 or more months of antibiotics with little effect Sepsis in the absence of a known risk (e.g., indwelling vascular catheter, neutropenia) Bacterial meningitis Pneumonia with empyema Resistant superficial or oral candidiasis	Failure to gain weight or grow normally Family history of immunodeficiency or unexplained early deaths Lymphopenia in infancy Complications from a live vaccine Part of a syndrome complex [(e.g., Wiskott-Aldrich (with thrombocytopenia, eczema), DiGeorge syndrome (with facial dysmorphism, congenital cardiac disease, hypoparathyroidism)]

Adapted from Stiehm ER. Approach to the child with recurrent infections. Up to Date 2015. http://www.uptodate.com.

TABLE 15.2
EVALUATION OF SUSPECTED IMMUNODEFICIENCY

Suspected Functional Abnormality	Clinical Findings	Initial Tests	More Advanced Tests
Antibody (e.g., common variable immunodeficiency, X-linked agammaglobulin-emia, IgA deficiency)	Sinopulmonary and systemic infections (pyogenic bacteria) Enteric infections (enterovirus, other viruses, *Giardia* spp.) Autoimmune diseases (immune thrombocytopenia, hemolytic anemia, inflammatory bowel disease)	Immunoglobulin levels (IgG, IgM, IgA) Antibody levels to T-cell–dependent protein antigens (e.g., tetanus or pneumococcal conjugate vaccines) Antibody levels to T-cell–independent polysaccharide antigens in a child ≥2 yr (e.g., pneumococcal polysaccharide vaccine such as Pneumovax)	B-cell enumeration Immunofixation electrophoresis

Continued

TABLE 15.2
EVALUATION OF SUSPECTED IMMUNODEFICIENCY—cont'd

Suspected Functional Abnormality	Clinical Findings	Initial Tests	More Advanced Tests
Cell-mediated immunity (e.g., severe combined immunodeficiency, DiGeorge syndrome)	Pneumonia (pyogenic bacteria, fungi, *Pneumocystis jiroveci*, viruses)	TRECs newborn screening* Total lymphocyte counts HIV ELISA/Western blot/PCR	T-cell enumeration (CD3, CD4, CD8) In vitro T-cell proliferation to mitogens, antigens, or allogeneic cells FISH 22q11 for DiGeorge deletion
Phagocytosis (chronic granulomatous disease, leukocyte adhesion deficiency, Chédiak-Higashi syndrome)	Cutaneous infections, abscesses, lymphadenitis (staphylococci, enteric bacteria, fungi, mycobacteria), poor wound healing	WBC/neutrophil count and morphology	Nitroblue tetrazolium (NBT) test or dihydro-rhodamine (DHR) reduction test Chemotactic assay Phagocytic assay
Spleen	Bacteremia/hematogenous infection (pneumococcus, other streptococci, *Neisseria* spp.)	Peripheral blood smear for Howell-Jolly bodies Hemoglobin electrophoresis (HbSS)	Technetium-99 spleen scan or sonogram
Complement	Bacterial sepsis and other bloodborne infections (encapsulated bacteria, especially *Neisseria* spp.) Lupus, glomerulonephritis Angioedema	CH50 (total hemolytic complement)	Alternative pathway assay (AH50) Mannose-binding lectin level Individual complement component assays

*Newborn screening using TRECs has now been implemented in multiple states. TRECs identify lymphopenia in children and prompt further testing for SCID or other immunodeficiencies associated with lymphopenia.

ELISA, enzyme-linked immunosorbent assay; FISH, fluorescent in situ hybridization; HIV, human immunodeficiency virus; PCR, polymerase chain reaction; TRECs, T-cell receptor excision circles; WBC, white blood cell.

From Lederman HM. Clinical presentation of primary immunodeficiency diseases. In: McMillan J. Oski's Pediatrics. Philadelphia: Lippincott Williams & Wilkins; 2006:2441-2444.

b. Immune thrombocytopenic purpura (see Chapter 14):
   (1) Initially given on a single day or in divided doses over 2–5 consecutive days.
   (2) Maintenance dose given every 3–6 weeks based on clinical response and platelet count.
c. Kawasaki disease (see Chapter 7):
   (1) Initial dose given over 8–12 hr.
   (2) If signs and symptoms persist, consider second dose.
   (3) Doses should be started within first 10 days of symptoms.
d. Pediatric human immunodeficiency virus (HIV) infection with antibody deficiency (IgG concentration <400 mg/dL, failure to form antibodies to common antigens, recurrent serious bacterial infections, or measles prophylaxis): Dosing same as for antibody-deficient disorders mentioned previously.
e. Bone marrow transplantation:
   (1) Adjust dosing to maintain trough IgG level of at least 400 mg/dL.
   (2) May decrease incidence of infection and death but not acute graft-versus-host disease.
f. Other potential uses:
   (1) Guillain-Barré syndrome
   (2) Refractory dermatomyositis and polymyositis
   (3) Chronic inflammatory demyelinating polyneuropathy

2. **Precautions and adverse reactions:**
a. Severe systemic symptoms (hemodynamic changes, respiratory difficulty, anaphylaxis)
b. Less-severe systemic reactions (headache, myalgia, fever, chills, nausea, vomiting) may be alleviated by decreasing infusion rate or premedication with intravenous corticosteroids, and/or antipyretics.
c. Aseptic meningitis syndrome
d. Acute renal failure (increased risk with preexisting renal insufficiency and with sucrose-containing IVIG)
e. Acute venous thrombosis (increased risk with sucrose-containing IVIG)
f. Use with caution in patients with undetectable IgA levels only if it is known that the patient has anti-IgA IgG antibodies

B. Intramuscular Immunoglobulin (IMIG)

1. **Indications:**
a. Hepatitis A prophylaxis: Immunoglobulin is not needed if at least one dose of hepatitis A vaccine was given at ≥1 month before exposure.
b. Measles prophylaxis: Within 6 days of exposure in immunocompetent patient and immediately following exposure in immunocompromised patients.
c. Rubella prophylaxis: Within 72 hours of exposure.
d. Rabies prophylaxis: As soon as possible after exposure with the first dose of rabies vaccine.

e. Varicella-Zoster prophylaxis (independent of HIV status): Single dose within 72 hours of exposure.
2. **Precautions and adverse reactions:**
a. Severe systemic symptoms (hemodynamic changes, anaphylaxis)
b. Local symptoms at injection site increase with repeated use; risk of local tissue injury
c. High risk for anaphylactoid reactions if given intravenously
d. Use with caution in patients with undetectable IgA levels only if it is known that the patient has anti-IgA IgG antibodies
3. **Administration:**
a. No more than 5 mL should be given at one site in an adult or large child.
b. Smaller amounts per site (1–3 mL) for smaller children and infants
c. Administration of >15 mL at one time is essentially never warranted.
d. Peak serum levels achieved by 48 hours; immune effect lasts 3–4 weeks
e. Intravenous or intradermal use of IMIG is absolutely contraindicated.

C. Subcutaneous Immunoglobulin

1. **Indication:** Replacement therapy for antibody deficiency.
2. **Dose:**
a. See Part IV, "Formulary," for dosages.
b. Can be given via manual push or via syringe-drive pump.
   (1) Rapid infusion rates have been demonstrated to be well tolerated.
   (2) Most children can tolerate 15–20 cc in a single site.
c. Larger doses can be given simultaneously in multiple sites or more frequently than once weekly.
d. Using the same areas for injections improves tolerability.
3. **Precautions and adverse reactions:** Systemic side effects are rare because of the small volumes given and the slow absorption rate.
a. Local redness and swelling are expected, and generally decrease with every infusion.
b. Correct infusion supplies (e.g., needle length and gauge) are critical for ensuring success.
4. **Considerations:** Does not require venous access or special nursing (parents can administer) but may require multiple needlesticks in larger children, depending on the volume to be infused.

D. Specific Immunoglobulins

1. **Hyperimmune globulins:**
a. Prepared from donors with high titers of specific antibodies
b. Includes hepatitis B immune globulin, varicella-zoster immune globulin, cytomegalovirus immune globulin, Rho(D) immune globulin, and others
2. **Monoclonal antibody preparations** (rituximab, palivizumab, and others)

VI. IMMUNOLOGIC REFERENCE VALUES

A. Serum IgG, IgM, IgA, and IgE Levels (Table 15.3)

B. Serum IgG, IgM, IgA, and IgE Levels for Low Birth Weight Preterm Infants (Table 15.4)

C. Lymphocyte Enumeration (Table 15.5)

D. Serum Complement Levels (Table 15.6)

VII. COMPLEMENT PATHWAY

See Fig. 15.3.

TABLE 15.3
SERUM IMMUNOGLOBULIN LEVELS*

Age	IgG (mg/dL)	IgM (mg/dL)	IgA (mg/dL)	IgE (IU/ml)
Cord blood (term)	1121 (636–1606)	13 (6.3–25)	2.3 (1.4–3.6)	0.22 (0.04–1.28)
1 mo	503 (251–906)	45 (20–87)	13 (1.3–53)	
6 wk				0.69 (0.08–6.12)
2 mo	365 (206–601)	46 (17–105)	15 (2.8–47)	
3 mo	334 (176–581)	49 (24–89)	17 (4.6–46)	0.82 (0.18–3.76)
4 mo	343 (196–558)	55 (27–101)	23 (4.4–73)	
5 mo	403 (172–814)	62 (33–108)	31 (8.1–84)	
6 mo	407 (215–704)	62 (35–102)	25 (8.1–68)	2.68 (0.44–16.3)
7–9 mo	475 (217–904)	80 (34–126)	36 (11–90)	2.36 (0.76–7.31)
10–12 mo	594 (294–1069)	82 (41–149)	40 (16–84)	
1 yr	679 (345–1213)	93 (43–173)	44 (14–106)	3.49 (0.80–15.2)
2 yr	685 (424–1051)	95 (48–168)	47 (14–123)	3.03 (0.31–29.5)
3 yr	728 (441–1135)	104 (47–200)	66 (22–159)	1.80 (0.19–16.9)
4–5 yr	780 (463–1236)	99 (43–196)	68 (25–154)	8.58 (1.07–68.9)[†]
6–8 yr	915 (633–1280)	107 (48–207)	90 (33–202)	12.89 (1.03–161.3)[‡]
9–10 yr	1007 (608–1572)	121 (52–242)	113 (45–236)	23.6 (0.98–570.6)[§]
14 yr				20.07 (2.06–195.2)
Adult	994 (639–1349)	156 (56–352)	171 (70–312)	13.2 (1.53–114)

*Numbers in parentheses are the 95% confidence intervals (CIs).
[†]IgE data for 4 yr
[‡]IgE data for 7 yr
[§]IgE data for 10 yr

Data from Kjellman NM, Johansson SG, Roth A. Serum IgE levels in healthy children quantified by a sandwich technique (PRIST). Clin Allergy. 1976;6:51-59; Jolliff CR, Cost KM, Stivrins PC, et al. Reference intervals for serum IgG, IgA, IgM, C3, and C4 as determined by rate nephelometry. Clin Chem. 1982;28:126-128; and Zetterström O, Johansson SG. IgE concentrations measured by PRIST in serum of healthy adults and in patients with respiratory allergy: a diagnostic approach. Allergy. 1981;36:537-547.

TABLE 15.4
SERUM IMMUNOGLOBULIN LEVELS FOR LOW BIRTH WEIGHT PRETERM INFANTS

Age (mo)	Plasma Ig Concentrations in 25- to 28-Wk Gestation Infants			Plasma Ig Concentrations in 29- to 32-Wk Gestation Infants		
	IgG (mg/dL)*	IgM (mg/dL)*	IgA (mg/dL)*	IgG (mg/dL)*	IgM (mg/dL)*	IgA (mg/dL)*
0.25	251 (114–552)[†]	7.6 (1.3–43.3)	1.2 (0.07–20.8)	368 (186–728)[†]	9.1 (2.1–39.4)	0.6 (0.04–1.0)
0.5	202 (91–446)	14.1 (3.5–56.1)	3.1 (0.09–10.7)	275 (119–637)	13.9 (4.7–41)	0.9 (0.01–7.5)
1.0	158 (57–437)	12.7 (3.0–53.3)	4.5 (0.65–30.9)	209 (97–452)	14.4 (6.3–33)	1.9 (0.3–12.0)
1.5	134 (59–307)	16.2 (4.4–59.2)	4.3 (0.9–20.9)	156 (69–352)	15.4 (5.5–43.2)	2.2 (0.7–6.5)
2.0	89 (58–136)	16.0 (5.3–48.9)	4.1 (1.5–11.1)	123 (64–237)	15.2 (4.9–46.7)	3.0 (1.1–8.3)
3	60 (23–156)	13.8 (5.3–36.1)	3.0 (0.6–15.6)	104 (41–268)	16.3 (7.1–37.2)	3.6 (0.8–15.4)
4	82 (32–210)	22.2 (11.2–43.9)	6.8 (1.0–47.8)	128 (39–425)	26.5 (7.7–91.2)	9.8 (2.5–39.3)
6	159 (56–455)	41.3 (8.3–205)	9.7 (3.0–31.2)	179 (51–634)	29.3 (10.5–81.5)	12.3 (2.7–57.1)
8–10	273 (94–794)	41.8 (31.1–56.1)	9.5 (0.9–98.6)	280 (140–561)	34.7 (17–70.8)	20.9 (8.3–53)

*Geometric mean
[†]Numbers in parentheses are ±2 SD

From Ballow M, Cates KL, Rowe JC, et al. Development of the immune system in very low birth weight (less than 1500 g) premature infants: concentrations of plasma immunoglobulins and patterns of infections. Pediatr Res. 1986;9:899-904.

TABLE 15.5
T AND B LYMPHOCYTES IN PERIPHERAL BLOOD

Age	CD3 (Total T Cell) Count*,[†] (%)[†]	CD4 Count*,[†] (%)[†]	CD8 Count*,[†] (%)[†]	CD19 (B Cell) Count*,[†] (%)[†]
0–3 mo	2.50–5.50 (53–84)	1.60–4.00 (35–64)	0.56–1.70 (12–28)	0.30–2.00 (6–32)
3–6 mo	2.50–5.60 (51–77)	1.80–4.00 (35–56)	0.59–1.60 (12–23)	0.43–3.00 (11–41)
6–12 mo	1.90–5.90 (49–76)	1.40–4.30 (31–56)	0.50–1.70 (12–24)	0.61–2.60 (14–37)
1–2 yr	2.10–6.20 (53–75)	1.30–3.40 (32–51)	0.62–2.00 (14–30)	0.72–2.60 (16–35)
2–6 yr	1.40–3.70 (56–75)	0.70–2.20 (28–47)	0.49–1.30 (16–30)	0.39–1.40 (14–33)
6–12 yr	1.20–2.60 (60–76)	0.65–1.50 (31–47)	0.37–1.10 (18–35)	0.27–0.86 (13–27)
12–18 yr	1.00–2.20 (56–84)	0.53–1.30 (31–52)	0.33–0.92 (18–35)	0.11–0.57 (6–23)
Adult[‡]	0.70–2.10 (55–83)	0.30–1.40 (28–57)	0.20–0.90 (10–39)	

*Absolute counts (number of cells per microliter ×10^{-3})
[†]Normal values (10th to 90th percentile)
[‡]From Comans-Bitter WM, de Groot R, van den Beemd R, et al. Immunotyping of blood lymphocytes in childhood. Reference values for lymphocyte subpopulations. J Pediatr. 1997;130:388-393.

From Shearer WT, Rosenblatt HM, Gelman RS, et al. Lymphocyte subsets in healthy children from birth through 18 years of age: the Pediatric AIDS Clinical Trials Group P1009 study. J Allergy Clin Immunol. 2003;112:973-980.

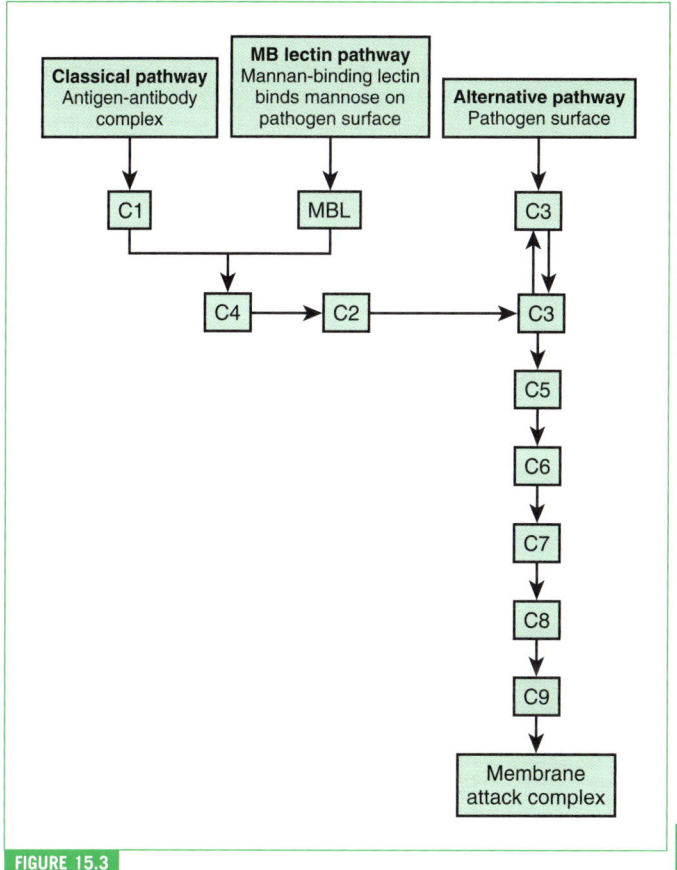

FIGURE 15.3
Complement pathway. MB, mannan-binding; MBL, mannan-binding lectin

TABLE 15.6
SERUM COMPLEMENT LEVELS*

Age	C3 (mg/dL)	C4 (mg/dL)
Cord blood (term)	83 (57–116)	13 (6.6–23)
1 mo	83 (53–124)	14 (7.0–25)
2 mo	96 (59–149)	15 (7.4–28)
3 mo	94 (64–131)	16 (8.7–27)
4 mo	107 (62–175)	19 (8.3–38)
5 mo	107 (64–167)	18 (7.1–36)
6 mo	115 (74–171)	21 (8.6–42)
7–9 mo	113 (75–166)	20 (9.5–37)
10–12 mo	126 (73–180)	22 (12–39)
1 yr	129 (84–174)	23 (12–40)
2 yr	120 (81–170)	19 (9.2–34)
3 yr	117 (77–171)	20 (9.7–36)
4–5 yr	121 (86–166)	21 (13–32)
6–8 yr	118 (88–155)	20 (12–32)
9–10 yr	134 (89–195)	22 (10–40)
Adult	125 (83–177)	28 (15–45)

*Numbers in parentheses are the 95% confidence intervals (CIs)
Modified from Jolliff CR, Cost KM, Stivrins PC, et al. Reference intervals for serum IgG, IgA, IgM, C3, and C4 as determined by rate nephelometry. Clin Chem. 1982;28:126-128.

REFERENCES

1. Gentile D, Bartholow A, Valovirta E, et al. Current and future directions in pediatric allergic rhinitis. *J Allergy Clin Immunol.* 2013;1 (in practice):214-226.
2. Blaiss MS. Antihistamines: treatment selection criteria for pediatric seasonal allergic rhinitis. *Allergy Asthma Proc.* 2005;26:95-102.
3. Garavello DW, DiBerardino F, Romagnoli M, et al. Nasal rinsing with hypertonic solution: an adjunctive treatment for pediatric seasonal allergic rhinoconjunctivitis. *Int Arch Allergy Immunol.* 2005;137:310-314.
4. Gelfand EW. Pediatric allergic rhinitis: factors affecting treatment choice. *Ear Nose Throat J.* 2005;84:163-168.
5. Hamrah P, Dana R. Allergic conjunctivitis: management. Up to Date 2015. Available at <www.uptodate.com>.
6. Wallace DV, Dykewicz MS, Bernstein DI, et al. The diagnosis and management of rhinitis: an updated practice parameter. *J Allergy Clin Immunol.* 2008;122(suppl 2):S1-S84.
7. Burks W. Diagnostic evaluation of food allergy. Up to Date 2015. Available at <www.uptodate.com>.
8. Chapman JA. Food allergy: a practice parameter. *Ann Allergy Asthma Immunol.* 2006;96(3 suppl 2):S1-S68.
9. Lake AM. Food protein-induced proctitis/colitis and enteropathy of infancy. Up to Date 2015. Available at <www.uptodate.com>.
10. Burks AW, Jones SM, Boyce JA, et al. NIAID-Sponsored 2010 guidelines for managing food allergy: applications in the pediatric population. *Pediatrics.* 2011;128:955-965.

11. Sicherer SH, Wood RA. Allergy testing in childhood: using allergen-specific IgE testing. *Pediatrics*. 2012;129:193-197.
12. Robbins KA, Wood RA. Clinical value of component-derived diagnostics in peanut-allergic patients. *Pediatrics*. 2013;132(suppl 1):S16-S17.
13. Solensky R. Penicillin allergy: immediate reactions. Up to Date 2015. Available at <www.uptodate.com>.
14. Solensky R, Khan DA. Drug allergy: an updated practice parameter. *Ann Allergy Asthma Immunol*. 2010;105:259-273.
15. Bonilla FA, Bernstein IL, Khan DA, et al. Practice parameters for the diagnosis and management of primary immunodeficiency. *Ann Allergy Asthma Immunol*. 2005;94(5 suppl 1):S1-S63.
16. Bonilla FA, Geha RS. Primary immunodeficiency diseases. *J Allergy Clin Immunol*. 2003;111(suppl 2):S571-S581.
17. Bonilla FA, Geha RS. Update on primary immunodeficiency diseases. *J Allergy Clin Immunol*. 2006;117(suppl 2 Mini–Primer):S435-S441.
18. Fleisher TA. Back to basics: primary immune deficiencies: windows into the immune system. *Pediatr Rev*. 2006;27:363-372.
19. Geha RS, Notarangelo LD, Casanova JL, et al; International Union of Immunological Societies Primary Immunodeficiency Diseases Classification Committee. Primary immunodeficiency diseases: an update from the International Union of Immunological Societies Primary Immunodeficiency Diseases Classification Committee. *J Allergy Clin Immunol*. 2007;120:776-794.
20. Lederman HM. Clinical presentation of primary immunodeficiency diseases. In: McMillan J, ed. *Oski's Pediatrics*. Philadelphia: Lippincott Williams & Wilkins; 2006:2441-2444.
21. Stiehm ER. Approach to the child with recurrent infections. Up to Date 2014. Available at <www.uptodate.com>.
22. Stiehm ER, Ochs HD, Winkelstein JA. Immunodeficiency disorders: general considerations. In: Stiehm ER, Ochs HD, Winkelstein JA, eds. *Immunologic Disorders in Infants and Children*. 5th ed. Philadelphia: Elsevier/Saunders; 2004.
23. Puck JM. Laboratory technology for population-based screening for SCID in neonates: The winner is T-cell receptor excision circles (TRECs). *J Allergy Clin Immunol*. 2012;129(3):607-616.
24. Garcia-Lloret M, McGhee S, Chatila TA, et al. Immunoglobulin replacement therapy in children. *Immunol Allergy Clin North Am*. 2008;28:833-849.
25. Moore ML, Quinn JM. Subcutaneous immunoglobulin replacement therapy for primary antibody deficiency: advancements into the 21st century. *Ann Allergy Asthma Immunol*. 2008;101:114-121.
26. Orange J, Hossny EM, Weiler CR, et al. Use of intravenous immunoglobulin in human disease: a review of evidence by members of the Primary Immunodeficiency Committee of the American Academy of Allergy, Asthma, and Immunology. *J Allergy Clin Immunol*. 2006;117(4 suppl):S525-S553.
27. Shapiro R. Subcutaneous immunoglobulin therapy given by subcutaneous rapid push vs. infusion pump: a retrospective analysis. *Ann Allergy Asthma Immunol*. 2013;111(1):51-55.

Chapter 16

Immunoprophylaxis

Alejandra Ellison-Barnes, MD

See additional content on Expert Consult

I. WEB RESOURCES

- American Academy of Pediatrics: *Red Book: 2015 Report of the Committee on Infectious Diseases,* 30th edition. 2015: http://redbook.solutions.aap.org/
- Centers for Disease Control and Prevention: Travelers' Health: http://www.cdc.gov/travel/
- Centers for Disease Control and Prevention: Vaccines and Immunization (including immunization schedules and *Morbidity and Mortality Weekly Reports* pertaining to vaccines): http://www.cdc.gov/vaccines/
- The Children's Hospital of Philadelphia: Vaccine Education Center: http://vec.chop.edu/
- Influenza vaccines A and B: http://www.cdc.gov/flu/professionals/antivirals/
- U.S. Food and Drug Administration: Vaccines Licensed for Immunization and Distribution in the US with Supporting Documents (including all package inserts): http://www.fda.gov/BiologicsBloodVaccines/Vaccines/ApprovedProducts/
- Vaccine Adverse Event Reporting System: http://vaers.hhs.gov/
- World Health Organization: Immunization, Vaccines and Biologicals: http://www.who.int/immunization/

II. IMMUNIZATION SCHEDULES

Recommended Childhood Immunization Schedule (Fig. 16.1) and Catch-up Immunization Schedules, with minimum age for initial vaccination and minimum intervals between doses (Fig. 16.2), vaccines that may be indicated for specific medical indications (Fig. EC 16.A), and accompanying footnotes (Fig. 16.3)[1]

III. IMMUNIZATION GUIDELINES

A. Vaccine Informed Consent

Current forms for the vaccine information statement (VIS) can be obtained from the Centers for Disease Control and Prevention (CDC). The most recent VIS must be provided to the patient (non-minor) or parent/guardian, with documentation of version date and date on which vaccine was administered.

Text continued on p. 419

Vaccine	Birth	1 mo	2 mos	4 mos	6 mos	9 mos	12 mos	15 mos	18 mos	19-23 mos	2-3 yrs	4-6 yrs	7-10 yrs	11-12 yrs	13-15 yrs	16 yrs	17-18 yrs
Hepatitis B[1] (HepB)	1st dose	←2nd dose→			←3rd dose→												
Rotavirus[2] (RV) RV1 (2-dose series); RV5 (3-dose series)			1st dose	2nd dose	See footnote 2												
Diphtheria, tetanus, & acellular pertussis[3] (DTaP: <7 yrs)			1st dose	2nd dose	3rd dose			←4th dose→				5th dose					
Haemophilus influenzae type b[4] (Hib)			1st dose	2nd dose	See footnote 4		←3rd or 4th dose, See footnote 4→										
Pneumococcal conjugate[5] (PCV13)			1st dose	2nd dose	3rd dose		←4th dose→										
Inactivated poliovirus[6] (IPV: <18 yrs)			1st dose	2nd dose	←3rd dose→							4th dose					
Influenza[7] (IIV)					Annual vaccination (IIV) 1 or 2 doses								Annual vaccination (IIV) 1 dose only				
Measles, mumps, rubella[8] (MMR)					See footnote 8		←1st dose→					2nd dose					
Varicella[9] (VAR)							←1st dose→					2nd dose					
Hepatitis A[10] (HepA)							←2-dose series, See footnote 10→										
Meningococcal[11] (Hib-MenCY ≥6 weeks; MenACWY-D ≥9 mos; MenACWY-CRM ≥2 mos)			See footnote 11											1st dose		2nd dose	
Tetanus, diphtheria, & acellular pertussis[12] (Tdap: ≥7 yrs)														Tdap			
Human papillomavirus[13] (HPV)														See footnote 13			
Meningococcal B[11]													See footnote 11				
Pneumococcal polysaccharide[5] (PPSV23)											See footnote 5						

Legend: Range of recommended ages for all children; Range of recommended ages for catch-up immunization; Range of recommended ages for certain high-risk groups; Range of recommended ages for non-high-risk groups that may receive vaccine, subject to individual clinical decision making; No recommendation

NOTE: The above recommendations must be read along with the footnotes of this schedule.

FIGURE 16.1 Recommended immunization schedule for persons aged 0 through 18 years—United States, 2017. *(From Centers for Disease Control and Prevention. Recommended Immunization Schedules for Persons Aged 0 Through 18 Years—United States, 2017. Available online at http://www.cdc.gov/vaccines/schedules/.)*

Vaccine	Minimum Age for Dose 1	Dose 1 to Dose 2	Dose 2 to Dose 3	Dose 3 to Dose 4	Dose 4 to Dose 5
Children age 4 months through 6 years					
Hepatitis B[1]	Birth	4 weeks	8 weeks and at least 16 weeks after first dose. Minimum age for the final dose is 24 weeks.		
Rotavirus[2]	6 weeks	4 weeks	4 weeks[2]		6 months[2]
Diphtheria, tetanus, and acellular pertussis[3]	6 weeks	4 weeks	4 weeks	6 months	6 months[3]
Haemophilus influenzae type b[4]	6 weeks	4 weeks if first dose was administered before the 1st birthday. 8 weeks (as final dose) if first dose was administered at age 12 through 14 months. No further doses needed if first dose was administered at age 15 months or older.	4 weeks[4] if current age is younger than 12 months **and** first dose was administered at younger than age 7 months, **and** at least 1 previous dose was PRP-T (ActHib, Pentacel, Hiberix) or unknown. **OR** 8 weeks **and age 12 through 59 months** (as final dose)[4] • If current age is younger than 12 months **and** first dose was administered at age 7 through 11 months; **OR** • If current age is 12 through 59 months **and** first dose was administered before the 1st birthday, **and** second dose was administered at younger than 15 months; **OR** • If both doses were PRP-OMP (PedvaxHIB, Comvax) **and** were administered before the 1st birthday. No further doses needed if previous dose was administered at age 15 months or older.	8 weeks (as final dose) This dose only necessary for children age 12 through 59 months who received 3 doses before the 1st birthday.	
Pneumococcal[5]	6 weeks	4 weeks if first dose was administered before the 1st birthday. 8 weeks (as final dose for healthy children) if first dose was administered at the 1st birthday or after. No further doses needed for healthy children if first dose was administered at age 24 months or older.	4 weeks if current age is younger than 12 months and previous dose given at <7 months old; 8 weeks (as final dose for healthy children) if previous dose given between 7-11 months (wait until at least 12 months old); **OR** if current age is 12 months or older and at least 1 dose was given before age 12 months. No further doses needed for healthy children if previous dose administered at age 24 months or older.	8 weeks (as final dose) This dose only necessary for children aged 12 through 59 months who received 3 doses before age 12 months or for children at high risk who received 3 doses at any age.	
Inactivated poliovirus[6]	6 weeks	4 weeks	4 weeks[6]	6 months[6] (Minimum age 4 years for final dose).	
Measles, mumps, rubella[7]	12 months	4 weeks			
Varicella[8]	12 months	3 months			
Hepatitis A[9]	12 months	6 months			
Meningococcal[10] (Hib-MenCY ≥6 weeks; MenACWY-CRM ≥2 mos; MenACWY-D ≥9 mos)	6 weeks	8 weeks[10]	See footnote 11		
Children and adolescents age 7 through 18 years					
Meningococcal[10] (MenACWY-D ≥9 mos; MenACWY-CRM ≥2 mos)	Not Applicable (N/A)	8 weeks[10]			
Tetanus, diphtheria/tetanus, diphtheria, and acellular pertussis[3]	7 years[3]	4 weeks	4 weeks if first dose of DTaP/DT was administered before the 1st birthday. 6 months (as final dose) if first dose of DTaP/DT or Tdap/Td was administered at or after the 1st birthday.	6 months if first dose of DTaP/DT was administered before the 1st birthday.	
Human papillomavirus[11]	9 years	Routine dosing intervals are recommended.[11]			
Hepatitis A[9]	N/A	6 months			
Hepatitis B[1]	N/A	4 weeks	8 weeks **and at least 16 weeks after first dose**.		
Inactivated poliovirus[6]	N/A	4 weeks	6 months[6]		
Measles, mumps, rubella[7]	N/A	4 weeks			
Varicella[8]	N/A	3 months if younger than age 13 years. 4 weeks if age 13 years or older.			

NOTE: The above recommendations must be read along with the footnotes of this schedule.

FIGURE 16.2
Catch-up immunization schedule for persons aged 4 months through 18 years who start late or who are more than 1 month behind—United States, 2017. (From Centers for Disease Control and Prevention. *Recommended Immunization Schedules for Persons Aged 0 Through 18 Years—United States, 2017.* Available online at http://www.cdc.gov/vaccines/schedules/.)

Footnotes — Recommended Immunization Schedule for Children and Adolescents Aged 18 Years or Younger, UNITED STATES, 2017

For further guidance on the use of the vaccines mentioned below, see: www.cdc.gov/vaccines/hcp/acip-recs/index.html.
For vaccine recommendations for persons 19 years of age and older, see the Adult Immunization Schedule.

Additional information

- For information on contraindications and precautions for the use of a vaccine and for additional information regarding that vaccine, vaccination providers should consult the ACIP General Recommendations on Immunization and the relevant ACIP statement, available online at www.cdc.gov/vaccines/hcp/acip-recs/index.html.
- For purposes of calculating intervals between doses, 4 weeks = 28 days. Intervals of 4 months or greater are determined by calendar months.
- Vaccine doses administered ≤4 days before the minimum interval are considered valid. Doses of any vaccine administered ≥5 days earlier than the minimum interval or minimum age should not be counted as valid and should be repeated as age-appropriate. The repeat dose should be spaced after the invalid dose by the recommended minimum interval. For further details, see Table 1, Recommended and minimum ages and intervals between vaccine doses, in MMWR, General Recommendations on Immunization and Reports / Vol. 60 / No. 2 available online at www.cdc.gov/mmwr/pdf/rr/rr6002.pdf.
- Information on travel vaccine requirements and recommendations is available at www.cdc.gov/travel.
- For vaccination of persons with primary and secondary immunodeficiencies, see Table 13, Vaccination of persons with primary and secondary immunodeficiencies, in General Recommendations on Immunization (ACIP), available at www.cdc.gov/mmwr/pdf/rr/rr6002.pdf, and Immunization in Special Clinical Circumstances, (In: Kimberlin DW, Brady MT, Jackson MA, Long SS, eds. Red Book: 2015 report of the Committee on Infectious Diseases. 30th ed. Elk Grove Village, IL: American Academy of Pediatrics, 2015:68-107.
- The National Vaccine Injury Compensation Program (VICP) is a no-fault alternative to the traditional legal system for resolving vaccine injury petitions. Created by the National Childhood Vaccine Injury Act of 1986, it provides compensation to people found to be injured by certain vaccines. All vaccines within the recommended childhood immunization schedule are covered by VICP except for pneumococcal polysaccharide vaccine (PPSV23). For more information, see www.hrsa.gov/vaccinecompensation/index.html.

1. **Hepatitis B (HepB) vaccine. (Minimum age: birth)**
   Routine vaccination:
   At birth:
   - Administer monovalent HepB vaccine to all newborns within 24 hours of birth.
   - For infants born to hepatitis B surface antigen (HBsAg)-positive mothers, administer HepB vaccine and 0.5 mL of hepatitis B immune globulin (HBIG) within 12 hours of birth. These infants should be tested for HBsAg and antibody to HBsAg (anti-HBs) at age 9 through 12 months (preferably at the next well-child visit) or 1 to 2 months after completion of the HepB series if the series was delayed.
   - If mother's HBsAg status is unknown, within 12 hours of birth, administer HepB vaccine regardless of birth weight. For infants weighing less than 2,000 grams, administer HBIG in addition to HepB vaccine within 12 hours of birth. Determine mother's HBsAg status as soon as possible and, if mother is HBsAg-positive, also administer HBIG to infants weighing 2,000 grams or more as soon as possible, but no later than age 7 days.

   Doses following the birth dose:
   - The second dose should be administered at age 1 or 2 months. Monovalent HepB vaccine should be used for doses administered before age 6 weeks.
   - Infants who did not receive a birth dose should receive 3 doses of a HepB-containing vaccine on a schedule of 0, 1 to 2 months, and 6 months, starting as soon as feasible (see Figure 2).
   - Administer the second dose 1 to 2 months after the first dose (minimum interval of 4 weeks); administer the third dose at least 8 weeks after the second dose AND at least 16 weeks after the first dose. The final (third or fourth) dose in the HepB vaccine series should be administered **no earlier than age 24 weeks**.
   - Administration of a total of 4 doses of HepB vaccine is permitted when a combination vaccine containing HepB is administered after the birth dose.

   Catch-up vaccination:
   - Unvaccinated persons should complete a 3-dose series.
   - A 2-dose series (doses separated by at least 4 months) of adult formulation Recombivax HB is licensed for use in children aged 11 through 15 years.
   - For other catch-up guidance, see Figure 2.

2. **Rotavirus (RV) vaccines. (Minimum age: 6 weeks for both RV1 [Rotarix] and RV5 [RotaTeq])**
   Routine vaccination:
   Administer a series of RV vaccine to all infants as follows:
   1. If Rotarix is used, administer a 2-dose series at ages 2 and 4 months.
   2. If RotaTeq is used, administer a 3-dose series at ages 2, 4, and 6 months.
   3. If any dose in the series was RotaTeq or vaccine product is unknown for any dose in the series, a total of 3 doses of RV vaccine should be administered.

   Catch-up vaccination:
   - The maximum age for the first dose in the series is 14 weeks, 6 days; vaccination should not be initiated for infants aged 15 weeks, 0 days, or older.
   - The maximum age for the final dose in the series is 8 months, 0 days.
   - For other catch-up guidance, see Figure 2.

3. **Diphtheria and tetanus toxoids and acellular pertussis (DTaP) vaccine. (Minimum age: 6 weeks. Exception: DTaP-IPV [Kinrix, Quadracel]: 4 years)**
   Routine vaccination:
   - Administer a 5-dose series of DTaP vaccine at ages 2, 4, 6, 15 through 18 months, and 4 through 6 years. The fourth dose may be administered as early as age 12 months, provided at least 6 months have elapsed since the third dose.
   - Inadvertent administration of fourth DTaP dose early: If the fourth dose of DTaP was administered at least 4 months after the third dose of DTaP and the child was 12 months of age or older, it does not need to be repeated.

   Catch-up vaccination:
   - The fifth dose of DTaP vaccine is not necessary if the fourth dose was administered at age 4 years or older.
   - For other catch-up guidance, see Figure 2.

4. **Haemophilus influenzae type b (Hib) conjugate vaccine. (Minimum age: 6 weeks for PRP-T [ActHIB, DTaP-IPV/Hib (Pentacel), Hiberix], PRP-OMP [PedvaxHIB])**
   Routine vaccination:
   - Administer a 2- or 3-dose Hib vaccine primary series and a booster dose (dose 3 or 4, depending on vaccine used in primary series) at age 12 through 15 months to complete a full Hib vaccine series.
   - The primary series with ActHIB, MenHibrix, Hiberix, or Pentacel consists of 3 doses and should be administered at ages 2, 4, and 6 months. The primary series with PedvaxHIB consists of 2 doses and should be administered at ages 2 and 4 months; a dose at age 6 months is not indicated.
   - One booster dose (dose 3 or 4, depending on vaccine used in primary series) of any Hib vaccine should be administered at age 12 through 15 months.
   - For recommendations on the use of MenHibrix in patients at increased risk for meningococcal disease, refer to the meningococcal vaccine footnotes and also to MMWR February 28, 2014 / 63(RR01):1-13, available at www.cdc.gov/mmwr/pdf/rr/rr6301.pdf.

FIGURE 16.3

Footnotes—Recommended immunization schedule for persons aged 0 through 18 years—United States, 2017. *(From Centers for Disease Control and Prevention. Recommended Immunization Schedules for Persons Aged 0 Through 18 Years—United States, 2017. Available online at http://www.cdc.gov/vaccines/schedules/.)*

Continued

For further guidance on the use of the vaccines mentioned below, see: www.cdc.gov/vaccines/hcp/acip-recs/index.html

Catch-up vaccination:
- If dose 1 was administered at ages 12 through 14 months, administer a second (final) dose at least 8 weeks after dose 1, regardless of Hib vaccine used in the primary series.
- If both doses were PRP-OMP (PedvaxHIB or COMVAX) and were administered before the first birthday, the third (and final) dose should be administered at age 12 through 59 months and at least 8 weeks after the second dose.
- If the first dose was administered at age 7 through 11 months, administer the second dose at least 4 weeks later and a third (and final) dose at age 12 through 15 months or 8 weeks after second dose, whichever is later.
- If first dose is administered before the first birthday and second dose administered at younger than 15 months, a third (and final) dose should be administered 8 weeks later.
- For unvaccinated children aged 15–59 months, administer only 1 dose.
- For other catch-up guidance, see Figure 2. For catch-up guidance related to MenHibrix, see the meningococcal vaccine footnotes and also MMWR February 28, 2014 / 63(RR01):1–13, available at www.cdc.gov/mmwr/PDF/rr/rr6301.pdf

Vaccination of persons with high-risk conditions:
- Children aged 12 through 59 months who are at increased risk for Hib disease, including chemotherapy recipients and those with anatomic or functional asplenia (including sickle cell disease), human immunodeficiency virus (HIV) infection, immunoglobulin deficiency, or early component complement deficiency, who have received either no doses or only 1 dose of Hib vaccine before age 12 months, should receive 2 additional doses of Hib vaccine 8 weeks apart; children who received 2 or more doses of Hib vaccine before age 12 months should receive 1 additional dose.
- For patients younger than age 5 years undergoing chemotherapy or radiation treatment who received a Hib vaccine dose(s) within 14 days of starting therapy or during therapy, repeat the dose(s) at least 3 months following therapy completion.
- Recipients of hematopoietic stem cell transplant (HSCT) should be revaccinated with a 3-dose regimen of Hib vaccine starting 6 to 12 months after successful transplant, regardless of vaccination history; doses should be administered at least 4 weeks apart.
- A single dose of any Hib-containing vaccine should be administered to unimmunized* children and adolescents 15 months of age and older undergoing an elective splenectomy; if possible, vaccine should be administered at least 14 days before procedure.
- Hib vaccine is not routinely recommended for patients 5 years or older. However, 1 dose of Hib vaccine should be administered to unimmunized* persons aged 5 years or older who have anatomic or functional asplenia

(including sickle cell disease) and unimmunized* persons 5 through 18 years of age with HIV infection.
*Patients who have not received a primary series and booster dose or at least 1 dose of Hib vaccine after 14 months of age are considered unimmunized.

5. **Pneumococcal vaccines. (Minimum age: 6 weeks for PCV13, 2 years for PPSV23)**

Routine vaccination with PCV13:
- Administer a 4-dose series of PCV13 at ages 2, 4, and 6 months and at age 12 through 15 months.

Catch-up vaccination with PCV13:
- Administer 1 dose of PCV13 to all healthy children aged 24 through 59 months who are not completely vaccinated for their age.
- For other catch-up guidance, see Figure 2.

Vaccination of persons with high-risk conditions with PCV13 and PPSV23:
- All recommended PCV13 doses should be administered prior to PPSV23 vaccination if possible.
- For children aged 2 through 5 years with any of the following conditions: chronic heart disease (particularly cyanotic congenital heart disease and cardiac failure); chronic lung disease (including asthma if treated with high-dose oral corticosteroid therapy); diabetes mellitus; cerebrospinal fluid leak; cochlear implant; sickle cell disease and other hemoglobinopathies; anatomic or functional asplenia; HIV infection; chronic renal failure; nephrotic syndrome; diseases associated with treatment with immunosuppressive drugs or radiation therapy, including malignant neoplasms, leukemias, lymphomas, and Hodgkin disease; solid organ transplantation; or congenital immunodeficiency:
  1. Administer 1 dose of PCV13 if any incomplete schedule of 3 doses of PCV13 was received previously.
  2. Administer 2 doses of PCV13 at least 8 weeks apart if unvaccinated or any incomplete schedule of fewer than 3 doses of PCV13 was received previously.
  3. The minimum interval between doses of PCV13 is 8 weeks.
- For children aged 6 through 18 years with no history of PPSV23 vaccination, administer PPSV23 at least 8 weeks after the most recent dose of PCV13.
- For children aged 6 through 18 years with: cerebrospinal fluid leak; cochlear implant; sickle cell disease and other hemoglobinopathies; anatomic or functional asplenia; congenital or acquired immunodeficiencies; HIV infection; chronic renal failure; nephrotic syndrome; diseases associated with treatment with immunosuppressive drugs or radiation therapy, including malignant neoplasms, leukemias, lymphomas, and Hodgkin disease; generalized malignancy; solid organ transplantation; or multiple myeloma:
  1. If neither PCV13 nor PPSV23 has been received previously, administer 1 dose of PCV13 now and 1 dose of PPSV23 at least 8 weeks later.

  2. If PCV13 has been received previously but PPSV23 has not, administer 1 dose of PPSV23 at least 8 weeks after the most recent dose of PCV13.
  3. If PPSV23 has been received but PCV13 has not, administer 1 dose of PCV13 at least 8 weeks after the most recent dose of PPSV23.
- For children aged 6 through 18 years with chronic heart disease (particularly cyanotic congenital heart disease and cardiac failure), chronic lung disease (including asthma if treated with high-dose oral corticosteroid therapy), diabetes mellitus, alcoholism, or chronic liver disease, who have not received PPSV23, administer 1 dose of PPSV23. If PCV13 has been received previously, then PPSV23 should be administered at least 8 weeks after any prior PCV13 dose.
- A single revaccination with PPSV23 should be administered 5 years after the first dose to children with sickle cell disease or other hemoglobinopathies; anatomic or functional asplenia; congenital or acquired immunodeficiencies; HIV infection; chronic renal failure; nephrotic syndrome; diseases associated with treatment with immunosuppressive drugs or radiation therapy, including malignant neoplasms, leukemias, lymphomas, and Hodgkin disease; generalized malignancy; solid organ transplantation; or multiple myeloma.

6. **Inactivated poliovirus vaccine (IPV). (Minimum age: 6 weeks)**

Routine vaccination:
- Administer a 4-dose series of IPV at ages 2, 4, 6 through 18 months, and 4 through 6 years. The final dose in the series should be administered on or after the fourth birthday and at least 6 months after the previous dose.

Catch-up vaccination:
- In the first 6 months of life, minimum age and minimum intervals are only recommended if the person is at risk of imminent exposure to circulating poliovirus (i.e., travel to a polio-endemic region or during an outbreak).
- If 4 or more doses are administered before age 4 years, an additional dose should be administered at age 4 through 6 years and at least 6 months after the previous dose.
- A fourth dose is not necessary if the third dose was administered at age 4 years or older and at least 6 months after the previous dose.
- If both oral polio vaccine (OPV) and IPV were administered as part of a series, a total of 4 doses should be administered, regardless of the child's current age. If only OPV was administered, and all doses were given prior to age 4 years, 1 dose of IPV should be given at 4 years or older, at least 4 weeks after the last OPV dose.
- IPV is not routinely recommended for U.S. residents aged 18 years or older.
- For other catch-up guidance, see Figure 2.

FIGURE 16.3, cont'd

For further guidance on the use of the vaccines mentioned below, see: www.cdc.gov/vaccines/hcp/acip-recs/index.html

7. **Influenza vaccines. (Minimum age: 6 months for inactivated influenza vaccine [IIV], 18 years for recombinant influenza vaccine [RIV])**

   Routine vaccination:
   - Administer influenza vaccine annually to all children beginning at age 6 months. For the 2016–17 season, use of the attenuated influenza vaccine (LAIV) is not recommended.

   For children aged 6 months through 8 years:
   - For the 2016–17 season, administer 2 doses (separated by at least 4 weeks) to children who are receiving influenza vaccine for the first time or who have not previously received 2 doses of trivalent or quadrivalent influenza vaccine before July 1, 2016. For additional guidance, follow dosing guidelines in the 2016–17 ACIP influenza vaccine recommendations (see MMWR August 26, 2016;65(5):1-54, available at www.cdc.gov/mmwr/volumes/65/rr/pdfs/rr6505.pdf).
   - For the 2017–18 season, follow dosing guidelines in the 2017–18 ACIP influenza vaccine recommendations.

   For persons aged 9 years and older:
   - Administer 1 dose.

8. **Measles, mumps, and rubella (MMR) vaccine. (Minimum age: 12 months for routine vaccination)**

   Routine vaccination:
   - Administer a 2-dose series of MMR vaccine at ages 12 through 15 months and 4 through 6 years. The second dose may be administered before age 4 years, provided at least 4 weeks have elapsed since the first dose.
   - Administer 1 dose of MMR vaccine to infants aged 6 through 11 months before departure from the United States for international travel. These children should be revaccinated with 2 doses of MMR vaccine, the first dose at age 12 months through 15 months (12 months if the child remains in an area where disease risk is high), and the second dose at least 4 weeks later.
   - Administer 2 doses of MMR vaccine to children aged 12 months and older before departure from the United States for international travel. The first dose should be administered on or after age 12 months and the second dose at least 4 weeks later.

   Catch-up vaccination:
   - Ensure that all school-aged children and adolescents have had 2 doses of MMR vaccine; the minimum interval between the 2 doses is 4 weeks.

9. **Varicella (VAR) vaccine. (Minimum age: 12 months)**

   Routine vaccination:
   - Administer a 2-dose series of VAR vaccine at ages 12 through 15 months and 4 through 6 years. The second dose may be administered before age 4 years, provided at least 3 months have elapsed since the first dose. If the second dose was administered at least 4 weeks after the first dose, it can be accepted as valid.

   Catch-up vaccination:
   - Ensure that all persons aged 7 through 18 years without evidence of immunity (see MMWR 2007;56[No. RR-4], available at www.cdc.gov/mmwr/pdf/rr/rr5604.pdf) have 2 doses of varicella vaccine. For children aged 7 through 12 years, the recommended minimum interval between doses is 3 months (if the second dose was administered at least 4 weeks after the first dose, it can be accepted as valid); for persons aged 13 years and older, the minimum interval between doses is 4 weeks.

10. **Hepatitis A (HepA) vaccine. (Minimum age: 12 months)**

    Routine vaccination:
    - Initiate the 2-dose HepA vaccine series at ages 12 through 23 months; separate the 2 doses by 6 to 18 months.
    - Children who have received 1 dose of HepA vaccine before age 24 months should receive a second dose 6 to 18 months after the first dose.
    - For any person aged 2 years and older who has not already received the HepA vaccine series, 2 doses of HepA vaccine separated by 6 to 18 months may be administered if immunity against hepatitis A virus infection is desired.

    Catch-up vaccination:
    - The minimum interval between the 2 doses is 6 months.

    Special populations:
    - Administer 2 doses of HepA vaccine at least 6 months apart to previously unvaccinated persons who live in areas where vaccination programs target older children, or who are at increased risk for infection. This includes persons traveling to or working in countries that have high or intermediate endemicity of infection; men having sex with men; users of injection and non-injection illicit drugs; persons who work with HAV-infected primates or with HAV in a research laboratory; persons with clotting-factor disorders; persons with chronic liver disease; and persons who anticipate close, personal contact (e.g., household or regular babysitting) with an international adoptee during the first 60 days after arrival in the United States from a country with high or intermediate endemicity. The first dose should be administered as soon as the adoption is planned, ideally, 2 or more weeks before the arrival of the adoptee.

11. **Meningococcal vaccines. (Minimum age: 6 weeks for Hib-MenCY [Menhibrix], 2 months for MenACWY-CRM [Menveo], 9 months for MenACWY-D [Menactra], 10 years for serogroup B meningococcal [MenB] vaccines: MenB-4C [Bexsero] and MenB-FHbp [Trumenba])**

    Routine vaccination:
    - Administer a single dose of Menactra or Menveo vaccine at age 11 through 12 years, with a booster dose at age 16 years.
    - For children aged 2 months through 10 years with high-risk conditions, see "Meningococcal conjugate ACWY vaccination of children at increased risk for meningococcal disease" and "Meningococcal B

    vaccination of persons with high-risk conditions and other persons at increased risk of disease" below.

    Catch-up vaccination:
    - Administer Menactra or Menveo vaccine at age 13 through 18 years if not previously vaccinated.
    - If the first dose is administered at age 13 through 15 years, a booster dose should be administered at age 16 through 18 years, with a minimum interval of at least 8 weeks between doses.
    - If the first dose is administered at age 16 years or older, a booster dose is not needed.
    - For other catch-up guidance, see Figure 2.

    Clinical discretion:
    - Young adults aged 16 through 23 years (preferred age range is 16 through 18 years) who are not at increased risk for meningococcal disease may be vaccinated with a 2-dose series of either Bexsero (0, ≥1 month) or Trumenba (0, 6 months) vaccine to provide short-term protection against most strains of serogroup B meningococcal disease. The two MenB vaccines are not interchangeable; the same vaccine product must be used for all doses.
    - If the second dose of Trumenba is given at an interval of <6 months, a third dose should be given at least 6 months after the first dose; the minimum interval between the second and third doses is 4 weeks.

    Meningococcal conjugate ACWY vaccination of persons with high-risk conditions and other persons at increased risk:

    Children with anatomic or functional asplenia (including sickle cell disease), children with HIV infection, or children with persistent complement component deficiency (includes persons with inherited or chronic deficiencies in C3, C5-9, properdin, factor D, factor H, or taking eculizumab [Soliris]):
    - **Menveo**
      o Children who initiate vaccination at 8 weeks: Administer doses at ages 2, 4, 6, and 12 months.
      o Unvaccinated children who initiate vaccination at 7 through 23 months: Administer 2 primary doses, with the second dose at least 12 weeks after the first dose AND after the first birthday.
      o Children 24 months and older who have not received a complete series: Administer 2 primary doses at least 8 weeks apart.
    - **MenHibrix**
      o Children who initiate vaccination at 6 weeks: Administer doses at ages 2, 4, 6, and 12 through 15 months.
      o If the first dose of MenHibrix is given at or after age 12 months, a total of 2 doses should be given at least 8 weeks apart to ensure protection against serogroups C and Y meningococcal disease.

FIGURE 16.3, cont'd

Continued

For further guidance on the use of the vaccines mentioned below, see: www.cdc.gov/vaccines/hcp/acip-recs/index.html.

- **Menactra**
  - **Children with anatomic or functional asplenia or HIV infection**
    - Children 24 months and older who have not received a complete series: Administer 2 primary doses at least 8 weeks apart. If Menactra is administered to a child with asplenia (including sickle cell disease) or HIV infection, do not administer Menactra until age 2 years, and at least 4 weeks after the completion of all PCV13 doses.
  - **Children with persistent complement component deficiency**
    - Children 9 through 23 months: Administer 2 primary doses at least 12 weeks apart.
    - Children 24 months and older who have not received a complete series: Administer 2 primary doses at least 8 weeks apart.
  - **All high-risk children**
    - If Menactra is to be administered to a child at high risk for meningococcal disease, it is recommended that Menactra be given either before or at the same time as DTaP.

Meningococcal B vaccination of persons with high-risk conditions and other persons at increased risk of disease: Children with anatomic or functional asplenia (including sickle cell disease) or children with persistent complement component deficiency (includes persons with inherited or chronic deficiencies in C3, C5-9, properdin, factor D, factor H, or taking eculizumab [Soliris]):
- **Bexsero or Trumenba**
  - Persons 10 years or older who have not received a complete series: Administer a 2-dose series of Bexsero, with doses at least 1 month apart, or a 3-dose series of Trumenba, with the second dose at least 1-2 months after the first. The two MenB vaccines are not interchangeable; the same vaccine product must be used for all doses.

For children who travel to or reside in countries in which meningococcal disease is hyperendemic or epidemic, including countries in the African meningitis belt or the Hajj:
- Administer an age-appropriate formulation and series of Menactra or Menveo for protection against serogroups A and W meningococcal disease. Prior receipt of MenHibrix is not sufficient for children traveling to the meningitis belt or the Hajj because it does not contain serogroups A or W.

For children at risk during an outbreak attributable to a vaccine serogroup:
- For serogroup A, C, W, or Y: Administer or complete an age- and formulation-appropriate series of MenHibrix, Menactra, or Menveo.

- For serogroup B: Administer a 2-dose series of Bexsero, with doses at least 1 month apart, or a 3-dose series of Trumenba, with the second dose at least 1-2 months after the first and the third dose at least 6 months after the second. The two MenB vaccines are not interchangeable; the same vaccine product must be used for all doses.

For MenACWY booster doses among persons with high-risk conditions, see MMWR 2013;62(RR02):1-22, at www.cdc.gov/mmwr/preview/mmwrhtml/rr6202a1.htm, MMWR June 20, 2014 / 63(24):527-530, at www.cdc.gov/mmwr/pdf/wk/mm6324.pdf, and MMWR November 4, 2016 / 65(43):1189-1194, at www.cdc.gov/mmwr/volumes/65/wr/pdfs/mm6543a3.pdf.

For other catch-up recommendations for these persons and complete information on use of meningococcal vaccines, including guidance related to vaccination of persons at increased risk of infection, see meningococcal MMWR publications, available at: www.cdc.gov/vaccines/hcp/acip-recs/vacc-specific/mening.html.

12. **Tetanus and diphtheria toxoids and acellular pertussis (Tdap) vaccine. (Minimum age: 10 years for both Boostrix and Adacel)**

    Routine vaccination:
    - Administer 1 dose of Tdap vaccine to all adolescents aged 11 through 12 years.
    - Tdap may be administered regardless of the interval since the last tetanus and diphtheria toxoid-containing vaccine.
    - Administer 1 dose of Tdap vaccine to pregnant adolescents during each pregnancy (preferably during the early part of gestational weeks 27 through 36), regardless of time since prior Td or Tdap vaccination.

    Catch-up vaccination:
    - Persons aged 7 years and older who are not fully immunized with DTaP vaccine should receive Tdap vaccine as 1 dose (preferably the first) in the catch-up series; if additional doses are needed, use Td vaccine. For children 7 through 10 years who receive a dose of Tdap as part of the catch-up series, an adolescent Tdap vaccine dose at age 11 through 12 years may be administered.
    - Persons aged 11 through 18 years who have not received Tdap vaccine should receive a dose, followed by tetanus and diphtheria toxoids (Td) booster doses every 10 years thereafter.
    - Inadvertent doses of DTaP vaccine:
      - If administered inadvertently to a child aged 7 through 10 years, the dose may count as part of the catch-up series. This dose may be counted as the adolescent Tdap booster, or the child may receive a Tdap booster dose at age 11 through 12 years.
      - If administered inadvertently to an adolescent aged 11 through 18 years, the dose should be counted as the adolescent Tdap booster.
    - For other catch-up guidance, see Figure 2.

13. **Human papillomavirus (HPV) vaccines. (Minimum age: 9 years for HPV9 [Gardasil 9] and HPV [Gardasil 9])**

    Routine and catch-up vaccination:
    - Administer a 2-dose series of HPV vaccine on a schedule of 0, 6-12 months to all adolescents aged 11 or 12 years. The vaccination series can start at age 9 years.
    - Administer HPV vaccine to all adolescents through age 18 years who were not previously adequately vaccinated. The number of recommended doses is based on age at administration of the first dose.
    - For persons initiating vaccination before age 15, the recommended immunization schedule is 2 doses of HPV vaccine at 0, 6-12 months.
    - For persons initiating vaccination at age 15 years or older, the recommended immunization schedule is 3 doses of HPV vaccine at 0, 1-2, 6 months.
    - A vaccine dose administered at a shorter interval should be readministered at the recommended interval.
      - In a 2-dose schedule of HPV vaccine, the minimum interval is 5 months between the first and second dose. If the second dose is administered at a shorter interval, a third dose should be administered a minimum of 12 weeks after the second dose and a minimum of 5 months after the first dose.
      - In a 3-dose schedule of HPV vaccine, the minimum intervals are 4 weeks between the first and second dose, 12 weeks between the second and third dose, and 5 months between the first and third dose. If a vaccine dose is administered at a shorter interval, it should be readministered after another minimum interval has been met since the most recent dose.

    Special populations:
    - For persons with history of sexual abuse or assault, administer HPV vaccine beginning at age 9 years.
    - Immunocompromised persons*, including those with human immunodeficiency virus (HIV) infection, should receive a 3-dose series at 0, 1-2, and 6 months, regardless of age at vaccine initiation.
    - Note: HPV vaccination is not recommended during pregnancy, although there is no evidence that the vaccine poses harm. If a woman is found to be pregnant after initiating the vaccination series, no intervention is needed; the remaining vaccine doses should be delayed until after the pregnancy. Pregnancy testing is not needed before HPV vaccination.

    *See MMWR December 16, 2016;65(49):1405-1408, available at www.cdc.gov/mmwr/volumes/65/wr/pdfs/mm6549a5.pdf.

FIGURE 16.3, cont'd

B. Vaccine Administration

1. **Preferred sites of administration of intramuscular (IM) and subcutaneous (SQ) vaccines:**
a. <18 months old: Anterolateral thigh
b. Toddlers: Anterolateral thigh or deltoid (deltoid preferred if large enough)
c. Children, adolescents, and young adults: Deltoid
2. **Route:**
a. IM: Deep into muscle to avoid tissue damage from adjuvants, usually with a 22 G–25 G needle, ⅝- to 1-inch in infants and toddlers and 1- to 2-inch in adolescents and young adults
b. SQ: Into pinched skin fold with a 23 G–25 G, ⅝- to ¾-inch needle
3. **Simultaneous administration:**
a. Routine childhood vaccines are safe and effective when administered simultaneously at different sites, generally 1–2 inches apart. This includes inactivated and live vaccines.
b. If live vaccines are not given at the same visit, an interval of 28 days should be allotted between them.

C. Vaccine Types

1. **Live vaccines:** Influenza (intranasal); measles, mumps, and rubella (MMR); polio (oral); rotavirus; tuberculosis [Bacille Calmette–Guérin (BCG)]; typhoid (oral); varicella; yellow fever
2. **Nonlive vaccines:** Diphtheria, tetanus, pertussis combination vaccines (DTaP/DT/Td/Tdap); hepatitis A (HepA); hepatitis B (HepB); *Haemophilus influenzae* type b (Hib); human papillomavirus (HPV); influenza (injectable); Japanese encephalitis (JE); meningococcal; pneumococcal; rabies; typhoid (injectable)

D. General Indications and Precautions for All Vaccines

This information is based on the Advisory Committee on Immunization Practices (ACIP) and the Committee on Infectious Diseases of the American Academy of Pediatrics (AAP) and may vary from that listed on the manufacturers' inserts.[2] See vaccination-specific information in Section V.

1. **Contraindications**
a. Anaphylactic reaction to a vaccine or a vaccine constituent contraindicates further doses of that vaccine or vaccines containing that substance
2. **Precautions:** If risks are believed to outweigh benefits, immunization should be withheld; if benefits are believed to outweigh risks (e.g., during an outbreak, for foreign travel), immunization should be given.
a. Moderate or severe illnesses with or without a fever
b. Anaphylactic latex allergy (vaccines supplied in vials or syringes that contain natural rubber; a list is available from the CDC at http://www.cdc.gov/vaccines/pubs/pinkbook/downloads/appendices/B/latex-table.pdf)

3. **Not considered contraindications:** Vaccines should be given in the circumstances below, as well as those listed in the specific vaccine sections.
   a. Mild acute illness with or without low-grade fever, current antimicrobial therapy, or convalescent phase of illness
   b. Mild-to-moderate local reaction (soreness, redness, swelling) after a dose of an injectable antigen; low-grade or moderate fever after a previous vaccine dose
   c. Allergy to products not present in vaccine (e.g., penicillin) or allergy that is not anaphylactic (e.g., contact allergy to latex)
   d. Malnutrition
   e. Family history of adverse event to immunization
   f. Unimmunized or immunodeficient household contact; exceptions are smallpox in nonemergent situations and live attenuated influenza virus (LAIV) in close contacts of persons with severe immunosuppression requiring a protected environment
   g. Pregnancy of mother or household contact
   h. Breastfeeding (nursing infant or lactating mother); exception is yellow fever vaccine, which is a precaution

E. Misconceptions

1. Misconceptions about the need for and safety of recommended immunizations have been associated with underimmunization and/or delay in immunization.
2. The CDC and AAP publish Provider Resources for Vaccine Conversations with Parents with up-to-date vaccine information and resources to effectively communicate with parents regarding vaccines (available at http://www.cdc.gov/vaccines/hcp/patient-ed/conversations/).

IV. IMMUNOPROPHYLAXIS GUIDELINES FOR SPECIAL HOSTS[2,3]

A. Children at High Risk for Pneumococcal Disease[4]

1. **Definition:**
   a. Immunocompetent: Chronic heart disease, chronic lung disease (CLD), diabetes mellitus, cerebrospinal fluid (CSF) leak, cochlear implant
   b. Immunocompromised: Functional or anatomic asplenia including sickle cell disease, human immunodeficiency virus (HIV) infection, chronic renal failure or nephrotic syndrome, malignancy, immunosuppressive therapy, congenital immunodeficiency
2. All recommended doses of pneumococcal conjugate vaccine (PCV13) should be administered prior to PPSV23 vaccination, if possible.
3. **For those younger than 6 years at high risk,** complete primary series with PCV13.

4. **For those aged 2 years and older at high risk**, give one dose of PPSV23 at least 8 weeks after the last dose of PCV13.
5. **For those aged 6 years and older with immunocompromise, CSF leak, or cochlear implant** who have never received PCV13, give one dose of PCV13 (minimum interval from PPSV23 8 weeks). If the patient has never received PPSV23, give one dose of PPSV23 at least 8 weeks after the PCV13 dose.
6. **For those aged 6 years and older with immunocompromise**, a single booster of PPSV23 is indicated 5 years after the first dose but should not be repeated.

B. Children at High Risk for Meningococcal Disease[5]

1. **Definition:** Functional or anatomic asplenia, HIV infection, persistent complement deficiency, travel to or residence in areas with hyperendemic or epidemic meningococcal disease, or residence in a community with a meningococcal outbreak.
2. **For those younger than 2 years**, refer to Table 16.1. Note that MenHibrix is not sufficient for children traveling to parts of sub-Saharan Africa or the Hajj in Saudi Arabia as it does not contain serotypes A or W.
3. **For those aged 2 years and older**, give two-dose primary series of MenACWY-D or MenACWY-CRM at an interval of 8–12 weeks. Give MenACWY-D at least 4 weeks after completion of PCV13 series.
4. **Boosters**: If the most recent dose was prior to age 7 years, a booster dose should be given 3 years after completion of the primary series and then every 5 years thereafter. If the most recent dose was at age

TABLE 16.1

MENINGOCOCCAL VACCINATION OF CHILDREN AGED 2–23 MONTHS AT INCREASED RISK

Vaccine	Schedule
Men ACWY-CRM (Menveo)	8 weeks–6 months: Doses at 2, 4, 6, and 12 months of age 7–23 months (and unvaccinated): Two doses with second dose at 12-week interval or after the first birthday (whichever is later)
Hib-MenCY (MenHibrix) (Not for international travel)	6 weeks–18 months: Doses at 2, 4, 6, and 12–15 months. If first dose is given after 12 months of age, a total of two doses should be given 8 weeks apart.
MenACWY-D (Menactra) (For persistent complement deficiency or travel/exposure only; do not use for asplenia or HIV under age 2 years)	9–23 months: Two doses at 12-week interval, though 8-week interval acceptable if being given prior to travel.

Modified from Centers for Disease Control and Prevention. Use of MenACWY-CRM Vaccine in Children Aged 2 through 23 Months at Increased Risk for Meningococcal Disease: Recommendations of the Advisory Committee on Immunization Practice, 2013. MMWR. 2014;63:527-530.

7 years or older, a booster dose should be given every 5 years. Only MenACWY-CRM or MenACWY-D should be used.

5. **For those aged 10 years and older with asplenia or persistent complement deficiency**, give a two-dose series of MenB-4C or a three-dose series of MenB-FHbp in addition to MCV4 series.[6] The two MenB vaccines are not interchangeable; the same product must be used for all doses in a series.

C. Children at High Risk for Hib Disease

1. **Definition:** Functional or anatomic asplenia, HIV infection, immunoglobulin deficiency, early component complement deficiency, or chemotherapy/radiation.
2. **For those younger than 12 months,** give primary series.
3. **For those aged 12 through 59 months** who are unimmunized or received one dose prior to age 12 months, give two doses at 8-week interval. If two doses were received before age 12 months, give one additional dose.
4. **For those aged 5 years and older** who are not fully immunized and have asplenia or HIV, give one dose.

D. Functional or Anatomic Asplenia (Including Sickle Cell Disease)

1. **Penicillin prophylaxis:** See Chapter 14.
2. **Pneumococcal vaccines:** See Section IV.A.
3. **Meningococcal vaccines:** See Section IV.B.
4. **Hib vaccines:** See Section IV.C.
5. **Children aged 2 years and older** undergoing elective splenectomy should ideally receive pneumococcal and meningococcal vaccines at least 2 weeks before surgery for optimal immune response, and may also benefit from another dose of Hib.

E. Congenital Immunodeficiency Disorders

1. **Live vaccines are generally contraindicated.** (See Table 1.15 in the *AAP Red Book*[2] for details regarding individual immunodeficiencies.)
2. **Inactivated vaccines should be given** according to the routine schedule. Immune response may vary and may be inadequate; titers can be used to assess response.
3. **Immunoglobulin (Ig) therapy** may be indicated.
4. **Household contacts should be immunized** according to the routine schedule. Exceptions are LAIV if immunocompromise is severe [severe combined immunodeficiency (SCID), hematopoietic stem cell transplantation (HSCT) within 2 months, graft-versus-host disease (GVHD) requiring therapy] and oral poliovirus (OPV).

F. Known or Suspected HIV Disease

1. **Inactivated vaccines should be given** according to the routine immunization schedule. Influenza vaccine should be given annually.

a. Pneumococcal vaccines: See Section IV.A.
b. Meningococcal vaccines: See Section IV.B.
c. Hib vaccines: See Section IV.C.
2. **Live vaccines:**
a. Rotavirus vaccines should be given according to routine schedule.
b. MMR and varicella vaccines should be given to clinically stable patients with CD4+ count >200 cells/mm^3 (or percentage ≥15% if under age 5 years). Do not administer the measles, mumps, rubella, and varicella (MMRV) combination vaccine.
c. Do not administer LAIV. OPV and BCG vaccine are generally not given except in areas where risk of disease is thought to outweigh possibility of vaccine-associated disease.
3. **Passive immunoprophylaxis or chemoprophylaxis should be considered** after exposures.

G. Oncology Patients

Refer to specialized guidelines or consult with the patient's oncologist.
1. **During maintenance chemotherapy, inactivated vaccines may be considered** but should not be counted toward series unless titers show adequate response.
2. **All live vaccines should be delayed** at least 3 months after immunosuppressive therapy has been discontinued. Live vaccines may need to be readministered if titers have fallen below protective levels.
3. **Hematopoietic stem cell transplant recipients** should receive all routinely recommended vaccines prior to transplant if they are not already immunosuppressed and if the interval to the start of conditioning is at least 2 weeks for inactivated vaccines and 4 weeks for live vaccines. Patients will need reimmunization against vaccine-preventable illnesses after transplantation; refer to specialized guidelines.

H. Solid Organ Transplant Recipients

All vaccinations should be given based on routine schedules prior to transplant. PCV13 and PCV23 should also be administered as indicated (see Section IV.A). Inactivated vaccine administration may resume 2–6 months after transplant; live vaccines are generally not administered after transplant.

I. Patients on Corticosteroids

Only live vaccines are potentially contraindicated. See Table 16.2 for recommendations.

J. Patients on Biological Response Modifier Therapy (Cytokine Inhibitors)

Administer live vaccines a minimum of 4 weeks and inactivated vaccines a minimum of 2 weeks before initiating therapy, according to routine schedules. Live vaccines are contraindicated during therapy and

TABLE 16.2
LIVE VACCINE IMMUNIZATION FOR PATIENTS RECEIVING CORTICOSTEROID THERAPY

Steroid Dose	Recommended Guidelines
Topical, inhaled, or local injection of steroids	Live vaccines can generally be given unless there is clinical evidence of immunosuppression
Low-dose steroids (<2 mg/kg/day or <20 mg/day of prednisone equivalent), including physiologic doses	Live vaccines may be given
High-dose steroids (≥2 mg/kg/day or ≥20 mg/day of prednisone equivalent)	
Duration of therapy <14 days	Live vaccines may be given immediately after cessation of therapy (but consider 2-week delay)
Duration of therapy ≥14 days	Delay live vaccines until 4 weeks after discontinuation of therapy
Systemic or local steroids in patients with underlying disease affecting immune response (e.g., lupus) or receiving other immunosuppressant medication	Do not administer live vaccines

Data from American Academy of Pediatrics. Red Book: 2015 Report of the Committee on Infectious Diseases. *30th ed. Elk Grove Village, IL: AAP; 2015.*

for weeks to months after discontinuation; inactivated vaccines may be given.

K. Pregnancy

1. **Give Tdap during each pregnancy**, preferably at 27–36 weeks gestation, regardless of prior immunization status.
2. **Give inactivated influenza vaccine** regardless of trimester; do not give LAIV.
3. Other inactivated vaccines are considered precautionary and generally deferred until after the pregnancy.
4. **Live vaccines are generally contraindicated** during pregnancy. Yellow fever vaccine may be considered if travel to a high-risk area cannot be postponed.

L. Preterm and Low-Birth-Weight Infants

1. **Immunize according to chronologic age, using regular vaccine dosage.** Defer rotavirus vaccine until discharge from the hospital due to risk of nosocomial spread.
2. **HepB:** For infants <2 kg born to hepatitis B surface antigen (HBsAg)–negative mothers, delay first vaccine dose until 1 month of age or hospital discharge (whichever is first). For management of low-birth-weight infants of mothers with positive or unknown HepB status, see Fig. 16.4.

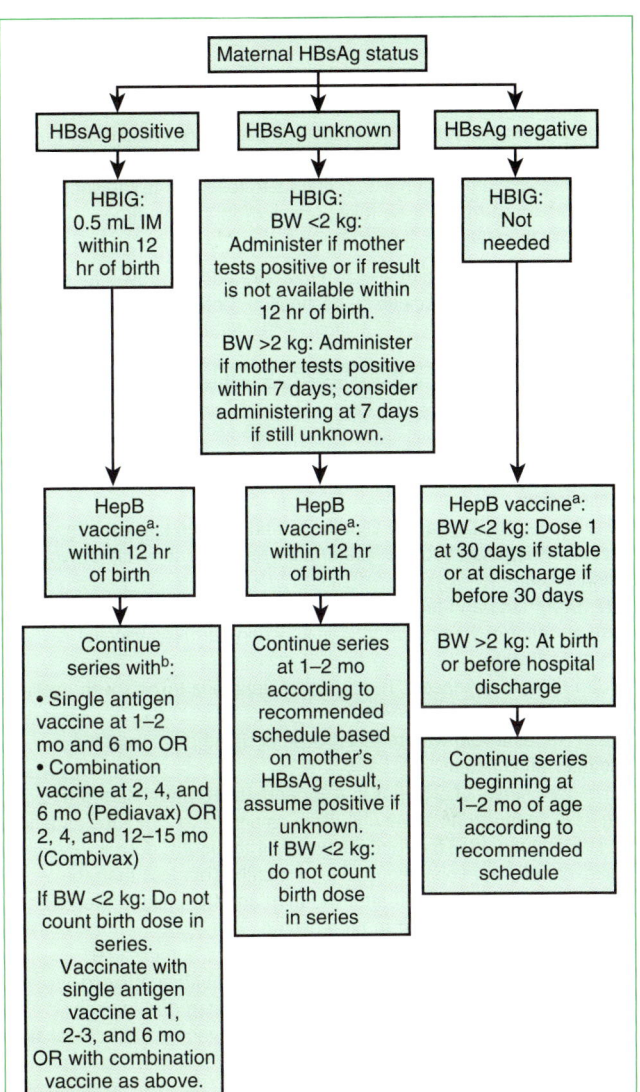

FIGURE 16.4

Management of neonates born to mothers with unknown or positive hepatitis B surface antigen (HbsAg) status. BW, Birth weight; HBIG, hepatitis B immune globulin; HepB, hepatitis B virus. [a]Only single antigen vaccine should be used. [b]Reimmunization may be required based on anti-HBs; test for HBsAg and anti-HBs at age 9–12 months or 1–2 months after completion of HepB series if delayed. (Modified from American Academy of Pediatrics. Red Book: 2015 Report of the Committee on Infectious Diseases. 30th ed. Elk Grove Village, IL: AAP; 2015.)

M. Patients Treated with Immunoglobulin or Other Blood Products

See Table EC 16.A for suggested intervals between any immunoglobulin or blood product administration (including packed red blood cells) and MMR or varicella immunization. The delay allows a decrease in passive antibodies so children will have an adequate response to the vaccine; however, children may not be fully protected during this time.

N. Travelers to Foreign Countries

See CDC's Travelers' Health site at http://www.cdc.gov/travel/ for specific recommendations on vaccines by destination. Consider referral to a travel clinic.

V. IMMUNOPROPHYLAXIS GUIDELINES FOR SPECIFIC DISEASES[2,7]

Refer to Fig. 16.2 and Fig. 16.3 for information on catch-up vaccination schedules.

A. Diphtheria/Tetanus/Pertussis Vaccines and Tetanus Immunoprophylaxis

1. **Description:**
   a. DTaP (Infanrix, Daptacel): Diphtheria and tetanus toxoids with acellular pertussis vaccine; preferred formulation for children younger than 7 years.
   b. DT: Diphtheria and tetanus toxoids without pertussis vaccine; use in children younger than 7 years when pertussis vaccine is contraindicated.
   c. Tdap (Boostrix, Adacel): Tetanus and diphtheria toxoids with acellular pertussis vaccine.
   d. Td: Tetanus toxoid with reduced dose of diphtheria toxoid.
2. **Routine vaccination:**
   a. Five-dose series of DTaP at 2, 4, 6, and 15–18 months, and 4–6 years. The fourth dose may be given as early as 12 months as long as it is 6 months after the third. However, if the fourth dose is inadvertently administered at least 4 months (but less than the recommended 6 months) after the third and the child is over 12 months, it does not need to be repeated.
   b. One dose of Tdap at age 11–12 years. May be administered regardless of interval since last tetanus and diphtheria toxoid-containing vaccine. Administer one dose of Tdap during each pregnancy (ideally 27–36 weeks gestation) regardless of interval since last Td or Tdap vaccination.
3. **Catch-up vaccination:**
   a. See CDC job aid at http://www.cdc.gov/vaccines/schedules/downloads/child/job-aids/dtap.pdf.
4. **Contraindications:** Encephalopathy within 7 days of administration of previous dose of DTaP/Tdap not attributable to another identifiable cause
   a. Precautions
      (1) Evolving/progressive neurologic disorder including uncontrolled seizures: Defer DTaP/Tdap temporarily; use DT or Td instead in

children aged 1 year and older. Reconsider pertussis immunization at each visit (i.e., if condition stabilized).
(2) Guillain–Barré syndrome (GBS) within 6 weeks of previous dose
(3) History of Arthus-type hypersensitivity reaction after tetanus or diphtheria toxoid-containing vaccine: Defer vaccination for 10 years after last administration.
(4) Personal or family history of febrile seizures, including seizures after previous dose of DTaP: Consider antipyretic use for 24 hours after vaccination.
(5) Temperature of 40.5°C (104.8°F) within 48 hours after immunization with a previous dose of DTaP (precaution does not apply to Tdap)
(6) Collapse or shock-like state (hypotonic–hyporesponsive episode) within 48 hours of receiving a previous dose of DTaP (precaution does not apply to Tdap)
(7) Persistent, inconsolable crying lasting 3 hours within 48 hours of receiving a previous dose of DTaP (precaution does not apply to Tdap)
b. Conditions that are not precautions or contraindications:
(1) Stable neurologic condition
(2) Extensive limb swelling after prior dose that was not an Arthus reaction
5. **Side effects:** Substantially decreased with DTaP compared to previously used DTP. Local reaction (common), fever ≥38.0°C (up to 30%), drowsiness (up to 50%), vomiting (4%–7%), crying ≥1 hour (1%–2%). Severe side effects of allergic reactions, persistent crying >3 hours, hypotonic–hyporesponsive episode, seizures, and body temperature >40.5°C that were more common with DTP vaccine are very rare with DTaP.[8,9]
6. **Administration:**
a. DTaP, DT, Td, or TdaP: Dose is 0.5 mL IM.
b. Tetanus Ig (TIG): Postexposure prophylaxis dose is 250 units IM once.
7. **Special considerations:**
a. Tetanus prophylaxis in wound management (Table 16.3)
b. Pertussis exposure:
(1) Immunize all unimmunized or partially immunized close contacts based on the recommended schedule.
(2) Postexposure chemoprophylaxis with azithromycin, erythromycin, or clarithromycin is recommended for household contacts and other close contacts. Alternatives include trimethoprim–sulfamethoxazole. (See Table 3.49 of the 2015 *Red Book* for details.[2])

B. *Haemophilus influenzae* Type B Immunoprophylaxis

1. **Description:** The three licensed vaccines consist of a capsular polysaccharide antigen (PRP) conjugated to a carrier protein. It is not necessary to use the same formulation for the entire series.

TABLE 16.3
INDICATIONS FOR TETANUS PROPHYLAXIS

Prior Tetanus Toxoid Doses	Clean, Minor Wounds		All Other Wounds	
	Tetanus Vaccine*	TIG	Tetanus Vaccine*	TIG
Unknown or <3	Yes	No	Yes	Yes
≥3, last <5 yr ago	No	No	No	No[†]
≥3, last 5–10 yr ago	No	No	Yes	No[†]
≥3, last >10 yr ago	Yes	No	Yes	No[†]

*DTaP preferred under age 7 years; Tdap preferred over age 7 years (DT or Td if pertussis is contraindicated).
[†]Any child with HIV infection or other severe immunodeficiency should receive TIG for any tetanus-prone wound, regardless of vaccination status.
Modified from American Academy of Pediatrics. Red Book: 2015 Report of the Committee on Infectious Diseases. 30th ed. Elk Grove Village, IL: AAP; 2015.

    a. PRP-OMP (PedvaxHIB): Conjugated to outer membrane protein of *Neisseria meningitidis*.
    b. PRP-T (ActHIB): Conjugated to tetanus toxoid.
    c. PRP-T (Hiberix): Conjugated to tetanus toxoid.
2. **Routine vaccination:** Two- or three-dose primary series at 2, 4, and 6 months (if indicated), with booster dose at 12–15 months. Primary series is three doses with ActHIB, Hiberix, MenHibrix, or Pentacel or two doses with PedvaxHIB (PRP-OMP, no 6-month dose). See Section IV.C for children with high-risk conditions.
3. **Contraindications:** None
4. **Side effects:** Local pain, redness, and swelling in 25% of recipients (mild, lasting <24 hours).
5. **Administration:** Dose is 0.5 mL IM.
6. **Special considerations:**
    a. See Section IV.C.
    b. Children with invasive Hib disease at age <24 months: Begin Hib immunization 1 month after acute illness and continue as if previously unimmunized. Vaccination is not required if invasive disease develops after age 24 months. Consider immunologic workup for any child with invasive Hib disease after completing the immunization series.
    c. Invasive Hib exposure: Rifampin prophylaxis is recommended for household contacts in certain circumstances. (See Table 3.9 of the 2015 *Red Book* for details.[2])

C. Hepatitis A Virus Immunoprophylaxis

1. **Description:** Havrix and Vaqta, licensed for children older than 12 months.
2. **Routine vaccination:** Two-dose series starting at age 12–23 months with 6–18-month interval.
3. **Contraindications:** Anaphylactic reaction to aluminum hydroxyphosphate sulfate, aluminum hydroxide, or neomycin.

4. **Side effects:** Local reactions are typically mild and include injection site tenderness (19%–37%) or redness (21%–29%). Other common effects are irritability (42%), drowsiness (28%), fever (16%–27%), and headache (<9%).[10,11]
5. **Administration:**
a. HepA vaccine: Dose is 0.5 mL IM for age 1–18 years and 1 mL IM for age 19 years and older.
b. Intramuscular immune globulin (IMIG): Dose is 0.02 mL/kg IM (do not administer more than 3–5 mL per site).
6. **Special considerations:**
a. Pre-exposure immunoprophylaxis for travelers
   (1) For travelers age 12 months and older, HepA vaccine is preferred; a single dose usually provides adequate immunity if time does not allow a second dose before travel.
   (2) For travelers younger than 12 months, IMIG is protective for up to 3 months (5 months with higher dose) and can be given without vaccine.
b. Postexposure immunoprophylaxis
   (1) If ≤2 weeks since exposure: Children younger than 12 months should receive IMIG. Children aged 12 months and older should receive HepA vaccine (or IMIG if immunocompromised).
   (2) If >2 weeks since exposure: No prophylaxis is indicated for children younger than 12 months. Children aged 12 months and older may receive HepA vaccine if exposure will be ongoing.

D. Hepatitis B Virus Immunoprophylaxis

1. **Description:**
a. HepB vaccine: Engerix-B and Recombivax HB, produced by recombinant DNA technology. Monovalent formulations may be used interchangeably.
b. Hepatitis B immune globulin (HBIG): Prepared from plasma containing high-titer anti-HBsAg antibodies.
2. **Routine vaccination:** Three-dose series at birth, 1–2 months, and 6–18 months. Administer monovalent Hep B vaccine to all newborns within 24 hours of birth. Refer to Fig. 16.4 if mother's HBsAg status is positive or unknown. A four-dose series is acceptable when combination vaccinations are used after the birth dose.
3. **Contraindications:** Anaphylactic reaction to yeast
4. **Side effects:** Pain at injection site (3%–29%) or fever >37.7°C (1%–6%).
5. **Administration:**
a. Recombivax: Dose is 5 mcg IM (0.5 mL pediatric formulation) for patients younger than 20 years, 10 mcg IM (1 mL adult formulation) for age 20 years and older or for two-dose adolescent series, and 40 mcg IM (1 mL dialysis formulation) for adult dialysis patients.

TABLE 16.4
HEPATITIS B VIRUS PROPHYLAXIS AFTER PERCUTANEOUS EXPOSURE TO BLOOD

Exposed Person	HBsAg Status of Source of Blood		
	Positive	Negative	Unknown
UNIMMUNIZED	HBIG and HBV series	HBV series	HBV series
PREVIOUSLY IMMUNIZED			
Known responder	No treatment	No treatment	No treatment
Known nonresponder	HBIG and HBV series (or HBIG ×2 at 1 month interval if already received two HBV series without response)	No treatment	Treat as if positive if known high-risk source
Response unknown	Test exposed person for anti-HBs: If adequate*, no treatment If inadequate, HBIG ×1 and HBV booster	No treatment	Test exposed person for anti-HBs: If adequate, no treatment If inadequate, HBV booster dose and recheck titer in 1–2 months

*Adequate anti-HBs is ≥10 mIU/mL.
Modified from American Academy of Pediatrics. Red Book: 2015 Report of the Committee on Infectious Diseases. 30th ed. Elk Grove Village, IL: AAP; 2015.

b. Engerix-B: Dose is 10 mcg IM (0.5 mL) for patients younger than 20 years, 20 mcg IM (1 mL) for age 20 years and older, and 40 mcg IM (2 mL) for adult dialysis patients.
c. HBIG: Dose is 0.5 mL IM for infants younger than 12 months and 0.06 mL/kg IM for children older than 12 months.

6. **Special considerations:**
a. Infants of mothers who are HBsAg–positive or of unknown status will have a different schedule, see Fig. 16.4.
b. See Table 16.4 for HepB prophylaxis after percutaneous exposure to blood.

E. Human Papillomavirus Immunoprophylaxis

1. **Description:**
a. HPV9 (Gardasil 9): Protects against HPV types 6, 11, 16, 18, 31, 33, 45, 52, and 58.
b. HPV4 (Gardasil): Protects against HPV types 6, 11, 16, and 18.
2. **Routine vaccination:** Two-dose series on a schedule of 0 and 6–12 months to all adolescents aged 11–12 years. Vaccination may be started at age 9 years. For persons initiating vaccination at age 15 years or older, three doses should be given at 0, 1–2, and 6 months. In a two-dose schedule, the minimum dose interval is 5 months; if the second dose is administered early it should be re-administered at least 12 weeks after the second dose and 5 months after the first dose. In a three-dose schedule, the second dose must be given a minimum of

4 weeks after the first, and the third dose must be given a minimum of 5 months after the first with a minimum interval of 12 weeks from the second dose.
3. **Contraindications:** Anaphylaxis to yeast, pregnancy
4. **Side effects:** Pain, swelling, and erythema at injection site (up to 90%, 48%, and 34% respectively), headache (11%–15%), and syncope. Observation for syncope for 15 minutes after administration is recommended.[12]
5. **Administration:** Dose is 0.5 mL IM.
6. **Special considerations:**
a. Females or males with evidence of current HPV infection such as cervical dysplasia, warts, or a positive HPV DNA test should still be immunized.
b. Children with a history of sexual abuse or assault should start the series at age 9 years.
c. Immunocompromised persons should receive a three-dose series.
d. HPV vaccination is not recommended during pregnancy, though there is no evidence that it poses harm.

F. Influenza Immunoprophylaxis[13]

Influenza strains can change year to year, particularly during times of pandemic flu; refer to the CDC for up-to-date guidelines at http://www.cdc.gov/flu/professionals/acip/.
1. **Description:** Activated and inactivated influenza vaccines contain multiple viral strains (including both type A and type B strains) based on expected prevalent influenza strains for the upcoming winter.
a. Inactivated (IIV): Subvirion or purified surface-antigen vaccines; given IM for children age 6 months and older; cell culture-based (ccIIV3) and recombinant (RIV3) vaccines available for age 18 years and older
b. Live attenuated (LAIV): Intranasal vaccine for healthy children aged 2 years and older. Was not recommended in 2016–2017 due to poor efficacy compared to injectable.
2. **Routine vaccination:** Annual administration starting at age 6 months. Children through age 8 years who have not previously received at least two total doses (regardless of interval) should receive two doses at a 4-week interval; see annual ACIP recommendations.
3. **Contraindications:** Anaphylaxis to eggs, anaphylaxis to gelatin (present in some influenza vaccines, check package insert). Contraindications specific to LAIV are pregnancy, asthma, children younger than 5 years with wheezing in the past 12 months, immunocompromise, aspirin treatment, or use of antivirals in previous 48 hours.
a. **Precautions:** GBS within 6 weeks after a previous influenza vaccine dose
b. Conditions that are not precautions or contraindications:
   (1) Less severe or local manifestations of allergy to egg
   (2) Pregnancy (use IIV)

4. **Side effects:** Local reactions, fever within 24 hours after immunization in children younger than 2 years (10%–35%). Possible association with GBS; however, the risk is rare, at fewer than 1–2 cases per million doses.
5. **Administration:**
a. Inactivated: Dose is 0.25 mL IM for ages 6–35 months and 0.5 mL IM for age 3 years and older.
b. Live attenuated: Dose is 0.2 mL intranasally.
6. **Special considerations:**
a. **Chemoprophylaxis for influenza A and B:** Due to high rates of resistance to adamantanes (amantadine and rimantadine), neuraminidase inhibitors (oseltamivir) have generally been recommended. However, recommendations may vary by season and location. Please refer to http://www.cdc.gov/flu/professionals/antivirals/.
    (1) Indications for chemoprophylaxis following exposure:
        (a) Unimmunized high-risk children, including those for whom the vaccine is contraindicated or children immunized <2 weeks before exposure
        (b) Unimmunized individuals in close contact with high-risk individuals
        (c) Immunodeficient individuals unlikely to have protective response to vaccine
        (d) Control of outbreaks in a closed setting
        (e) Immunized high-risk individuals if vaccine strain different from circulating strain
    (2) Chemoprophylaxis is not a substitute for immunization and does not interfere with the immune response to the inactivated virus vaccine. LAIV should not be administered until >48 hours after completing antiviral therapy for influenza. Do not administer chemoprophylaxis until at least 2 weeks after administration of LAIV.
b. Infants younger than 6 months cannot be immunized. Close contacts should receive the vaccine.

G. Japanese Encephalitis (JE) Immunoprophylaxis

See Expert Consult for more information.

H. Measles/Mumps/Rubella Immunoprophylaxis

1. **Description:**
a. MMR: Combination vaccine composed of live attenuated viruses
b. Rubella Ig: Does not prevent infection or viremia. To be used in pregnancy only when termination is not being considered.[2]
2. **Routine vaccination:** Two-dose series at 12–15 months and 4–6 years. The second dose may be given prior to age 4 years as long as there has been a 4-week interval. For children

aged 6–11 months traveling internationally, one dose should be given prior to departure. These children should be revaccinated with two doses, the first at age 12–15 months (12 months if in high-risk area) and the second at least 4 weeks later. For children aged 12 months and older traveling internationally, two doses should be given at 4-week interval prior to departure.

3. **Contraindications:** Anaphylactic reaction to neomycin or gelatin, immunocompromise, or pregnancy
  a. **Precautions:**
     (1) Recent (within 3–11 months, depending on product and dose) blood product administration, see Table EC 16.A.
     (2) Thrombocytopenia or history of thrombocytopenic purpura
     (3) Tuberculosis or positive purified protein derivative (PPD) tuberculin test. In individuals with untreated tuberculosis infection, antituberculosis treatment should be initiated prior to MMR administration.
     (4) Personal or family history of seizures (precaution for MMRV only)
  b. **Conditions that are not precautions or contraindications:**
     (1) PPD testing may be done on the day of immunization but otherwise should be postponed 4–6 weeks because of suppression of response.
     (2) Immunodeficiency or pregnancy of a household member
     (3) HIV infection
     (4) Breastfeeding
     (5) Nonanaphylactic reactions to gelatin or neomycin or anaphylactic reaction to egg (consider observation for 90 minutes; skin testing not predictive)
4. **Side effects:** High fever (>39.4°C) develops in 5%–15% of immunized persons, usually 6–12 days after immunization, and may last up to 5 days. Febrile seizures may occur 5–12 days after the first dose (rare). Other reactions include transient rash (5%), transient thrombocytopenia (1 in 22,000 to 40,000), encephalitis and encephalopathy (<1 in 1 million).[2]
5. **Administration:**
  a. MMR vaccine: Dose is 0.5 mL SQ.
  b. IMIG: 0.50 mL/kg (maximum dose 15 mL) IM
6. **Special considerations:**
  a. Measles postexposure immunoprophylaxis:
     (1) Vaccine prevents or modifies disease if given within 72 hours of exposure; it is the intervention of choice for measles outbreak.
     (2) IMIG or intravenous immune globulin (IVIG) prevents or modifies disease if given within 6 days of exposure. IMIG is indicated

in children younger than 1 year or nonimmune individuals who cannot receive the vaccine. IVIG is the recommended preparation for nonimmune pregnant women and severely immunocompromised hosts (including HIV-infected children) regardless of immunization status. Additional therapy not required if IVIG received within 3 weeks before exposure.
b. Rubella postexposure immunoprophylaxis: May be considered in rubella-susceptible women exposed to confirmed rubella early in pregnancy if termination of the pregnancy is refused.

I. Meningococcal Immunoprophylaxis

1. **Description:**
a. HibMenCY (MenHibrix): Conjugate vaccine against Hib and meningococcus groups C and Y for patients aged 6 weeks through 18 months.
b. MenACWY-D (Menactra): Quadrivalent conjugate vaccine against groups A, C, Y, and W for patients aged 9 months and older.
c. MenACWY-CRM (Menveo): Quadrivalent conjugate vaccine against groups A, C, Y, and W for patients aged 2 months and older.
d. MPSV4: Quadrivalent polysaccharide vaccine against groups A, C, Y, and W for patients aged 2 years and older.
e. MenB-FHbp (Trumenba): Serogroup B vaccine for ages 10–25 years.
f. MenB-4C (Bexsero): Serogroup B vaccine for ages 10–25 years.
2. **Routine vaccination:** Primary dose of quadrivalent conjugate vaccine at age 11–12 years with booster at age 16 years. May also consider vaccination with two-dose series of MenB to provide short-term protection for young adults aged 16 through 23, even if not at increased risk for meningococcal disease. Dose interval for Bexsero is 1 month and for Trumenba is 6 months; vaccines are not interchangeable. See Section IV.B for children with high-risk conditions, including HIV.
3. **Contraindications:** Anaphylaxis to tetanus toxoid or diphtheria toxoid
4. **Side effects:**
a. MenACWY: Mild localized tenderness (10%–41%) or erythema (11%–15%), irritability (18%–57%), sleepiness (14%–50%), headache (11%–30%)[15]
b. HibMenCY: Injection-site pain, redness, and swelling (15%–46%); irritability (62%–71%); drowsiness (49%–63%); loss of appetite (30%–34%) and fever (11%–26%)[16]
c. MenB: Injection-site pain (85%), fatigue (35%–40%), headache (35%), and muscle pain (30%–48%)[17,18]
5. **Administration:** Dose is 0.5 mL IM for MenACWY, HibMenCY, and MenB, and 0.5 mL SQ for MPSV4.
6. **Special considerations:**
a. See Sections IV.B and IV.F.

b. Postexposure prophylaxis:
   (1) Chemoprophylaxis is indicated for people who have been directly exposed to an infected person's oral secretions (including unprotected healthcare workers) or who had close contact in the 7 days prior to onset of disease including child care, preschool, and household contacts and passengers seated next to the index patient during airline flights longer than 8 hours. Chemoprophylaxis should be initiated within 24 hours of index patient diagnosis. (See Table 3.41 of the 2015 *Red Book* for details.[2])
   (2) Immunoprophylaxis is indicated as an adjunct to chemoprophylaxis when an outbreak is caused by a vaccine-preventable serogroup.

J. Pneumococcal Immunoprophylaxis

1. **Description:**
a. PCV13: Pneumococcal conjugate vaccine containing 13 purified capsular polysaccharides of *Streptococcus pneumoniae*, each coupled to a variant of diphtheria toxin. PCV7 had serotypes 4, 6B, 9V, 14, 18C, 19F, and 23F. Serotypes 1, 3, 5, 6A, 7F, and 19A were added to generate PCV13.
b. PPSV23: Purified capsular polysaccharide from 23 serotypes (1, 2, 3, 4, 5, 6B, 7F, 8, 9N, 9V, 10A, 11A, 12F, 14, 15B, 17F, 18C, 19A, 19F, 20, 22F, 23F, and 33F) of *S. pneumoniae*. Approved for children aged 2 years and older with certain underlying medical conditions.
2. **Routine vaccination:** Four-dose series of PCV13 at 2, 4, 6, and 12–15 months. See Section IV.A for children with high-risk conditions.
3. **Contraindications:** Anaphylaxis to diphtheria toxoid (PCV13 only)
4. **Side effects:** Pain or erythema at injection site (>50%), irritability (20%–70%), decreased appetite (20%–40%), decreased sleep (up to 40%), increased sleep (up to 40%), fever (up to 20%)[19]
5. **Administration:** Dose for both PCV13 and PPSV23 is 0.5 mL IM. Concurrent administration of PCV13 and PPSV23 vaccines is not recommended.
6. **Special considerations:**
a. See Section IV.A.

K. Poliomyelitis Immunoprophylaxis

1. **Description:**
a. IPV: Inactivated injectable vaccine containing three types of poliovirus.
b. OPV: Live attenuated oral vaccine with three types of poliovirus. No longer available in the United States.
2. **Routine vaccination:** Four-dose series at 2, 4, and 6–18 months, and 4–6 years.
3. **Contraindications:** Anaphylactic reactions to neomycin, streptomycin, polymyxin B, 2-phenoxyethanol, and formaldehyde. OPV should generally not be given to immunocompromised children.

4. **Side effects:** Local reactions (up to 30%), irritability (up to 65%), tiredness (up to 61%), fever ≥39°C (up to 4%)[20]
5. **Administration:** Dose is 0.5 mL IM or SQ.

L. Rabies Immunoprophylaxis

1. **Description:**
   a. HDCV (Imovax): Human diploid cell vaccine
   b. PCECV (RabAvert): Purified chicken embryo cell vaccine
   c. Human rabies immune globulin (RIG): Antirabies Ig prepared from plasma of donors hyperimmunized with rabies vaccine
2. **Routine vaccination:** Preexposure prophylaxis is indicated for high-risk groups, including veterinarians, animal handlers, laboratory workers, children living in high-risk environments, those traveling to high-risk areas, and spelunkers. Series is three injections of HDCV or PCECV on days 0, 7, and 21 or 28. Rabies serum antibody titers should be followed at 6-month intervals for those at continuous risk and at 2-year intervals for those at risk of frequent exposure; give booster doses only if titers are nonprotective.
3. **Contraindications:** Anaphylaxis to gelatin (present in some vaccines, check package insert). PCECV can be used if there is a serious allergic reaction to HDCV.
4. **Side effects:** Uncommon in children. In adults, local reactions occur in 15%–25%, mild systemic reactions (e.g., headache, abdominal pain, nausea, muscle aches, dizziness) in 10%–20%. Immune complex–like reaction (urticaria, arthralgia, angioedema, vomiting, fever, malaise) 2–21 days after immunization with HDCV is rare in primary series, but 6% after booster dose.
5. **Administration:**
   a. Rabies vaccines: Dose is 1 mL IM. Do not administer in same part of body or in same syringe as RIG.
   b. RIG: Dose is 20 IU/kg. Infiltrate around the wound, and give remainder IM.
6. **Special considerations:**
   a. Postexposure prophylaxis (Table 16.5): Indicated for infectious exposures including bites, scratches, or contamination of open wound or mucous membrane with infectious material of a potentially rabid animal or human.
      (1) General wound management: Clean immediately with soap and water and flush thoroughly. Avoid suturing wound unless indicated for functional reasons. Consider tetanus prophylaxis and antibiotics if indicated. Report all patients suspected of rabies infection to public health authorities.
      (2) Active and passive immunization:
         (a) Unimmunized: Give vaccine on days 0, 3, 7, and 14 with one dose of RIG on day 0. If the person is immunosuppressed, a fifth dose should be given on day 28.

TABLE 16.5
RABIES POSTEXPOSURE PROPHYLAXIS

Animal Type	Evaluation and Disposition of Animal	Postexposure Prophylaxis Recommendations
Dogs, cats, ferrets	Healthy and available for 10 days' observation	Do not begin prophylaxis unless animal develops signs of rabies
	Rabid or suspected rabid: euthanize animal and test brain	Provide immediate immunization and RIG†
	Unknown (escaped)	Consult public health officials
Skunk, raccoon, bat*, fox, woodchuck, most other carnivores	Regard as rabid unless geographic area is known to be free of rabies or until animal is euthanized and proven negative by testing	Provide immediate immunization and RIG†
Livestock, rodents, rabbit, other mammals	Consider individually	Consult public health officials; these bites rarely require treatment

*In the case of direct contact between a human and a bat, consider prophylaxis even if a bite, scratch, or mucous membrane exposure is not apparent.
†Treatment may be discontinued if animal fluorescent antibody is negative.
Modified from American Academy of Pediatrics. Red Book: 2015 Report of the Committee on Infectious Diseases. *30th ed. Elk Grove Village, IL: AAP; 2015.*

     (b) Previously immunized (including preexposure and postexposure): Booster doses on days 0 and 3. Do not give RIG.
  (3) Vaccine and RIG should be given jointly in unimmunized individuals. If vaccine is not immediately available, give RIG alone and vaccinate later. If RIG is unavailable, give vaccine alone. RIG may be given within 7 days after initiating immunization.

M. Respiratory Syncytial Virus (RSV) Immunoprophylaxis[21]

1. **Description:** Palivizumab is a humanized mouse Ig G1 monoclonal antibody to RSV.
2. **Routine vaccination:** Palivizumab should be given every 30 days during RSV season (timing varies regionally) for up to five doses. Indications are as follows:
a. Preterm infants born prior to 29 weeks, 0 days gestation who are younger than 12 months at the start of RSV season
b. Preterm infants with CLD of prematurity (i.e., gestational age <32 weeks, 0 days and requiring >21% oxygen for at least 28 days after birth) during the first year of life
c. Preterm infants with CLD of prematurity requiring ongoing medical support (e.g., chronic corticosteroid therapy, diuretic therapy, or supplemental oxygen) during the second year of life in the 6-month period prior to the start of RSV season

d. Certain children younger than 12 months with hemodynamically significant congenital heart disease. Children receiving prophylaxis who undergo a surgical procedure with cardiopulmonary bypass may require a postoperative dose.
    (1) Acyanotic heart disease requiring medication to control congestive heart failure with plan for surgical procedures
    (2) Moderate-to-severe pulmonary hypertension
    (3) Cyanotic heart defect (discuss with cardiologist)
    (4) Cardiac transplantation (younger than 2 years)
e. Children younger than 12 months with anatomic pulmonary abnormality or neuromuscular disorder that impairs ability to clear secretions from upper airway
f. Children younger than 2 years with profound immunocompromise
3. **Contraindications:** None
4. **Side effects:** Fever and rash
5. **Administration:** Dose is 15 mg/kg IM.

N. Rotavirus Immunoprophylaxis

1. **Description:**
a. RotaTeq (RV5): Pentavalent live attenuated oral vaccine containing five reassortant human and bovine rotavirus strains
b. Rotarix (RV1): Monovalent live attenuated oral vaccine
2. **Routine vaccination:** Administer Rotarix at 2 and 4 months of age, or RotaTeq at 2, 4, and 6 months of age. If any dose is administered as RotaTeq or is unknown, three doses should be given.
3. **Contraindications:** SCID, history of intussusception, severe allergic reaction to latex (RV1 only)
a. **Precautions:** Concern for altered immunocompetence, preexisting chronic gastrointestinal disease, spina bifida, or bladder exstrophy
b. **Conditions that are not precautions or contraindications:** Breastfeeding, immunodeficient or pregnant family member/contact, receipt of blood products (including antibody-containing blood products)
4. **Side effects:** There may be a small risk of intussusception associated with the rotavirus vaccines (1 excess case per 30,000–100,000 vaccinated infants); it usually occurs within 1 week of vaccination. Common side effects are diarrhea (24%), vomiting (15%), otitis media (14.5%), nasopharyngitis (7%), and bronchospasm (1%); rates are similar to placebo.[22]
5. **Administration:**
a. RotaTeq: Dose is 2 mL orally (PO). Vaccine is packaged in single-dose tubes to be administered without dilution. Do not readminister if infant spits out or vomits dose.
b. Rotarix: Dose is 1 mL PO. Vaccine is packaged to be reconstituted only with the accompanying diluent. If the infant spits out or vomits a dose, a single replacement dose at the same visit may be considered.

6. **Special considerations:**
a. Preterm infants should be immunized on the routine schedule, but initiation should be deferred if still hospitalized to prevent nosocomial spread.

O. Tuberculosis Immunoprophylaxis

See Expert Consult for more information.

P. Typhoid Fever Immunoprophylaxis

1. **Description:** Two typhoid vaccines are available and induce a protective response in 50%–80% of recipients.
a. ViCPS (Typhim Vi): Vi capsular polysaccharide vaccine administered IM for age 2 years and older
b. Ty21a (Vivotif): Oral live attenuated vaccine for age 6 years and older
2. **Routine vaccination:** Immunization is indicated for travelers to areas with risk of exposure to *Salmonella* serovar Typhi, people with frequent close contact with a documented carrier, laboratory workers in contact with *Salmonella* serovar Typhi, and people living in areas with endemic infection. For ViCPS, administer one dose at least 2 weeks prior to exposure; reimmunize every 2 years. For Ty21a, one dose is taken by mouth every other day for a total of four doses at least 1 week prior to exposure; reimmunize every 5 years.
3. **Contraindications:** Immunocompromise (Ty21a only)
a. **Precautions:** Active gastrointestinal tract illness (Ty21a only), certain antibiotics or antimalarials that would be active against *Salmonella* serovar Typhi or interfere with immunogenicity (Ty21a only)
4. **Side effects:** For Ty21a, mild reactions including abdominal pain, nausea, diarrhea, vomiting, fever, or headache. For ViCPS, reactions include local discomfort or erythema (up to 14%), subjective fever (3%), and decreased activity (2%).[24]
5. **Administration:**
a. ViCPS: Dose is 0.5 mL IM.
b. Ty21a: Each dose is one enteric-coated capsule. Must be kept refrigerated and taken with cool liquid approximately 1 hour before meal.

Q. Varicella Immunoprophylaxis

1. **Description:**
a. Varivax: Cell-free live attenuated varicella virus vaccine
b. Varicella-zoster immune globulin (VariZIG): Prepared from plasma containing high-titer antivaricella antibodies
2. **Routine vaccination:** Two-dose series at 12–15 months and 4–6 years. The second dose may be administered before age 4 years as long as there has been a 3-month interval; however, a second dose given at least 4 weeks after the first is valid.
3. **Contraindications:** Anaphylactic reaction to neomycin or gelatin, immunocompromise, pregnancy, or concurrent febrile illness

a. **Precautions:**
   (1) Recent (within 3–11 months, depending on product and dose) blood product administration (see Section IV.M)
   (2) Receipt of acyclovir, famciclovir, or valacyclovir within 24 hours before vaccination (also avoid for 21 days after vaccination)
b. **Conditions that are not precautions or contraindications:** Household contact with immunodeficiency (including HIV infection) or who is pregnant
4. **Side effects:** Injection site reactions (20%–25%) and fever (10%–15%). Mild varicelliform rash within 5–26 days of vaccine administration (3%–5%) may occur, though not all postimmunization rashes are attributable to vaccine. Vaccine rash is often very mild, but patient may be infectious.[25]
5. **Administration:**
a. Varicella vaccine: Dose is 0.5 mL SQ.
b. VariZIG: Dose is by weight, administered IM. Give 62.5 units (0.5 vial) for ≤2.0 kg; 125 units (1 vial) for 2.1 to 10 kg; 250 units (2 vials) for 10.1 to 20 kg; 375 units (3 vials) for 20.1 to 30 kg; 500 units (4 vials) for 30.1 to 40 kg; and 625 units (5 vials) for >40 kg. If VariZIG is unavailable, can give IVIG 400 mg/kg IV.
6. **Special considerations:**
a. Avoid salicylates for 6 weeks after vaccine administration if possible. Avoid antiviral treatment for 21 days after vaccination. Do not give vaccine concurrently with or for 5 months after VariZIG.
b. Vaccinate nonimmune household contacts of immunocompromised hosts. If a rash develops in the immunized person, avoid direct contact if possible.
c. Postexposure prophylaxis:
   (1) Immunocompetent, nonimmune people older than 12 months should receive varicella vaccine as soon as possible after exposure, preferably within 3 days. However, since not all exposures result in infection, vaccination should still be given after this time for protection against subsequent exposures.
   (2) VariZIG may be considered for significant exposures to varicella in individuals with no immunity and a high likelihood of complications from infection including immunocompromised people, pregnant women, and certain newborn infants. (See Fig. 3.14 of the 2015 *Red Book* for details.[2]) It should be given as soon as possible and within 10 days of exposure. IVIG may be used if VariZIG is not available.
   (3) If VariZIG or IVIG are not available, consider prophylaxis with acyclovir or valacyclovir beginning 7–10 days after exposure and continuing for 7 days in immunocompromised, nonimmune patients.

R. Yellow Fever Immunoprophylaxis

1. **Description:** Live attenuated (17D strain) vaccine approved for children older than 9 months.
2. **Routine vaccination:** Indicated for travelers to endemic areas including parts of sub-Saharan Africa and South America. Vaccine is required by some countries as a condition of entry. Give a single dose at least 10 days prior to travel. Booster doses are generally not needed unless immune response is limited (e.g., pregnancy, stem cell transplant, HIV infection) or if at increased risk of disease due to location or duration of exposure (e.g., prolonged travel or lab workers).
3. **Contraindications:** Anaphylaxis to eggs or gelatin, immunocompromise, younger than 6 months
   a. **Precautions:**
      (1) Age 6–8 months: Risk of vaccine-associated encephalitis
      (2) Pregnant or breastfeeding: Rare cases of *in utero* or breastfeeding transmission of the vaccine virus
      (3) Asymptomatic HIV infection with CD4+ counts 200 to 499/mm^3 (or 15% to 24% of total lymphocytes for those younger than 6 years)
4. **Side effects:** Rare viscerotropic disease (multiple-organ system failure) and neurotropic disease (encephalitis). Increased risk of adverse events in persons of any age with thymic dysfunction and an increased risk of postvaccine encephalitis in children younger than 9 months.
5. **Administration:** Dose is 0.5 mL IM.
6. **Special considerations:**
   a. Vaccine is available in the United States only in designated centers. A list of centers that provide yellow fever vaccine (and usually other travel vaccines) can be found at http://wwwnc.cdc.gov/travel/yellow-fever-vaccination-clinics/search/.

S. Combination Vaccines

1. **Kinrix = DTaP/IPV:** Ages 4 to 6 years, used as fifth dose of DTaP and fourth dose of IPV
2. **Pediarix = DTaP/HepB/IPV:** Ages 6 weeks through 6 years
   a. Higher rates of fever are reported with combination vaccine than the vaccines administered separately.
3. **Pentacel = DTaP/IPV/PRP-T (Hib):** Ages 6 weeks through 4 years
4. **ProQuad = MMR/Varicella:** Ages 12 months to 12 years
   a. Unless caregiver prefers MMRV vaccine, CDC recommends that MMR and varicella vaccines be administered separately for the first dose in 12- to 47-month-old children due to increased risk for febrile seizure with combination vaccine in this age group. Combination MMRV vaccine can be used for second dose or as first dose for children aged 48 months and older

5. **Quadracel = DTaP/IPV:** Ages 4 to 6 years, used as fifth dose of DTaP and fourth or fifth dose of IPV
6. **Twinrix = HepA/HepB:** Age 18 years and older. Administered in a three-dose schedule given at 0, 1, and 6 months; dose is 1 mL.
7. **MenHibrix = Hib/MenCY:** Ages 6 weeks to 18 months

REFERENCES

1. Centers for Disease Control and Prevention. Recommended Immunization Schedules for Persons Aged 0 Through 18 Years—United States, 2017. Available online at <http://www.cdc.gov/vaccines/schedules>.
2. American Academy of Pediatrics. *Red Book: 2015 Report of the Committee on Infectious Diseases*. 30th ed. Elk Grove Village, IL: AAP; 2015.
3. Rubin LG, Levin MJ, Ljungman P, et al. 2013 IDSA Clinical Practice Guideline for Vaccination of the Immunocompromised Host. *Clin Infect Dis*. 2014;58:e44-e100.
4. AAP Committee on Infectious Diseases. Immunization for Streptococcus pneumoniae Infections in High-Risk Children. *Pediatrics*. 2014;134:1230-1233.
5. American Academy of Pediatrics Committee on Infectious Diseases. Updated recommendations on the use of meningococcal vaccines. *Pediatrics*. 2014;134:400-403.
6. Folaranmi T, Rubin L, Martin SW, et al. Centers for Disease Control and Prevention. Use of Serogroup B Meningococcal (MenB) Vaccines in Persons Aged ≥10 Years at Increased Risk for Serogroup B Meningococcal Disease: Recommendations of the Advisory Committee on Immunization Practice. *MMWR Morb Mortal Wkly Rep*. 2015;64:608-612.
7. Centers for Disease Control and Prevention. Vaccines and immunizations. 2015. Available online at <http://www.cdc.gov/vaccines/>.
8. Sanofi Pasteur package insert for Daptacel.
9. GlaxoSmithKline package insert for Infanrix.
10. GlaxoSmithKline package insert for Havrix.
11. Merck package insert for Vaqta.
12. Merck package insert for Gardasil 9.
13. Centers for Disease Control and Prevention. Prevention and Control of Influenza with Vaccines: Recommendations of the Advisory Committee on Immunization Practices, United States, 2015-16 Influenza Season. *MMWR Morb Mortal Wkly Rep*. 2015;64(30):818-825.
14. Novartis package insert for IXIARO.
15. Novartis package insert for Menveo.
16. GlaxoSmithKline package insert for MenHibrix.
17. Novartis package insert for Bexsero.
18. Pfizer package insert for Trumenba.
19. Pfizer package insert for Prevnar 13.
20. Sanofi Pasteur package insert for IPOL (poliovirus vaccine inactivated).
21. AAP Committee on Infectious Diseases and Bronchiolitis. Updated guidance for palivizumab prophylaxis among infants and young children at increased risk of hospitalization for respiratory syncytial virus infection. *Pediatrics*. 2014;134(2):415-420.
22. Merck package insert for RotaTeq.
23. Organon package insert for BCG.
24. Sanofi Pasteur package insert for Typhoid Vi Polysaccharide Vaccine.
25. Merck package insert for Varivax.

Chapter 17
Microbiology and Infectious Disease
Devan Jaganath, MD, MPH, and Rebecca G. Same, MD

See additional content on Expert Consult

I. MICROBIOLOGY

A. Collection of Specimens for Blood Culture

1. **Preparation:** To minimize contamination, clean venipuncture site with 70% isopropyl ethyl alcohol. Apply tincture of iodine or 10% povidone–iodine and allow skin to dry for at least 1 minute, or scrub site with 2% chlorhexidine for 30 seconds and allow skin to dry for 30 seconds. Clean blood culture bottle injection site with alcohol only.
2. **Collection:** Two sets of cultures from two different sites of equal blood volume should be obtained for each febrile episode, based on patient weight: <8 kg, 1–3 mL each; 8–13 kg, 4–5 mL; 14–25 kg, 10–15 mL each; >25 kg, 20–30 mL each.[1] Peripheral sites preferred. If concern for central line infection, collect one from central access site, second from peripheral.

B. Rapid Microbiologic Identification of Common Aerobic Bacteria (Fig. 17.1) and Anaerobic Bacteria (Fig. 17.2)

C. Choosing Appropriate Antibiotic Based on Sensitivities

1. **Minimum inhibitory concentration (MIC):** Lowest concentration of an antimicrobial agent that prevents visible growth; MICs are unique to each agent, and there are standards to determine if susceptible, intermediate, or resistant. Antibiotic selection should generally be based on whether an agent is "susceptible" rather than the MIC.
2. **See** Tables 17.1 through 17.6 **for spectrum of activity of commonly used antibiotics.**[2,3]
   Note: Antibiotic sensitivities can vary greatly with local resistance patterns. Follow published institutional guidelines and culture results for individual patients and infections. When possible, always use agent with narrowest spectrum of activity, particularly when organism susceptibilities are known.

II. INFECTIOUS DISEASE

A. Fever without Localizing Source: Evaluation and Management Guidelines[4,5]

1. **Age <28 days:** Hospitalize for full evaluation (Fig. 17.3). Owing to the greater risk of serious bacterial infections in young infants with fever, a conservative approach is warranted.
2. **Age 29–90 days:** Well-appearing infants who meet low-risk criteria can potentially be managed as outpatients if reliable follow-up and monitoring is ensured.
3. **Age >90 days:** The marked decline in invasive infections due to *Haemophilus influenzae* type b and *Streptococcus pneumoniae*, since introduction of conjugate vaccines, has reduced the likelihood of

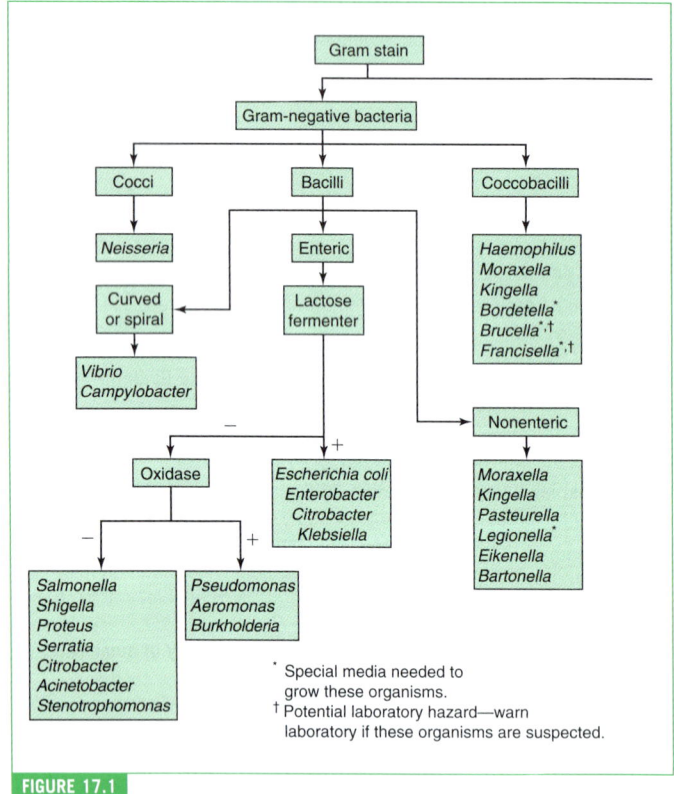

FIGURE 17.1
Algorithm demonstrating identification of aerobic bacteria.

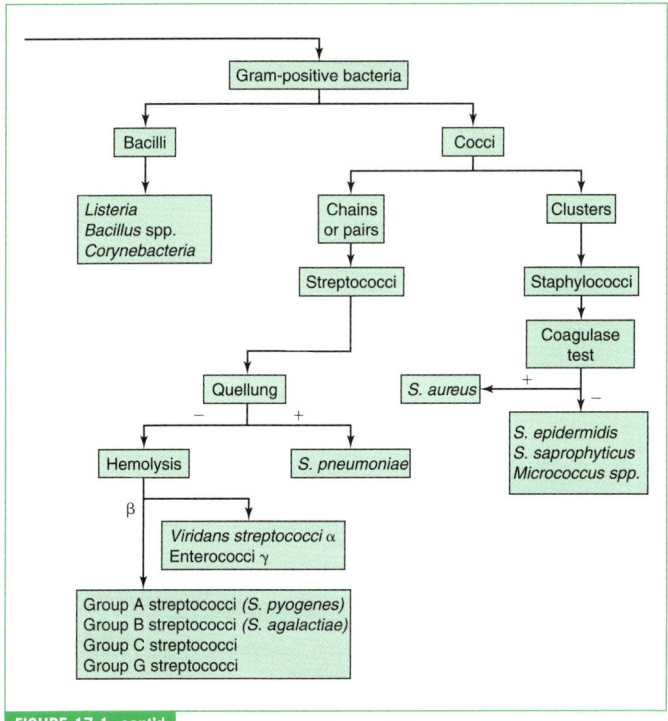

FIGURE 17.1, cont'd

serious bacterial infection in a well-appearing child within this age group:
a. If ill-appearing without source of infection identified, consider admission and empirical antimicrobial therapy.
b. If source of infection identified, treat accordingly.
c. If well-appearing and without foci of infection, many experts advocate urinalysis and urine culture as the only routine diagnostic test if reliable follow-up and monitoring is ensured, including all females and uncircumcised males aged <2 years, all circumcised males aged <6 months, and all children with known genitourinary tract abnormalities.
4. **Fever of unknown origin**[6,7]
a. Generally defined as fever >38.3°C for 2 or more weeks
b. Often an unusual presentation of a common disease
c. Broad differential, such as infectious (including deep-seated bone infections or abscesses), neoplasms, collagen vascular disease (i.e., juvenile idiopathic arthritis), drug fever, and Kawasaki syndrome

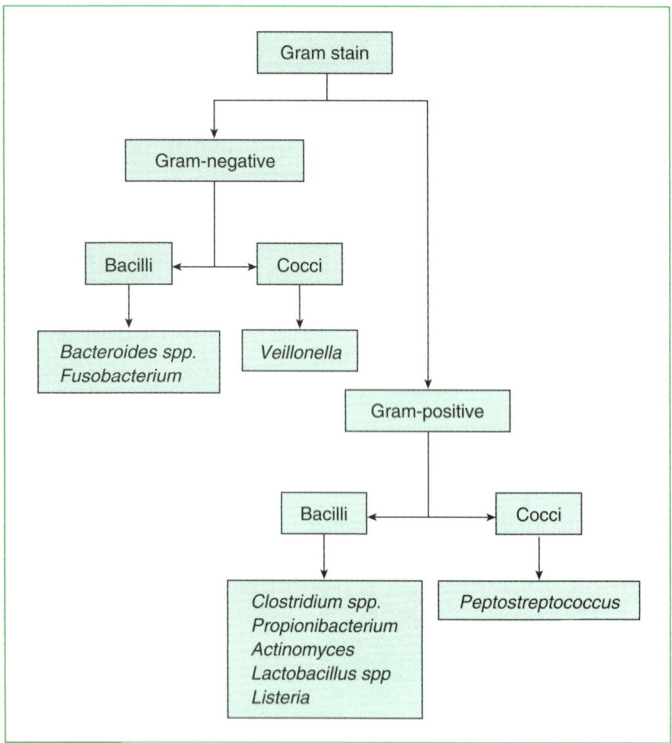

FIGURE 17.2
Algorithm demonstrating identification of anaerobic bacteria.

d. Confirmation of fever is essential, thorough history of fever pattern, associated signs/symptoms, family history, ethnic/genetic background, environmental and animal exposures, and complete physical exam
e. Labs and imaging will be guided by history and physical, and corresponding category of differential (i.e., infectious vs. oncologic vs. autoimmune/rheumatologic vs. immunodeficiency)

B. Evaluation of Lymphadenopathy[8]

1. **Etiology**
a. Reactive lymph nodes (LNs): Majority of lymphadenopathy
b. Direct infection of LN: Suppurative lymphadenitis (typically due to *Staphylococcus aureus* or *Streptococcus pyogenes*) or indolent lymphadenitis (e.g., *Bartonella henselae*, atypical *Mycobacterium*)
c. Malignancy: Can be observed with leukemia, and lymphoma

Text continued on p. 452

TABLE 17.1

β-LACTAMS: INHIBIT CELL WALL SYNTHESIS

	Gram-Positive Organisms	Gram-Negative Organisms	Anaerobes	Spirochetes
PENICILLINS				
Natural penicillins (Pen G or Pen V)	Streptococcus pyogenes, Streptococcus agalactiae, Streptococcus pneumoniae (with about 10%–20% resistance depending on local epidemiology), Viridans streptococcus, Listeria monocytogenes, Corynebacterium diphtheriae	Neisseria meningitidis	Oral anaerobes	Borrelia burgdorferi, Leptospira interrogans, Treponema pallidum
Anti-*Staphylococcus*–resistant penicillins: Nafcillin, oxacillin, dicloxacillin	MSSA, CoNS (high levels of resistance)			
Aminopenicillins: Amoxicillin, ampicillin	S. pyogenes, S. agalactiae, S. pneumoniae, Viridans streptococcus, L. monocytogenes, Enterococcus faecalis	Non–β-lactamase–producing Escherichia coli, other Gram-negative enterics, and non–β-lactamase–producing respiratory Gram-negatives such as Haemophilus influenzae	Oral anaerobes	B. burgdorferi, L. interrogans, T. pallidum
Extended-spectrum β-lactamase inhibitors without pseudomonal activity: Amoxicillin/clavulanic acid, ampicillin/sulbactam	Organisms covered by amoxicillin/ ampicillin plus MSSA	β-Lactamase–producing Gram-negative intestinal (E. coli) and respiratory organisms (H. influenzae)	Oral and intestinal anaerobes	

Continued

TABLE 17.1
β-LACTAMS: INHIBIT CELL WALL SYNTHESIS—cont'd

	Gram-Positive Organisms	Gram-Negative Organisms	Anaerobes	Spirochetes
Extended-spectrum β-lactamase inhibitors with pseudomonal activity: Piperacillin/tazobactam	E. faecalis, MSSA, S. pyogenes, S. agalactiae	E. coli and other Enterobacteriaceae and enterics, Pseudomonas aeruginosa (percent susceptibility varies based on local epidemiology)	Oral and intestinal anaerobes	
CEPHALOSPORINS				
Do not cover LAME [Listeria, Atypicals such as Mycoplasma and Chlamydia, MRSA (except for ceftaroline), and Enterococci]				
First-generation: Cephalexin, cefazolin	MSSA, S. pyogenes, S. agalactiae	Very good coverage of enteric Gram-negative organisms (e.g., E. coli, Klebsiella)		
Second-generation: cefuroxime and the cephamycins (cefotetan and cefoxitin)	Cefuroxime: same as first-generation; cephamycins: little activity	β-Lactamase–producing Gram-negative organisms (E. coli, H. influenzae, Klebsiella spp., Proteus spp., Moraxella catarrhalis), Enterobacter, some Neisseria spp.	Cephamycins have good oral anaerobic activity but generally poor intestinal anaerobic activity	
Third-generation: IV/IM: Ceftriaxone, cefotaxime, ceftazidime Enteral: Cefixime, cefpodoxime, cefdinir *Good CNS penetration*	S. pneumoniae (majority), S. pyogenes, S. agalactiae, Viridans streptococcus	Ceftriaxone/cefotaxime and orals: β-lactamase–producing Gram-negatives (E. coli, H. influenzae, M. catarrhalis, Klebsiella, Proteus, Neisseria Ceftazidime: β-lactamase-producing Gram-negative spp.		B. burgdorferi
Fourth-generation: Cefepime *Good CNS penetration*	Same as third-generation plus MSSA	β-Lactamase–producing Gram-negatives, P. aeruginosa		
Fifth-generation: Ceftaroline	Same as third-generation plus MRSA			

TABLE 17.1
β-LACTAMS: INHIBIT CELL WALL SYNTHESIS—cont'd

	Gram-Positive Organisms	Gram-Negative Organisms	Anaerobes	Spirochetes
CARBAPENEMS				
Meropenem, imipenem, doripenem	MSSA, *S. pneumoniae*, *S. pyogenes*, *S. agalactiae*, Enterococcus	β-Lactamase-producing Gram-negatives, including some very resistant *Pseudomonas* spp., *Acinetobacter* spp., *Serratia* spp., *Klebsiella* spp., *E. coli*, *Burkholderia cepacia*	Oral and intestinal (not *Clostridium difficile*)	
Ertapenem	MSSA	β-Lactamase-producing Gram-negatives (poor activity against *Pseudomonas* and *Acinetobacter* than other carbapenems)	All oral and intestinal (not *C. difficile*)	
MONOBACTAMS				
Aztreonam		Covers most aerobic Gram-negative bacilli, including ~70% of *Pseudomonas* spp.		

CNS, Central nervous system; CoNS, coagulase-negative Staphylococci; IM, intramuscular; IV, intravenous; MRSA, methicillin-resistant *Staphylococcus aureus*; MSSA, methicillin-sensitive *Staphylococcus aureus*

TABLE 17.2
FLUOROQUINOLONES[a]: INHIBIT DNA TOPOISOMERASES

	Gram-Positive Organisms	Gram-Negative Organisms	Anaerobes	Other
Ciprofloxacin, Ofloxacin	*Bacillus anthracis, Staphylococcus saprophyticus*	Broad coverage, including *Shigella* spp., *Pseudomonas aeruginosa*; emerging *Neisseria* resistance		
Levofloxacin	Excellent *Streptococcus pneumoniae* coverage	Similar coverage as ciprofloxacin		Great atypical coverage, including *Mycoplasma pneumoniae, Chlamydia pneumoniae, Legionella* spp.
Moxifloxacin	Same as levofloxacin	Good enteric coverage; poor *Pseudomonas* coverage	Best anaerobic coverage of quinolones	Good for MTB and atypical *Mycobacteria*

[a]The American Academy of Pediatrics does not generally recommend fluoroquinolones for patients younger than 18 years unless no alternative options or for specific situations such as multidrug resistance, *Pseudomonas*, and *Mycobacterium* (Bradley and Jackson, 2011).
MSSA, Methicillin-sensitive *Staphylococcus aureus*; MTB, *Mycobacterium tuberculosis*

TABLE 17.3
MACROLIDES: INHIBIT PROTEIN SYNTHESIS, BIND 50S RIBOSOMAL SUBUNIT

	Gram-Positive Organisms	Atypicals	Others
Clarithromycin	Reasonably good against *Streptococcus pneumoniae* (50%–70%)	*Mycoplasma pneumoniae, Chlamydia pneumoniae, Legionella* spp.	*Bartonella henselae, Bordetella pertussis, Campylobacter, Borrelia burgdorferi, H. influenza*, MAI and other atypical *Mycobacteria*
Erythromycin	Same as clarithromycin	Above and *Chlamydia trachomatis*	*Haemophilus ducreyi, Moraxella catarrhalis*
Azithromycin	Same as clarithromycin	Same as above	*B. henselae, H. ducreyi, Neisseria gonorrhoeae*

MAI, *Mycobacterium avium* subsp. *intracellulare*

TABLE 17.4
TETRACYCLINES: INHIBIT PROTEIN SYNTHESIS, BIND 30S RIBOSOMAL SUBUNIT

	Gram-Positive Organisms	Atypicals	Others
Doxycycline and tetracycline	*Streptococcus pneumoniae*, MSSA, MRSA, *Propionibacterium acnes*	*Mycoplasma, Chlamydia, Legionella*	*Haemophilus influenzae, Helicobacter pylori, Vibrio* spp., some anaerobic activity, *Borrelia burgdorferi, Coxiella burnetii, Francisella tularensis, Rickettsia, Treponema pallidum, Yersinia pestis*

MRSA, Methicillin-resistant *Staphylococcus aureus*; MSSA, methicillin-sensitive *Staphylococcus aureus*

TABLE 17.5
AMINOGLYCOSIDES: INHIBIT PROTEIN SYNTHESIS, BIND 30S RIBOSOMAL SUBUNIT

	Gram-Negative Organisms
Gentamicin and streptomycin	Almost all Gram-negative organisms; synergy with ampicillin for *Enterococcus* endocarditis
Tobramycin and amikacin	Almost all Gram-negative organisms

TABLE 17.6
SINGLE DRUG CLASS

	Gram-Positive Organisms	Gram-Negative Organisms	Other
Clindamycin (Binds 50S ribosomal subunit)	Broad Gram-positive coverage: MRSA, MSSA, *Streptococcus* spp.		Oral anaerobes
Linezolid (Binds 50S ribosomal subunit)	MRSA, MSSA, *Enterococcus* (including VRE), CoNS, *Streptococcus* spp., Viridans streptococci		*Mycobacterium* spp., *Nocardia*
Metronidazole (Inhibits nucleic acid synthesis)	Anaerobic Gram-positive organisms: *Clostridium* spp., *Peptostreptococcus* spp.	Broad anaerobic coverage	*Entamoeba histolytica*, *Giardia lamblia*, *Trichomonas vaginalis*, and *Gardnerella vaginalis*
Nitrofurantoin (Damages intracellular macromolecules)	*Enterococcus faecalis*, *Staphylococcus saprophyticus*	*Citrobacter* spp., *Escherichia coli*, some *Klebsiella* spp., some *Enterobacter* spp.	
Trimethoprim + Sulfamethoxazole (Inhibits folate synthesis)	MRSA, MSSA, *Listeria* (second choice if PCN allergy)	Many Gram-negative bacilli, including *Stenotrophomonas*, *Maltophilia*, *Burkholderia cepacia*	*Pneumocystis jirovecii*, *Toxoplasma gondii*, *Nocardia*
Vancomycin (Inhibits peptidoglycan synthesis)	MRSA, MSSA, *Enterococcus* (except VRE), CoNS, *Streptococcus* spp., Viridans streptococci, *C. difficile* (orally)		

CoNS, Coagulase-negative staphylococci; MRSA, methicillin-resistant *Staphylococcus aureus*; MSSA, methicillin-sensitive *Staphylococcus aureus*; PCN, penicillin; VRE, vancomycin-resistant *Enterococcus*

d. Other causes: Autoimmune disorders, drug reactions, serum sickness, acute human immunodeficiency virus (HIV)

2. **Physical findings**

a. Size: Cervical and axillary LN are typically <1 cm in size. Inguinal LN are typically <1.5 cm in size. Cervical LN >2 cm or palpable supraclavicular LN are associated with higher risk for malignancy.

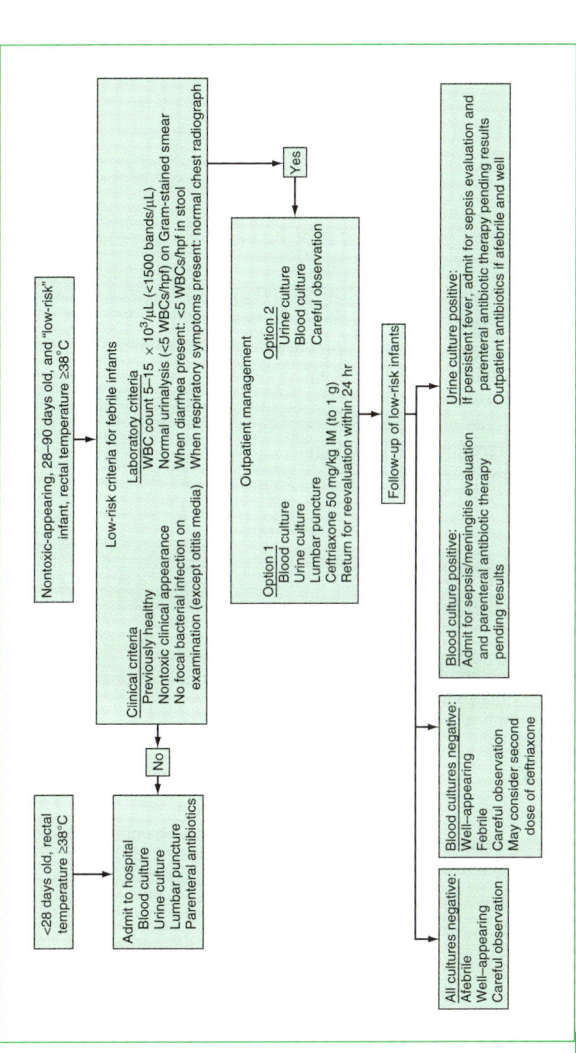

FIGURE 17.3

Algorithm for management of a previously healthy infant aged ≤90 days, with a fever without localizing signs. This algorithm is a suggested but not exhaustive approach. hpf, High-power field. (Modified from Baraff LJ. Management of fever without source in infants and children. *Ann Emerg Med.* 2000;36:602-614 and Baraff LJ. Management of infants and young children with fever without source. *Pediatr Ann.* 2008;37:673-679.)

b. Palpation: Tenderness is more common with reactive or infected LN but does not exclude malignancy. Fluctuance, warmth, and/or overlying erythema are more common in lymphadenitis. Hard, rubbery, fixed, or matted LN are suspicious for malignancy and require further investigation (see Section 22.III for features of malignant LN).
c. If reactive lymphadenopathy is suspected, consider observation, with expected decrease in size over 4–6 weeks and resolution in 8–12 weeks.
d. If lymphadenitis is suspected, consider a 5–7-day trial of antibiotics with streptococcal and staphylococcal coverage.
e. Laboratory studies: Complete blood cell count (CBC) with differential, erythrocyte sedimentation rate (ESR), lactate dehydrogenase (LDH), specific serologies based on exposures and symptoms [*B. henselae*, Epstein–Barr virus (EBV), HIV], tuberculin skin testing (TST).
f. Imaging: Chest x-ray, consider ultrasound if etiology unclear. CT may be needed to evaluate anatomy for excision or evaluation of retropharyngeal abscess.[8]
g. Excision/fine needle aspiration: See Section 22.III for criteria.
3. **Cervical Lymphadenopathy in Children**[8,9]
a. Differential diagnosis of enlarged cervical LN (Fig. 17.4)

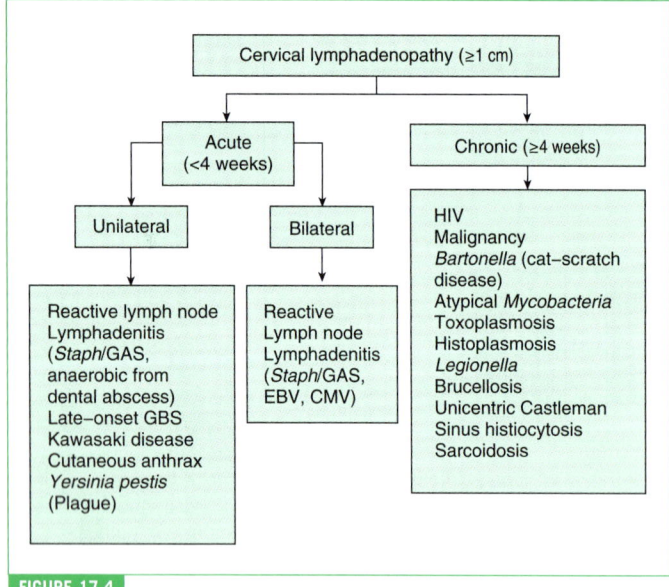

FIGURE 17.4
Differential diagnosis of cervical lymphadenopathy.

b. Correlate location of nodes and drainage patterns of head and neck (Fig. EC 17.A).
c. Rule out other causes of cervical masses including branchial cleft cysts, epidermoid cysts, thyroglossal duct cysts, thyroid nodule, cystic hygroma, fibroma, cervical rib, and lymphatic malformation.

C. Intrauterine and Perinatal Infections

1. **Intrauterine (congenital) infections:** The acronym TORCH [toxoplasmosis, other, rubella, cytomegalovirus (CMV), herpes simplex virus (HSV)] is used to describe a group of infections (including a large number that fall under "other") outlined individually in Table 17.7. These infections often present in the neonate with overlapping findings: intrauterine growth retardation (IUGR), hematologic insult, ocular abnormalities, central nervous system (CNS) signs, and other organ system involvement (e.g., pneumonitis, myocarditis, nephritis, and hepatitis).[10-12] Workup and management of these infections are detailed in Table 17.7.
2. **Perinatal viral infections:** Perinatal varicella-zoster virus (VZV), HSV, lymphocytic choriomeningitis virus and CMV infections can be severe, with profound morbidity and mortality. It can be difficult to clinically distinguish neonatal VZV and HSV lesions.[14] Workup and management of these infections are also detailed in Table 17.7.
3. **Group B streptococcal (GBS) infection:**
a. Adequate maternal intrapartum prophylaxis is intravenous (IV) penicillin, ampicillin, or cefazolin ≥4 hours before delivery.[13] Fig. 17.5 shows an algorithm for secondary prevention of early-onset GBS disease in newborns.
b. Late-onset GBS: See Table 17.8.

D. Common Neonatal and Pediatric Bacterial Infections: Guidelines for Initial Management (See Table 17.8)

1. **Deep neck infections**[19,20]
a. **Submandibular**. Ludwig angina, causes rapidly progressive indurated cellulitis and swelling of the floor of mouth, significant risk of airway compromise; often caused by dental infection. Treat with antibiotics targeting oral flora, such as ampicillin–sulbactam or clindamycin AND ceftriaxone, surgical decompression, and drainage.
b. **Parapharyngeal**. Posterior compartment infection by *Fusobacterium* tonsillitis can lead to suppurative jugular thrombophlebitis or Lemierre syndrome. This can cause bloodstream infection, septic emboli, and intracranial venous thrombosis. Signs include neck pain and swelling around sternocleidomastoid, torticollis, and increased intracranial pressure. Consider magnetic resonance imaging or computed tomography (CT) with contrast of the neck. Requires at least 2 weeks of IV antibiotics with anaerobic coverage.

Text continued on p. 470

TABLE 17.7
CONGENITAL AND PERINATAL INFECTIONS

Infective Agent	Clinical Findings	Diagnostic Testing	Therapy
Toxoplasmosis	May be asymptomatic at birth. Major clinical signs: chorioretinitis, cerebral calcifications, hydrocephalus. Additional signs: maculopapular rash, generalized lymphadenopathy, hepatosplenomegaly, jaundice, pneumonitis, petechiae, thrombocytopenia, microcephaly, seizures, and hearing loss	Test for IgM, IgA, IgG. Presence of IgM after 5 days or IgA after 10 days or persistence of IgG beyond 12 months is diagnostic. Positive PCR in CSF, blood, or urine is also diagnostic. Eye examination. Cerebral calcifications best seen on CT	Pyrimethamine + sulfadiazine with folinic acid for at least 12 months
Syphilis*	Early signs: hepatosplenomegaly, snuffles (copious nasal secretions), lymphadenopathy, mucocutaneous lesions, pneumonia, osteochondritis, hemolytic anemia, or thrombocytopenia. Skin lesions and secretions are highly infectious. If untreated, may develop late manifestations affecting CNS, bones and joints, teeth, eyes, or skin	All women should be screened prenatally. If maternal serology positive, screen infant using nontreponemal test such as VDRL or RPR. Confirmatory test using treponemal test such as FTA-ABS or MHA-TP.† See Table EC 17.A.	For abnormal neonatal testing/physical examination: aqueous penicillin G **or** procaine penicillin G. For negative neonatal testing: benzathine penicillin G (see Formulary for dosing)
Rubella*	IUGR, cataracts, cardiac anomalies, deafness, "blueberry muffin rash"	IgM–positive at birth–3 months. Eye examination. Echocardiogram	Supportive care for newborn. Ensure mother is immunized

Cytomegalovirus (CMV)	90% asymptomatic at birth IUGR, jaundice, hepatosplenomegaly, microcephaly, thrombocytopenia, intracranial calcifications, hearing loss (may develop later in life), retinitis. Developmental delay is common.	Isolation of virus in culture or by PCR from urine, oral fluids, respiratory tract secretions, blood, or CSF within 2–4 weeks of birth	Treatment not indicated for asymptomatic CMV 6 months of valganciclovir improves audiologic and neurodevelopmental outcomes at 2 years of age in infants with symptomatic disease May use ganciclovir if unable to absorb enterally
Parvovirus B19	Fetal hydrops, IUGR, intellectual disability, isolated pleural and pericardial effusions Risk of fetal death when infection occurs during pregnancy is 2%–6%, greatest risk in first half of pregnancy	Positive serum IgM suggests infection occurred 2–4 months earlier	Supportive care
Herpes simplex virus (HSV)	HSV can present any time within the first 1–4 weeks of life as: 1. Disease localized to SEM (45%) 2. Localized CNS infection (30%) 3. Disseminated disease (25%) with severe pneumonitis and hepatitis as well as CNS involvement in 60%–75% Consider HSV in neonates with sepsis, liver dysfunction, or consumptive coagulopathy.	Surface culture: conjunctiva, nasopharynx, mouth, rectum, skin vesicles PCR: blood, CSF, skin vesicles +/− other surface sites Ancillary: CMP for elevated transaminases; CXR for pneumonitis	Acyclovir • 14 days for skin, eye, and mouth disease • 21 days with up to 6 months prophylaxis for CNS involvement or disseminated disease

Continued

TABLE 17.7
CONGENITAL AND PERINATAL INFECTIONS—cont'd

Infective Agent	Clinical Findings	Diagnostic Testing	Therapy

Varicella[14]	Maternal infection during first or early second trimester may result in fetal death or in varicella embryopathy: limb hypoplasia, cutaneous scarring, eye anomalies, and CNS damage (congenital varicella syndrome)
	Maternal infection from 5 days prior or 2 days after delivery can result in severe neonatal infection in first 2 weeks. Can include pneumonitis, encephalitis, purpura fulminans, bleeding, death.
	Maternal infection >5 days before delivery and GA >28 weeks causes milder disease
		DFA of vesicle scraping
		PCR from vesicle or CSF
			VZIG (or IVIG if VZIG unavailable) should be administered to:
			• All neonates if mother developed primary varicella (not zoster) between 5 days before and 2 days after delivery
			• To hospitalized preterm infants if mother has active lesions at delivery (regardless of duration):
			  • <28 weeks or <1000 g
			  • >28 weeks if mother lacks historical or serologic evidence of immunity
			Acyclovir: If lesions develop, some consider treating if giving VZIG

Enterovirus	Hepatitis, myocarditis, meningitis, encephalitis, pneumonitis, coagulopathy	RNA PCR from throat, stool, rectal swab, urine, blood, or CSF	IVIG
Hepatitis B virus (HBV)[15]	*In utero* transmission accounts for <2% of vertical transmission. Perinatal transmission is much more efficient, and 90% develop chronic hepatitis B. Appropriate prophylaxis can prevent 95% of vertical transmission.	ALT is usually normal at birth. Testing for HBsAg and anti-HBs should be done at 9 and 18 months in infants with HBsAg-positive mothers	For HBIG and HBV vaccine guidelines, see Fig. 16.4. Breastfeeding not contraindicated.

Hepatitis C virus (HCV)	Risk of perinatal transmission is 5% and occurs only from women who are HCV RNA–positive at time of delivery. Maternal co-infection with HIV is associated with increased risk of perinatal transmission.	HCV RNA can be detected in serum or plasma within 1–2 weeks after exposure. Maternal anti-HCV antibodies can persist up to 18 months.	No therapy until HCV status ascertained Peginterferon plus ribavirin approved in children aged 3–17 years, but no data for neonates. Refer to pediatric hepatitis specialist Breastfeeding not contraindicated
Human immunodeficiency virus (HIV)[§]	Most mother-to-child transmission occurs perinatally, with lower rates of transmission occurring *in utero* and postnatally through breastfeeding. Greater viral exposure, especially maternal VL, increases risk, as does longer duration of ruptured membranes, more months of breastfeeding, vaginal delivery, or laboring before cesarean section.	See Table 17.12.	See Table 17.12. Breastfeeding contraindicated where safe infant feeding alternatives are available, including in the United States

[*] See 2015 American Academy of Pediatrics *Red Book* for isolation recommendations[12]
[†] All mothers should be screened prenatally for rubella immune status and syphilis.
[‡] Link to diagnostic algorithm for syphilis: http://redbook.solutions.aap.org/data/Books/1484/fig3-12.jpeg
[§] From Panel on Treatment of HIV-Infected Pregnant Women and Prevention of Perinatal Transmission. Recommendations for use of antiretroviral drugs in pregnant HIV-1-infected women for maternal health and interventions to reduce perinatal HIV transmission in the United States. Available at https://aidsinfo.nih.gov/contentfiles/lvguidelines/perinatalgl.pdf. Accessed Sep 22, 2015

ALT, Alanine aminotransferase; CMP, comprehensive metabolic panel; CNS, central nervous system; CSF, cerebrospinal fluid; CT, computed tomography; CXR, chest x-ray; DFA, direct fluorescent antibody; FTA-ABS, fluorescent treponemal antibody absorption test; GA, gestational age; HBIG, hepatitis B immune globulin; IM, intramuscular; IUGR, intrauterine growth retardation; IV, intravenous; IVIG, intravenous immunoglobulin; MHA-TP, microhemagglutination assay for *Treponema pallidum* antibodies; PCR, polymerase chain reaction; sAg, surface antigen; RPR, rapid plasma reagin; SEM, skin, eyes, mouth; VDRL, Venereal Disease Research Laboratory test; VL, viral load; VZIG, varicella-zoster immune globulin

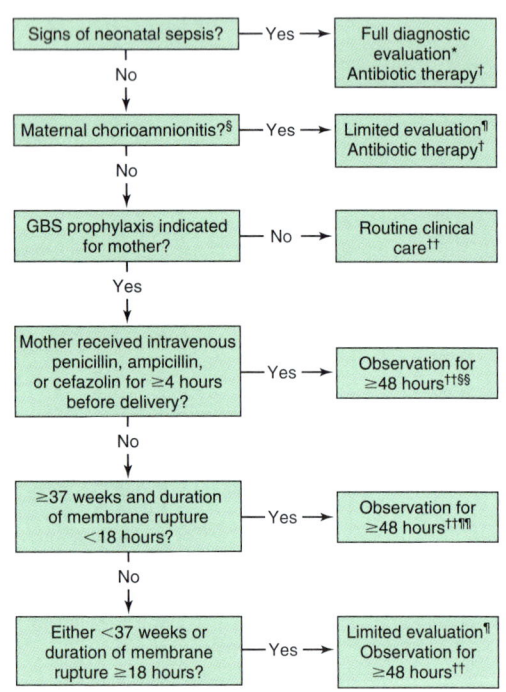

FIGURE 17.5

Algorithm for secondary prevention of early-onset group B streptococcal (GBS) disease among newborns. (From Verani JR, McGee L, Schrag SJ. Division of Bacterial Diseases, National Center for Immunization and Respiratory Diseases, Centers for Disease Control and Prevention (CDC). Prevention of perinatal group B streptococcal disease: Revised guidelines from CDC, 2010. MMWR Recomm Rep. 2010;59:1-36.)

TABLE 17.8
COMMON PEDIATRIC AND NEONATAL INFECTIONS: GUIDELINES FOR INITIAL MANAGEMENT

Infectious Syndrome	Usual Etiology	Suggested Empirical Therapy	Suggested Length of Therapy/Comments
BITES			
Human	Streptococcus spp., Staphylococcus aureus, oral anaerobes, Eikenella corrodens, Haemophilus spp.	PO: amoxicillin/clavulanate Alt: clindamycin + (third-generation cephalosporin or TMP/SMX) IV: ampicillin/sulbactam Alt: TMP/SMX + clindamycin	For all bites, cleaning, irrigation, and debridement are critical. Human: 5–7 days. Assess immunization status (tetanus, hepatitis B) and HIV risk.
Dog/cat	Add Pasteurella multocida, Streptococcus spp., Capnocytophaga, oral anaerobes	Same	Animal: 7–10 days Assess tetanus immunization status, risk of rabies
CATHETER-RELATED BLOODSTREAM INFECTIONS	S. aureus, CoNS, enteric Gram-negative bacilli including Pseudomonas, Candida spp.	Immunocompetent: vancomycin +/− (third-generation cephalosporin OR aminoglycoside) Immunocompromised: vancomycin + (piperacillin/tazobactam OR cefepime OR ceftazidime) +/− aminoglycoside	Remove catheter
CELLULITIS	Nonsuppurative: GAS, MSSA Suppurative: GAS, MSSA, and MRSA	PO: nonsuppurative: cephalexin Suppurative or PCN allergy: clindamycin TMP/SMX has poor activity against GAS	5 days Incision and drainage alone may be adequate for abscess and should be performed when indicated; obtain cultures for susceptibility. Hospitalize for severe infections, limb-threatening infections, immunocompromised status

Continued

TABLE 17.8
COMMON PEDIATRIC AND NEONATAL INFECTIONS: GUIDELINES FOR INITIAL MANAGEMENT—cont'd

Infectious Syndrome	Usual Etiology	Suggested Empirical Therapy	Suggested Length of Therapy/Comments
CONJUNCTIVITIS			
Neonatal Exudative conjunctivitis	*Chlamydia trachomatis*	Saline irrigation regardless of etiology PO/IV Erythromycin OR azithromycin	Onset 3–10 days Topical treatment ineffective
	Neisseria gonorrhoeae	Ceftriaxone OR cefotaxime	Onset 2–4 days. Admit for evaluation and treatment of possible disseminated disease
Suppurative, non-neonatal	*Streptococcus pneumoniae, Haemophilus influenzae, Moraxella, S. aureus,* viral *N. gonorrhoeae, C. trachomatis*	Ophthalmic polymyxin B/TMP drops Alt: FQ drops, erythromycin ointment Ceftriaxone + doxycycline	5 days Ointments preferred for infants or young children Ophthalmic consult if suspected gonorrhea
DACRYOCYSTITIS	*S. pneumoniae, H. influenzae, S. aureus,* CoNS, *Streptococcus pyogenes, Pseudomonas aeruginosa*	Initial management: warm compresses PO: oxacillin OR cephalexin OR clindamycin	Consider ophthalmologic evaluation to relieve obstruction.
DENTAL ABSCESSES	Oral flora, including anaerobes	Amoxicillin/clavulanic acid	Consider dental evaluation for surgical drainage.

GASTROENTERITIS (BACTERIAL)	*Escherichia coli*	Antibiotics discouraged because of possible increased risk of HUS occurring in patients with *E. coli* O157:H7 treated with antibiotics[16] Azithromycin or ciprofloxacin for traveler's diarrhea	Rehydration is the most important component of therapy for diarrhea, regardless of etiology
	Salmonella spp.	Ceftriaxone Alt: azithromycin, ampicillin, amoxicillin, or TMP/SMX for susceptible strains	7–10 days for infants aged <3 months, bacteremia, toxic appearance, hemoglobinopathy, or immunosuppressed. Antibiotics generally not indicated otherwise
	Shigella spp.	Ceftriaxone, azithromycin, or FQ	5 days for dysentery, immunosuppressed, or to prevent spread in mild disease. Otherwise, treatment not indicated. Oral cephalosporins not useful. High rates of resistance with amoxicillin or TMP/SMX
	Yersinia spp.	Ceftriaxone, TMP/SMX, aminoglycosides, FQ, or tetracycline	Usually no antibiotic therapy is recommended except for bacteremia, extraintestinal infections, or in neonates or immunocompromised hosts.
	Campylobacter spp.	Azithromycin or erythromycin	5 days; shortens duration of fecal shedding
	Clostridium difficile	Metronidazole Oral vancomycin for severe infection	10 days Stop the precipitating antibiotic therapy
INTRA-ABDOMINAL INFECTIONS	*E. coli, Enterococcus, Bacteroides* spp., *Clostridium* spp., *Peptostreptococcus, P. aeruginosa, S. aureus*, other Gram-negative bacilli	Previously healthy: ceftriaxone AND metronidazole Healthcare-associated: piperacillin–tazobactam (ciprofloxacin AND metronidazole if PCN allergy)	4 days after source control procedure For patients with healthcare-associated infection, consider MRSA coverage. May use ciprofloxacin for severe PCN allergy

Continued

TABLE 17.8
COMMON PEDIATRIC AND NEONATAL INFECTIONS: GUIDELINES FOR INITIAL MANAGEMENT—cont'd

Infectious Syndrome	Usual Etiology	Suggested Empirical Therapy	Suggested Length of Therapy/Comments
LYMPHADENITIS	Viruses, GAS, S. aureus, anaerobes, atypical mycobacteria, Actinomyces, Bartonella henselae (cat-scratch disease), Mycobacterium tuberculosis	PO: amoxicillin/clavulanate; clindamycin if MRSA prevalent Alt: cephalexin or dicloxacillin IV: oxacillin or cefazolin; clindamycin if MRSA prevalent	Surgical excision with M. tuberculosis, atypical mycobacteria Needle aspiration with B. henselae If allergic to PCN: cefdinir, cefuroxime, or vancomycin
MASTOIDITIS (ACUTE)	S. pneumoniae, S. pyogenes, S. aureus, H. influenzae	Vancomycin OR clindamycin	4 weeks Surgical management required; definitive therapy should be guided by culture obtained at surgery
MENINGITIS			
Neonatal	GBS, E. coli, Listeria monocytogenes Consider S. aureus, resistant enteric GNRs, and Candida in patients with prolonged hospitalization	Ampicillin + cefotaxime	Treat 10 days for GBS infection, 21 days for Listeria For Gram-negative organisms: cefotaxime for 21 days
Non-neonatal (age >1 month)	S. pneumoniae, Neisseria meningitidis, H. influenzae	Ceftriaxone + vancomycin For severe PCN allergy, consider chloramphenicol + vancomycin	Duration depends on organism See Red Book: 2015[2] for chemoprophylaxis recommendations for contacts of meningococcal and Hib disease. Dexamethasone use, except for with H. influenzae, is controversial.
ORBITAL CELLULITIS	S. pneumoniae, H. influenzae, Moraxella catarrhalis, S. aureus, GAS With trauma: anaerobes, GNRs	Ampicillin/sulbactam OR ceftriaxone + vancomycin	10 days Recommend ophthalmologic consultation; CT to evaluate intracranial extension

OSTEOMYELITIS			
Uncomplicated		S. aureus, GAS, Streptococcus spp. (including GBS in neonates), GNRs such as Kingella (≤4 years)	Oxacillin, nafcillin, or clindamycin Alt: vancomycin	4–6 weeks (consider conversion to oral antibiotics after improvement observed) Clindamycin ineffective as monotherapy for Kingella
Foot puncture		Add P. aeruginosa coverage	Ceftazidime OR antipseudomonal PCN + aminoglycoside	
Sickle cell disease		Add Salmonella spp. coverage	Add ceftriaxone	
OTITIS MEDIA (ACUTE)[17]		S. pneumoniae, H. influenzae (nontypeable), M. catarrhalis	High-dose amoxicillin 80–90 mg/kg/day If child has received amoxicillin within the past 30 days or has concurrent purulent conjunctivitis, amoxicillin/clavulanate is recommended Alt/PCN Allergy: cefdinir, cefpodoxime, ceftriaxone For treatment failure with high-dose amoxicillin (persistent symptoms 48–72 hours after initial treatment): amoxicillin/clavulanate or ceftriaxone (IM daily ×3 days) Alt: clindamycin + third-generation cephalosporin	10 days Consider 5–7 days for children aged ≥2 years with mild–moderate symptoms Consider watchful waiting in patients 6–23 months with unilateral, nonsevere symptoms or in patients >2 years with unilateral or bilateral and nonsevere symptoms. Severe symptoms: toxic-appearing, otalgia >48 h, Temperature ≥39°C, or uncertain follow-up Always give analgesia, whether or not antibiotics are prescribed
OTITIS EXTERNA (UNCOMPLICATED)		Pseudomonas	Eardrops: ciprofloxacin or polymyxin–neomycin	7 days Analgesics for pain

Continued

TABLE 17.8
COMMON PEDIATRIC AND NEONATAL INFECTIONS: GUIDELINES FOR INITIAL MANAGEMENT—cont'd

Infectious Syndrome	Usual Etiology	Suggested Empirical Therapy	Suggested Length of Therapy/Comments
PAROTITIS	*S. aureus* most common; also oral flora, Gram-negative rods, viruses (including mumps, HIV, EBV), or noninfectious causes	PO: clindamycin *Alt: nafcillin/oxacillin* In neonates: vancomycin + (aminoglycoside or ceftriaxone)	Local heat, gentle massage of gland from posterior to anterior, and hydration provide symptomatic relief. Surgical drainage may be required. Consider HIV in chronic parotitis.
PERIORBITAL CELLULITIS (PRESEPTAL)	GAS and *Streptococcus* spp., *S. aureus*, *H. influenzae* (nontypeable), *M. catarrhalis*	Ampicillin/sulbactam or amoxicillin/clavulanate or third-generation cephalosporin Consider adding vancomycin, TMP/SMX, or clindamycin if concern for MRSA	10 days If secondary to local trauma and not associated with sinusitis, treat as staph./strep. cellulitis (clindamycin)
PERTUSSIS	*Bordetella pertussis*	Azithromycin, erythromycin Azithromycin for age <1 month *Alt: TMP-SMX, limited evidence*	5 days for azithromycin 7 days for erythromycin Chemoprophylaxis for close contacts
PHARYNGITIS	GAS, group C and G streptococci, *Arcanobacterium haemolyticum*, viruses (including Coxsackie virus, other enteroviruses, EBV)	For GAS: PCN V or amoxicillin or benzathine PCN G × 1 *Alt: clindamycin, macrolide, or cephalosporin*	10 days to prevent acute rheumatic fever 50 mg/kg amoxicillin daily is as effective as BID PCN V or BID amoxicillin Supportive treatment only for viral pharyngitis
PNEUMONIA			
Neonatal	GBS, *E. coli*	Ampicillin + gentamicin	7–10 days, depending on severity Obtain blood cultures Effusions should be drained; Gram stain and culture collected from fluid
	C. trachomatis	Erythromycin *Alt: azithromycin for 5 days*	14 days Presents up to 5 months of life with staccato cough, tachypnea, rales, bilateral infiltrates, and hyperinflation on CXR; usually afebrile

Age >3 months	*S. pneumoniae*, *Mycoplasma*, *Chlamydia pneumoniae*, GAS, *S. aureus*, viruses are most common, including influenza	Outpatient: amoxicillin (high dose) ± azithromycin (atypical coverage) Inpatient: ampicillin ± azithromycin *Alt:* clindamycin *Alt:* ceftriaxone + azithromycin Consider influenza antiviral therapy during influenza season	10 days Atypical organisms (*Mycoplasma*, *Chlamydia*) are more likely in children aged >5 years. Addition of azithromycin should be considered. Add vancomycin or clindamycin if severe illness or features suggestive of *S. aureus* (pleural effusion, cavitation)
Nonimmunized child (for *H. influenzae*, *S. pneumoniae*)	See above	Ceftriaxone or cefotaxime ± azithromycin	Consider vancomycin or clindamycin for MRSA coverage.
RETROPHARYNGEAL OR PERITONSILLAR ABSCESS	GAS, other streptococci, *S. aureus*, oral anaerobes	Ampicillin/sulbactam OR (ceftriaxone or cefotaxime) + clindamycin	Surgical drainage may be required.
SPINAL FUSION INFECTIONS	*Staphylococcus*, *Streptococcus* spp.; enteric or genitourinary Gram-negative organisms	Vancomycin + piperacillin/tazobactam	Greater than 3 months Consider washout of wound initially. Deep tissue culture of wound may direct treatment. Removal of instrumentation may be necessary.
SEPTIC ARTHRITIS			
Neonatal	*S. aureus*, GBS, Gram-negative bacilli	(Cefotaxime or gentamicin) + (nafcillin or oxacillin)	Incision and drainage necessary
Age <5 years	*S. aureus*, GAS, *S. pneumoniae*, *Kingella kingae* (≤4 years), *Haemophilus* spp., *Borrelia burgdorferi*	(Clindamycin or oxacillin) + cefotaxime For all ages, consider amoxicillin or doxycycline in areas with endemic *Borrelia*	3 weeks Aspiration of affected joint recommended Therapy should be guided by culture results Convert to oral therapy when improvement observed

Continued

TABLE 17.8

COMMON PEDIATRIC AND NEONATAL INFECTIONS: GUIDELINES FOR INITIAL MANAGEMENT—cont'd

Infectious Syndrome	Usual Etiology	Suggested Empirical Therapy	Suggested Length of Therapy/Comments
Age ≥5 years	S. aureus, Streptococcus spp., Borrelia burgdorferi	Nafcillin, oxacillin, or clindamycin Alt: vancomycin	Switch to oral antibiotics after improvement observed
Adolescent	S. aureus, Streptococcus spp., Borrelia burgdorferi, N. gonorrhoeae	Add ceftriaxone if N. gonorrhoeae present	If gonorrhea suspected, always treat for chlamydia and test for other STIs
SINUSITIS[18]			
Acute	S. pneumoniae, H. influenzae, M. catarrhalis	Amoxicillin ± clavulanate Alt: cefpodoxime or cefixime PCN allergy: levofloxacin If no improvement in 3–5 days, broaden coverage	7 days Antibiotics indicated for severe onset or worsening course If severe/fails to respond, consider imaging ± drainage
Chronic	Add S. aureus, anaerobes	Amoxicillin/clavulanate ± clindamycin Alt: ceftriaxone OR cefotaxime ± clindamycin OR vancomycin	10–14 days Consider culture to guide therapy.
Seriously ill or immunocompromised	Add Pseudomonas, Gram-negative bacilli, Mucor, Rhizopus, Aspergillus	Cefepime OR piperacillin/tazobactam + amphotericin B	Surgical intervention needed
TRACHEITIS	S. aureus, S. pneumoniae, GAS, M. catarrhalis, H. influenzae, Pseudomonas	Ceftriaxone if community-acquired Cefepime if ventilator or tracheostomy-dependent	5 days Antibiotics will treat the acute illness but will not eliminate the organism if endotracheal tube is present

UTI			
Cystitis	*E. coli*, Enterobacteriaceae, *Enterococcus* spp., *Proteus* spp., *Staphylococcus saprophyticus*	PO: cephalexin, TMP/SMX *Alt: nitrofurantoin or ciprofloxacin*	5 days
Pyelonephritis	*E. coli*, Enterobacteriaceae, *Proteus* spp.	Ceftriaxone	7 days Consider oral cephalexin (or therapy as guided by susceptibility results) as soon as able to tolerate enteral antibiotics
Abnormal host/urinary tract	Add *Pseudomonas*, resistant Gram-negative organisms	Cefepime (ciprofloxacin as oral step-down therapy or for patients with PCN allergy)	7 days
VENTRICULOPERITONEAL SHUNT, INFECTED	*Staphylococcus epidermidis*, *S. aureus*, Gram-negative organisms (including *Pseudomonas*)	Vancomycin + cefepime	14–21 days, depending on organism and response Shunt removal or revision is required for successful treatment.

First antibiotics listed indicate treatment of choice. *Alternative treatment regimens are listed in italics.* Cultures should be obtained when clinically appropriate; antibiotic coverage should be narrowed once organism and susceptibility information is available.

Alt., Alternative; BID, twice daily; CoNS, coagulase-negative staphylococci; CSF, cerebrospinal fluid; CT, computed tomography; CXR, chest x-ray; EBV, Epstein-Barr virus; FQ, fluoroquinolone; GAS, group A streptococcus; GBS, group B streptococcus; GNR, Gram-negative rods; *Haemophilus influenzae* type b; HIV, human immunodeficiency virus; IM, intramuscular; IV, intravenous; MRSA, methicillin-resistant *Staphylococcus aureus*; MSSA, methicillin-sensitive *Staphylococcus aureus*; PCN, penicillin; PO, by mouth; QID, four times daily; STI, sexually transmitted infection; TMP/SMX, trimethoprim/sulfamethoxazole; UTI, urinary tract infection

Recommendations modified from American Academy of Pediatrics. In: Kimberlin DW, Brady MT, Jackson MA, Long SS, eds. *Red Book®. 2015 REPORT OF THE COMMITTEE ON INFECTIOUS DISEASES. American Academy of Pediatrics*; 2015 and McMillan JA, Lee CKK, Sberry GK, Carroll KC. *The Harriet Lane Handbook of Pediatric Antimicrobial Therapy.* Philadelphia, PA: Saunders Elsevier; 2014.

c. **Peritonsillar abscess**. Involves space surrounding palatine tonsil and is most common deep neck infection. Presents with sore throat, muffled voice, odynophagia, dysphagia, trismus, drooling, cervical lymphadenopathy, and uvular deviation. More likely unilateral, but can be bilateral. Most common in adolescents and young adults. Requires drainage and antibiotic coverage against β-lactamase–producing bacteria and anaerobes. Treat for about 5–7 days after drainage.
d. **Retropharyngeal abscess**. Most common in ages 2–4 years, when space has small LNs that atrophy in adolescents. Etiology often polymicrobial, including *S. aureus, S. pyogenes,* viridans streptococci, *Haemophilus,* and anaerobes. Symptoms include sore throat, odynophagia, dysphagia, neck pain, swelling, reduced range of motion, and deviation of lateral wall of the oropharynx to midline. Lateral neck x-ray can show widening of retropharyngeal space, although CT is most sensitive. Depending on clinical situation, IV antibiotics alone may be tried (polymicrobial coverage including for *S. aureus*, such as ampicillin–sulbactam or clindamycin AND ceftriaxone) and if not better within 24–48 hours, consider intraoral surgical or CT-guided drainage.

E. Selected Viral Infections: Table 17.9 and Fig. 17.6

Treatment for most viral illnesses is supportive care unless otherwise specified.

F. Selected Tickborne Infections[12]: Table 17.10

For all tickborne illnesses, infection typically occurs between spring and fall seasons.

G. Fungal and Yeast Infections

1. **Diagnosis**
a. Place specimen (nail or skin scrapings, biopsy specimens, fluids from tissues or lesions) in 10% potassium hydroxide (KOH) on glass slide to look for hyphae, pseudohyphae.
b. Germ tube screen of yeast (3 hours) for *Candida albicans*: All germ tube–positive yeast are *C. albicans,* but not all *C. albicans* are germ tube–positive.
2. **Common community-acquired fungal infections, etiology, and treatment** (Table 17.11)

H. Sexually Transmitted and Genitourinary Infections

For information about the diagnosis and treatment of common sexually transmitted infections as well as the evaluation and management of pelvic inflammatory disease, please see Chapter 5, Tables 5.3 and 5.4.

I. Human Immunodeficiency Virus (HIV) and Acquired Immunodeficiency Syndrome (AIDS)

Recommendations provided are current at the time of publication. Please see the Centers for Disease Control and Prevention (CDC) guidelines on

Text continued on p. 477

TABLE 17.9
SELECTED VIRAL INFECTIONS

Virus	Syndrome	Transmission	Diagnosis	Treatment/Comments
Measles	Fever, Koplik spots, cough, coryza, conjunctivitis, exanthem beginning on face and spreading downward	Aerosol; infectious 3 days before to 4–6 days after rash onset. Virus remains viable in air for 1 hour	Serum IgM levels	Prevalence increasing in areas of under-vaccination. No targeted therapy, but administration of vitamin A reduces morbidity and mortality
Rubella	Postnatal infection is mild, often indiscernible from other viral infections in children. Associated with suboccipital, postauricular, and anterior cervical lymphadenopathy. Rash starts on face and extends to torso and extremities	Direct or droplet contact from nasopharyngeal secretions	Serum IgM levels	See Table 17.7 for congenital rubella
Mumps	Nonspecific prodrome, parotitis, meningitis, meningoencephalitis, orchitis, oophoritis, pancreatitis, myocarditis, arthritis	Respiratory droplets, infectious 7 days before to 7 days after onset of symptoms	Viral culture, antigen testing by immunofluorescence, or PCR from respiratory tract, CSF, or urine	

Continued

TABLE 17.9
SELECTED VIRAL INFECTIONS—cont'd

Virus	Syndrome	Transmission	Diagnosis	Treatment/Comments

Polioviruses	Asymptomatic
	Abortive: nonspecific flu-like syndrome
	Nonparalytic: nuchal rigidity followed by changes (increase or decrease) in reflexes
	Paralytic:
	  Spinal paralysis
	  Bulbar
	  Polioencephalitis
		Fecal–oral transmission; isolated from feces from 2+ weeks before paralysis to several weeks after symptom onset	Virus isolated from stool. Samples should be sent to CDC or WHO laboratories for DNA analysis to distinguish wild type from vaccine-type	Vaccine strains can cause vaccine-associated paralytic poliomyelitis

Other enteroviruses: Multiple serotypes of Coxsackie A, Coxsackie B, echovirus, and Enteroviridae	Nonspecific febrile illness Hand-foot-mouth disease: Usually mild illness characterized by inflamed oropharynx with scattered vesicles that may ulcerate as well as maculopapular, vesicular, or pustular lesions on hands, feet, buttocks, groin. Caused by Coxsackie A, B, and some echoviruses Herpangina: Sudden onset fever, sore throat, dysphagia, posterior pharynx lesions Respiratory: Sore throat, coryza, wheezing, asthma exacerbations, pneumonia, otitis media, pleurodynia	Fecal–oral and respiratory transmission	Viral culture or PCR from CSF, serum, urine, conjunctival, nasopharyngeal, rectal, and stool specimens	IVIG has been used with variable success in neonatal infections and in neurologic and cardiopulmonary disease. Epidemic peak in summer/fall in temperate climates

	Ocular: Acute hemorrhagic conjunctivitis Myocarditis Gastroenteritis Meningitis Neonatal infection			
Parvovirus B19	Erythema infectiosum (fifth disease): prodrome of low-grade fever and URI symptoms followed by slapped-cheek rash and then spread to trunk and extremities, usually sparing palms and soles Arthropathy Transient aplastic crisis because of infection of erythroid precursors and arrest of erythropoiesis Chronic infection in immunocompromised hosts can cause chronic anemia Fetal infection (see Table 17.7)	Respiratory	Diagnosis of erythema infectiosum is based on clinical presentation. B19-specific IgM is the best marker of acute infection. It is rapidly detectable after infection and for 6–8 weeks. PCR for B19 DNA required for diagnosis in immunocompromised patients	Some success with IVIG in anemia and bone marrow failure in immunocompromised children and red blood cell aplasia Seasonal peaks in late winter and spring

Continued

TABLE 17.9
SELECTED VIRAL INFECTIONS—cont'd

Virus	Syndrome	Transmission	Diagnosis	Treatment/Comments
Varicella-zoster virus (VZV)	Primary infection: Varicella (chickenpox): Fever, malaise, headache followed by pruritic macules that evolve into vesicles Predisposes to severe GAS and *S. aureus* infections, encephalitis, pneumonia Herpes zoster: reactivation of latent VZV. Vesicles clustered in 1–2 adjacent dermatomes. Can be complicated by postherpetic neuralgia. 20–30% lifetime risk in those with history of varicella Congenital infection: see Table 17.7	Airborne spread or direct contact with fluid of skin lesions. 10–21-day incubation period.	Primarily clinical diagnosis Also via direct fluorescence or PCR amplification from vesicular fluid or scabs	For varicella: oral valacyclovir or intravenous acyclovir in individuals at risk of moderate-to-severe infection. Antiviral therapy not recommended as routine treatment for uncomplicated varicella because of usual benign self-limited course. For herpes zoster: acyclovir, famciclovir, and valacyclovir reduce duration of illness and risk of postherpetic neuralgia. IV acyclovir for varicella and herpes zoster in immunocompromised children.
Epstein–Barr virus	Infectious mononucleosis: prodrome of fever, fatigue, exudative pharyngitis, headache, myalgia. Cervical and submandibular lymphadenopathy, splenomegaly; hepatomegaly Can have maculopapular rash, especially if given β-lactam Also associated with oncogenesis	Oral secretions Sexual transmission	Heterophile antibody positive in the first week for 75%, second week for 90%–95%, only present in 50% of children <4 yr. EBV-specific Ab testing appropriate if infectious mononucleosis suspected with negative heterophile	Supportive care Avoid contact sports or strenuous athletic activities during splenomegaly and/or first 2–3 weeks of infection

Cytomegalovirus (CMV)	Immunocompetent: Usually asymptomatic, or mononucleosis-like syndrome with fatigue and cervical lymphadenopathy, can have mildly elevated transaminases and thrombocytopenia Immunocompromised: Proportionate to degree of compromise Less severe: Fever, leukopenia, thrombocytopenia, mild hepatocellular dysfunction. Disseminated infection can involve liver, lung, GI tract, and rarely CNS Congenital/neonatal: See Table 17.7	Infection is ubiquitous. Virus intermittently shed throughout life after infection. Community exposure: Through saliva and urine. Breastmilk is most common source in early childhood Sexual transmission is most common source in adolescence and early adulthood Nosocomial: Via blood or organ transplantation Congenital: Intrauterine transmission	See Fig. 17.6 for changes in EBV antibodies over time in acute mononucleosis Because virus can be shed throughout life, diagnosis in immunocompetent individuals depends on signs of acute infection, usually combined with CMV-specific IgG seroconversion or CMV-specific IgM may persist for months depending on assay. PCR-based detection of virus in urine, saliva, blood, and tissue can also be helpful and can allow for monitoring of treatment in immunocompromised hosts. Congenital: see Table 17.7	Immunocompromised: Ganciclovir, foscarnet, also used for prophylaxis in allograft transplant recipients Infants: Treatment with valganciclovir or ganciclovir may limit hearing loss and improve neurologic development.

Continued

TABLE 17.9
SELECTED VIRAL INFECTIONS—cont'd

Virus	Syndrome	Transmission	Diagnosis	Treatment/Comments
Influenza	Often abrupt onset of systemic symptoms (myalgias, chills, headache, malaise, anorexia). Respiratory symptoms may include URI, croup, bronchiolitis, pneumonia. Complications include AOM, secondary bacterial pneumonia (especially S. aureus and S. pneumoniae), rarely myositis, myocarditis, or CNS complications including encephalitis, myelitis, Guillain–Barré syndrome.	Via respiratory droplets. Incubation 12–72 hours. Seasonal peaks during colder months in temperate climates	May diagnose clinically; laboratory confirmation not required for treatment. Diagnosis options include rapid diagnostic tests with low sensitivity, DFA/IFA (antibody staining), PCR with high sensitivity, and rapid or conventional cell culture.	Oseltamivir PO for 5 days Recommendations change yearly. See http://www.cdc.gov/flu/ for most up-to-date recommendations. Most effective within 48 hours of onset of symptoms; may initiate therapy later in hospitalized patients or others with severe or complicated illness

Ab, Antibody; AOM, acute otitis media; CDC, Centers for Disease Control and Prevention; CNS, central nervous system; CSF, cerebrospinal fluid; DFA, direct immunofluorescence; EBV, Epstein–Barr virus; GI, gastrointestinal; IFA, indirect immunofluorescence; IgG, immunoglobulin G; IgM, immunoglobulin M; PCR, polymerase chain reaction; PO, by mouth; S. aureus, Staphylococcus aureus; URI, upper respiratory tract infection; WHO, World Health Organization

Modified from Kliegman RE, Stanton B, St Geme J, et al. Nelson Textbook of Pediatrics. 20th ed. Philadelphia, PA: Elsevier, 2016.

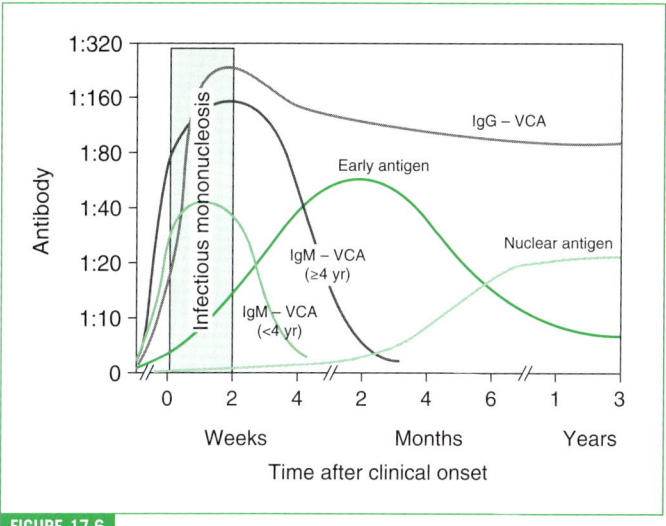

FIGURE 17.6

Graphic representation of the development of antibodies to Epstein–Barr virus antigens as a function of time from infection. Antibody titers are calculated as geometric mean values expressed as reciprocals of the serum dilution. The immunoglobulin M (IgM) response to viral capsid antigen (VCA) varies according to age of the patient. IgG, Immunoglobulin G. (From Jenson HB. Epstein-Barr Virus. In: Kliegman RE, Stanton B, St Geme J, et al. Nelson Textbook of Pediatrics. 20th ed. Philadelphia, PA: Elsevier; 2016.)

the diagnosis and management of children with HIV infection at www.aidsinfo.nih.gov/ for the most up-to-date recommendations.
1. **Clinical presentation**[12,21]
   a. Acute infection with nonspecific findings, including intermittent fever, diarrhea, failure to thrive, parotitis, malaise, myalgia, hepatosplenomegaly, lymphadenopathy, rash, oral ulcers, leukopenia, thrombocytopenia, elevated transaminases
   b. May present with opportunistic infections, including *Pneumocystis jirovecii* pneumonia, candidiasis, herpes zoster, varicella, toxoplasmosis, cryptosporidiosis
   c. Thorough history essential, including *in utero* exposure, injection drug use, unprotected sexual intercourse, and international adoption
   d. If abnormal findings or confirmed diagnosis, consult pediatric HIV specialist

TABLE 17.10
SELECTED TICKBORNE ILLNESSES

Disease	Geographic Distribution	Presentation	Transmission	Diagnosis	Treatment
Lyme disease	New England Middle Atlantic Upper Midwest Pacific Northwest	Early localized: Up to 1 month after tick bite. Erythema migrans, fever, headache, myalgia, malaise Early disseminated: 3–10 weeks after bite. Secondary erythema migrans with multiple smaller target lesions, cranioneuropathy (especially facial nerve palsy), systemic symptoms, lymphadenopathy, 1% develop carditis with heart block or aseptic meningitis Late disease: 2–12 months from initial bite. Pauciarticular arthritis of large joints in 7% of untreated, peripheral neuropathy, encephalopathy	Spirochete *Borrelia burgdorferi* carried by deer tick, *Ixodes scapularis* or *Ixodes pacificus*; requires 24–48 hr of tick attachment. Disseminates systemically through blood and lymphatics	Early: Clinical diagnosis. Tests are insensitive and not recommended in first 4 weeks of infection Early disseminated and late disease: EIA or IFA for antibodies. IgM detectable for first 30 days, IgG detectable by week 6. False positives occur with viral infections, other spirochetes, and autoimmune disease. If antibody negative, no further testing required. If positive, confirm with western blot. Perform LP as clinically indicated for CNS involvement.	No antibiotics recommended for ticks attached <24–48 hr Early localized: Doxycycline for 14 days for children ≥8 years. Amoxicillin or cefuroxime for 14 days for younger children Early disseminated or late onset: same medications for 14–21 days See AAP Redbook for more details on treatment course for complications

Rocky Mountain spotted fever	Widespread; most common in South Atlantic, Southeastern, and South Central United States	Incubation period is ~1 week (range 2–14 days) Fever, headache, myalgia, nausea, anorexia, abdominal pain, diarrhea Rash: Usually appears by day 6; initially erythematous and macular; progresses to maculopapular and petechial due to vasculitis. Usually appears on wrists and ankles and spreads proximally. Palms and soles are often involved. Laboratory manifestations: Thrombocytopenia, hyponatremia, and anemia. White blood cell count usually normal Severe disease may manifest in CNS, cardiac, pulmonary, gastrointestinal tract, renal involvement, disseminated intravascular coagulation (DIC), and shock leading to death. 20%–80% case fatality if untreated	*Rickettsia rickettsii*, an obligate intracellular Gram-negative bacillus transmitted to humans by a tick bite	Identification of *R. rickettsii* DNA by PCR in blood and serum specimens, preferably within the first week of symptoms and within 24 hours of starting antibiotics Gold standard is indirect fluorescent antibody; IgG and IgM increase around 7–10 days. Negative result (PCR or antibody testing) does not rule out the diagnosis	Doxycycline is recommended for children of any age and should be started as soon as the diagnosis is suspected. Duration: 7 days and continue until patient is afebrile for ≥3 days and has demonstrated clinical improvement

Continued

TABLE 17.10
SELECTED TICKBORNE ILLNESSES—cont'd

Disease	Geographic Distribution	Presentation	Transmission	Diagnosis	Treatment
Ehrlichiosis	Southeastern, South Central, East Coast, and Midwestern United States	Systemic febrile illness with headache, chills, rigors, malaise, myalgia, nausea. Rash is variable in location and appearance Laboratory manifestations: Leukopenia, anemia, and transaminitis. CSF with lymphocytic pleocytosis or elevated protein More severe disease: Pulmonary infiltrates, bone marrow hypoplasia, respiratory failure, encephalopathy, meningitis, DIC, spontaneous hemorrhage, and renal failure	*Ehrlichia chaffeensis* (human monocytic ehrlichiosis) and *Ehrlichia ewingii* associated with the bite of a Lone Star tick (*Amblyomma americanum*), although other tick species may be vectors. Mammalian reservoirs include white-tailed deer and white-footed mice.	Identification of DNA by PCR from whole blood is highly sensitive and specific. Isolation in culture must be done at CDC specialty labs from samples prior to initiation of antibiotics.	Doxycycline for at least 3 days after defervescence, for a minimum total course of 7 days
Anaplasmosis	North Central, and Northeastern United States, Northern California	Same as *Ehrlichia*	*Anaplasma phagocytophilum*, transmitted by the deer tick (*Ixodes scapularis*) or western black-legged tick (*Ixodes pacificus*)	Same as *Ehrlichia*	Same as *Ehrlichia*

CDC, Centers for Disease Control and Prevention; CNS, central nervous system; CSF, cerebrospinal fluid; EIA, enzyme immunoassay; Hr, Hour; IFA, immunofluorescent assay; IgG, immunoglobulin G; IgM, immunoglobulin M; PCN, penicillin; PCR, polymerase chain reaction

Data from American Academy of Pediatrics. In: Kimberlin DW, Brady MT, Jackson MA, Long SS, eds. Red Book®. 2015 Report of the Committee on Infectious Diseases. American Academy of Pediatrics; 2015.

TABLE 17.11
COMMON COMMUNITY-ACQUIRED FUNGAL INFECTIONS

Disease	Usual Etiology	Suggested Therapy	Suggested Length of Therapy
Tinea capitis (ringworm of scalp)	Trichophyton tonsurans, Microsporum canis, Microsporum audouinii, Microsporum gypseum, Trichophyton mentagrophytes, Trichophyton violacea, Trichophyton soudanense	Oral griseofulvin (ultramicro) or terbinafine Alt: 2–4 weeks of itraconazole or fluconazole (once weekly) Fungal shedding decreased with selenium sulfide or ketoconazole shampoo, but shampoo alone is not sufficient treatment	4–8 weeks or 2 weeks after clinical resolution Addition of corticosteroid may augment treatment of kerion
Tinea corporis/pedis/cruris (ringworm of body/feet/genital region)	Epidermophyton floccosum, Trichophyton rubrum, T. mentagrophytes, M. canis	Topical antifungal (miconazole, clotrimazole, ketoconazole) once daily or BID; terbinafine BID Alt: griseofulvin, itraconazole, fluconazole	4 weeks for tinea corporis 1–4 weeks for tinea pedis 4–6 weeks for tinea cruris
Oral candidiasis (thrush) in immunocompetent patients	Candida albicans, Candida tropicalis	Nystatin suspension or clotrimazole troche (only nystatin for infants)	7–10 days, then continue 3 days after clinical resolution
Candidal skin infections (intertriginous)	C. albicans	Topical nystatin, miconazole, clotrimazole	7 days
Tinea unguium (ringworm of nails)	T. mentagrophytes, T. rubrum, E. floccosum	Itraconazole or terbinafine	6–12 weeks

BID, Twice daily
Modified from McMillan JA, Lee CKK, Siberry GK, Carroll KC. The Harriet Lane Handbook of Pediatric Antimicrobial Therapy. Philadelphia, PA: Elsevier; 2014. See Table 1.4 in The Harriet Lane Handbook of Pediatric Antimicrobial Therapy for further details regarding treatment of fungal infections.

2. **Diagnosis**
   a. Counseling: Legal requirements for consent vary by state. Counseling includes informed consent for testing, implications of positive test results, and prevention of transmission.
   b. Testing
      (1) Perinatal: See Table 17.12 for diagnosis in perinatal period.[22]

TABLE 17.12
DIAGNOSIS AND MANAGEMENT FOR INFANTS WITH *IN UTERO* HIV EXPOSURE

Age	Laboratory Tests*	Next Steps
Prenatal/Labor	Opt-out testing of all pregnant women HIV antibody testing in third trimester, before 36 weeks' gestation preferred Rapid HIV testing with confirmation if unknown HIV status during labor	Start ART in mother If viral load RNA >1000 copies/mL or unknown at labor, start IV zidovudine and consider cesarean section if greater than 38 weeks' gestation
Newborn	HIV DNA PCR if maternal status unknown, or high risk of infection Baseline CBC with differential	Start ZDV within 6–12 hours of delivery Nevirapine if no maternal ART; three doses: first dose within 48 hours of birth, second dose 48 hours after first dose, third dose 96 hours after second dose
2–3 weeks	HIV DNA PCR (or RNA assay) CBC with differential	Check ZDV dosing and administration Assess psychosocial needs, consider case management referral
4–6 weeks	HIV DNA PCR (or RNA assay) CBC with differential	Discontinue ZDV regardless of PCR result (ZDV monotherapy is used during first 6 weeks for prophylaxis only) Presumptively exclude HIV infection if results of ≥2 weeks PCR and ≥4 weeks PCR both negative. No TMP-SMX needed If PCR results not yet known, begin *Pneumocystis jirovecii* pneumonia prophylaxis, such as TMP-SMX
2 months		Discontinue TMP-SMX if DNA or RNA testing negative
4–6 months	HIV DNA PCR (or RNA assay)	Definitively exclude HIV infection: Two negative PCRs at ≥1 month and ≥4 months, as long as no signs/symptoms of HIV infection
18–24 months	Antibody testing may be performed to confirm clearance of maternal HIV antibodies. If present, need to use nucleic acid testing	

*Any abnormal result requires prompt pediatric HIV specialist consultation.
ART, Antiretroviral therapy; CBC, complete blood cell count; HIV, human immunodeficiency virus; IV, intravenous; PCR, polymerase chain reaction; TMP-SMX, trimethoprim–sulfamethoxazole; ZDV, zidovudine
Modified from Department of Health and Human Services guidelines for pediatric and perinatal HIV infection (see www.aidsinfo.nih.gov for more detailed information).

(2) Children >24 months[23]: HIV antibody testing possible as maternal antibodies likely cleared. If concern for breastmilk exposure, test immediately, then 4–6 weeks, 3 months, and 6 months after stopping breastfeeding.

(3) Adolescents[24]: HIV screening with antigen/antibody assay with opt-out consent as part of routine clinical care. If positive, confirm with HIV-1/HIV-2 immunoassay; if indeterminate, HIV-1 nucleic acid testing.

3. **Management**[21-24]

a. Perinatal exposure

(1) See Table 17.12 for management during perinatal period.

b. Criteria for starting antiretroviral therapy (ART) in HIV-positive patients: U.S. Department of Health and Human Services Guidelines[22-24]

(1) <12 months: All HIV-infected infants, regardless of immunologic, virologic, or clinical status

(2) 12 months to 18 years: Urgently start if CDC Stage 3 defining opportunistic infections or Stage 3 immunodeficiency (<500 cells/mm^3 if age 1 to <6 years, <200 cells/mm^3 if ≤6 years). Recommended if moderate symptoms (CDC stage 2), viral load >100,000 copies/mL, and Stage 2 CD4 counts (500–999 cells/mm^3 for 1 to <6 years, 200–499 cells/mm^3 if ≤6 years). Milder symptoms and greater CD4 counts can be considered on a case-by-case basis.

(3) Adolescents 18 years and older: Initiate ART regardless of CD4 count at diagnosis.

(4) Note: World Health Organization guidelines recommend treatment for all individuals diagnosed with HIV.[25]

c. Therapy: Mainstay is combination ART of at least three drugs from at least two different classes. Go to http://www.aidsinfo.nih.gov/ for most current therapy recommendations.

4. **Lab monitoring**

a. Absolute CD4 count is now preferred over percentage.

b. At diagnosis: CD4 count, plasma HIV RNA viral load, genotype resistance. If starting therapy, HLA-B*5701 (for abacavir) and hepatitis B.

c. Not on ART: Every 3–4 months, CD4 count, plasma HIV RNA viral load, CBC with differential, complete metabolic panel with glucose, renal function, albumin, transaminases, lipid panel. Every 6–12 months, obtain urinalysis to evaluate for nephropathy. Other testing should be performed based on concern for opportunistic infections.

d. On ART: At 2–4 weeks after initiation or switching therapy, CD4, viral load, and labs according to possible toxicities of ART. Then similar testing as above every 3–4 months.

e. Once viral suppression achieved, CD4 improved, good adherence, and otherwise stable for 2–3 years, can space to every 6–12 months.

f. Latent tuberculosis skin testing starting at age 3 to 12 months, and then annually.

J. Tuberculosis (TB)
1. **Clinical presentation**[12]
   a. Infection often asymptomatic (latent TB).
   b. Can progress to TB disease 1–6 months after infection with nonspecific findings including fever, cough, lymphadenopathy, weight loss, failure to thrive, night sweats, and chills. Cavitation and necrosis is uncommon in children. Infants and postpubescent adolescents are at greater risk of progression.
   c. Extrapulmonary involvement can include any organ.
2. **Diagnosis**
   a. **Screening guidelines**[12,26]**:** The American Academy of Pediatrics recommends risk assessment questionnaire, testing for infection in at-risk individuals at first well-child visit and then every 6 months in first year of life, and then routine care (at least annually). Screening questions include:
      (1) Born outside the United States in countries with endemic infection
      (2) Traveled outside United States in countries with endemic infection for ≥1 week
      (3) Family member with positive TST
      (4) Exposed to someone who had TB disease
      (5) Special populations including children with HIV, organ transplant, and those on immunosuppressive therapies including tumor necrosis factor blockers/antagonists
   b. **Latent TB infection (LTBI)**
      (1) IGRA (interferon gamma release assay): Similar sensitivity to TST but higher specificity [because antigens used are not found in bacillus Calmette–Guérin (BCG) or most pathogenic nontuberculous *Mycobacteria*]. Preferred for children 5 years or older, BCG-positive individuals, those unlikely to return for TST read, and if TST negative and still at high risk.
      (2) TST
         i. Inject five tuberculin units of purified protein derivative (0.1 mL) intradermally with a 27-gauge needle on the volar aspect of the forearm to form a 6- to 10-mm wheal. Results of skin testing should be read 48–72 hours later.
         ii. Definition of positive Mantoux test (regardless of whether BCG has been previously administered): Box 17.1
         iii. The incubation period from TB infection to a positive TST or IGRA is approximately 2–10 weeks.
         iv. Measles vaccine can suppress tuberculin for 4–6 weeks.
   c. **Active TB disease**
      (1) If positive for LTBI, obtain chest x-ray
      (2) If symptoms indicate TB disease, determine source

> **BOX 17.1**
>
> **DEFINITIONS OF POSITIVE TUBERCULIN SKIN TESTING**[12]
>
> **Induration ≥5 mm**
>
> - Children in close contact with known or suspected contagious cases of tuberculosis
> - Children suspected to have tuberculosis based on clinical or radiographic findings
> - Children on immunosuppressive therapy or with immunosuppressive conditions (including HIV infection)
>
> **Induration ≥10 mm**
>
> - Children at increased risk for dissemination based on young age (<4 yr) or with other medical conditions (cancer, diabetes mellitus, chronic renal failure, or malnutrition)
> - Children with increased exposure: Those born in or whose parents were born in endemic countries; those with travel to endemic countries; those exposed to HIV-infected adults, homeless persons, illicit drug users, nursing home residents, or incarcerated or institutionalized persons
>
> **Induration ≥15 mm**
>
> - Children ≥4 yr without any risk factors

(3) Specimen sources include sputum, bronchial washings, gastric aspirates (three mornings before feeding/ambulation), pleural fluid, cerebrospinal fluid, urine, tissue biopsy.
  i. Solid media culture can take as long as 10 weeks, liquid media 1–6 weeks. Nucleic acid amplification testing can provide more rapid diagnosis.
(4) Lumbar puncture to assess TB meningitis depending on signs and symptoms. Strongly consider in children aged <24 months with confirmed TB as it is difficult to assess for TB meningitis.

3. **Treatment**
a. Latent TB infection
  (1) Indications:
    i. Children with positive tuberculin tests but no evidence of clinical disease
    ii. Recent contacts, especially with HIV-infected children, of people with TB disease, even if tuberculin test and clinical evidence are not indicative of disease
  (2) Isoniazid susceptible: 9 months of isoniazid daily [if daily therapy not possible, alternative is DOT (directly observed therapy) twice weekly for 9 months] or 12 weeks of weekly isoniazid and rifapentine by DOT for those aged 12 years and older
  (3) Isoniazid resistant: Rifampin daily for 4 months

b. Active TB disease: Consult infectious disease specialist. Includes 6-month regimen, including 2 months RIPE (rifampin, isoniazid, pyrazinamide, ethambutol) followed by 4 months of rifampin/isoniazid. See Red Book 2015 for more details on different regimens, including for meningitis.
c. Multidrug resistance (MDR): Consult infectious disease specialist. At least isoniazid and rifampin resistant. Will require four or five anti-TB drugs for 12–24 months, including an injectable for 4–6 months. Extensively drug resistant (XDR) if also resistant to at least a fluoroquinolone and at least one of the parenteral drugs.

K. Exposures to Bloodborne Pathogens and Prophylaxis

1. **General practice**[27]
a. Always practice universal precautions, use personal protective equipment, and safely dispose of sharps to reduce chance of transmission.
b. Regardless of status of patient, if you experience a needlestick or splash exposure, immediately wash with soap/water, irrigate, report to supervisor, and seek medical assistance.
c. There is an increased risk of transmission if large volume of blood, prolonged exposure, high viral titer, deep injury, or advanced disease.
d. Initial testing: Source should be tested for HIV antibody, hepatitis C antibody, and hepatitis B surface antigen. Exposed person should be tested for HIV antibody, hepatitis C antibody, hepatitis B surface antibody (to look for immune status), and hepatitis B surface antigen.
e. For assistance, contact Clinicians' Postexposure Prophylaxis (PEP) Line at 1-888-448-4911.
2. **HIV:** Updated guidelines may be found at aidsinfo.nih.gov:
a. Pre-exposure prophylaxis (PrEP)[28]: Studies have all been conducted in individuals 18 years and older. Current CDC guidelines recommend PrEP (tenofovir, disoproxil, fumarate, and emtricitabine) as an option for HIV prevention for individuals 18 years and older who are at high risk for HIV acquisition. For adolescent minors, they recommend considering risks, benefits, and that local laws and rules about autonomy vary by state.
b. Postexposure prophylaxis (PEP)[29,30]
    (1) Indications for occupational PEP: Consider with percutaneous, mucosal, or skin exposure to blood or bodily fluids from a patient with known HIV or if unknown, at high suspicion of infection.
    (2) Indications for nonoccupational (nPEP): Consider with unprotected vaginal/anal intercourse, oral sex with ejaculation or blood exposure, needle sharing, or injuries with blood exposure from an individual with known HIV or unknown status.
    (3) Regimen: Initiate as soon as possible (lower likelihood of efficacy at greater than 72 hours), three-drug (or more) ART regimen for 28 days. Preferred tenofovir and entricitabine with raltegravir or

dolutegravir. Consult infectious disease expert for alternative regimens.
(4) Follow-up testing can occur at 6 weeks, 12 weeks, and 6 months; if fourth–generation testing available, can be done at 6 weeks and 4 months.
3. **Hepatitis B**[31]**:** Risk of transmission 37%–62% if surface antigen and e-antigen positive, 23%–37% if surface antigen positive, e-antigen negative. Postexposure management includes hepatitis B immune globulin and initiation of hepatitis B vaccine series depending on immune status. For details, see Chapter 16.
4. **Hepatitis C**[31]**:** Risk of transmission about 1.8%. No preventive therapy available. Serologic testing and follow-up are important to document if infection occurs.

REFERENCES

1. Kaditis AG, O'Marcaigh AS, Rhodes KH, et al. Yield of positive blood cultures in pediatric oncology patients by a new method of blood culture collection. *Pediatr Infect Dis J*. 1996;15:615-620.
2. The Johns Hopkins POC-IT ABX Guide. Bartlett JG, Auewaerter PG, Pham P, eds. Baltimore: POC-IT Center; 2015.
3. McMillan JA, Lee CKK, Siberry GK, et al. *The Harriet Lane Handbook of Pediatric Antimicrobial Therapy*. 2nd ed. Philadelphia: Mosby Elsevier; 2014.
4. Shapiro ED. Fever without localizing signs. In: Long SS, Pickering LK, Prober CG, eds. *Principles and Practice of Pediatric Infectious Disease*. 3rd ed. Philadelphia, PA: Churchill Livingstone; 2008.
5. Arora R, Mahajan P. Evaluation of child with fever without source: review of literature and update. *Pediatr Clin North Am*. 2013;60(5):1049-1062.
6. Long SS. Distinguishing among prolonged, recurrent, and periodic fever syndromes: approach of a pediatric infectious diseases subspecialist. *Pediatr Clin North Am*. 2005;52(3):811-835, vii.
7. Antoon JW, Potisek NM, Lohr JA. Pediatric fever of unknown origin. *Pediatr Rev*. 2015;36(9):380-391.
8. Sahai S. Lymphadenopathy. *Pediatr Rev*. 2013;34(5):216-227.
9. Healy CM, Baker CJ. Cervical lymphadenitis. In: Cherry JD, Harrison GJ, Kaplan SL, Steinbach WJ, Hotez PJ, eds. *Feigin and Cherry's Textbook of Pediatric Infectious Diseases*. 7th ed. Philadelphia, PA: 2014.
10. Kliegman RE, Stanton B, St Geme J, et al. *Nelson Textbook of Pediatrics*. 20th ed. Philadelphia, PA: Elsevier; 2016.
11. Del Pizzo J. Focus on diagnosis: congenital infections (TORCH). *Pediatr Rev*. 2011;32:537-542.
12. American Academy of Pediatrics. *Red Book: 2015 Report of the Committee on Infectious Diseases*. 30th ed. Elk Grove Village, III: AAP; 2015.
13. Verani JR, McGee L, Schrag SJ, Division of Bacterial Diseases, National Center for Immunization and Respiratory Diseases, Centers for Disease Control and Prevention (CDC). Prevention of perinatal group B streptococcal disease—revised guidelines from CDC, 2010. *MMWR Recomm Rep*. 2010;59(RR–10):1-36.
14. Centers for Disease Control and Prevention. Updated recommendations for use of variZIG–United States, 2013. *MMWR Morb Mortal Wkly Rep*. 2013;62(28):574-576.

15. Wong VC, Reesink HW, Lelie PN, et al. Prevention of the HBsAg carrier state in newborn infants of mothers who are chronic carriers of HBsAg and HBeAg by administration of hepatitis-B vaccine and hepatitis-B immunoglobulin: double-blind randomized placebo-controlled study. *Lancet.* 1984;1:921-926.
16. Wong CS, Jelacic S, Habeeb RL, et al. The risk of hemolytic-uremic syndrome after antibiotic treatment of Escherichia coli O157:H7 infections. *N Engl J Med.* 2000;342:1930-1936.
17. Lieberthal AS, Carroll AE, Chonmaitree T, et al. The diagnosis and management of acute otitis media. *Pediatrics.* 2013;131:e964-e999.
18. Wald ER, Applegate KE, Bordley C, et al. Clinical practice guideline for the diagnosis and management of acute bacterial sinusitis in children aged 1 to 18 years. *Pediatrics.* 2013;132(1):e262-e280.
19. Thorell EA. Cervical lymphadenitis and neck infections. In: Long SS, Pickering LK, Prober CG, eds. *Principles and Practice of Pediatric Infectious Disease.* 4th ed. Philadelphia, PA: Elsevier; 2012:135-147.
20. Tebruegge M, Curtis N. Infections related to the upper and middle airways. In: Long SS, Pickering LK, Prober CG, eds. *Principles and Practice of Pediatric Infectious Disease.* 4th ed. Philadelphia: Elsevier; 2012:205-213.
21. Seeborg FO, Paul ME, Shearer WT. Human immunodeficiency virus and acquired immunodeficiency syndrome. In: Cherry JD, Harrison GJ, Kaplan SL, Steinbach WJ, Hotez PJ, eds. *Feigin and Cherry's Textbook of Pediatric Infectious Diseases.* 7th ed. Philadelphia, PA: 2014.
22. Panel on Treatment of HIV-Infected Pregnant Women and Prevention of Perinatal Transmission. Recommendations for Use of Antiretroviral Drugs in Pregnant HIV-1-Infected Women for Maternal Health *and* Interventions to Reduce Perinatal HIV Transmission in the United States. Available at <https://aidsinfo.nih.gov/contentfiles/lvguidelines/perinatalgl.pdf>. Accessed Oct 1, 2015.
23. Panel on Antiretroviral Therapy and Medical Management of HIV-Infected Children. Guidelines for the Use of Antiretroviral Agents in Pediatric HIV Infection. Available at <http://aidsinfo.nih.gov/contentfiles/lvguidelines/pediatricguidelines.pdf>. Accessed Oct 1, 2015.
24. Panel on Antiretroviral Guidelines for Adults and Adolescents. Guidelines for the Use of Antiretroviral Agents in HIV-1-Infected Adults and Adolescents. Department of Health and Human Services. Available at <http://www.aidsinfo.nih.gov/ContentFiles/AdultandAdolescentGL.pdf>. Accessed Oct 1, 2015.
25. World Health Organization (WHO). Guideline on when to start antiretroviral therapy and on pre-exposure prophylaxis for HIV. Geneva: WHO, 2015.
26. Pediatric Tuberculosis Collaborative Group. Targeted tuberculin skin testing and treatment of latent tuberculosis infection in children and adolescents. *Pediatrics.* 2004;114(S4):1175-1201.
27. Siegel JD, Rhinehart E, Jackson M, et al. 2007 Guideline for Isolation Precautions: Prevention Transmission of Infectious Agents in Healthcare Settings. Available at <http://www.cdc.gov/ncidod/dhqp/pdf/isolation2007.pdf>. Accessed Oct 1, 2015.
28. Smith DK, Koenig LJ, Martin M, et al. Preexposure prophylaxis for the prevention of HIV infection – 2014: a clinical practice guideline. Available at: <http://stacks.cdc.gov/view/cdc/23109>. Accessed Oct 1, 2015.
29. Chapman LE, Sullivent EE, Grohskopf LA, et al. Recommendations for postexposure interventions to prevent infection with hepatitis B virus,

hepatitis C virus, or human immunodeficiency virus, and tetanus in persons wounded during bombings and other mass-casualty events–United States, 2008: recommendations of the Centers for Disease Control and Prevention (CDC). *MMWR Recomm Rep*. 2008;57(RR–6):1-21.
30. Kuhar DT, Henderson DK, Struble KA, et al. Updated US Public Health Service guidelines for the management of occupational exposures to human immunodeficiency virus and recommendations for postexposure prophylaxis. *Infect Control Hosp Epidemiol*. 2013;34(9):875-892.
31. U.S. Public Health Service. Updated U.S. Public Health Service Guidelines for the Management of Occupational Exposures to HBV, HCV, and HIV and Recommendations for Postexposure Prophylaxis. *MMWR Recomm Rep*. 2001;50(RR–11):1-52.

Chapter 18

Neonatology

Jennifer Fundora, MD

See additional content on Expert Consult

I. WEB RESOURCES

- www.nicuniversity.org
- Outcomes calculator: http://www.nichd.nih.gov/about/org/der/branches/ppb/programs/epbo/pages/epbo_case.aspx
- Neonatal dermatology: http://www.adhb.govt.nz/newborn/TeachingResources/Dermatology/Dermatology.htm
- Premature growth chart and calculator: http://peditools.org/fenton2013
- Bilitool: bilitool.org
- Neofax: http://micromedex.com/neofax-pediatric

II. FETAL ASSESSMENT

See Expert Consult.

III. NEWBORN RESUSCITATION

A. Neonatal Advanced Life Support Algorithm for Neonatal Resuscitation (Fig. 18.1)

Please see the 7th Edition of the Neonatal Resuscitation Program text for additional details of newborn resuscitation.

1. Prior to delivery, the following equipment checks should be made: radiant warmer on, pre-warmed blankets, hat, bag-and-mask equipment, functional laryngoscope, and an appropriate size endotracheal tube +/− stylet. A suction device and bulb syringe should be available.
2. Based on the seventh edition of the Neonatal Resuscitation Program (NRP)[1]: For infants with meconium-stained amniotic fluid (both vigorous and nonvigorous infants), routine intrapartum oropharyngeal/nasopharyngeal suctioning and endotracheal intubation for suctioning are not recommended.
3. Cord clamping should be delayed for at least 30–60 seconds for the most vigorous term and preterm infants, as long as no contraindications are present. There is not enough evidence to suggest an approach for cord clamping in infants requiring resuscitation at birth.

B. Endotracheal Tube Size and Depth of Insertion (Table 18.1)

C. Ventilatory Support (see Chapter 4)

D. Vascular Access (See Chapter 3 for Umbilical Venous Catheter and Umbilical Artery Catheter Placement)

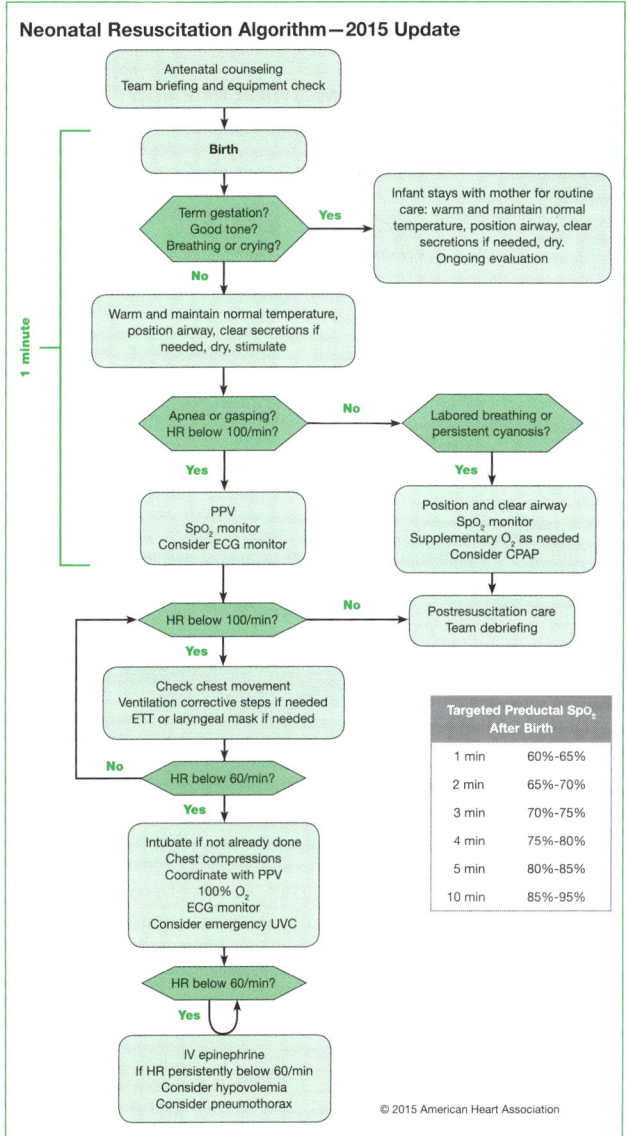

FIGURE 18.1

Overview of resuscitation in the delivery room. CPAP, continuous positive airway pressure; HR, heart rate; IV, intravenous; PPV, positive pressure ventilations; SpO$_2$, oxygen saturation by pulse oximetry

From Wykoff M, Aziz K, Escobedo M. et al. Part 15: neonatal resuscitation: 2015 American Heart Association guidelines for cardiopulmonary resuscitation and emergency cardiovascular care. Circulation. 2015;132(2):S543-560.

TABLE 18.1
PREDICTED ENDOTRACHEAL TUBE SIZE AND DEPTH BY BIRTH WEIGHT AND GESTATIONAL AGE

Gestational Age (wk)	Weight (g)	ETT Size (mm)	ETT Depth of Insertion (cm from Upper Lip)
23–24	500–600	2.5	5.5
25–26	700–800	2.5	6
27–29	900–1000	2.5	6.5
30–32	1100–1400	2.5–3.0	7
33–34	1500–1800	3.0	7.5
35–37	1900–2400	3.0–3.5	8
38–40	2500–3100	3.5	8.5

NOTE: Based on Tochen's 1979 study, the "7-8-9-10" rule recommended that 1-, 2-, 3-, or 4-kg babies were to be intubated at a "tip to lip" distance of 7, 8, 9, or 10 cm, respectively. However, recent literature suggests that these guidelines may better represent the appropriate depth of insertion of endotracheal tube (ETT).
Data from Peterson J, Johnson N, Deakins K, et al. Accuracy of the 7-8-9 rule for endotracheal tube placement in the neonate. J Perinatol. *2006;26:333-336.*

NOTE: During the initial resuscitation, an umbilical venous catheter (UVC) should be inserted just far enough to obtain blood return; no measurement or verified placement is needed initially.

IV. ROUTINE NEWBORN CARE OF A TERM INFANT

A. General Care for the Full-term Healthy Newborn With Uncomplicated Delivery

NOTE: Protocols vary by hospital.
1. Drying, removal of wet blankets. Then, preferably skin-to-skin contact with mother[3] or otherwise placed under warmer.
2. Feeding—Preferably breastfeeding soon after birth and on demand thereafter. Breastfed newborns should feed 8–12 times daily. See Chapter 21 for more information about benefits of breastfeeding. Formula-fed newborns should be offered a bottle soon after birth.
3. Vitamin K for prevention of hemorrhagic disease of the newborn.
4. Antibiotic ophthalmic ointment for prophylaxis against gonococcal infection.
5. Monitor clinically for jaundice, accounting for newborn's risk factors for hyperbilirubinemia. Transcutaneous bilirubin monitoring may be useful as a screening tool but does not replace plasma level.[4] Obtain plasma bilirubin level if warranted. See Section X for more information and management.
6. Consider blood glucose monitoring if infant is at increased risk or is symptomatic of hypoglycemia (see Fig. 18.4 for management).
7. Monitor for stool/urine output. Most infants should have 1 void and 1 meconium stool within first 24 hours.[5]
8. Monitor for significant weight loss in neonate.

TABLE 18.2
APGAR SCORES

Score	0	1	2
Heart rate	Absent	<100 bpm	>100 bpm
Respiratory effort	Absent, irregular	Slow, crying	Good
Muscle tone	Limp	Some flexion of extremities	Active motion
Reflex irritability (nose suction)	No response	Grimace	Cough or sneeze
Color	Blue, pale	Acrocyanosis	Completely pink

Data from Apgar V. Proposal for a new method of evaluation of the newborn infant. Anesth Analg. 1953;32:260.

B. Prior to Discharge

1. Newborn metabolic screening: If term infant, first screen should typically be performed within first 72 hours of life (at least 24 hours after initiation of feeding). (See Chapter 13 for more information.)
2. Vaccinations: Hepatitis B vaccine +/− other vaccinations, taking into account the risk factors, geographical location. See Chapter 16 for more information.
3. Critical congenital heart disease screening: Measure post-ductal oxygen saturation. (See Chapter 7 for more details.)

V. NEWBORN ASSESSMENT

A. Vital Signs and Birth Weight

1. **Normal vital signs:** Heart rate 120–160 bpm, respiratory rate (RR) 40–60 breaths/min, rectal temperature 36.5°–37.5°C
2. **Arterial blood pressure:** Related to birth weight, gestational age (see Chapter 7)
3. **Weight:**
a. By birth weight: Extremely low birth weight (ELBW): <1000 g, very low birth weight (VLBW): <1500 g, low birth weight (LBW): <2500 g.
b. By gestational age: Small for gestational age (SGA): <10% for gestational age, large for gestational age (LGA): >90% for gestational age.
c. See Chapter 21 for growth charts for the premature infant.

B. Apgar Scores (Table 18.2)

Assess at 1 and 5 minutes. Repeat at 5-minute intervals if 5-minute score is <7.[6]

C. New Ballard Gestational Age Estimation

The Ballard score is most accurate when performed between the age of 12 and 20 hours.[7] Approximate gestational age is calculated based on the sum of the neuromuscular and physical maturity ratings (Fig. 18.2).

1. **Neuromuscular maturity:**
a. Posture: Observe infant quiet and supine. Score 0 for arms, legs extended; 1 for starting to flex hips and knees, arms extended; 2 for

Neuromuscular maturity

Neuromuscular maturity sign	Score							Record score here
	−1	0	1	2	3	4	5	
Posture 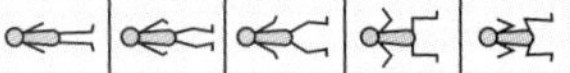								
Square window (wrist) 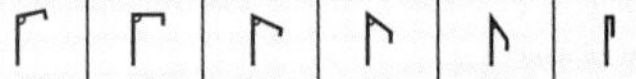	> 90°	90°	60°	45°	30°	0°		
Arm recoil 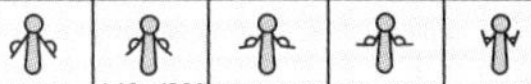			180°	140–180°	110–140°	90–110°	< 90°	
Popliteal angle 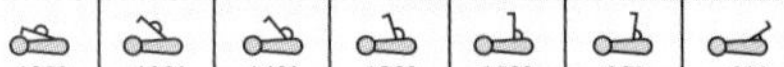	180°	160°	140°	120°	100°	90°	< 90°	
Scarf sign 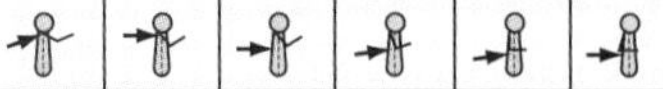								
Heel to ear 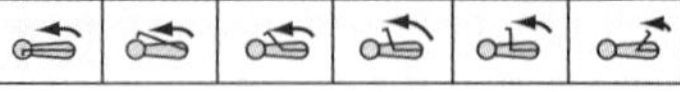								

TOTAL NEUROMUSCULAR MATURITY SCORE

Physical maturity

Physical maturity sign	Score							Record score here
	−1	0	1	2	3	4	5	
Skin	Sticky, friable, transparent	Gelatinous, red, translucent	Smooth, pink, visible veins	Superficial peeling and/or rash, few veins	Cracking, pale areas, rare veins	Parchment, deep cracking, no vessels	Leathery, cracked, wrinkled	
Lanugo	None	Sparse	Abundant	Thinning	Bald areas	Mostly bald		
Plantar surface	Heel-toe: 40–50 mm: −1; <40 mm: −2	>50 mm, no crease	Faint red marks	Anterior transverse crease only	Creases anterior two thirds	Creases over entire sole		
Breast	Imperceptible	Barely perceptible	Flat areola, no bud	Stippled areola, 1–2 mm bud	Raised areola, 3–4 mm bud	Full areola, 5–10 mm bud		
Eye/ear	Lids fused: loosely: −1 tightly: −2	Lids open, pinna flat, stays folded	Sl. curved pinna, soft, slow recoil	Well-curved pinna, soft but ready recoil	Formed and firm, instant recoil	Thick cartilage, ear stiff		
Genitals (male)	Scrotum flat, smooth	Scrotum empty, faint rugae	Testes in upper canal, rare rugae	Testes descending, few rugae	Testes down, good rugae	Testes pendulous, deep rugae		
Genitals (female)	Clitoris prominent and labia flat	Prominent clitoris and small labia minora	Prominent clitoris and enlarging minora	Majora and minora equally prominent	Majora large, minora small	Majora cover clitoris and minora		

TOTAL PHYSICAL MATURITY SCORE

Score
Neuromuscular___
Physical___
Total___

Maturity rating

Score	−10	−5	0	5	10	15	20	25	30	35	40	45	50
Weeks	20	22	24	26	28	30	32	34	36	38	40	42	44

Gestational age (weeks)
By dates___
By ultrasound___
By exam___

FIGURE 18.2

Neuromuscular and physical maturity (New Ballard Score).
(Modified from Ballard JL et al. New Ballard Score, expanded to include extremely premature infants. J Pediatr. 1991;119:417-423.)

stronger flexion of legs, arms extended; 3 for arms slightly flexed, legs flexed and abducted; and 4 for full flexion of arms and legs.
  b. Square window: Flex hand on forearm enough to obtain fullest possible flexion without wrist rotation. Measure angle between hypothenar eminence and ventral aspect of forearm.
  c. Arm recoil: With infant supine, flex forearms for 5 seconds, fully extend by pulling on hands, then release. Measure the angle of elbow flexion to which arms recoil.
  d. Popliteal angle: Hold infant supine with pelvis flat, thigh held in knee-chest position. Extend leg by gentle pressure and measure popliteal angle.
  e. Scarf sign: With baby supine, pull infant's hand across the neck toward opposite shoulder. Determine how far elbow will reach across. Score 0 if elbow reaches opposite axillary line, 1 if past midaxillary line, 2 if past midline, and 3 if elbow unable to reach midline.
  f. Heel-to-ear maneuver: With baby supine, draw foot as near to head as possible without forcing it. Observe distance between foot and head and degree of extension at knee.
2. **Physical maturity:** Based on developmental stage of eyes, ears, breasts, genitalia, skin, lanugo, and plantar creases (see Fig. 18.2)

D. Birth Trauma

1. **Extradural fluid collections** (Table 18.3 and Fig. 18.3).
2. **Fractured clavicle:** Possible crepitus/deformity on day 1 ± swelling/discomfort on day 2.
3. **Brachial plexus injuries:** Erb palsy (C5–6) most common, but also possible to have Klumpke (C8-T1; least common) and total brachial plexus palsy (C5–T1). See Section XII.

TABLE 18.3
BIRTH-RELATED EXTRADURAL FLUID COLLECTIONS

	Caput Succedaneum	Cephalohematoma	Subgaleal Hemorrhage
LOCATION	At point of contact; can extend across sutures	Usually over parietal bones; does not cross sutures	Beneath epicranial aponeurosis; may extend to orbits or nape of neck
FINDINGS	Vaguely demarcated; pitting edema, shifts with gravity	Distinct margins; initially firm, more fluctuant after 48 hr	Firm to fluctuant, ill-defined borders; may have crepitus or fluid waves
TIMING	Maximal size/firmness at birth; resolves in 48–72 hr	Increases after birth for 12–24 hr; resolution over weeks	Progressive after birth; resolution over weeks
SIZE	Minimal	Rarely severe	May be severe, especially in the setting of associated coagulopathy

Data from DJ Davis. Neonatal subgaleal hemorrhage: diagnosis and management. CMAJ. 2001;164:1452.

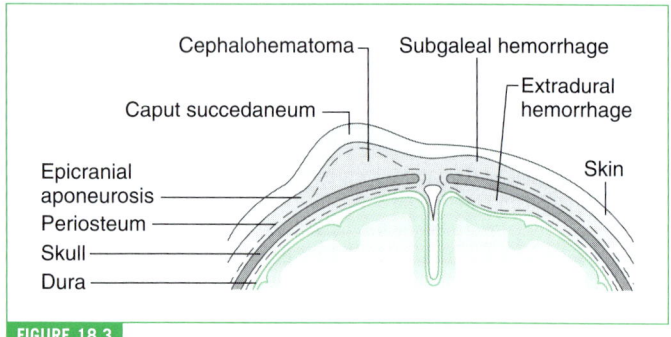

FIGURE 18.3

Types of extradural fluid collections seen in newborn infants.

E. Selected Anomalies, Syndromes, and Malformations (See Chapter 13 for Common Syndromes/Genetic Disorders)

1. **VATER association: V**ertebral anomalies, **A**nal anomalies and anal atresia, **T**racheoesophageal fistula, **E**sophageal atresia, and **R**adial and/or **R**enal defects. May also include vascular (cardiac) defects.
2. **CHARGE syndrome** (associated with mutations in gene *CHD7* on chromosome 8q12): **C**oloboma, **H**eart disease, choanal **A**tresia, **R**etarded growth and development [may include central nervous system (CNS) anomalies], **G**enital anomalies (may include hypogonadism), and **E**ar abnormalities or deafness.
3. **Infant of a diabetic mother:** Increased risk of sacral agenesis, femoral hypoplasia, heart defects, and cleft palate. May also include preaxial radial defects, microtia, cleft lip, microphthalmos, holoprosencephaly, microcephaly, anencephaly, spina bifida, hemivertebrae, urinary tract defects, and polydactyly.
4. **Fetal alcohol syndrome:** SGA, short palpebral fissures, epicanthal folds, flat nasal bridge, long philtrum, thin upper lip, small hypoplastic nails. May be associated with cardiac defects.

V. FLUIDS, ELECTROLYTES, AND NUTRITION

A. Fluids

1. **Insensible water loss in preterm infants** (Table EC 18.B)
2. **Water requirements of newborns** (Table 18.4)

B. Glucose

1. **Requirements:** Preterm neonates require approximately 5–6 mg/kg/min of glucose (40–100 mg/dL).[8] Term neonates require approximately 3–5 mg/kg/min of glucose. The formula to calculate the glucose infusion rate (GIR) is as follows:

TABLE 18.4
WATER REQUIREMENTS OF NEWBORNS

Birth Weight (g)	Water Requirements (mL/kg/24 hr) by Age		
	1–2 Days	3–7 Days	7–30 Days
<750	100–250	150–300	120–180
750–1000	80–150	100–150	120–180
1000–1500	60–100	80–150	120–180
>1500	60–80	100–150	120–180

Data from Taeusch HW, Ballard RA, eds. Schaeffer and Avery's Diseases of the Newborn. 7th ed. Philadelphia: WB Saunders; 1998.

$$\text{GIR (mg/kg/min)} = [(\% \text{ glucose in solution} \times 10) \times (\text{rate of infusion per hour})]/[60 \times \text{weight (kg)}]$$
$$= 0.167 \times (\% \text{ glucose}) \times \text{infusion rate (mL/hr)}/\text{weight (kg)}$$

2. **Management of hyperglycemia and hypoglycemia:** Table 18.5 and Fig. 18.4.[8] Also see Chapter 10.

C. Electrolytes, Minerals, and Vitamins

1. **Electrolyte requirements** (Table 18.6)
2. **Mineral and vitamin requirements:**
a. Infants born at <34 weeks' gestation have higher calcium, phosphorus, sodium, iron, and vitamin D requirements, and require breast-milk fortifier or special preterm formulas with iron. Fortifier should be added to breast milk only after the second week of life.
b. Iron: Enterally fed preterm infants require an elemental iron supplementation of 2 mg/kg/day after age 4–8 weeks.

D. Nutrition

1. **Growth and caloric requirements:** Table 18.7
2. Total parenteral nutrition (see Chapter 21)

VI. CYANOSIS IN THE NEWBORN

A. Differential Diagnosis

1. **General:** Hypothermia, hypoglycemia, sepsis, shock
2. **Neurologic:** Central apnea, central hypoventilation, intraventricular hemorrhage (IVH), meningitis
3. **Respiratory:** Persistent pulmonary hypertension of the newborn (PPHN), diaphragmatic hernia, pulmonary hypoplasia, choanal atresia, pneumothorax, respiratory distress syndrome (RDS), transient tachypnea of the newborn, pneumonia, meconium aspiration
4. **Cardiac:** Congestive heart failure, congenital cyanotic heart disease
5. **Hematologic:** Polycythemia, methemoglobinemia
6. **Medications:** Respiratory depression from maternal medications (e.g., magnesium sulfate, narcotics)

TABLE 18.5
MANAGEMENT OF HYPERGLYCEMIA AND HYPOGLYCEMIA[a]

	Hypoglycemia	Hyperglycemia
Definition	Serum glucose <40 mg/dL in term and late preterm infants	Serum glucose >125 mg/dL in term infants, >150 mg/dL in preterm infants
Differential diagnosis	Insufficient glucose delivery Decreased glycogen stores Increased circulating insulin (infant of a diabetic mother, maternal drugs, Beckwith-Wiedemann syndrome, tumors) Endocrine and metabolic disorders Sepsis or shock Hypothermia, polycythemia, or asphyxia	Excess glucose administration Sepsis Hypoxia Hyperosmolar formula Neonatal diabetes mellitus Medications
Evaluation	Assess for symptoms and calculate glucose delivery to infant. Laboratory evaluation: serum glucose (bedside); complete blood cell count with differential; electrolytes; blood, urine, ± cerebrospinal fluid cultures; urinalysis; insulin and C-peptide levels if warranted	
Management	(See Fig. 18.4.) If glucose <40 and symptomatic, treat with intravenous glucose (dose = 200 mg/kg, which is equivalent to dextrose 10% at 2 mL/kg). Change dextrose infusion rates gradually. Generally, no more than 2 mg/kg/min in a 2-hr interval (See Chapter 10 for further guidelines.) Monitor glucose levels every 30–60 min until normal.	Gradually decrease glucose infusion rate if receiving >5 mg/kg/min Monitor glucosuria. Consider insulin infusion for persistent hyperglycemia.

TABLE 18.6
ELECTROLYTE REQUIREMENTS

	Before 48 Hours of Life	After 48–72 Hours of Life
Sodium	None unless serum sodium <135 mEq/L, without evidence of volume overload	Term infants: 2–3 mEq/kg/day Preterm infants: 3–5 mEq/kg/day
Potassium	None	1–2.5 mEq/kg/day if adequate urine output is established and serum level <4.5 mEq/L

B. Evaluation

1. **Physical examination:** Note central vs. peripheral and persistent vs. intermittent cyanosis, respiratory effort, single vs. split S_2, presence of heart murmur. Acrocyanosis is often a normal finding in newborns.
2. **Clinical tests:** Hyperoxia test (see Chapter 7), preductal/postductal arterial blood gases or pulse oximetry to assess for right-to-left shunt, and transillumination of chest for possible pneumothorax.
3. **Other data:** Complete blood cell count (CBC) with differential, serum glucose, chest radiograph, electrocardiogram (ECG),

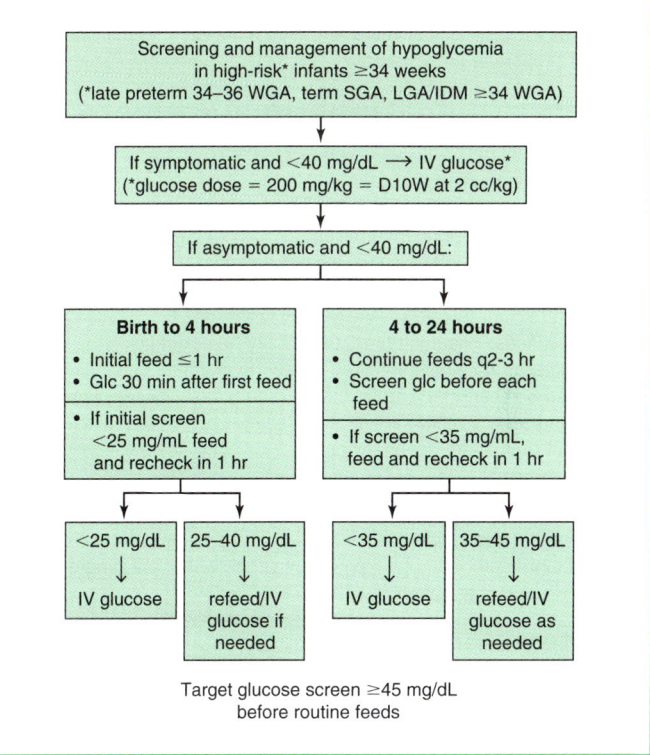

FIGURE 18.4

Screening for and management of postnatal glucose homeostasis in late-preterm (34–36 6/7 weeks), and term small-for-gestational-age and large-for-gestational-age infants of diabetic mothers.

D10W, 10% dextrose in water; glc, glucose; IDM, infant of diabetic mother; IV, intravenous; LGA, large for gestational age; SGA, small for gestational age; WGA, weeks gestational age

(Modified from Adamkin D., Committee on the Fetus and Newborn. Postnatal glucose homeostasis in late-preterm and term infants. Pediatrics. 2011;127:575-579).

TABLE 18.7
AVERAGE CALORIC REQUIREMENTS AND GROWTH FOR PRETERM AND TERM INFANTS

	Preterm Infant	Term Infant
Caloric requirements (kcal/kg/day)	115–130 (up to 150 for VLBW infants)	100–120
Growth after 10 days of life (g/kg/day)	15–20	10

echocardiography. Consider blood, urine, and cerebrospinal fluid cultures if sepsis is suspected and methemoglobin level if cyanosis is out of proportion to hypoxemia.

VII. RESPIRATORY DISEASES

A. General Respiratory Considerations

1. **Exogenous surfactant therapy:**
   a. Indications: RDS in preterm infants, meconium aspiration, pneumonia, persistent pulmonary hypertension
   b. Administration: If infant is ≤26 weeks' gestation, first dose is typically given in delivery room or as soon as stabilized; repeat dosing may follow at 6-hour intervals
   c. Complications: Pneumothorax, pulmonary hemorrhage
2. **Supplemental O_2:** Adjust inspired oxygen to maintain O_2 saturation between 85% and 94% until retina are fully vascularized, between 94% and 98% if retinas are mature (see Section XIII) and >97% in cases of pulmonary hypertension

B. Respiratory Distress Syndrome

1. **Definition:** Deficiency of pulmonary surfactant (a phospholipid protein mixture that decreases surface tension and prevents alveolar collapse). Surfactant is produced by type II alveolar cells in increasing quantities from 32 weeks' gestation.
   a. Antenatal maternal administration of steroids has been shown to decrease neonatal morbidity and mortality. Risk for RDS is decreased in babies born >24 hours and <7 days after maternal steroid administration.
   b. Other factors that accelerate lung maturity include maternal hypertension, sickle cell disease, narcotic addiction, intrauterine growth retardation, prolonged rupture of the membranes, and fetal stress.
2. **Incidence:**
   a. <30 weeks' gestation: 60% without antenatal steroids, 35% in those who received antenatal steroids
   b. 30–34 weeks' gestation: 25% without antenatal steroids, 10% in those who received antenatal steroids
   c. >34 weeks' gestation: 5%
3. **Risk factors:** Prematurity, maternal diabetes, cesarean section without antecedent labor, perinatal asphyxia, second twin, previous infant with RDS
4. **Clinical presentation:** Respiratory distress worsens during first few hours of life, progresses over 48–72 hours, and subsequently improves:
   a. Recovery is accompanied by brisk diuresis.
   b. Chest x-ray findings: *Reticulogranular* pattern in the lung fields; may obscure heart borders.

5. **Management:**
   a. Ventilatory and oxygenation support
   b. Surfactant therapy

C. Persistent Pulmonary Hypertension of the Newborn

1. **Etiology:** Idiopathic or secondary to conditions leading to increased pulmonary vascular resistance. PPHN is most commonly seen in term or postterm infants, infants born by cesarean section, and infants with a history of fetal distress and low Apgar scores. It usually presents within 12–24 hours of birth:
   a. Vasoconstriction secondary to hypoxemia and acidosis (e.g., neonatal sepsis)
   b. Interstitial pulmonary disease (meconium aspiration syndrome, pneumonia)
   c. Hyperviscosity syndrome (polycythemia)
   d. Pulmonary hypoplasia, either primary or secondary to congenital diaphragmatic hernia or renal agenesis
2. **Diagnostic features:**
   a. Severe hypoxemia (PaO_2 <35–45 mmHg in 100% O_2) disproportionate to radiologic changes.
   b. Structurally normal heart with right-to-left shunt at foramen ovale and/or ductus arteriosus; decreased postductal oxygenation compared with preductal (difference of at least 7–15 mmHg between preductal and postductal PaO_2 is significant).
   c. Must be distinguished from cyanotic heart disease. Infants with heart disease will have an abnormal cardiac examination and show little to no improvement in oxygenation with increased fraction of inspired O_2 (FIO_2) and hyperventilation. See Chapter 7 for interpretation of oxygen challenge (hyperoxia) test.
3. **Principles of therapy:**
   a. **Improve oxygenation:** Supplemental oxygen (FIO_2) to improve alveolar oxygenation. Optimize oxygen-carrying capacity with blood transfusions as needed.
   b. **Minimize pulmonary vasoconstriction:**
      (1) Minimal handling of infant and limited invasive procedures. Sedation and occasionally paralysis of intubated neonates may be necessary.
      (2) Avoid severe hypocarbia (PCO_2 <30 mmHg), which can be associated with myocardial ischemia and decreased cerebral blood flow. Hyperventilation may result in barotrauma, predisposing to chronic lung disease, so it should be minimized if possible. Consider high-frequency ventilation.
   c. **Maintenance of systemic blood pressure and perfusion:** Reversal of right-to-left shunt through volume expanders and/or inotropes
   d. **Consider pulmonary vasodilator therapy:**

(1) Inhaled nitric oxide (NO): Reduces pulmonary vascular resistance (PVR). Blended with ventilatory gases and titrated to effect. Typical starting dose is 20 parts per million (ppm). Unlikely to be efficacious at >40 ppm. Complications include methemoglobinemia (reduce NO dose for methemoglobin >4%), NO_2 poisoning (reduce NO dose for NO_2 concentration >1–2 ppm).

(2) Prostaglandin I_2 (prostacyclin): A complex molecule made from arachidonic acid; major endogenous pulmonary vasodilator. Normally produced by lung when lung vessels are constricted.

e. **Broad-spectrum antibiotics:** Sepsis is a common underlying cause of PPHN.

f. **Consider extracorporeal membrane oxygenation (ECMO):** Reserved for cases of severe cardiovascular instability, oxygenation index (OI) >40 for >3 hour, or alveolar-arterial gradient (A-aO_2) ≥610 for 8 hours (see Chapter 4 for calculation of OI and A-aO_2; PaO_2 should be postductal). Infants typically need to be >2000 g and at >34 weeks' gestation; should have head ultrasound and EEG before initiating ECMO.

4. **Mortality depends on underlying diagnosis:** Mortality rates are generally lower for RDS and meconium aspiration, but higher in sepsis and diaphragmatic hernia.

D. Spontaneous Pneumothorax

1. Seen in 1%–2% of normal newborns.
2. Associated with use of high inspiratory pressures and underlying diseases such as RDS, meconium aspiration, and pneumonia.
3. Patients should be monitored in a neonatal intensive care unit (NICU) setting.
4. See Chapter 3 for an overview of chest tube placement and thoracentesis.

VIII. APNEA AND BRADYCARDIA

A. Apnea[9]

1. **Definition:** Respiratory pause >20 seconds or a shorter pause associated with cyanosis, pallor, hypotonia, or bradycardia <100 bpm. In preterm infants, apnea may be central (no diaphragmatic activity), obstructive (upper airway obstruction), or mixed central and obstructive. Common causes of apnea in the newborn are listed in Fig. 18.5.
2. **Incidence:** Apnea of prematurity occurs in most infants born at <28 weeks' gestation, ≈50% of infants born at 30–32 weeks' gestation, and <7% of infants born at 34–35 weeks' gestation. Usually resolves by 34–36 weeks' postconceptual age, but may persist after term in infants born at <25 weeks' gestation.
3. **Management:**
a. Consider pathologic causes for apnea.
b. Pharmacotherapy with caffeine or other stimulants.

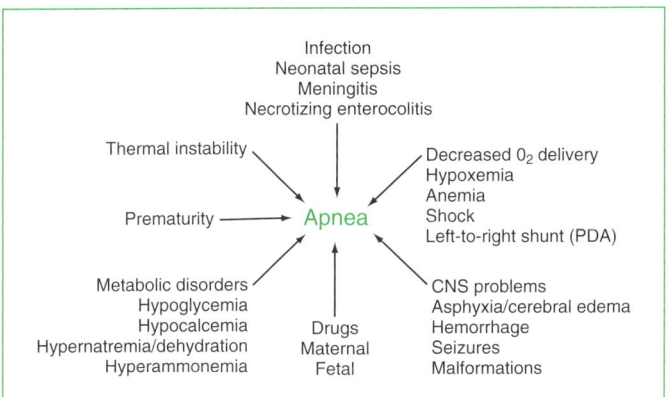

FIGURE 18.5
Causes of apnea in the newborn. CNS, central nervous system; PDA, patent ductus arteriosus.
(From Klaus MH, Fanaroff AA. Care of the High-Risk Neonate. 5th ed. Philadelphia: WB Saunders;2001:268.)

  c. Continuous positive airway pressure or mechanical ventilation (see Chapter 4).

B. Bradycardia Without Central Apnea

Etiologies include obstructive apnea, mechanical airway obstruction, gastroesophageal reflux, increased intracranial pressure, increased vagal tone [defecation, yawning, rectal stimulation, and placement of nasogastric (NG) tube], electrolyte abnormalities, heart block

IX. CARDIAC DISEASES

A. Patent Ductus Arteriosus (PDA)

1. **Definition:** Failure of ductus arteriosus to close in first few days of life or reopening after functional closure. Typically results in left-to-right shunting of blood once PVR has decreased. If PVR remains high, blood may be shunted right to left, resulting in hypoxemia (see Section VII.C).
2. **Incidence:** Up to 60% in preterm infants weighing <1500 g and higher in those weighing <1000 g. Female-to-male ratio is 2:1. Obligatory PDA is found in 10% of infants with congenital heart disease.
3. **Risk factors:** Most often related to hypoxia and immaturity. Term infants with PDA usually have structural defects in ductal vessel walls.
4. **Diagnosis:**
a. Examination: Systolic murmur that may be continuous and best heard at the left upper sternal border or left infraclavicular area. May have apical diastolic rumble due to increased blood flow across mitral valve

in diastole. Bounding peripheral pulses with widened pulse pressure if large shunt. Hyperactive precordium and palmar pulses may be present.
b. ECG: Normal or left ventricular hypertrophy in small to moderate PDA; Biventricular hypertrophy in large PDA.
c. Chest radiograph: May show cardiomegaly and increased pulmonary vascular markings, depending on size of shunt.
d. Echocardiogram

5. **Management:**
a. Ongoing controversy over indications for treatment, timing of intervention, and best management strategy
b. Indomethacin: Prostaglandin synthetase inhibitor; 80% closure rate in preterm infants:
   (1) For dosage information and contraindications, see Part IV, Formulary.
   (2) Complications: Transient decrease in glomerular filtration rate and decreased urine output, transient gastrointestinal bleeding [not associated with an increased incidence of necrotizing enterocolitis (NEC)], a prolonged bleeding time, and disturbed platelet function for 7–9 days independent of platelet count (not associated with increased incidence of intracranial hemorrhage). Spontaneous isolated intestinal perforations are seen with indomethacin use. Rates are higher with concomitant hydrocortisone use.
c. Ibuprofen[9,10]: As effective as indomethacin but fewer renal adverse effects
d. Surgical ligation of the duct

B. Cyanotic Heart Disease
See Chapter 7.

X. HEMATOLOGIC DISEASES

A. Unconjugated Hyperbilirubinemia in the Newborn[11]

1. **Overview:**
a. During first 3–4 days of life, serum bilirubin increases from 1.5 mg/dL (cord blood) to 6.5 ± 2.5 mg/dL.
b. Maximum rate of bilirubin increase for normal infants with nonhemolytic hyperbilirubinemia: 5 mg/dL/24 hr or 0.2 mg/dL/hr.
c. Consider pathologic cause: Visible jaundice or total bilirubin concentration >5 mg/dL on first day of life.
d. Risk factors: Birth weight <2500 g, breast-feeding, prematurity.

2. **Evaluation:**
a. Maternal prenatal testing: ABO and Rh (D) typing and serum screen for isoimmune antibodies
b. Infant or cord blood: Blood smear, direct Coombs test, blood and Rh typing (if maternal blood type is O, Rh negative, or prenatal blood typing was not performed)

3. **Management:**
a. Phototherapy: Ideally, intensive phototherapy should produce a total serum bilirubin (TSB) level decline of 1–2 mg/dL within 4–6 hours, with further subsequent decline:
   (1) Preterm newborn (Table 18.8)
   (2) Term newborn (Fig. 18.6)
b. Intravenous immunoglobulin (IVIG) (>35 weeks' gestational age): In isoimmune hemolytic disease, IVIG administration (0.5–1 g/kg over 2 hours) is recommended if TSB is rising despite intensive phototherapy or TSB level is within 2–3 mg/dL of exchange level. Repeat in 12 hours if needed. (See Chapter 15 for adverse effects of IVIG.)
c. Neonatal double-volume exchange transfusion (see Table 18.8 and Fig. 18.7):

TABLE 18.8

GUIDELINES FOR THE USE OF PHOTOTHERAPY IN PRETERM INFANTS AGED <1 WEEK

Weight (g)	Phototherapy (mg/dL)	Consider Exchange Transfusion (mg/dL)
500–1000	5–7	12–15
1000–1500	7–10	15–18
1500–2500	10–15	18–20
>2500	>15	>20

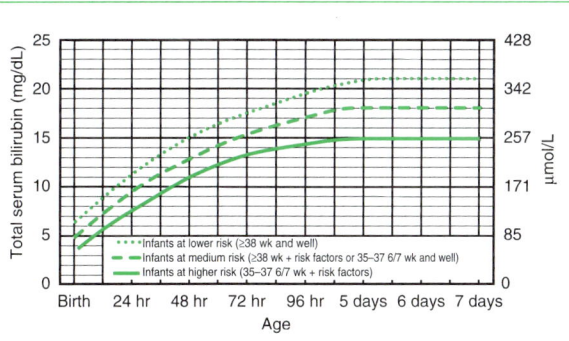

- Use total bilirubin. Do not subtract direct reacting or conjugated bilirubin.
- Risk factors: Isoimmune hemolytic disease, G6PD deficiency, asphyxia, significant lethargy, temperature instability, sepsis, acidosis, or albumin <3.0 g/dL (if measured)
- For well infants 35–37 6/7 wk can adjust TSB levels for intervention around the medium risk line. It is an option to intervene at lower TSB levels for infants closer to 35 wk and at higher TSB levels for those closer to 37 6/7 wk.
- It is an option to provide conventional phototherapy in hospital or at home at TSB levels 2–3 mg/dL (35–50 mmol/L) below those shown, but home phototherapy should not be used in any infant with risk factors.

FIGURE 18.6

Guidelines for phototherapy in infants born at 35 weeks of gestation or more. G6PD, glucose-6-phosphate dehydrogenase; TSB, total serum bilirubin

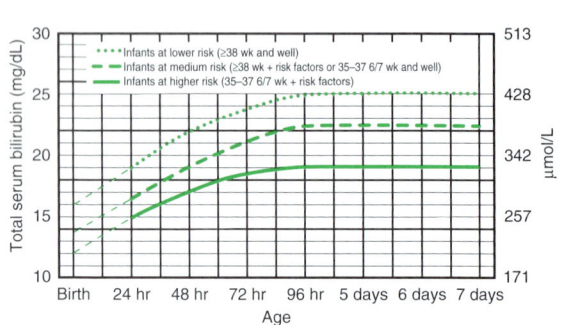

- The dashed lines for the first 24 hours indicate uncertainty due to a wide range of clinical circumstances and a range of responses to phototherapy.
- Immediate exchange transfusion is recommended if infant shows signs of acute bilirubin encephalopathy (hypertonia, arching, retrocollis, opisthotonos, fever, high-pitched cry) or if TBS is ≥5 mg/dL (85 µmol/L) above these lines.
- Risk factors: Isoimmune hemolytic disease, G6PD deficiency, asphyxia, significant lethargy, temperature instability, sepsis, acidosis.
- Measure serum albumin and calculate B/A ratio.
- Use total bilirubin. Do not subtract direct reacting or conjugated bilirubin.
- If infant is well and 35–37 6/7 wk (median risk) can individualize TSB levels for exchange based on actual gestational age.

FIGURE 18.7

Guidelines for exchange transfusion in infants born at 35 weeks of gestation or more. B/A, bilirubin/albumin; G6PD, glucose-6-phosphate dehydrogenase; TSB, total serum bilirubin

(1) Volume: 160 mL/kg for full-term infant, 160–200 mL/kg for preterm infant.
(2) Route: During exchange, blood is removed through umbilical arterial catheter (UAC) and an equal volume is infused through UVC. If UAC is unavailable, use a single venous catheter.
(3) Rate: Exchange in 15-mL increments for vigorous full-term infants. Exchange at 2–3 mL/kg/min in premature/less stable infants to avoid trauma to red blood cells.
(4) Complications: Emboli, thromboses, hemodynamic instability, electrolyte disturbances, coagulopathy, infection, death.

NOTE: CBC, reticulocyte count, peripheral smear, bilirubin, Ca^{2+}, glucose, total protein, infant blood type, Coombs test, and newborn screen should be performed on a *preexchange sample* of blood; they are of no diagnostic value on postexchange blood. If indicated, save preexchange blood for serologic or chromosome studies.

B. Conjugated Hyperbilirubinemia

1. **Definition:** Direct bilirubin >2.0 mg/dL and >10% of TSB

2. **Etiology:** Biliary obstruction/atresia, choledochal cyst, hyperalimentation, α_1-antitrypsin deficiency, hepatitis, sepsis, infections (especially urinary tract infections), hypothyroidism, inborn errors of metabolism, cystic fibrosis, red blood cell abnormalities
3. **Management:** Ursodiol for infants on full feeds; consider supplementation with fat-soluble vitamins (A, D, E, K)

C. Polycythemia

1. **Definition:** Venous hematocrit >65% confirmed on two consecutive samples. May be falsely elevated when sample obtained by heel stick. Arterial hematocrit samples may be lower and should not be used to evaluate polycythemia.
2. **Etiologies:** Delayed cord clamping, twin-twin transfusion, maternal-fetal transfusion, intrauterine hypoxia, Beckwith-Wiedemann syndrome, maternal gestational diabetes, neonatal thyrotoxicosis, congenital adrenal hyperplasia, trisomy 13, 18, or 21.
3. **Clinical findings:** Plethora, respiratory distress, cardiac failure, tachypnea, hypoglycemia, irritability, lethargy, seizures, apnea, jitteriness, poor feeding, thrombocytopenia, hyperbilirubinemia.
4. **Complications:** Hyperviscosity predisposes to venous thrombosis and CNS injury. Hypoglycemia may result from increased erythrocyte utilization of glucose.
5. **Management:** Partial exchange transfusion for symptomatic infants, with isovolemic replacement of blood with isotonic fluid. Blood is exchanged in 10- to 20-mL increments to reduce hematocrit to <55%. (See Chapter 14 to calculate amount of blood to be exchanged. Use birth weight (kg) × 90 mL/kg for estimated blood volume in mL.)

XI. GASTROINTESTINAL DISEASES

A. Necrotizing Enterocolitis

1. **Definition:** Serious intestinal inflammation and injury thought to be secondary to bowel ischemia, immaturity, and infection.
2. **Incidence:** More common in preterm (3%–4% of infants weighing <2000 g) and African–American infants. Occurs principally in infants who have been fed.
3. **Risk factors:** Prematurity, asphyxia, hypotension, polycythemia–hyperviscosity syndrome, umbilical vessel catheterization, exchange transfusion, bacterial and viral pathogens, enteral feeds, PDA, congestive heart failure, cyanotic heart disease, RDS, intrauterine cocaine exposure.
4. **Clinical findings:** See Table EC 18.C.
a. Systemic: Temperature instability, apnea, bradycardia, metabolic acidosis, hypotension, disseminated intravascular coagulopathy (DIC).
b. Intestinal: Elevated pregavage residuals with abdominal distention, blood in stool, absent bowel sounds, and/or abdominal tenderness or

mass. Elevated pregavage residuals in the absence of other clinical symptoms rarely raise a suspicion of NEC.
  c. Radiologic: Ileus, intestinal pneumatosis, portal vein gas, ascites, pneumoperitoneum.
5. **Management:** Nothing by mouth, NG tube decompression, maintain adequate hydration and perfusion, antibiotics for 7–14 days, surgical consultation. Surgery is performed for signs of perforation or necrotic bowel.
6. **Minimizing risk for NEC:**
  a. There have been several studies linking the use of probiotics and a decreased risk of NEC.[12] However, variations among formulations of probiotics, dosing, and lack of long-term studies on outcome have prevented the standard use of probiotics in the NICU.[13]
  b. Additionally, the exclusive use of human milk including donor breast milk has been shown to decrease the risk of NEC and associated mortality.[14]

B. Bilious Emesis Differential
See Table EC 18.D.
See Chapter 12.
1. **Mechanical:** Annular pancreas, intestinal atresia/duplication/malrotation/obstruction (including adjacent organomegaly), meconium plug or ileus, Hirschsprung disease, imperforate anus.
2. **Functional (i.e., poor motility):** NEC, electrolyte abnormalities, sepsis.
  NOTE: Must eliminate malrotation as an etiology because its complication (volvulus) is a surgical emergency.

C. Abdominal Wall Defects
See Table EC 18.E.

XII. NEUROLOGIC DISEASES

A. Neonatal Hypoxic-Ischemic Encephalopathy (HIE): Initial Management[15]
1. **Hypothermia protocol:** Infants with evidence of HIE shortly after birth who are >36 weeks' gestation should be considered for hypothermia. Protocol should be initiated within 6 hours of delivery.
2. **Criteria for hypothermia vary by center but typically include one or more of the following:**
  a. Cord gas or blood gas in the first hour of life with a pH of <7.0 or base deficit of >16. For infants with a pH of 7.01–7.15 or base deficit of 10–15.9, additional criteria should be met (e.g., significant perinatal event).
  b. 10-minute APGAR ≤5.
  c. Evidence of moderate to severe encephalopathy.
  d. Need for assisted ventilation at birth for at least 10 minutes.
3. **Severity and outcome of HIE in full-term neonate:** Table 18.9.

TABLE 18.9
SEVERITY AND OUTCOME OF HYPOXIC-ISCHEMIC ENCEPHALOPATHY IN FULL-TERM NEONATE

Severity	Level of Consciousness	Seizures	Primitive Reflexes	Brain Stem Dysfunction	Elevated Intracranial Pressure	Duration	Poor Outcome (%)*
Mild	Increased irritability, hyperalertness	(−); Jitteriness	Exaggerated	(−)	(−)	<24 h	0
Moderate	Lethargy	Variable	Supressed	(−)	(−)	>24 h (variable)	20–40
Severe	Stupor or coma	(+)	Absent	(+)	Variable	>5 days	100

*Poor outcome is defined by presence of mental retardation, cerebral palsy, or seizures
(+), common; (−), rare
Data from MacDonald M, Mullett, M. Severity and outcome of hypoxic-ischemic encephalopathy in full term neonate. In: Avery's Neonatology. 6th edition. Philadelphia, Lippincott Williams & Wilkins; 2005.

B. Intraventricular Hemorrhage

1. **Definition:** IVH usually arising in the germinal matrix and periventricular regions of the brain
2. **Incidence:**
   a. 30%–40% of infants <1500 g; 50%–60% of infants <1000 g
   b. Highest incidence within first 72 hours of life: 60% within 24 hours, 85% within 72 hours, and <5% after 1 week of age
3. **Diagnosis and classification:**
Ultrasonography; grade is based on maximum amount of hemorrhage seen by age 2 weeks:
   a. Grade I: Hemorrhage in germinal matrix only
   b. Grade II: IVH without ventricular dilation
   c. Grade III: IVH with ventricular dilation (30%–45% incidence of motor and cognitive impairment)
   d. Grade IV: IVH with periventricular hemorrhagic infarct (60%–80% incidence of motor and cognitive impairment)
4. **Screening:** Indicated in infants <32 weeks' gestational age within first week of life; repeat in second week
5. **Prophylaxis:** Maintain acid–base balance and avoid fluctuations in blood pressure. Indomethacin is considered for IVH prophylaxis in some newborns (<28 weeks' gestation, birth weight <1250 g) and is most efficacious if given within first 6 hours of life; however, it has not been shown to impact long-term outcome.[16]
6. **Outcome:** Infants with grade III and IV hemorrhages have a higher incidence of neurodevelopmental disabilities and an increased risk for posthemorrhagic hydrocephalus.

C. Periventricular Leukomalacia

1. **Definition and ultrasound findings:** Ischemic necrosis of periventricular white matter, characterized by CNS depression within first week of life and ultrasound findings of cysts with or without ventricular enlargement caused by cerebral atrophy
2. **Incidence:** More common in preterm infants but also occurs in term infants; 3.2% in infants <1500 g
3. **Etiology:** Primarily ischemia-reperfusion injury, hypoxia, acidosis, hypoglycemia, acute hypotension, slow cerebral blood flow
4. **Outcome:** Commonly associated with cerebral palsy with or without sensory and cognitive deficits

E. Neonatal Seizures (see Chapter 20)

F. Neonatal Abstinence Syndrome

Onset of symptoms usually occurs within first 24–72 hours of life (methadone may delay symptoms until 96 hours or later). Symptoms may last weeks to months. Box 18.1 shows signs and symptoms of opiate withdrawal.

BOX 18.1
OPIATE WITHDRAWAL
Signs and Symptoms of Opiate Withdrawal

- W Wakefulness
- I Irritability, insomnia
- T Tremors, temperature variation, tachypnea, twitching (jitteriness)
- H Hyperactivity, high-pitched cry, hiccoughs, hyperreflexia, hypertonia
- D Diarrhea (explosive), diaphoresis, disorganized suck
- R Rub marks, respiratory distress, rhinorrhea, regurgitation
- A Apnea, autonomic dysfunction
- W Weight loss
- A Alkalosis (respiratory)
- L Lacrimation (photophobia), lethargy
- S Seizures, sneezing, stuffy nose, sweating, sucking (nonproductive)

TABLE 18.10
PLEXUS INJURIES

Plexus Injury	Spinal Level Involved	Clinical Features
Erb-Duchenne palsy (90% of cases)	C5–C6 Occasionally involves C4	Adduction and internal rotation of arm. Forearm is pronated; wrist is flexed. Diaphragm paralysis may occur if C4 is involved.
Total palsy (8%–9% of cases)	C5–T1 Occasionally involves C4	Upper arm, lower arm, and hand involved. Horner syndrome (ptosis, anhidrosis, and miosis) exists if T1 is involved.
Klumpke paralysis (<2% of cases)	C7–T1	Hand flaccid with little control. Horner syndrome if T1 is involved.

G. Peripheral Nerve Injuries

1. **Etiology:** Result from lateral traction on shoulder (vertex deliveries) or head (breech deliveries).
2. **Clinical features** (Table 18.10).
3. **Management:** Evaluate for associated trauma (clavicular and humeral fractures, shoulder dislocation, facial nerve injury, cord injuries). Full recovery is seen in 85%–95% of cases in first year of life.

XIII. RETINOPATHY OF PREMATURITY (ROP)[17]

A. Definition
Interruption of normal progression of retinal vascularization.

B. Etiology
Exposure of the immature retina to high oxygen concentrations can result in vasoconstriction and obliteration of the retinal capillary network, followed by vasoproliferation. Risk is greatest in the most immature infants.

C. Diagnosis—Dilated Funduscopic Examination

Dilated funduscopic examination should be performed in the following patients:
1. All infants born ≤30 weeks gestation
2. Infants born >30 weeks gestation with unstable clinical course, including those requiring cardiorespiratory support
3. Any infant with a birth weight ≤1500 g

D. Timing[18]

1. For all infants ≤27 weeks gestation at birth, initial ROP screening examination should be performed at 31 weeks' postmenstrual age.
2. For all infants ≥28 weeks gestation at birth, initial ROP screening examination should be performed at 4 weeks' chronologic age.
3. For infants born before 25 weeks gestation, consider earlier screening at 6 weeks chronologic age (even if before 31 weeks' postmenstrual age) on the basis of severity of comorbidities. This may enable earlier detection and treatment of aggressive posterior ROP, which is a severe form of rapidly progressive ROP.

E. Classification

1. **Stage** See Fig EC 18-A:
a. Stage 1: Demarcation line separates avascular from vascularized retina
b. Stage 2: Ridge forms along demarcation line
c. Stage 3: Extraretinal, fibrovascular proliferation tissue forms on ridge
d. Stage 4: Partial retinal detachment
e. Stage 5: Total retinal detachment
2. **Zone** (Fig. 18.8)

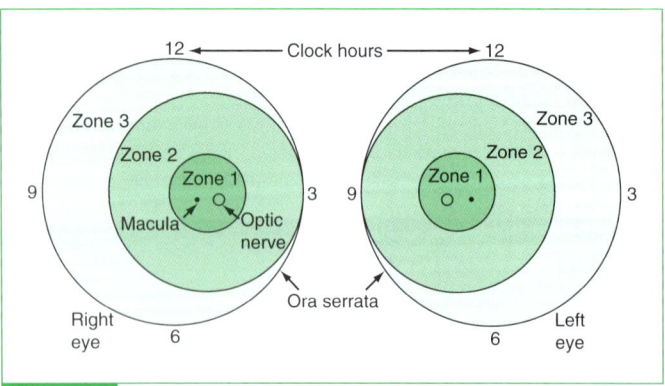

FIGURE 18.8

Zones of the retina. *(From American Academy of Pediatrics. Screening examination of premature infants for retinopathy of prematurity, AAP policy statement. Pediatrics. 2013;131:189-195.)*

3. **Plus disease:** Abnormal dilation and tortuosity of posterior retinal blood vessels in two or more quadrants of retina; may be present at any stage
4. **Number of clock hours or 30-degree sectors involved**

F. Management[17]

1. **Type 1 ROP:**
Peripheral retinal ablation should be considered. Type 1 ROP classified as:
   a. Zone I: Any stage ROP with plus disease
   b. Zone I: Stage 3 ROP without plus disease
   c. Zone II: Stage 2 or 3 ROP with plus disease
2. **Type 2 ROP:**
Serial examinations rather than retinal ablation should be considered. Type 2 ROP classified as:
   a. Zone I: Stage 1 or 2 ROP without plus disease
   b. Zone II: Stage 3 ROP without plus disease
3. Follow-up (Table EC 18.F)

XIV. CONGENITAL INFECTIONS

See Chapter 17.

XV. COMMONLY USED MEDICATIONS IN THE NEONATAL INTENSIVE CARE UNIT

See Table 18.11. For neonatal specific drug dosing, refer to Formulary.

TABLE 18.11

DOSING OF COMMONLY USED ANTIMICROBIALS IN THE NEONATAL INTENSIVE CARE UNIT, BASED ON POSTMATERNAL AND POSTNATAL AGE

Drug	Dosing (IV)
Acyclovir	HSV infection: 20 mg/kg/dose
Ampicillin	Typical dosing: 25–50 mg/kg/dose; GBS meningitis: 300 mg/kg/day
Cefotaxime	50 mg/kg/dose (gonococcal infections: 25 mg/kg/dose; GC ophthalmia prophylaxis if maternal GC infection: 100 mg/kg × 1 dose)
Fluconazole[†]	Invasive candidiasis: loading 12–25 mg/kg/dose; maintenance 6–12 mg/kg/dose
Gentamicin	See chart below See Formulary for recommendations for therapeutic monitoring.
Metronidazole	Loading dose: 15 mg/kg/dose; maintenance: 7.5 mg/kg/dose
Oxacillin	25–50 mg/kg/dose; Use higher dose for meningitis
Vancomycin	Bacteremia: 10 mg/kg/dose; meningitis: 15 mg/kg/dose See Formulary for recommendations for therapeutic monitoring.

Dosing Interval Chart: Ampicillin, cefotaxime, oxacillin			Dosing Interval Chart: Vancomycin			Dosing Interval Chart: Metronidazole		
PMA (Weeks)	Postnatal (Days)	Interval (Hours)	PMA (Weeks)	Postnatal (Days)	Interval (Hours)	PMA (Weeks)	Postnatal (Days)	Interval (Hours)
≤29	0–28	12	≤29	0–14	18	≤29	0–28	48
	>28	8		>14	12		>28	24

Continued

TABLE 18.11
DOSING OF COMMONLY USED ANTIMICROBIALS IN THE NEONATAL INTENSIVE CARE UNIT, BASED ON POSTMATERNAL AND POSTNATAL AGE—cont'd

Dosing Interval Chart: Ampicillin, cefotaxime, oxacillin			Dosing Interval Chart: Vancomycin			Dosing Interval Chart: Metronidazole		
PMA (Weeks)	Postnatal (Days)	Interval (Hours)	PMA (Weeks)	Postnatal (Days)	Interval (Hours)	PMA (Weeks)	Postnatal (Days)	Interval (Hours)
30–36	0–14	12	30–36	0–14	12	30–36	0–14	24
	>14	8		>14	8		>14	12
37–44	0–7	12	37–44	0–7	12	37–44	0–7	24
	>7	8		>7	8		>7	12
≥45	All	6	≥45	All	6	≥45	All	8

Dosing and Interval Chart: Gentamicin				Dosing Interval Chart: Fluconazole			Dosing Interval Chart: Acyclovir		
PMA (weeks)	Postnatal (Days)	Dose (mg/kg)	Interval (Hours)	Gest. Age (Weeks)	Postnatal (Days)	Interval (Hours)	Gest. Age (Weeks)	Postnatal (Days)	Interval (Hours)
≤29*	0–7	5	48	≤29	0–14	48			
	8–28	4	36		>14	24			
	≥29	4	24	≥30	0–7	48	<30	All	12
30–34	0–7	4.5	36		>7	24	≥30	All	8
	≥8	4	24						
≥35	All	4	24						

*Or significant asphyxia, PDA, or treatment with indomethacin
†Thrush = 6 mg/kg/dose on day 1, then 3 mg/kg/dose orally (PO) Q24 hr, regardless of gestational or postnatal age.
See Online Neofax: http://micromedex.com/neofax-pediatric
GBS, Group B *Streptococcus*; GC, gonococcus; Gest., gestational; IV, intravenous; PDA, patent ductus arteriosus; PMA, postmenstrual age

REFERENCES

1. AAP, Weiner GM, AHA. *Textbook of neonatal resuscitation.* 7th ed. AAP; 2016.
2. Cell-free DNA screening for fetal aneuploidy. Committee Opinion No. 640. American College of Obstetricians and Gynecologists. *Obstet Gynecol.* 2015;126:e31-e37.
3. Moore ER, Anderson GC, Bergman N, et al. Early skin-to-skin contact for mothers and their healthy newborn infants. *Cochrane Database Syst Rev.* 2012;(5): CD003519, DPO: 10.1102/14651858. CD003519.pub3.
4. Bosschaart N, Kok J, Newsum A, et al. Limitations and opportunities of transcutaneous bilirubin measurements. *Pediatrics.* 2012;129:689-694.
5. Laing I. General Care. In: MacDonald M, Mullett M, Seshia M, eds. *Avery's Neonatology.* 6th ed. Philadelphia.: Lippincott Williams and Wilkins; 2005.
6. Apgar V. A proposal for a new method of evaluation of the newborn infant. *Anesth Analg.* 1953;32:260-267.
7. Ballard JL, Khoury JC, Wedig K, et al. New Ballard Score, expanded to include extremely premature infants. *J Pediatr.* 1991;119:417-423.
8. Cornblath M. Neonatal hypoglycemia. In: Donn SM, Fisher CW, eds. *Risk Management Techniques in Perinatal and Neonatal Practice.* Armonk, NY: Futura; 1996.
9. Klaus MH, Fanaroff AA. *Care of the High-Risk Neonate.* 5th ed. Philadelphia: Saunders; 2001.

10. Ohlsson A, Walia R, Shah SS. Ibuprofen for the treatment of patent ductus arteriosus in preterm and/or LBW infants. *Cochrane Database Syst Rev.* 2008;(1):CD003481.
11. American Academy of Pediatrics: Subcommittee on Hyperbilirubinemia. Management of hyperbilirubinemia in the newborn infant 35 or more weeks of gestation. *Pediatrics.* 2004;114(1):297-316. Erratum in Pediatrics. 2004;114(4):1138.
12. AlFaleh K, Anabrees J. Probiotics for prevention of necrotizing enterocolitis in preterm infants. *Cochrane Database Syst Rev.* 2014;(4):10.1002/14651858.CD005496.pub4. Art. No.: CD005496
13. Neu J. Routine Probiotics for Premature Infants: Let's be Careful! *J Pediatr.* 2011;158(4):672-674.
14. American Academy of Pediatrics Section on Breastfeeding. Breastfeeding and the use of human milk. *Pediatrics.* 2012;129:e827-841.
15. Tagin MA, Woolcott CG, Vincer MJ, et al. Hypothermia for neonatal hypoxic ischemic encephalopathy: an updated systemic review and meta-analysis. *Arch Pediatr Adolesc Med.* 2012;166:558-566.
16. Schmidt B, Davis P, Moddemann D, et al. Long-term effects of indomethacin prophylaxis in ELBW infants. *N Engl J Med.* 2001;344:1966-1972.
17. Good WV, Early Treatment for Retinopathy of Prematurity Cooperative Group. Revised indications for the treatment of retinopathy of prematurity: results of the early treatment for retinopathy of prematurity randomized trial. *Arch Ophthalmol.* 2003;121:1684-1694.
18. Fierson WM, American Academy of Pediatrics Section on Ophthalmology, American Academy of Ophthalmology; American Association for Pediatric Ophthalmology and Strabismus; American Association of Certified Orthoptists. Screening examination of premature infants for retinopathy of prematurity. *Pediatrics.* 2013;131:189-195.

Chapter 19
Nephrology
Riddhi Desai, MD, MPH

I. WEB RESOURCES
- The International Pediatric Hypertension Association: www.pediatrichypertension.org
- American Academy of Pediatrics (AAP) Urinary Tract Infection (UTI) Practice Guidelines for Children 2–24 months: UTI Guidelines 2011
- National Kidney Disease Education Program: NKDEP Website
- National Kidney Foundation: www.kidney.org

II. URINALYSIS, URINE DIPSTICK, AND MICROSCOPY[1]

Urinalysis (UA) components are useful in clinical evaluation but rarely diagnostic in isolation. The clinician should be mindful of the possibility of false-positive and false-negative results, particularly with the dipstick, owing to a variety of factors.

Best if urine specimen is evaluated within 1 hour of voiding. Annual screening UAs are not recommended by the American Academy of Pediatrics (AAP).

A. Color
Normal urine varies in color from almost colorless to amber.

B. Turbidity
Cloudy urine can be normal; it is most often the result of crystal formation at room temperature. Uric acid crystals form in acidic urine and phosphate crystals form in alkaline urine. Cellular material and bacteria can also cause turbidity.

C. Specific Gravity
1. **Purpose:** Used as a measurement of a kidney's ability to concentrate urine. Easily determined surrogate of osmolality.
2. **Normal findings:** Between 1.003 and 1.030
3. **Special circumstances:**
   a. Isosthenuria: Excretion of urine with osmolality equal to plasma (neither concentrated or diluted). Typically a specific gravity of 1.010.
   b. Disease states affecting the kidney's ability to concentrate urine may have a urine specific gravity fixed at 1.010 (i.e., chronic kidney disease).
   c. Glucose, abundant protein, and iodine-containing contrast materials can give false high readings.

D. pH

1. **Purpose:** Used in determining the renal tubules' ability to maintain normal hydrogen ion concentration.
2. **Findings:** Normal ranges from 4.5–8, with an average range of 5–6. Urine pH must be interpreted in the context of serum pH.

E. Protein

1. **Purpose:** Used for screening and monitoring proteinuria. Should be quantified more precisely when needed for diagnostic purposes (see Section VII and related figures).
2. **Findings:** Dipstick provides readings of negative, trace, 1+ (~30 mg/dL), 2+ (~100 mg/dL), 3+ (~300 mg/dL), and 4+ (>1000 mg/dL).

F. Sugars

1. **Purpose:** Used to detect sugar in urine; glucosuria is always abnormal.
2. **Findings:** Glucosuria is suggestive but not diagnostic of diabetes mellitus or proximal renal tubular disease (see Section VIII). Blood glucose level at which kidney tubular reabsorption is exceeded is typically between 160 and 180 mg/dL.
3. **Special circumstances:** Different tests are available to detect glucose/sugars. Reduction tests (e.g., Clinitest) will detect other sugars such as galactose, lactose, fructose, pentoses, and glucose. Enzyme tests (e.g., Clinistix) are specific for glucose only.

G. Ketones

1. **Purpose:** Used to detect altered metabolism by detecting breakdown of fatty acids and fats. Useful in patients with diabetes and altered carbohydrate metabolism.
2. **Findings:** Except for trace amounts, ketonuria suggests ketoacidosis usually due to diabetes mellitus or catabolism induced by inadequate intake. Neonatal ketoacidosis may occur with metabolic defects (e.g., propionic acidemia, methylmalonic aciduria, glycogen storage disease).

H. Nitrite

See Section III.E.1.a.

I. Leukocyte Esterase

See Section III.E.1.b.

J. Hemoglobin and Myoglobin

1. **Purpose:** Used to detect glomerular or urologic injury.
2. **Findings:** Dipstick reads positive with intact red blood cells [as few as 3–4 red blood cells (RBCs)/high-power field (hpf)], hemoglobin, or myoglobin. Hemoglobinuria is seen with intravascular hemolysis or in a hematuric urine that has been standing for an extended period. Myoglobinuria is seen in crush injuries, vigorous exercise, major motor seizures, fever, malignant hyperthermia, electrocution, snake bites, and ischemia.

TABLE 19.1
URINALYSIS FOR BILIRUBIN/UROBILINOGEN

	Normal	Hemolytic Disease	Hepatic Disease	Biliary Obstruction
Urine urobilinogen	Normal	Increased	Increased	Decreased
Urine bilirubin	Negative	Negative	±	Positive

K. Bilirubin, Urobilinogen (Table 19.1)

Dipstick measures each individually
1. **Urine bilirubin:** Positive with conjugated hyperbilirubinemia; in this form, bilirubin is water soluble and excreted by the kidney
2. **Urobilinogen:** Increased in all cases of hyperbilirubinemia in which there is no obstruction to enterohepatic circulation

L. Red Blood Cells

1. **Purpose:** Used to differentiate the presence of hemoglobinuria/myoglobinuria from intact RBCs
2. **Findings:** Centrifuged urine normally contains <5 RBCs/hpf. Examination of RBC morphology may help to localize the source of bleeding, i.e., dysmorphic RBCs suggest a glomerular origin, whereas normal RBCs suggest lower tract bleeding. See Section VI for further definitions and evaluation of persistent hematuria.

M. White Blood Cells

1. **Purpose:** Used to detect infection or inflammation anywhere in the genitourinary tract.
2. **Findings:** ≥5 white blood cells (WBCs)/hpf of a properly spun urine specimen is suggestive of UTI. Relative to UTI, sterile pyuria is much less common in the pediatric population. If sterile pyuria is present, it is usually transient and accompanies systemic infectious or inflammatory disorders (e.g., Kawasaki disease).

N. Epithelial Cells

1. **Purpose:** Squamous epithelial cells are used as an index of possible contamination by vaginal secretions in females or by the foreskin in uncircumcised males.
2. **Findings:** Any amount indicates possible contamination.

O. Sediment

Using light microscopy, unstained, centrifuged urine can be examined for formed elements, including casts, cells, and crystals.

P. Urine Gram Stain

Gram stain is used to screen for UTIs. One organism/hpf in uncentrifuged urine represents at least 10^5 colonies/mL.

III. EVALUATION AND MANAGEMENT OF URINARY TRACT INFECTIONS[3]

A. History
Obtain voiding history (stool, urine), stream characteristics in toilet-trained children, sexual intercourse, sexual abuse, circumcision, masturbation, pinworms, prolonged baths, bubble baths, evaluation of growth curve, recent antibiotic use, and family history of vesicoureteral reflux (VUR), recurrent UTIs, or chronic kidney disease.

B. Physical Examination
Vital signs (especially blood pressure), abdominal examination for flank masses, bowel distention, evidence of impaction, meatal stenosis or circumcision in males, vulvovaginitis or labial adhesions in females, neurologic examination of lower extremities, perineal sensation and reflexes, and rectal and sacral examination (for anteriorly placed anus)

C. Risk Factors
Recent AAP guidelines[3] for children 2–24 months provide resources to help clinicians stratify the risk of UTI in the absence of another source of infection in a febrile child.
1. Females are at higher risk for UTI than males.
2. Uncircumcised males are at higher risk.
3. Other risk factors include nonblack race, fever ≥39°C, and fever >1–2 days.

D. Method of Obtaining Urine Sample
1. **If a child is 2 months to 2 years old, has a fever, and appears sufficiently ill to warrant immediate antibiotics**, obtain UA and urine culture by transurethral catheterization.
2. **If a child is 2 months to 2 years old, has a fever, and does not appear ill enough to warrant immediate antibiotics**, obtain urine by catheterization or the most convenient method available. If UA does not suggest UTI, it is reasonable to avoid antimicrobial therapy. If UA does suggest UTI, urine culture should be obtained by catheterization.

E. Diagnosis
1. **To establish the diagnosis of UTI,** both UA results suggestive of infection and positive urine culture are recommended.
a. Nitrite test:
   (1) Purpose: Used to detect nitrites produced by reduction of dietary nitrates by urinary gram-negative bacteria (especially *Escherichia coli, Klebsiella,* and *Proteus*).
   (2) Findings: Positive test is strongly suggestive of a UTI because of high specificity. Nitrite sensitivity is 15%–82% and specificity is 90%–100%.
   (3) Special circumstances: False-negative (low sensitivity) results commonly occur with insufficient time for conversion of urinary

nitrates to nitrites (age-dependent voiding frequency) and inability of bacteria to reduce nitrates to nitrites (many gram-positive organisms such as *Enterococcus, Mycobacterium* spp., and fungi).
b. Leukocyte esterase test:
    (1) Purpose: Used to detect esterases released from broken-down leukocytes. An indirect test for WBCs.
    (2) Findings: Positive test is more sensitive (67%–84%) than specific (64%–92%) for a UTI.
c. Pyuria is defined at a threshold of ≥5 WBCs/hpf. Absence of pyuria is rare if a true UTI is present.
d. Urine culture:
    (1) Suprapubic aspiration: >50,000 colony-forming units (CFUs) necessary to diagnose a UTI. Some resources do consider <50,000 CFUs diagnostic of a UTI. Recommend clinical correlation.
    (2) Transurethral catheterization: >50,000 CFUs necessary to diagnose a UTI.
    (3) Clean catch: >100,000 CFUs necessary to diagnose a UTI.
    (4) Bagged specimen: Positive culture cannot be used to document a UTI.
    (5) Catheter-associated (indwelling urethral or suprapubic): No specific data for pediatric patients. Adult Infectious Diseases Society of America guidelines define it as presence of symptoms and signs compatible with UTI and >1000 CFU/mL of one or more bacterial species in a single catheter urine specimen or in a midstream voided urine specimen from a patient whose catheter has been removed within previous 48 hours.[2]

F. Culture-Positive UTI

Treatment: Based on urine culture and sensitivities if possible; for empirical therapy, see Chapter 17
1. **Upper versus lower UTI:** Fever, systemic symptoms, and costovertebral angle tenderness suggest pyelonephritis (upper UTI) rather than cystitis (lower UTI). Fever that persists for >48 hours after initiating appropriate antibiotics is also suggestive of pyelonephritis. Although a ^{99m}Tc-dimercaptosuccinic acid (DMSA) scan is the gold standard to diagnose pyelonephritis, infants with febrile UTI are assumed to have pyelonephritis and are treated as such.
2. **Organisms:** *E. coli* is the most common cause of pediatric UTI. Other common pathogens include *Klebsiella, Proteus* spp., *Staphylococcus saprophyticus,* and *Staphylococcus aureus.* Group B streptococci and other bloodborne pathogens are important in neonatal UTIs, whereas *Enterococcus* and *Pseudomonas* are more prevalent in abnormal hosts (e.g., recurrent UTI, abnormal anatomy, neurogenic bladder, hospitalized patients, or those with frequent bladder catheterizations).

3. **Treatment considerations:**
a. Hospitalize all febrile children aged <4 weeks and treat with intravenous (IV) antibiotics, owing to risk for bacteremia and meningitis.
b. Parenteral antibiotics for children who are toxic, dehydrated, or unable to tolerate oral medication due to vomiting or noncompliance. Studies comparing duration are inconclusive, but experts traditionally recommend 7–10 days for uncomplicated cases and 14 days for toxic children and those with pyelonephritis. Some studies have shown that 2–4 days of oral antibiotics in uncomplicated lower tract UTIs are as effective as 7–10 days of oral treatment.[4]
4. **Inadequate response to therapy:** Repeat urine culture in children with expected response is controversial but generally thought to be unnecessary. Repeat culture, as well as renal ultrasound to rule out an abscess or urinary obstruction, is indicated in children with a poor response to therapy. Repeat cultures should also be considered in patients with recurrent UTIs to rule out persistent bacteriuria.
5. **Imaging studies** (Fig. 19.1):
a. Anatomic evaluation: New guidelines for children aged 2–24 months continue to recommend obtaining an ultrasound of the kidneys and bladder after the first UTI is diagnosed. In a change from prior recommendations, a voiding cystourethrogram (VCUG) is recommended after a second UTI is diagnosed or as indicated by an abnormal kidney and bladder ultrasound [hydronephrosis, scarring, or other findings to suggest either high-grade VUR or obstructive uropathy].[3]
    (1) Kidney and bladder ultrasonography: To evaluate for gross structural defects, obstructive lesions, positional abnormalities, and kidney size and growth. Should be done at the earliest convenient time unless the child fails to demonstrate expected clinical response, which should prompt a more immediate kidney sonogram.
    (2) VCUG: To evaluate bladder anatomy, emptying, and VUR. May be substituted with radionuclide cystogram (RNC), which has 1/100 the radiation exposure of VCUG and increased sensitivity for transient reflux. RNC does not visualize urethral anatomy, is not sensitive for low-grade reflux, and cannot grade reflux.
b. Abdominal radiograph: If indicated, to evaluate stool pattern and for spinal dysraphism.
c. DMSA: ^{99m}Tc-DMSA scan can detect areas of decreased uptake that may represent acute pyelonephritis or chronic kidney scarring; does not differentiate between the two. Routine use not recommended; may be indicated in patients with an abnormal VCUG or kidney sonography or in patients with history of asymptomatic bacteriuria and fever. Repeat in 3–6 months if initial study is positive to evaluate for persistent infection and kidney scarring if clinically indicated.

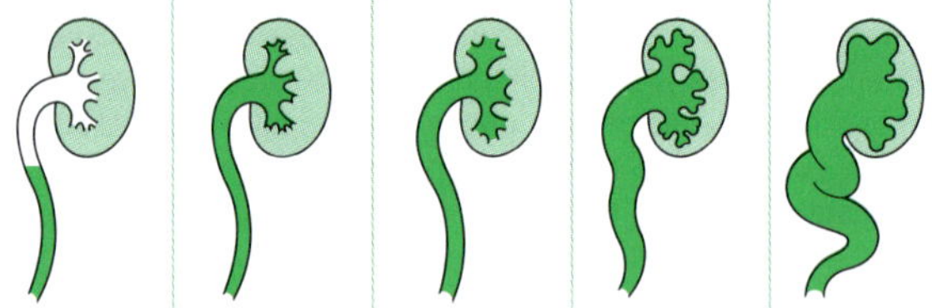

Grade I	Grade II	Grade III	Grade IV	Grade V
Ureter only	Ureter, pelvis, calyces; no dilatation, normal calyceal fornices	Mild or moderate dilatation and/or tortuosity of ureter; mild or moderate dilatation of the pelvis, but no or slight blunting of the fornices	Moderate dilatation and/or tortuosity of the ureter; mild dilatation of renal pelvis and calyces; complete obliteration of sharp angle of fornices, but maintenance of papillary impressions in majority of calyces	Gross dilatation and tortuosity of ureter; gross dilatation of renal pelvis and calyces; papillary impressions are no longer visible in majority of calyces

FIGURE 19.1

International classification of vesicoureteral reflux. *(Modified from Rushton H. Urinary tract infections in children: epidemiology, evaluation, and management. Pediatr Clin North Am. 1997;44:5 and International Reflux Committee. Medical vs. surgical treatment of primary vesicoureteral reflux: report of the International Reflux Study Committee. Pediatrics. 1981;67:392.)*

d. Diethylenetriamine pentaacetic acid (DTPA)/mercaptoacetyl triglycine (MAG-3): In the setting of hydronephrosis, can be used to assess drainage of the urinary collecting system to characterize possible upper urologic tract obstructions at ureteropelvic or ureterovesical junction. May also be used for indications listed above for DMSA.

6. **Management of VUR:**
a. Antibiotic prophylaxis: Conventionally, low-dose antibiotic prophylaxis has been recommended in all children with VUR and obstructive disease. However, the 2011 AAP UTI guidelines questioned the efficacy of antibiotic prophylaxis in preventing UTI and subsequent kidney disease in the setting of VUR.[3] The Randomized Intervention for the Management of Vesicoureteral Reflux (RIVUR) study, published

in 2014, is the largest randomized, double-blinded, placebo-controlled, multicenter clinical trial that has been published to date evaluating the clinical utility of antibiotic prophylaxis for VUR. The RIVUR study showed that prophylactic trimethoprim/sulfamethoxazole reduced the risk of UTI recurrence by 50% compared to placebo, but with no significant difference in renal scarring. Some experts suggest that the study was insufficiently powered to detect a difference in the relatively rare outcome of renal scarring, and thus recommend shifting guideline recommendations from "no prophylaxis" to "selective prophylaxis" in certain groups of patients.[5,6]
b. Surgical intervention: Persistence/grade of VUR is typically monitored annually, often in consultation with a pediatric urologist. Higher-grade VUR that persists as the child grows may ultimately require surgical intervention, the timing of which may be affected by factors such as presence of bilateral VUR, kidney scarring, other underlying urologic disease, recurrent kidney infections, and/or ease of family follow-up. No model predicting the resolution of VUR has been verified.
7. **Asymptomatic bacteriuria:** Defined as bacteria in urine on microscopy and Gram stain in an afebrile, asymptomatic patient without pyuria. Antibiotics not necessary if voiding habits and urinary tract are normal. DMSA may be helpful in differentiating pyelonephritis from fever and coincidental bacteriuria.
8. **Referral to pediatric urology:** Consider in children with abnormal voiding patterns based on history or imaging, neurogenic bladder, abnormal anatomy, recurrent UTI, or poor response to appropriate antibiotics.

IV. KIDNEY FUNCTION TESTS

A. Tests of Glomerular Function

1. **Glomerulogenesis is complete at 36 weeks' gestation.** Glomerular filtration rate (GFR) increases over the first few years of life related to glomerular maturation.
2. **Normal GFR values, as measured by inulin clearance (gold standard)** are shown in Table 19.2.
3. **Creatinine clearance (CCr):**
Timed urine specimen: Standard measure of GFR; closely approximates inulin clearance in the normal range of GFR. When GFR is low, CCr overestimates GFR. Usually inaccurate in children with obstructive uropathy or problems with bladder emptying

$$CCr\ (mL/min/1.73\ m^2) = [U \times (V/P)] \times 1.73/BSA,$$

where U (mg/dL) = urinary creatinine concentration; V (mL/min) = total urine volume (mL) divided by the duration of the collection (min) (24 hours = 1440 minutes); P (mg/dL) = serum creatinine concentration (may average two levels); and BSA (m^2) = body surface area.
4. **Estimated GFR (eGFR) from plasma creatinine:** Convenient estimate of kidney function in clinical setting is challenging to determine if

TABLE 19.2
NORMAL VALUES OF GLOMERULAR FILTRATION RATE

Age	GFR (Mean) (mL/min/1.73 m^2)	Range (mL/min/1.73 m^2)
Neonates <34 wk gestational age		
2–8 days	11	11–15
4–28 days	20	15–28
30–90 days	50	40–65
Neonates >34 wk gestational age		
2–8 days	39	17–60
4–28 days	47	26–68
30–90 days	58	30–86
1–6 mo	77	39–114
6–12 mo	103	49–157
12–19 mo	127	62–191
2 yr–adult	127	89–165

From Holliday MA, Barratt TM. Pediatric Nephrology. Baltimore: Williams & Wilkins; 1994:1306.

creatinine is normal, given variation related to body size/muscle mass. If body habitus is markedly abnormal or precise measurement of GFR is needed, consider determining GFR by methods other than estimation. Creatinine must be in steady state to estimate GFR; use caution in the setting of acute kidney injury. Two equations to calculate estimated GFR:

a. Bedside Chronic Kidney Disease in Children (CKiD) cohort: Newly developed equation based on current laboratory methodologies to determine creatinine. Recommended for eGFR determination in children aged 1–16 years. Estimated GFRs of ≥75 mL/min/1.73 m^2 determined by this equation likely represents normal kidney function; clinical correlation is recommended as always with GFR estimation[7]

$$\text{eGFR (mL/min/1.73 m}^2\text{)} = 0.413 \times (L/Pcr),$$

where *0.413* is the proportionality constant, *L* = height (cm), and *Pcr* = plasma creatinine (mg/dL).

b. Schwartz equation: Traditional equation for eGFR. However, given changes in the laboratory assays used to determine creatinine, this equation systemically overestimates GFR and should be considered when applying clinically:

$$\text{eGFR (mL/min/1.73 m}^2\text{)} = kL/Pcr,$$

where *k* = proportionality constant; *L* = height (cm); and *Pcr* = plasma creatinine (mg/dL) (Table 19.3).

c. Modification of Diet in Renal Disease (MDRD) and Chronic Kidney Disease Epidemiology Collaboration (CKD-EPI): Used to calculate GFR in those >18 years old. (See NKDEP website)

TABLE 19.3
PROPORTIONALITY CONSTANT FOR CALCULATING GLOMERULAR FILTRATION RATE

Age	k Values
Low birth weight during first year of life	0.33
Term AGA during first year of life	0.45
Children and adolescent girls	0.55
Adolescent boys	0.70

AGA, appropriate for gestational age.
Data from Schwartz GJ, Brion LP, Spitzer A. The use of plasma creatinine concentration for estimating glomerular filtration rate in infants, children, and adolescents. Pediatr Clin North Am. 1987;34:571.

5. **Other measurements of GFR:** May be used when more precise determination of GFR is needed (e.g., dosing of chemotherapy). These methods include iothalamate, DTPA, and iohexol.

B. Tests of Kidney Tubular Function

1. **Proximal tubule:**
a. Proximal tubule reabsorption: Proximal tubule is responsible for reabsorption of electrolytes, glucose, and amino acids. Studies to evaluate proximal tubular function compare urine and blood levels of specific compounds, arriving at a percentage of tubular reabsorption (Tx):

$$Tx = 1 - [(Ux/Px)/(UCr/PCr)] \times 100\%,$$

where Ux = concentration of compound in urine; Px = concentration of compound in plasma; Ucr = concentration of creatinine in urine; and Pcr = concentration of creatinine in plasma. This formula can be used for amino acids, electrolytes, calcium, and phosphorus. For example, in the setting of hypophosphatemia, a tubular reabsorption of phosphorus near 100% would be expected in a kidney with preserved proximal tubular function.

b. Calculation of fractional excretion of sodium (FENa) is derived from the following equation[8]:

$$FENa = [(UNa/PNa)/(UCr/PCr)] \times 100\%$$

FENa is usually <1% in prerenal azotemia or glomerulonephritis, and >1% (usually >3%) in acute tubular necrosis (ATN) or postrenal azotemia. Infants have diminished ability to reabsorb sodium; FENa in volume-depleted infants is <3%. Recent diuretic use may give inaccurate results. The fractional excretion of urea (FEurea) may be useful in certain clinical scenarios:

$$FEurea = [(Uurea/Purea)/(UCr/PCr)] \times 100\%$$

FEurea is usually <35% in prerenal azotemia and >50% in ATN.[8]

c. Glucose reabsorption: Glucosuria must be interpreted in relation to simultaneously determined plasma glucose concentration. If plasma

glucose concentration is <160 mg/dL and glucose is present in urine, this implies abnormal tubular reabsorption of glucose and proximal renal tubular disease (see Section II.F).
d. Bicarbonate reabsorption: Majority occurs in proximal tubule. Abnormalities in reabsorption lead to type 2 renal tubular acidosis (RTA; see Table 19.9).

2. **Distal tubule:**
a. Urine acidification: A urine acidification defect (distal RTA) should be suspected when random urine pH values are >6 in the presence of moderate systemic metabolic acidosis. Confirm acidification defects by simultaneous venous or arterial pH, plasma bicarbonate concentration, and determination of the pH of fresh urine.
b. Urine concentration occurs in the distal tubule: Urine osmolality, ideally on a first morning urine specimen, can be used to evaluate capacity to concentrate urine. (For more formal testing, see the water deprivation test in Chapter 10.)
c. Urine calcium: Hypercalciuria may be seen with distal RTA, vitamin D intoxication, hyperparathyroidism, immobilization, excessive calcium intake, use of steroids or loop diuretics, or idiopathic. Diagnosis is as follows:
   (1) 24-hour urine: Calcium >4 mg/kg/24 hr (gold standard)
   (2) Spot urine: Determine calcium/creatinine (Ca/Cr) ratio. Normal urine Ca/Cr ratio does not rule out hypercalciuria. Correlate clinically and follow elevated spot urine Ca/Cr ratio with a 24-hr urine calcium determination if indicated (Table 19.4).[9]

V. ACUTE KIDNEY INJURY[10,11]

A. Definition
Sudden decline in kidney function, clinically represented by rising creatinine, with or without changes in urine output

B. Etiology (Table 19.5)
Causes are generally subdivided into three categories:
1. **Prerenal:** Impaired perfusion of kidneys, the most common cause of acute kidney injury (AKI) in children. Volume depletion is a common cause of prerenal AKI.
2. **Renal:**
a. Parenchymal disease due to vascular or glomerular lesions
b. ATN: Typically a diagnosis of exclusion when no evidence of renal parenchymal disease is present and prerenal and postrenal causes have been eliminated if possible
3. **Postrenal:** Obstruction of the urinary tract, commonly due to inherited anatomic abnormalities in children

C. Clinical Presentation
Pallor, decreased urine output, edema, hypertension, vomiting, and lethargy. The hallmark of early kidney failure is often oliguria.

TABLE 19.4
AGE-ADJUSTED CALCIUM/CREATININE RATIOS

Age	Ca^{2+}/Cr Ratio (mg/mg) (95th Percentile for Age)
<7 mo	0.86
7–18 mo	0.60
19 mo–6 yr	0.42
Adults	0.22

From Sargent JD, Stukel TA, Kresel J, et al. Normal values for random urinary calcium-to-creatinine ratios in infancy. J Pediatr. 1993;123:393.

TABLE 19.5
ETIOLOGIES OF ACUTE KIDNEY INJURY

PRERENAL	**DECREASED TRUE INTRAVASCULAR VOLUME:** Hemorrhage, volume depletion, sepsis, burns **DECREASED EFFECTIVE INTRAVASCULAR VOLUME:** Congestive heart failure, hepatorenal syndrome **ALTERED GLOMERULAR HEMODYNAMICS:** NSAIDs, ACE inhibitors (when renal perfusion is already low)
INTRINSIC RENAL	**ACUTE TUBULAR NECROSIS:** Hypoxic/ischemic insults Drug-induced—aminoglycosides, amphotericin B, acyclovir, chemotherapeutic agents (ifosfamide, cisplatin) Toxin-mediated—endogenous toxins (myoglobin, hemoglobin); exogenous toxins (ethylene glycol, methanol) **INTERSTITIAL NEPHRITIS:** Drug-induced—β-lactams, NSAIDs (may be associated with high-grade proteinuria), sulfonamides, PPIs Idiopathic **URIC ACID NEPHROPATHY** Tumor lysis syndrome **GLOMERULONEPHRITIS:** In most severe degree, presents as rapidly progressive glomerulonephritis (RPGN) **VASCULAR LESIONS:** Renal artery thrombosis, renal vein thrombosis, cortical necrosis, hemolytic uremic syndrome **HYPOPLASIA/DYSPLASIA:** Idiopathic or exposure to nephrotoxic drugs in utero
POSTRENAL	**OBSTRUCTION IN A SOLITARY KIDNEY** **BILATERAL URETERAL OBSTRUCTION** **URETHRAL OBSTRUCTION** **BLADDER DYSFUNCTION**

ACE, angiotensin-converting enzyme; NSAIDs, nonsteroidal antiinflammatory drugs; PPIs, proton pump inhibitors
Data from Andreoli SP. Acute kidney injury in children. Pediatr Nephrol. 2009;24:253-263.

1. **Oliguria:** Urine output <300 mL/m^2/24 hr, or <0.5 mL/kg/hr in children and <1.0 mL/kg/hr in infants. May be a reflection of intrinsic or obstructive kidney disease. Always interpret urine output in the context of physical exam, clinical scenario and fluid delivery. For example, low urine output may be appropriate (physiologic response to water depletion in a prerenal state) and "normal" urine output may be inappropriate in a volume-depleted patient (potentially representing kidney tubular damage or another pathologic state).
    a. Blood urea nitrogen/creatinine (BUN/Cr) ratio (both in mg/dL): Interpret ratios with caution in small children with low serum creatinine.
        (1) 10–20 (normal ratio): Suggests intrinsic renal disease in the setting of oliguria
        (2) >20: Suggests volume depletion, prerenal azotemia, or gastrointestinal bleeding
        (3) <5: Suggests liver disease, starvation, inborn error of metabolism
    b. Laboratory differentiation of oliguria (Table 19.6)

D. Acute Tubular Necrosis

Clinically defined by three phases:
1. **Oliguric phase:** Period of severe oliguria that may last days. If oliguria or anuria persists for longer than 3–6 weeks, kidney recovery from ATN is less likely.
2. **High urine output phase:** Begins with increased urine output and progresses to passage of large volumes of isosthenuric urine containing sodium levels of 80–150 mEq/L.
3. **Recovery phase:** Signs and symptoms usually resolve rapidly, but polyuria may persist for days to weeks.

E. Treatment Considerations

1. **Placement of indwelling catheter to monitor urine output**
2. **Prerenal and postrenal factors** should be excluded, and intravascular volume maintained with appropriate fluids in consultation with a pediatric nephrologist.

F. Complications

Often dependent on clinical severity; usually includes fluid overload [hypertension, congestive heart failure (CHF), or pulmonary edema],

TABLE 19.6

LABORATORY DIFFERENTIATION OF OLIGURIA

Test	Prerenal	Renal
FENa	≤1%	>3%
BUN/Cr ratio	>20:1	<10:1
Urine specific gravity	>1.015	<1.010

electrolyte disturbances (hyperkalemia), metabolic acidosis, hyperphosphatemia, and uremia

G. Acute Dialysis

1. **Indications:**

When metabolic or fluid derangements are not controlled by aggressive medical management alone. Generally accepted criteria include the following, although a nephrologist should always be consulted, if possible:
a. **Acidosis:** Intractable metabolic acidosis
b. **Electrolyte abnormalities:** Hyperkalemia >6.5 mEq/L despite restriction of delivery and medical management. Calcium and phosphorus imbalance (e.g., hypocalcemia with tetany, seizures in the presence of a very high serum phosphate level). Derangements implicated in neurologic abnormalities.
c. **Ingestion or accumulation of dialyzable toxins or poisons:** Lithium, ammonia, alcohol, barbiturates, ethylene glycol, isopropanol, methanol, salicylates, theophylline. When available, poison control centers can provide guidance and expertise.
d. **Volume overload:** Evidence of pulmonary edema or hypertension
e. **Uremia:** BUN >150 mg/dL (lower if rising rapidly), uremic pericardial effusion, neurologic symptoms

2. **Techniques:**
a. Peritoneal dialysis: Requires catheter to access peritoneal cavity, as well as adequate peritoneal perfusion. May be used acutely or chronically.
b. Intermittent hemodialysis: Requires placement of special vascular access catheters. May be method of choice for certain toxins (e.g., ammonia, uric acid, poisons) or when there are contraindications to peritoneal dialysis.
c. Continuous arteriovenous hemofiltration/hemodialysis (CAVH/D) and continuous venovenous hemofiltration/hemodialysis (CVVH/D):
   (1) Requires special vascular access catheter
   (2) Lower efficiency of solute removal compared with intermittent hemodialysis, but higher efficiency is not necessary because of the continuous nature of this form of dialysis
   (3) Sustained nature of dialysis allows for more gradual removal of volume/solutes, which is ideal for patients with hemodynamic or respiratory instability

H. Radiographic Imaging Considerations in AKI/CKD

1. To prevent radiographic contrast-induced nephropathy, select radiographic studies that do not require administration of a radiographic iodinated contrast media (RICM) if possible, particularly in high-risk populations such as patients with AKI or CKD.[12]
2. If RICM is required, use of low or iso-osmolality contrast media is preferred.[12]

3. Hydration has been found to be effective in preventing or minimizing contrast-induced nephropathy in some studies of high–risk populations. Intravenous hydration 6 hours prior to and 6 to 12 hours after contrast administration has been studied.[12]
4. Use of N-acetylcysteine is controversial in preventing contrast-induced nephropathy.[12]
5. Gadolinium and nephrogenic systemic fibrosis: The triad of gadolinium use, a pro-inflammatory state, and renal impairment (GFR <30 mL/min per 1.73 m^2, peritoneal or hemodialysis) is associated with nephrogenic systemic fibrosis. Gadolinium is contraindicated in patients with GFR <30 mL/min per 1.73 m^2, and caution should be used at GFR levels between 30 and 60 mL/min per 1.73 m^2.[13]

VI. HEMATURIA AND ASSOCIATED DISORDERS[14,15]

A. Definitions
1. **Gross hematuria:** Blood in urine visible to the naked eye
2. **Microscopic hematuria:** Blood not visible to naked eye, but ≥5 RBCs/hpf
3. **Red urine that is not hematuria:** Hemoglobinuria, myoglobinuria, brick dust urine (precipitated urates in typically acidic urine of neonates)
4. **Persistent hematuria:** Three positive urinalyses, based on dipstick and microscopic examination over at least a 2- to 3-week period, warranting further evaluation
5. **Extraglomerular hematuria:** No RBC casts, minimal if any proteinuria
6. **Glomerular hematuria:** Most often tea-colored urine but may be red/pink, RBC casts, dysmorphic RBCs, associated with proteinuria
7. **Acute nephritic syndrome:** Classically tea-colored urine, facial or body edema, hypertension, and oliguria

B. Etiologies (Table 19.7)

C. Evaluation (Fig. 19.2)
1. **Differentiate glomerular and extraglomerular hematuria:** Examine urine sediment looking for RBC casts and protein
a. Glomerular hematuria
   (1) Determine whether isolated kidney disease or multisystem disease: Complete blood cell count (CBC) with differential and smear, serum electrolytes with Ca, BUN/Cr, serum protein/albumin, and other testing driven by history and exam, including ANA, hepatitis B and C serologies, HIV, family history, audiology screen if indicated
   (2) Consider other studies to determine underlying diagnosis: C3/C4, antineutrophil antibody (c- and p-antineutrophil cytoplasmic antibodies), anti–double-stranded DNA
b. Extraglomerular hematuria
   (1) Rule out infection: Urine culture, gonorrhea, chlamydia
   (2) Rule out trauma: History, consider imaging of abdomen/pelvis

TABLE 19.7
CAUSES OF HEMATURIA IN CHILDREN

Kidney-related disease	Isolated glomerular disease	IgA nephropathy, Alport syndrome, thin glomerular basement membrane nephropathy, postinfectious/poststreptococcal glomerulonephritis, membranous nephropathy, membranoproliferative glomerulonephritis, focal segmental glomerulosclerosis, antiglomerular basement membrane disease
	Multisystem disease involving glomerulus	Systemic lupus erythematosus nephritis, Henoch-Schönlein purpura nephritis, granulomatosis with polyangiitis, polyarteritis nodosa, Goodpasture syndrome, hemolytic-uremic syndrome, sickle cell glomerulopathy, HIV nephropathy
	Tubulointerstitial disease	Pyelonephritis, interstitial nephritis, papillary necrosis, acute tubular necrosis
	Vascular	Arterial or venous thrombosis, malformations (aneurysms, hemangiomas), nutcracker syndrome, hemoglobinopathy (sickle cell trait/disease)
	Anatomical	Hydronephrosis, cystic kidney disease, polycystic kidney disease, multicystic dysplasia, tumor, trauma
Urinary tract disease		Inflammation (cystitis, urethritis)
		Urolithiasis
		Trauma
		Coagulopathy
		Arteriovenous malformations (AVMs)
		Bladder tumor
		Factitious syndrome

Data from Kliegman RM, Stanton BF, St. Geme JW, et al. Nelson Textbook of Pediatrics. 19th ed. Philadelphia: Saunders; 2011:1779.

   (3) Investigate other potential causes: Urine Ca/Cr ratio or 24-hour urine for kidney stone risk analysis, sickle cell screen, kidney/bladder ultrasound. Consider serum electrolytes with Ca, prothrombin time/partial thromboplastin time.
D. Management (Fig. 19.3)

VII. PROTEINURIA AND ASSOCIATED DISORDERS[15,16]

A. Methods of Detection
1. **Urinalysis:** See Section II.E. Proteinuria on a urine dipstick should be verified by a protein/creatinine ratio in an appropriately collected first morning urine specimen.

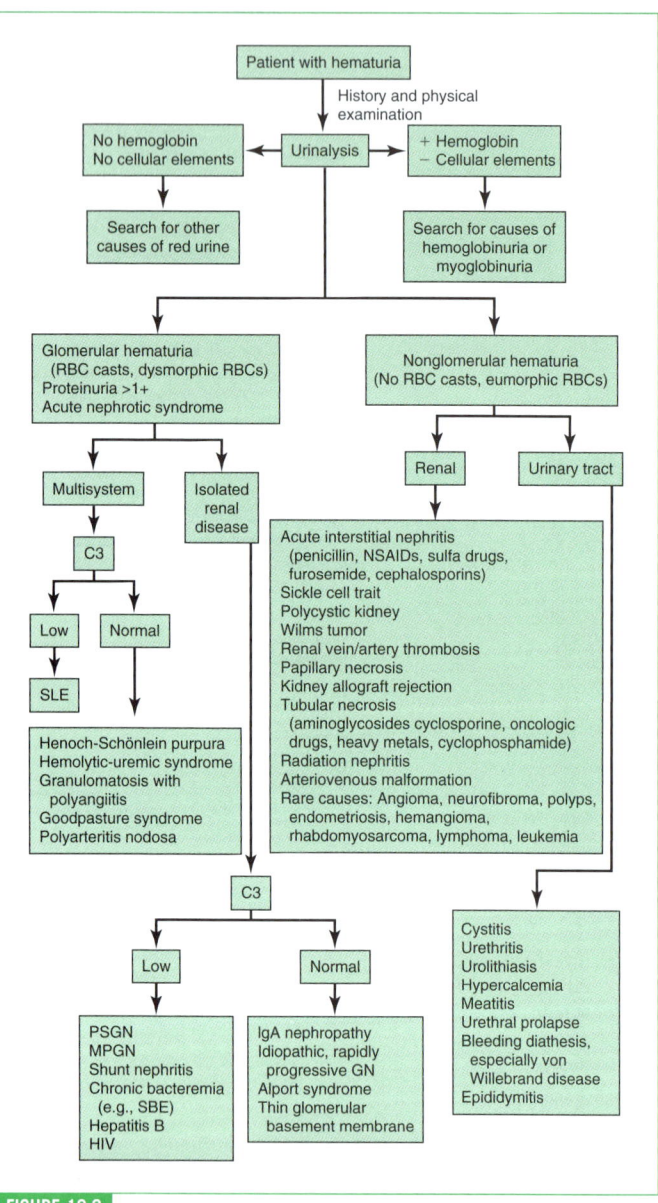

FIGURE 19.2

Diagnostic strategy for hematuria. GN, glomerulonephritis; HIV, human immunodeficiency virus; MPGN, membranoprolifcrative glomerulonephritis; NSAIDs, nonsteroidal antiinflammatory drugs; PSGN, poststreptococcal glomerulonephritis; RBC, red blood cell; SBE, subacute bacterial endocarditis; SLE, systemic lupus erythematosus

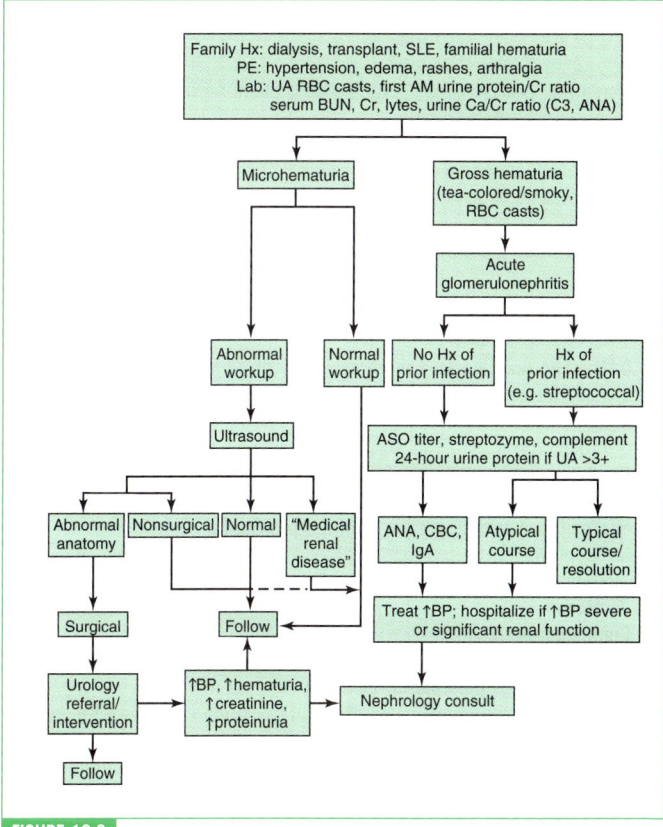

FIGURE 19.3

Management algorithm for hematuria. *(Data from Hay WM, Levin MJ, Deterding RR, Azbug MJ, Sondheimer JM. CURRENT Diagnosis & Treatment Pediatrics. 21st edition. Available at www.accessmedicine.com, Fig. 24.1.)*

2. **First morning urine protein/creatinine ratio:** Approximates 24-hour urine collections well and has additional benefit of minimizing detection of proteinuria from orthostatic proteinuria.
Appropriate collection of a first morning urine sample is very important for accurate results. A child must empty the bladder before going to bed. If the child gets up during the night, they should empty their bladder before returning to bed. When the child wakes up in the morning, they should provide a urine sample immediately.

a. Normal ratios:
   (1) <2 years old: <0.5 mg/mg
   (2) >2 years old: <0.2 mg/mg
   b. Abnormal ratios (mg/mg): Significant proteinuria detected on a first morning protein/creatinine ratio should prompt verification of appropriate collection. Repeat specimen should be analyzed within 1–2 weeks, or sooner based on clinical scenario (e.g., edema, hypertension, or symptom of concern would prompt a more expedited workup).
3. **24-hour urine protein:** Can have a contribution from benign orthostatic proteinuria, which cannot be ruled out without a fractional urine collection. Protein level >4 mg/m^2/hr is considered significant.

B. Definitions

1. **Orthostatic proteinuria:** Excretion of insignificant amounts of protein in the supine position, but in the standing position, protein excretion increases to significant range. A benign condition and common cause of proteinuria in children and adolescents.
2. **Fixed proteinuria:** Proteinuria found on first morning urine void over several consecutive days. Suggestive of kidney disease.
3. **Microalbuminuria:** Presence of albumin in urine below detectable range of dipsticks. In adults, defined as 30–300 mg/g creatinine. Most often used in screening for kidney disease secondary to diabetes.
4. **Significant proteinuria:** UPr:UCr ratio 0.2–2.0 mg/mg or 4–40 mg/m^2/hr in a 24-hour collection.
5. **Nephrotic-range proteinuria:** UPr:UCr ratio >2 mg/mg or >40 mg/m^2/hr in a 24-hour collection. In adults, 24-hour urine protein excretion of 3000 mg/24 hr.
6. **Nephrotic syndrome:** Nephrotic-range proteinuria, hypoalbuminemia, and edema. Also associated with hyperlipidemia (cholesterol >200 mg/dL).

C. Etiologies (Box 19.1)

See Section VII.E for information about nephrotic syndrome.

D. Evaluation[17]

Further evaluation is necessary if proteinuria is significant and not secondary to orthostatic proteinuria (Box 19.2).

E. Nephrotic Syndrome[18]

Manifestation of a glomerular disorder secondary to primary kidney disease, a systemic disorder resulting in glomerular injury, or rarely certain drugs. Idiopathic nephrotic syndrome is the most common form, representing approximately 90% of cases in children between the ages of 1 and 10 years. Minimal change disease is the most commonly found renal pathology found among children with idiopathic nephrotic syndrome in this age group.

BOX 19.1
CAUSES OF PROTEINURIA

Transient proteinuria: Caused by fever, exercise, dehydration, cold exposure, seizure, stress

Orthostatic proteinuria

Glomerular diseases with isolated proteinuria: Idiopathic (minimal change disease) nephrotic syndrome, focal segmental glomerulosclerosis, mesangial proliferative glomerulonephritis, membranous nephropathy, membranoproliferative glomerulonephritis, amyloidosis, diabetic nephropathy, sickle cell nephropathy

Glomerular diseases with proteinuria as a prominent feature: Acute postinfectious glomerulonephritis, immunoglobulin A nephropathy

Tubular disease: Cystinosis, Wilson disease, acute tubular necrosis, tubulointerstitial nephritis, polycystic kidney disease, renal dysplasia

Data from Kliegman RM, Stanton BF, St. Geme JW, et al. Nelson Textbook of Pediatrics. 19th ed. Philadelphia: Saunders; 2011:1801.

BOX 19.2
BASIC EVALUATION OF SIGNIFICANT (NEPHROTIC AND NON-NEPHROTIC) PROTEINURIA

Complete metabolic panel with phosphorus
C3 and C4
Antinuclear antibody, anti–double-stranded DNA antibody
Hepatitis B, C, and HIV in high-risk populations
Antineutrophil antibodies (c- and p-ANCA)
Kidney and bladder ultrasonography
Referral to nephrologist

1. **Clinical manifestations**
   Hypoalbuminemia and decrease in oncotic pressure results in generalized edema. Initial swelling commonly occurs on the face (especially periorbital), as well as in the pretibial area. Eye swelling is often mistaken for allergic reactions or seasonal allergies.
2. **Etiologies** (Table 19.8 and Box 19.3)
3. **Management of idiopathic nephrotic syndrome of childhood:** Empirical corticosteroid treatment without kidney biopsy is recommended for children without atypical features. Hospitalization recommended for children with overwhelming edema or infection.
a. Steroid-responsive: Approximately 95% of patients with minimal change disease (MCD) and 20% with focal segmental glomerulosclerosis (FSGS) achieve remission within 4–8 weeks of starting prednisone. Response to corticosteroids is the best prognostic indicator, including the likelihood of underlying MCD. Treatment of the

TABLE 19.8
ETIOLOGIES OF NEPHROTIC SYNDROME

Primary Causes (90%)	Secondary Causes (10%)
Minimal change nephrotic syndrome (MCNS): 85% of idiopathic causes in children	Infections (HIV, hepatitis B, hepatitis C)
Focal segmental glomerulosclerosis (FSGS)	Systemic lupus erythematosus
Membranous nephropathy	Diabetes mellitus
IgA nephropathy	Drugs
Genetic disorders involving the slit diaphragm	Malignancy (leukemias, lymphomas)

BOX 19.3
FACTORS SUGGESTING DIAGNOSIS OTHER THAN IDIOPATHIC MINIMAL CHANGE NEPHROTIC SYNDROME

Age <1 year or >10 years
Family history of kidney disease
Extrarenal disease (arthritis, rash, anemia)
Chronic disease of another organ or systemic disease
Symptoms due to intravascular volume expansion (hypertension, pulmonary edema)
Kidney failure
Active urine sediment (red blood cell casts)

---

initial presentation of idiopathic nephrotic syndrome involves prolonged use of corticosteroid therapy based on literature demonstrating reduced risk/frequency of relapse with such regimens. The duration of a particular therapy varies according to the center and the consensus body. One regimen by the Children's Nephrotic Syndrome Consensus includes prednisone 60 mg/m^2 or 2 mg/kg/day (maximum dose, 60 mg/day) for 6 weeks, followed by 40 mg/m^2 or 1.5 mg/kg on alternate days for 6 weeks.[17] Relapses of idiopathic nephrotic syndrome are treated with a shorter duration of corticosteroids and regimens also vary according to the center and the consensus body. The Children's Nephrotic Syndrome Consensus recommends prednisone 60 mg/m^2 or 2 mg/kg/day (maximum dose, 60 mg/day) until urine protein is negative for 3 consecutive days, followed by 40 mg/m^2 or 1.5 mg/kg on alternate days for 4 weeks.

b. Frequently relapsing: Defined as two or more relapses within 6 months of initial response, or four or more relapses in any 12-month period.
c. Steroid-dependent: Defined as two consecutive relapses during tapering or within 14 days of cessation of steroids. Some patients can be managed with low-dose steroids, given daily or on alternate days, but many still relapse. Second-line treatments for frequently relapsing and steroid-dependent nephrotic syndrome: Cyclophosphamide,

mycophenolate mofetil (MMF), calcineurin inhibitors, levamisole, or rituximab.
d. **Steroid-resistant:** Lack of remission or partial remission after 8 weeks of corticosteroids. Second-line agents, including calcineurin inhibitors or MMF, are often introduced once steroid resistance is confirmed.
e. **Further evaluation:** Biopsy recommended for macroscopic hematuria, persistent creatinine elevation, low complement levels, and persistent proteinuria after 4–8 weeks of adequate steroid treatment.
f. **Complications:** AKI, thromboembolic disease, infection, and side effects of systemic steroids.

VIII. TUBULAR DISORDERS

A. Renal Tubular Acidosis (Table 19.9)[8,19]

A group of transport defects resulting in abnormal urine acidification; due to deficiencies in reabsorption of bicarbonate (HCO_3^-), excretion of hydrogen ions (H^+), or both. Results in a persistent nonanion-gap metabolic acidosis accompanied by hyperchloremia. RTA syndromes often do not progress to kidney failure but are instead characterized by a normal GFR. Clinical presentation may be characterized by failure to thrive, polyuria, constipation, vomiting, and dehydration.

1. **Fractional excretion of bicarbonate ($FeHCO_3$) should be checked after a HCO_3 load.** Can help differentiate the types of RTA. Equation is based on the same concept found in Section IV.B.1:

$$FeHCO_3 = ([UHCO_3/PHCO_3]/[UCr/PCr]) \times 100\%$$

2. **Urine anion gap (UAG) is also useful in differentiating between the types of RTA;** however, it should not be used when a patient is volume depleted or has an anion-gap metabolic acidosis.

$$UAG = UNa + UK - UCl$$

B. Type 3 (Combined Proximal and Distal) RTA

Infants with mild type 1 and mild type 2 defects were previously classified as type 3 RTA. Studies have shown that this is not a genetic entity itself, which has resulted in reclassification as a subtype of type 1 RTA that occurs primarily in premature infants.

C. Fanconi Syndrome

Generalized dysfunction of the proximal tubule resulting not only in bicarbonate loss but also in variable wasting of phosphate, glucose, and amino acids. May be hereditary, as in cystinosis and galactosemia, or acquired through toxin injury and other immunologic factors. Clinically characterized by rickets and impaired growth.

D. Nephrogenic Diabetes Insipidus

1. **Water conservation is dependent on antidiuretic hormone (ADH) and its effects on the distal renal tubules.** Polyuria, a hallmark of nephrogenic

TABLE 19.9
BIOCHEMICAL AND CLINICAL CHARACTERISTICS OF VARIOUS TYPES OF RENAL TUBULAR ACIDOSIS

	Type 1 (Distal)	Type 2 (Proximal)	Type 4 (Hypoaldosteronism)
Mechanism	Impaired distal acidification	Impaired bicarbonate absorption	Decreased aldosterone secretion or aldosterone effect
Etiology	Hereditary Sickle cell Toxins/drugs Cirrhosis Obstructive uropathy Connective tissue disorder	Hereditary Metabolic disease Fanconi syndrome Prematurity Toxins/heavy metals Amyloidosis PNH	Absolute mineralocorticoid deficiency Adrenal failure CAH DM Pseudohypoaldosteronism Interstitial nephritis
Minimal urine pH	>5.5	<5.5 (urine pH can be >5.5 with a bicarbonate load)	<5.5
Fractional excretion of bicarbonate (FeHCO₃)	↓ (<5%)	↑ (>15%)	↓ (<5%)
Plasma K⁺ concentration	Normal or ↓	Usually ↓	↑
Urine anion gap	Positive	Positive or negative	Positive
Nephrocalcinosis/nephrolithiasis	Common	Rare	Rare
Treatment	1–3 mEq/kg/day of HCO₃ (5–10 mEq/kg/day if bicarb wasting)	5–20 mEq/kg/day of HCO₃	1–5 mEq/kg/day of HCO₃ May add Fludrocortisone and potassium binders

CAH, congenital adrenal hyperplasia; DM, diabetes mellitus; PNH, paroxysmal nocturnal hemoglobinuria
Adapted from Holiday MA et al. Pediatric Nephrology. Baltimore: Williams & Wilkins, 1994:650.

diabetes insipidus (NDI), is due to diminished or lack of response of the ADH receptor in the distal renal tubules. Hereditary defects of ADH receptor or acquired insults (e.g., interstitial nephritis, sickle cell disease, lithium toxicity, CKD) may underlie NDI.

2. **Must be differentiated from other causes of polyuria:**
a. Central diabetes insipidus: ADH deficiency that may be idiopathic or acquired (through infection or pituitary trauma)
b. Diabetes mellitus
c. Psychogenic polydipsia
d. Cerebral salt wasting

IX. CHRONIC KIDNEY DISEASE[20]

Kidney damage for >3 months, as defined by structural or functional abnormalities, with or without decreased GFR. Classified as:

Stage I: Kidney injury with normal or increased GFR
Stage II: GFR 60–89 mL/min/1.73 m^2
Stage III: GFR 30–59 mL/min/1.73 m^2
Stage IV: GFR 15–29 mL/min/1.73 m^2
Stage V: GFR <15 mL/min/1.73 m^2 or dialysis

A. Etiology

There is a close association with age at which kidney failure is first detected. CKD in children <5 years is most commonly due to congenital abnormalities (e.g., kidney hypoplasia/dysplasia, urologic malformations), whereas older children more commonly have acquired glomerular diseases (e.g., glomerulonephritis, FSGS) or hereditary disorders (e.g., Alport syndrome).

B. Clinical Manifestations (Table 19.10)

1. **Edema:**

Secondary to excessive accumulation of both Na$^+$ and water. Causes of generalized edema include:
   a. Inability to excrete Na$^+$ with or without water (e.g., glomerular diseases resulting in decreased GFR)
   b. Decreased oncotic pressure (e.g., nephrotic syndrome, protein-losing enteropathy, hepatic failure, CHF)
   c. Reduced cardiac output (e.g., CHF, pericardial disease)
   d. Mineralocorticoid excess (e.g., hyperreninemia, hyperaldosteronism)
2. **See Table 19.10 for additional manifestations.**

X. CHRONIC HYPERTENSION[21-23]

NOTE: For the management of acute hypertension and normal BP parameters, see Chapters 4 and 7.

A. Definition

1. **Normal blood pressure (BP):** Systolic and diastolic BP <90th percentile for age, gender, and height (See Tables 7.1 and 7.2.)
2. **High-normal BP (prehypertension):** Systolic and/or diastolic BP between 90th and 95th percentiles for age, gender, and height, or if BP exceeds 120/80 mmHg (even if <90th percentile for age, gender, and height)
3. **Hypertension:** Systolic and/or diastolic BPs >95th percentile for age, gender, and height on three separate occasions
4. **Measurement of BP in children:**
   a. Children ≥3 years should have BP measured at all routine and emergency visits. Children aged <3 years with risk factors (e.g., history of prematurity/low birth weight, congenital heart disease, kidney disease or family history of kidney disease, history of malignancy, solid organ or bone marrow transplant) should have BP measured.
   b. BP should be measured in a seated position, 5 minutes after resting quietly; auscultation is preferred.

TABLE 19.10

CLINICAL MANIFESTATIONS OF CHRONIC KIDNEY DISEASE

Manifestation	Mechanisms
Uremia	Decline in GFR
Acidosis	Urinary bicarbonate wasting
	Decreased excretion of NH_4 and acid
Sodium wasting	Solute diuresis, tubular damage
	Aldosterone resistance
Sodium retention	Nephrotic syndrome
	CHF
	Reduced GFR
Urinary concentrating defect	Solute diuresis, tubular damage
	ADH resistance
Hyperkalemia	Decline in GFR, acidosis
	Aldosterone resistance
Renal osteodystrophy	Impaired production of 1,25 (OH) vitamin D
	Decreased intestinal calcium absorption
	Impaired phosphorus excretion
	Secondary hyperparathyroidism
Growth retardation	Protein-calorie deficiency
	Renal osteodystrophy
	Acidosis
	Anemia
	Inhibitors of insulin-like growth factors
Anemia	Decreased erythropoietin production
	Low-grade hemolysis
	Bleeding, iron deficiency
	Decreased erythrocyte survival
	Inadequate folic acid intake
	Inhibitors of erythropoiesis
Bleeding tendency	Thrombocytopenia
	Defective platelet function
Infection	Defective granulocyte function
	Glomerular loss of immunoglobulin/opsonins
Neurologic complaints	Uremic factors
Gastrointestinal ulceration	Gastric acid hypersecretion/gastritis
	Reflux
	Decreased motility
Hypertension	Sodium and water overload
	Excessive renin production
Hypertriglyceridemia	Diminished plasma lipoprotein lipase activity
Pericarditis and cardiomyopathy	Unknown
Glucose intolerance	Tissue insulin resistance

ADH, antidiuretic hormone; CHF, congestive heart failure; GFR, glomerular filtration rate; NH_4, ammonium
Adapted from Brenner BM. Brenner and Rector's The Kidney. 6th ed. Philadelphia: WB Saunders; 2000.

c. Appropriate cuff size has a bladder width at least 40% of upper arm circumference at midway point. Bladder length should cover 80%–100% of arm circumference. Cuffs that are too small may result in falsely elevated BPs. Choose a larger-sized cuff if there is a choice between two.

B. Etiologies of Hypertension in Neonates, Infants, and Children (Table 19.11)

C. Evaluation of Chronic Hypertension

1. **Rule out factitious causes of hypertension** [improper cuff size or measurement technique (e.g., manual vs. oscillometric)], nonpathologic causes of hypertension (e.g., fever, pain, anxiety, muscle spasm), and iatrogenic mechanisms (e.g., medications, excessive fluid administration).
2. **History:** Headache, blurred vision, dyspnea on exertion, edema, obstructive sleep apnea symptoms, endocrine symptoms (diaphoresis, flushing, constipation, weakness, etc.), history of neonatal intensive care unit stay, rule out pregnancy, history of UTIs, history of medications and supplements, illicit drug use, or any family history of kidney dysfunction or hypertension.
3. **Physical examination:** Four-extremity pulses and BPs, endocrine disease stigmata, edema, hypertrophied tonsils, skin lesions, abdominal mass, or abdominal bruit.
4. **Clinical evaluation of confirmed hypertension:**

TABLE 19.11
CAUSES OF HYPERTENSION BY AGE GROUP

Age	Most Common	Less Common
Neonates/infants	Renal artery thrombosis after umbilical artery catheterization Coarctation of aorta Renal artery stenosis	Bronchopulmonary dysplasia Medications Patent ductus arteriosus Intraventricular hemorrhage
1–10 yr	Renal parenchymal disease Coarctation of aorta	Renal artery stenosis Hypercalcemia Neurofibromatosis Neurogenic tumors Pheochromocytoma Mineralocorticoid excess Hyperthyroidism Transient hypertension Immobilization-induced Sleep apnea Essential hypertension Medications
11 yr–adolescence	Renal parenchymal disease Essential hypertension	All diagnoses listed in this table

Modified from Sinaiko A. Hypertension in children. N Engl J Med. *1996;335:26.*

a. Laboratory studies: UA with microscopic evaluation, urine culture, serum electrolytes, CBC, Cr, BUN, fasting glucose, and lipid panel.
b. Imaging: Kidney and bladder ultrasonography and echocardiography. Consider renovascular imaging as indicated.
c. Consider (as indicated) thyroid function tests, urine catecholamines, plasma and urinary steroids, plasma renin, aldosterone, and toxicology screen. Consider polysomnography and retinal examination.

5. **Consider referral to specialist in hypertension**

D. Treatment of Hypertension

1. **Nonpharmacologic:** Aerobic exercise, sodium restriction, smoking cessation, and weight loss indicated in all patients with hypertension. Reevaluate BP after lifestyle interventions, and begin pharmacologic therapy if hypertension persists.
2. **Pharmacologic:** Indications include secondary hypertension, symptomatic hypertension, target-organ damage, diabetes mellitus, and persistent hypertension despite nonpharmacologic measures.

E. Classification of Hypertension in Children and Adolescents, With Measurement Frequency and Therapy Recommendations (Table 19.12)

F. Antihypertensive Drugs for Outpatient Management of Hypertension in Children 1–17 Years of Age (Table 19.13)

XI. NEPHROLITHIASIS[24-26]

A. Epidemiology

Lower incidence than adults but increasingly recognized

B. Risk Factors

Congenital and structural urologic abnormalities (urinary stasis), hypercalciuria, hyperoxaluria/oxalosis, hypocitraturia, other metabolic abnormalities

C. Presentation

Microscopic hematuria (90%), flank/abdominal pain (50%–75%), gross hematuria (30%–55%), and concomitant UTI in up to 20%. Have higher likelihood than adults of having asymptomatic stones, especially younger children.

D. Diagnosis

Ultrasonography is an effective and preferred modality, particularly at centers with expertise, given benefit of avoiding radiation exposure. In certain scenarios (radiolucent stones such as uric acid stones, ureteral stones, and lack of ultrasonographic expertise), noncontrast helical CT may be preferred to improve diagnostic sensitivity.

E. Management

1. **Pain control, urine culture, hydration.** Some centers initiate α-blockers to facilitate stone passage, although evidence of benefit in children is equivocal.

TABLE 19.12
CLASSIFICATION OF HYPERTENSION IN CHILDREN AND ADOLESCENTS AND THERAPY RECOMMENDATIONS

	SBP or DBP Percentile	Frequency of BP Measurement	Pharmacologic Therapy (in Addition to Lifestyle Modifications)
Normal	<90th percentile	Recheck at next physical examination	None
Prehypertension	90th to <95th percentile or if BP exceeds 120/80 mmHg even if <90th percentile	Recheck in 6 months	None unless compelling indications: CKD, DM, heart failure, or LVH
Stage 1 hypertension	95th–99th percentile plus 5 mmHg	Recheck in 1–2 weeks, sooner if patient is symptomatic; if persistently elevated on 2 additional occasions, evaluate or refer	Initiate therapy based on symptoms, secondary hypertension, end-organ damage, diabetes, persistent hypertension despite nonpharmacologic measures
Stage 2 hypertension	>99th percentile plus 5 mmHg	Evaluate or refer within 1 week or immediately if the patient is symptomatic	Initiate therapy

CKD, chronic kidney disease; DBP, diastolic blood pressure; DM, diabetes mellitus; LVH, left ventricular hypertrophy; SBP, systolic blood pressure
Modified from National High Blood Pressure Education Program Working Group on High Blood Pressure in Children and Adolescents: The fourth report on the diagnosis, evaluation, and treatment of high blood pressure in children and adolescents. Pediatrics. 2004;114:555-576.

2. **Urologic intervention** (extracorporeal shock wave lithotripsy, ureteroscopy, and percutaneous nephrolithotomy). May be necessary in setting of unremitting pain or urinary obstruction, especially in the setting of AKI or at-risk patients (e.g., solitary kidney, etc.).
3. **Collect and analyze stone composition to aid in prevention of future stones.**

F. Workup

Up to 75% of children with a kidney stone will have a metabolic abnormality (e.g., hypercalciuria, hyperoxaluria, hyperuricosuria, cystinuria). Workup should include analysis of the stone (if possible), urinalysis, basic metabolic panel, and phosphate, magnesium, and uric acid levels. If evidence of elevated calcium or phosphate, obtain parathyroid hormone (PTH) level and consider checking 25- and

TABLE 19.13

ANTIHYPERTENSIVE DRUGS FOR OUTPATIENT MANAGEMENT OF HYPERTENSION IN CHILDREN 1–17 YEARS OF AGE

Class	Drug	Comments
Angiotensin-converting enzyme (ACE) inhibitor	Benazepril Captopril Enalapril Fosinopril Lisinopril Quinapril	Blocks angiotensin I to angiotensin II Decreases proteinuria while preserving renal function Contraindicated in pregnancy, compromised renal perfusion Check serum potassium and creatinine periodically to monitor for hyperkalemia and uremia Monitor for cough and angioedema
Angiotensin-II receptor blocker (ARB)	Irbesartan Losartan	Contraindicated in pregnancy Check serum potassium and creatinine periodically to monitor for hyperkalemia and uremia
α- and β-Blockers	Labetalol Carvedilol	Cause decreased peripheral resistance and decreased heart rate Contraindications: asthma, heart failure, insulin-dependent diabetes Heart rate is dose-limiting May impair athletic performance
β-Blocker	Atenolol Metoprolol Propranolol	Decreases heart rate, cardiac output, and renin release Noncardioselective agents (e.g., propranolol) are contraindicated in asthma and heart failure Metoprolol and atenolol are β_1 selective Heart rate is dose-limiting May impair athletic performance Should not be used in insulin-dependent diabetics
Calcium channel blocker	Amlodipine Felodipine Isradipine Extended-release nifedipine	Acts on vascular smooth muscles Renal perfusion/function is minimally affected; generally few side effects Amlodipine and isradipine can be compounded into suspensions May cause tachycardia
Central α-agonist	Clonidine	Stimulates brainstem α_2 receptors and decreases peripheral adrenergic drive May cause dry mouth and/or sedation ($\downarrow$ opiate withdrawal) Transdermal preparation also available Sudden cessation of therapy can lead to severe rebound hypertension

TABLE 19.13

ANTIHYPERTENSIVE DRUGS FOR OUTPATIENT MANAGEMENT OF HYPERTENSION IN CHILDREN 1–17 YEARS OF AGE—cont'd

Class	Drug	Comments
Diuretic	Furosemide Bumetanide	Side effects are hyponatremia, hypokalemia, and ototoxicity
	Hydrochlorothiazide Chlorthalidone	Side effects are hypokalemia, hypercalcemia, hyperuricemia, and hyperlipidemia
	Spironolactone Triamterene	Useful as add-on therapy in patients being treated with drugs from other drug classes
	Amiloride	Potassium-sparing diuretics are modest antihypertensives. They may cause severe hyperkalemia, especially if given with ACE inhibitor or ARB
Peripheral α-antagonist	Doxazosin Prazosin Terazosin	May cause hypotension and syncope, especially after first dose
Vasodilator	Hydralazine	Hydralazine can cause a lupus-like syndrome Directly acts on vascular smooth muscle and is very potent Tachycardia, Na retention, and water retention are common side effects
	Minoxidil	Used in combination with diuretics or β-blockers Minoxidil is usually reserved for patients with hypertension resistant to multiple drugs

Modified from National High Blood Pressure Education Program Working Group on High Blood Pressure in Children and Adolescents. The fourth report on the diagnosis, evaluation, and treatment of high blood pressure in children and adolescents. Pediatrics. 2004;114:568-569; Hospital for Sick Children. The HSC Handbook of Pediatrics. 9th ed. St. Louis: Mosby, 1997; Sinaiko A. Treatment of hypertension in children. Pediatr Nephrol. 1994;8:603-609; and Khattak S et al. Efficacy of amlodipine in pediatric bone marrow transplant patients. Clin Pediatr. 1998:37:31-35.

1,25(OH) vitamin D levels. A 24-hour urine collection should be obtained several weeks after the stone has passed, and urine sodium, calcium, urate, oxalate, citrate, creatinine, and cystine should be evaluated.

G. Prevention

1. **Recurrence of a kidney stone in children is common.**
2. **All children with history of stones should increase fluid intake** (e.g., at least 2 L/day in those aged >10 years old).
3. **Targeted interventions of any identified metabolic abnormalities** (e.g., low-sodium diet in those with hypercalciuria). Pharmacologic interventions are also available in certain scenarios (e.g., citrate supplementation).
4. **Dietary Modifications:** Long–term adherence (5 years) to normal calcium, low–sodium diet may decrease recurrence of stones in people with idiopathic hypercalciuria with recurrent nephrolithiasis.[26]

REFERENCES

1. Fischbach FT, Dunning MB. *A Manual of Laboratory and Diagnostic Tests*. 8th ed. Philadelphia: Lippincott Williams & Wilkins; 2008.
2. Hooton T, Bradley SF, Cardenas DD, et al. Diagnosis, Prevention, and Treatment of Catheter-Associated Urinary Tract Infections in Adults: 2009 International Clinical Practice Guidelines from the Infectious Disease Society of America. *Clin Infect Dis*. 2010;50:625-663.
3. Subcommittee on Urinary Tract Infection, Steering Committee on Quality Improvement and Management. Urinary tract infection: clinical practice guidelines for the diagnosis and management of the initial UTI in febrile infants and children 2 to 24 months. *Pediatrics*. 2011;128:595-610.
4. Michael M, Hodson EM, Craig JC, et al. Short versus standard duration oral antibiotic therapy for acute urinary tract infection in children. *Cochrane Database Syst Rev*. 2003;(1):CD003966, Art. No.: CD003966. doi:10.1002/14651858.
5. Cara-Fuentes G, Gupta N, Garin EH. The RIVUR study: a review of its findings. *Pediatr Nephrol*. 2015;30:703-706. doi:10.1007/s00467-014-3021-2.
6. RIVUR Trial Investigators, Hoberman A, Greenfield SP, et al. Antimicrobial prophylaxis for children with vesicoureteral reflux. *N Engl J Med*. 2014;370(25):2367-2376.
7. Schwartz GJ, Munoz A, Schneider MF. New equations to estimate GFR in children with CKD. *J Am Soc Nephrol*. 2009;20:629-637.
8. Carmody JB. Focus on diagnosis: urine electrolytes. *Pediatr Rev*. 2011;32:65-68.
9. Sargent JD, Stukel TA, Kresel J, et al. Normal values for random urinary calcium to creatinine ratios in infancy. *J Pediatr*. 1993;123:393-397.
10. Whyte DA, Fine RN. Acute renal failure in children. *Pediatr Rev*. 2008;29:299-306.
11. Andreoli SP. Acute kidney injury in children. *Pediatr Nephrol*. 2009;24: 253-263.
12. Ellis JH, Cohan RH. Prevention of contrast-induced nephropathy: an overview. *Radiol Clin North Am*. 2009;47(5):801-811.
13. Schlaudecker JD, Bernheisel CR. Gadolinium-associated nephrogenic systemic fibrosis. *Am Fam Physician*. 2009;80(7):711-714.
14. Massengill SF. Hematuria. *Pediatr Rev*. 2008;29:342-348.
15. Kliegman RM, Stanton BF. *Nelson Textbook of Pediatrics*. 19th ed. Philadelphia: Saunders; 2011.
16. Cruz C, Spitzer A. When you find protein or blood in urine. *Contemp Pediatr*. 1998;15:89.
17. Gipson DS, Massengill SF, Yao L, et al. Management of childhood-onset nephrotic syndrome. *Pediatrics*. 2009;124:747-757.
18. Gordillo R, Spitzer A. The nephrotic syndrome. *Pediatr Rev*. 2009;30:94-104.
19. Soriano JR. Renal tubular acidosis: the clinical entity. *J Am Soc Nephrol*. 2002;13:2160-2170.
20. Whyte DA, Fine RN. Chronic kidney disease in children. *Pediatr Rev*. 2008;29:335-341.
21. Sinaiko A. Hypertension in children. *N Engl J Med*. 1996;335:26.
22. National High Blood Pressure Education Program Working Group on High Blood Pressure in Children and Adolescents. The fourth report on the diagnosis, evaluation, and treatment of high blood pressure in children and adolescents. *Pediatrics*. 2004;114(2 Suppl 4th Report):555-576.

23. Brady TM, Solomon B, Siberry G. Pediatric hypertension: a review of proper screening, diagnosis, evaluation, and treatment. *Contemp Pediatr.* 2008;25:46-56.
24. Tanaka ST, Pope JC 4th. Pediatric stone disease. *Curr Urol Rep.* 2009;10:138-143.
25. McKay CP. Renal stone disease. *Pediatr Rev.* 2010;31:179-188.
26. Escribano J, Balaguer A, Roqué i Figuls M, Feliu A, Ferre N. Dietary interventions for preventing complications in idiopathic hypercalciuria. *Cochrane Database Syst Rev.* 2014;(2):CD006022.

Chapter 20
Neurology
Clare Stevens, MD

See additional content on Expert Consult

I. WEB RESOURCES
- Child Neurology Society: www.childneurologysociety.org
- American Academy of Neurology Practice Guidelines: www.aan.com/Guidelines/
- American Heart Association Statement on Management of Stroke in Infants and Children: www.stroke.ahajournals.org

II. NEUROLOGIC EXAMINATION

A. Mental Status
Evaluate alertness and orientation to time, person, place, and current situation. Assess attentiveness and behavior in infants. Play interests are a window into development.

B. Cranial Nerves (Table 20.1)

C. Motor
1. **Muscle bulk**
2. **Tone:** Infants with low tone will slip when held under their arms.
   a. Passive movements: Resting resistance to examiner's movement
   b. Active movements: Regulation of power with defined movements (e.g., posture, gait, pull to stand).
3. **Power/strength:** Assess and quantify activity [e.g., rising from the floor, distance of standing broad jump, time to run 30 feet or climb 10 stairs (Box 20.1)].

D. Sensory (Fig. 20.1 and Table 20.2)
1. **Spinal cord level:** Best assessed with pinprick and temperature. If concerned about spinal cord impairment, ask about continence. Compare lower with upper, check both anterior and posterior trunk.
2. **Intraspinal lesions:**
   a. Anterior pathways: Pinprick and temperature
   b. Posterior pathways: Vibratory and joint position sense
3. **Root/plexus/nerve impairment:** Pin sensibility; consult dermatomal/nerve maps (see Fig. 20.1).
4. **Polyneuropathy:** Large fiber (vibration and position sense) vs. small fiber (pinprick and temperature). Compare distal with proximal sites in a limb and lower with upper extremities.

TABLE 20.1

CRANIAL NERVES

Function/Region	Cranial Nerve	Test/Observation
Olfactory	I	Smell (e.g., coffee, vanilla, peppermint)
Vision	II	Acuity, fields, fundus
Pupils	II, III	Sympathetic activity, size, reaction to light, accommodation
Eye movements and eyelids	III, IV, VI	Range and quality of eye movements, saccades, pursuits, nystagmus, ptosis
Sensation	V	Corneal reflexes, facial sensation
Muscles of mastication	V	Clench teeth
Facial strength	VII	Degree of expression of emotions; strength of eye closure, smile, and puffing out cheeks; facial symmetry
Hearing	VIII	Localize sound, attend to finger rub, audiologic testing
Mouth, pharynx	IX, X	Swallowing, speech quality, symmetrical palatal elevation, gag reflex
Head control	XI	Lateral head movement, shoulder shrug
Tongue movement	XII	Tongue protrusion, push tongue against inner cheek

TABLE 20.2

UPPER AND LOWER MOTOR NEURON FINDINGS

On Examination	Upper	Lower
Power	Decreased	Decreased
Reflexes	Increased	Decreased
Tone	Increased	Normal or decreased
Babinski	Upgoing (present)	Downgoing (normal)
Fasciculations	Absent	Present
Muscle wasting	Absent	Present

BOX 20.1

STRENGTH RATING SCALE

0/5: No movement (i.e., no palpable tension at tendon)
1/5: Flicker of movement
2/5: Movement in a gravity-neutral plane
3/5: Movement against gravity but not resistance
4/5: Subnormal strength against resistance
5/5: Normal strength against resistance

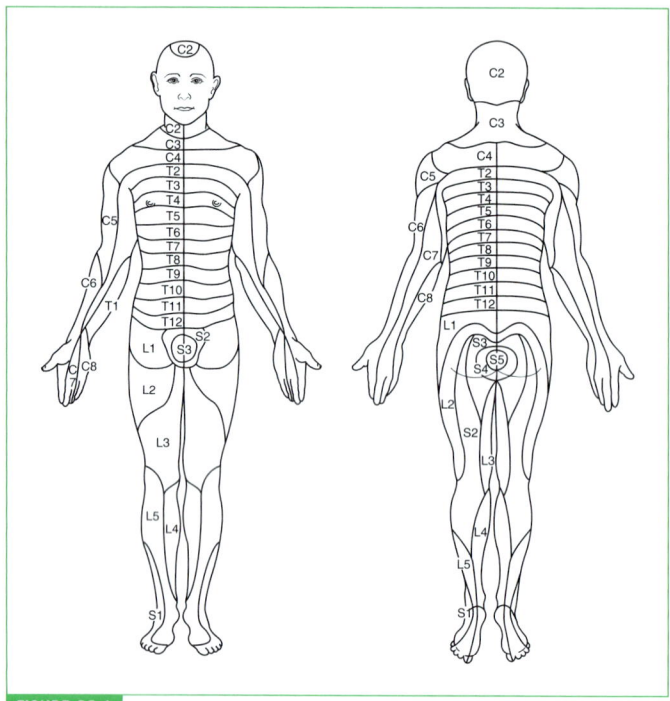

FIGURE 20.1

Dermatomes. *(From Athreya BH, Silverman BK. Pediatric physical diagnosis. Norwalk, CT: Appleton-Century-Crofts; 1985:238-239.)*

BOX 20.2

REFLEX RATING SCALE

0: None
1+: Diminished (need use of clasped hands/gritting teeth to engage reflex)
2+: Normal
3+: Increased (reflexes cross neighboring joint or cross to other side)
4+: Hyperactive with clonus

E. Tendon Reflexes

This assessment is most helpful in localizing other abnormalities, especially in the presence of weakness or asymmetry. Compare right with left sides, upper with lower extremities, and distal with proximal reflexes (Box 20.2 and Table EC 20.A on Expert Consult).

1. **Isolated abnormality of reflexes:** Little significance in the setting of normal strength and coordination
2. **Brisk reflexes combined with weakness:** Indicate upper motor neuron disorder
3. **Absent reflexes:**
  a. Muscle disease: Reflexes usually diminished commensurate with power
  b. Selective reflex dropout: Spinal cord, root, or nerve lesion

F. Coordination and Movement

1. **Evaluate general coordination while watching activities** (e.g., throwing a ball, dressing, writing, drawing)
2. **Tests for cerebellar function:** Rapid alternating movements, finger-to-nose, heel-to-shin, walking, running
3. **Extra movements:** Quality and conditions under which they are enhanced or suppressed (tremor, dystonia, chorea, athetosis, tics, myoclonus)

III. HEADACHES[1-3]

A. Evaluation of Headaches

1. **Classification:** Primary versus secondary[4]
  a. Primary headaches: Migraines, tension-type, cluster, trigeminal autonomic cephalgias (TACs)
  b. Secondary headaches: Caused by other underlying pathologies. Differential diagnoses in Boxes 20.3 and 20.4
2. **History and physical examination:** See Boxes 20.5 and 20.6 and Table EC 20.B on Expert Consult.

BOX 20.3

DIFFERENTIAL DIAGNOSIS OF ACUTE HEADACHE

Evaluation of the first acute headache should exclude pathologic causes listed here before more common etiologies are considered.
1. Increased intracranial pressure (ICP): Trauma, hemorrhage, tumor, hydrocephalus, pseudotumor cerebri, abscess, arachnoid cyst, cerebral edema
2. Decreased ICP: After ventriculoperitoneal shunt, lumbar puncture, cerebrospinal fluid leak from basilar skull fracture
3. Meningeal inflammation: Meningitis, leukemia, subarachnoid or subdural hemorrhage
4. Vascular: Vasculitis, arteriovenous malformation, hypertension, cerebrovascular accident
5. Bone, soft tissue: Referred pain from scalp, eyes, ears, sinuses, nose, teeth, pharynx, cervical spine, temporomandibular joint
6. Infection: Systemic infection, encephalitis, sinusitis, etc.
7. First migraine

BOX 20.4
DIFFERENTIAL DIAGNOSIS OF RECURRENT OR CHRONIC HEADACHES

1. Migraine (with or without aura)
2. Tension
3. Analgesic rebound
4. Caffeine withdrawal
5. Sleep deprivation (e.g., in children with sleep apnea) or chronic hypoxia
6. Tumor
7. Psychogenic: conversion disorder, malingering, depression, acute stress, mood disorder
8. Cluster headache
9. Chronic daily headache

BOX 20.5
HEADACHE WARNING SIGNS ON HISTORY

1. Pain that awakens child from sleep
2. Age < 3 years
3. Pain made worse with straining or Valsalva
4. Explosive onset
5. Focal deficits
6. Headache associated with persistent emesis or upon awakening
7. Changes in chronic pattern or steady worsening of headaches
8. Altered mental status: Changes in mood, personality, school performance
9. Concurrent fever

BOX 20.6
IMPORTANT HISTORICAL INFORMATION IN EVALUATING HEADACHE

1. Age at onset
2. Associated trauma
3. Presence or absence of aura
4. Change in weight or other constitutional symptoms
5. Change in vision or any other neurologic symptoms
6. Frequency, severity, and duration of headaches (ask about school absences)
7. Quality, site, and radiation of pain (focal occipital pain is concerning for secondary headaches)
8. Associated symptoms such as weakness, tingling, photophobia, phonophobia
9. Triggers and alleviating/exacerbating factors
10. Family history of migraine
11. Changes and new stressors in school or at home

> **BOX 20.7**
>
> **LUMBAR PUNCTURE**[33]
> - Indications: Fever, infection, concern for pseudotumor cerebri or other causes of increased intracranial pressure after negative imaging.
> - Contraindications: Elevated intracranial pressure or mass effect, owing to concern for herniation. Obtain a head CT before lumbar puncture if this is a concern.
> - Standard tests: Cell counts + differential, Gram stain, cerebrospinal fluid (CSF) culture, protein, glucose. Consider viral studies (herpes simplex virus, enterovirus, etc.).
> - Special tests: Manometer for opening pressure if concern for pseudotumor cerebri. Performed in a lateral decubitus position with legs extended.
> - Correction for white blood cells (WBCs): Expected CSF WBC count = [red blood cells (RBCs) CSF/RBCs serum] × WBCs serum.
> - Xanthochromia: Yellow or pink discoloration of CSF due to breakdown of hemoglobin. If CSF is xanthochromic, suspect subarachnoid hemorrhage.

3. **Studies**[2]
a. Neuroimaging: Not indicated if there are no red flags on history and neurologic and funduscopic exams are normal. Computed tomography (CT) without contrast or magnetic resonance imaging (MRI) should be obtained for focal neurologic findings, suspected increased intracranial pressure (ICP), abnormal level of consciousness, atypical or progressive headaches, seizures, and abrupt-onset severe headaches. CT provides poor imaging of the posterior fossa (see Chapter 25 for more detailed advantages of each modality).
b. Laboratory studies: Not routinely indicated if no red flags.
c. Lumbar puncture: Not routinely indicated if no red flags (Box 20.7).
d. Electroencephalogram (EEG): Not routinely indicated if no red flags.

B. Migraine Headache

1. **Box 20.8 lists diagnostic criteria.** Migraines are typically throbbing, pulsatile, or pressure-like in children. They are usually bifrontal in children and unilateral in adolescents and adults. There are many potential triggers (e.g., stress, caffeine, menses, sleep disruption).
2. **Classification**[4]:
a. With aura: *Aura* is any neurologic symptom that occurs prior to onset of a migraine (e.g., visual aberrations, paresthesias, numbness, dysphasia).
b. Without aura
3. **Precursors to migraines and close associations include** cyclic vomiting, abdominal migraines, recurrent abdominal pain, paroxysmal vertigo of childhood, paroxysmal torticollis of infancy, and motion sickness.
4. **Treatment**[5,6,7,8]: Includes reassurance and education regarding lifestyle modification (e.g., sleep, hygiene, exercise, stress reduction, fluids,

> **BOX 20.8**
>
> **DIAGNOSTIC CRITERIA FOR PEDIATRIC MIGRAINE WITHOUT AURA**[4,34]
>
> At least five attacks fulfilling the following criteria:
> 1. Headache 2–72 hours in children younger than 18 years (untreated or unsuccessfully treated)
> 2. At least two of the following characteristics:
>   a. Unilateral or bilateral
>   b. Pulsating quality
>   c. Moderate to severe in intensity
>   d. Aggravated by or causing avoidance of routine physical activities
> 3. At least one of the following occur during the headache:
>   a. Nausea and/or vomiting
>   b. Photophobia and phonophobia (which may be inferred from behavior)
> 4. Not better accounted for by another diagnosis

TABLE 20.3

ABORTIVE TRIPTANS FOR MIGRAINE[‡]

Medication	Dose (Preparation)	Duration[†]
Sumatriptan (Imitrex)	6 mg (SQ); 5, 20 mg (NS); 25, 50, 100 mg (T)	Short
Rizatriptan (Maxalt) 6 years and older	5, 10 mg (T); 5, 10 mg (D)	Short
Zolmitriptan (Zomig) 12 years and older	2.5, 5 mg (NS)	Short
Almotriptan (Axert) 12 years and older	6.25, 12.5 mg (T)	Short
Eletriptan (Relpax)*	20, 40 mg (T)	Short
Naratriptan (Amerge)*	1, 2.5 mg (T)	Long
Frovatriptan (Frova)*	2.5 mg (T)	Long

*Safety and efficacy not established in children aged <18 years, although, still widely used clinically
[†]Short (4-hr half-life); long (12- to 24-hr half-life).
[‡]See Formulary for specific dosing.
D, dissolvable tablet; NS, nasal spray; SQ, subcutaneous; T, tablet

not missing meals). Refer any child with focal neurologic deficits to a pediatric neurologist.

a. Acute symptomatic: Avoid medication overuse (>2–3 doses/week); it can lead to rebound headache.
b. Outpatient setting
   (1) Dark, quiet room, and sleep.
   (2) Nonsteroidal antiinflammatory drugs (NSAIDs) (e.g., naproxen, ibuprofen, ketorolac, and acetaminophen).
   (3) Caffeine (e.g., coffee, tea, soda).
   (4) Triptans (Table 20.3). Objective data support nasal sumatriptan, which has been studied in children as young as 5 years of age. In 2009, the U.S. Food and Drug Administration (FDA) approved

almotriptan for migraine treatment in adolescents aged 12–17 years. Only effective at onset of migraine; typically not used in emergency room or inpatient setting.
- (5) Antidopaminergics (e.g., metoclopramide, prochlorperazine, promethazine) have antiemetic properties, though effective even if nausea is not a predominant factor. Prochlorperazine shown to be superior to metoclopramide.
- c. Emergency room/inpatient setting
  - (1) Often helpful to combine medications and administer intravenous (IV) "migraine cocktail"—typically a NSAID (i.e., ketorolac), antidopaminergic (prochlorperazine, metoclopramide), antihistamine (diphenhydramine) along with IV normal saline bolus.
  - (2) Steroids (e.g., methylprednisolone) may be useful in intractable cases, although evidence is lacking.
  - (3) Magnesium may be useful in intractable cases, although evidence is lacking.
  - (4) Dihydroergotamine.
  - (5) Sodium valproate.
- d. Chronic treatment (if less than three migraines per month and if migraines interfere with daily functioning or school):
  - (1) Avoid triggers and stress. Balanced diet restrictive of certain migraine-causing foods (especially caffeine). Headache journal to help identify potential triggers. Encourage aerobic exercise and regular sleep. Keep hydrated.
  - (2) Offer counseling when appropriate; also consider biofeedback, acupuncture, yoga, and massage therapy if parents are interested.
  - (3) Consider medications (Table 20.4).

IV. PAROXYSMAL EVENTS

A. Differential Diagnosis of Recurrent Events That Mimic Epilepsy in Childhood (Table 20.5)

B. Seizures: First and Recurrent[9,10]

1. **Seizure:** Paroxysmal synchronized discharge of cortical neurons resulting in alteration of function (motor, sensory, cognitive)
2. **Causes of seizures**
- a. Diffuse brain dysfunction: Fever, metabolic compromise, toxin or drugs, hypertension
- b. Focal brain dysfunction: Stroke, neoplasm, focal cortical dysgenesis, trauma
3. **Febrile illness–associated seizures**[11]
- a. Definitions:
  - (1) Simple febrile seizure: Primary generalized seizure associated with fever in a child 6–60 months of age that is nonfocal, lasts for <15 minutes, and does not recur in a 24-hour period

TABLE 20.4
PREVENTIVE THERAPIES FOR MIGRAINE*

Medications	Adverse Effects	Consider in Patients With the Following Comorbidities
ANTICONVULSANT MEDICATIONS		
Divalproex sodium (Depakote)	Dizziness, drowsiness, weight gain, gastrointestinal upset, teratogenicity, potential liver injury	Bipolar, epilepsy, underweight
Topiramate (Topamax)	Cognitive changes, weight loss, sensory changes, paresthesias, kidney stones	Obesity, epilepsy
ANTIDEPRESSANT MEDICATIONS		
Amitriptyline (Elavil)	Sedation, dry mouth, constipation	Depression, insomnia
Nortriptyline	Sedation, dry mouth, constipation	Depression, insomnia
ANTIHISTAMINE MEDICATION		
Cyproheptadine (Periactin)	Sedation, increased appetite	Seasonal allergies, poor appetite, insomnia
β-BLOCKER		
Propranolol (Inderal)	Hypotension, exacerbates exercise-induced asthma, masks hypoglycemia	Hypertension

*See Formulary for specific dosing.

(2) Complex febrile seizure: Seizure associated with a fever in a child 6–60 months of age that is focal, lasts for >15 minutes, or recurs within a 24-hour period
b. No further workup is necessary for a simple febrile seizure in a neurologically intact child who appears well, has a normal neurologic examination, is fully immunized, and has no meningeal signs.
c. Neuroimaging and EEG are not routinely recommended in previously healthy children who have had a simple febrile seizure. Further studies should be directed toward ascertaining the source of the fever.
d. Perform a lumbar puncture in any child with seizures and meningeal signs or symptoms (e.g., nuchal rigidity, Kernig's and/or Brudzinski signs, etc.).
e. Consider lumbar puncture in these circumstances:
   (1) Infant 6–12 months of age with incomplete or unknown *Haemophilus influenzae* or *Streptococcus pneumoniae* immunizations
   (2) Febrile seizure in a child pretreated with antibiotics. Antibiotics can mask signs and symptoms of meningitis
4. **Evaluation of nonfebrile seizures**
a. If clinically indicated, check glucose, Na, K, Ca, Phos, blood urea nitrogen, creatinine, complete blood cell count toxicology screen.

TABLE 20.5
DIFFERENTIAL DIAGNOSIS OF RECURRENT EVENTS THAT MIMIC EPILEPSY IN CHILDHOOD[9]

Event	Differentiation From Epilepsy
Nonepileptic event (formerly pseudoseizure)	No EEG changes except movement artifact during event; movements thrashing rather than clonic; brief/absent postictal period; most likely to occur in patient with epilepsy
Paroxysmal vertigo (toddler)	Patient frightened and crying; no loss of awareness; staggers and falls, vomiting, dysarthria
GER in infancy, childhood	Paroxysmal dystonic posturing associated with meals (Sandifer syndrome)
Breath-holding spells (18 mo–3 yr)	Loss of consciousness and generalized convulsions, always provoked by an event that makes child cry
Syncope	Loss of consciousness with onset of dizziness and clouded or tunnel vision; slow collapse to floor; triggered by postural change, heat, emotion, etc.
Cardiogenic syncope	Abnormal ECG/Holter monitor finding (e.g., prolonged QT, atrioventricular block, other arrhythmias); exercise a possible trigger; episodic loss of consciousness without consistent convulsive movement
Cough syncope	Prolonged cough spasm during sleep in asthmatic, leading to loss of consciousness, often with urinary incontinence
Paroxysmal dyskinesias	May be precipitated by sudden movement or startle; not accompanied by change in alertness
Shuddering attacks	Brief shivering spells with continued awareness
Night terrors (4–6 yr)	Brief nocturnal episodes of terror without typical convulsive movements
Rages (6–12 yr)	Provoked and goal-directed anger
Tics/habit spasms	Involuntary, nonrhythmic, repetitive movements not associated with impaired consciousness; suppressible
Narcolepsy	Sudden loss of tone secondary to cataplexy; emotional trigger; no postictal state or loss of consciousness; EEG with recurrent REM sleep attacks
Migraine (confusional)	Headache or visual changes that may precede attack; family history of migraine; autonomic or sensory changes that can mimic focal seizure; EEG with regional area of slowing during attack
Myoclonus	Involuntary muscle jerking or twitch

ECG, electrocardiography; EEG, electroencephalography; GER, gastroesophageal reflux; REM, rapid eye movement

- b. EEG is recommended in all children with first nonfebrile seizure to evaluate for an epilepsy syndrome.[12] Routine interictal EEGs may be normal in children with focal epilepsies. Repeat EEGs, prolonged EEG monitoring with video, or studies done with sleep deprivation or photic stimulation may be more informative (if clinically indicated).
- c. If this is not the first seizure and patient is receiving anticonvulsant therapy, a change in seizure pattern should prompt a drug level (see Table 20.7 for therapeutic drug levels).

d. Imaging: Although not required for diagnosis, MRI and CT can detect focal brain abnormalities that may predispose to focal seizures.
   (1) Head ultrasound may be used in early infancy and requires open fontanelles.
   (2) Head CT without contrast: Can detect mass lesions, acute hemorrhage, hydrocephalus, and calcifications secondary to congenital disease such as cytomegalovirus infection. Obtain a head CT only when concerned about a mass or bleed or in an emergency situation (due to radiation risk).
   (3) Brain MRI without contrast: Obtain in infants with epilepsy and children with recurrent partial seizures, focal neurologic deficits, or developmental delay. Not routinely indicated when evaluating a first-time seizure.
5. **Seizure disorders (epilepsy):** Assess seizure type (Table 20.6), epilepsy classification (Box 20.9), and severity of disorder

---

BOX 20.9
INTERNATIONAL CLASSIFICATION OF EPILEPTIC SEIZURES[10]

I. Partial Seizures (Seizures With Focal Onset)

1. Simple partial seizures (consciousness unimpaired)
   a. With motor signs
   b. With somatosensory or special sensory symptoms
   c. With autonomic symptoms or signs
   d. With psychic symptoms (higher cerebral functions)
2. Complex partial seizures (consciousness impaired)
   a. Starting as simple partial seizures
      (a) Without automatisms
      (b) With automatisms (e.g., lip smacking, drooling, dazed-eyes look)
   b. With impairment of consciousness at onset
      (a) Without automatisms
      (b) With automatisms
3. Partial seizures evolving into secondary generalized seizures

II. Generalized Seizures

1. Absence seizures: Brief lapse in awareness without postictal impairment (atypical absence seizures may have mild clonic, atonic, tonic, automatism, or autonomic components)
2. Myoclonic seizures: Brief, repetitive, symmetrical muscle contractions
3. Clonic seizures: Rhythmic jerking, flexor spasm of extremities
4. Tonic seizures: Sustained muscle contraction
5. Tonic–clonic seizures
6. Atonic seizures: Abrupt loss of muscle tone

III. Unclassified Epileptic Seizures

TABLE 20.6
SPECIAL SEIZURE SYNDROMES[9,20,32]

Syndrome	Etiology	Evaluation	Treatment	Comment
Neonatal seizures	Brain malformation, hypoxic–ischemic encephalopathy, intracranial hemorrhage, inborn errors of metabolism, CNS infection, cerebral infarction, hypoglycemia, hypocalcemia, hypomagnesemia	Screen for electrolyte and metabolic abnormalities and pyridoxine deficiency, workup for sepsis, LP, head ultrasound, CT or MRI, EEG	Treat underlying abnormality, consider pyridoxine ± EEG, phenobarbital (± additional agents).	Occurs within first 28 days of life; may be myoclonic, tonic, clonic, or subtle; presents as blinking, chewing, bicycling, or apnea; distinguished from jitteriness by vital sign changes and inability to provoke or inhibit movements
Infantile spasms	Symptomatic—67%. May be secondary to CNS malformation, acquired infantile brain injury, tuberous sclerosis, Down syndrome, inborn errors of metabolism Cryptogenic—33%	EEG (shows hypsarrhythmia), MRI	High-dose steroids, vigabatrin, topiramate, ketogenic diet	Usual onset after age 2 mos, peak onset 4–6 mos; initiate treatment as soon as possible. Presents as sudden flexion or extension of the trunk and extremities, often in clusters
Absence seizures	Unknown	EEG (sudden generalized 3-Hz spike and slow-wave discharges)	Ethosuximide, valproic acid, lamotrigine	Age of onset 4–8 years; provoked by hyperventilation; staring spells ± automatisms (eye blinking, mouth movements); often resolves spontaneously by puberty; good neurologic outcome

Continued

TABLE 20.6
SPECIAL SEIZURE SYNDROMES—cont'd

Syndrome	Etiology	Evaluation	Treatment	Comment
Benign rolandic epilepsy/BECTS (benign epilepsy of childhood with centrotemporal spikes)	Unknown	EEG (characteristic pattern of centrotemporal spikes)	Treatment is not always necessary; avoid sleep deprivation; if seizures are frequent, may use levetiracetam or oxcarbazepine.	Age of onset 2–13 years; seizures are nocturnal and consist of hemisensory or motor phenomena of the face, motor findings in limbs; most patients outgrow by age 16–18 years.
Juvenile myoclonic epilepsy	Unknown genetic predisposition	Clinical history, sleep-deprived EEG (reveals generalized spike and wave discharges with normal background activity)	Levetiracetam, valproate, lamotrigine, other meds for generalized seizure	Adolescent onset; morning myoclonus; 75%–95% have GTC seizures; good intellectual outcome, no progressive deterioration
Panayiotopoulos syndrome	Benign age-related focal seizure disorder. Prolonged seizure with predominantly autonomic symptoms	EEG (shifting and/or multiple foci, often occipital spikes)	Often not treated owing to benign nature of condition, but occasionally oxcarbazepine and levetiracetam used	Syndrome specific to childhood; symptoms include vomiting, pallor, eye deviation, sweating, ± convulsions
Lennox-Gastaut syndrome	Cryptogenic or symptomatic	Interictal EEG (reveals slow spike and wave discharges)	Pharmacologic and nonpharmacologic treatments have varying degrees of effectiveness. Ketogenic diet helpful.	Age of onset 1–8 years; multiple seizure types, often intractable; intellectual disability

CNS, central nervous system; CT, computed tomography; EEG, electroencephalography; GTC, generalized tonic–clonic; LP, lumbar puncture; MRI, magnetic resonance imaging

6. **Breakthrough seizures**[13]: Causes of seizures in a child with known, typically well-controlled epilepsy including missed medications or outgrowing weight-based dosing, lack of sleep, stress, drugs/alcohol, physical exertion, excessive screen time (television, video games), illness, dehydration, flickering lights, menses, and drug interactions (common ones include tricyclic antidepressants, certain antibiotics, over-the-counter cold preparations, diphenhydramine, herbal supplements, all of which may lower seizure threshold).
7. **Status epilepticus**[14]: Traditionally defined as continuous or recurrent seizures lasting ≥30 minutes without the patient regaining consciousness. For treatment purposes, status epilepticus can be diagnosed after 5 minutes of continuous seizure or at least two discrete seizures without complete recovery of consciousness between them. See Chapter 1 for treatment guidelines.
8. **Treatment**[12,15,16]
a. If patient's first seizure, seizure was nonfocal, and patient has returned to baseline: No anticonvulsant medication indicated. Overall recurrence of seizure varies from 14%–65% in the first year, but is usually about 50%. Most recurrences occur within 1–2 years after the initial event. Epileptiform abnormalities on EEG indicate a higher chance of recurrence.
b. Educate parents and patient (as age–appropriate) regarding epilepsy basics.[17] Review seizure first aid. Recommend supervision during bathing or swimming. Know driver's license laws in the state. Advocate teacher and school awareness.
c. Pharmacotherapy (Table 20.7): Weigh risk of future seizures without therapy against risk for treatment side effects plus residual seizures despite therapy. Reserve pharmacotherapy for recurrent afebrile seizures.
d. Dietary therapies
    (1) Ketogenic diet[18]: High-fat, low-carbohydrate therapy typically used for intractable seizures. Especially effective for infantile spasms, GLUT1 deficiency, Doose syndrome, pyruvate dehydrogenase deficiency, Dravet syndrome, tuberous sclerosis complex, and others. Urine ketones can be monitored to assess compliance. Side effects include acidosis with bicarbonate value as low as 10–15 mEq/L, kidney stones, growth disturbance, and constipation. Typically used for 2 years, but can be maintained for longer.
    (2) Modified Atkins diet[19]: Low-carbohydrate, high-fat but less restrictive. No limits to calories or protein, no need to weigh food, may be started as outpatient. Carbohydrates 10–20 grams per day. Similar efficacy, tends to be used in adolescents and adults.

TABLE 20.7
COMMONLY USED ANTICONVULSANTS

Anticonvulsant (Trade Name)	Standard Therapeutic Levels (mg/dL)	Efficacy (Generalized/Partial)	IV Preparation Available?	Side Effects
Carbamazepine (Tegretol/Carbatrol)	8–12	P	No	Sedation, ataxia, diplopia, Stevens-Johnson syndrome, blood dyscrasias, hepatotoxicity, may worsen generalized seizures
Clobazam (Onfi)	n/a	G/P	No	Sedation, dizziness
Clonazepam (Klonopin)	n/a	G/P	No	Sedation, drooling, dependence
Ethosuximide (Zarontin)	40–100	G (absence)	No	Gastrointestinal upset
Felbamate (Felbatol)	40–100	G/P	No	Weight loss, hepatotoxicity, sleep disturbances, aplastic anemia (1:7900)
Gabapentin (Neurontin)	3–18	P	No	Weight gain, leg edema, dizziness
Lacosamide (Vimpat)	n/a	P	Yes	Sedation, reduced benefit with sodium channel drugs
Lamotrigine (Lamictal)	3–18	G/P	No	Rash (increased risk in combination with valproate). OCPs significantly decrease level.
Levetiracetam (Keppra)	30–60	G/P	Yes	Behavioral changes, irritability, rare psychosis
Oxcarbazepine (Trileptal)	MHD level (5–40)	P	No	Hyponatremia

Perampanel (Fycompa)	n/a	G/P	No	Irritability, dizziness
Phenobarbital (Luminal)	15–40	G/P	Yes	Altered cognition, sedation
Phenytoin (Dilantin)	10–20	P	Yes	Hirsutism, gingival hyperplasia, teratogenicity, rash, purple-glove syndrome with infusion
Pregabalin (Lyrica)	n/a	P	No	Peripheral edema, weight gain, constipation, dizziness, ataxia, sedation
Rufinamide (Banzel)	n/a	G (Lennox-Gastaut syndrome)	No	Shortened QT interval, nausea, dizziness, sedation, headache. Interacts with valproate.
Tiagabine (Gabitril)	n/a	P	No	Can worsen generalized seizures
Topiramate (Topamax)	2–20	G/P	No	Cognitive side effects, weight loss, renal stones, acidosis, glaucoma
Valproic acid (Depakote, Depakene)	75–100	G/P	Yes	Weight gain, alopecia, hepatotoxicity, pancreatitis, PCOS, teratogenicity
Vigabatrin (Sabril)	n/a	G (infantile spasms)	No	Rash, weight gain, irritability, dizziness, sedation, visual field defects (requires ophthalmology evaluations)
Zonisamide (Zonegran)	20–40	G/P	No	Renal stones, weight loss; rare: Stevens-Johnson syndrome, aplastic anemia

G, generalized; IV, intravenous; MHD, 10-monohydroxy metabolite; n/a, not available; OCP, oral contraceptive pill; P, partial; PCOS, polycystic ovarian syndrome
Data based on personal communication with Eric Kossoff, MD, Johns Hopkins Pediatric Neurology.

e. Surgical therapies
   (1) Hemispherectomy, focal resection, corpus callosotomy, vagus nerve stimulation

C. Special Seizure Syndromes[17,20]

See Table 20.6 for seizure types, etiologies, evaluation, and treatment of many common seizure syndromes.

V. HYDROCEPHALUS[21]

A. Diagnosis[21]

Assess increasing head circumference, misshapen skull, frontal bossing, bulging large anterior fontanelle, increased ICP (*setting-sun* eye sign due to upward gaze paresis, increased tone/reflexes, vomiting, irritability, papilledema), and developmental delay. Obtain neuroimaging if increase in head circumference crosses more than two percentile lines or if patient is symptomatic. Differentiate hydrocephalus from megalencephaly or hydrocephalus *ex vacuo*.

B. Treatment

1. **Medical:**
a. Emergently manage acute increase of ICP (see Chapter 4).
b. Slowly progressive hydrocephalus: Acetazolamide and furosemide may provide temporary relief by decreasing the rate of cerebrospinal fluid (CSF) production (see Formulary for dosing).
2. **Surgical:** CSF shunting
a. Shunts: Ventriculoperitoneal shunts used most commonly.
   (1) Shunt dysfunction may be caused by infection, obstruction (clogging or kinking), disconnection, and migration of proximal and distal tips. Patient will develop signs of increased ICP with shunt malfunction.
   (2) Evaluation of shunt integrity: Obtain ultrafast MRI of the head, if available, or head CT (See Chapter 25) to evaluate shunt position, ventricular size, and evidence of increased ICP. Obtain shunt series (skull, neck, chest, and abdominal radiographs) to look for kinking or disconnection. Referral to a neurosurgeon is then warranted to test shunt function and for possible percutaneous shunt drainage.
b. Endoscopic third ventriculostomy may be used to avoid ventricular shunting.

VI. ATAXIA[22,23]

A. Ataxia Definition: Impaired Coordination of Movement and Balance

B. Differential Diagnosis of Acute Ataxia (Box 20.10)

C. Evaluation (Box 20.11)

BOX 20.10
DIFFERENTIAL DIAGNOSIS OF ACUTE ATAXIA

1. Drug ingestion (e.g., phenytoin, carbamazepine, sedatives, hypnotics, phencyclidine) or intoxication (e.g., alcohol, ethylene glycol, hydrocarbon fumes, lead, mercury, thallium)
2. Postinfectious [cerebellitis (e.g., varicella), acute disseminated encephalomyelitis]
3. Head trauma (cerebellar contusion or hemorrhage, posterior fossa hematoma, vertebrobasilar dissection, postconcussive syndrome)
4. Basilar migraine
5. Benign paroxysmal vertigo (migraine equivalent)
6. Intracranial mass lesion (tumor, abscess, vascular malformation)
7. Opsoclonus–myoclonus: Chaotic eye movements combined with ataxia and myoclonus of either postinfectious or paraneoplastic (neuroblastoma or other neural crest tumors) etiology
8. Hydrocephalus
9. Infection (e.g., labyrinthitis)
10. Seizure (ictal or postictal)
11. Vascular events (e.g., cerebellar hemorrhage or stroke)
12. Guillain-Barré syndrome or Miller-Fisher variant (ataxia, ophthalmoplegia, and areflexia). Warning: If bulbar signs present, patient may lose ability to protect airway.
13. Rare inherited paroxysmal ataxias
14. Inborn errors of metabolism (e.g., mitochondrial disorders, aminoacidopathies, urea cycle defects) (See Chapter 13 for workup.)
15. Multiple sclerosis
16. Somatoform disorders (conversion)

BOX 20.11
EVALUATION OF ACUTE ATAXIA (BASED ON CLINICAL SCENARIO)

1. Complete blood cell count, electrolytes, urine and serum toxicology
2. Imaging (computed tomography and/or magnetic resonance imaging)
3. Lumbar puncture
4. Electroencephalography
5. If neuroblastoma is suspected (opsoclonus–myoclonus), obtain urine vanillylmandelic acid and homovanillic acid, and imaging of chest and abdomen.

VII. STROKE[24-27, 28,29,30]

A. Etiology

1. Risk factors for childhood stroke: Congenital heart disease, cerebral arteriopathies, hematologic disorders (sickle cell disease, prothrombotic state), serious systemic infection (meningitis, sepsis), head or neck trauma causing arterial dissection, and drugs.

> **BOX 20.12**
> **DIFFERENTIAL DIAGNOSIS OF ACUTE-ONSET FOCAL NEUROLOGIC DEFICIT**
> 1. Hemiplegic migraine
> 2. Focal seizure
> 3. Postictal (Todd) paralysis
> 4. Cervical spinal cord injury (deficits spare face)
> 5. Ischemic stroke
> 6. Hemorrhagic stroke

> **BOX 20.13**
> **INITIAL WORKUP OF ACUTE STROKE**
> 1. Imaging: Diffusion weighted MRI is the gold standard for diagnosing acute ischemic stroke. In cases where MRI is not readily available or intracranial hemorrhage is suspected, a head CT can be obtained more quickly but may not show an ischemic stroke in the early stages. In addition, vessel imaging should always be obtained by either MR angiography, CT angiography, or, in special circumstances, conventional digital subtraction angiography.
> 2. Initial laboratory studies: Complete blood cell count, comprehensive metabolic panel, erythrocyte sedimentation rate, prothrombin time, partial thromboplastin time, international normalized ratio, type and screen, urine toxicology screen
> 3. Echocardiogram
> 4. Hypercoagulability workup
> 5. Other studies to consider on a case-by-case basis: Fasting lipid panel, rheumatologic and metabolic studies, hemoglobin electrophoresis, and HIV testing

2. Risk factors for prenatal, perinatal, and neonatal stroke: Maternal chorioamnitis, IUGR, PPROM, preeclampsia, maternal diabetes, birth trauma, infant pulmonary hypertension, extracorporeal membrane oxygenation, fetal or maternal prothrombotic disorders.

B. Differential Diagnosis (Box 20.12)

Stroke should be considered in the differential diagnosis for any child who presents with acute-onset focal neurologic deficits, focal seizures with prolonged postictal paralysis, new-onset refractory focal status epilepticus, altered mental status, or unexplained encephalopathy.

C. Initial Workup (Box 20.13)

D. Management[26]

1. **Supportive care is critical** and should proceed rapidly and parallel with initial workup. Ensure airway patency, provide supplemental oxygen to maintain $SaO_2 > 94\%$ and start maintenance IV fluids.

2. **Optimize cerebral perfusion pressure:** Ensure adequate fluid volume and maintenance of median blood pressure (BP) for age. Treatment of hypertension is controversial. Unless BP is extremely elevated, *do not* use acute antihypertensive therapy because hypertension may be a compensatory reaction to maintain cerebral perfusion.
3. **Monitoring:** Assess neurologic status frequently. Aim for normoglycemia (blood glucose 60–120 mg/dL). Treat fevers, with goal core temperature < 37°C. Treat seizures aggressively. Correct dehydration and anemia.
4. **Deep venous thrombosis (DVT) prophylaxis for immobilized patients.**
5. **Antiplatelet and anticoagulation therapy:** If no evidence of hemorrhage, aspirin is typically recommended (1–5 mg/kg/day). Long-term anticoagulation with low-molecular-weight heparin or warfarin may be considered by a specialist on a case-by-case basis in children with substantial risk of recurrent cardiac embolism and cerebral venous sinus thrombosis, and in selected hypercoagulable states.
6. **Children with sickle cell disease:** Hydration and urgent exchange transfusion to reduce sickle hemoglobin to <30% is recommended. Consult a hematologist. Transcranial Doppler now used as means of screening/preventing stroke in patients with sickle cell disease.
7. **Urgent neurology consultation,** along with transfer to a tertiary care center with expertise in childhood stroke.
8. **Thrombolytic therapy**[31]: Thrombolytic therapy may be considered under appropriate circumstances in centers with extensive pediatric stroke experience (American Heart Association guidelines).

REFERENCES

1. Forsyth R, Farrell K. Headache in childhood. *Pediatr Rev*. 1999;20:39-45.
2. Lewis DW, Ashwal S, Dahl G, et al. Practice parameter: evaluation of children and adolescents with recurrent headaches. *Neurology*. 2002;59:490-498.
3. Brenner M, Oakley C, Lewis D. The evaluation of children and adolescents with headache. *Curr Pain Headache Rep*. 2008;12(5):361-366.
4. Headache Classification Committee of the International Headache Society (IHS). The International Classification of Headache Disorders, 3rd edition (beta version). *Cephalalgia*. 2013;33(9):629-808.
5. Lewis D, Ashwal S, Hershey A, et al. Practice parameter: pharmacological treatment of migraine headache in children and adolescents. *Neurology*. 2004;63:2215-2224.
6. Hershey AD, Kabbouche MA, Powers SW. Treatment of pediatric and adolescent migraine. *Pediatr Ann*. 2010;39:416-423.
7. O'Brien HL, Kabbouche MA, Hershey AD. Treating pediatric migraine: an expert opinion. *Expert Opin Pharmacother*. 2012;13(7):959-966.
8. Toldo I, De Carlo D, Bolzonella B, et al. The pharmacological treatment of migraine in children and adolescents: an overview. *Expert Rev Neurother*. 2012;12(9):1133-1142.
9. Murphy JV. Dehkharghani F. Diagnosis of childhood seizure disorders. *Epilepsia*. 1994;35(suppl 2):S7-S17.

10. Committee on Classification and Terminology of the International League against Epilepsy. Classification of epilepsia: its applicability and practical value of different diagnostic categories. *Epilepsia*. 1996;38:1051-1059.
11. Subcommittee on Febrile Seizures, American Academy of Pediatrics. Neurodiagnostic evaluation of the child with a simple febrile seizure. *Pediatrics*. 2011;127:389-394.
12. Hirtz D, Berg A, Bettis D, et al. Practice parameter: treatment of the child with a first unprovoked seizure. *Neurology*. 2003;60:166-175.
13. Schacter SC, Shafer PO, Sirven JI. "Triggers of Seizures." Epilepsy Foundation, Aug. 2013. Web. 3 Oct 2015. <www.epilepsy.com/learn/triggers-seizures>.
14. Lowenstein DH, Bleck T, Macdonald RL. It's time to revise the definition of status epilepticus. *Epilepsia*. 1999;40:120-122.
15. Baumann RJ, Duffner PK. Treatment of children with simple febrile seizures: the AAP practice parameter. American Academy of Pediatrics. *Pediatr Neurol*. 2000;23:11-17.
16. Joshi SM, Singh RK, Shellhaas RA. Advanced treatments for childhood epilepsy: beyond antiseizure medications. *JAMA Pediatr*. 2013;167(1):76-83.
17. Freeman JM, Vining EP, Pillas DJ. *Seizures and Epilepsy in Childhood: A Guide*. 3rd ed. Baltimore: Johns Hopkins Press; 2002.
18. Kossoff EH, Hartman AL. Ketogenic diets: new advances for metabolism-based therapies. *Curr Opin Neurol*. 2012;25:173-178.
19. Kossoff E. "Treating seizures and Epilepsy: Dietary Therapies." Epilepsy Foundation, Oct. 2013. Web. 3 Oct 2015. <http://www.epilepsy.com/learn/treating-seizures-and-epilepsy/dietary-therapies>.
20. Scher MS. Seizures in the newborn infant: diagnosis, treatment and outcomes. *Clin Perinatol*. 1997;24:735-772.
21. Kliegman RM, Stanton BF. In: Kliegman RM, et al., eds. *Nelson Textbook of Pediatrics*, Chapter 585, "Congenital Anomalies of the Central Nervous System," Section 585.11 Hydrocephalus. 19th ed. Philadelphia: Saunders; 2011.
22. Dinolfo EA. Evaluation of ataxia. *Pediatr Rev*. 2001;22:177-178.
23. Ryan M. Acute ataxia in childhood. *J Child Neurol*. 2003;18:309-316.
24. Ichord R. Treatment of pediatric neurologic disorders. In: Singer H, Kossoff EH, Hartman AL, et al., eds. *Treatment of Pediatric Neurologic Disorders*. Boca Raton, FL: Taylor & Francis Group; 2005.
25. Monagle P, Chalmers E, Chan AK, et al. Antithrombotic therapy in neonates and children: ACCP evidence-based clinical practice guidelines. *Chest*. 2008;1336(suppl 6):887S-968S.
26. Roach ES, Golomb M, Adams R, et al. Management of stroke in infants and children: a scientific statement from a Special Writing Group of the American Heart Association Stroke Council and the Council on Cardiovascular Disease in the Young. *Stroke*. 2008;39:2644-2691.
27. Royal College of Physicians of London. Pediatric Stroke Working Group. *Stroke in Childhood: Clinical Guidelines for Diagnosis, Management and Rehabilitation*. London: Royal College of Physicians; 2004.
28. Fox CK, Fullerton HJ. Recent Advances in Childhood Arterial Ischemic Stroke. *Curr Atheroscler Rep*. 2010;12(4):217-224.
29. Mazumdar M, Heeney MM, Sox CM, Lieu TA. Preventing stroke among children with sickle cell anemia: an analysis of strategies that involve transcranial Doppler testing and chronic transfusion. *Pediatrics*. 2007;120(4):e1107-e1116.

30. Chalmers EA. Perinatal stroke: risk factors and management. *Br J Haematol.* 2005;130(3):333-343.
31. Adams HP Jr, Brott TG, Furlan AJ, et al. Guidelines for thrombolytic therapy for acute stroke: a supplement to the guidelines for the management of patients with acute ischemic stroke. A statement for healthcare professionals from a Special Writing Group of the Stroke Council, American Heart Association. *Circulation.* 1996;94(5):1167-1174.
32. Singer HS, Kossoff EH. In: *Treatment of Pediatric Neurological Disorders.* Boca Raton, FL: Taylor & Francis Group; 2005.
33. Fishman RA. *Cerebrospinal Fluid in Diseases of the Nervous System.* 2nd ed. Philadelphia: Saunders; 1992:190.
34. Blume HK. Pediatric headache: a review. *Pediatr Rev.* 2012;33:562-576.

Chapter 21
Nutrition and Growth
Brandon Smith, MD,
and Jenifer Thompson, MS, RD, CSP

See additional content on Expert Consult

I. WEB RESOURCES

A. Professional and Government Organizations
- Growth Charts and Nutrition Information: http://www.cdc.gov
- American Academy of Pediatrics (AAP) Children's Health Topics: http://www.healthychildren.org
- Academy of Nutrition and Dietetics: http://www.eatright.org
- American Society for Parenteral and Enteral Nutrition: http://www.nutritioncare.org
- National Institute of Child Health and Human Development – Breastfeeding: https://www.nichd.nih.gov/health/topics/breastfeeding/Pages/default.aspx
- U.S. Department of Agriculture Healthy Eating Guidelines: http://www.choosemyplate.gov

B. Infant and Pediatric Formula Company Websites
For complete and up-to-date product information regarding more specialized and metabolic formulas, see these websites:
- Enfamil, Enfacare, Nutramigen, and Pregestimil: http://www.meadjohnson.com
- Carnation, Good Start, Nutren, Peptamen, Vivonex, Boost, Alfamino, and Resource: https://www.nestlehealthscience.us/ and http://medical.gerber.com/
- Alimentum, EleCare, Ensure, NeoSure, PediaSure, Pedialyte, Alfamino, and Similac: http://www.abbottnutrition.com
- Bright Beginnings: http://www.brightbeginnings.com
- America's Store Brand: http://www.storebrandformula.com
- KetoCal, Neocate, and Pepdite: http://www.nutricia-na.com

II. ASSESSMENT OF NUTRITIONAL STATUS

A. Elements of Nutritional Assessment
1. **Anthropometric measurements** [weight, length/height, head circumference, body mass index (BMI), skin folds]: Data plotted on growth charts according to age and compared with a reference population

2. **Clinical assessment** [general appearance (e.g., hair, skin, oral mucosa) and gastrointestinal symptoms of nutritional deficiencies]
3. **Dietary evaluation** (feeding history, current intake)
4. **Physical activity and exercise**
5. **Laboratory findings** (comparison with age-based norms)

B. Indicators of Nutritional Status[1] (Growth Charts) (Figs. 21.1 to 21.9; Figs. EC 21.A to 21.C on Expert Consult)

1. **Growth:** Ideally, should be evaluated over time, but one measurement can be used for screening. Height (or length), weight, and weight for height should be plotted on a growth chart for every patient.
2. **BMI:** Defined as an index of healthy weight and a predictor of morbidity and mortality risk. Used to classify underweight and overweight individuals.[2] BMI should be determined and plotted for children ≥2 years. Use this formula to calculate BMI:

$$BMI = wt\ (kg)/[height\ (m)^2]$$

or

$$BMI = wt\ (lb)/[height\ (in)^2] \times 703$$

   NOTE: Height indicates height measured by stadiometer, not recumbent length.

3. **BMI percentile:** BMI percentile is plotted on the Centers for Disease Control and Prevention (CDC) growth charts for children ≥2 years. Although not a direct measure of body fat, it is highly correlated with amount of body fat in most children and adolescents.[2]
4. **Interpretation of growth charts:**
  a. Stunting: Length or height for age <5th percentile
  b. Underweight:
     (1) Children <2 years: weight for height <5th percentile
     (2) Children ≥2 years: BMI for age <5th percentile
  c. Healthy weight: BMI for age 5th percentile to <85th percentile
  d. Overweight:
     (1) Children <2 years: weight for height >95th percentile
     (2) Children ≥2 years: BMI for age 85th to <95th percentile
  e. Obese:
     (1) Children <2 years: no consensus definition exists
     (2) Children ≥2 years: BMI for age ≥95th percentile or BMI ≥30 kg/m^2
5. **Growth charts:** For boys and girls, including weight, height, head circumference, BMI, and height velocity (see Figs. 21.1 to 21.9; Figs. EC 21.A to 21.C on Expert Consult). *CDC recommends that clinicians in the United States use the 2006 World Health Organization (WHO) international growth charts rather than the CDC growth charts for children <24 months.* Growth charts for children aged 0–20 years, including 2000 CDC growth charts for ages 0–36 months and 2006 WHO growth charts for ages 0–24 months, can be downloaded from http://www.cdc.gov/growthcharts/.

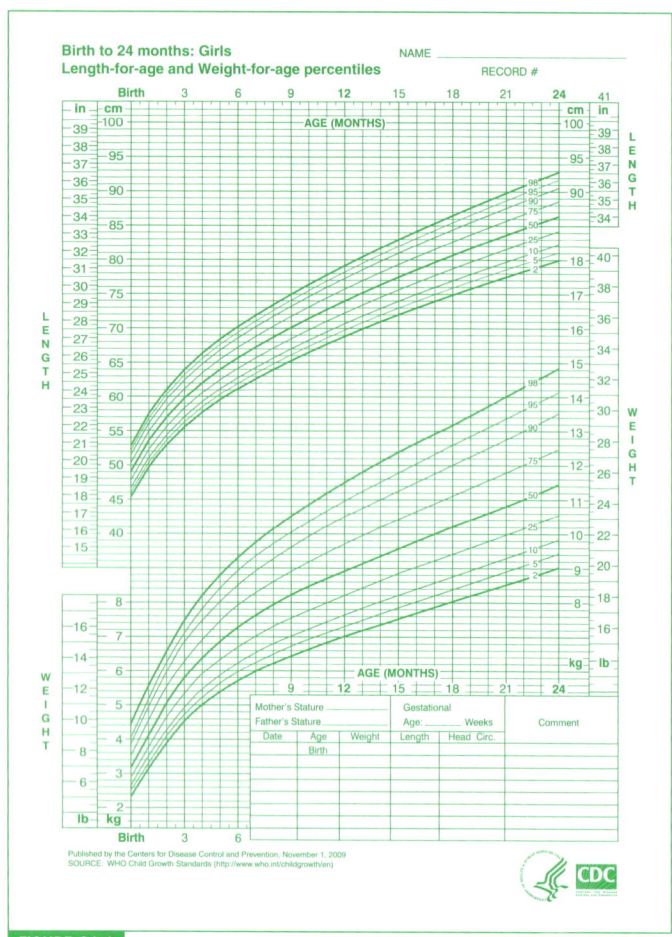

FIGURE 21.1

Length and weight for girls, birth to age 24 months. *(Published by the Centers for Disease Control and Prevention, November 1, 2009. SOURCE: WHO Child Growth Standards at http://www.who.int/childgrowth/en.)*

6. **Growth charts for special populations:**
a. Due to limited reference data, the current CDC recommendation is to use CDC growth charts in all cases; however, condition-specific growth charts do exist and may be useful for illustrative purposes.
7. **Waist circumference and waist/height ratio:** Both waist circumference (WC) and waist/height ratio are indicators of visceral fat or abdominal

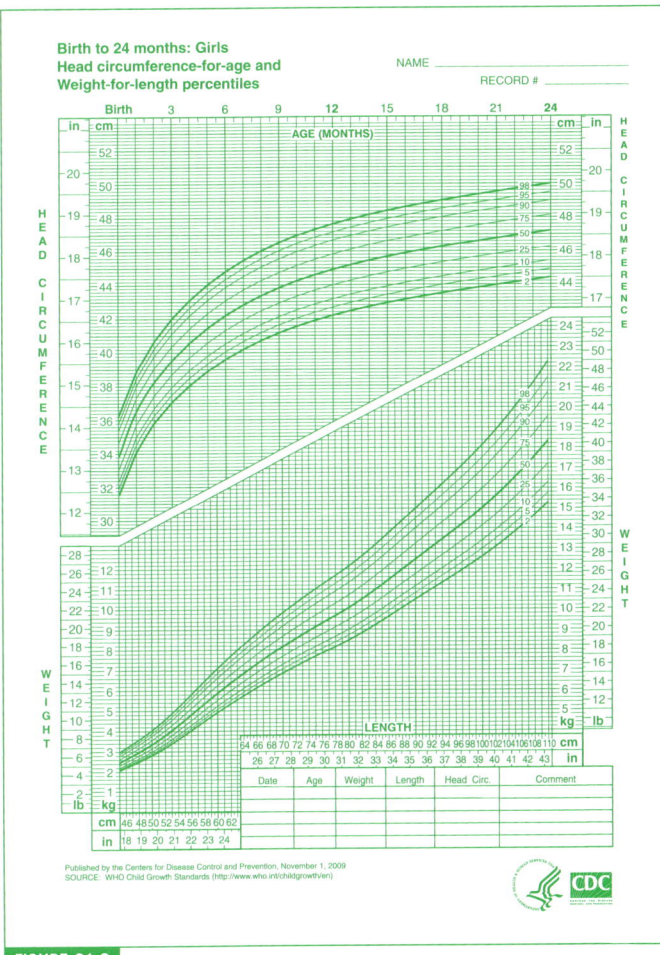

FIGURE 21.2

Head circumference and length-to-weight ratio for girls, birth to age 24 months. *(Published by the Centers for Disease Control and Prevention, November 1, 2009. SOURCE: WHO Child Growth Standards at http://www.who.int/childgrowth/en.)*

obesity in children and adolescents aged 2–19 years. Increased visceral adiposity measured by WC increases the risk of obesity-related morbidity and mortality. WC should be measured at the high point of the iliac crest when the individual is standing and at minimal respiration. Waist/height ratio is calculated as a ratio of WC (cm) and

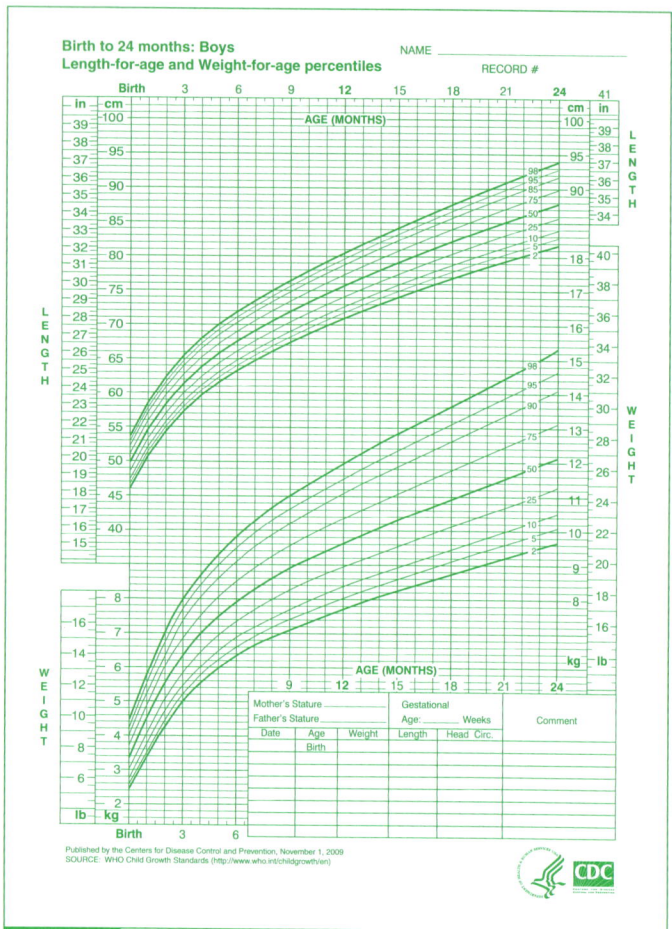

FIGURE 21.3

Length and weight for boys, birth to age 24 months. *(Published by the Centers for Disease Control and Prevention, November 1, 2009. SOURCE: WHO Child Growth Standards at http://www.who.int/childgrowth/en.)*

height (cm).[3] See CDC WC tables for individuals aged 2–19 years (http://www.cdc.gov/nchs/data/nhsr/nhsr010.pdf; Table 18).

C. Recommendations for Management of Overweight and Obese Children
(Fig. EC 21.D on Expert Consult)[4]

1. Management is three-tiered and focused on identification, assessment, and prevention:

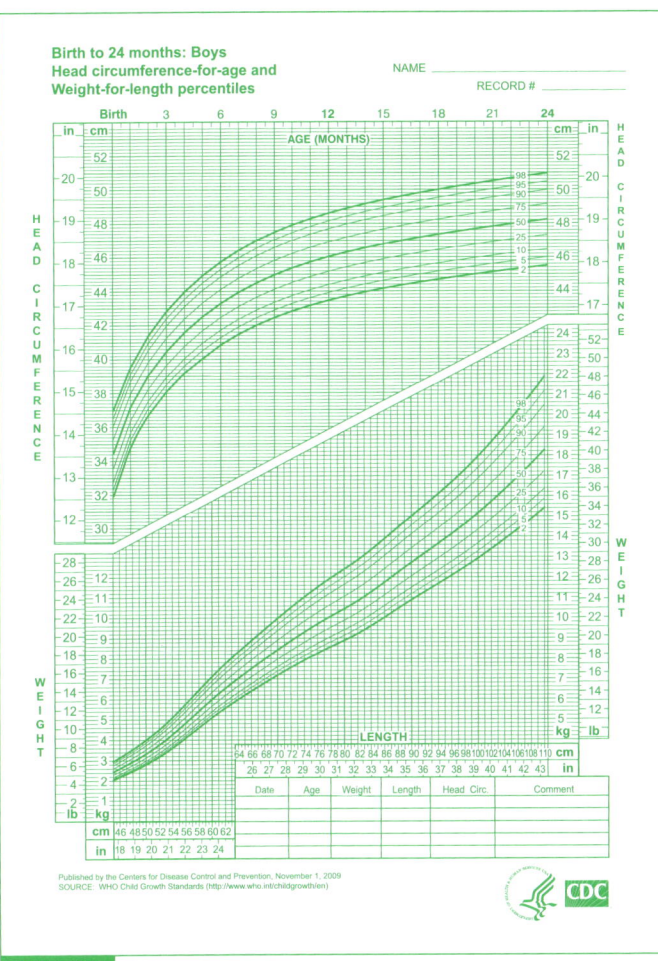

FIGURE 21.4

Head circumference and length-to-weight ratio for boys, birth to age 24 months. *(Published by the Centers for Disease Control and Prevention, November 1, 2009. SOURCE: WHO Child Growth Standards at http://www.who.int/childgrowth/en.)*

    a. Identification: Calculate BMI at each well-child visit
    b. Assessment: Medical risk, behavior risk, and attitude
    c. Prevention: Targeted at behaviors and treatment interventions based on BMI stratification
  2. AAP recommendations[4]:

576 Part II Diagnostic and Therapeutic Information

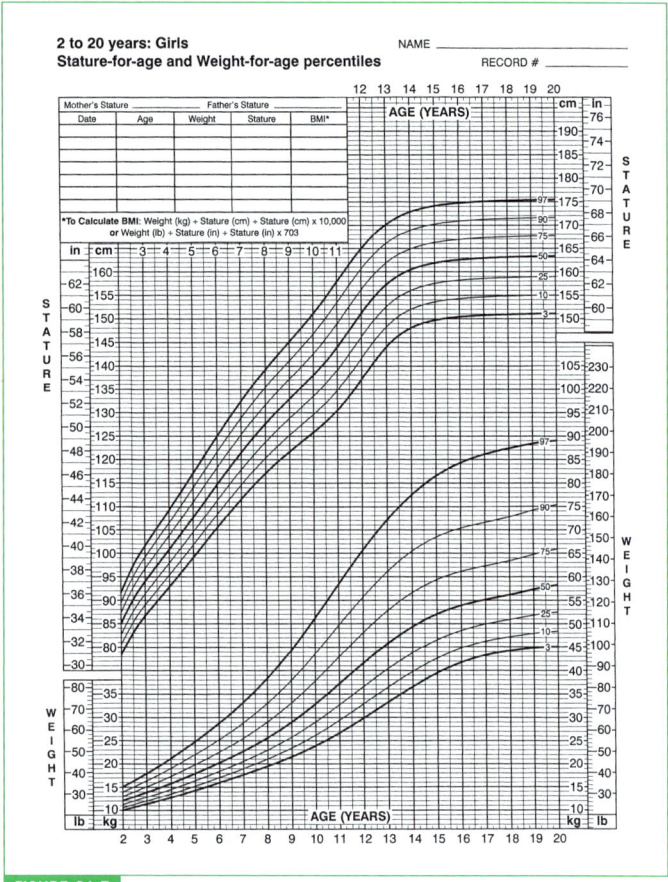

FIGURE 21.5

Stature and weight for girls aged 2–20 years. *(Developed by the National Center for Health Statistics in collaboration with the National Center for Chronic Disease Prevention and Health Promotion, 2000.)*

a. Exclusive breastfeeding until 6 months of age and then maintenance of breastfeeding until 12 months and beyond
b. Encourage daily breakfast and family meal times
c. Limit sugary beverages, fast food, energy-dense foods, and encourage fruits and vegetables
d. Reduce screen time to 0 hours for <2 years old and maximum of 2 hours for >2 years old

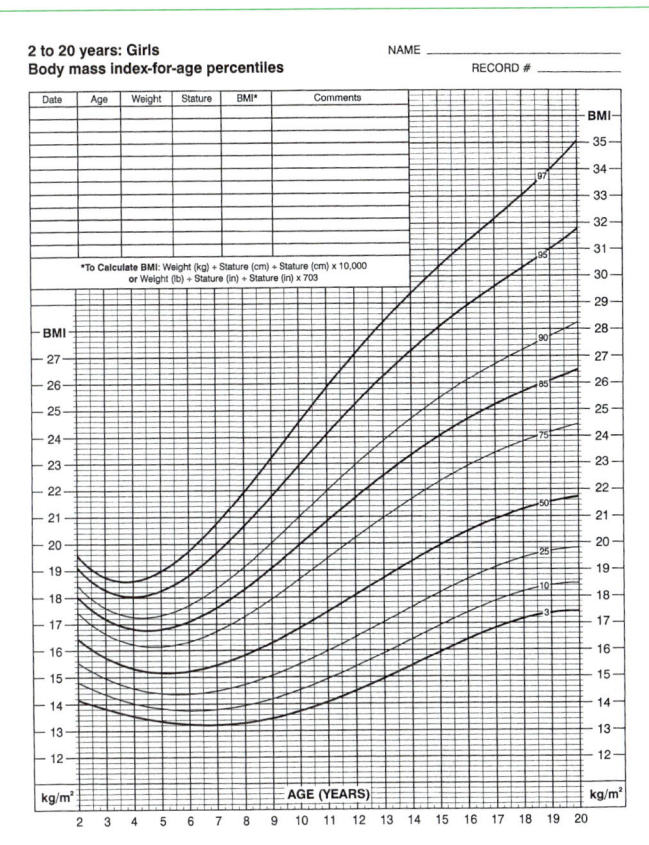

FIGURE 21.6

Body mass index for girls aged 2–20 years. *(Developed by the National Center for Health Statistics in collaboration with the National Center for Chronic Disease Prevention and Health Promotion, 2000.)*

 e. Sixty minutes of moderate-to-vigorous exercise a day
 f. If no improvement after 3–6 months, then refer to structured weight management program. If further interventions are warranted, the next step is a comprehensive, multidisciplinary approach beyond the primary care office. Finally, the last option is evaluation at a tertiary care center for medication management and weight reduction surgery.
3. Based on expert committee opinions, the Childhood Obesity Action Network has also developed an implementation guide for assessment and management of childhood obesity.[5]

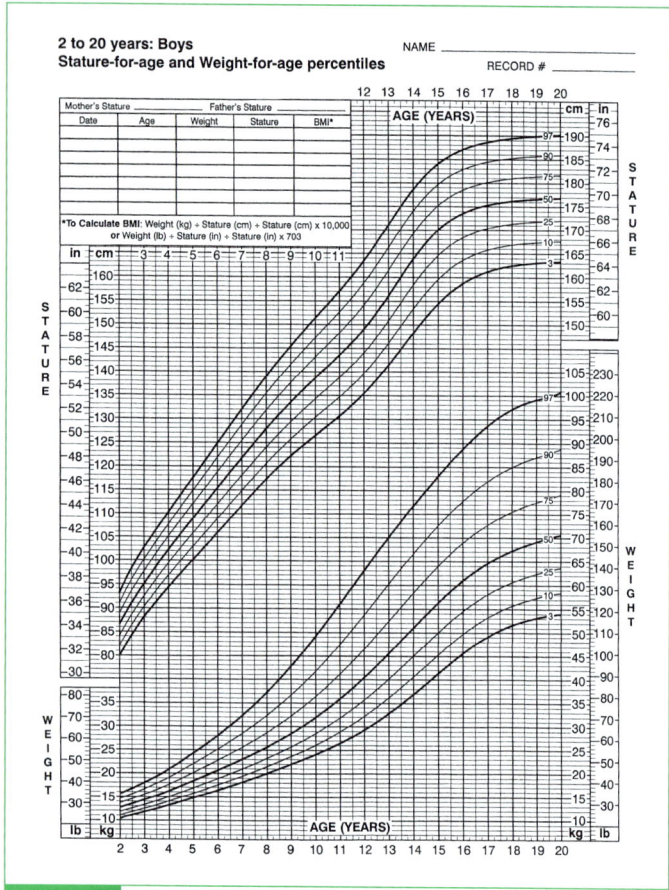

FIGURE 21.7

Stature and weight for boys aged 2–20 years. *(Developed by the National Center for Health Statistics in collaboration with the National Center for Chronic Disease Prevention and Health Promotion, 2000.)*

III. ESTIMATING ENERGY NEEDS

A. Definitions of Energy Needs[6]

1. **Basal metabolic rate (BMR):** Rate of energy expenditure after an overnight fast, resting comfortably, supine, awake, and motionless in a thermoneutral environment.
2. **Basal energy expenditure (BEE):** BMR over 24 hours.

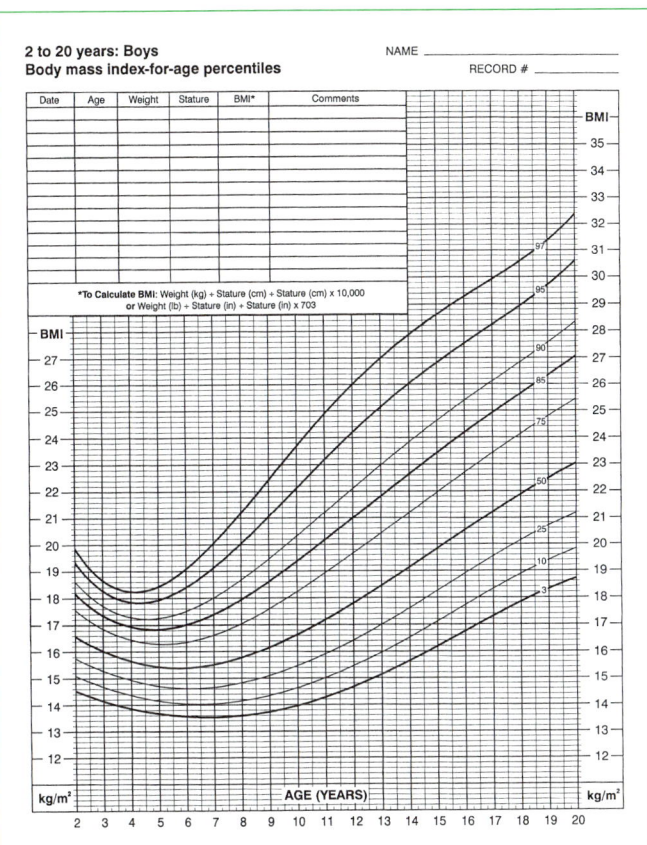

FIGURE 21.8

Body mass index for boys aged 2–20 years. *(Developed by the National Center for Health Statistics in collaboration with the National Center for Chronic Disease Prevention and Health Promotion, 2000.)*

3. **Thermic effect of food (TEF):** Increase in energy expenditure elicited by food consumption.
4. **Energy deposition:** Energy requirement for growth.
5. **Total energy expenditure (TEE):** Sum of BEE, TEF, physical activity, thermoregulation, and energy expended in depositing new tissues and/or producing milk.
6. **Physical activity level (PAL):** Ratio of total to basal daily energy expenditure (TEE/BEE). Describes and accounts for physical activity habits.

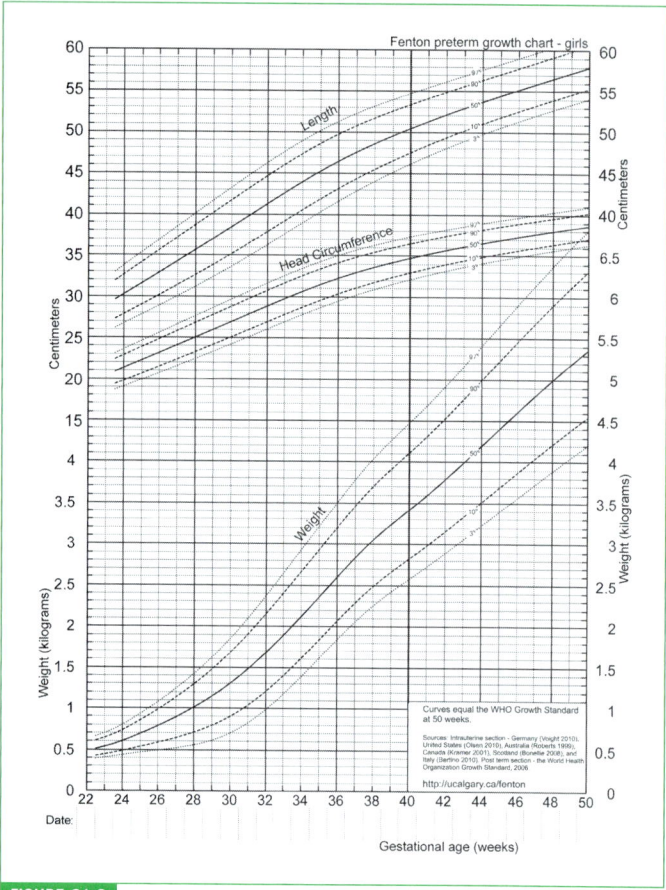

FIGURE 21.9

Length, weight, and head circumference for preterm infants. *(From Fenton RT, Kim HJ. A systematic review and meta-analysis to revise the Fenton growth chart for preterm infants.* BMC Pediatrics. *2013;13:59.)*

7. **Physical activity coefficient (PA):** The physical activity coefficient that correlates with PAL (see Table EC 21.A on Expert Consult) can be used to calculate estimated energy requirements (EER).
8. **Estimated energy requirements (EER):** Dietary energy intake predicted to maintain energy balance in a healthy individual. In children, EER includes the needs associated with growth.

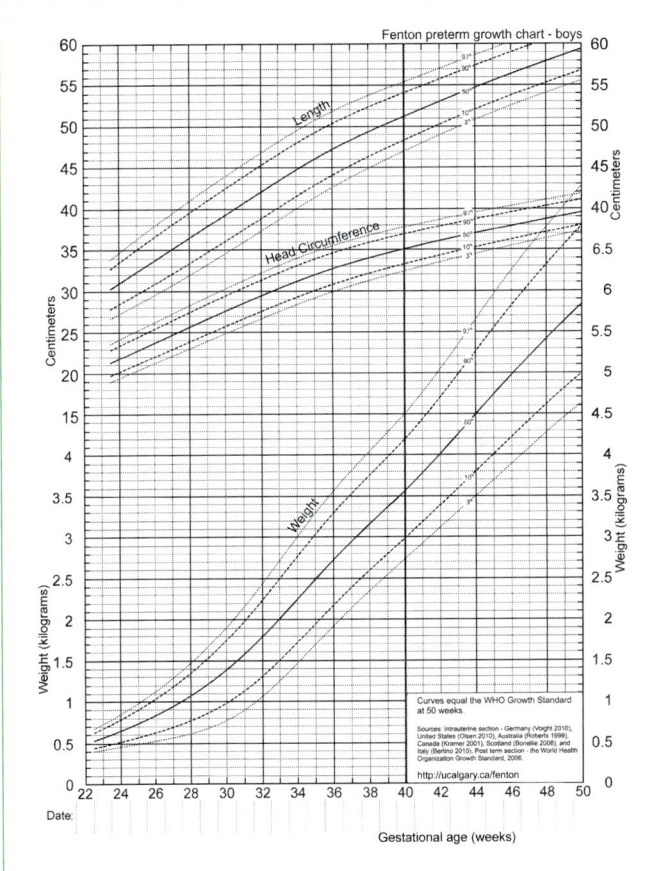

FIGURE 21.9, cont'd

a. For infants, children, and adolescents, EER (kcal/day) = TEE + energy deposition
b. For most hospitalized patients, it can be assumed PAL = sedentary, PA = 1
c. Table 21.1[6] contains the estimated EER for healthy boys and girls of median weight (weight for age at 50th percentile) at both sedentary and active PAL levels

B. Estimated Energy Requirement Calculations[6]

See Expert Consult for more information (sections B and C).

TABLE 21.1

SAMPLE ESTIMATED ENERGY REQUIREMENTS FOR HEALTHY BOYS AND GIRLS OF MEDIAN WEIGHT AND HEIGHT*

Age	Boys EER (kcal/kg/day)	Girls EER (kcal/kg/day)
0–2 mo	107	104
3 mo	95	95
4–35 mo	82	82

	Boys			Girls		
	Median Weight, Boys (kg)	Sedentary[†] (kcal/kg/d)	Active[†] (kcal/kg/d)	Median Weight, Girls (kg)	Sedentary[†] (kcal/kg/d)	Active[†] (kcal/kg/d)
3 yr	14.3	80	104	13.9	76	100
4 yr	16.2	74	97	15.8	70	93
5 yr	18.4	68	90	17.9	65	87
6 yr	20.7	63	84	20.2	61	81
7 yr	23.1	59	80	22.8	56	75
8 yr	25.6	56	75	25.6	52	71
9 yr	28.6	53	71	29.0	48	65
10 yr	31.9	49	67	32.9	44	60
11 yr	35.9	46	63	37.2	41	56
12 yr	40.5	44	60	41.6	38	52
13 yr	45.6	42	57	45.8	36	50
14 yr	51.0	40	55	49.4	34	47
15 yr	56.3	39	54	52.0	33	45
16 yr	60.9	38	52	53.9	32	44
17 yr	64.6	36	50	55.1	31	43
18 yr	67.2	35	49	56.2	30	42

*Weight and height for age at 50th percentile.
[†]See definition of sedentary and active PAL for further information.
EER, Estimated energy requirements; PAL, physical activity level.
From Otten JJ, Hellwig JP, Meyers LD, eds. Dietary Reference Intakes: The Essential Guide to Nutrient Requirements. Washington, DC: National Academies Press; 2006.

D. Catch-Up Growth Requirement for Malnourished Infants and Children (<3 years)[7]

1. **Growth failure** (also known as *failure to thrive*)[8]: Condition of undernutrition generally identified in the first 3 years of life. Can be described by the following growth scenarios: Weight for age <5th percentile, weight for length (or height) <5th percentile, or decreased growth velocity resulting in weight falling more than two major percentiles over 3–6 months.
2. **Catch-up growth:** Time period of accelerated growth as a result of caloric provision in excess of the recommended dietary allowances (RDAs). Approximately 20%–30% more energy may be required to achieve catch-up growth in children. Protein needs also increase. This

BOX 21.1
DETERMINING CATCH-UP GROWTH REQUIREMENTS
1. Plot the child's height and weight on the appropriate growth charts.
2. Determine recommended calories needed for age [recommended dietary allowances (RDA)].
3. Determine the ideal weight (50th percentile) for child's height.*
4. Multiply the RDA calories by ideal body weight for height (kg).
5. Divide this value by the child's actual weight (kg).
   For example, for a 12-month-old boy whose weight is 7 kg and length is 72 cm, RDA for age would be 98 kcal/kg/day, and ideal body weight for height is 9 kg (50th percentile weight for height). Thus his catch-up growth requirement would be as follows:

   $$98 \text{ kcal/kg/day} \times (9 \text{ kg}/7 \text{ kg}) = 126 \text{ kcal/kg/day}$$

*Ideal weight can be 10th–85th percentile weight for height, depending on past growth trends; clinical judgment should be used.

should continue until the previous growth percentiles are regained. Catch-up in linear growth may lag several months behind that in weight. Box 21.1 lists the steps for determining catch-up growth requirements.

NOTE: Aggressive refeeding in the severely malnourished child can result in metabolic alterations, vomiting, diarrhea, and circulatory decompensation known as *refeeding syndrome* (hypophosphatemia, hypokalemia, hypomagnesemia, and glucose and/or fluid imbalance).[9,10]

IV. DIETARY REFERENCE INTAKES FOR INDIVIDUALS[6]

A. Dietary Reference Intakes
DRIs are reference values based on quantitative estimates of nutrient intakes and are measured in several ways:
1. **Recommended dietary allowance (RDA):** The daily nutrient intake level estimated to meet the requirement of 97%–98% of healthy individuals in a particular life stage and gender group
2. **Adequate intake (AI):** Observed range of intakes in a healthy population; used when data are insufficient to calculate RDA
3. **Tolerable upper intake level (UL):** Highest daily nutrient intake level likely to pose no risk for adverse health effects to almost all individuals in the general population

B. Protein Requirements (Table 21.2)[6]

C. Fat Requirements (Table 21.3)[6]

D. Vitamin Requirements (Table 21.4)[6]

TABLE 21.2
PROTEIN REQUIREMENTS

Age	RDA (g/kg/day)
0–6 mo	1.52 (AI)*
7–12 mo	1.2
1–3 yr	1.05
4–8 yr	0.95
9–13 yr	0.95
14–18 yr	0.85
Pregnancy (first half)	Unchanged
Pregnancy (second half)	1.1
Lactation	1.3

*If sufficient scientific evidence is not available to establish RDA (recommended dietary allowance), an AI (adequate intake) is usually developed. For healthy breast-fed infants, the AI is the mean intake.

From Otten JJ, Hellwig JP, Meyers LD, eds. Dietary Reference Intakes: The Essential Guide to Nutrient Requirements. Washington, DC: National Academies Press; 2006.

1. **Vitamin D supplementation**[11]
   a. Breast-fed and partially breast-fed infants should be supplemented with 400 IU/day of vitamin D beginning in the first few days of life until the age of 12 months. Supplementation should be continued unless the infant is taking 1000 mL/day of vitamin D–fortified formula.
   b. For children and adolescents aged 1–18 years, RDA of vitamin D increases to 600 IU/day if the child is ingesting <1000 mL/day of vitamin D–fortified milk or not taking that amount through fortified foods (cereals, egg yolks).
2. **Examples of multivitamins for infants and children** (Tables 21.5 and 21.6)

E. Mineral Requirements (Table 21.7)[6]

1. **Iron supplementation**[12]
   a. Breast-fed term infants: Should receive 1 mg/kg of an oral iron supplement beginning at 4 months of age, preferably from iron-fortified cereal or, alternatively, elemental iron
   b. Breast-fed preterm infants: Should receive 2 mg/kg/day by 1 month of age, which should be continued until the infant is weaned to iron-fortified formula or begins eating complementary foods
   c. Formula-fed term infants: Receive adequate iron from fortified formula (4–12 mg/L) from birth to age 12 months
   d. Formula-fed preterm infants: Need an additional supplementation of 1 mg/kg/day to get total daily dose of 2 mg/kg/day
   e. Universal screening for iron-deficiency anemia recommended at 12 months

TABLE 21.3
FAT REQUIREMENTS: ADEQUATE INTAKE (AI)*

Age	Total Fat (g/day)	Linoleic Acid (g/day)	α-Linolenic Acid (g/day)
0–6 mo	31	4.4 (n-6 PUFA)	0.5 (n-3 PUFA)
7–12 mo	30	4.6 (n-6 PUFA)	0.5 (n-3 PUFA)
1–3 yr	†	7	0.7
4–8 yr	†	10	0.9
9–13 yr, boys	†	12	1.2
9–13 yr, girls	†	10	1.0
14–18 yr, boys	†	16	1.6
14–18 yr, girls	†	11	1.1
Pregnancy	†	13	1.4
Lactation	†	13	1.3

*If sufficient scientific evidence is not available to establish RDA (recommended dietary allowance), an AI (adequate intake) is usually developed. For healthy breast-fed infants, the AI is the mean intake. The AI for other life stage and gender groups is believed to cover the needs of all healthy individuals in the group, but a lack of data or uncertainty in the data prevents from being able to specify with confidence the percentage of individuals covered by this intake.
†No AI, estimated average requirement (EAR), or RDA established.
PUFA, Polyunsaturated fatty acid.
From Otten JJ, Hellwig JP, Meyers LD, eds. Dietary Reference Intakes: The Essential Guide to Nutrient Requirements. Washington, DC: National Academies Press; 2006.

2. **Fluoride supplementation**[13]
    a. Supplementation not needed during the first 6 months of life. Thereafter, 0.5 mg/day is recommended for exclusively breast-fed infants.
    b. Consider fluoride supplementation for those patients who use bottled water and home filtration systems. Most bottled water does not contain adequate amounts of fluoride. Some home water treatment systems can reduce fluoride levels.
    c. Fluoridated toothpaste is recommended for all children starting at tooth eruption, using a smear (grain of rice size) until age 3 and then a pea-sized amount after that time. Fluoride varnish is recommended every 3–6 months in the primary care setting starting after tooth eruption until the establishment of a dental home. Children younger than 6 years should not use over-the-counter fluoride rinse.

F. **Fiber Requirements** (Table 21.8)[6]

V. BREASTFEEDING AND THE USE OF HUMAN MILK[14]

A. Breastfeeding Recommendations
1. Exclusive breastfeeding is recommended for first 6 months of life with continuation until 1 year or longer as desired by mother and infant.
2. All exclusively breastfed infants should be started on vitamin D supplementation of 400 IU/day starting at hospital discharge.

B. Associated with Decreased Risk of[14]
1. Otitis media, lower respiratory tract infections including respiratory syncytial virus (RSV) bronchiolitis and pneumonia

TABLE 21.4
DIETARY REFERENCE INTAKES: RECOMMENDED INTAKES FOR INDIVIDUALS—VITAMINS

Life Stage	Vit. A[a] (IU)	Vit. C (mg/day)	Vit. D[b,c] (IU)	Vit. E[d] (IU)	Vit. K (mcg/day)	Thiamin (mg/day)	Riboflavin (mg/day)	Niacin[e] (mg/day)	Vit. B$_6$ (mg/day)	Folate[f] (mcg/day)	Vit. B$_{12}$ (mcg/day)	Pantothenic Acid (mg/day)	Biotin (mcg/day)	Choline[g] (mg/day)
INFANTS														
0–6 mo	1333	40*	400	4*	2.0*	0.2*	0.3*	2*	0.1*	65*	0.4*	1.7*	5*	125*
7–12 mo	1666	50*	400	5*	2.5*	0.3*	0.4*	4*	0.3*	80*	0.5*	1.8*	6*	150*
CHILDREN														
1–3 yr	1000	15	600	6	30*	0.5	0.5	6	0.5	150	0.9	2*	8*	200*
4–8 yr	1333	25	600	7	55*	0.6	0.6	8	0.6	200	1.2	3*	12*	25*
MALES														
9–13 yr	2000	45	600	11	60*	0.9	0.9	12	1.0	300	1.8	4*	20*	375*
14–18 yr	3000	75	600	15	75*	1.2	1.3	16	1.3	400	2.4	5*	25*	550*
19–30 yr	3000	90	600	15	120*	1.2	1.3	16	1.3	400	2.4	5*	30*	550*
FEMALES														
9–13 yr	2000	45	600	11	60*	0.9	0.9	12	1.0	300	1.8	4*	20*	375*
14–18 yr	2333	65	600	15	75*	1.0	1.0	14	1.2	400	2.4	5*	25*	400*
19–30 yr	2333	75	600	15	90*	1.1	1.1	14	1.3	400	2.4	5*	30*	425*
PREGNANCY														
<18 yr	2500	80	600	15	75*	1.4	1.4	18	1.9	600	2.6	6*	30*	450*
19–30 yr	2567	85	600	15	90*	1.4	1.4	18	1.9	600	2.6	6*	30*	450*

LACTATION

<18 yr	4000	115	600	19	75*	1.4	1.6	17	2.0	500	2.8	7*	35*	550*
19–30 yr	4333	120	600	19	90*	1.4	1.6	17	2.0	500	2.8	7*	35*	550*

NOTE: This table (taken from the Dietary Reference Intakes reports; see www.nap.edu) presents recommended dietary allowances (RDAs) in **bold type** and adequate intakes (AIs) in regular type followed by an asterisk (*). RDAs and AIs may both be used as goals for individual intake. RDAs are set to meet the needs of almost all (97%–98%) individuals in a group. For healthy breast-fed infants, the AI is the mean intake. The AI for other life stage and gender groups is believed to cover needs of all individuals in the group, but lack of data or uncertainty in the data prevent from being able to specify with confidence the percentage of individuals covered by this intake.

[a] One International Unit (IU) = 0.3 mcg retinol equivalent.
[b] One mcg cholecalciferol = 40 IU vitamin D.
[c] In the absence of adequate exposure to sunlight.
[d] One IU = 1 mg vitamin E.
[e] As niacin equivalents (NE). 1 mg of niacin = 60 mg of tryptophan; 0–6 months = preformed niacin (not NE).
[f] As dietary folate equivalents (DFE). 1 DFE = 1 mcg food folate = 0.6 mcg of folic acid from fortified food or as a supplement consumed with food = 0.5 mcg of a supplement taken on an empty stomach. In view of evidence linking folate with neural tube defects in the fetus, it is recommended that all women capable of becoming pregnant consume 400 mcg from supplements or fortified foods in addition to intake of food folate from a varied diet. It is assumed that women will continue consuming 400 mcg from supplements or fortified food until their pregnancy is confirmed and they enter prenatal care, which ordinarily occurs after the end of the periconceptual period—the critical time for formation of the neural tube.
[g] Although AIs have been set for choline, there are few data to assess whether a dietary supply of choline is needed at all life stages, and it may be that the choline requirement can be met by endogenous synthesis at some of these stages.

Modified from Otten JJ, Hellwig JP, Meyers LD, eds. Dietary Reference Intakes: The Essential Guide to Nutrient Requirements. Washington, DC: National Academies Press; 2006.

TABLE 21.5
INFANT MULTIVITAMIN DROPS ANALYSIS (PER ML)*

Nutrient	Poly-Vi-Sol Multivitamin [w/iron]	Tri-Vi-Sol [w/iron]	AquADEKs[†‡]	D Vi-Sol	Fer-In-Sol
Vitamin A (IU)	750	750	5751	—	—
Vitamin D (IU)	400	400	400	400	—
Vitamin E (IU)	5	—	50	—	—
Vitamin C (mg)	35	35	45	—	—
Thiamin (mg)	0.5	—	0.6	—	—
Riboflavin (mg)	0.6	—	0.6	—	—
Niacin (mg)	8	—	6	—	—
Vitamin B_6 (mg)	0.4	—	0.6	—	—
Vitamin B_{12} (mcg)	2	—	—	—	—
Vitamin K (mcg)	—	—	400	—	—
Iron (mg)	[10]	[10]	—	—	15
Fluoride (mg)	—	—	—	—	—
Zinc (mg)	—	—	5	—	—

*Standard dose = 1 mL.
[†]Also contains biotin, 15 mcg; pantothenic acid, 3 mg; 87% vitamin A as β-carotene; coenzyme Q_{10}, 2 mg; selenium, 10 mcg.
[‡]Recommended for use in infants with fat malabsorption, such as cystic fibrosis, liver disease.

2. Necrotizing enterocolitis (NEC), celiac disease, inflammatory bowel disease
3. Obesity, diabetes mellitus types 1 and 2
4. Allergies, asthma, atopic dermatitis
5. Sudden infant death syndrome (SIDS)

C. Breastfeeding Resources

1. LactMed is an online resource from the National Library of Medicine/National Institutes of Health (NIH) that provides information on the safety of maternal medications and breastfeeding: http://toxnet.nlm.nih.gov/newtoxnet/lactmed.htm.
2. Video instruction on breastfeeding techniques from Stanford Newborn Nursery: http://newborns.stanford.edu/Breastfeeding/FifteenMinuteHelper.html.

D. Contraindications to Breastfeeding (Table 21.9)[14]

1. Tobacco smoking is not contraindicated but strongly discouraged because of increased rates of SIDS, respiratory disease, and infections.
2. Alcohol should be limited to occasional intake of 2-oz liquor, 8-oz wine, or two beers for the average 60-kg woman, >2 hours prior to the onset of nursing.
3. Methadone use is not contraindicated if the mother is in a stable and reliable maintenance program.

TABLE 21.6
MULTIVITAMIN TABLETS (ANALYSIS/TABLET)

	Flintstones Sour Gummies	Centrum Kids	Flintstones Complete	Centrum Tablet*	AquADEKs (Softgel)	Vitamax (Chewable)	Phlexy-Vits (7-g Packet)	NanoVM 1–3 yrs (Two Scoops)	NanoVM 4–8 yrs (Two Scoops)	NanoVM 9–13 yrs (Four Scoops)	NanoVM 14–18 yrs (Five Scoops)
Vitamin A (IU)	2000	3500	3000	3500	18,167	5000[a]	2664	1000	1332	2000[a]	2476[a]
Vitamin D (IU)	600	400	600	1000	1200	400	400	600	600	600	744
Vitamin E (IU)	18	30	30	30	150	200	13.5	9	10	11	11.8
Vitamin K (mcg)	—	10	55	25	700	150	70	30	55	60	74
Vitamin C (mg)	30	60	60	60	75	60	50	15	25	45	56
Thiamin (mg)	—	1.5	1.5	1.5	1.5	1.5	1.2	0.5	0.6	0.9	1.1
Riboflavin (mg)	—	1.7	1.7	1.7	1.7	1.7	1.4	0.5	0.6	0.9	1.1
Niacin (mg)	—	20	15	20	10	20	20	6	8	12	15
Vitamin B_6 (mg)	1	2	2	2	1.9	2	1.6	0.5	0.6	1	1.2
Folate (mcg)	200	400	400	400	100	200	700	150	200	300	371
Vitamin B_{12} (mcg)	3	6	6	6	12	6	5	0.9	1.2	1.8	2.2
Biotin (mcg)	75	45	40	30	100	300	150	8	12	20	25

Continued

TABLE 21.6
MULTIVITAMIN TABLETS (ANALYSIS/TABLET)—cont'd

	Flintstones Sour Gummies	Centrum Kids	Flintstones Complete	Centrum Tablet*	AquADEKs (Softgel)	Vitamax (Chewable)	Phlexy-Vits (7-g Packet)	NanoVM 1–3 yrs (Two Scoops)	NanoVM 4–8 yrs (Two Scoops)	NanoVM 9–13 yrs (Four Scoops)	NanoVM 14–18 yrs (Five Scoops)
Pantothenic acid (mg)	5	10	10	10	12	10	5	2	3	4	5
Calcium (mg)	—	108	100	200	—	—	1000	700	1000	1300	1609
Phosphorus (mg)	—	50	—	20	—	—	775	460	500	979	1212
Iron (mg)	—	18	18	18	—	—	15.1	7	10	8	10
Iodine (mcg)	30	150	150	150	—	—	150	90	90	120	149
Magnesium (mg)	—	40	20	50	—	—	300	65	110	240	297
Zinc (mg)	2.5	15	12	11	10	—	11.1	3	5	8	10
Copper (mg)	—	2	2	0.5	—	—	1.5	0.34	0.44	0.7	867
Manganese (mg)	—	1	—	2.3	—	—	1.5	1.2	1.5	1.9	2.4
Chromium (mcg)	—	20	—	35	—	—	30	11	15	25	31
Molybdenum (mcg)	—	20	—	45	—	—	70	17	22	34	42
Selenium (mcg)	—	—	—	55	75	—	75	20	30	40	49.5
Sodium (mg)	—	—	10	—	10	—	8.8	—	—	—	—
Potassium (mg)	—	—	—	80	—	—	<1.4	575	775	1960	1960
Chloride	—	—	—	72	—	—	<0.35	—	—	—	—

[a]Vitamin A as 50% acetate and 50% β-carotene.
*Contains boron, nickel, silicon, and tin.
NOTE: Fluoride and choline not included in listed multivitamins.

TABLE 21.7
DIETARY REFERENCE INTAKES: RECOMMENDED INTAKES—ELEMENTS

Life Stage	Calcium (mg/day)	Chromium (mcg/day)	Copper (mcg/day)	Fluoride (mg/day)	Iodine (mcg/day)	Iron (mg/day)	Magnesium (mg/day)	Manganese (mg/day)	Molybdenum (mcg/day)	Phosphorus (mg/day)	Selenium (mcg/day)	Zinc (mg/day)
INFANTS												
0–6 mo	200*	0.2*	200*	0.01*	110*	0.27*	30*	0.003*	2*	100*	15*	2*
7–12 mo	260*	5.5*	220*	0.5*	130*	11	75*	0.6*	3*	275*	20*	3
CHILDREN												
1–3 yr	700	11*	340	0.7*	90	7	80	1.2*	17	460	20	3
4–8 yr	1000	15*	440	1.0*	90	10	130	1.5*	22	500	30	5
MALES												
9–13 yr	1300	25*	700	2*	120	8	240	1.9*	34	1250	40	8
14–18 yr	1300	35*	890	3*	150	11	410	2.2*	43	1250	55	11
19–30 yr	1000	35*	900	4*	150	8	400	2.3*	45	700	55	11
FEMALES												
9–13 yr	1300	21*	700	2*	120	8	240	1.6*	34	1250	40	8
14–18 yr	1300	24*	890	3*	150	15	360	1.6*	43	1250	55	9
19–30 yr	1000	25*	900	3*	150	18	310	1.8*	45	700	55	8
PREGNANCY												
<18 yr	1300	29*	1000	3*	220	27	400	2.0*	50	1250	60	13
19–30 yr	1000	30*	1000	3*	220	27	350	2.0*	50	700	60	11
LACTATION												
<18 yr	1300	44*	1300	3*	290	10	360	2.6*	50	1250	70	14
19–30 yr	1000	45*	1300	3*	290	9	310	2.6*	50	700	70	12

NOTE: This table presents recommended dietary allowances (RDAs) in **bold type** and adequate intakes (AIs) in ordinary type followed by an asterisk (*). RDAs and AIs may both be used as goals for individual intake. RDAs are set to meet the needs of almost all (97%–98%) individuals in a group. For healthy breast-fed infants, the AI is the mean intake. The AI for other life stage and gender groups is believed to cover needs of all individuals in the group, but lack of data or uncertainty in the data prevent from being able to specify with confidence the percentage of individuals covered by this intake.

Modified from Otten JJ, Hellwig JP, Meyers LD, eds. Dietary Reference Intakes: The Essential Guide to Nutrient Requirements. Washington, DC: National Academies Press; 2006. Includes updates from Ross AC, Taylor CL, Yaktine AL, Del Valle HB, eds. Dietary Reference Intakes for Calcium and Vitamin D. Washington, DC: National Academies Press; 2011.

TABLE 21.8
FIBER REQUIREMENTS: ADEQUATE INTAKE*

Age	Total Fiber (g/day)
0–12 mo	Not determined
1–3 yr	19
4–8 yr	25
9–13 yr, boys	31
9–13 yr, girls	26
14–18 yr, boys	38
14–18 yr, girls	26
Pregnancy	28
Lactation	29

*Adequate intake (AI). If sufficient scientific evidence unavailable to establish recommended dietary allowance (RDA), an AI is usually developed. For healthy breast-fed infants, the AI is the mean intake. AI for other life stage and gender groups is believed to cover the needs of all healthy individuals in the group, but a lack of data or uncertainty in the data prevents from being able to specify with confidence the percentage of individuals covered by this intake.
Modified from Otten JJ, Hellwig JP, Meyers LD, eds. *Dietary Reference Intakes: The Essential Guide to Nutrient Requirements*. Washington, DC: National Academies Press; 2006.

TABLE 21.9
CONTRAINDICATIONS TO BREASTFEEDING

Infant galactosemia
Maternal human T-cell lymphotropic virus I/II infection
Maternal untreated brucellosis
Maternal HIV (developed countries)
Maternal active, untreated tuberculosis (may give expressed BM)
Maternal active HSV lesions on breast (may give expressed BM)
Maternal varicella infection 5 days before through 2 days after delivery (may give expressed BM)
Maternal use of diagnostic or therapeutic radioactive isotopes, antimetabolites, or chemotherapeutic agents
Illicit street drugs such as cannabis, cocaine, phencyclidine, etc.

Modified from American Academy of Pediatrics, Section on Breastfeeding. Policy Statement - Breastfeeding and the Use of Human Milk. *Pediatrics*. 2012;129:e827-e841.

VI. ENTERAL NUTRITION[15]

A. Mixing Instructions for Full-Term Standard and Soy-Based Infant Formulas (Table 21.10)

B. Common Caloric Modulars (Table 21.11)

For the child who needs additional protein, carbohydrate, fat, or a combination

C. Enteral Formulas, Including Their Main Nutrient Components (Table 21.12)

A comprehensive (but not complete) list. Most of these formulas are cow's milk–based and designed for normal digestive tracts.

Text continued on p. 602

TABLE 21.10

PREPARATION OF INFANT FORMULAS FOR MOST FULL-TERM STANDARD AND SOY FORMULAS*

Formula Type	Caloric Concentration (kcal/oz)	Amount of Formula	Water (oz)
Liquid concentrates (40 kcal/oz)	20	13 oz	13 oz
	24	13 oz	8.5 oz
	27	13 oz	6.3 oz
	30	13 oz	4.3 oz
Powder (approx 44 kcal/scoop)**	20	1 scoop	2 oz
	24	3 scoops	5 oz
	27	3 scoops	4.25 oz
	30	3 scoops	4 oz

*Does not apply to Enfacare, Neocate Infant, Alfamino Infant, or NeoSure. Enfamil A.R. and Similac Sensitive for Spit-Up should not be concentrated greater than 24 kcal/oz. Use a packed measure for Nutramigen and Pregestimil; all others unpacked powder.
**Slight variations in brands, range 40–45 kcal/scoop.

TABLE 21.11

COMMON CALORIC MODULARS*

Component	Calories
PROTEIN	
Beneprotein (powder)	25 kcal/scoop (6 g protein)
ProSource protein powder	30 kcal/scoop (6 g protein)
Complete Amino Acid Mix (powder)	3.28 kcal/g (0.82 g protein)
	2.9 g/teaspoon (9.5 kcal, 2.38 g protein)
Abbott Liquid Protein Fortifier	0.67 kcal/mL (0.167 g protein/mL)
CARBOHYDRATE	
SolCarb	3.75 kcal/g; 23 kcal/tbsp
FAT	
MCT oil[†]	7.7 kcal/mL
Vegetable oil	8.3 kcal/mL
Microlipid (emulsified LCT)	4.5 kcal/mL
Liquigen (emulsified MCT)[†]	4.5 kcal/mL
FAT AND CARBOHYDRATE	
Duocal (powder)	42 kcal/tbsp; 25 kcal/scoop (59% carb, 41% fat, 35% fat as MCT)

*Use these caloric supplements when you want to increase protein or when you have reached the maximum concentration tolerated and wish to further increase caloric density.
[†]Medium-chain triglyceride (MCT) oil is unnecessary unless there is fat malabsorption.

TABLE 21.12
ENTERAL NUTRITION COMPONENTS (PER LITER)
A. INFANT FORMULAS

	Kcal/oz	Protein (g)	Fat (g)	Carbs (g)	Na (mEq)	K (mEq)	Ca (mg)	P (mg)	Fe (mg)	Osmolality
HUMAN MILK										
Term	20	11	39	72	8	14	279	143	0.3	286
Preterm	20	14	39	66	11	15	248	128	1.2	290
HUMAN MILK AND FORTIFIERS ANALYSIS										
Enfamil HMF Liquid + Preterm Human Milk (5 mL + 25 mL breast milk)	24	32	48	65	20	20	1150	650	15	322
Similac HMF + Preterm Human Milk (1 pkt/25 mL)	24	23	41	82	17	30	1381	777	4.6	N/A
PRETERM FORMULAS										
Enfamil EnfaCare	22	21	39	77	11	7.2	890	490	13.3	280
Enfamil Premature 20	20	20	34	74	17	17	1100	553	12	240
Enfamil Premature 24	24	27	41	88	25	21	1340	730	15	280
Enfamil Premature 24 High Protein	24	28	41	89	20	21	1340	670	15	300
Enfamil Premature 30	30	30	52	112	26	27	1670	840	18	300
Gerber Good Start Premature 20	20	20	35	71	16	21	1110	570	12	229
Gerber Good Start Premature 24	24	29	42	79	19	25	1330	690	15	299
Gerber Good Start Premature 30 High Protein	30	30	53	107	24	31	1660	860	18	341
Similac NeoSure	22	21	41	75	11	27	781	461	13.4	250
Similac Special Care 20	20	20	37	70	13	22	1217	676	12.2	235

Similac Special Care 24 High Protein	24	27	44	81	15	27	1461	812	14.6	280
Similac Special Care 30	30	30	67	78	19	34	1826	1014	18.3	325
COW'S MILK–BASED FORMULAS										
Enfamil Infant	20	14	36	74	8	19	520	287	12	300
Enfamil Newborn	20	14	36	74	8	19	520	287	12	300
Enfamil A.R.	20	17	34	74	12	19	520	353	12	230 (240*)
Enfamil LactoFree	20	14	36	73	9	19	547	307	12	200
Enfagrow Toddler Transitions	20	18	36	70	10	23	1300	867	13.4	270
Evap. Milk (13 oz + 19 oz water + 30 mL corn syrup)	20	27	31	72	21	32	1066	832	0.8	N/A
Organic Milk–Based Infant Formula	20	15	36	71	7	15	420	280	12	294
Parent's Choice Premium Infant Formula	20	14	36	74	8	19	523	287	12	295
Similac Advance	19 (20)	13 (14)	36 (38)	69 (72)	7	18	527	283	12	310
Similac Go and Grow Milk-Based Formula	19	20	35	66	8	25	1268	845	13	300
Similac Sensitive	19 (20)	14 (15)	35 (37)	72 (75)	9	18	566 (568)	379	12.2	200
Similac Advance Organic	19 (20)	13 (14)	36 (38)	69 (71)	7	18	527 (530)	283 (285)	12.2	225
Similac PM 60/40	20	15	38	69	7	14	379	189	4.7	280
Similac for Spitup	20	14	37	72	9	19	568	379	12.2	180

Continued

TABLE 21.12
ENTERAL NUTRITION COMPONENTS (PER LITER)—cont'd

A. INFANT FORMULAS—cont'd

	Kcal/oz	Protein (g)	Fat (g)	Carbs (g)	Na (mEq)	K (mEq)	Ca (mg)	P (mg)	Fe (mg)	Osmolality
SOY BASED										
America's Store Brand Soy (also w/ ARA/DHA)	20	17	36	71	11	21	700	460	12	164
Enfamil ProSobee	20	17	36	71	11	21	700	460	12	170
Enfagrow Soy Toddler	20	22	30	79	11	21	1307	871	13.3	230
Gerber Graduates Soy	20	17	34	75	12	20	704	422	12.1	180
Similac Soy Isomil	19 (20)	16 (17)	35 (37)	67 (70)	13	18 (19)	707 (710)	507	12.2	200
Similac for Diarrhea	20	18	37	68	13	19	710	507	12.2	240
Similac Go and Grow Soy-Based Formula	20	17	34	67	13	19	1014	676	13.5	200
CASEIN, EXTENSIVELY HYDROLYZED										
Alimentum	20	19	37	69	13	20	710	507	12.2	320
Nutramigen	20	19	36	69	14	19	627	347	12	300 (320*)
Nutramigen with Enflora LGG	20	19	36	69	14	19	627	347	12	300
Pregestimil	20	19	38	69	14	19	627	347	12.2	320
WHEY, EXTENSIVELY HYDROLYZED										
Gerber Extensive HA	20	17	34	73	11	17	603	422	12	220
WHEY, PARTIALLY HYDROLYZED										
Gerber Good Start Gentle	20	15	34	78	8	19	450	260	10.1	250
Gerber Graduates Gentle	20	15	34	78	8	19	1273	710	13.4	180
Gerber Good Start Soothe	20	15	34	75	8	19	480	270	10	195
Similac Total Comfort	19	15	35	71	13	20	675	450	12.2	200

WHEY AND CASEIN, PARTIALLY HYDROLYZED									
Enfamil Gentlease	20	15	36	72	10	19	547	307	12	230
Enfamil Reguline	20	15	35	74	10	19	549	308	10.1	230
AMINO ACID BASED									
EleCare Infant	20	20	32	72	13	26	780	568	12	350
Neocate Infant	20	21	30	78	11	27	830	624	12.4	375
PurAmino	20	19	36	69	14	19	627	347	12	350
Alfamino Infant	20	19	34	74	12	17	797	523	12	330
SPECIALIZED									
3232A	20	19	28	89	9	19	627	422	12.5	250
RCF	20	20	36	68	13	19	704	503	12.2	168
Enfaport	30	35	54	102	13	29	940	520	18	280
B. TODDLER AND YOUNG CHILD 1–10 YEARS									
COW'S MILK–BASED FORMULAS									
Boost Kid Essentials	30	30	38	135	24	30	1181	886	14	550/600/570
Boost Kid Essentials 1.5 (w/ fiber)	45	42	75	165	30	33	1300	990	14	390 (405)
Carnation Instant Breakfast Essentials	24	43	16	105	24	27	1539	1539	13.8	N/A
Compleat Pediatric	30	38	39	132	33	42	1440	1000	14	380
Cow's Milk, 2%	15	35	20	50	22	41	1258	979	0.5	N/A
Cow's Milk, whole	19	34	34	48	22	40	1226	956	0.5	285
KetoCal 3:1	30	22	97	10	18	35	1140	801	16	180
KetoCal 4:1	43	30	144	6	26	55	1600	1600	22	197
Monogen	30	27	28	163	21	22	617	480	10.1	370
Nutren Junior (also w/ fiber)	30	30	50	110	20	34	1000	800	14	350
PediaSure Enteral (also w/ fiber)	30	30	38	139	17	38	1050	845	14	335 (345)

Continued

TABLE 21.12
ENTERAL NUTRITION COMPONENTS (PER LITER)—cont'd
A. INFANT FORMULAS—cont'd

	Kcal/oz	Protein (g)	Fat (g)	Carbs (g)	Na (mEq)	K (mEq)	Ca (mg)	P (mg)	Fe (mg)	Osmolality
PediaSure 1.5 (also w/ fiber)	45	59	67	160 (165)	17	42	1476	1054	11	370 (390)
PediaSure SideKicks	19	30	21	89	17	42	1055	844	11	420
PediaSure Vanilla (also w/ fiber)	30	30	38	139	17	34	972	845	14	490 (480)
Portagen	30	34	46	110	22	29	900	680	18	350
SOY BASED										
Bright Beginnings Soy Pediatric Drink	30	30	50	109	17	40	1050	690	18	350
SEMI-ELEMENTAL, HYDROLYZED										
Peptamen Junior Fiber	30	30	39	137	20	34	1000	800	14	390
Peptamen Junior with Prebio	30	30	39	137	20	34	1000	800	14	365
Peptamen Junior, unflavored (w/ fiber, vanilla–flavored)	30	30	39	138	20	34	1000	800	14	260 (390)
Peptamen Junior 1.5	45	45	68	180	30	51	1652	1352	20.8	450
PediaSure Peptide (also flavored)	30	30	41	134	31	35	1060	844	14	250 (390)
PediaSure Peptide 1.5	45	45	61	201	47	52	1580	1265	21	450
SOY AND PORK, HYDROLYZED										
Pepdite Junior, Unflavored	30	31	50	106	18	35	1130	940	14	430
AMINO ACID BASED										
EleCare Jr, Unflavored and Vanilla	30	31	49	107	20	39	1174	854	18	590
E028 Splash	30	25	35	146	9	24	620	620	7.7	820
Neocate Junior Flavored	30	35	47	110	19	36	1200	738	16	690
Neocate Junior Unflavored	30	33	50	104	18	35	1130	697	15	590
Alfamino Junior	30	33	44	122	21	36	1200	840	18	590
Vivonex Pediatric	24	24	24	130	17	31	970	800	10	360

C. OLDER CHILDREN AND ADULT STANDARD FORMULAS

COW'S MILK–BASED FORMULAS

	Kcal/oz	Protein (g)	Fat (g)	Carbs (g)	Na (mEq)	K (mEq)	Ca (mg)	P (mg)	Fe (mg)	Osmolality
Boost	30	40	17	171	24	43	1250	1250	19	625
Boost Glucose Control	32	59	50	84	48	29	1160	928	15	400
Boost High Protein	30	63	25	138	31	41	1459	1250	19	650
Boost Plus	45	59	59	188	31	41	1459	1250	19	670
Compleat	32	48	40	128	43	44	760	760	14	340
Ensure Clear	30	35	0	215	6.5	0	0	0	9	700
Ensure Immune Health	32	38	25	177	37	40	1266	1055	19	620
Ensure Plus	45	55	46	215	40	43	1266	1266	19	680
Glucerna 1.0 Cal	30	42	54	96	41	40	705	705	13	355
Jevity 1 Cal	32	44	35	155	40	40	910	760	14	300
Jevity 1.2 Cal	36	56	39	169	59	47	1200	1200	18	450
Jevity 1.5 Cal	45	64	50	216	61	55	1200	1200	18	525
Nepro	54	81	96	161	46	27	1060	720	19	745
Novasource Renal	60	74	100	200	39	21	1300	650	18	700/960
Nutren 1.0, vanilla (w/ fiber)	30	40	38	127	38	32	668	668	12	370 (410)
Nutren 1.5, unflavored	45	60	68	169	51	48	1000	1000	18	430
Nutren 2.0	60	80	104	196	57	49	1340	1340	24	745
Osmolite 1 Cal	32	44	35	144	40	40	760	760	14	300
Osmolite 1.2 Cal	36	56	39	158	58	46	1200	1200	18	360
Osmolite 1.5 Cal	45	63	49	204	61	46	1000	1000	18	525
Promote (w/ fiber)	30	63	26	130	44	51	1200	1200	18	340 (380)
Pulmocare	45	63	93	106	57	50	1060	1060	19	475

Continued

TABLE 21.12

ENTERAL NUTRITION COMPONENTS (PER LITER)—cont'd

Product									
Renalcal	60	35	83	291	0	0	0	0	600
Replete, unflavored	30	63	34	113	39	39	1000	1000	300/350
Resource 2.0	60	84	88	217	35	39	1042	1042	790
Resource Breeze	32	38	0	230	15	1	42	633	18.8	750
Suplena	54	45	96	196	35	29	1055	717	11	780
TwoCal HN	60	84	91	219	64	63	1050	1050	19	725

SOY BASED

Product									
Fibersource HN	36	53	39	160	52	51	1000	1000	17	490
Isosource 1.5 CAL	45	68	65	170	56	58	1070	1070	19	650/585
Isosource HN	36	53	39	160	48	49	1200	1200	15	490

SEMI-ELEMENTAL HYDROLYZED

Product									
Peptamen, unflavored	30	40	39	127	25	39	800	700	18	270
Peptamen with Prebio	30	40	39	127	25	39	800	700	18	300
Peptamen 1.5, unflavored	45	68	56	188	45	48	1000	1000	27	550
Peptamen AF	36	76	55	107	35	41	800	800	14.4	390
Peptamen Bariatric	30	93	38	78	29	34	670	670	12	345
Perative	39	67	37	180	45	44	870	870	16	460
Pivot 1.5	45	94	51	172	61	51	1000	1000	18	595
Vital 1.0 Cal	30	40	38	130	46	36	705	705	13	390
Vital AF 1.2 Cal	35.6	75	54	111	55	43	844	844	15	425
Vital 1.5 Cal	45	67.5	57	187	65	51	1000	1000	18	610

AMINO ACID BASED

Product									
Tolerex	30	21	1.5	230	20	30	560	560	10	550
Vivonex RTF	30	50	12	175	29	31	670	670	12	630
Vivonex Plus	30	45	7	190	27	27	560	560	10	650
Vivonex T.E.N.	30	38	3	210	26	24	500	500	9	630

*Liquid formulation.

TABLE 21.13
FORMULAS FOR SPECIAL CLINICAL CIRCUMSTANCES

A. INFANTS

Preterm	
Predischarge	Enfamil Premature 20, 24 HP, 30 Similac Special Care Advance 20, 24 HP, 30 Gerber Good Start Premature 20, 24 HP, 30
Postdischarge (through 12 mo)	Enfamil EnfaCare Similac NeoSure
Lactose intolerance	Enfamil LactoFree Similac Sensitive Similac for Diarrhea
Vegetarian, lactose intolerance, or galactosemia	America's Store Brand Soy Infant Formula Gerber Graduates Soy Similac Go and Grow Soy-Based Formula (9–24 mo) Similac Soy Isomil Enfagrow Soy NEXT STEP (9–24 mo) Enfamil ProSobee
Protein (e.g., cow's milk) allergy/intolerance and/or fat malabsorption	Alimentum EleCare Infant Neocate Infant Nutramigen PurAmino Pregestimil Gerber Extensive HA Alfamino Infant
Severe carbohydrate intolerance	3232A RCF
Requiring lower calcium and phosphorus	Similac PM 60/40

B. TODDLERS AND YOUNG CHILDREN AGES 1–10 YR

Vegetarian, lactose intolerance, or milk protein intolerance	Bright Beginnings Soy Pediatric Drink
Protein allergy/intolerance and/or fat malabsorption	PediaSure Peptide (and 1.5) Pepdite Junior Peptamen Junior (with and without Prebio) Vivonex Pediatric EleCare Junior Neocate Junior (Unflavored and Flavored) E028 Splash Alfamino Junior
Fat malabsorption, intestinal lymphatic obstruction, chylothorax	Portagen Monogen Enfaport
Increased caloric needs	Boost Kids Essentials Carnation Instant Breakfast Essentials Nutren Junior (also with fiber) PediaSure (also with fiber)
Requiring clear liquid diet	Resource Breeze Ensure Clear PediaSure SideKicks Clear
Intractable epilepsy	KetoCal (3:1 and 4:1)

Continued

TABLE 21.13
FORMULAS FOR SPECIAL CLINICAL CIRCUMSTANCES—cont'd

C. OLDER CHILDREN AND ADULTS

Enteral Nutrition (tube feeding)	
For malabsorption of protein and/or fat	Peptamen, Peptamen w/ Prebio, Peptamen 1.5 Perative Tolerex Vital High Protein Vital 1.0 Cal and AF 1.2 Cal, 1.5 Cal Vivonex Plus and Vivonex T.E.N.
For critically ill and/or malabsorption	Pulmocare Pivot 1.5 Cal Perative
For impaired glucose tolerance	Glucerna Glytrol Store-brand diabetic nutritional drink
For dialysis patients	Magnacal Renal Nepro NutriRenal
For patients with acute renal failure not on dialysis	Renalcal Suplena
Increased caloric needs (oral)	
With a normal gastrointestinal (GI) tract	Boost, Boost with fiber Boost Plus, Boost High Protein Carnation Instant Breakfast Essentials with whole milk Ensure Original NUTRA Shake
For clear liquid diet	Resource Breeze Ensure Clear PediaSure SideKicks Clear Ensure Enlive
For patients with cystic fibrosis (CF)	Scandishake with whole milk

D. Clinical Conditions Requiring Special Diets and Suggested Formula(s) (Table 21.13)

A comprehensive (but not complete) list of special clinical conditions (e.g., cow's milk allergy or intolerance) and the growing number of formulas designed for these conditions

E. Common Oral Rehydration Solutions (Table 21.14)

VII. PARENTERAL NUTRITION[16]

Necessary to adequately support the pediatric patient with insufficient enteral intake

TABLE 21.14
ORAL REHYDRATION SOLUTIONS

Solution	Kcal/mL (kcal/oz)	Carbohydrate (g/L)	Na (mEq/L)	K (mEq/L)	Osmolality (mOsm/kg H_2O)
CeraLyte-50	0.16 (4.9)	Rice digest (40)	50	20	N/A
CeraLyte-70	0.16 (4.9)	Rice digest (40)	70	20	N/A
CeraLyte-90	0.16 (4.9)	Rice digest (40)	90	20	N/A
Enfalyte	0.12 (3.7)	Rice syrup solids (30)	50	25	160
Oral Rehydration Salts (WHO)	0.06 (2)	Dextrose (20)	90	20	330
Pedialyte (unflavored)	0.1 (3)	Dextrose (25)	45	20	250

TABLE 21.15
INITIATION AND ADVANCEMENT OF PARENTERAL NUTRITION*

Nutrient	Initial Dose	Advancement	Maximum
Glucose	5%–10%	2.5%–5%/day	12.5% peripheral 18 mg/kg/min (maximum rate of infusion)
Protein	1–1.5 g/kg/day	0.5–1 g/kg/day	3–4 g/kg/day 10%–16% of calories
Fat[†]	0.5–1 g/kg/day	1 g/kg/day	4 g/kg/day 0.17 g/kg/hr (maximum rate of infusion)

*Acceptable osmolarity of parenteral nutrition through a peripheral line varies between 900 and 1050 osm/L by institution. An estimate of the osmolarity of parenteral nutrition can be obtained with the following formula: Estimated osmolarity = (dextrose concentration $\times$ 50) + (amino acid concentration $\times$ 100) + (mEq of electrolytes $\times$ 2). Consult individual pharmacy for hospital limitations.

[†]Essential fatty acid deficiency may occur in fat-free parenteral nutrition within 2–4 weeks in infants and children and as early as 2–14 days in neonates. A minimum of 2%–4% of total caloric intake as linoleic acid and 0.25%–0.5% as linolenic acid is necessary to meet essential fatty acid requirements.

Modified from Baker RD, Baker SS, Davis AM. Pediatric Parenteral Nutrition. New York: Chapman and Hall; 1997 and Cox JH, Melbardis IM. Parenteral nutrition. In: Samour PQ, King K, eds. Handbook of Pediatric Nutrition. 4th ed. Boston: Jones and Bartlett Learning; 2012.

A. Situations Where Parenteral Nutrition (PN) Is Suggested

1. Inability to feed enterally or when alimentation via gastrointestinal tract is restricted > 3–5 days (or earlier for premature infants and neonates)
2. Chronic gastrointestinal dysfunction and/or malabsorption
3. Increased gastrointestinal losses or requirements

B. Suggested Formulations for Initiation and Advancement of PN
(Table 21.15)

Suggested glucose, protein, and fat during initiation, as well as recommendations for advancement and maximum allowable amounts

TABLE 21.16
PARENTERAL NUTRITION FORMULATION RECOMMENDATIONS

Component	Preterm	Term Infants	1–3 yr	4–6 yr	7–10 yr	11–18 yr
Energy (kcal/kg/day)	85–105	90–108	75–90	65–80	55–70	30–55
Protein (g/kg/day)	2.5–4	2.5–3.5	1.5–2.5	1.5–2.5	1.5–2.5	0.8–2
Sodium (mEq/kg/day)	2–4	2–4	2–4	2–4	2–4	60–150 mEq/day
Potassium (mEq/kg/day)	2–4	2–4	2–4	2–4	2–4	70–180 mEq/day
Calcium (mg/kg/day)	50–60	20–40	10–20	10–20	10–20	200–800 mg/day
Phosphorus (mg/kg/day)	30–45	30–45	15–40	15–40	15–40	280–900 mg/day
Magnesium (mEq/kg/day)	0.5–1	0.25–1	0.25–0.5	0.25–0.5	0.25–0.5	8–24 mEq/day
Zinc (mcg/kg/day)	325–400	100–250	100	100	50	2–5 mg/day
Copper (mcg/kg/day)*	20	20	20	20	5–20	200–300 mcg/day
Manganese (mcg/kg/day)*	1	1	1	1	1	40–50 mcg/day
Selenium (mcg/kg/day)	2	2	2	2	1–2	40–60 mcg/day

*Copper and manganese needs may be lowered in cholestasis.
Modified from Baker RD, Baker SS, Davis AM. Pediatric Parenteral Nutrition. New York: Chapman and Hall; 1997; Cox JH, Melbardis IM. Parenteral nutrition. In: Samour PQ, King K, eds. Handbook of Pediatric Nutrition. 4th ed. Boston: Jones and Bartlett Learning; 2012; and American Society for Parenteral and Enteral Nutrition (ASPEN). Safe practices for parenteral nutrition. JPEN J Parenter Enteral Nutr. 2004;28(6):S39-S70.

C. Recommended Parenteral Formulations (Table 21.16)
Based on age groups; includes recommendations for electrolytes, elements, and minerals

D. Suggested Monitoring Schedule for Patients Receiving PN (Table 21.17)

TABLE 21.17
MONITORING SCHEDULE FOR PATIENTS RECEIVING PARENTERAL NUTRITION*

Variable	Initial Period[†]	Later Period[‡]
GROWTH		
Weight	Daily	2 times/week
Height	Weekly (infants)	
	Monthly (children)	Monthly
Head circumference (infants)	Weekly	Monthly[§]
LABORATORY STUDIES		
Electrolytes and glucose	Daily until stable	Weekly
BUN/creatinine	Twice weekly	Weekly
Albumin or prealbumin	Weekly	Weekly
Ca^{2+}, Mg^{2+}, P	Twice weekly	Weekly
ALT, AST, ALP	Weekly	Weekly
Total and direct bilirubin	Weekly	Weekly
CBC	Weekly	Weekly
Triglycerides	With each increase	Weekly
Vitamins	—	As indicated
Trace minerals	—	As indicated

ALP, Alkaline phosphatase; ALT, alanine transaminase; AST, aspartate transaminase; BUN, blood urea nitrogen; CBC, complete blood cell count.
*For patients on long-term parenteral nutrition, monitoring every 2–4 weeks is adequate in most cases.
[†]The period before nutritional goals are reached or during any period of instability.
[‡]When stability is reached, no changes in nutrient composition.
[§]Weekly in preterm infants.

REFERENCES

1. Centers for Disease Control and Prevention (CDC). Growth Charts. Available at <http://www.cdc.gov/growthcharts/>.
2. Centers for Disease Control and Prevention (CDC), Division of Nutrition, Physical Activity, and Obesity. Body Mass Index (BMI). Available at <http://www.cdc.gov/healthyweight/assessing/bmi/>.
3. Li C, Ford ES, Mokdad AH, et al. Recent trends in waist circumference and waist-height ratio among US children and adolescents. *Pediatrics*. 2006;118:e1390-e1398.
4. Barlow SE, Expert Committee. Expert Committee recommendations regarding the prevention, assessment, and treatment of child and adolescent overweight and obesity: summary report. *Pediatrics*. 2007;120(Suppl 4):S164-S192.
5. Childhood Obesity Action Network. Expert Committee Recommendations on the Assessment, Prevention and Treatment of Child and Adolescent Overweight and Obesity - 2007. Available at <http://obesity.nichq.org/resources/expert%20committee%20recommendation%20implementation%20guide>.
6. Otten JJ, Hellwig JP, Meyers LD, eds. *Dietary Reference Intakes: The Essential Guide to Nutrient Requirements*. Washington, DC: National Academies Press; 2006.
7. Corrales KM, Utter SL. Growth failure. In: Samour PQ, King K, eds. *Handbook of Pediatric Nutrition*. Boston: Jones and Bartlett Publishers; 2005:391-406.

8. Shah MD. Failure to thrive in children. *J Clin Gastroenterol.* 2002;35(5):371-374.
9. Solomon SM, Kirby DF. The refeeding syndrome: a review. *JPEN J Parenter Enteral Nutr.* 1990;14:90-96.
10. Kraft MD, Btaiche IF, Sacks GS. Review of the refeeding syndrome. *Nutr Clin Pract.* 2005;20:625-633.
11. Golden NH, Abrams SA, AAP Committee on Nutrition. Optimizing bone health in children and adolescents. *Pediatrics.* 2014;134:e1229-e1243.
12. Baker RD, Greer FR, AAP Committee on Nutrition. Diagnosis and prevention of iron deficiency and iron-deficiency anemia in infants and young children 0 through 3 years. *Pediatrics.* 2010;126:1040-1050.
13. Clark MB, Slayton RL, AAP Section on Oral Health. Fluoride use in caries prevention in the primary care setting. *Pediatrics.* 2014;134:626-633.
14. American Academy of Pediatrics, Section on Breastfeeding. Policy Statement - Breastfeeding and the use of human milk. *Pediatrics.* 2012;129:e827-e841.
15. Enteral Nutrition Practice Recommendations Task Force, Bankhead R, Boullata J, et al. Enteral nutrition practice recommendations. *JPEN J Parenter Enteral Nutr.* 2009;33(2):122-167.
16. American Society for Parenteral and Enteral Nutrition (ASPEN). Safe practices for parenteral nutrition. *JPEN J Parenter Enteral Nutr.* 2004;28(6):S39-S70. Available at: <http://www.ashp.org/DocLibrary/BestPractices/2004ASPEN.aspx>.

Chapter 22
Oncology
Chelsea Kotch, MD, and Zarah Yusuf, MD

See additional content on Expert Consult

I. WEB RESOURCES

- National Cancer Institute (NCI): http://www.cancer.gov/cancertopics/pdq/pediatrictreatment
- SEER (Surveillance, Epidemiology, and End Results) data from the NCI: http://seer.cancer.gov/
- Long-term follow-up guidelines for survivors of pediatric cancer: http://www.survivorshipguidelines.org/
- NCI Clinical Trial Database: www.cancer.gov/clinicaltrials
- Children's Oncology Camping Association, International: http://www.cocai.org/

II. PRESENTING SIGNS AND SYMPTOMS OF PEDIATRIC MALIGNANCIES (Tables 22.1 and 22.2)

NOTE: Common presenting signs and symptoms of many malignancies include weight loss, failure to thrive, anorexia, malaise, fever, pallor, and lymphadenopathy.

III. FEATURES OF A PATHOLOGIC LYMPH NODE

A. Size
<2 cm usually insignificant unless >1 cm in supraclavicular fossa or increase in size over time >2 weeks.

B. Consistency
Rubber (classically lymphoma), hard (malignant, granulomatous infectious).

C. Sensation
Nontender more concerning for malignancy.

D. Evaluation if Concern for Malignancy

1. Laboratory studies: Complete blood count (CBC) with differential, erythrocyte sedimentation rate, lactate dehydrogenase
2. Specific serologies based on potential exposures: HIV, hepatitis B surface antigen, syphilis (rapid plasma reagin), tuberculosis (purified protein derivative), Epstein–Barr virus
3. Other options: Chest x-ray (CXR), excisional biopsy

TABLE 22.1
PRESENTING SIGNS AND SYMPTOMS OF PEDIATRIC MALIGNANCIES[3,10]

Malignancy	Signs and Symptoms	Initial Workup*	Peak Incidence by Age, Prognosis
ALL	Anorexia, fatigue, malaise, irritability, pallor, low-grade fevers, bone pain/limp ± bone tenderness, bruising/bleeding, petechiae, hepatosplenomegaly, lymphadenopathy, painless testicular enlargement/mass	CBC with differential, peripheral blood smear, complete metabolic panel, calcium, phosphate, pregnancy test, prothrombin time, activated partial prothrombin time, lactate dehydrogenase, uric acid, blood type and screen, chest x-ray, ECG, echocardiogram, HIV, bone marrow biopsy, blood and urine cultures if febrile	Peaks at age 2–5 years; overall cure rate exceeds 80%–90% (pre-B ALL best prognosis, prognosis worsens with age >14 years)
AML	Similar to ALL; may also have subcutaneous nodules, gingival hyperplasia, chloromas (masses)	Same initial workup as ALL plus DIC testing, HLA typing, CSF for staging, ophthalmologic exam	Peaks in first year of life, declines until age 4 years, risk increases again after adolescence; cure rate ~50% (cytogenetics determines prognosis, acute promyelocytic leukemia best prognosis)
Lymphoma (HD, NHL)	Painless lymphadenopathy, hepatosplenomegaly, stridor, cough, fever, weight loss, night sweats, fatigue, anorexia, pruritus, intussusception, focal neurologic symptoms, alcohol-induced pain	CBC with differential, peripheral smear, electrolytes, LFTs, ESR, ferritin, uric acid, LDH, CSF, CXR, bilateral bone marrow biopsy, echocardiogram, ECG, CT/PET	HD peak incidence occurs in bimodal distribution (15–34 year old and >55 years); NHL no sharp peak but most common in second decade of life; HD has 95% survival with stage I disease and 75% for stage IV; NHL prognosis varies widely with histology and stage
Brain tumors (see Table 22.2)	Headache, irritability, emesis, gait changes, focal neurologic symptoms, cranial nerve palsies, changes in vision, personality changes, diabetes insipidus, precocious puberty	MRI of brain and spine, ophthalmology examination, CSF, PFTs, CrCl, audiology, endocrine workup if pituitary dysfunction is suspected	Higher incidence in children <5 years; prognosis widely variable by subtype, however, brain tumors are leading cause of cancer death in children 0 through 14 years of age

Neuroblastoma	Abdominal mass, anorexia, vomiting, change in bowel habits, hepatomegaly, fever, irritability, bone pain, limp, subcutaneous nodules, SVC syndrome, Horner syndrome, periorbital ecchymosis, opsoclonus-myoclonus syndrome, secretory diarrhea (vasoactive intestinal peptide effect)	Abdominal ultrasound, CT chest/abdomen/pelvis, urine HVA and VMA	Peaks at age <2 years; 5-year survival for age <1 year, 83%; between 1 and 4 years, 55%; and 5–9 years, 40% (poor prognosis if >1 year old with Stage III or IV disease, high Shimada rating, N-myc amplification)
Wilms tumor	Abdominal mass (may be asymptomatic), abdominal pain, anorexia, vomiting, hypertension, hematuria, anemia (bleeding within the tumor)	Abdominal ultrasound, abdominal CT or MRI, urinalysis, CBC	Peaks at age 2–5 years (5% incidence with Beckwith–Wiedemann syndrome); >90% patient survive 4 years after diagnosis (poor prognosis with diffuse anaplasia)
Bone sarcoma (Osteosarcoma, Ewing sarcoma)	Longbone pain not relieved with conservative treatment; limp, swelling, fracture; distal femur and proximal tibia most common sites	X-ray of primary site, CT of chest	Peaks at age 10–20 years; osteosarcoma >70% survival with nonmetastatic disease, worse prognosis in primary tumor of axial skeleton; initial management involves neoadjuvant chemotherapy with assessment of tumor necrosis at resection, with poorer prognosis if poor necrosis at time of resection; Ewing sarcoma have poorer prognosis if metastatic disease and/or axial primary tumors
Rhabdomyosarcoma (soft tissue malignant tumor of skeletal muscle origin)	Localized symptoms based on location of tumor, most common sites are head, neck, or orbit; may see painful or painless mass, proptosis, hearing loss, urinary obstruction, hematuria	CT or MRI of primary site	Peaks at age <6 years and in adolescence: prognosis based on stage, extent of surgical resection, and histopathology (alveolar histopathology poorer prognosis than embryonal). 5 year survival of patients with metastases at diagnosis is <30%.
Retinoblastoma (Rb)	Leukocoria (retrolental mass), strabismus, hyphema, irregular pupil(s)	Ophthalmology referral, MRI of brain to evaluate pineal gland if bilateral	Peaks at age 2 years; survival at 5 years >90%; bilateral Rb implies germ-line Rb1 mutation

Continued

TABLE 22.1
PRESENTING SIGNS AND SYMPTOMS OF PEDIATRIC MALIGNANCIES—cont'd

Malignancy	Signs and Symptoms	Initial Workup*	Peak Incidence by Age, Prognosis
Liver cancer (hepatoblastoma, hepatocellular carcinoma)	Painless abdominal mass, anorexia, emesis, abdominal pain, fever (hepatoblastoma may be associated with anemia, thrombocytosis)	CBC, LFTs, AFP, hep B and C titers, abdominal ultrasound	Hepatoblastoma peaks at age <3 years, HCC peaks after 12 years of age (associated with hep B and hep C); hepatoblastoma 5-year survival is 75% (poorer prognosis if low AFP at diagnosis), HCC 5-year survival is 25%
Histiocytic disease	Scaly papular rash, fever, weight loss, gingival hyperplasia, diarrhea, pituitary dysfunction, precocious puberty, polydipsia, polyuria, long bone pain	Skeletal survey, CXR, CBC, LFTs, LDH, ferritin, uric acid, triglycerides, urine osmolality, skin biopsy	Variable
Gonadal tumor	Testicular masses, scrotal swelling. Ovarian tumors are typically asymptomatic until quite large	Ultrasound, CT or MRI, AFP, β-hCG, LDH	Peaks in adolescence

AFP, α-Fetoprotein; ALL, acute lymphocytic leukemia; AML, acute myeloid leukemia; β-hCG, beta human chorionic gonadotropin; CBC, complete blood cell count; CSF, cerebrospinal fluid; CT, computed tomography; CXR, chest x-ray; DIC, disseminated intravascular coagulation; ECG, electrocardiogram; ESR, erythrocyte sedimentation rate; hep, hepatitis; HD, Hodgkin disease; HIV, human immunodeficiency virus; HLA, human leukocyte antigen; HVA/VMA, homovanillic acid/vanillylmandelic acid (urine catecholamines); LDH, lactate dehydrogenase; LFTs, liver function tests; MRI, magnetic resonance imaging; NHL, non-Hodgkin lymphoma; PET, positron emission tomography; PFTs, pulmonary function tests; SVC, superior vena cava.

*Laboratory test and imaging suggestions are meant as a guide for evaluation of a potential malignancy. Patients warranting definitive testing should be referred to an oncologist.

TABLE 22.2
PRESENTING SIGNS AND SYMPTOMS OF PEDIATRIC BRAIN TUMORS[1,2]

Tumor Location	Ped Brain Tumor Subtype	Symptoms Based on Location*
Suprasellar/ Chiasmatic	Optic glioma, craniopharyngioma, germinoma, prolactinoma, pituitary adenoma, astrocytoma, LCH	Headache, visual field deficit, precocious/delayed puberty, anorexia, DI
Cortex	Low/high grade glioma, astrocytoma, DNET, PNET, oligodendroglioma, ganglioglioma, pleomorphic xanthoastrocytoma	Headache, seizures, papilledemia, weakness, altered language, encephalopathy, visual field deficit, hemiplegia
Pineal gland/ midbrain	Low/high grade glioma, teratoma, pineoblastoma, pineocytoma, germinoma, PNET	Upgaze paralysis, vomiting, nystagmus, diplopia, tremor
Pons	DIPG, focal low/high grade glioma	Diplopia, facial weakness, drooling, weakness, incoordination, disconjugate gaze
Basal ganglia/ thalamus	Low/high grade glioma, germinoma, oligodendroglioma	Abnormal movements, weakness, hemi-sensory deficit, visual field deficit
Cerebellum	Medulloblastoma[†], JPA, ependymoma, ATRT, high grade glioma, hemangioblastoma, dysplastic gangliocytoma of cerebellum	Vomiting, ataxia, tremor, dysmetria, papilledema, nystagmus
Ventricular system	Choroid plexus papilloma/carcinoma, subependymal giant cell astrocytoma, ependymoma, ATRT, DIG	Early morning vomiting, recurring headache, macrocephaly
Meninges	Meningioma	

*Children <1 year old are challenging to diagnose clinically, may present with macrocephaly, vomiting, irritability, lethargy, failure to thrive, early handedness, head tilt.
[†]Medulloblastoma is the most common malignant brain tumor in children.
ATRT, atypical teratoid rhaboid tumor; DNET dysembryoplastic neuroepithelial tumor; DI, diabetes insipidus; DIG, desmoplastic infantile glioma; DIPG, diffuse intrapontine glioma; JPA, juvenile pilocytic astrocytoma; LCH, Langerhans Cell Histiocytosis; PNET, primitive neuroectodermal tumor.
Modified from Crawford J. Childhood Brain Tumors. Pediatrics In Review 2013; 34:1-7 and Wilne, S, et al. Presentation of Childhood CNS tumours: a systematic review and meta-analysis. Lancet Oncology. 2007; 8(3):685-695.

E. Consider Lymph Node Biopsy

1. Size: >2 cm, increasing over 2 weeks, no decrease in size of node after 4 weeks
2. Location: Supraclavicular lymph node
3. Associated features: Abnormal chest radiograph with hilar adenopathy or mediastinal widening, fever, weight loss, hepatosplenomegaly

IV. GENERAL MANAGEMENT OF NEWLY DIAGNOSED PEDIATRIC BRAIN TUMORS

A. Initial Approach
1. Airway, breathing, circulation stabilization
2. Neurosurgery/neuro-oncology consultation
3. Take nothing by mouth (NPO)

B. Laboratory Evaluation
1. Presurgical laboratory tests (electrolytes, CBC, coagulation studies, blood type and cross-matching)
2. Preoperative endocrine laboratory tests for suprasellar tumors
3. Lumbar puncture for cerebrospinal fluid (CSF) cytology and tumor markers [for medulloblastoma and suspected central nervous system (CNS) germinoma, respectively] performed 7–10 days postoperatively if no contraindications

C. Imaging
Magnetic resonance imaging (MRI) of brain and spine with/without intravenous (IV) contrast.

D. Medication Management
1. IV steroids (dexamethasone) with gastrointestinal (GI) protective agent (i.e., ranitidine)
2. Seizure prophylaxis for those at high risk of seizures or seizure history

E. Additional Consults
1. Ophthalmologic examination
2. Social work consultation
3. Child life consultation

V. COMMONLY USED CHEMOTHERAPEUTIC DRUGS AND ASSOCIATED ACUTE TOXICITIES (Table 22.3)

VI. ONCOLOGIC EMERGENCIES[3-5]

A. Hyperleukocytosis/Leukostasis
1. **Etiology:** Elevated white blood cell (WBC) count (>100,000/μL) in leukemia patients, leading to leukostasis in the microcirculation and diminished tissue perfusion (notably in CNS and lungs). Leukostasis occurs more commonly and at lower WBC counts (>100,000/μL) in acute myeloid leukemia [AML (especially M4 and M5)] than in acute lymphocytic leukemia [ALL (typically requiring a WBC count >300,000/μL)]. Leukostasis is very common in chronic myeloid leukemia (CML) but at WBC counts >300,000/μL.
2. **Presentation:** Hypoxia, tachypnea, and dyspnea from pulmonary leukostasis. Mental status changes, headaches, seizures, papilledema from cerebral leukostasis. May also see GI bleeding, abdominal pain, renal insufficiency, priapism, and/or intracranial hemorrhage. Hyperleukocytosis may be asymptomatic.

TABLE 22.3
CHARACTERISTICS OF CHEMOTHERAPEUTIC AGENTS

Drug Name (Drug Class)	Toxicity*	Monitoring and Supportive Care
Asparaginase (L-Asp, PEG-Asp, Elspar, Erwinia) (Enzyme)	Pancreatitis, hypersensitivity reactions (both acute and delayed), coagulopathy (thrombosis and bleeding), hyperammonemia	Avoid premedication (hypersensitivity reaction dictates change in formulation), monitor coagulation studies, consider amylase/lipase for abdominal pain
Bleomycin (Blenoxane) (DNA strand breaker)	Anaphylaxis, pneumonitis, pulmonary fibrosis	Monitor PFTs
Busulfan (Myleran) (Alkylator)	Significant myelosuppression, seizures, veno-occlusive disease, acute/chronic lung injury	Seizure prophylaxis; monitor weight/abdominal girth/bilirubin
Carboplatin (CBDCA, Paraplatin) (DNA cross-linker)	Thrombocytopenia, nephrotoxicity, ototoxicity, peripheral neuropathy	Monitor creatinine, adjust dose based on creatinine clearance, audiology evaluation
Cisplatin (cis-platinum, CDDP, Platinol) (DNA cross-linker)	Tubular and glomerular nephrotoxicity (related to cumulative dose), severe emesis, hypomagnesemia, hypophosphatemia, ototoxicity	Monitor creatinine, magnesium, phosphate; audiology evaluation; aggressive antiemetic regimen
Clofarabine (Clolar) (Purine analog)	Capillary leak syndrome, veno-occlusive disease, nephrotoxicity, hyperbilirubinemia	Monitor creatinine; monitor weight, abdominal girth, bilirubin
Cyclophosphamide (CTX, Cytoxan) (Alkylator prodrug)	Cardiomyopathy, hemorrhagic cystitis, severe emesis, SIADH, leukoencephalopathy	Hyperhydration and mesna; ECG
Cytarabine (Ara-C) (Nucleotide analog)	Significant myelosuppression, cytarabine syndrome (rash, fever), conjunctivitis, severe mucositis, ataxia, respiratory distress rapidly progressing to pulmonary edema	Corticosteroid eye drops; antibiotic coverage for viridans streptococci with infectious concerns or fever, systemic steroids for Ara-C syndrome
Dactinomycin (actinomycin D) (Antibiotic)	Rash, hypocalcemia, radiation recall, veno-occlusive disease	Monitor calcium; monitor weights, abdominal girth, and bilirubin
Daunorubicin (daunomycin) and doxorubicin (Adriamycin) (Anthracyclines)	Arrhythmia, congestive heart failure (related to cumulative dose), cardiomyopathy, severe mucositis, severe emesis, red urine and bodily fluids, radiation recall	Limit cumulative dose; echocardiogram; consider dexrazoxane
Etoposide (VP-16, VePesid) (Topoisomerase inhibitor)	Anaphylaxis (rare), hypotension, transient cortical blindness, hyperbilirubinemia, transaminitis, secondary malignancy (AML)	Slow infusion if hypotension; change formulation to etoposide phosphate if anaphylaxis; monitor bilirubin and transaminases

Continued

TABLE 22.3
CHARACTERISTICS OF CHEMOTHERAPEUTIC AGENTS—cont'd

Drug Name (Drug Class)	Toxicity*	Monitoring and Supportive Care
Fludarabine (Fludara) (Nucleotide analog)	Significant myelosuppression, elevation of transaminases, neurotoxicity	Monitor creatinine (decreased clearance results in increased risk of neurotoxicity)
Ifosfamide (isophosphamide, Ifex) (Alkylator prodrug)	Mental status changes, encephalopathy (rarely progressing to death), renal tubular damage, hemorrhagic cystitis, Fanconi syndrome	Monitor creatinine, magnesium, phosphate, potassium; mesna
Lomustine (CCNU) (Alkylating agent)	Significant emesis, disorientation, fatigue	Aggressive antiemetic regimen
Melphalan (L-PAM, Alkeran) (Alkylator)	Prolonged leukopenia, severe mucositis, diarrhea, severe emesis, pulmonary fibrosis, infertility, cataracts	Aggressive oral hygiene, ophthalmologic examination, aggressive antiemetic regimen
Mercaptopurine (6-MP) (Nucleotide analog)	Headache, hepatotoxicity (increased risk in hypometabolizers)	Monitor transaminases, liver function tests
Methotrexate (MTX, amethopterin, Folex, Mexate) (Folate antagonist)	Mucositis, diarrhea, renal dysfunction, encephalopathy, ventriculitis (intrathecal), photosensitivity, leukoencephalopathy, osteoporosis	Leucovorin with high-dose therapy; oral hygiene; monitor neurologic examination and developmental milestones
Mitoxantrone (dihydroxyanthracenedione dihydrochloride, Novantrone) (DNA intercalator)	Myelosuppression, cardiomyopathy, severe mucositis, blue–green urine	Aggressive oral hygiene; consider dexrazoxane
Procarbazine (Matulane) (Alkylating agent)	Encephalopathy, significant thrombocytopenia, adverse effects with tyramine-rich foods, ethanol, MAOIs, meperidine, and many other drugs, infertility	Avoid selective serotonin reuptake inhibitors and maintain a diet low in tyramine (avoid aged cheese, beer, soy sauce)
Temozolomide (Temodar) (Alkylating agent)	Myelosuppression, constipation, headache, seizures	
Thioguanine (6-TG, 6-thioguanine) (Nucleotide analog)	Severe mucositis, diarrhea, hepatotoxicity, dermatitis	Aggressive oral hygiene; monitor liver function tests
Thiotepa (Alkylating agent)	Cognitive impairment, significant myelosuppression, rash, burns, desquamation of skin, impaired fertility, lower extremity weakness	Frequent bathing

TABLE 22.3
CHARACTERISTICS OF CHEMOTHERAPEUTIC AGENTS—cont'd

Drug Name (Drug Class)	Toxicity*	Monitoring and Supportive Care
Vinblastine (BVL, vincaleukoblastine, Velban) and Vincristine (VCR, Oncovin) *(Microtubule inhibitors)*	Constipation, bone and jaw pain, peripheral and autonomic sensory and motor neuropathy, foot drop, SIADH (rare)	Bowel regimen; monitor for neuropathy; fatal if given intrathecally
Vinorelbine (Navelbine) *(Microtubule inhibitor)*	Peripheral neuropathy, asthenia, hyperbilirubinemia, constipation, diarrhea	Monitor liver function tests and bilirubin
MOLECULARLY TARGETED CHEMOTHERAPEUTIC AGENTS		
Alemtuzumab (Campath) *(Monoclonal Ab binds CD52 on mature lymphocytes)*	Hypotension, bronchospasm, acute respiratory distress syndrome, cardiac arrhythmia	
Brentuximab (Adcetris) *(Chimeric monoclonal Ab binds CD30)*	Peripheral neuropathy, diarrhea	
Dinutuximab *(Monoclonal Ab binds GD-2; for use in neuroblastoma)*	Severe infusion reactions (26% of patients experience bronchospasm, facial edema, hypotension, stridor), neuropathy, hyponatremia, hepatotoxicity, hypocalcemia, capillary leak syndrome	Monitor sodium, calcium, liver function tests
Imatinib (Gleevec) *(Tyrosine kinase inhibitor)*	Congestive heart failure, edema, pleural effusions, rash, night sweats	ECG, consider serial echocardiograms
Rituximab (Rituxan) *(Chimeric monoclonal Ab binds CD20 on B cells)*	Infusion reaction, arrhythmia, urticaria, cytokine release syndrome, progressive multifocal leukoencephalopathy	
CHEMOTHERAPY ADJUNCTS		
Amifostine	Indication: Reduces toxicity of radiation Side effects: Hypotension (62%), nausea and vomiting, flushing, chills, dizziness, somnolence, hiccups, sneezing, hypocalcemia in susceptible patients (<1%), rigors (<1%), mild skin rash	
Dexrazoxane	Indication: Protective agent for anthracycline-induced cardiotoxicity Side effects: Myelosuppression	
Leucovorin	Indication: Reduces methotrexate toxicity Side effects: Allergic sensitization (rare)	
Mesna	Indication: Reduces risk of hemorrhagic cystitis Side effects: Headache, limb pain, abdominal pain, diarrhea, rash	

*All chemotherapeutic medications may cause nausea, vomiting, fever, immunosuppression, mucositis, gastrointestinal upset.

AML, Acute myeloid leukemia; ECG, electrocardiogram; MAOI, monoamine oxidase inhibitor; PEG, polyethylene glycol; PFTs, pulmonary function tests; SIADH, syndrome of inappropriate antidiuretic hormone.

Data from Physician's Desk Reference. 64th ed. Montvale, NJ: Medical Economics; 2010; Taketomo CK, Hodding JH, Kraus DM. American Pharmaceutical Association Pediatric Dosage Handbook. 16th ed. Hudson, OH: Lexi-Comp; 2009; and Micromedex 2.0.

3. **Management:**
a. Consider leukapheresis or exchange transfusion if CNS or pulmonary leukostasis.
b. Transfuse platelets as needed to keep count above 20,000/µL.
c. Avoid red blood cell (RBC) transfusions because they will raise viscosity (keep hemoglobin ≤10 g/dL). If RBCs are required, consider partial exchange transfusion.
d. Hydration, alkalinization, and allopurinol should be initiated (as discussed in Section VI.B).
e. Administer fresh frozen plasma (FFP) and vitamin K for coagulopathy.
f. Start disease treatment as soon as patient is clinically stable.

B. Tumor Lysis Syndrome

1. **Etiology:** Rapid lysis of tumor cells releases intracellular contents into the blood stream spontaneously before diagnosis or during early stages of chemotherapy (especially Burkitt lymphoma, T-cell ALL).
2. **Presentation:** Classic triad: hyperuricemia, hyperkalemia, hyperphosphatemia. Also hypocalcemia. Can lead to acute kidney injury due to precipitation of uric acid crystals and/or calcium phosphate crystals in renal tubules and microvasculature, respectively.
3. **Prevention and management:**
a. Hydration: Dextrose 5% (D_5) 1/4 normal saline (NS) ± 40 mEq/L $NaHCO_3$ (without K) at two times maintenance rate. Keep urine-specific gravity <1.010 and urine output >100 mL/m^2/hr.
b. Hyperuricemia: Allopurinol inhibits formation of uric acid and can be given orally (PO) or IV (see Formulary for dosing). Rasburicase converts uric acid to the more soluble allantoin. Use in higher-risk patients, especially those with uric acid >7.5 mg/dL.
c. Monitor K^+, Ca^{2+}, phosphate, uric acid, and urinalysis closely (up to Q2 hr for high-risk patients). There is an increased risk of calcium phosphate precipitation when Ca × Phos > 60.
d. Manage abnormal electrolytes as described in Chapter 11. See Chapter 19 for dialysis indications.
e. Consider stopping alkalinization after uric acid levels return to normal to facilitate calcium phosphate excretion.

C. Spinal Cord Compression

1. **Etiology:** Intrinsic or extrinsic compression of spinal cord; occurs most commonly with drop metastases from brain tumors, spinal tumors, soft tissue sarcomas, leukemia with lymphomatous involvement, lymphoma, and neuroblastoma.
2. **Presentation:** Back pain (localized or radicular), weakness, sensory loss, change in bowel or bladder function. Prognosis for recovery based on duration and level of disability at presentation.
3. **Diagnosis:** MRI (preferred) or computed tomography (CT) scan of spine. A plain film of spine has good specificity but detects only two-thirds of abnormalities.

4. **Management:** (NOTE: Steroids may prevent accurate diagnosis of leukemia/lymphoma; plan diagnostic procedure as soon as possible)
a. Consult neurosurgery if suspicious for compression.
b. In the presence of neurologic abnormalities, strong history, and rapid progression of symptoms, immediately start bolus dexamethasone 1–2 mg/kg/day IV and obtain an emergent MRI of the spine.
c. With back pain but less acute symptoms and no anatomic level of dysfunction, consider lower dose of dexamethasone, 0.25–0.5 mg/kg/day PO, divided Q6 hr. Perform MRI of spine within 24 hours.
d. If cause of tumor is known, emergent radiotherapy or chemotherapy is indicated for sensitive tumors; otherwise, emergent neurosurgery consultation is warranted.
e. If cause of tumor is unknown or debulking may remove most or all of tumor, surgery is indicated to decompress the spine.

D. Increased Intracranial Pressure

1. **Etiology:** Ventricular obstruction or impaired CSF flow. Most commonly seen with brain tumors but also with brain bleed, meningeal involvement by tumor or infection, decreased venous return, etc.
2. **Presentation:** Headaches, altered mental status, irritability, lethargy, emesis (especially if projectile); Cushing triad and pupillary changes occur late.
3. **Diagnosis:**
a. Evaluate for vital sign changes [i.e., Cushing triad (↓ heart rate, ↑ systolic blood pressure, irregular respirations)].
b. Funduscopic evaluation for papilledema.
c. Obtain CT or MRI of the head (MRI more sensitive for diagnosis of posterior fossa tumors).
4. **Management:**
a. See Chapter 4 for basic intracranial pressure (ICP) management.
b. Obtain emergent neurosurgical consultation.
c. If tumor is the cause, start IV dexamethasone: 1–2 mg/kg as first dose, then 0.5 mg/kg Q6 hr (discuss final dosing with neurosurgeon).
d. Consider mannitol for altered mental status and/or cardiovascular instability.

E. Cerebrovascular Accident

1. **Etiology:** Hyperleukocytosis, coagulopathy, thrombocytopenia, radiation (fibrosis) or chemotherapy-related (e.g., L-asparaginase–induced hemorrhage or thrombosis, methotrexate). Most common in patients with leukemia.
2. **Diagnosis and management:**
a. Emergent consultation with neurologist
b. Platelet transfusions (and likely increase threshold for transfusion), FFP as needed to replace factors (e.g., if depleted by L-asparaginase)

c. Brain CT with contrast, MRI, magnetic resonance angiography (MRA), or magnetic resonance venography (MRV) if venous thrombosis is suspected
d. Administer heparin acutely, followed by warfarin, for thromboses (if no venous hemorrhage observed on MRI)
e. Avoid L-asparaginase
f. Leukapheresis for hyperleukocytosis

F. Respiratory Distress and Superior Vena Cava Syndrome

1. **Etiology:** Mediastinal mass, edema, or thrombosis; typically seen with Hodgkin disease, non-Hodgkin lymphoma (e.g., lymphoblastic lymphoma), ALL (T-lineage), germ cell tumors
2. **Presentation:** Orthopnea, headaches, facial swelling, dizziness, plethora, acute respiratory distress or failure
3. **Diagnosis:** Chest radiograph. Consider CT or MRI to assess airway. Attempt diagnosis of malignancy (if not known) by least invasive method possible. Avoid sedation or general anesthesia if unstable, high risk.
4. **Management:**
a. Control airway
b. Biopsy (e.g., bone marrow, pleurocentesis, lymph node biopsy) before therapy if patient can tolerate sedation or general anesthesia
c. Empiric therapy: Radiotherapy, steroids, chemotherapy

G. Typhlitis (Neutropenic Enterocolitis)

1. **Etiology:** Inflammation of bowel wall, usually localized to cecum. Occurs most often in association with prolonged neutropenia.
2. **Presentation:** Right lower quadrant abdominal pain, nausea, diarrhea, fever (may be absent early in course; neutropenic patient with abdominal pain warrants evaluation for typhlitis and empiric antibacterial coverage). Risk for perforation.
3. **Diagnosis:**
a. Careful serial abdominal examinations
b. X-ray or ultrasound of abdomen (may show pneumatosis intestinalis, bowel wall edema)
c. CT (IV and PO contrast) most sensitive imaging; may reveal bowel wall thickening, pneumatosis intestinalis
4. **Management:**
a. NPO, IV fluids; consider nasogastric decompression
b. Broad anaerobic and Gram-negative antibiotic coverage (consider coverage for *Clostridium difficile*)
c. Follow closely with surgery consult

H. Fever and Neutropenia

1. **Etiology:** Presumed infection (bacterial, viral, or fungal) in a neutropenic host. Bacterial infection is the most common

documented infection. Occasionally, fevers may be due to medications.
2. **Presentation:** Fever, fatigue, chills, rigors, listlessness, lethargy, tachypnea, tachycardia, localized pain. May deteriorate after initial doses of antibiotics.
3. **Diagnosis:** Fever [temperature (T) > 38.3°C or T > 38.0°C for >1 hour] in the setting of neutropenia (absolute neutrophil count < 500 cells/µL or <1000 cells/µL but expected to drop to <500 cells/µL in the next 48 hours).
4. **Management:** Constitutes a medical emergency. Antibiotics should be administered within 60 minutes of presentation to medical facility (Fig. 22.1).

VII. HEMATOPOIETIC STEM CELL TRANSPLANTATION (HSCT)[3,6]

A. Goal
Administer healthy functioning hematopoietic stem cells from the bone marrow, peripheral blood, or umbilical cord blood to a patient whose bone marrow is diseased (from hematologic malignancy) or depleted (after treatment with myeloablative chemotherapy). HSCT is also used for some congenital and acquired hematologic, immunologic, and metabolic disorders.

B. Preparative Regimens
1. **Myeloablative:** Ablation of recipient's diseased marrow with high-dose chemotherapy or chemotherapy plus total body irradiation (TBI).
2. **Nonmyeloablative:** Host marrow is not destroyed. Provides sufficient immune suppression to prevent graft rejection, but also allows host and graft marrow competition.
3. **Reduced intensity:** Conditioning regimen that uses less chemotherapy and/or radiation than the conventional myeloablative regimen. Aims to provide some disease control, yet reducing regimen-related morbidity and mortality.

C. Types of HSCT
1. **Allogeneic:**
a. Recipient is transfused with donor stem cells after a myeloablative preparative regimen that includes chemotherapy and often also radiation. Donors are screened for human leukocyte antigen (HLA) subtype matching to recipient. Possible donors include HLA-matched sibling, matched unrelated donors, umbilical cord stem cells, and haploidentical (half-matched) related donors.
b. Increased level of mismatch between donor and recipient increases graft-versus-tumor effect, but also increases risk for graft-versus-host complications and graft rejection.
c. Used commonly for AML, ALL (high–risk/relapse), myelodysplastic syndrome, juvenile myelomonocytic leukemia (JMML),

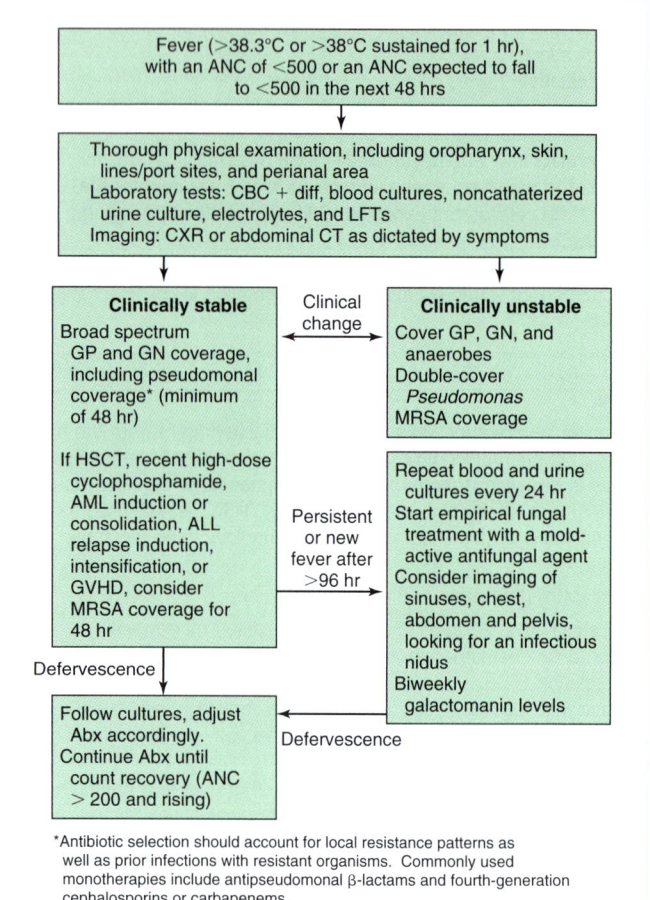

FIGURE 22.1

Guideline for management of fever and neutropenia in children with cancer and/or undergoing hematopoietic stem cell transplantation. Abx, Antibiotics; ALL, acute lymphocytic leukemia; AML, acute myeloid leukemia; ANC, absolute neutrophil count; CBC, complete blood cell count; CT, computed tomography; CXR, chest x-ray; diff, differential; GN, Gram-negative; GP, Gram-positive; GVHD, graft-versus-host disease; HSCT, hematopoietic stem cell transplantation; LFTs, liver function tests; MRSA, methicillin-resistant *Staphylococcus aureus*.

(Data from Lehrnbecher T, Phillips R, Alexander S, et al. Guideline for the management of fever and neutropenia in children with cancer and/or undergoing hematopoietic stem-cell transplantation. *J Clin Oncol.* 2012;30:4427-4438; Freifeld AG, Bow EJ, Sepkowitz KA, et al. Clinical practice guideline for the use of antimicrobial agents in neutropenic patients with cancer: 2010 update by the Infectious Diseases Society of America. *Clin Infect Dis.* 2011;52:e56-e93.)

hemophagocytic lymphohistiocytosis, and a number of nonmalignant hematologic, immunologic, and metabolic disorders.

2. **Autologous:**
a. Donor is recipient. After several cycles of conventional chemotherapy, stem cells from patient are harvested (often with assistance of growth factors such as granulocyte colony-stimulating factor [GCSF] to mobilize), stored, and given back (rescue) after the patient has received myeloablative doses of chemotherapy and radiation.
b. Avoids the complication of graft-versus-host disease (GVHD).
c. Used for high-risk neuroblastoma, lymphoma, and various high-risk solid tumors.

D. Engraftment
1. Recipient's bone marrow is repopulated with donor stem cells that proliferate and mature.
2. Usually starts within 2–4 weeks of transplant, and presents with an inflammatory response but can be significantly delayed with certain conditions, medications, or infection.

VIII. COMMON COMPLICATIONS OF BONE MARROW TRANSPLANTATION[3,6]

A. Acute Graft-Versus-Host Disease (aGVHD)
1. **Etiology:** Donor T-cell–mediated reaction to "foreign" (recipient) antigens. Risk factors include HLA disparity, source of stem cells (peripheral blood > bone marrow > umbilical cord blood).
2. **Presentation:** Classically occurs within 100 days of transplantation, most commonly within 6 weeks, but may occur or persist beyond this time point.
a. Maculopapular skin rash: Can progress to bullous lesions and toxic epidermal necrolysis
b. Laboratory findings: Abnormal liver enzymes (direct hyperbilirubinemia and elevated alkaline phosphatase)
c. Upper GI symptoms: Anorexia, dyspepsia, nausea, vomiting
d. Lower GI symptoms: Abdominal cramping, diarrhea
3. **Diagnosis:** Triad of rash, abdominal cramping with diarrhea, hyperbilirubinemia. Tissue biopsy of skin or mucosa can provide histologic confirmation. Clinical staging is performed by organ system and dictates the clinical grading of aGVHD (Table EC 22.A).
4. **Prevention and management:**
a. Prophylaxis: Immunosuppression with cyclosporine or tacrolimus; adjuvants are methotrexate and prednisone
b. First-line treatment: Steroids commonly used
c. Second-line agents: Cyclosporine, tacrolimus, sirolimus, antithymocyte globulin, mycophenolate mofetil, psoralens plus ultraviolet A photopheresis (PUVA) and pentostatin

B. Chronic Graft-Versus-Host Disease (cGVHD)

1. **Etiology:** Chronic activation of donor immune cells against host antigens. Primary risk factor is prior/current aGVHD. Other risk factors are the same as for aGVHD.
2. **Presentation:** Traditionally presents >100 days after transplant, but may occur earlier either alone or in conjunction with aGVHD:
a. Skin is most commonly affected organ, with lichenoid changes on the face, palms, and soles and scleroderma-like changes, predominantly on extremities.
b. Cholestasis and hepatitis can be seen with elevated alkaline phosphatase, bilirubin, aspartate aminotransferase, and alanine aminotransferase (AST/ALT).
c. GI involvement results in lichenoid changes of oral mucosa, with painful ulcerations that may result in dysphagia. Esophageal strictures, chronic diarrhea, and malabsorption may also be seen.
d. Dyspnea and cough may indicate lung involvement, with inflammation and fibrosis that can culminate in bronchiolitis obliterans.
e. Xerophthalmia with chronically dry eyes, keratoconjunctivitis, and uveitis.
3. **Diagnosis:** Clinically diagnosed by classic findings in skin and GI system, as well as evidence of cholestasis. Skin and/or oral mucosa biopsies may be obtained for confirmation. Liver biopsy may be necessary in patients with suspected hepatic cGVHD.
4. **Prevention and management:**
a. Treatment should be targeted to affected tissues if cGVHD is limited to a single organ system.
b. Steroids continue to be first-line treatment.
c. Second-line agents are similar to those used in aGVHD.
d. Patients with cGVHD are functionally asplenic and immunosuppressed. They should receive four doses of pneumococcal conjugate vaccine 13 (PCV13) after transplant.

C. Veno-Occlusive Disease (Sinusoidal Obstruction Syndrome)

1. **Etiology:** Occlusive fibrosis of terminal intrahepatic venules and sinusoids; occurs as a consequence of hematopoietic cell transplantation, hepatotoxic chemotherapy, and/or high-dose liver radiation. Typically occurs within 3 weeks of the insult, most common at the end of the first week after transplant.
2. **Presentation:** Tender hepatomegaly, jaundice, edema, ascites, and sudden weight gain.
3. **Diagnosis:** Based on one of two established clinical diagnostic criteria.
a. Modified Seattle Criteria: Two or more of the following events within 20 days of HSCT:
   (1) Serum total bilirubin concentration greater than 2 mg/dL
   (2) Hepatomegaly or right upper quadrant pain
   (3) Weight gain >2% from baseline body weight

b. Baltimore Criteria: Bilirubin >2 mg/dL within 21 days of HSCT plus at least two of the following:
   (1) Hepatomegaly
   (2) Ascites
   (3) Weight gain >5% from pre-HSCT weight
4. **Prevention and Treatment**
a. Fluid and sodium restriction to limit third space fluid collection
b. Defibrotide has been shown to be successful in 35%–50% of patients with veno-occlusive disease.

D. Thrombotic Microangiopathy: Thrombotic Thrombocytopenic Purpura (TTP) or Hemolytic Uremic Syndrome (HUS)

1. **Etiology:** Post-HSCT, associated with immunosuppressants (cyclosporine, tacrolimus).
2. **Presentation:** Both TTP and HUS present with microangiopathic hemolytic anemia and thrombocytopenia. HUS completes the triad with renal insufficiency/failure, whereas TTP can be associated with neurologic symptoms.
3. **Diagnosis:** Anemia and thrombocytopenia on CBC, schistocytes on peripheral blood smear, hematuria, proteinuria, casts on urinalysis, elevated lactate dehydrogenase, decreased haptoglobin, impaired renal function, elevated D-dimer on coagulation panel.
4. **Prevention and treatment**: Urgent plasma exchange if TTP is suspected; blood products, fluid management, dialysis.

E. Hemorrhagic Cystitis

1. **Etiology:** Pretransplant conditioning regimens (specifically those that include cyclophosphamide, pelvic or total body irradiation [TBI]) or viral (adenovirus, BK virus).
2. **Presentation:** Hematuria, dysuria, difficulty voiding.
3. **Diagnosis:** Urine viral polymerase chain reaction (PCR) assay, bacterial cultures, bladder ultrasound, CBC, coagulation studies.
4. **Prevention and management:** Hydration and mesna with preparative regimen. Treatment with aggressive hydration, blood products as indicated, cystoscopy, bladder irrigation, clot evacuation.

F. Idiopathic Pneumonia Syndrome

1. **Etiology:** Widespread alveolar injury in the absence of infection or other known etiology. Thought to occur from a variety of insults, including toxic effects of the conditioning regimen, immunologic cell–mediated injury, and inflammation secondary to cytokine release. Most commonly occurs within the first 120 days after transplant.
2. **Presentation:** Dry cough, dyspnea, hypoxemia, and diffuse radiographic opacities
3. **Diagnosis:** Imaging, transbronchial biopsy if tolerated
4. **Prevention and management:** Supportive care together with broad-spectrum antibiotics, IV corticosteroids, and occasionally, a tumor necrosis factor-alpha inhibitor such as etanercept.

G. Viral Infections in Bone Marrow Transplantation (BMT) Patients

See Table EC 22.B.

IX. COMMON CHEMOTHERAPY COMPLICATIONS AND SUPPORTIVE CARE[3]

NOTE: Transfuse only irradiated and leukoreduced packed red blood cells (PRBCs) and single-donor platelets, cytomegalovirus (CMV)-negative or leukofiltered PRBCs/platelets for CMV-negative patients. Use leukofiltered PRBCs/platelets for those who may undergo BMT in the future to prevent alloimmunization, or for those who have had nonhemolytic febrile transfusion reactions. Many oncology patients have nonhemolytic reactions (temperature elevation, rash, hypotension, respiratory distress) to PRBCs and/or platelet transfusion and should subsequently be premedicated with diphenhydramine and/or acetaminophen for future transfusions.

A. Anemia

1. **Etiology:** Blood loss, chemotherapy, marrow infiltration, hemolysis
2. **Management:**
a. See Chapter 14 for specific details on PRBC transfusions.
b. Hematocrit thresholds for PRBC transfusions in cancer patients are based on clinical status and symptoms and are not uncommonly <30 g/dL.

B. Thrombocytopenia

1. **Etiology:** Chemotherapy, marrow infiltration, consumptive coagulopathy, medications
2. **Management:**
a. See Chapter 14 for specific details on platelet transfusions.
b. In general, maintain platelet count above 10,000/μL unless patient is actively bleeding or febrile, or before selected procedures (e.g., intramuscular injection). Consider maintaining platelet counts at higher levels for patients who have brain tumors, recent brain surgery, or history of stroke.

C. Neutropenia

1. **Etiology:** Chemotherapy, marrow infiltration, radiation
2. **Management:**
a. Broad-spectrum antibiotics with concomitant fever (see Fig. 22.1)
b. GCSF to assist in recovery of neutrophils
c. Granulocyte transfusion can be performed in settings of infection or declining clinical status.

D. Mucositis

1. **Etiology:** Damage to endothelial cells of the GI tract from chemotherapy, leading to breakdown of the mucosa. In BMT patients, typically peaks in the first 1–2 weeks after transplant.
2. **Presentation:** Oropharyngeal pain, abdominal pain, nausea, vomiting, diarrhea, intolerance of PO intake.

3. **Prevention and management:** Supportive care aimed at pain control and nutrition. Local pain control with lidocaine-containing mouthwashes and bicarbonate rinses. Systemic pain control usually requires patient-controlled analgesia (PCA) infusion. Total parenteral nutrition (TPN) is commonly required.

E. Nausea and Emesis

1. **Etiology**: Usual cause is chemotherapy treatment. Also suspect opiate therapy, GI and CNS radiotherapy, obstructive abdominal process, elevated ICP, certain antibiotics, or hypercalcemia.
2. **Presentation**
   a. Acute: Emesis within 24 hours of starting chemotherapy; occurs in one third of patients despite treatment.
   b. Delayed: Emesis occurring >24 hours after chemotherapy. Risk factors include female gender, prior acute emesis, highly emetogenic agents (e.g., cisplatin).
   c. Anticipatory: Emesis before chemotherapy administration.
3. **Therapy** (Table 22.4)**:** Hydration plus one or more antiemetic medications (see Part IV, Formulary, for dosages)[7]

X. ANTIMICROBIAL PROPHYLAXIS IN ONCOLOGY PATIENTS (Table 22.5)

Treatment length and dosage may vary per protocol.

XI. BEYOND CHILDHOOD CANCER: TREATING A CANCER SURVIVOR[3,8,9]

A. Understand the Treatment Regimen

1. **Identify all components of therapy received:** Comprehensive treatment summary from oncologist, summarizing:
   a. Diagnosis: Site/stage, date, relapse
   b. Chemotherapy: Cumulative doses, high dose vs. low dose for methotrexate and cytarabine
   c. Radiation: Locations, cumulative dose
   d. Surgeries: Dates, sites, resection
   e. BMT: Preparation regimen, source of donor cells (including degree of HLA mismatch), GVHD, complications
   f. Investigational treatments
   g. Adverse drug reactions or allergies
2. **Follow up with any investigational treatments used.**
3. **Determine any potential problems by organ system**, and devise plan for routine evaluation (Table EC 22.C).

B. Common Late Effects[3,8,10]:

See Table EC 22.C and www.survivorshipguidelines.org.

C. Vaccinations in Oncology Patients: See Chapter 16 and Expert Consult.

TABLE 22.4
ANTIEMETIC THERAPIES

Antiemetic Classes	Common Agents	Common Adverse Effects
Serotonin (5-HT$_3$) antagonists	Ondansetron, granisetron	QT prolongation, QRS widening
Histamine-1 antagonist	Diphenhydramine, scopolamine	Sedation, urinary retention, blurred vision
Benzodiazepines	Lorazepam	Sedation
Dopamine antagonists	Metoclopramide, prochlorperazine, promethazine	Sedation, extrapyramidal effects, QT prolongation; rarely, seizures or neuroleptic malignant syndrome. Consider diphenhydramine to reduce risk of extrapyramidal symptoms.
Substance P receptor antagonists	Aprepitant	Exercise caution with agents metabolized by CYP3A4
Steroids (helpful in patients with brain tumors and prophylaxis for delayed symptoms)	Dexamethasone	Hypertension, hyperglycemia, bradycardia
Cannabinoids (useful in patients with large tumor burden, also an appetite stimulant)	Dronabinol	Hallucinations, dizziness
Antipsychotics (used rarely in adolescent patients with refractory vomiting)	Olanzapine	Weight gain, sedation; rarely, extrapyramidal side effects

TABLE 22.5
ANTIMICROBIAL PROPHYLAXIS IN ONCOLOGY PATIENTS

Organism	Medication	Indication
Pneumocystis jirovecii	TMP-SMX, atovaquone, dapsone, or pentamidine	Chemotherapy and BMT per protocol (usually at least 6 mo after chemotherapy, 12 mo after BMT)
HSV, CMV, VZV	Acyclovir or valacyclovir (dosing is different for zoster, varicella, and mucocutaneous HSV)	After BMT if patient or donor is HSV or CMV–positive; recurrent zoster
Candida albicans	Fluconazole (alternatives: voriconazole or micafungin)	Patients with leukemia or after BMT (usually at least 28 days)
Gram-positive organisms	Penicillin	After BMT (usually at least 1 mo)

BMT, Bone marrow transplantation; CMV, cytomegalovirus; HSV, herpes simplex virus; TMP-SMX, trimethoprim–sulfamethoxazole; VZV, varicella zoster virus.

REFERENCES

1. Crawford J. Childhood Brain Tumors. *Pediatrics In Review*. 2013;34:1-7.
2. Wilne S, et al. Presentation of Childhood CNS tumours: a systematic review and meta-analysis.. *Lancet Oncology*. 2007;8(3):685-695.
3. Poplack D, Pizzo P. *Principles and Practice of Pediatric Oncology*. 6th ed. Philadelphia: Lippincott, Williams & Wilkins; 2011.
4. Lehrnbecher T, Phillips R, Alexander S, et al. Guideline for the management of fever and neutropenia in children with cancer and/or undergoing hematopoietic stem-cell transplantation. *J Clin Oncol*. 2012;30:4427-4438.
5. Freifeld AG, Bow EJ, Sepkowitz KA, et al. Clinical practice guideline for the use of antimicrobial agents in neutropenic patients with cancer: 2010 update by the Infectious Diseases Society of America. *Clin Infect Dis*. 2011;52:e56-e93.
6. Bishop MR, ed. *Hematopoietic Stem Cell Transplantation*. New York: Springer; 2009.
7. Dupuis LL, Boodhan S, Holdsworth M, et al. Guideline for the prevention of acute nausea and vomiting due to antineoplastic medication in pediatric cancer patients. *Pediatr Blood Cancer*. 2013;60:1073-1082.
8. Meck MM, Leary M, Sills RH. Late effects in survivors of childhood cancer. *Pediatr Rev*. 2006;27:257-262.
9. Pickering LK, American Academy of Pediatrics. *Red Book: 2012 Report of the Committee on Infectious Diseases*. 29th ed. Elk Grove Village, III: AAP; 2012.
10. Kliegman RM, Behrman RE, Stanton BF, et al. *Nelson Textbook of Pediatrics*. 19th ed. Philadelphia: Saunders; 2011.
11. Tomblyn M, Chiller T, Einsele H, et al. Guidelines for preventing infectious complications among hematopoietic cell transplantation recipients: a global perspective. *Biol Blood Marrow Transplant*. 2009;15:1143-1238.

Chapter 23
Palliative Care
Daniel Hindman, MD

I. WEB RESOURCES
- The American Academy of Hospice and Palliative Medicine at: www.aahpm.org
- The National Hospice and Palliative Care Organization at: www.nhpco.org

II. PALLIATIVE CARE
A. Definition[1,2]
Palliative care is the active total care of the child's body, mind, and spirit with the intent to prevent and relieve suffering. It supports the best quality of life for the child and family beginning at diagnosis of a life-limiting condition and continuing regardless of whether the child receives treatment. Hospice care is a form of palliative care that focuses on the end of life and bereavement. Effective palliative care requires an interdisciplinary approach that works with child and family to determine goals of care. This is best accomplished when the palliative care team is involved as early in the child's course of illness as possible (Fig. 23.1).

B. Palliative Care Team Composition
1. **Child and family**
2. **Physician:** Primary care physician, specialist attending physician, fellow, resident, intern
3. **Nurses:** Primary nurse, charge nurse, home care nurse, hospice nurse
4. **Pain specialist and hospice palliative care specialist**
5. **Social worker**
6. **Child life specialist**
7. **Pastoral care**
8. **Patient care coordinator and case manager**
9. **Bereavement coordinator**
10. **Community resources:** School, faith community, hospice program

III. COMMUNICATION AND DECISION MAKING
A. Decision-Making Tools (DMTs)[3]
1. See www.seattlechildrens.org/pdf/Decision_Making_Tool.pdf.
2. **Provides consistent, reliable format for discussion and formulation of plan of care.** Patients, families, and healthcare providers all participate in the process.

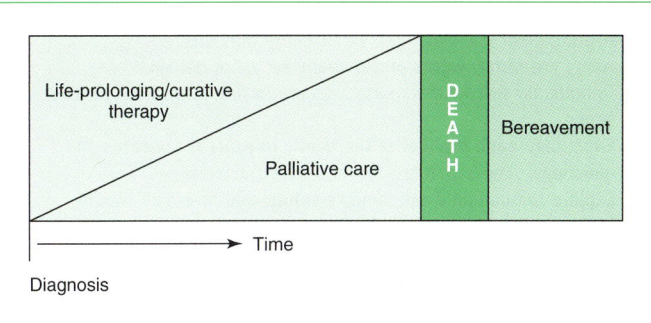

FIGURE 23.1

Current accepted model for palliative care.

3. **Four domains of DMT should be updated regularly,** especially during "noncrisis" periods
a. Medical indications: Diagnosis, symptoms, risk/benefits of treatment, cure/relapse rate, complications
b. Patient and family preferences: Information, decision-making, desire for autonomy and privacy
c. Quality of life: Important activities of child, important relationships, emotional/spiritual well-being
d. Contextual issues: Identifying family unit, home environment, financial barriers, legal issues, cultural and spiritual beliefs

B. Family Meetings[4]

1. **Prepare the people and the messages.**
a. Why are you having the meeting?
b. Do you have all the information you need?
c. Are all clinicians in agreement about the patient's condition and the recommendations?
d. Are there decisions to be made?
e. Who should attend? Patient, parents, other important individuals? Which clinicians?
f. Who will take the lead role as the facilitator?
2. **Choose a private location with minimal distraction.**
3. **Always have water and tissues available.**
4. **Begin by introducing all participants and the purpose of the meeting.**
a. Check whether any additional issues for discussion have arisen.
5. **Assess what the family knows and expects.**
a. What is their current understanding of the patient's condition?
b. What have they already been told?

6. **Describe the clinical situation.**
   a. A brief, clear overview first: What is the big picture?
   b. Ask if the family wants and is ready for more details.
   c. Periodically ask whether what you are saying is clear and makes sense.
7. **Encourage each member of the family to express concerns and questions.** Ask until there are no more questions.
8. **Explore the patient's and family's values and how they should influence decision-making.**
   a. Has there been any prior experience with serious medical decisions for this patient or another family member?
   b. How does the family decide what is best?
   c. Are there guides or principles that help the family decide?
      (1) FICA acronym[5]
         i. **F**aith and belief: "Do you consider yourself spiritual or religious?"
         ii. **I**mportance in life: "What importance does your faith or belief have in your life?"
         iii. **C**ommunity: "Are you a part of a spiritual or religious community?"
         iv. **A**ddress in care: "How would you like me, your healthcare provider, to address these issues in your healthcare?"
9. **Propose goals for the patient's care that reflect the stated values.**
   a. Begin with what treatments or interventions you recommend as beneficial and that support the goals of care.
   b. If there are treatments you would not recommend because they do not support the overall goals of care, mention them later with your clinical reasoning.
   c. Be prepared to listen compassionately and negotiate.
10. **Provide a concrete follow-up plan.**
    a. Summarize the plan for care.
    b. Agree on when to talk or meet again.

C. Communication Tools for Difficult Conversations

1. NURSE
   a. **N**aming—state the emotion that is present
   b. **U**nderstanding—try to put yourself in the family's or patient's situation
   c. **R**especting—express appreciation
   d. **S**upporting—articulate your continued commitment
   e. **E**xploring—focus in on particular concerns
2. Ask-Tell-Ask[6]
   a. **Ask** the patient or family to describe their understanding of the situation or issue
   b. **Tell** them what you need to communicate in a straightforward manner
   c. **Ask** them questions to assess their understanding
3. "Tell me more"
4. "I wish" statements

Chapter 23 Palliative Care 631

TABLE 23.1

CONCEPTUALIZATION OF DEATH IN CHILDREN

Age Range	Characteristics	Concepts of Death	Interventions
0–2 yr	Achieve object permanence May sense something is wrong	None	Provide maximal comfort with familiar persons and favorite toys.
2–6 yr	Magical thoughts	Believes death is temporary Does not personalize death Believes death can be caused by thoughts	Minimize separation from parents; correct perceptions that the illness is punishment.
6–12 yr	Concrete thoughts	Understands death can be personal Interested in details of death	Be truthful, evaluate fears, provide concrete details if requested, allow participation in decision making.
12–18 yr	Reality becomes objective Capable of self-reflection	Searches for meaning, hope, purpose, and value of life	Be truthful, allow expression of strong feelings, allow participation in decision making.

5. For more on helpful communication tools, please see www.vitaltalk.org/quick-guides

D. Child Participation

1. **Development of death concepts in children**[7-10] (Table 23.1)
2. **Child's capacity to participate in healthcare decisions.** Minor children can participate meaningfully in decision making if they demonstrate all of the following:
   a. Communicate understanding of the medical information
   b. State his or her preference
   c. Communicate understanding of the consequences of decisions

E Advance Directive

1. **Adolescents aged 18 years and older** can name another adult to make healthcare decisions if they are unable to speak for themselves.
2. **Healthcare team can help patients voice their preferences** for future healthcare decisions.

IV. LEGACY AND MEMORY MAKING

A. Memory Making

1. **Provide opportunities for the family to participate in memory making** (e.g., create memory boxes/packets; take lock of hair, foot/hand molds or prints, videos, photographs).

2. **Older children may have specific wishes for funeral, memorial, or distribution of personal belongings.**
a. Voicing my choices: A planning guide for adolescents with terminal illness and their families. More information can be found at https://www.agingwithdignity.org/voicing-my-choices.php

B. Rituals
Allow for culturally important rituals to be performed by the family (e.g., baptism, bathing, music, faith ceremonies, and prayer).

C. Being at Home
For many children and families, the opportunity to be at home together, especially as a child approaches the end of life, is a top priority. Be sure to ask families about this early, before it is too late to transfer the patient, and assess what preparations have to be made.

V. DECISIONS TO LIMIT INTERVENTIONS

A. Do Not Attempt Resuscitation (DNAR)
1. **In the event of cardiorespiratory arrest,** cardiopulmonary resuscitation (CPR) is automatically initiated in hospitals by healthcare teams and in community settings by first responders. For patients with life-threatening conditions, CPR may not prolong or enhance quality of life, making it inconsistent with goals of care. The healthcare team should offer patients and families the option of forgoing CPR and other resuscitative interventions as part of an overall care plan that emphasizes comfort and quality of living.
2. **If this option is desired,** physician must write a specific order *not* to attempt CPR (e.g., "In the event of cardiopulmonary arrest, do not attempt resuscitation"). Orders must follow local emergency medical services (EMS) policies for patients at home.

B. Do Not Escalate Treatment
When escalation of treatment no longer supports the goals of care, offer patients and families the option to forgo treatment changes even as the patient's condition worsens. Because death is expected, DNAR must also be discussed. Examples of such requests include:
1. **Do not increase the dose of current medications** (e.g., vasopressors).
2. **Do not add new medications** (e.g., antibiotics).
3. **Do not initiate new interventions** (e.g., dialysis, mechanical ventilation).
4. **Initiate and increase interventions** to treat pain and reduce suffering.

C. Discontinuing Current Interventions
When death is expected regardless of intervention, especially if current interventions are prolonging the dying process, patients and families can be offered the option of discontinuing these interventions (e.g., "Discontinue blood products, monitors, mechanical ventilation, medically provided hydration or nutrition"). Because death is expected, DNAR must also be discussed.

D. State Forms

MOLST (Medical Orders for Life-Sustaining Treatment) and POLST (Physician Orders for Life-Sustaining Treatment) Forms

1. **These are portable and enduring medical order forms** completed by patients or their authorized decision makers and signed by a physician. They contain orders regarding CPR and other life-sustaining treatments.
2. **If a state offers one of these forms,** the orders are valid for EMS providers as well as all healthcare providers and facilities within that state.
3. **A copy must be provided to the patient or authorized decision maker** within 48 hours of completion, or sooner if the patient is to be transferred.
4. **Please refer to your state's laws prior to completion of any documentation.** Additional information can be found at www.polst.org.

VI. BODY, MIND, AND SPIRIT CHANGES AS DEATH APPROACHES[11]

A. Physical Changes

1. **Cardiac:** Blood pressure decreases, heart rate increases, and pulse becomes weaker.
2. **Circulation:** Cool extremities; cyanosis of fingers, nails, lips; mottling of skin
3. **Gastrointestinal:** Metabolism slows and appetite gradually decreases. Liquids are preferred to solids. The body will become naturally dehydrated, and fevers may occur as death approaches. Provide relief with ice chips, moist mouth swabs, antipyretic per rectum.
4. **Respiratory:** Variable pattern of breathing (tachypnea followed by periods of apnea); congestion secondary to secretion build-up; provide relief as follows:
a. Turn patient every few hours, elevate head of bed, provide frequent mouth care, hyoscyamine as needed.
b. Relief of air hunger: Morphine and lorazepam as needed, oxygen for comfort.
c. **NOTE:** Deep suctioning is not helpful.
5. **Sensation changes:** Senses become overactive. Bright lights, noise, or television may be upsetting. Hearing is typically the last sense to diminish. Provide relief by dimming lights, reducing noise, and providing soft background music.
6. **Sleep:** Need for sleep increases as death approaches. Occasionally, the child exhibits a surge of energy to play, eat, or socialize.

B. Emotional Changes

Detachment from the outside world: Reduced need to socialize leads to pulling inward of thoughts, emotions, and fears. Listen and reassure family about decreased interactions.

C. Mental Changes

Mental status: Confusion, restlessness, agitation, delirium. Provide relief by keeping child oriented to surroundings, surrounding him/her with family as a way to reinforce safety, and speaking in calm tones. Use lorazepam and haloperidol as needed.

D. Spiritual Changes

Spiritual: Child may call out or reach out for loved ones who are not physically present. Reassure the family that this is not unusual during the dying process.

VII. LAST HOURS: MEDICATION AND MANAGEMENT[12]

See Table 23.2.

VIII. DEATH PRONOUNCEMENT[13]

Residents may be called to pronounce the death of a patient in the hospital. This important task should be carried out with competence, compassion, and respect.

TABLE 23.2
COMMON MEDICATIONS USED FOR SYMPTOMATIC RELIEF IN PALLIATIVE CARE

Indication	Medication	Initial Regimen
Pain	Morphine	0.3 mg/kg/dose PO, SL, PR Q2–4 hr* 0.1–0.2 mg/kg/dose IV Q2–4 hr* **NOTE:** Morphine should be titrated to symptomatic relief.
Dyspnea	Morphine	0.1–0.25 mg/kg/dose PO, SL, PR Q2–4 hr 0.05–0.1 mg/kg/dose IV Q2–4 hr 2.5–5 mg/3 mL normal saline nebulizer Q4 hr **NOTE:** Nebulized morphine can cause severe bronchospasm and worsen dyspnea. Nebulized fentanyl may be preferred.
Agitation	Lorazepam Haloperidol	0.05 mg/kg/dose PO, IV, SL, PR Q4–8 hr 0.01–0.02 mg/kg/dose PO, SL, PR Q8–12 hr
Pruritus	Diphenhydramine	0.5–1 mg/kg/dose PO, IV Q6–8 hr
Nausea and vomiting	Prochlorperazine Ondansetron	0.1–0.15 mg/kg/dose PO, PR Q6–8 hr 0.15 mg/kg/dose PO, IV Q6–8 hr
Seizures	Diazepam Lorazepam	0.3–0.5 mg/kg/dose PR Q2–4 hr 0.05–0.1 mg/kg/dose IV Q2–4 hr
Secretions	Hyoscyamine	0.03–0.06 mg/kg/dose PO, SL Q4 hr (if <2 yr) 0.06–0.12 mg/kg/dose PO, SL Q4 hr (if 2–12 yr) 0.12–0.25 mg/kg/dose PO, SL Q4 hr (if >12 yr)

IV, Intravenous; PO, oral; PR, rectal; SL, sublingual.
*Infants <6 mo should receive one-third to one-half the dose. For adolescents, consider starting adult dosing of PO: 10–30 mg/dose, IV: 2–15 mg/dose.
Note: For adult-sized patients, please see formulary for adult dosing recommendations.
Adapted from Himelstein BP, Hilden JM, Boldt AM, et al. Pediatric palliative care. *N Engl J Med.* 2004;350:1752-1762.

A. Preparation

1. **Know the child's name and gender.**
2. **Be prepared to answer simple pertinent questions** from family and friends.
3. **Consult with nursing staff for relevant information:** recent events, family response, family dynamics
4. **Determine the need and call for interdisciplinary support:** social work, child life, pastoral care, bereavement coordinator

B. Entering the Room

1. **Enter quietly and respectfully** along with the primary nurse.
2. **Introduce yourself and identify your role:**
a. "I am Dr. _____, the doctor on call."
b. Determine the relationships of those in the room.
c. Inform the family of the purpose of your visit ("I am here to examine your child"), and invite them to remain in the room.

C. Procedure for Pronouncement

1. **Check ID bracelet and pulse.**
2. **Respectfully check response to tactile stimuli.**
3. **Check for spontaneous respirations.**
4. **Check for heart sounds.**
5. **Record the time of death.**
6. **Inform the family of death.**
7. **Offer to contact other family members.**
8. **Remember to convey sympathy:** "I am so sorry for your loss."

D. Document Death in the Chart

1. **Write date, time of death, and the provider pronouncing the death.**
2. **Document absence of pulse, respirations, and heart sounds.**
3. **Identify family members who were present and informed of death.**
4. **Document notification of attending physician.**

E. Death Certificate

1. **Locate a copy of a sample death certificate for reference.**
2. **Use BLACK INK ONLY and complete *Physician sections*.**
a. **NOTE:** Do *NOT* use abbreviations (e.g., spell out the month: January 31 and not 1/31).
b. **NOTE:** Do *NOT* cross out or use correction fluid; you must begin again if mistakes are made.
c. **NOTE:** Cardiopulmonary or respiratory arrest is *not* an acceptable primary cause of death.
3. For specific instructions for your state and/or institution, contact the Office of Decedent Affairs at your institution.

F. Autopsy Consent

1. **Obtain family consent if indicated.**
2. **Plan follow-up to contact and review autopsy results.**

IX. AFTER DEATH—BEREAVEMENT[13]

A. Etiquette

Families want to know that their children are not forgotten. Sending condolence cards, attending funerals, and contacting the family weeks to months later are all appropriate physician activities that are deeply valued by bereaved families. Respectful listening to families and sharing memories of the child help provide support during bereavement.

B. Available Services[14]

Be familiar with available services: Pastoral care, social work, bereavement coordinator, community support groups, counseling services, bereavement follow-up programs.

REFERENCES

1. Sepulveda C, Marlin A, Yoshida T, et al. Palliative care: World Health Organization's global perspective. *J Pain Symptom Manage*. 2002;24:91-96.
2. Nelson R. Palliative care for children: policy statement. *Pediatrics*. 2007;119:351-357.
3. Hays RM, Valentine J, Haynes G, et al. The Seattle Pediatric Palliative Care Project: effects on family satisfaction and health-related quality of life. *J Palliat Med*. 2006;9:716-728.
4. Back A, Arnold R, Tulsky J. *Mastering Communication with Seriously Ill Patients: Balancing Honesty with Empathy and Hope*. New York: Cambridge University Press; 2009:85-88.
5. Puchalski CM. Spirituality and end-of-life care: a time for listening and caring. *J Palliat Med*. 2002;5:289-294.
6. Back AL, Arnold RM, Baile WF, et al. Approaching difficult communication tasks in oncology. *CA Cancer J Clin*. 2005;55(3):164-177. doi:10.3322/canjclin.55.3.164.
7. Sourkes BM. *Armfuls of Time: The Psychological Experience of Children with Life-Threatening Illnesses*. Pittsburgh: University of Pittsburgh Press; 1995.
8. Corr CA. Children's understanding of death: striving to understand death. In: Doka KJ, ed. *Children Mourning, Mourning Children*. Washington, DC: Hospice Foundation of America; 1995:8-10.
9. Corr CA, Balk DE, eds. *Handbook of Adolescent Death and Bereavement*. New York: Springer; 1996.
10. Faulkner K. Children's understanding of death. In: Armstrong-Dailey A, Zarbock S, eds. *Hospice Care for Children*. 2nd ed. New York: Oxford University Press; 2001:9-22.
11. Sigrist D. *Journey's End: A Guide to Understanding the Final Stages of the Dying Process*. Rochester, NY: Hospice of Rochester and Hospice of Wayne and Seneca Counties, Genesee Region Home Care; 1995.
12. Himelstein BP, Hilden JM, Boldt AM, et al. Pediatric palliative care. *N Engl J Med*. 2004;350:1752-1762.
13. Bailey A. *The Palliative Response*. Birmingham, AL: Menasha Ridge Press; 2003.
14. AAP Policy Statement. Committee on Bioethics and Committee on Hospital Care: palliative care for children. *Pediatrics*. 2000;106(2 Pt 1):351-357.

Chapter 24
Pulmonology
Jason Gillon, MD

See additional content on Expert Consult

I. WEB RESOURCES
- American Lung Association: http://www.lung.org
- Cystic Fibrosis Foundation: http://www.cff.org
- American Academy of Allergy, Asthma and Immunology: http://www.aaaai.org
- National Heart Lung and Blood Institute: National Asthma Education and Prevention Program: http://www.nhlbi.nih.gov
- American Thoracic Society: http://www.thoracic.org

II. RESPIRATORY PHYSICAL EXAMINATION

A. Normal Respiratory Rates in Children (Table 24.1)

B. Inspection
Evaluate for chest wall abnormalities (barrel chest, pectus excavatum, or pectus carinatum), symmetry, accessory muscle use, cyanosis of lips, skin, or nails, or digital clubbing.

C. Palpation and Percussion

D. Auscultation (Table 24.2)

III. EVALUATION OF PULMONARY GAS EXCHANGE

A. Pulse Oximetry[1-5]
1. Pulse oximetry (SpO_2) is an indirect measurement of arterial O_2 saturation (SaO_2) estimated by light absorption characteristics of oxygenated and deoxygenated hemoglobin through the skin in peripheral blood.
2. Important uses:
a. Rapid and continuous assessment of oxygenation in acutely ill patients or patients requiring oxygen therapy
b. Assessment of oxygen requirements during feeding, sleep, exercise, or sedation
c. Monitoring of physiologic effects of apnea and bradycardia
3. Limitations:
a. Measures oxygen saturation, not O_2 delivery to tissues. A marginally low saturation in an anemic patient may be more significant because of their reduced O_2-carrying capacity.

TABLE 24.1
NORMAL RESPIRATORY RATES IN CHILDREN

Age (yr)	Respiratory Rate (breaths/min)
0–1*	24–38
1–3	22–30
4–6	20–24
7–9	18–24
10–14	16–22
14–18	14–20

*Slightly higher respiratory rates (i.e., 40–50 breaths/min) in the neonatal period may be normal in the absence of other signs and symptoms.
Data from Bardella IJ. Pediatric advanced life support: a review of the AHA recommendations. Am Fam Physician. 1999;60:1743-1750.

TABLE 24.2
RESPIRATORY AUSCULTATION

Sound	Description	Possible Causes
Crackles (rales)	Intermittent scratchy, bubbly noises Heard predominantly on inspiration Produced by reopening of airways closed on previous expiration	Bronchiolitis, pulmonary edema, pneumonia, asthma
Wheezes	Continuous, high-pitched, musical sound predominantly on expiration	Asthma, bronchiolitis, foreign body
Rhonchi	Continuous, low-pitched, nonmusical sound	Pneumonia, cystic fibrosis
Stridor	High-pitched, harsh, blowing sound Heard predominantly on inspiration	Croup, laryngomalacia, subglottic stenosis, allergic reaction, vocal cord dysfunction

b. Insensitive to hyperoxia because of the sigmoid shape of the oxyhemoglobin curve (Fig. 24.1).
c. Artificially increased: Carboxyhemoglobin levels >1%–2% (e.g., in chronic smokers or with smoke inhalation).
d. Artificially decreased: Patient motion, intravenous dyes (methylene blue, indocyanine green), opaque nail polish, and methemoglobin levels >1%.
e. Unreliable when pulse signal is poor: Hypothermia, hypovolemia, shock, edema, or movement artifact.
f. SpO_2 reading often does not correlate with PaO_2 in sickle cell disease.[6]
4. Oxyhemoglobin dissociation curve (see Fig. 24.1)

B. Capnography

1. Measures CO_2 concentration of expired gas by infrared spectroscopy or mass spectroscopy.
2. End-tidal CO_2 ($ETCO_2$) correlates with $PaCO_2$ (usually within 5 mmHg in healthy subjects).

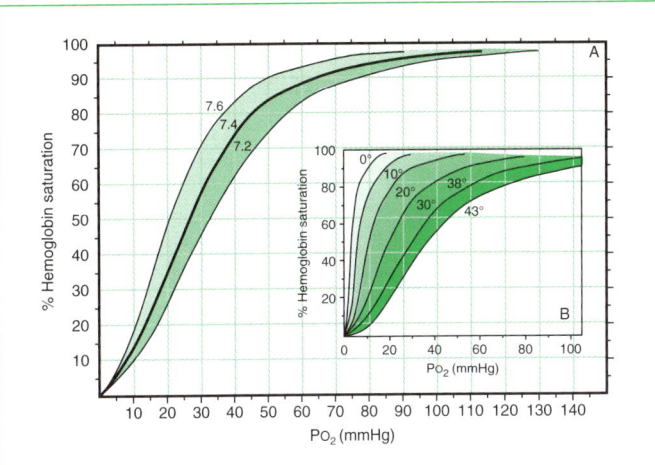

FIGURE 24.1

Oxyhemoglobin dissociation curve. **A,** Curve shifts to the left as pH increases. **B,** Curve shifts to the left as temperature decreases. *(Data from Lanbertsten CJ. Transport of oxygen, CO_2, and inert gases by the blood. In: Mountcastle VB, ed. Medical Physiology. 14th ed. St Louis: Mosby; 1980.)*

3. Can be used for demonstrating proper placement of an endotracheal tube, continuous monitoring of CO_2 trends in ventilated patients, and monitoring ventilation during polysomnography.

C. Blood Gases

1. Arterial blood gas (ABG): Most accurate way to assess oxygenation (PaO_2), ventilation ($PaCO_2$), and acid–base status (pH and HCO_3^-). (See Chapter 27 for normal mean values.)
2. Venous blood gas (VBG): $PvCO_2$ averages 6–8 mmHg higher than $PaCO_2$, and venous pH is slightly lower than arterial pH. Measurement is strongly affected by the local circulatory and metabolic environment.
3. Capillary blood gas (CBG): Correlation with ABG is generally best for pH, moderate for PCO_2, and worst for PO_2.

D. Analysis of Acid–Base Disturbances[7-9]

1. Determine primary disturbance, then assess for mixed disorder by calculating expected compensatory response (Fig. 24.2 and Table 24.3).

IV. PULMONARY FUNCTION TESTS

Provide objective and reproducible measurements of airway function and lung volumes. Used to characterize disease, assess severity, and follow response to therapy.

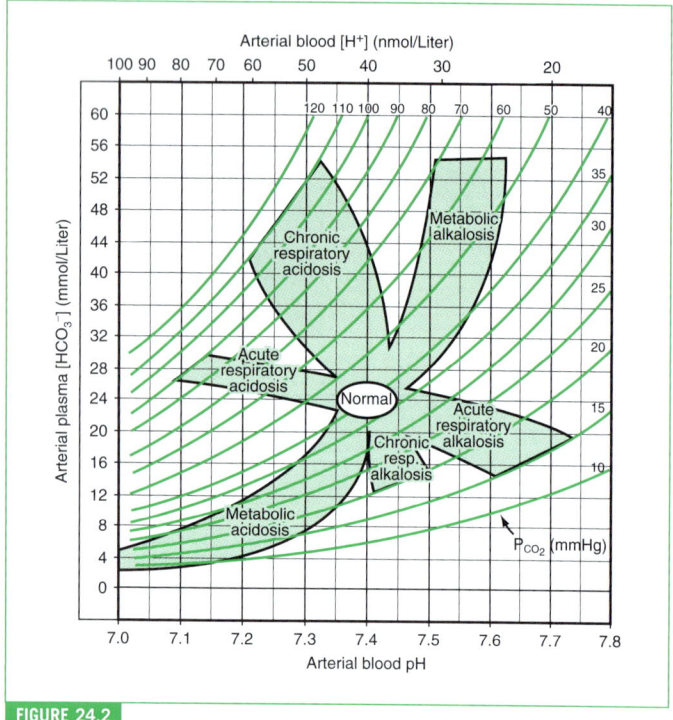

FIGURE 24.2

Interpretation of arterial blood gases. *(Modified from Siggaard-Anderson O. The Acid-Base Status of the Blood. 4th ed. Copenhagen: Munksgaard; 1976.)*

A. Peak Expiratory Flow Rate (PEFR)

Maximal flow rate generated during a forced expiratory maneuver.

1. Often used to follow the course of asthma and response to therapy by comparing a patient's PEFR with the previous "personal best" and the normal predicted value.
a. Limitations: Normal predicted values vary across different racial groups. Measurement is effort dependent and cannot be done reliably by many young children. PEFR is also insensitive to small airway function.
2. Normal predicted PEFR values for children (Table 24.4)

B. Maximal Inspiratory and Expiratory Pressures[10,11]

Maximal pressure generated during inhalation and exhalation against a fixed obstruction.

TABLE 24.3
CALCULATION OF EXPECTED COMPENSATORY RESPONSE

Disturbance	Primary Change	pH*	Expected Compensatory Response
Acute respiratory acidosis	↑$PaCO_2$	↓pH	↑HCO_3^- by 1 mEq/L for each 10-mmHg rise in $PaCO_2$
Acute respiratory alkalosis	↓$PaCO_2$	↑pH	↓HCO_3^- by 1–3 mEq/L for each 10-mmHg fall in $PaCO_2$
Chronic respiratory acidosis	↑$PaCO_2$	↓pH	↑HCO_3^- by 4 mEq/L for each 10-mmHg rise in $PaCO_2$
Chronic respiratory alkalosis	↓$PaCO_2$	↑pH	↓HCO_3^- by 2–5 mEq/L for each 10-mmHg fall in $PaCO_2$
Metabolic acidosis	↓HCO_3^-	↓pH	↓$PaCO_2$ by 1–1.5 times fall in HCO_3^-
Metabolic alkalosis	↑HCO_3^-	↑pH	↑$PaCO_2$ by 0.25–1 times rise in HCO_3^-

*Pure respiratory acidosis (or alkalosis): 10-mmHg rise (fall) in $PaCO_2$ results in an average 0.08 fall (rise) in pH. Pure metabolic acidosis (or alkalosis): 10-mEq/L fall (rise) in HCO_3^- results in an average 0.15 fall (rise) in pH.
Data from Schrier RW. Renal and Electrolyte Disorders. 3rd ed. Boston: Little, Brown; 1986.

TABLE 24.4
PREDICTED AVERAGE PEAK EXPIRATORY FLOW RATES FOR NORMAL CHILDREN

Height Inches (cm)	PEFR (L/min)	Height Inches (cm)	PEFR (L/min)
43 (109)	147	56 (142)	320
44 (112)	160	57 (145)	334
45 (114)	173	58 (147)	347
46 (117)	187	59 (150)	360
47 (119)	200	60 (152)	373
48 (122)	214	61 (155)	387
49 (124)	227	62 (157)	400
50 (127)	240	63 (160)	413
51 (130)	254	64 (163)	427
52 (132)	267	65 (165)	440
53 (135)	280	66 (168)	454
54 (137)	293	67 (170)	467
55 (140)	307		

PEFR, Peak expiratory flow rate.
Data from Voter KZ. Diagnostic tests of lung function. Pediatr Rev. 1996;17:53-63.

1. Used as a measure of respiratory muscle strength.
2. Maximal inspiratory pressure (MIP) is in the range of 80–120 cm H_2O at all ages. Maximum expiratory pressure (MEP) increases with age and is greater in males.
3. A low MIP may be an indication for ventilatory support, and a low MEP correlates with decreased effectiveness of coughing.

C. Spirometry (for Children ≥6 Years)

Plot of airflow versus time during rapid, forceful, and complete expiration from total lung capacity (TLC) to residual volume (RV) is useful to

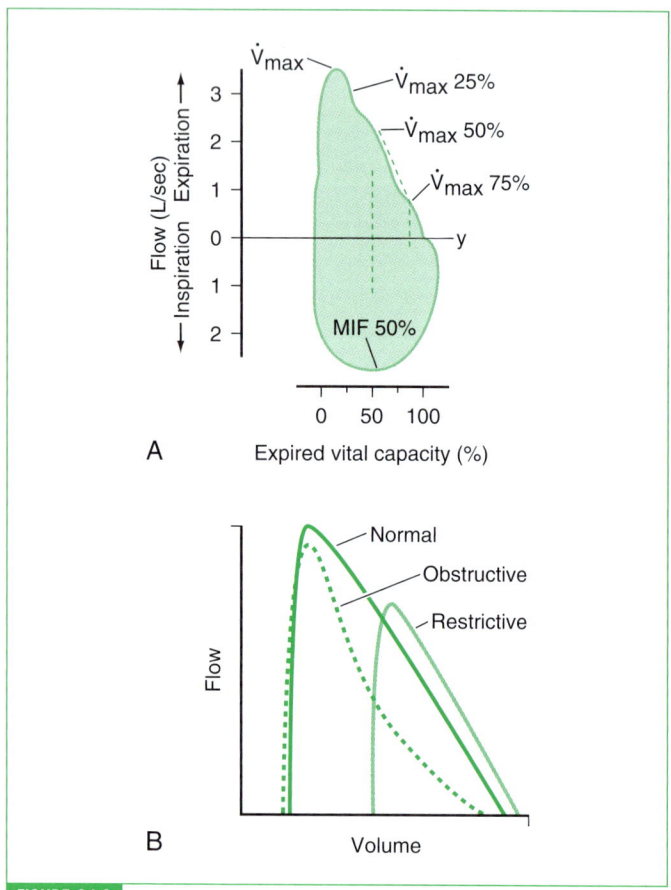

FIGURE 24.3

A, Normal flow–volume curve. **B,** Worsening intrathoracic airway obstruction as in asthma or cystic fibrosis. (***B*** *Data from Baum GL, Wolinsky E. Textbook of Pulmonary Diseases. 5th ed. Boston: Little, Brown; 1994.)*

characterize different patterns of airway obstruction (Fig. 24.3). Usually performed before and after bronchodilation to assess response to therapy or after bronchial challenge to assess airway hyperreactivity.
1. Important definitions (Fig. 24.4)
a. Forced vital capacity (FVC): Maximum volume of air exhaled from the lungs after a maximum inspiration. Bedside measurement of vital capacity with a handheld spirometer can be useful in confirming or predicting hypoventilation associated with muscle weakness.

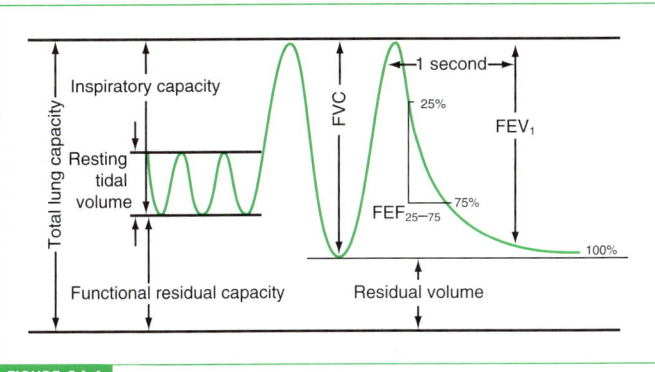

FIGURE 24.4

Lung volumes. FEF_{25-75}, forced expiratory flow between 25% and 75% of FVC; FEV_1, forced expiratory volume in 1 second; FVC, forced vital capacity.

TABLE 24.5

INTERPRETATION OF SPIROMETRY AND LUNG VOLUME READINGS

	Obstructive Disease (Asthma, Cystic Fibrosis)	Restrictive Disease (Interstitial Fibrosis, Scoliosis, Neuromuscular Disease)
SPIROMETRY		
FVC*	Normal or reduced	Reduced
FEV_1*	Reduced	Reduced§
FEV_1/FVC†	Reduced	Normal
FEF_{25-75}	Reduced	Normal or reduced§
PEFR*	Normal or reduced	Normal or reduced§
LUNG VOLUMES		
TLC*	Normal or increased	Reduced
RV*	Increased	Reduced
RV/TLC‡	Increased	Unchanged
FRC	Increased	Reduced

*Normal range: ±20% of predicted.
†Normal range: >85%.
‡Normal range: 20 ± 10%.
§Reduced proportional to FVC.
FEF_{25-75}, Forced expiratory flow between 25% and 75% of FVC; FEV_1, forced expiratory volume in 1 second; FRC, functional residual capacity; FVC, forced vital capacity; PEFR, peak expiratory flow rate; RV, residual volume; TLC, total lung capacity.

b. Forced expiratory volume in 1 second (FEV_1): Volume exhaled during the first second of the FVC maneuver.
c. Forced expiratory flow (FEF_{25-75}): Mean rate of airflow over the middle half of the FVC between 25% and 75% of FVC. Sensitive to medium and small airway obstruction.
2. Interpretation of spirometry and lung volume readings (Table 24.5).

V. BRIEF RESOLVED UNEXPLAINED EVENT (BRUE)[12-14]

A. Definition

Formerly termed an apparent life-threatening event (ALTE), a BRUE is defined as an event occurring in an infant younger than 1 year when the observer reports a sudden, brief (typically 20–30 seconds), and now resolved episode of at least one of the following:
1. Cyanosis or pallor
2. Absent, decreased, or irregular breathing
3. Marked change in tone (hyper- or hypotonia)
4. Altered level of responsiveness

B. Differential Diagnosis (Box 24.1)

In almost half of all cases of BRUEs, no cause is found. The three most common comorbid conditions (which account for roughly 50% of all diagnoses eventually made) are gastroesophageal reflux (GER), seizure, and lower respiratory tract infection.

C. Management

1. If the patient has symptoms or abnormal vital signs, or if an explanation for the event is identified (e.g., GER), the event is not a BRUE. Manage accordingly.
2. Risk-stratify the patient into lower or higher risk. The patient must meet all of the following criteria to be classified as lower risk:

a. Age >60 days
b. Born ≥32 weeks' gestation and corrected age ≥45 weeks

BOX 24.1
DIFFERENTIAL DIAGNOSIS OF BRIEF RESOLVED UNEXPLAINED EVENT

I. Gastroenterologic

Gastroesophageal reflux disease
Gastroenteritis
Esophageal dysfunction
Surgical abdomen
Dysphagia

II. Neurologic

Seizure
Central apnea/hypoventilation
Meningitis/encephalitis
Hydrocephalus
Brain tumor
Neuromuscular disorders
Vasovagal reaction

> **BOX 24.1**
>
> **DIFFERENTIAL DIAGNOSIS OF BRIEF RESOLVED UNEXPLAINED EVENT—cont'd**
>
> **III. Respiratory**
>
> Respiratory syncytial virus
> Pertussis
> Aspiration
> Respiratory tract infection
> Reactive airway disease
> Foreign body
>
> **IV. Otolaryngologic**
>
> Laryngomalacia
> Subglottic and/or laryngeal stenosis
> Obstructive sleep apnea
>
> **V. Cardiovascular**
>
> Congenital heart disease
> Cardiomyopathy
> Cardiac arrhythmias/prolonged QT syndrome
> Myocarditis
>
> **VI. Metabolic/Endocrine**
>
> Inborn error of metabolism
> Hypoglycemia
> Electrolyte disturbance
>
> **VII. Infectious**
>
> Sepsis
> Urinary tract infection
>
> **VIII. Other Diagnosis**
>
> Child maltreatment
> Shaken baby syndrome
> Breath-holding spell
> Choking
> Drug or toxin reaction
> Anemia
> Periodic breathing
> Factitious disorder imposed by another (Munchausen syndrome by proxy)

Modified from DeWolfe CC. Apparent life-threatening event: a review. Pediatr Clin North Am. 2005;52:1127-1146, ix.

    c. No cardiopulmonary resuscitation (CPR) by trained medical provider
    d. Event lasted <1 minute
    e. First event
  3. For lower risk patients, caregivers should be educated about BRUEs and offered resources for CPR training. Pertussis testing,

electrocardiogram (ECG), and monitoring of the patient with continuous pulse oximetry and serial observations may be considered. Further testing is not recommended.
4. For higher risk patients, there is a paucity of outcomes data to derive evidence-based recommendations. Individualize management after a careful history and physical examination.

VI. ASTHMA[15]

A. Definition

A chronic inflammatory disorder of the airways resulting in recurrent episodes of wheezing, breathlessness, chest tightness, and cough, particularly at night and in the early morning. These episodes are usually associated with obstruction of airflow in the lower airway and are reversible either spontaneously or with therapy. The inflammation causes increased airway hyperreactivity to a variety of stimuli: viral infections, cold air, exercise, emotions, and environmental allergens and pollutants.

B. Clinical Presentation

1. Cough, increased work of breathing (tachypnea, retractions, or accessory muscle use), wheezing, hypoxia, and hypoventilation. Crackles may also be present with asthma exacerbations.
2. No audible wheezing may indicate very poor air movement and severe bronchospasm.
3. Chest radiographs often show peribronchial thickening, hyperinflation, and patchy atelectasis.

C. Treatment

1. Acute management and status asthmaticus (see Chapter 1)
2. Initial classification and initiation of treatment for ages 0–4, 5–11, and ≥12 years (Figs. 24.5, 24.6, and 24.7)
3. Stepwise approach to continued management for ages 0–4, 5–11, and ≥12 years (Figs. 24.8, 24.9, and 24.10)

D. Prevention of Exacerbations

1. Ensure up-to-date immunizations, including influenza.
2. Create an asthma action plan (see http://www.nhlbi.nih.gov/files/docs/public/lung/asthma_actplan.pdf or http://phpa.dhmh.maryland.gov/mch/Documents/FINAL_AAP_WRITABLE_Nov2013.pdf).
3. Identify and minimize asthma triggers and environmental exposures, including tobacco smoke, mold, pollen, and dust mites.
4. Assess symptom control, inhaler technique, and medication adherence with regular clinical evaluations.
a. Consider specialist referral for formal pulmonary function testing (PFT), monitoring, and allergy testing.
b. For dosing guidelines on inhaled corticosteroids, see Table EC 24.A on Expert Consult.

Text continued on p. 653

CLASSIFYING ASTHMA SEVERITY AND INITIATING TREATMENT IN CHILDREN 0–4 YEARS OF AGE

Assessing severity and initiating therapy in children who are not currently taking long-term control medication

Components of severity		Classification of asthma severity (0–4 years of age)			
		Intermittent	Persistent Mild	Persistent Moderate	Persistent Severe
Impairment	Symptoms	≤2 days/week	>2 days/week but not daily	Daily	Throughout the day
	Nighttime awakenings	0	1–2×/month	3–4×/month	>1×/week
	Short-acting β_2-agonist use for symptom control (not prevention of EIB)	≤2 days/week	>2 days/week but not daily	Daily	Several times per day
	Interference with normal activity	None	Minor limitation	Some limitation	Extremely limited
Risk	Exacerbations requiring oral systemic corticosteroids	0–1/year	≥2 exacerbations in 6 months requiring oral systemic corticosteroids, or ≥4 wheezing episodes/1 year lasting >1 day AND risk factors for persistent asthma		
		Consider severity and interval since last exacerbation. Frequency and severity may fluctuate over time. Exacerbations of any severity may occur in patients in any severity category.			
Recommended step for initiating therapy (See Fig. 24-8 for treatment steps.)		Step 1	Step 2	Step 3 and consider short course of oral systemic corticosteroids	
		In 2–6 weeks, depending on severity, evaluate level of asthma control that is achieved. If no clear benefit is observed in 4–6 weeks, consider adjusting therapy or alternative diagnoses.			

Key: EIB, exercise-induced bronchospasm

Notes
- The stepwise approach is meant to assist, not replace, the clinical decision making required to meet individual patient needs.
- Level of severity is determined by both impairment and risk. Assess impairment domain by patient's/caregiver's recall of previous 2–4 weeks. Symptom assessment for longer periods should reflect a global assessment such as inquiring whether the patient's asthma is better or worse since the last visit. Assign severity to the most severe category in which any feature occurs.
- At present, there are inadequate data to correspond frequencies of exacerbations with different levels of asthma severity. For treatment purposes, patients who had ≥2 exacerbations requiring oral systemic corticosteroids in the past 6 months, or ≥4 wheezing episodes in the past year, and who have risk factors for persistent asthma may be considered the same as patients who have persistent asthma, even in the absence of impairment levels consistent with persistent asthma.

FIGURE 24.5

Guidelines for classifying asthma severity and initiating treatment in infants and young children (aged 0–4 years). *(Adapted from National Asthma Education and Prevention Program (NAEPP)—Expert Panel Report 3. Guidelines for the Diagnosis and Management of Asthma. August 2007. Available at http://www.nhlbi.nih.gov/guidelines/asthma/asthgdln.htm. August 2007. Accessed July 27, 2009.)*

CLASSIFYING ASTHMA SEVERITY AND INITIATING TREATMENT IN CHILDREN 5–11 YEARS OF AGE

Assessing severity and initiating therapy in children who are not currently taking long-term control medication

Components of severity		Classification of asthma severity (5–11 years of age)			
		Intermittent	Persistent		
			Mild	Moderate	Severe
Impairment	Symptoms	≤2 days/week	>2 days/week but not daily	Daily	Throughout the day
	Nighttime awakenings	≤2×/month	3–4×/month	>1×/week but not nightly	Often 7×/week
	Short-acting β_2-agonist use for symptom control (not prevention of EIB)	≤2 days/week	>2 days/week but not daily	Daily	Several times per day
	Interference with normal activity	None	Minor limitation	Some limitation	Extremely limited
	Lung function	• Normal FEV_1 between exacerbations • FEV_1 >80% predicted • FEV_1/FVC >85%	• FEV_1 = >80% predicted • FEV_1/FVC >80%	• FEV_1 = 60%–80% predicted • FEV_1/FVC = 75%–80%	• FEV_1 <60% predicted • FEV_1/FVC <75%
Risk	Exacerbations requiring oral systemic corticosteroids	0–1/year (see note)	≥2/year (see note)		
		Consider severity and interval since last exacerbation. Frequency and severity may fluctuate over time for patients in any severity category.			
		Relative annual risk of exacerbations may be related to FEV_1.			
Recommended step for initiating therapy (See Fig. 24-9 for treatment steps.)		Step 1	Step 2	Step 3, medium-dose ICS option	Step 3, medium-dose ICS option, or step 4 and consider short course of oral systemic corticosteroids
		In 2–6 weeks, evaluate level of asthma control that is achieved, and adjust therapy accordingly.			

Key: EIB, exercise-induced bronchospasm; FEV_1, forced expiratory volume in 1 second; FVC, forced vital capacity; ICS, inhaled corticosteroids

Notes
- The stepwise approach is meant to assist, not replace, the clinical decision making required to meet individual patient needs.
- Level of severity is determined by both impairment and risk. Assess impairment domain by patient's/caregiver's recall of previous 2–4 weeks and spirometry. Assign severity to the most severe category in which any feature occurs.
- At present, there are inadequate data to correspond frequencies of exacerbations with different levels of asthma severity. In general, more frequent and intense exacerbations (e.g., requiring urgent, unscheduled care, hospitalization, or ICU admission) indicate greater underlying disease severity. For treatment purposes, patients who had ≥2 exacerbations requiring oral systemic corticosteroids in the past year may be considered the same as patients who have persistent asthma, even in the absence of impairment levels consistent with persistent asthma.

FIGURE 24.6

Guidelines for classifying asthma severity and initiating treatment in children aged 5–11 years. (Adapted from National Asthma Education and Prevention Program (NAEPP)—Expert Panel Report 3. Guidelines for the Diagnosis and Management of Asthma. August 2007. http://www.nhlbi.nih.gov/guidelines/asthma/asthgdln.htm. Accessed July 27, 2009.)

CLASSIFYING ASTHMA SEVERITY AND INITIATING TREATMENT IN YOUTHS ≥12 YEARS OF AGE

Assessing severity and initiating treatment for patients who are not currently taking long-term control medications

Components of severity		Classification of asthma severity ≥12 years of age			
		Intermittent	Persistent		
			Mild	Moderate	Severe
Impairment Normal FEV_1/FVC: 8–19 yr 85% 20–39 yr 80% 40–59 yr 75% 60–80 yr 70%	Symptoms	≤2 days/week	>2 days/week but not daily	Daily	Throughout the day
	Nighttime awakenings	≤2×/month	3–4×/month	>1×/week but not nightly	Often 7×/week
	Short-acting β_2-agonist use for symptom control (not prevention of EIB)	≤2 days/week	>2 days/week but not daily, and not more than 1 time on any day	Daily	Several times per day
	Interference with normal activity	None	Minor limitation	Some limitation	Extremely limited
	Lung function	• Normal FEV_1 between exacerbations • FEV_1 >80% predicted • FEV_1/FVC normal	• FEV_1 >80% predicted • FEV_1/FVC normal	• FEV_1 >60% but <80% predicted • FEV_1/FVC reduced 5%	• FEV_1 <60% predicted • FEV_1/FVC reduced >5%
Risk	Exacerbations requiring oral systemic corticosteroids	0–1/year (see note)	≥2/year (see note)		
		Consider severity and interval since last exacerbation. Frequency and severity may fluctuate over time for patients in any severity category.			
		Relative annual risk of exacerbations may be related to FEV_1.			
Recommended step for initiating treatment (See Fig. 24-10 for treatment steps.)		Step 1	Step 2	Step 3	Step 4 or 5 and consider short course of oral systemic corticosteroids
		In 2–6 weeks, evaluate level of asthma control that is achieved and adjust therapy accordingly.			

Key: FEV_1, forced expiratory volume in 1 second; FVC, forced vital capacity; ICU, intensive care unit

Notes
- The stepwise approach is meant to assist, not replace, the clinical decision making required to meet individual patient needs.
- Level of severity is determined by both impairment and risk. Assess impairment domain by patient's/caregiver's recall of previous 2–4 weeks and spirometry. Assign severity to the most severe category in which any feature occurs.
- At present, there are inadequate data to correspond frequencies of exacerbations with different levels of asthma severity. In general, more frequent and intense exacerbations (e.g., requiring urgent, unscheduled care, hospitalization, or ICU admission) indicate greater underlying disease severity. For treatment purposes, patients who had ≥2 exacerbations requiring oral systemic corticosteroids in the past year may be considered the same as patients who have persistent asthma, even in the absence of impairment levels consistent with persistent asthma.

FIGURE 24.7

Guidelines for classifying asthma severity and initiating treatment in youth 12 years and older. *(Adapted from National Asthma Education and Prevention Program (NAEPP)—Expert Panel Report 3. Guidelines for the Diagnosis and Management of Asthma. August 2007. http://www.nhlbi.nih.gov/guidelines/asthma/asthgdln.htm. Accessed July 27, 2009.)*

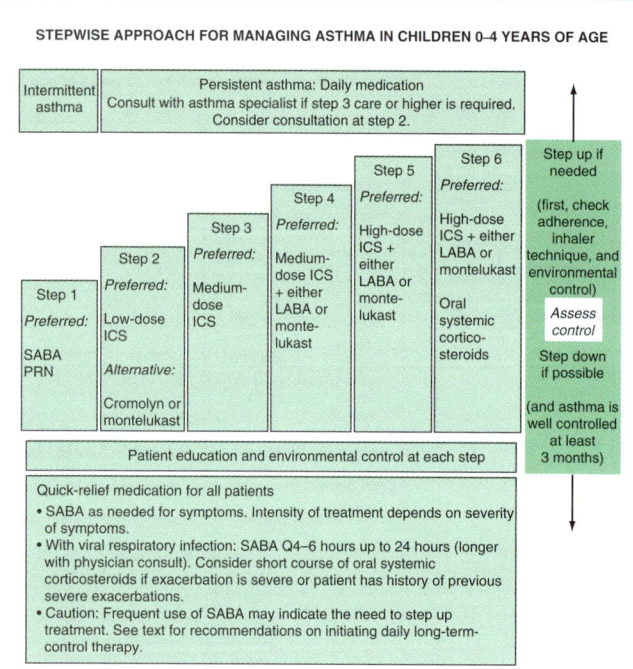

FIGURE 24.8

Stepwise approach for managing asthma in infants and young children (aged 0–4 years). *(Adapted from National Asthma Education and Prevention Program (NAEPP)—Expert Panel Report 3. Guidelines for the Diagnosis and Management of Asthma. August 2007. http://www.nhlbi.nih.gov/guidelines/asthma/asthgdln.htm. Accessed July 27, 2009.)*

STEPWISE APPROACH FOR MANAGING ASTHMA IN CHILDREN 5–11 YEARS OF AGE

Intermittent asthma	Persistent asthma: Daily medication Consult with asthma specialist if step 4 care or higher is required. Consider consultation at step 3.

Step 1	Step 2	Step 3	Step 4	Step 5	Step 6	Step up if needed
Preferred: SABA PRN	*Preferred:* Low-dose ICS *Alternative:* Cromolyn, LTRA, nedocromil, or theophylline	*Preferred:* EITHER: Low-dose ICS + either LABA, LTRA, or theophylline OR Medium-dose ICS	*Preferred:* Medium-dose ICS + LABA *Alternative:* Medium-dose ICS + either LTRA or theophylline	*Preferred:* High-dose ICS + LABA *Alternative:* High-dose ICS + either LTRA or theophylline	*Preferred:* High-dose ICS + LABA + oral systemic corticosteroid *Alternative:* High-dose ICS + either LTRA or theophylline + oral systemic corticosteroid	(first, check adherence, inhaler technique, environmental control, and comorbid conditions) *Assess control* Step down if possible (and asthma is well controlled at least 3 months)

Each step: Patient education, environmental control, and management of comorbidities.
Steps 2–4: Consider subcutaneous allergen immunotherapy for patients who have allergic asthma (see notes).

Quick-relief medication for all patients
- SABA as needed for symptoms. Intensity of treatment depends on severity of symptoms: up to 3 treatments at 20-minute intervals as needed. Short course of oral systemic corticosteroids may be needed.
- Caution: Increasing use of SABA or use >2 days a week for symptom relief (not prevention of EIB) generally indicates inadequate control and the need to step up treatment.

Key: Alphabetical order is used when more than one treatment option is listed within either preferred or alternative therapy. ICS, inhaled corticosteroid; LABA, long-acting inhaled β_2-agonist; LTRA, leukotriene receptor antagonist; PRN, as needed; SABA, short-acting inhaled β_2-agonist

Notes:
- The stepwise approach is meant to assist, not replace, the clinical decision making required to meet individual patient needs.
- If alternative treatment is used and response is inadequate, discontinue it and use the preferred treatment before stepping up.
- Theophylline is a less desirable alternative due to the need to monitor serum concentration levels.
- Step 1 and step 2 medications are based on Evidence A. Step 3 ICS + adjunctive therapy and ICS are based on Evidence B for efficacy of each treatment and extrapolation from comparator trials in older children and adults—comparator trials are not available for this age group; steps 4–6 are based on expert opinion and extrapolation from studies in older children and adults.
- Immunotherapy for steps 2–4 is based on Evidence B for house dust mites, animal danders, and pollens; evidence is weak or lacking for molds and cockroaches. Evidence is strongest for immunotherapy with single allergens. The role of allergy in asthma is greater in children than in adults. Clinicians who administer immunotherapy should be prepared and equipped to identify and treat anaphylaxis that may occur.

FIGURE 24.9

Stepwise approach for managing asthma in children 5–11 years. *(Adapted from National Asthma Education and Prevention Program (NAEPP)—Expert Panel Report 3. Guidelines for the Diagnosis and Management of Asthma. August 2007. http://www.nhlbi.nih.gov/guidelines/asthma/asthgdln.htm. Accessed July 27, 2009.)*

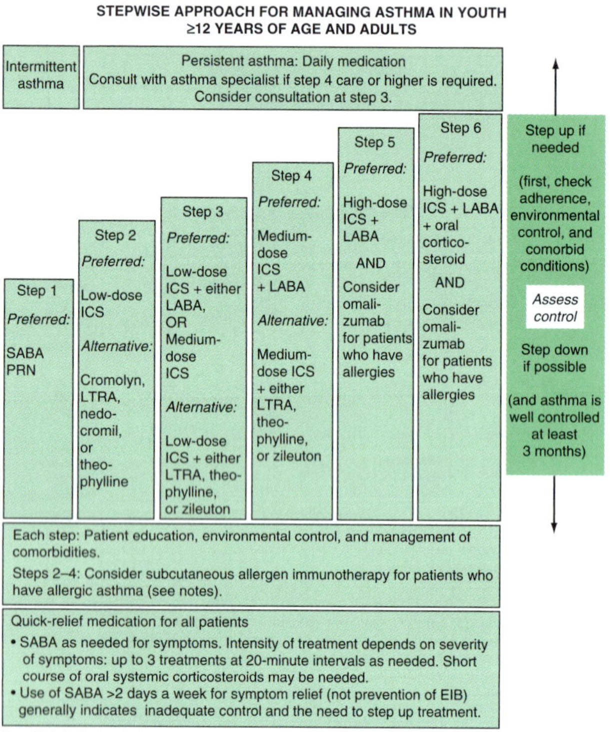

STEPWISE APPROACH FOR MANAGING ASTHMA IN YOUTH ≥12 YEARS OF AGE AND ADULTS

Intermittent asthma	Persistent asthma: Daily medication Consult with asthma specialist if step 4 care or higher is required. Consider consultation at step 3.

Step 1	Step 2	Step 3	Step 4	Step 5	Step 6
Preferred: SABA PRN	*Preferred:* Low-dose ICS *Alternative:* Cromolyn, LTRA, nedocromil, or theophylline	*Preferred:* Low-dose ICS + either LABA, OR Medium-dose ICS *Alternative:* Low-dose ICS + either LTRA, theophylline, or zileuton	*Preferred:* Medium-dose ICS + LABA *Alternative:* Medium-dose ICS + either LTRA, theophylline, or zileuton	*Preferred:* High-dose ICS + LABA AND Consider omalizumab for patients who have allergies	*Preferred:* High-dose ICS + LABA + oral corticosteroid AND Consider omalizumab for patients who have allergies

Step up if needed

(first, check adherence, environmental control, and comorbid conditions)

Assess control

Step down if possible

(and asthma is well controlled at least 3 months)

Each step: Patient education, environmental control, and management of comorbidities.
Steps 2–4: Consider subcutaneous allergen immunotherapy for patients who have allergic asthma (see notes).

Quick-relief medication for all patients
- SABA as needed for symptoms. Intensity of treatment depends on severity of symptoms: up to 3 treatments at 20-minute intervals as needed. Short course of oral systemic corticosteroids may be needed.
- Use of SABA >2 days a week for symptom relief (not prevention of EIB) generally indicates inadequate control and the need to step up treatment.

Key: Alphabetical order is used when more than one treatment option is listed within either preferred or alternative therapy. EIB, exercise-induced bronchospasm; ICS, inhaled corticosteroid; LABA, long-acting inhaled β_2-agonist; LTRA, leukotriene receptor antagonist; PRN, as needed; SABA, short-acting inhaled β_2-agonist

Notes:
- The stepwise approach is meant to assist, not replace, the clinical decision making required to meet individual patient needs.
- If alternative treatment is used and response is inadequate, discontinue it and use the preferred treatment before stepping up.
- Zileuton is a less-desirable alternative due to limited studies as adjunctive therapy and the need to monitor liver function. Theophylline requires monitoring of serum concentration levels.
- In step 6, before oral systemic corticosteroids are introduced, a trial of high-dose ICS + LABA + either LTRA, theophylline, or zileuton may be considered, although this approach has not been studied in clinical trials.
- Step 1, 2, and 3 preferred therapies are based on Evidence A; step 3 alternative therapy is based on Evidence A for LTRA, Evidence B for theophylline, and Evidence D for zileuton. Step 4 preferred therapy is based on Evidence B, and alternative therapy is based on Evidence B for LTRA and theophylline and Evidence D for zileuton. Step 5 preferred therapy is based on Evidence B. Step 6 preferred therapy is based on Expert Panel Report 2 (1997) and Evidence B for omalizumab.
- Immunotherapy for steps 2–4 is based on Evidence B for house dust mites, animal danders, and pollens; evidence is weak or lacking for molds and cockroaches. Evidence is strongest for immunotherapy with single allergens. The role of allergy in asthma is greater in children than in adults.
- Clinicians who administer immunotherapy or omalizumab should be prepared and equipped to identify and treat anaphylaxis that may occur.

FIGURE 24.10

Stepwise approach for managing asthma in youth 12 years and older. (*Adapted from National Asthma Education and Prevention Program (NAEPP)—Expert Panel Report 3. Guidelines for the Diagnosis and Management of Asthma, August 2007. http://www.nhlbi.nih.gov/guidelines/asthma/asthgdln.htm. Accessed July 27, 2009.*)

VII. BRONCHIOLITIS[16]

Bronchiolitis is a lower respiratory tract infection common in infants and children aged 2 years and younger. It is characterized by acute inflammation, edema, and necrosis of airway epithelium, leading to increased mucus production and bronchospasm. It is most commonly caused by respiratory syncytial virus (RSV), but can also be seen with other viruses including: parainfluenza, adenovirus, mycoplasma, and human metapneumovirus.

A. Clinical Presentation

1. Signs and symptoms typically begin with rhinitis and cough, which may progress to tachypnea, wheezing, rales, use of accessory muscles, and/or nasal flaring. Transient apnea may also be seen.
2. Radiographic findings: Hyperinflation and atelectasis
a. Radiographs (or laboratory studies) should not be routinely obtained, as bronchiolitis is primarily a clinical diagnosis.

B. Treatment

Mainstay is supportive care.
1. Assess risk factors for severe disease, such as age less than 12 weeks, a history of prematurity, underlying cardiopulmonary disease, or immunodeficiency, when making decisions about evaluation and management.
2. Clinicians should not administer albuterol, epinephrine, systemic corticosteroids, chest physiotherapy, or antibiotics (unless with concomitant bacterial infection) to previously healthy infants and children with a diagnosis of bronchiolitis.
3. Nebulized hypertonic saline should not be administered to infants and children with a diagnosis of bronchiolitis in the emergency department but may be administered if hospitalized.
4. Evidence supporting continuous pulse oximetry and supplemental O_2 when SpO_2 is greater than 90% is currently lacking.
5. Nasogastric or intravenous fluid is necessary when bronchiolitic infants cannot maintain oral hydration. Consider holding oral feedings in infants that are very tachypneic to minimize risk of aspiration.
6. Ensure RSV immunoprophylaxis with palivizumab for high-risk infants (see Chapter 16).

VIII. BRONCHOPULMONARY DYSPLASIA (BPD)[17-20]

Also known as chronic lung disease of prematurity or chronic lung disease of infancy, BPD is a chronic pulmonary condition that usually evolves after premature birth, characterized by the need for oxygen supplementation >21% for at least 28 days after birth. Thought to be a result of airway inflammation, damage from hyperoxia, hypoxia, or mechanical ventilation; results in interference with normal lung alveolar, airway, and vascular development. Earlier gestational age in preterm infants is associated with a higher likelihood of BPD development.

A. Clinical Presentation

Children with BPD may have persistent respiratory symptoms, airway hyperreactivity, and supplemental oxygen requirements, especially during intercurrent illness.

B. Diagnosis

1. Severity based on oxygen requirement at time of assessment and characterized as mild if on room air, moderate if requiring <30% oxygen, or severe if requiring >30% oxygen and/or positive pressure
a. If gestational age at birth was <32 weeks: Assess infant at 36 weeks' postmenstrual age or at discharge to home, whichever comes first
b. If gestational age at birth >32 weeks: Assess infant at 28–56 days postnatal age or at discharge to home, whichever comes first

C. Treatment

1. Children with BPD often require some combination of the following for their lung disease:
a. Bronchodilators
b. Antiinflammatory agents
c. Supplemental oxygen therapy
d. Diuretics
e. Tracheostomy and prolonged mechanical ventilation for severe cases
f. RSV and influenza prophylaxis, if indicated (see Chapter 16)
2. Children with BPD need close monitoring for complications, which can affect additional organ systems: pulmonary or systemic hypertension, electrolyte abnormalities, nephrocalcinosis (from chronic diuretics), neurodevelopmental or growth delay, aspiration from dysphagia and/or GER, and more severe superinfections with RSV or influenza

IX. CYSTIC FIBROSIS (CF)[21-23]

An autosomal recessive disorder in which mutations of the cystic fibrosis transmembrane conductance regulator (*CFTR*) gene reduce the function of a chloride channel that usually resides within mucosal epithelial cells in the airways, pancreatic ducts, biliary tree, intestine, vas deferens, and sweat glands. Most patients have chronic progressive obstructive pulmonary disease, pancreatic exocrine insufficiency with protein and fat malabsorption, and abnormally high sweat electrolyte concentrations.

A. Clinical Manifestations (Table 24.6)

B. Diagnosis

More than half of patients are diagnosed by age 6 months, three fourths by 2 years
1. Quantitative pilocarpine iontophoresis (sweat chloride) test: Gold standard for diagnosis

TABLE 24.6
MAJOR CLINICAL MANIFESTATIONS OF CYSTIC FIBROSIS BY ORGAN SYSTEM

Respiratory	Chronic productive cough, hemoptysis
	Bronchiectasis, bronchitis, pneumonia
	Obstructive lung disease
	Sinusitis
	Nasal polyposis
Gastrointestinal	Meconium ileus
	Rectal prolapse
	Pancreatic insufficiency
	Liver disease including cirrhosis
	Obstructive cholestasis
	Distal intestinal obstruction syndrome
	Fat-soluble vitamin deficiency (A, D, E, K)
Genitourinary	Infertility (male) and decreased fertility (female)
	Absence of vas deferens
Miscellaneous	Diabetes
	Increased sweat electrolytes
	Hypokalemic alkalosis
	Digital clubbing
	Pulmonary hypertrophic osteoarthropathy
	Failure to thrive

 a. Positive for CF: >60 mEq/L (mEq/L = mmol/L)
 b. Indeterminant:
    (1) Infants <6 months: Indeterminant if 30–60 mEq/L
    (2) Children >6 months: Indeterminant if 40–60 mEq/L
 c. Normal:
    (1) Infants <6 months: Normal if <30 mEq/L
    (2) Children >6 months: Normal if <40 mEq/L
2. DNA testing is becoming increasingly important in diagnosis. Over 1800 mutations have been described; most common is F508del (present in 70% of those with CF).
3. Many states have adopted universal newborn screening (NBS) by measuring infants' immunoreactive trypsinogen (IRT) levels and/or DNA testing for most common mutations. A confirmatory sweat chloride test should be performed promptly in those patients who have a positive NBS result.
4. Clinical pearl: Elevated sweat chloride levels can be from other disorders, including untreated adrenal insufficiency, glycogen storage disease type 1, fucosidosis, hypothyroidism, nephrogenic diabetes insipidus, ectodermal dysplasia, malnutrition, mucopolysaccharidosis, panhypopituitarism, or poor testing technique.

C. Treatment

1. Pulmonary
a. Airway clearance therapy (ACT) to mobilize airway secretions and facilitate expectoration: Often manual/mechanical percussion and postural drainage. Older children may use high-frequency chest wall compression device (vest therapy), mechanical chest percussors, or oscillatory positive expiratory pressure (PEP) handheld devices (e.g., flutter valve and acapella).
b. Aerosolized medications to increase mucociliary clearance: Recombinant human DNAase (dornase alfa), which cleaves nucleic material, and hypertonic saline nebs to hydrate airway mucus and stimulate cough
c. Chronic antibiotics: If *Pseudomonas aeruginosa* is persistently present in culture of airways, consider aerosolized aminoglycosides and/or chronic oral macrolide therapy.
d. Intermittent use of IV antibiotics when hospitalized for exacerbations. Common bacteria that cause exacerbations include *P. aeruginosa* and *Staphylococcus aureus*.
   NOTE: All CF patients should be managed within an accredited CF care center.
2. Nonpulmonary
a. Pancreatic disease
   (1) Pancreatic enzyme replacement therapy (PERT) prior to meals to improve digestion and intestinal absorption of dietary protein and fat.
   (2) Nutritional supplementation to maintain body mass index (BMI) ≥50th percentile.
   (3) Monitoring for CF-induced diabetes or liver disease.
b. Infertility
   (1) Absence of the vas deferens; however, assisted fertilization is possible using aspiration of viable sperm from testes.
   (2) Women may have trouble becoming pregnant because of mucus-associated obstruction of the cervix.
c. Decreased life expectancy; survival continues to improve, and median predicted survival age is more than 37 years.

X. OBSTRUCTIVE SLEEP APNEA SYNDROME (OSAS)[24-27]

Part of the spectrum of sleep-disordered breathing; characterized by prolonged partial and/or intermittent partial or complete upper airway obstruction with accompanying hypoxemia, hypercapnia, and/or sleep disruption. Alternate names include *obstructive hypoventilation*, *upper airway resistance syndrome*.

A. Clinical Presentation

1. Snoring sometimes accompanied by snorts, gasps, or intermittent pauses in breathing

2. Increased respiratory effort during sleep, disturbed or restless sleep with increased arousals and awakenings
3. Daytime cognitive and/or behavioral problems. (Young children rarely present with daytime sleepiness.)
4. Long-term complications include neurocognitive impairment, behavioral problems, poor growth, and systemic and pulmonary hypertension.
5. Risk factors include adenotonsillar hypertrophy, obesity, family history of OSAS, craniofacial or laryngeal anomalies, prematurity, nasal/pharyngeal inflammation, cerebral palsy, and neuromuscular disease.

B. Diagnosis

1. All children and adolescents should be screened for snoring.
2. If a child snores on a regular basis and has any of the complaints or findings shown in Box 24.2, clinicians should obtain a polysomnogram or, if polysomnography is not available, refer the patient to a sleep specialist or otolaryngologist for more extensive evaluation.
a. Polysomnography includes measurement of electroencephalography (EEG), electrooculography (EOG), and electromyography (EMG) to monitor sleep stage and movement; ECG; chest wall and abdominal

---

BOX 24.2

SYMPTOMS AND SIGNS OF OBSTRUCTIVE SLEEP APNEA SYNDROME

I. History

Frequent snoring (≥3 nights/week)
Labored breathing during sleep
Gasping/snorting noises or observed episodes of apnea
Sleep enuresis (especially secondary enuresis)
Sleeping in a seated position or with the neck hyperextended
Cyanosis
Headache on awakening
Daytime sleepiness
Attention–deficit/hyperactivity disorder
Learning problems

II. Physical Examination

Underweight or overweight
Tonsillar hypertrophy
Adenoidal facies
Micrognathia/retrognathia
High-arched palate
Failure to thrive
Hypertension

Adapted from Marcus CL, Brooks LJ, Draper KA, et al. Diagnosis and management of childhood obstructive sleep apnea syndrome. Pediatrics. 2012;130:575-584.

movement to assess respiratory effort; nasal/oral airflow; and transcutaneous or $ETCO_2$ (ventilation) and pulse oximetry (oxygenation).
  b. Diagnosis of OSAS by polysomnography is based on obstructive apnea–hypopnea index (AHI) and gas exchange abnormalities resulting from upper airway obstruction. Polysomnography is used to differentiate OSAS from benign snoring and other disorders that may disrupt sleep, including central hypoventilation syndrome, sleep-related respiratory failure related to neuromuscular or lung disease, and nocturnal seizures.

C. Treatment

1. Adenotonsillectomy is recommended as the first-line treatment of patients with adenotonsillar hypertrophy. Patients should be reevaluated postoperatively to determine whether further treatment is required.
2. Continuous positive airway pressure is recommended as treatment if adenotonsillectomy is not performed or if OSAS persists postoperatively.
3. Weight loss is recommended in patients who are overweight or obese.
4. Intranasal corticosteroids may be considered as an option for children with mild OSAS (AHI < 5). Follow-up is needed to assess for recurrence of OSAS or possible adverse effects of long-term intranasal steroids.

XI. CHILDHOOD SLEEP PROBLEMS[28,29]

Sleep concerns are common in childhood. Inadequate or poor quality sleep can have negative impacts on health, behavior, and learning. Snoring children should be evaluated for OSAS. Other common sleep concerns include:

A. Inadequate Sleep

Inadequate sleep due to social, school, and family schedules is common. Fig. 24.11 shows typical sleep duration by age.

B. Insomnia

1. Difficulty falling asleep, staying asleep, or both.
2. In younger children, the common behavioral insomnias of childhood include limit-setting (bedtime resistance) and sleep-onset association disorder (night wakings).
  a. Treatment includes bedtime limits and appropriate sleep hygiene.
3. In older children, psychosocial or primary insomnia is characterized by excessive worry about sleep and the consequences of inadequate sleep.
  a. Managed with behavioral interventions.
4. Insomnia can be secondary to another sleep or medical disorder. A comprehensive evaluation is required. Referral to a sleep specialist or behavioral psychologist may be useful.

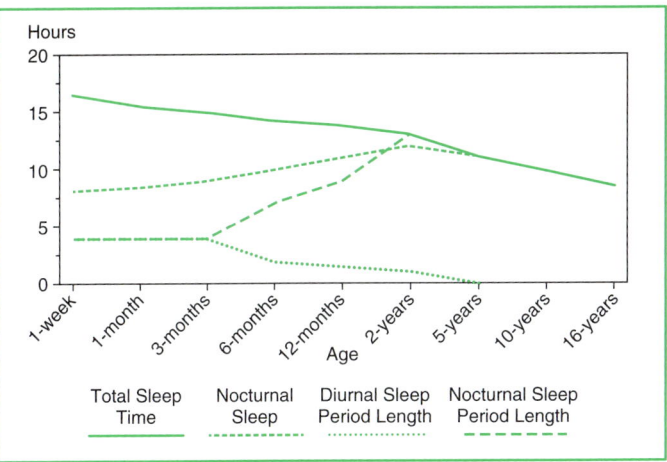

FIGURE 24.11

Change in hours of daytime and nighttime sleep with increasing age. (*From Sheldon SH, Spire JP, Levy HB:* Pediatric Sleep Medicine. *Philadelphia, WB Saunders, 1992, p. 21.*)

C. Nighttime Fears

1. Common and parallel cognitive development
2. Characterized by tearful, fearful behavior at bedtime
3. Relieved by sleeping with member of household
4. Treatment involves reassurance, teaching coping skills, and security objects. Consider evaluation for anxiety disorder in older children/adolescents.

D. Nightmares

1. Frightening dreams that result in awakening from sleep
2. Part of normal development
3. Peak at age 6–10 years
4. May be reduced by reducing stressors, avoiding exposure to frightening images, and ensuring adequate sleep

E. Delayed Sleep Phase Syndrome

1. A circadian rhythm with a persistent, intractable shift in the sleep–wake cycle. Patients move to a late bedtime and late awakening.
2. Seen most commonly in adolescent and young adults
3. Patients have daytime sleepiness and tardiness/absenteeism when unable to sleep during the day.
4. Treatment includes behavioral therapy, bright light exposure, and melatonin. Consider evaluation by a sleep specialist.

F. Parasomnias

1. Common and benign disorders of arousal.
2. Includes sleepwalking, night terrors, and confusional arousals.
3. Onset typically at age 4–6 years and usually disappear by adolescence.
4. Characterized by agitation and confusion. Child avoids comfort and does not recall event.
5. Usually occur in the first few hours of the night.
6. Treatment involves keeping child safe, ensuring adequate sleep, and avoiding triggers. Discourage parental intervention during an episode.

XI. SUDDEN INFANT DEATH SYNDROME[30,31]

Sudden death of an infant younger than 1 year that remains unexplained after a thorough case investigation, including performance of complete autopsy, examination of death scene, and review of clinical history. Thought to be caused when a genetically vulnerable infant is exposed to an exogenous stressor during a critical developmental period when there is immaturity of the cardiorespiratory system, autonomic nervous system, immune system, and arousal pathways, together with a failure of arousal responsiveness from sleep.

A. Epidemiology

1. Incidence is 0.56 per 1000 in the United States, two to three times higher in African-American and Native American populations.
2. Peak incidence is at age 2–4 months, with a male predominance.

B. Risk Factors and Protective Factors (Box 24.3)

BOX 24.3

FACTORS ASSOCIATED WITH SUDDEN INFANT DEATH SYNDROME (SIDS)

Risk Factors	Protective Factors
Side and prone sleeping	Sleeping in supine position
Sleeping on a soft surface or bedding	Sleeping on a firm surface
Smoke exposure during pregnancy or after birth	Living and sleeping in a smoke-free environment
Alcohol or illicit drug use during pregnancy or after birth	Avoiding alcohol or illicit drugs
Bedsharing	Sleeping in same room (but not bed) as caregivers
Overheating	Avoiding overbundling
Prematurity	Breastfeeding
Recent infection	Pacifier use during sleep
Siblings with SIDS	Up-to-date immunizations*
Low socioeconomic factors	Observed tummy time while awake*

*U.S. Preventive Services Task Force level B recommendations. All other protective factors listed are level A recommendations.[31]

REFERENCES

1. Murray CB, Loughlin GM. Making the most of pulse oximetry. *Contemp Pediatr*. 1995;12:45-52, 55-57, 61-62.
2. Comber JT, Lopez BL. Examination of pulse oximetry in sickle cell anemia patients presenting to the emergency department in acute vasoocclusive crisis. *Am J Emerg Med*. 1996;14:16-18.
3. Salyer JW. Neonatal and pediatric pulse oximetry. *Respir Care*. 2003;48:386-396, discussion 397-398.
4. Committee on Fetus and Newborn. American Academy of Pediatrics. Apnea, sudden infant death syndrome and home monitoring. *Pediatrics*. 2003;111(4 Pt 1):914-917.
5. Taussig L. *Pediatric Respiratory Medicine*. 2nd ed. Philadelphia: Mosby; 2008.
6. Blaisdell CJ, Goodman S, Clark K, et al. Pulse oximetry is a poor predictor of hypoxemia in stable children with sickle cell disease. *Arch Pediatr Adolesc Med*. 2000;154:900-903.
7. Schrier RW. *Renal and Electrolyte Disorders*. 7th ed. Philadelphia: Wolters Kluwer/Lippincott Williams & Wilkins; 2010.
8. Brenner BM, ed. *Brenner & Rector's The Kidney*. 8th ed. Philadelphia: Saunders; 2007.
9. Lanbertsten CJ. Transport of oxygen, CO_2, and inert gases by the blood. In: Mountcastle VB, ed. *Medical Physiology*. 14th ed. St Louis: Mosby; 1980.
10. Panitch HB. The pathophysiology of respiratory impairment in pediatric neuromuscular diseases. *Pediatrics*. 2009;123(Suppl 4):S215-S218.
11. Domènech-Clar R, López-Andreu JA, Compte-Torrero L, et al. Maximal static respiratory pressures in children and adolescents. *Pediatr Pulmonol*. 2003;35:126-132.
12. AAP Clinical Practice Guideline. Brief resolved unexplained events (formerly apparent life-threatening events) and evaluation of lower-risk infants. *Pediatrics*. 2016;doi:10.1542/peds.2016-0591.
13. McMillan JA, Feigin RD, DeAngelis CD, et al. *Oski's Pediatrics: Principles and Practice*. 4th ed. Philadelphia: Lippincott Williams & Wilkins; 2006.
14. Fu LY, Moon RY. Apparent life-threatening events: an update. *Pediatr Rev*. 2012;33:361-369.
15. National Asthma Education and Prevention Program (NAEPP)—Expert Panel Report 3. Guidelines for the diagnosis and management of asthma. August 2007. Available at <http://www.nhlbi.nih.gov/guidelines/asthma/asthgdln.htm>. Accessed July 27, 2009.
16. Ralston SL, Lieberthal AS, Meissner HC, et al. Clinical practice guideline: the diagnosis, management, and prevention of bronchiolitis. *Pediatrics*. 2014;134:e1474-e1502.
17. Kair L, Leonard D, Anderson J. Bronchopulmonary dysplasia. *Pediatr Rev*. 2012;33(6):255-264.
18. Jobe A, Bancalari E. Bronchopulmonary dysplasia. *Am J Respir Crit Care Med*. 2001;163:1723-1729.
19. Allen J, Zwerdling R, Ehrenkranz R, et al; American Thoracic Society. Statement on the care of the child with chronic lung disease of infancy and childhood. *Am J Respir Crit Care Med*. 2003;168:356-396.
20. Ehrenkranz RA, Walsh MC, Vohr BR, et al. Validation of the National Institutes of Health consensus definition of bronchopulmonary dysplasia. *J Pediatr*. 2005;116:1353-1360.
21. Montgomery G, Howenstine M. Cystic fibrosis. *Pediatr Rev*. 2009;30:302-310.

22. Farrell PM, Rosenstein BJ, White TB, et al. Guidelines for diagnosis of cystic fibrosis in newborns through older adults: Cystic Fibrosis Foundation Consensus Report. *J Pediatr.* 2008;153:S4-S14.
23. Flume PA, O'Sullivan BP, Robinson KA, et al. Cystic fibrosis pulmonary guidelines: chronic medicines for maintenance of lung health. *Am J Respir Crit Care Med.* 2007;176:957-969.
24. Marcus CL, Brooks LJ, Draper KA, et al. Diagnosis and management of childhood obstructive sleep apnea syndrome. *Pediatrics.* 2012;130:576-584.
25. AAP Clinical Practice Guideline. Diagnosis and management of childhood obstructive sleep apnea syndrome. *Pediatrics.* 2012;130:576-584.
26. Carroll JL. Obstructive sleep-disordered breathing in children: new controversies, new directions. *Clin Chest Med.* 2003;24:261-282.
27. Wagner MH, Torrez DM. Interpretation of the polysomnogram in children. *Otolaryngol Clin North Am.* 2007;40:745-759.
28. Bhargava S. Diagnosis and management of common sleep problems in children. *Pediatr Rev.* 2011;32:91-98.
29. Mindel JA, Owens JA. *A Clinical Guide to Pediatric Sleep: Diagnosis and Management of Sleep Problems.* Philadelphia, PA: Lippincott Williams & Wilkins; 2003.
30. Moon R, Horne R, Hauck F. Sudden infant death syndrome. *Lancet.* 2007;370:1578-1587.
31. Task Force on Sudden Infant Death Syndrome, Moon RY. SIDS and other sleep-related infant deaths: expansion of recommendations for a safe infant sleeping environment. *Pediatrics.* 2001;128:e1341-e1367.

Chapter 25
Radiology
Kameron Lockamy Rogers, MD

See additional content on Expert Consult

I. WEB RESOURCES
- American College of Radiology Appropriateness Criteria: http://www.acr.org/Quality-Safety/Standards-Guidelines/Practice-Guidelines-by-Modality/Pediatric
- Image Gently Alliance: www.imagegently.org
- Society for Pediatric Radiology: http://www.pedrad.org

II. GENERAL PEDIATRIC PRINCIPLES

A. Limit Radiation Exposure
The amount of radiation children receive from medical sources is increasing. Considerations unique to the pediatric population include greater lifetime exposure than previous generations, increased radiosensitivity (e.g., thyroid, breast tissue, gonads), and a longer lifespan in which to manifest radiation-related cancer. One computed tomography (CT) scan of the chest, for example, can be equivalent to about 68 chest x-rays.[1]

B. Employ Judicious Use of CT: Consider Ultrasound (US) or Magnetic Resonance Imaging (MRI) Whenever Possible

1. To limit exposure, use child-size protocols to decrease tube voltage (kVp) and tube current (mA).
2. One scan (single phase) is often enough.
3. Scan only the indicated areas (e.g., do not include pelvis if only abdomen is required).
4. Body CT scans *without* intravenous (IV) contrast are helpful in delineating fine bony details, calcifications, and lung parenchyma, but almost nothing else. If your clinical question concerns something other than these areas, and you cannot use IV contrast, then consider US as a substitute for CT.

III. CHOOSING THE RIGHT STUDY (Table 25.1)
Provide the radiologist with adequate clinical details. The clinical scenario is important in both allowing the radiologist to choose the right study/sequences to properly visualize desired structures and ensures particular attention is paid to conditions for which the study was ordered. Pay attention to whether contrast is indicated (or paramount) to visualize what

TABLE 25.1
ADVANTAGES AND DISADVANTAGES OF IMAGING MODALITIES

Modality	Advantages	Disadvantages
X-ray *	Fast; portable; readily available; relatively inexpensive	Poor soft-tissue contrast; 2D imaging only
Fluoroscopy *	Real-time imaging; useful in operating room; ±portable, ±readily available	No cross-sectional imaging
CT *	Delineation of bones, soft tissues, calcifications; multi-planar and 3D reconstructions; minimally-invasive (CT angiography); assists in procedures	Intermediate to high radiation dose; relatively expensive; side effects from IV contrast (nephrotoxicity, anaphylaxis); weight limit
MRI	Excellent soft tissue characterization; functional imaging; multi-planar imaging; minimally-invasive (MR angiography); assists in procedures	Less readily available; expensive; lengthy exams; limited use in unstable patients; potential need for sedation/anesthesia; contraindicated with certain implanted devices; side effects from gadolinium if renally impaired; weight limit
Ultrasound	Portable; real-time imaging; multi-planar imaging; Doppler evaluation of blood flow; differentiates cystic vs. solid masses; least-expensive cross-sectional imaging modality	Highly operator–dependent; bone/gas can obscure anatomy; difficult in obese and immobile patients
Nuclear medicine *	Readily available; Functional/molecular imaging	Intermediate to high radiation dose; expensive; potential need for sedation; radioactive urine and body fluids

*Denotes radiation exposure.
Modified from Zitelli and Davis' Atlas of Pediatric Physical Diagnosis. 6th ed. Philadelphia: Saunders; 2012.

you want to find. When you are unsure of which study is best to order, consult your radiologist.

IV. HEAD[2]

Most intracranial processes, malformations, and tumors are best imaged with MRI. MRI is useful for neurodegenerative and demyelination disorders, diffuse axonal injury, neurocutaneous syndromes, structural lesions in focal seizure disorders, and vascular lesions. Compared to CT, MRI is more useful in detecting lesions in the posterior fossa.

A. Germinal Matrix Hemorrhage

Head US should be performed in premature infants to detect intraventricular hemorrhage and periventricular leukomalacia, and to screen for hydrocephalus and congenital abnormalities.[3]

B. Congenital Malformations

Head US can be used as long as the fontanelle can still be felt. Once detected on US, malformations are best further defined with MRI.

C. Congenital Infections

1. Congenital infections such as herpes simplex virus (HSV) are best imaged with MRI.
2. Calcifications consistent with toxoplasmosis and cytomegalovirus (CMV) infection may be best detected with CT. Calcifications in toxoplasmosis have a predilection for the basal ganglia and tend to be more diffuse than those of CMV, which primarily affect the periventricular region.

D. Head Trauma

1. Best imaged using noncontrast CT to reveal skull fractures and subdural and epidural hematomas. To prevent unnecessary radiation exposure, PECARN criteria should be utilized to determine trauma patients unlikely to benefit from CT (see Chapter 4).
2. Skull radiography is of limited value.
3. MRI is useful to delineate multiple hemorrhages of various ages. This is most often obtained subsequent to head CT.

E. Ventriculoperitoneal (VP) Shunt Malfunction

1. Ultrafast MRI is the preferred imaging modality to grossly evaluate ventricular size (if the child is beyond the age where head US can be done).[4,5]
2. Noncontrast CT can be obtained in the event that ultrafast MRI is not available, or if contraindications precluding MRI exist.
3. If signs of shunt malfunction are noted, a radiographic shunt series should be performed to assess the entire length of tubing for position and patency.[6] Determine where the shunt ends (e.g., atrium, cava, pleural space, peritoneum) to request the appropriate views.

F. Craniosynostosis

Suture examination is best done initially with radiographs of the skull. If there are changes consistent with craniosynostosis, three-dimensional CT reconstructions should be obtained.

V. EYES[7]

When deciding between CT and MRI, remember that CT is best used to delineate the bony orbit while MRI is better for orbital soft tissues and surrounding structures.

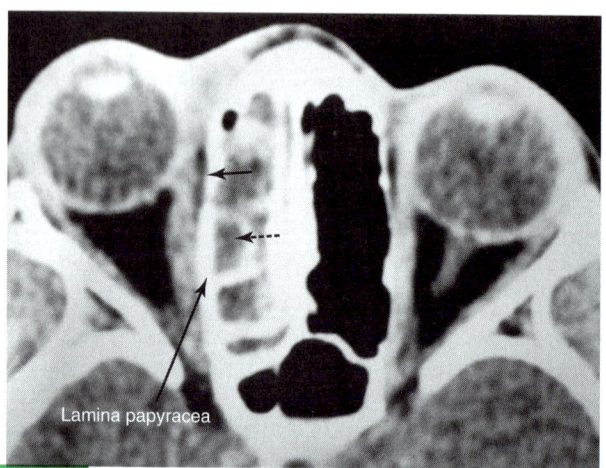

FIGURE 25.1

Orbital cellulitis with subperiosteal abscess. Preseptal (*dashed arrow*) and extracoronal portions of the medial right orbit are involved. Medial rectus muscle is slightly thickened and displaced, and a small focal fluid collection *(arrow)* representing a subperiosteal abscess is present. *(From Slovis TL. Caffey's Pediatric Diagnostic Imaging. 11th ed. Philadelphia: Mosby; 2008. Courtesy Kenneth D. Hopper, MD, Hershey, Pa.)*

A. Orbital Cellulitis (Fig. 25.1)

1. Best imaged with contrast-enhanced CT with orbital cuts to appreciate the orbital septum, the anterior reflection of the orbital wall periosteum into the tarsal plate.
2. Infection is preseptal (periorbital) when inflammation is anterior to the orbital septum, or orbital when posterior to the orbital septum. A line is drawn from the medial to the lateral bony walls of the orbit on transverse cuts.

VI. SPINE

A. Cervical Spine Trauma[8,9]

1. After immobilization in a collar, lateral and anteroposterior (AP) radiographs of the cervical spine (C-spine) should be performed in all children who have sustained significant head trauma, deceleration injury, or undergone unwitnessed trauma. The C7 vertebral body and the C7–T1 junction must be visualized. C-spine injuries are most common from the occiput to C3 in children (especially subluxation at the atlanto-occipital joint or atlantoaxial joint in infants and toddlers) and in the lower C-spine in older children and adults.
2. Flexion-extension radiographs may be helpful, especially in patients with Down syndrome, who are at risk for atlantoaxial subluxation.

3. Odontoid views may be helpful in older children with suspected occipitocervical injury (e.g., whiplash) only if the odontoid cannot be seen on the lateral C-spine view.

B. Reading C-Spine Films[8,9]

The following ABCDDS (or ABCDs) mnemonic is useful:
1. Alignment: Anterior vertebral body line, posterior vertebral body line, facet line, and spinous process line should each form a continuous line with smooth contour and no step-offs (Fig. 25.2)
2. Bones: Assess each bone looking for chips or fractures
3. Count: Must see C7 body in its entirety
4. Dens: Examine for chips or fractures
5. Disk spaces: Should see consistent distance between each vertebral body
6. Soft tissue: Assess for swelling, particularly in prevertebral area

C. Spinal Cord Injury Without Radiographic Abnormality[9,10]

1. Should be suspected in the setting of normal C-spine images when clinical signs or symptoms (e.g., point tenderness, focal neurologic symptoms) suggest C-spine injury.
2. If neurologic symptoms persist despite normal C-spine and flexion-extension views, MRI is indicated to rule out swelling, contusion, or intramedullary hemorrhage of the cord.

D. Spinal Dysraphism (e.g., myelocele, myelomeningocele)

Screening often performed with spinal US based on clinical findings (age < 3 months corrected age). Plain radiographs should be obtained if the patient is too old for US. Positive results should be confirmed by MRI.

E. Scoliosis

Best evaluated by erect AP radiograph of the spine. Posteroanterior (PA) views can be used in postpubertal girls to decrease breast radiation dose.

VII. AIRWAY[8]

A. Importance of Lateral Radiographs

1. Lateral radiograph of the upper airway is the most useful film for evaluating a child with stridor. Ideally, should be obtained on inspiration.
2. A radiologic workup should always include AP and lateral radiographs of the chest, with inclusion of upper airway in the lateral view. Diagnosis is based on airway radiologic examination in conjunction with clinical presentation (Table 25.2, Figs. 25.3 and 25.4).

B. Vascular Rings

1. Vascular rings and other extrinsic masses that obstruct the lower airways can be imaged with contrast-enhanced CT or MRI.
2. Tracheomalacia and intrinsic masses can be studied with bronchoscopy.

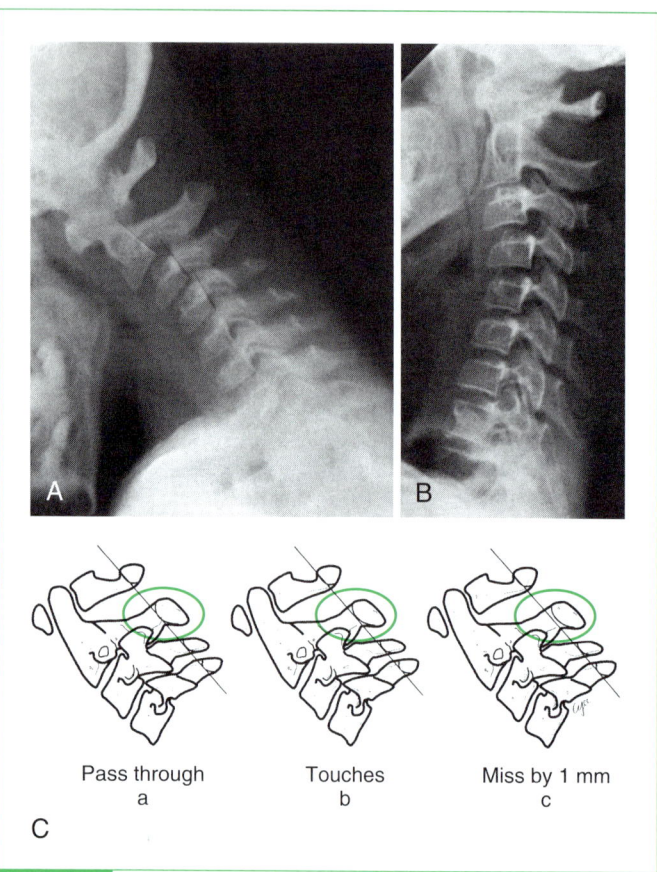

FIGURE 25.2

Normal cervical spine mobility in children. **A,** Normal forward shift of C2 on C3 in an asymptomatic 3-year-old girl. **B,** Normal forward shift of C3 on C4 (pseudosubluxation) in an asymptomatic 5-year-old girl. **C,** Normal limits of the posterior cervical line. Normal posterior cervical line can pass through or just behind the anterior cortex of C2 (*a*), touch the anterior cortex of C2 (*b*), or come within 1 mm of the anterior aspect of C2 (*c*). (***A** and **B** from Sullivan CR, Bruwer AJ, Harris LE. Hypermobility of the cervical spine in children: a pitfall in the diagnosis of cervical dislocation.* Am J Surg. *1958;95:636-640;* ***C** from Kuhns LR.* Imaging of Spinal Trauma in Children: An Atlas and Text. *Hamilton Ontario: BC Decker; 1998:31.*)

TABLE 25.2
DIAGNOSIS OF DISEASES BASED ON AIRWAY RADIOLOGIC EXAMINATION

Diagnosis	Findings on Airway Films
Croup	AP and lateral radiographs with subglottic narrowing (*steeple sign*)
Epiglottitis	Enlarged, indistinct epiglottis on lateral film (*thumbprint sign*)
Vascular ring	AP and lateral radiographs with airway narrowing; double or right aortic arch
Retropharyngeal abscess or pharyngeal mass	Soft tissue air or persistent enlargement of prevertebral soft tissues (more than half of a vertebral body width above C3 and more than one vertebral body width below C3)
Immunodeficiency	Absence of adenoidal and tonsillar tissue after age 6 mo

AP, Anteroposterior

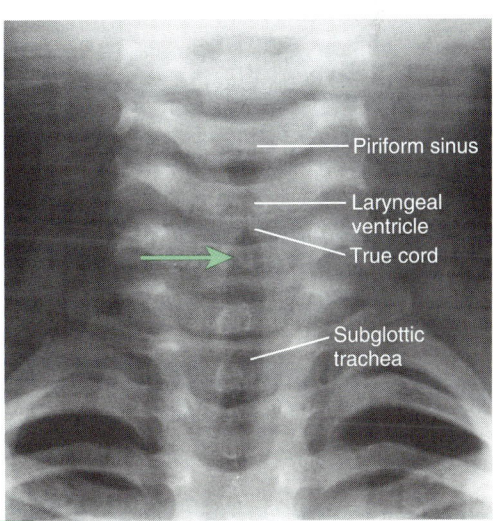

FIGURE 25.3
Anteroposterior (AP) neck film with normal anatomy including "Bordeaux bottle" appearance of the subglottic region (*arrow*). *(Figure modified from Blickman JG, Van Die L. Pediatric Radiology: The Requisites. 3rd ed. Philadelphia: Elsevier; 2009. Fig. 2.17B.)*

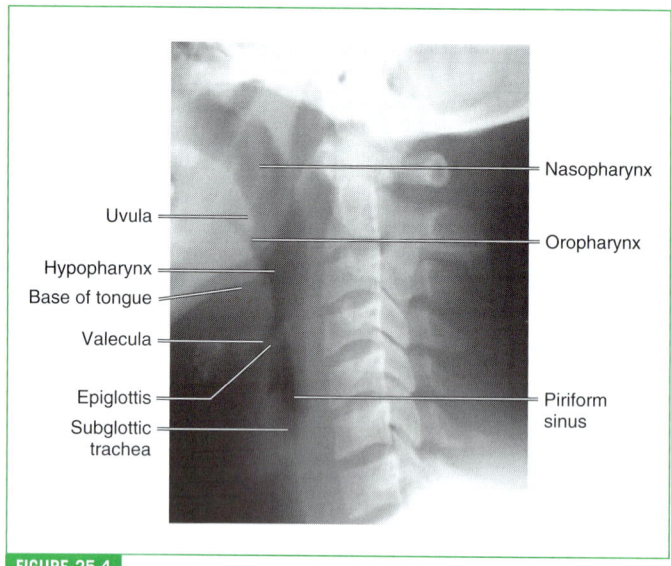

FIGURE 25.4

Lateral neck film with normal anatomy on lateral airway view.

C. Foreign Bodies

1. Lower airway foreign bodies: In the absence of a radiopaque foreign body, radiologic findings include air trapping, hyperinflation, atelectasis, consolidation, pneumothorax, and pneumomediastinum. Further studies should include expiratory radiographs (in a cooperative patient), bilateral decubitus chest radiographs (in an uncooperative patient), or airway fluoroscopy.
2. Esophageal foreign bodies: Usually lodged at one of three locations—thoracic inlet, level of aortic arch and left mainstem bronchus, or gastroesophageal junction. Evaluation should include:
a. Lateral airway radiograph (include nasopharynx)
b. AP radiograph of chest and abdomen (including supraclavicular region)
c. Contrast study of esophagus if other studies are normal. If perforation is suspected, use nonionic water-soluble contrast.

VIII. CHEST[6,8,9]

A. Posteroanterior and Lateral Radiographs

First images obtained when studying the chest (Figs. 25.5 and 25.6).

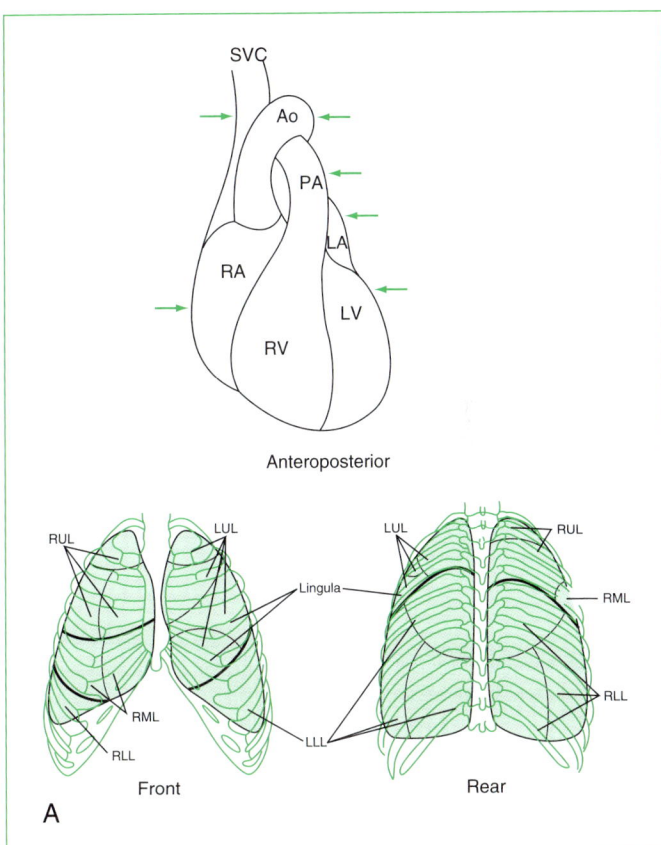

FIGURE 25.5

A, Normal lung and cardiac anatomy as seen on an anteroposterior chest radiograph. Arrows indicate contours seen on anteroposterior chest radiographs **(B)**. Ao, Aorta; LA, left atrium; LLL, left lower lobe; LUL, left upper lobe; LV, left ventricle; PA, pulmonary artery; RA, right atrium; RLL, right lower lobe; RML, right middle lobe; RUL, right upper lobe; RV, right ventricle; SVC, superior vena cava. *(Heart diagram modified from Kirks DR, Griscom NT. Practical Pediatric Imaging: Diagnostic Radiology of Infants and Children. 3rd ed. Philadelphia: Lippincott-Raven; 1998.)*

Continued

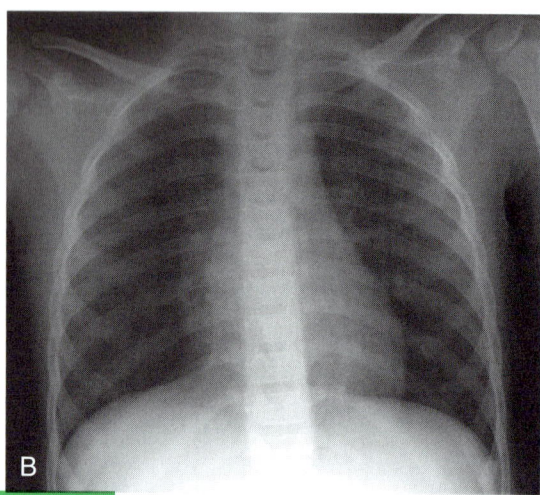

FIGURE 25.5, cont'd

B. Pneumonia

1. Lobar or segmental consolidation suggests bacterial infection.
2. Hyperinflation, bilateral patchy or streaky densities, and peribronchial thickening is more typical of nonbacterial disease.

C. Atelectasis vs. Infiltrate

1. Atelectasis: When air is removed from the lung, tissue collapses, resulting in volume loss on chest radiographs. If severe enough, mediastinum and/or diaphragm are pulled toward the lesion. Air may still remain in larger bronchi, creating air bronchograms on radiograph. Collapse and re-expansion can occur quickly.
2. Infiltrate: Fluid (blood, pus, edema) that invades one of the compartments of the lung (bronchoalveolar air space or peribronchial interstitial space), seen as a density on radiograph. When alveolar air is displaced by fluid but air remains in bronchi, classic pneumonic infiltrate with air bronchograms is seen. When infiltrate is interstitial, its borders can be vague and bronchial walls may be thickened. Typically, infiltrates resolve in 2–6 weeks.

D. Parapneumonic Effusions and Empyema

Initially, PA and lateral radiographs are obtained. Lateral decubitus radiographs may also be helpful. Ultrasound is often the best modality

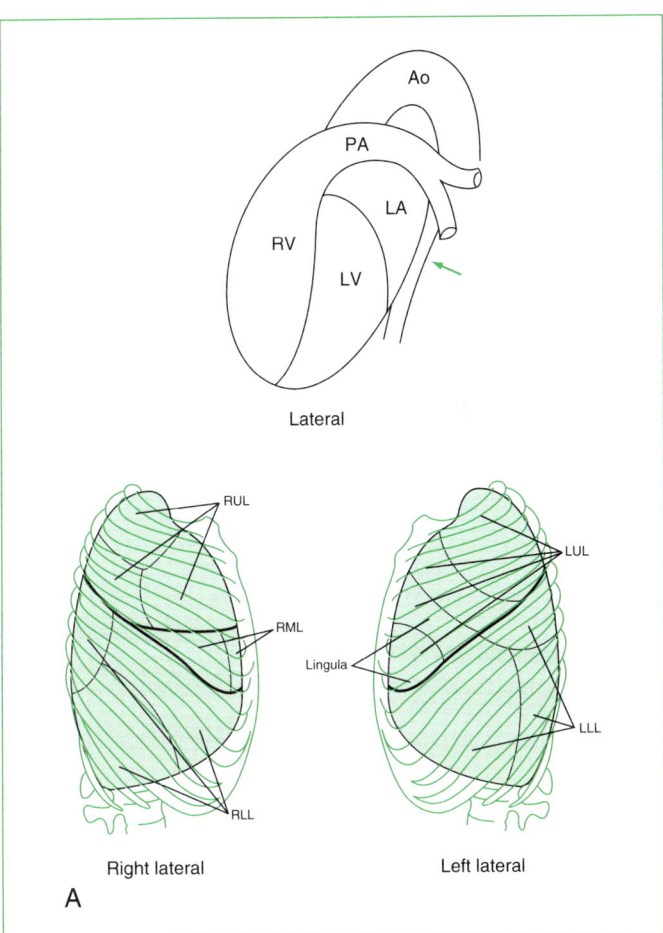

FIGURE 25.6

A, Normal lung and cardiac anatomy as seen on lateral chest radiograph. Arrow indicates contours seen on lateral chest radiograph **(B)**. Ao, Aorta; LA, left atrium; LLL, left lower lobe; LUL, left upper lobe; LV, left ventricle; PA, pulmonary artery; RLL, right lower lobe; RML, right middle lobe; RUL, right upper lobe; RV, right ventricle. *(Heart diagram modified from Kirks DR, Griscom NT.* Practical Pediatric Imaging: Diagnostic Radiology of Infants and Children. *3rd ed. Philadelphia: Lippincott-Raven; 1998.)*

Continued

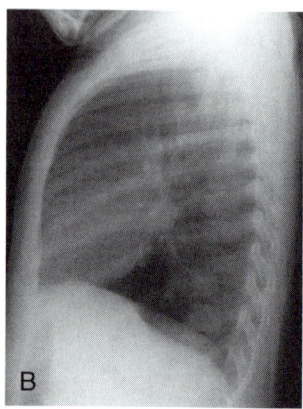

FIGURE 25.6, cont'd

for early identification of loculation, but a contrast-enhanced CT may be necessary to further delineate loculation. CT or color Doppler US can differentiate between pleural fluid and collapsed or consolidated tissue.

E. Parenchymal Findings

1. Contrast-enhanced CT: Lung abscess, cavitary necrosis, lung contusions.
2. Noncontrast CT: Pneumatocele, fungal infections, interstitial lung disease.

F. Mediastinal Masses

Mediastinal masses (thymus, lymphoma, bronchogenic cyst, neuroblastoma, neurofibroma) are initially imaged with plain films, followed by contrast-enhanced CT or MRI.

G. Central Line Placement

On chest radiographs, central venous catheters entering from the neck or arm are ideally placed with catheter tip at junction of superior vena cava and right atrium. Some extension into right atrium is acceptable, but if catheter is observed curving to patient's left on PA view, catheter may be positioned in right ventricle (Fig. 25.7). Catheters inserted below diaphragm should be placed with tips at level of diaphragm (Fig. 25.8).

H. Endotracheal Tube (ETT) Placement

On chest radiographs, end of the ETT should rest about midway between thoracic inlet and carina. Lung fields should show symmetric aeration.

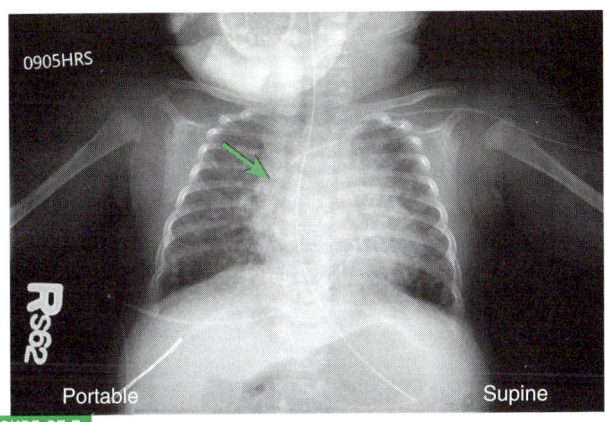

FIGURE 25.7

Central line placement on anteroposterior chest radiograph for line inserted in arm or neck. Arrow indicates termination of catheter at junction of superior vena cava (SVC) and right atrium.

IX. HEART AND VESSELS[8]

A. Congenital Heart Disease

Most clearly defined by echocardiography, but initial PA and lateral chest radiograph may yield important clues:

1. Position of aortic arch: Left or right (Fig. 25.9)
2. Situs: Noting positions of apex, stomach bubble, and liver
3. Heart size: With particular attention paid to lateral chest radiograph
4. Pulmonary vascularity: Increased or decreased flow in arteries and veins

B. Vessels

1. Moving blood is detected sonographically by frequency shifts (Doppler effect).
2. Color Doppler flow imaging: Can be used to evaluate deep vein thrombosis (DVT), vascular patency, intracranial blood flow [including transcranial Doppler (TCD) to screen for ischemic brain injury risk in sickle cell disease], cardiac shunt flow, transplant vascularity, veno-occlusive disease of the liver, and testicular perfusion in testicular torsion.
3. Power Doppler is particularly sensitive in detecting slow flow in small vessels (e.g., infant testes).

C. Vessel Abnormalities

Can be studied with echocardiography/US, CT, and MRI. Use these modalities to detect coarctation of the aorta, aortic stenosis, pulmonary artery and vein abnormalities, vascular rings, arteriovenous malformations,

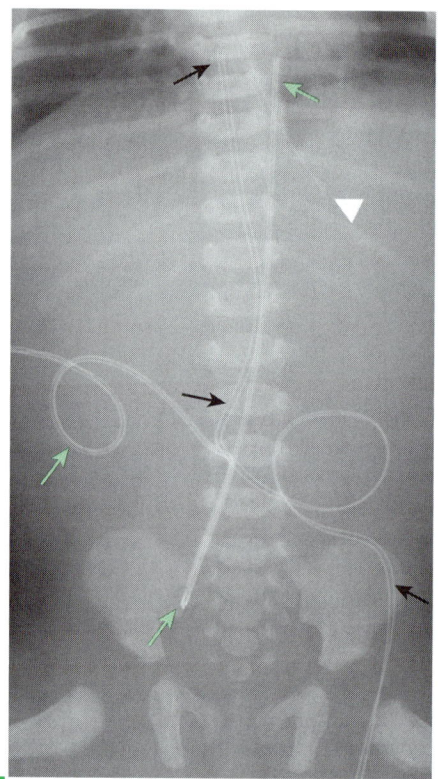

FIGURE 25.8

Central line placement on anteroposterior radiograph for line inserted below the diaphragm. This 3-day-old newborn has an umbilical venous line (*black arrow*) with the tip in the right atrium, an umbilical arterial line (*green arrow*) with the tip in the aorta at T8, and a nasogastric tube (*arrowhead*). (*From Tadros S, Sperling V, Kim S.* Zitelli and Davis' Atlas of Pediatric Physical Diagnosis. *6th ed. Philadelphia: Saunders; 2012. Fig. 24.15C.*)

hemangiomas, aneurysms, and postoperative complications like thrombosis and stenosis.

X. ABDOMEN[8,9,10]

A. Neonatal Enterocolitis (see Chapter 18)

Clinically diagnosed and followed by abdominal radiographs, which may show focal dilation, featureless loops, pneumatosis, and portal venous gas.

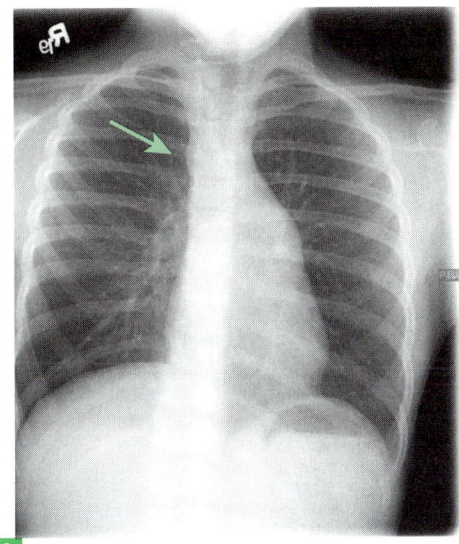

FIGURE 25.9
Right aortic arch as seen on anteroposterior chest radiograph.

B. Esophageal Atresia and Tracheoesophageal Fistula (Fig. EC 25.A)

Studied initially with chest radiographs, which may reveal the air-distended esophageal atretic pouch, nasogastric tube curled up in this pouch, or excessive dilation of stomach as a result of bronchial fistula communication.

C. High Intestinal Obstruction

1. Diagnosed with upper gastrointestinal (UGI) series, where oral contrast is ingested to allow visualization of the esophagus, stomach, and duodenum. Causes include esophageal webs and rings, masses, duodenal atresia or webs (Fig. EC 25.B), annular pancreas, midgut volvulus, and Ladd bands.
2. UGI can also help evaluate hiatal hernias, varices, gastric outlet obstruction, motility problems, ulcerations, and reflux.
3. During UGI, identifying duodenojejunal junction (ligament of Treitz) helps diagnose malrotation. Normally the junction is to the left of spine, at or above the level of duodenal bulb.

D. Pyloric Stenosis

1. US is the preferred examination because it directly visualizes the pyloric muscle. Normal pylorus is <17 mm in length, and its muscular wall is <3 mm in thickness (Fig. EC 25.C).

2. Radiographs: Show gastric distention.
3. UGI: Delayed gastric emptying and a narrow, elongated pyloric channel will be evident.

E. Bowel Obstruction

1. Determination of large or small bowel obstruction: Often aided by supine radiograph, prone radiograph, and either upright, supine cross-table lateral, or left lateral decubitus film to look for free air and air-fluid levels.
   Causes of obstruction: Adhesions, appendicitis, incarcerated inguinal hernias, Meckel's diverticulum, intussusception, malrotation/volvulus.
2. US can be helpful in thin patients and female patients who have ovarian pathology to further differentiate their abdominal pain.
3. CT with intravenous, oral, or rectal contrast is more useful with an obese patient or when looking for perforated appendicitis or abscess.
4. Contrast enemas with dilute water-soluble agents can also be useful in lower intestinal obstruction in the newborn.

F. Intussusception

1. On abdominal radiographs, particularly left lateral decubitus, findings include minimal gas in right abdomen and ascending colon.
2. US will show "target sign." Doppler will show flow in the intussuscepted mesentery, which will allow confirmation of the diagnosis as well as assessment of intussuscepted tissue viability. (Fig. 25.10).
3. For fluoroscopy-guided therapeutic enema, air insufflation is safest but other contrast agents may also be used. Reducing an intussusception with air or contrast is contraindicated if perforation is suspected.

G. Meckel Diverticulum

Suggested by painless lower GI bleeding; diagnosed by nuclear scintigraphy using technetium-99m (^{99m}Tc)-pertechnetate.

H. Abdominal Trauma

IV contrast-enhanced CT of abdomen and pelvis to detect solid organ injury, vascular extravasation, free fluid, bowel wall thickening, and organ laceration. (See Chapter 4 for FAST abdominal survey.)

I. Biliary Atresia

1. In neonates with jaundice, US initially to distinguish biliary atresia from hepatitis. Gallbladder will be small or absent with biliary atresia.
2. Hepatobiliary scintigraphy with ^{99m}Tc-iminodiacetate (HIDA) reveals absence of radionuclide in GI tract with biliary atresia.

J. Nasoduodenal (ND) Tube Placement

Visualize tube on an AP abdominal radiograph passing through stomach, crossing midline, and passing into duodenal bulb (where tip of tube will just begin to point inferiorly). If it remains unclear whether tube is in duodenum or coiled in stomach, a lateral film is indicated (a properly placed ND tube tip will lie posterior, near the spine).

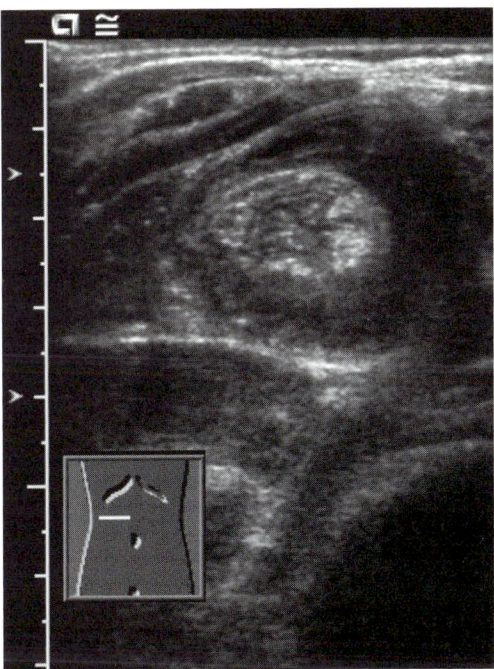

FIGURE 25.10

Ileocolic intussusception in the proximal transverse colon of a 2-year old. Ultrasound shows characteristic "target sign" on transverse section: hypoechoic ring with an echogenic center. *(From Tadros S, Sperling V, Kim S.* Zitelli and Davis' Atlas of Pediatric Physical Diagnosis. *6th ed. Philadelphia: Saunders; 2012. Fig. 24.20A.)*

XI. GENITOURINARY TRACT[8]

A. Urinary Tract Infection (UTI)[11]

1. Initial febrile UTIs in children aged <2 years requires renal/bladder ultrasound (RBUS) to look for congenital anomalies (e.g., posterior urethral valves, ureterocele, vesicoureteral reflux), baseline renal measurements, and damage to kidney cortices. Obtain during first 2 days of treatment if unusually severe or inadequate clinical recovery. Otherwise, avoid RBUS in acute infection and obtain after resolution.
2. RBUS may identify hydronephrosis, ureteropelvic junction obstruction, posterior urethral valves, multicystic dysplastic kidneys, chronic pyelonephritis, renal fusion (horseshoe kidney), and renal cysts.
3. Voiding cystourethrogram (VCUG): Indicated in evaluation of second episode of febrile UTI. For initial UTI, obtain only if RBUS reveals

hydronephrosis, scarring, or other findings concerning for high-grade VUR or obstructive nephropathy.
4. Rarely, a dimercaptosuccinic acid (DMSA) scan is used to follow renal cortical scarring over time. However, it remains more useful in research rather than clinical settings.

B. Uterine and Ovarian Pathology

US through a very full bladder should be performed if the clinical picture is suspicious for ovarian torsion, tubo-ovarian abscess (TOA), or hydrometroculpos. Transvaginal US can visualize the uterus and ovaries better (and the bladder does not have to be full), but evidence of coitarche is required.

C. Testicular Pathology[8]

US with Doppler allows for differentiation of acute scrotal pathology utilizing both intratesticular as well as peritesticular bloodflow.

XII. EXTREMITIES[8,10]

A. Trauma

1. Adequate evaluation requires AP and lateral radiographs. Restricting the image to the area of interest improves resolution (e.g., for a thumb injury, ask for an image of the thumb, not the hand).
2. Comparison films of the uninvolved extremity are not necessary but may be helpful, such as in the evaluation of joint effusions (particularly hip), suspected osteomyelitis, or pyarthrosis and/or evaluation of subtle fractures, especially in areas of multiple ossification centers such as the elbow. However, it is worthwhile to remember that ossification centers are not always symmetric.
3. Salter-Harris classification of growth-plate injury (Table 25.3).

TABLE 25.3

SALTER-HARRIS CLASSIFICATION OF GROWTH PLATE INJURY

Class I	Class II	Class III	Class IV	Class V
Fracture along growth plate	Fracture along growth plate with metaphyseal extension	Fracture along growth plate with epiphyseal extension	Fracture across growth plate, including metaphysis and epiphysis	Crush injury to growth plate without obvious fracture
I	II	III	IV	V

B. Stress Fractures

1. Occur most often at the tibia, fibula, metatarsals, and calcaneus.
2. Radiographs will show a band of sclerosis and new bone formation.
3. Skeletal scintigraphy is a sensitive method for making the diagnosis.

C. Osteomyelitis

1. Tends to occur at metaphysis of long bones and within flat bones.
2. Radiographs will show deep soft-tissue swelling and bony changes (may take 10 days to appear).
3. Skeletal scintigraphy and MRI will often be positive before radiographic changes are noticeable.

D. Hip Disorders

1. Developmental hip dysplasia (congenital hip dislocation) is imaged initially with US, typically around 6 weeks of age. Once femoral heads ossify (within 3–6 months), radiographs are more helpful (Fig. EC 25.D).
2. Legg-Calvé-Perthes disease (avascular necrosis of femoral head) can be imaged with AP and frog-leg lateral hip radiographs, as well as MRI and bone scintigraphy (Fig. EC 25.E).
3. Slipped capital femoral epiphysis (SCFE) will show femoral head displacement on frog-leg lateral and AP radiographs (Fig. EC 25.F).

E. Bone Lesions

Initially evaluated with radiographs, with further imaging guided by clinical suspicion of origin and need for additional information.

1. Osteochondroma: Benign lesion that arises from the metaphysis of a long bone, most frequently the distal femur, proximal humerus, and proximal tibia. Composed of cortical and medullary bone with a cap of hyaline cartilage and is continuous with the cortex and intramedullary cavity of the involved bone (Fig. EC 25.G).
2. Unicameral bone cyst: Benign lesion that appears on radiographs as a solitary, centrally located, lucent lesion located within the medullary portion of the bone and often extends to the physis. Tends to occur in the proximal femur or humerus (Fig. EC 25.H).
3. Nonossifying fibroma: Benign lesion that appears on radiographs as a lucency in the metaphyseal cortex, highlighted by a sclerotic, often scalloped border (Fig. EC 25.I).
4. Osteoid osteoma: Benign lesion that appears on radiographs as a small, oval lucency in the metaphysis or diaphysis. Most frequently occurs in the proximal femur and tibia, although any bone can be involved, including vertebrae. Often presents with gradually increasing pain that is worse at night (Fig. EC 25.J).
5. Osteosarcoma: Most common primary malignant bone tumor in children and adolescents aged >10 years. Lesion typically occurs at the metaphyses of long bones, and radiographs demonstrate amorphous sclerosis with a classic sunburst pattern (Fig. 25.11).

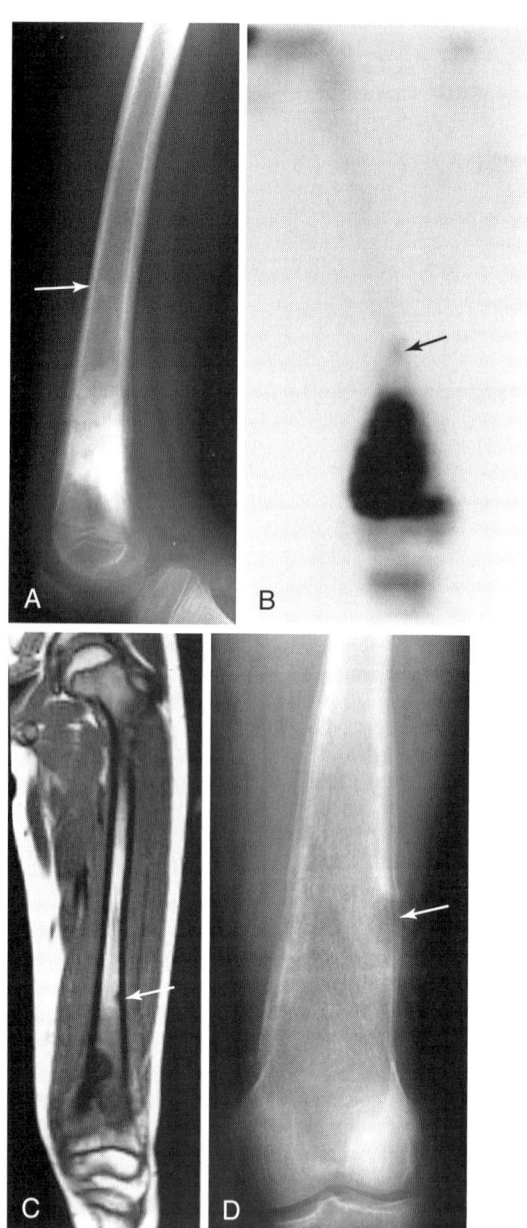

FIGURE 25.11

A, Lateral radiograph of femur of a 9-year-old boy with osteosarcoma shows a sclerotic intramedullary distal femoral tumor with slight periosteal new bone formation. A small, dense skip metastasis *(arrow)* is seen proximal to primary tumor of main tumor mass. Skip metastasis *(arrow)* is also seen on a technetium-99m methylene diphosphonate bone scan **(B)** and is shown as a cortical-based intramedullary lesion *(arrow)* on a coronal T1-weighted magnetic resonance image **(C). D,** Radiograph of femur of a 16-year-old boy with telangiectatic osteosarcoma shows large lesion in distal metadiaphysis extending into epiphysis. Tumor is lytic rather than bone forming. There is mild periosteal reaction. There has been a recent incisional biopsy *(arrow)*. *(From Slovis TL. Caffey's Pediatric Diagnostic Imaging. 11th ed. Philadelphia: Mosby; 2008.)*

6. Ewing sarcoma: Second most common primary malignant bone tumor in children and adolescents aged >10 years; most common primary malignant bone tumor in children younger than 10 years. Lesion is typically in the diaphyses of long and flat bones, and radiographs demonstrate a lytic lesion with periosteal reaction, creating a classic lamellar "onion-skinning" appearance. CT or MRI of lesion may demonstrate a soft-tissue mass (Fig. 25.12).

F. Bone Age
Obtain a PA view of the left hand and wrist.

G. Skeletal Survey
1. In cases of suspected child abuse, evaluation should include radiographs of the lateral skull, including C-spine, AP chest (bone technique), ribs (oblique views), AP pelvis, abdomen (bone technique) with lateral thoracic and lumbar spine, and AP views of individual limb segments, hands, and feet.
2. Classic findings: Multiple metaphyseal injuries (especially corner and bucket-handle fractures) and other coexisting fractures of various ages (Fig. 25.13). Suspicion should also be raised by fracture at unusual sites, such as posterior rib fractures or solitary spiral and transverse long-bone fractures with an inconsistent history of trauma (Fig. 25.14).

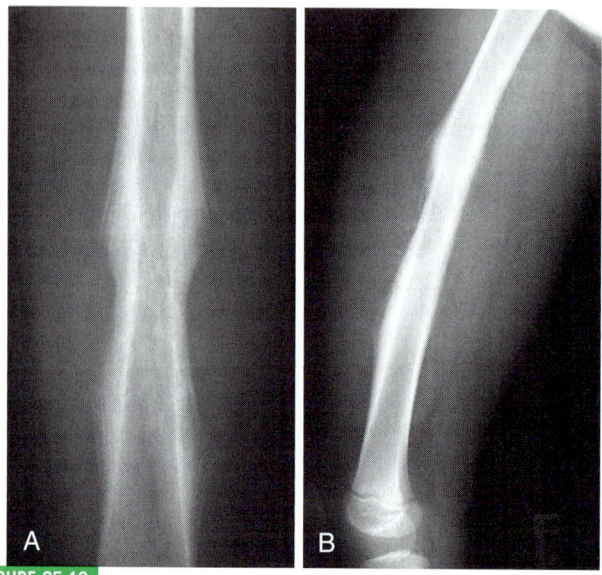

FIGURE 25.12

Anteroposterior **(A)** and lateral **(B)** radiographs of femur of a 6-year-old girl show a Ewing sarcoma arising from mid-diaphysis. Lamellar periosteal reaction and new bone formation are present, with Codman triangles at proximal and distal ends of tumor. Faint periosteal new bone extends perpendicularly into soft-tissue component of tumor. Medulla is not expanded. *(From Slovis TL.* Caffey's Pediatric Diagnostic Imaging. *11th ed. Philadelphia: Mosby; 2008.)*

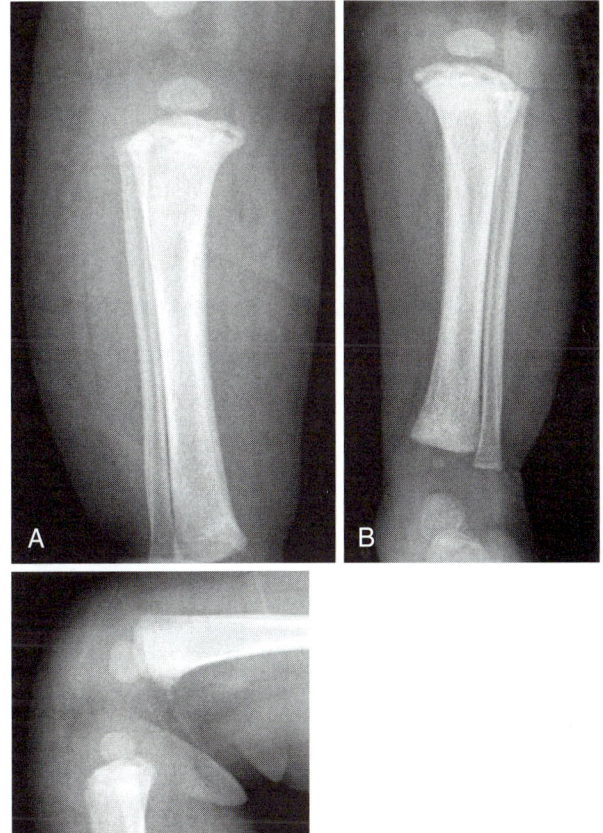

FIGURE 25.13

Anteroposterior right **(A)** and left **(B)** lower leg and lateral right **(C)** lower leg of 3-month-old male infant transferred with acute occipital skull fracture, classic metaphyseal lesions of distal femora and proximal and distal tibias, and 23 rib fractures. *(From Slovis TL. Caffey's Pediatric Diagnostic Imaging. 11th ed. Philadelphia: Mosby; 2008.)*

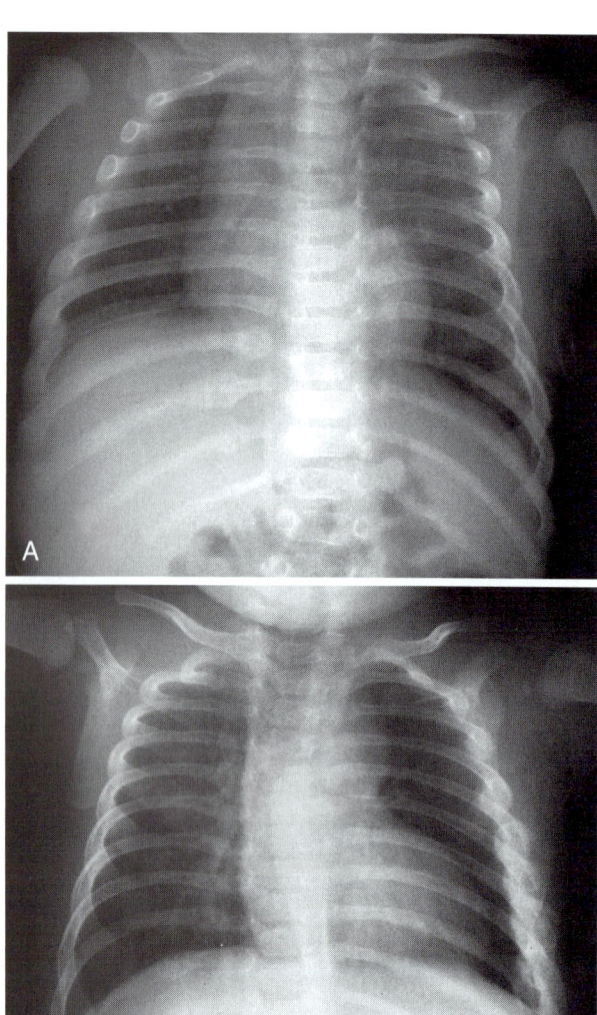

FIGURE 25.14

A 6-week-old male infant sent for an upper gastrointestinal series for evaluation of colicky pain was found to have healing rib fractures. **A,** Initial chest x-ray identifies healing fractures at the right 9th, 10th, and 11th ribs. **B,** Follow-up chest film 2 weeks later shows additional fractures, now healing, at lateral aspect of the left 3rd through 9th ribs. Father admitted to shaking the infant. *(From Slovis TL. Caffey's Pediatric Diagnostic Imaging. 11th ed. Philadelphia: Mosby; 2008.)*

REFERENCES

1. Frush DP, Donnelly LF, Rosen NS. Computed tomography and radiation risks: what pediatric health care providers should know. *Pediatrics.* 2003;112:951-957.
2. Kirks DR, Griscom NT. *Practical Pediatric Imaging: Diagnostic Radiology of Infants and Children.* 3rd ed. Philadelphia: Lippincott-Raven; 1998.
3. Orman G, Benson JE, Kweldam CF, et al. Neonatal head ultrasonography today: a powerful imaging tool. *J Neuroimaging.* 2015;25:e1-e55.
4. Iskandar BJ, Sansone JM, Medow J, et al. The use of quick-brain magnetic resonance imaging in the evaluation of shunt-treated hydrocephalus. *J Neurosurg Pediatr.* 2004;101(2):147-151.
5. Boyle TP, Paldino M, Amir A, et al. Rapid MRI versus CT for diagnosis of shunt malfunction. *AAP Grand Rounds.* 2014;134(1):47-54.
6. Pitteti R. Emergency department evaluation of shunt malfunction: is the shunt series really necessary? *Pediatr Emerg Care.* 2007;23(3):137-141.
7. Coley BD. *Caffey's Pediatric Diagnostic Imaging.* 12th ed. Philadelphia: Saunders; 2013.
8. Kuhn JP, Slovis T, Haller J. *Caffey's Pediatric Diagnostic Imaging.* 10th ed. St Louis: Mosby; 2003.
9. Donnelly LF. *Fundamentals of Pediatric Radiology.* Philadelphia: WB Saunders; 2001.
10. Slovis TL. *Caffey's Pediatric Diagnostic Imaging.* 11th ed. Philadelphia: Mosby; 2008.
11. Roberts KB. Urinary tract infection: clinical practice guidelines for the diagnosis and management of the initial UTI in febrile infants and children 2 to 24 months. *Pediatrics.* 2011;128:595-610.

Chapter 26
Rheumatology
Nayimisha Balmuri, MD

See additional content on Expert Consult

I. WEB RESOURCES
- American College of Rheumatology: http://www.rheumatology.org/

II. COMMON RHEUMATOLOGIC DISEASES

A. Arthritides

1. **Juvenile rheumatoid arthritis (JRA)**[1,2,3] **and Juvenile idiopathic arthritis (JIA)**[4]
   a. Definition of arthritis: Joint swelling or limitation/tenderness upon range of motion (ROM) lasting ≥ 6 weeks and not due to other identifiable cause.[5]
   b. Diagnosis:
      (1) Challenge of diagnosis: Children may not present with joint pain/swelling but other symptoms: morning stiffness, limp, refusal to walk, irritability, poor growth, or limb discrepancy.
      (2) Classical divisions: Based on clinical course over the first 6 months of illness in children aged <16 years, with arthritis present for at least 6 weeks.[1,2] Multiple classification systems exist; divisions used here are based on ACR classification (Table 26.1).
      NOTE: When evaluating a child with a history of chronic extremity pain (including nighttime awakenings due to pain), low white blood cell (WBC) count, and low normal platelets, consider in the differential malignancy such as acute lymphocytic leukemia (even without blasts seen on a peripheral smear). Bone marrow studies may be indicated.[6] For differential diagnosis of joint pain, see Table 26.2.
   c. Screening: Children with JIA/JRA have an increased risk of developing uveitis, which is often insidious and asymptomatic, so routine pediatric ophthalmology screening is required for children with JIA:
      (1) At diagnosis: First ophthalmologic examination should be within 1 month
      (2) Inactive disease: Frequency of examination varies based on ANA status, disease duration, and age at diagnosis[7]
      (3) Active disease: Ophthalmologic examination every 3 months, regardless of ANA status
2. **Psoriatic arthritis (PsA)**[8,9]
   a. Classification: Traditionally referred to as a *seronegative spondyloarthropathy*; ILAR classification considers PsA a subtype of JIA[5]

TABLE 26.1
CLASSICAL DIVISIONS OF JUVENILE IDIOPATHIC ARTHRITIS

	Pauciarticular	Polyarticular	Systemic-Onset
Frequency of cases	60%	30%	10%
Number of joints involved (in first 6 mo)	≤4	≥5	Variable
Age predominance	Type I: preschool age Type II: 9–11 years of age	2–5 years of age and 10–18 years of age	None
Gender ratio (female/male)	Type I: 4:1 Type II: 1:20	3:1	1:1
Involved joints	Knees and ankles	Larger joints, symmetric involvement	Any, including hips
Chronic uveitis	20% (higher with [+] ANA)	5%	Rare
Extraarticular manifestations	Uveitis	Mild fever, hepatosplenomegaly, lymphadenopathy, subcutaneous nodules	Once- to twice-daily high-spiking fevers, hepatosplenomegaly, lymphadenopathy, polyserositis, pericarditis, and characteristic macular rash
Seropositivity			
ANA	75%–85%	40%–50%	10%
RF	10% (increases with age)	75%–85%	10%
Destructive arthritis	Rare	>50%	>50%
Major morbidities	Uveitis, leg length discrepancy		Pericarditis, pleuropericarditis, secondary amyloidosis, macrophage activation syndrome*
Prognosis	Excellent apart from eyesight	Poorer prognosis with RF seropositivity and later onset	Moderate to poor

ANA, Antinuclear antibody; RF, rheumatoid factor.
*Macrophage activation syndrome (MAS) or reactive hematophagocytic lymphohistiocytosis: uncontrolled activation of T cells and macrophages, leading to rapid hepatic failure, encephalopathy, pancytopenia, purpura, mucosal bleeding, and renal failure. Paradoxically low erythrocyte sedimentation rate (ESR) with hypofibrinogenemia, elevated ferritin, and triglycerides, with disseminated intravascular coagulation (DIC).
Data from McMillan JA, Feigin RD, DeAngelis CD, et al. Oski's Pediatrics. 4th ed. Philadelphia: Lippincott Williams & Wilkins; 2006.

TABLE 26.2
DIFFERENTIAL DIAGNOSIS FOR JOINT OR EXTREMITY PAIN

Rheumatologic	JIA; SLE; juvenile dermatomyositis; polyarteritis; scleroderma; Sjögren syndrome; Behçet disease; granulomatosis with polyangiitis; sarcoidosis; HSP; chronic recurrent multifocal osteomyelitis; juvenile ankylosing spondylitis; psoriatic arthritis
Infectious	Bacterial: *Staphylococcus aureus, Streptococcus pneumoniae, Neisseria gonorrhoeae, Haemophilus influenzae* Viral: parvovirus, rubella, mumps, EBV, hepatitis B Fungal Other: spirochetes, mycobacterial, endocarditis, Lyme
Immunodeficiencies	Hypogammaglobulinemia; IgA deficiency; HIV
Congenital and metabolic	Gout and pseudogout; mucopolysaccharidoses; hypothyroidism or hyperthyroidism; vitamin C or D deficiency; connective tissue disease; lysosomal storage diseases: Fabry and Farber diseases; familial Mediterranean fever
Bone and cartilage	Trauma; patellofemoral syndrome; osteochondritis dissecans and avascular necrosis; SCFE; hypertrophic osteoarthropathy
Inflammatory and reactive	Kawasaki syndrome; IBD; acute rheumatic fever; reactive arthritis; toxic synovitis; serum sickness
Neurologic and pain syndromes	Peripheral neuropathy; carpal tunnel syndrome; Charcot joints; fibromyalgia; depression with somatization; reflex sympathetic dystrophy
Neoplastic	Leukemia and lymphoma; neuroblastoma; histiocytosis; synovial tumors Bone tumors: osteosarcoma, Ewing sarcoma, osteoid osteoma

EBV, Epstein-Barr virus; HIV, human immunodeficiency virus; HSP, Henoch-Schönlein purpura; IBD, Inflammatory bowel disease; IgA, immunoglobulin A; JIA, juvenile idiopathic arthritis; SCFE, slipped capital femoral epiphysis; SLE, systemic lupus erythematosus.
Modified from Kliegman RM, Stanton BF, St. Geme JW, et al. Nelson Textbook of Pediatrics. *19th ed. Philadelphia: Saunders Elsevier; 2011.*

---

b. History of psoriasis: Not required for diagnosis *(psoriatic arthritis sine psoriasis)*.
   (1) Patients often have a first-degree relative with psoriasis.
   (2) Patients may develop skin findings months or years after arthritis onset.
c. Presentation:
   (1) Mostly an oligoarthritis, but may be a polyarthritis or axial arthritis.
   (2) ±Sacroiliitis, inflammatory spinal pain/stiffness, synovitis, enthesitis, or dactylitis of toes or fingers (swelling beyond joint margins, producing a so-called sausage digit), especially the distal interphalangeal (DIP) joint.
   (3) Fingernails may show onycholysis or pitting.
d. Laboratory studies: No specific laboratory findings exist to suggest a diagnosis of psoriatic arthritis, although markers of inflammation (CRP, ESR) may be helpful in tracking activity of disease. RF is usually negative.

e. Radiographic findings: Blend of destruction and proliferation on plain films.
f. Prognosis: If left untreated, will result in a deforming combination of erosions and ankylosis within joints of digits.
g. Major morbidities: Chronic uveitis may develop; regular screening by an ophthalmologist recommended.

3. **Reactive arthritis**[2]
a. Definition: Diverse group of inflammatory arthritides that follow a bacterial or viral infection, particularly involving respiratory, gastrointestinal (GI), and genitourinary tracts.
b. Onset: Infection typically precedes development of arthritis by 1–4 weeks; ≈80% of cases are preceded by gastroenteritis.
c. Common precipitating organisms: *Mycoplasma, Chlamydia, Yersinia, Salmonella, Shigella, Campylobacter, Neisseria gonorrhoeae*, Epstein-Barr virus (EBV), parvovirus B19, and enteroviruses.
d. Presentation: Sometimes accompanied by constitutional signs and symptoms (fever, weight loss, fatigue), as well as dermatologic and ophthalmologic findings.
e. HLA-B27:
    (1) Strong association between HLA-B27 and susceptibility to developing reactive arthritis after an infection with a bacterial arthritogenic organism.
    (2) ≈50%–65% frequency seen in reactive arthritis.
f. Laboratory studies:
    (1) ±Evidence of systemic inflammation (leukocytosis, thrombocytosis, elevated ESR and CRP).
    (2) Autoantibodies are typically absent.
    (3) Stool cultures, serum *Chlamydia pneumoniae* and *Mycoplasma* titers, and urinary *Chlamydia* DNA probe can be helpful. Negative stool culture does not exclude diagnosis of reactive arthritis secondary to an enteric organism.
    (4) Complement-deficient patients are at risk for developing gonococcal arthritis, so complement levels should be measured in patients likely to be infected.
    (5) Consider enterovirus, EBV, and parvovirus B19 antibody titers.
    (6) Joint fluid analysis may be helpful to distinguish septic from reactive arthritis, especially in the case of *Salmonella* infection, where either a septic or reactive arthritis may develop (Fig. 26.1).
g. Prognosis: Arthritis can last weeks to months, with eventual remission or the development of recurrent episodes.

4. **Management of arthritis**
a. Pharmacologic agents[1,2,6,10]: See Formulary for dosing guidelines and Table EC 26.A for related side effects and laboratory surveillance.
    (1) Nonsteroidal antiinflammatory drugs (NSAIDs): First line (e.g., naproxen, ibuprofen).

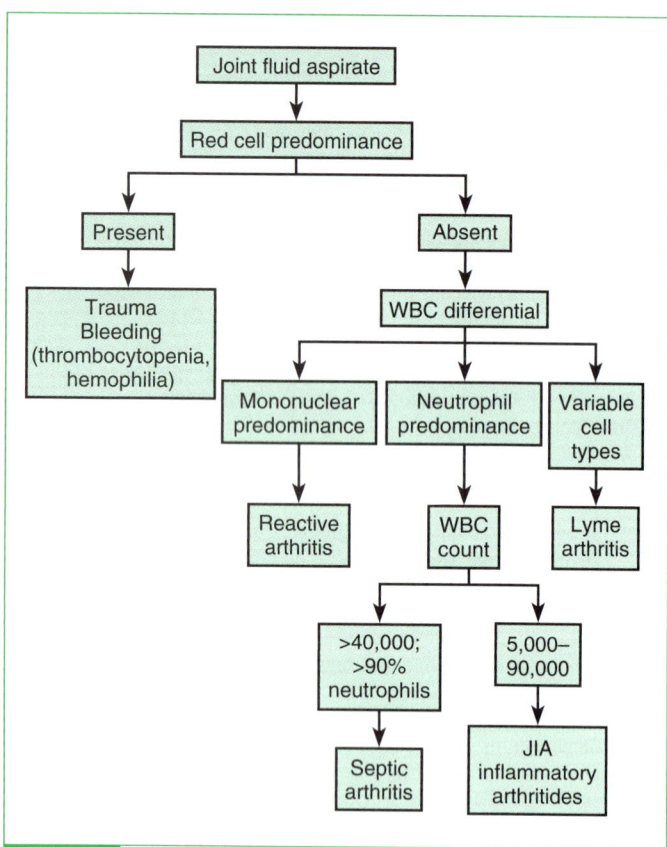

FIGURE 26.1

Joint fluid analysis algorithm. JIA, juvenile idiopathic arthritis; WBC, white blood cell. *(Data from Hay W, Levin M, Sondheimer J, et al.* Current Pediatric Diagnosis and Treatment. *17th ed. New York: Lange Medical/McGraw-Hill; 2005.)*

  (2) Disease-modifying antirheumatic drugs (DMARDs): Slow disease progression (e.g., methotrexate, sulfasalazine, hydroxychloroquine)
   (a) Biological immunomodulators: Tumor necrosis factor (TNF) inhibitors (e.g., etanercept, infliximab, adalimumab); rituximab (anti-CD20); abatacept (modulates T-cell activation); and interleukin (IL)-1 receptor antagonist (anakinra, canakinumab)
   (b) Cytotoxic and immunosuppressive drugs: Cyclosporine and mycophenolate mofetil
   (c) Corticosteroids: Can be systemic or intraarticular

b. Physical and occupational therapy: Important in maintaining joint ROM and strength of associated muscle groups, as well as decreasing pain and preventing joint deformities and contractures
c. Orthopedic surgery: Necessary in some cases for pain control, improvement in function, or contracture
5. **Health maintenance for patients with arthritis**[1,6,10-12]
a. Vaccines: Generally follow regular immunization schedule. Special considerations should be made for immunocompromised hosts (i.e., patients on biologic or immunosuppressive therapy; see Chapter 16). May have to postpone live viral vaccines.
b. Prevention or minimization of osteopenia: Adequate calcium and vitamin D intake and weight-bearing activities

B. Systemic Lupus Erythematosus (SLE)

An episodic multisystem autoimmune disease characterized by blood vessel and connective tissue inflammation. Apart from drug-induced SLE, the etiology remains unknown.

1. **American College of Rheumatology Classification Criteria** (Table 26.3)
   NOTE: These are not strict *diagnostic* criteria, but *classification* criteria for research purposes.[13,14]
2. **Diagnosis:**
a. Most often based on meeting 4 or more of the 11 classification criteria
b. Do not exclude the possibility of an SLE diagnosis for a pediatric patient who does not fully meet these criteria.
c. Majority of pediatric patients with *incomplete SLE* (<4 criteria) will likely completely fulfill these criteria in subsequent years
3. **Epidemiology:**
a. Females more commonly affected; onset usually at age 9–15 years (median age, 12 years)[13]
b. African Americans and Asian Americans more commonly affected than Caucasians[1]
4. **Laboratory studies and surveillance**[1,9]:
a. CBC with differential and direct Coombs.
b. Urinalysis and serum creatinine: See Table EC 26.B for World Health Organization (WHO) classification of SLE nephritis.[15]
c. ESR or CRP: May be increased with active disease; CRP levels may not correlate with disease activity.[16]
d. Complement levels (C3, C4): Serial levels most useful. Congenital complement deficiencies may also be seen in SLE, especially in males. Decreasing complement levels may indicate renal disease.
e. Autoantibodies (Table 26.4)
   (1) ANA: Most patients with positive ANA do not have SLE, but almost all patients with SLE have positive ANA.[17]

TABLE 26.3

1997 UPDATE OF THE 1982 AMERICAN COLLEGE OF RHEUMATOLOGY REVISED CRITERIA FOR CLASSIFICATION OF SYSTEMIC LUPUS ERYTHEMATOSUS

Criterion	
Malar rash	Fixed erythema (flat or raised) over malar eminences, tending to spare nasolabial folds; telangiectasias
Discoid rash	Erythematous raised patches with adherent keratotic scaling and follicular plugging; atrophic scarring may occur in older lesions
Photosensitivity	Rash due to unusual reaction to sunlight (by patient history or physician observation)
Oral ulcers	Oral or nasopharyngeal ulceration, usually painless, observed by physician
Nonerosive arthritis	Involving two or more peripheral joints, characterized by tenderness, swelling, or effusion
Pleuritis or pericarditis	1. Pleuritis: history of pleuritic pain or rubbing heard by physician, or evidence of pleural effusion AND/OR 2. Pericarditis: documented by electrocardiogram or rub or evidence of pericardial effusion
Renal disorder	1. Persistent proteinuria > 0.5 g/day or > 3+ if quantitation not performed AND/OR 2. Cellular casts: may be red cell, hemoglobin, granular, tubular, or mixed
Neurologic disorder	Seizures or psychosis: in the absence of offending drugs, hypertension, or known metabolic derangements
Hematologic disorder	1. Hemolytic anemia with reticulocytosis AND/OR 2. Leukopenia: < 4000/μL on ≥ two occasions AND/OR Lymphopenia: < 1500/μL on ≥ two occasions AND/OR 3. Thrombocytopenia: <100,000/μL in the absence of offending drugs
Autoimmune markers	1. Anti-DNA: antibody to native DNA in abnormal titer AND/OR 2. Anti-Smith (Sm): presence of antibody to Sm nuclear antigen
Positive antinuclear antibody	An abnormal titer of antinuclear antibody by immunofluorescence or an equivalent assay at any point in time in the absence of drugs

Data from http://www.rheumatology.org/, which was modified from Tan E, Cohen AS, Fries JF, et al. The 1982 revised criteria for the classification of systemic lupus erythematosus. Arthritis Rheum. 1982; 25: 1271-1277.

- (2) Anti-ds (double-stranded) DNA: Highly specific for SLE; seen in about 60% of patients. Titers rise/fall depending on disease activity and usually increase during development of lupus nephritis. Not associated with discoid or subacute cutaneous lupus.[17]
- (3) Anti-Sm: Highly specific for SLE; seen in ~10%–30% of patients.

TABLE 26.4
AUTOANTIBODIES ASSOCIATED WITH COMMON RHEUMATOLOGIC DISEASES

Disease Process	Associated AutoAntibodies
SLE	Anti-nuclear antibody (ANA)
	Anti-double stranded DNA
	Anti-Smith
	Anti-ribonucleoprotein (anti-RNP)
	Anti-microsomal
	Anti-phospholipids[†]
JIA*	Rheumatoid factor (RF)
	Anti–cyclic citrullinated peptide (anti-CCP)
	ANA
Vasculitis	Antineutrophil cytoplasmic antibody (ANCA)—cytoplasmic/proteinase-3 (PR3)
	ANCA—perinuclear/MPO (myeloperoxidase)
Polymyositis/Dermatomyositis	ANA
	Anti–Jo-1
Mixed connective tissue disease	ANA
	Anti-RNP
Scleroderma	ANA
	Anticentromere
	Anti-RNP
	Antitopoisomerase (anti–Scl-70)
Sjogren syndrome	ANA
	Anti-Ro
	Anti-La
Drug–induced lupus	Antihistone

*JIA is typically RF and CCP negative; when positive may indicate erosive disease.
[†]Antiphospholipids: anticardiolipin, lupus anticoagulant, and antiglycoprotein I.
Modified from Kliegman RM, Behrman RE, Jenson HB, et al. Nelson Textbook of Pediatrics. *18th ed.* Philadelphia: Saunders Elsevier; 2007.

5. **Treatment**[1]:
a. NSAIDs: Targeted to treat arthralgia and arthritis (use with caution; lupus patients more susceptible to renal toxicity with these agents).
b. Hydroxychloroquine: Treats milder manifestations (e.g., skin lesions, arthritis) and may lower lipid levels, decreasing risk for thromboembolic disease.
c. Corticosteroids: Used to treat symptoms and decrease autoantibody production.
d. Cytotoxic therapy: Reserved for more severe cases. Cyclophosphamide is used in patients with lupus nephritis, vasculitis, pulmonary hemorrhage, or central nervous system involvement.
e. DMARDs: Methotrexate, cyclosporine, mycophenolate mofetil. Biologics: Agents that target cytokine production; includes anti-CD20/22 monoclonal antibodies (i.e., rituximab).

6. **Drug-Induced SLE**[1,2]
   a. Pathogenesis:
      (1) Inciting drugs (including but not limited to): hydralazine, minocycline, ethosuximide, doxycycline, procainamide, isoniazid, chlorpromazine, phenytoin, carbamazepine
      (2) Usually resolves with discontinuation of drug
   b. Clinical and laboratory features:
      (1) Most frequent clinical manifestations are cutaneous and pleuropericardial involvement
      (2) Often associated with antihistone antibodies
7. **Neonatal SLE**[1,15]
   a. Pathogenesis: Neonates born to mothers with active SLE can develop a transient lupus-like syndrome in the perinatal period. Transplacental passage of anti-Ro (anti–SS-A) and anti-La (anti–SS-B) (also seen in Sjögren syndrome) mediate disease process. Mothers are often asymptomatic but carry antibodies and so are routinely screened for SS-A and SS-B.
   b. Clinical and laboratory features:
      (1) Thrombocytopenia, hemolytic anemia
      (2) Inflammatory features of neonatal lupus will resolve within 6 months as maternal autoantibodies are cleared
      (3) Congenital heart block (associated with anti-Ro): *Permanent* condition; usually requires pacemaker placement
      (4) Common cause of hydrops likely secondary to heart block or Coombs antibody-mediated immune anemia

C. Vasculitis

1. **General** (Table 26.5)[18]
   a. Definition: Inflammation of a blood vessel wall. Systemic vasculitis syndromes, although rare, are a concern in childhood.
   b. Clinical presentation: Variable, ranging from rash or fever of unknown origin to progressive multisystem failure[19]
   c. Initial laboratory tests: CBC, basic metabolic panel, liver function tests, acute phase reactants, stool guaiac, and complete urinalysis
   d. Diagnosis:
      (1) Small vessel vasculitis: Confirmed by biopsy. Magnetic resonance angiography (MRA) may also be helpful, but a negative test does not rule out disease.
      (2) Medium-large vessel vasculitis: MRA
2. **Henoch-Schönlein purpura**[1,2,20,21]
   a. Epidemiology:
      (1) Most common small-vessel vasculitis in children
      (2) More frequent in males than females
      (3) Typical age of onset 2–7 years
      (4) History of viral upper respiratory infection several weeks preceding onset of illness in half to two thirds of cases

TABLE 26.5
CHILDHOOD VASCULITIS SYNDROMES

Vessel Size	Vasculitis Syndrome	Clinical and Distinguishing Features
Large arteries	Takayasu arteritis	Aortic arch involvement leading to aneurysms, thrombosis, and stenosis Predominantly seen in young women Hypertension is most common sign
Aorta and large branches directed toward major body regions	Giant cell (temporal arteritis)	Granulomatous inflammation of aorta and major branches, with predilection for extracranial branches of carotid artery
Medium-sized arteries	Kawasaki disease	Arteritis including large, medium, and small arteries; associated with mucocutaneous lymph node syndrome (see Chapter 7)
Renal, hepatic, coronary, and mesenteric arteries	Polyarteritis nodosa	Cutaneous lesions include livedo reticularis, tender nodules, purpura Hypertension, renal failure, abdominal pain, intestinal infarction, and cerebrovascular accidents are common complications
Small arterioles and venules	Microscopic polyangiitis	Rare in pediatrics p-ANCA or myeloperoxidase (MPO) positive Glomerulonephritis and pulmonary capillaritis Associated with streptococcal infection or URIs
Venules, capillaries, arterioles, and intraparenchymal distal arteries	Henoch-Schönlein purpura	Most common pediatric vasculitis IgA-dominant immune deposits, palpable purpura involving buttocks and lower extremities, colicky abdominal pain, arthralgias/arthritis
	Granulomatosis with polyangiitis	Necrotizing granulomatous vasculitis of small and medium-sized vessels Presents with respiratory tract and kidney involvement c-ANCA or proteinase-3 (PR3) positive May also involve medium-sized vessels
	Churg-Strauss syndrome	Eosinophil-rich and granulomatous inflammation involving respiratory tract; associated with asthma

c–ANCA, Cytoplasmic antineutrophil cytoplasmic antibody; IgA, immunoglobulin A; p–ANCA, perinuclear antineutrophil cytoplasmic antibody; URI, upper respiratory infection
Data from Kliegman RM, Behrman, RE, Jenson HB, et al. Nelson Textbook of Pediatrics. 18th ed. Philadelphia: Saunders Elsevier; 2007; Cassidy J, Petty R. Textbook of Pediatric Rheumatology. 5th ed. Philadelphia: WB Saunders; 2005; Kim S, Dedeoglu F. Update on pediatric vasculitis. Curr Opin Pediatr. 2005;17:695-702; and Dillon M, Ozen S. A new international classification of childhood vasculitis. Pediatr Nephrol. 2006;21:1219-1222.

b. Presentation[19-21]:
   (1) Nonthrombocytopenic palpable purpura:
      (a) Most common and frequently presenting feature
      (b) Evolution of rash: Urticarial lesions progress to a maculopapular rash, followed by purpuric lesions involving ankles, buttocks, and elbows, beginning on lower extremities but can involve entire body
      (c) New lesions can appear over 2–4 weeks, leaving a mixed-stage appearance.
   (2) Migratory polyarthritis and/or polyarthralgias:
      (a) Presenting feature in 25% of cases: Very tender and painful periarticular joint swelling of ankles and knees (most often), without effusion
      (b) Joint involvement is transient with no permanent deformities.
   (3) Abdominal pain:
      (a) Colicky in nature, secondary to hemorrhage and edema of small intestine
      (b) Intussusception results in about 2% of cases (usually ileoileal)
      (c) Stool can be guaiac–positive without obvious signs of intestinal bleeding.
   (4) Glomerulonephritis:
      (a) Occurs in 20%–60% of patients; may develop months after onset or before development of rash
      (b) Renal biopsy: Typically consistent with IgA nephropathy, but crescentic glomerulonephritis may also be seen
      (c) More common in males, patients with GI bleeding, factor VIII activity <80%, and in patients aged <4 years[22]
   (5) Other features: Acute scrotal inflammation (2%–38% of male patients), dorsal edema of feet, occult pulmonary involvement
c. Diagnosis: Based on clinical characteristics[2,19,20]
d. Laboratory findings: Can help exclude other diagnoses and illuminate specific organ involvement:
   (1) Hematologic: Normal to elevated platelet count, normal platelet function tests and bleeding time, normal coagulation studies
   (2) Urinalysis: ±Proteinuria and hematuria, but casts uncommon
   (3) Antibodies: IgA levels may be elevated, especially in acute phase of disease
   (4) Stool guaiac: May be positive
   (5) Antistreptolysin O titer: May be elevated
   (6) Throat culture may be positive for group A β-hemolytic streptococcus, warranting antibiotic treatment
e. Treatment[19,20]:
   (1) Supportive care: Adequate hydration, analgesia for joint pain
   (2) Monitor vital signs because of GI bleeding and renal involvement
   (3) Serial urinalyses at routine office visits
   (4) Consider steroids, especially if GI and renal systems involved

(5) Prolonged immunosuppression may be necessary for renal disease (cyclophosphamide or azathioprine)
f. Prognosis: Typically self-limited course, but may recur in a minority (10%–20%) of cases
3. **Juvenile dermatomyositis**[1-3,23-26]
a. Pathogenesis:
   (1) Nonsuppurative vasculitis with inflammation of skin, GI tract, and striated muscle
   (2) Unlike adult-onset form, juvenile dermatomyositis is not related to malignancy
b. Epidemiology:
   (1) One study found the incidence to be 3.2 cases per million children per year; female/male ratio of 2.3:1
   (2) Peak age of onset for juvenile form is 5–14 years
c. Presentation:
   (1) Constitutional: Fever, fatigue, weight loss
   (2) Musculoskeletal: Symmetric proximal muscle pain or weakness involving shoulder and pelvic girdles
   (3) Dermatologic: **Required to diagnose dermatomyositis**. Heliotropic rash involving upper eyelids (or malar rash); Gottron papules (thickened, erythematous, scaly rash on extensor surfaces of elbows, knees, metacarpophalangeal and proximal interphalangeal joints). Dystrophic cutaneous calcifications or photosensitivity may be present.
   (4) Respiratory: Dyspnea/tachypnea may be present (restrictive lung disease due to respiratory muscle weakness), indicating more severe disease and poorer prognosis.
   (5) Other: Dysphagia, periorbital edema, nailfold or eyelid rim capillary abnormalities (dilation, aneurysms, dropout)
d. Laboratory studies:
   (1) Elevated muscle enzymes: AST, ALT, CK, LDH, and aldolase; may be normal at diagnosis.[25]
   (2) ANA may be positive; acute-phase reactants (ESR, CRP) are often normal.[24]
e. Diagnosis:
   (1) Muscle biopsy: Gold standard for definitive diagnosis.
   (2) MRI: Often used to demonstrate affected areas: T1-weighted images may show fibrosis, atrophy, and fatty infiltration; T2-weighted images may demonstrate active myositis
4. **Behçet disease**[1]:
a. Characteristics: Variable course with disease-free periods and exacerbations:
   (1) Oral ulcers: Most consistent symptom; painful, shallow, usually < 1 cm diameter, surrounded by erythema; develop on tongue, lips, buccal mucosa, and gingiva; last days to weeks and heal without scarring

(2) Genital ulcers: Similar to oral ulcers; may result in scaring; found on labia, scrotum, and penis
(3) Cutaneous pathergy: Traumatic injury (e.g., needlestick) results in development of a sterile pustule 24–48 hours later
(4) Ophthalmologic: Anterior or posterior uveitis, retinal vasculitis; more common in adults but often more severe in children; may result in blindness
(5) Arthritis: Usually recurrent, asymmetric, polyarticular, and involves large joints
(6) Other dermatologic findings: Erythema nodosum, papulopustular lesions, pseudofolliculitis, and acneiform nodules
(7) Others: GI manifestations include abdominal pain, dyspepsia, and mucosal ulcers. Neurologic include meningoencephalitis, cranial nerve palsies, and psychosis; usually occur in advanced disease. Rarely fever, orchitis, myositis, pericarditis, nephritis, splenomegaly, and amyloidosis. Increased risk for thrombophlebitis and venous thrombosis.
b. Diagnosis: Based on International Study Group criteria[27]:
(1) Recurrent oral ulcers: At least three times in a 12-month period
(2) Two or more of the following: Recurrent genital ulcers, eye lesions, other skin lesions, positive skin pathergy test
c. Treatment: Corticosteroids, colchicine, anti–TNF-α agents, chlorambucil, azathioprine, cyclosporine, tacrolimus, and interferon alfa-2a have been used. Symptomatic treatment of oral ulcers includes rinses with tetracycline, topical anesthetics, and/or chlorhexidine.

5. **Raynaud phenomenon (RP) and syndrome**[1,28,29]
a. Epidemiology[30]
(1) More common in women, younger age groups, and those with a family history of RP
(2) RP generally presents earlier in age compared to Raynaud syndrome
b. Clinical manifestation: Exaggerated vascular response to cold temperature or emotional stress manifested clinically by sudden onset sharply demarcated color changes in digits consisting of skin pallor (white attack) due to constricted blood flow, followed by cyanotic skin (blue attack), which indicates tissue hypoxia. The skin recovers, resulting in erythema of reperfusion.
(1) An attack typically begins in a single finger and then spreads to other digits symmetrically in both hands
(2) Cutaneous vasospasm is also common at other sites, including the skin of the ears, nose, face, knees, and nipples
c. Pathogenesis[28,29,31]
(1) Primary Raynaud phenomenon: Exaggeration of normal vasoconstriction to cold exposure with likely defect being an increase in alpha-2 adrenergic responses in the digital and cutaneous vessels

(2) Secondary Raynaud phenomenon or Raynaud syndrome: Clinical manifestations are secondary to another process such as:
- (a) Autoimmune rheumatic diseases including systemic sclerosis (scleroderma), systemic lupus erythematosus, mixed connective tissue disease, Sjögren syndrome and dermatomyositis/polymyositis
- (b) Various drugs or toxins such as amphetamines and chemotherapeutic agents
- (c) Hematologic abnormalities such as cryoglobulinemia, cold agglutinin disease and paraproteinemia
- (d) Occupational and environmental causes: vascular trauma, the use of vibrating tools, frostbite, and carpal tunnel syndrome
- (e) Hypothyroidism, improvement of cold induced vasospasm may occur with thyroid hormone replacement

d. Diagnosis[1,28,29]: Mostly based on physical exam and history, important to decipher between primary and secondary causes

e. Treatment: Efficacy of treatment depends upon severity of disease and presence or absence of an underlying disorder[32-34]
- (1) General measures: Maintaining body warmth, avoiding triggers, smoking cessation, avoidance of sympathomimetic medications
- (2) Behavioral therapies focusing on managing emotional stress
- (3) Initial pharmacotherapy: Calcium channel blockers for arterial vasodilation (nifedipine and diltiazem)

D. Granulomatous Disease:
See Expert Consult for information concerning granulomatous diseases

E. Other Rheumatologic Diseases:
See Expert Consult for information concerning other rheumatologic diseases.

III. LABORATORY STUDIES

Most laboratory studies used to diagnose rheumatic diseases are nonspecific, and results must be interpreted within the context of the full clinical picture. Once a diagnosis is established, however, they can be used to follow the condition's clinical course, indicating flares or remission of the rheumatic disease. Sensitivities and specificities of rheumatologic tests must be considered with any clinical decision (see Chapter 28).

A. Acute-Phase Reactants

1. **Overview:**
a. Indicate presence of inflammation when elevated
b. Elevation is nonspecific and can result from trauma, infection, rheumatic diseases, or malignancy.[1]
c. Markers include ESR, CRP, platelet count, ferritin, haptoglobin, fibrinogen, serum amyloid A, and complement.[1,2]

2. **ESR:**
   a. Measure of the rate of fall of red blood cells in anticoagulated blood within a vertical tube; reflects level of rouleaux formation caused by acute phase reactants[1]
   b. Can be falsely lowered in afibrinogenemia, anemia, and sickle cell disease; these states interfere with rouleaux formation[2]
   c. Levels vary depending on age, ethnicity, gender, and freshness of blood sample[1]
   d. Serial measurements may help in monitoring disease severity/activity in conditions such as SLE and JIA
3. **CRP**[1,41,42]:
   a. Synthesized by the liver; assists in clearance of pathologic bacteria and damaged cells via activation of complement-mediated phagocytosis; mediates acute inflammation by altering cytokine release and is thought to prevent autoimmunity by binding to and masking autoantigens
   b. Increases and decreases rapidly owing to short half-life (≈18 hours)
   c. Elevation is nonspecific, indicating only inflammation:
      (1) Most active phases of rheumatic disease result in elevation to 1–10 mg/dL
      (2) Level >10 mg/dL raises concern for bacterial infection or systemic vasculitis

B. Autoantibodies (see Table 26.4)

The positive predictive value of any autoantibody assay depends on clinical context. These studies can prove valuable in confirming clinical suspicion. However, in the absence of suspicion, they have low yield and may be misleading.

1. **Antinuclear antibody (ANA):**
   a. Nonspecific test for rheumatic disease[1]
   b. Positive in ≈60%–70% of children with an autoimmune disease, but can be seen in ≈15%–35% of normal persons
   c. If positive, consider ordering individual autoantibodies (see Table 26.4)
   d. Can be positive in nonrheumatic diseases:
      (1) Neoplasm
      (2) Infections (transiently positive): Mononucleosis, endocarditis, hepatitis, malaria
   e. If positive in pauciarticular JIA, there is increased risk of uveitis
2. **Rheumatoid factor (RF)**[1]:
   a. M antibodies to the Fc portion of IgG
   b. Positive in rheumatic and nonrheumatic diseases:
      (1) Rheumatic diseases: SLE, mixed cryoglobulinemia, JIA (rarely), mixed connective tissue disease, and Henoch-Schönlein purpura

(2) Infections: Hepatitis B, bacterial endocarditis, tuberculosis, and toxoplasmosis, other, rubella, cytomegalovirus, and herpes (TORCH) infections
c. Negative RF: Does not rule out rheumatic disease
d. Prognostic importance in polyarticular JIA: Positive RF suggests more progressive disease (see Section II)

3. **Anticyclic citrullinated peptide (anti-CCP) antibodies:**
a. Currently being explored as an RF adjunct,[10,17,43] but routine use in pediatric settings is not indicated until the full clinical significance in this population has been established
b. Although pediatric studies are scarce, anti-CCP has been shown to have a high sensitivity and specificity for adult rheumatoid arthritis
c. Anti-CCP–positive JRA patients are usually also RF–positive, as are females with late-onset polyarthritis[10]
d. Anti-CCP positivity correlates with erosive joint disease in JIA.[44]

C. Complement[1,3]

The complement system is composed of a series of plasma proteins and cellular receptors that function together to mediate host defense and inflammation. Inflammatory processes may increase complement protein synthesis or increase their consumption.

1. **Total hemolytic complement level (CH_{50}):**
a. General measure of complement; also an acute-phase reactant
b. Increased in the acute phase response of numerous inflammatory states
c. Useful screening test for homozygous complement deficiency states
d. Typically decreased in SLE

2. **C3 and C4:**
a. Most common complement proteins assayed
b. May be increased or decreased in rheumatic diseases/depending on disease stage or severity
c. Trends more instructive than isolated results

3. **Decreased levels of complement proteins:**
a. Indicator of immune complex formation:
    (1) Can occur in active SLE, some vasculitides, and multiple infections, including gram-negative sepsis, hepatitis, and pneumococcal infections
    (2) Decreased levels typically signify more severe SLE, particularly with regard to renal disease
b. Severe hepatic failure: Synthesis of complement proteins occurs primarily in the liver
c. Congenital complement deficiency, which may predispose to development of autoimmune disease

4. **Increased levels of complement proteins:**
   a. Indicates the active phase of most rheumatic diseases (e.g., SLE, JIA, dermatomyositis)
   b. May be seen in multiple infections (e.g., hepatitis, pneumococcal pneumonia) as part of the acute-phase response

D. Other Laboratory Studies

1. **Urinalysis:**
   a. Renal involvement occurs in many rheumatic diseases.
   b. Findings may include proteinuria, hematuria, or casts (see Chapter 19).
2. **Serum muscle enzymes**[2]**:**
   a. Including aspartate aminotransferase (AST), lactate dehydrogenase (LDH), aldolase, and creatine kinase (CK).
   b. Can be elevated in certain rheumatic diseases that cause muscle inflammation or destruction (e.g., dermatomyositis)
      NOTE: Patients with chronic ongoing myositis may have an elevated CK-MB fraction (noncardiac in origin) when serum CK levels are measured.
3. **Joint fluid analysis** (see Fig. 26.1)[45]**:**
   a. Important in the presence of an effusion, especially monoarticular disease
   b. Effusion can be seen in rheumatic and other disease processes (e.g., septic arthritis)

REFERENCES

1. Kliegman RM, Stanton BF, St. Geme JW, et al. *Nelson Textbook of Pediatrics*. 19th ed. Philadelphia: Elsevier; 2011.
2. Cassidy J, Petty R. *Textbook of Pediatric Rheumatology*. 5th ed. Philadelphia: Saunders; 2005.
3. Harris ED, Budd RC, Genovese MC, et al. *Kelley's Textbook of Rheumatology*. 7th ed. Philadelphia: Elsevier; 2005.
4. Prakken B, Albani S, Martini A. Juvenile idiopathic arthritis. *Lancet*. 2011;377:2138-2149.
5. Petty RE, Southwood TR, Manners P, et al. International League of Associations for Rheumatology classification of juvenile idiopathic arthritis: second revision, Edmonton; 2001. *J Rheumatol*. 2004;31: 390-392.
6. Jones OY, Spender CH, Bowyer SL, et al. A multicenter case-control study on predictive factors distinguishing childhood leukemia from juvenile rheumatoid arthritis. *Pediatrics*. 2006;117:840-844.
7. Cassidy J, Kivlin J, Lindsley C, et al. Ophthalmologic examinations in children with juvenile rheumatoid arthritis. *Pediatrics*. 2006;117:1843-1845.
8. Helliwell PS, Taylor WJ. Classification and diagnostic criteria for psoriatic arthritis. *Ann Rheum Dis*. 2005;64(Suppl 2):ii3-8.
9. Stoll ML, Zurakowski D, Nigrovic LE, et al. Patients with juvenile psoriatic arthritis comprise two distinct populations. *Arthritis Rheum*. 2006;54:3564-3572.

10. Habib HM, Mosaad YM, Youssef HM, et al. Anti-cyclic citrullinated peptide antibodies in patients with juvenile idiopathic arthritis. *Immunol Invest*. 2008;37:849-857.
11. Dell'Era L, Esposito S, Corona F. Vaccination of children and adolescents with rheumatic diseases. *Rheumatology* (Oxford). 2011;50:1358-1365.
12. Milojevic D, Ilowite N. Treatment of rheumatic diseases in children: special considerations. *Rheum Dis Clin North Am*. 2002;28:461-482.
13. Tan EM, Cohen AS, Fries JF, et al. The 1982 revised criteria for the classification of systemic lupus erythematosus. *Arthritis Rheum*. 1982;25:1271-1277.
14. Bader-Meunier B, Armengaud JB, Haddad E. Initial presentation of childhood-onset systemic lupus erythematosus: a French multicenter study. *J Pediatr*. 2005;146:648-653.
15. Petri M, Magder L. Classification criteria for systemic lupus erythematosus: a review. *Lupus*. 2004;13:829-837.
16. Williams RC, Harmon ME, Burlingame R. Studies of serum C-reactive protein in systemic lupus erythematosus. *J Rheumatol*. 2005;32:454-461.
17. Bosch X, Guilabert A, Font J. Antineutrophil cytoplasmic antibodies. *Lancet*. 2006;368:404-418.
18. Kim S, Dedeoglu F. Update on pediatric vasculitis. *Curr Opin Pediatr*. 2005;17:695-702.
19. Gross WL, Trabandt A, Reinhold-Keller T, et al. Diagnosis and evaluation of vasculitis. *Rheumatology* (Oxford). 2000;39:245-252.
20. Sundel R, Szer I. Vasculitis in childhood. *Rheum Dis Clin North Am*. 2002;28:625-654.
21. Saulsbury FT. Clinical update: Henoch-Schönlein purpura. *Lancet*. 2007;369:976-978.
22. Sano H, Izumida M, Ogawa Y, et al. Risk factors of renal involvement and significant proteinuria in Henoch-Schönlein purpura. *Eur J Pediatr*. 2002;161:196-201.
23. Mendez EP, Lipton R, Ramsey-Goldman R. US incidence of juvenile dermatomyositis, 1995-1998: results from the National Institute of Arthritis and Musculoskeletal and Skin Diseases Registry. *Arthritis Rheum*. 2003;49:300-305.
24. McCann LJ, Juggins AD, Maillard SM, et al. The Juvenile Dermatomyositis National Registry and Repository (UK and Ireland)—clinical characteristics of children recruited within the first 5 years. *Rheumatology*. 2006;45:1255-1260.
25. Ravelli A, Ruperto N, Trail L. Clinical assessment in juvenile dermatomyositis. *Autoimmunity*. 2006;39:197-203.
26. Feldman BM, Rider LG, Reed AM, et al. Juvenile dermatomyositis and other idiopathic inflammatory myopathies of childhood. *Lancet*. 2008;371:2201-2212.
27. International Study Group for Behçet's Disease. Criteria for diagnosis of Behçet's Disease. *Lancet*. 1990;335:1078-1080.
28. Linnemann B, Erbe M. Raynauds phenomenon: assessment and differential diagnoses. *Vasa*. 2015;44(3):166-177.
29. Boin F, Wigley FM. Understanding, assessing and treating Raynaud's phenomenon. *Curr Opin Rheumatol*. 2005;17:752-760.
30. Suter LG, Murabito JM, Felson DT, et al. The incidence and natural history of Raynaud's phenomenon in the community. *Arthritis Rheum*. 2005;52:1259-1263.

31. LeRoy EC, Medsger TA Jr. Raynaud's phenomenon: a proposal for classification. *Clin Exp Rheumatol.* 1992;10:485-488.
32. Thompson AE, Shea B, Welch V, et al. Calcium-channel blockers for Raynaud's phenomenon in systemic sclerosis. *Arthritis Rheum.* 2001;44:1841-1847.
33. Herrick AL. Contemporary management of Raynaud's phenomenon and digital ischaemic complications. *Curr Opin Rheumatol.* 2011;23:555-561.
34. Wigley FM. Clinical practice: Raynaud's Phenomenon. *N Engl J Med.* 2002;347:1001-1008.
35. Frosch M, Foell D. Wegener granulomatosis in childhood and adolescence. *Eur J Pediatr.* 2004;163:425-434.
36. Iannuzzi MC, Rybicki BA, Teirstein AS. Sarcoidosis. *N Engl J Med.* 2007;357:2153-2165.
37. Lindsley CB, Petty RE. Overview and report on international registry of sarcoid arthritis in children. *Curr Rheumatol Rep.* 2000;2:343-348.
38. Baumann R, Robertson W. Neurosarcoid presents differently in children than in adults. *Pediatrics.* 2003;112:e480-e486.
39. Nowak D, Widenka D. Neurosarcoidosis: a review of its intracranial manifestation. *J Neurol.* 2001;248:363-372.
40. McMillan JA, Feigin RD, DeAngelis CD, et al. *Oski's Pediatrics.* 4th ed. Philadelphia: Lippincott Williams & Wilkins; 2006.
41. Marnell L, Mold C, Du Clos TW, et al. C-reactive protein: ligands, receptors and role in inflammation. *Clin Immunol.* 2005;117:104-111.
42. Rhodes B, Fürnrohr B, Vyse T. C-reactive protein in rheumatology: biology and genetics. *Nat Rev Rheumatol.* 2011;7:282-289.
43. van Venrooij W, Zendman AJ. Anti-CCP2 antibodies: an overview and perspective of the diagnostic abilities of this serological marker for early rheumatoid arthritis. *Clin Rev Allergy Immunol.* 2008;34:36-39.
44. Gupta R, Thabah MM, Vaidya B. Anti-cyclic citrullinated peptide antibodies in juvenile idiopathic arthritis. *Indian J Pediatr.* 2010;77:41-44.
45. Hay W, Levin M, Sondheimer J, et al. *Current Pediatric Diagnosis and Treatment.* 17th ed. New York: Lange Medical/McGraw-Hill; 2007.

PART III

REFERENCE

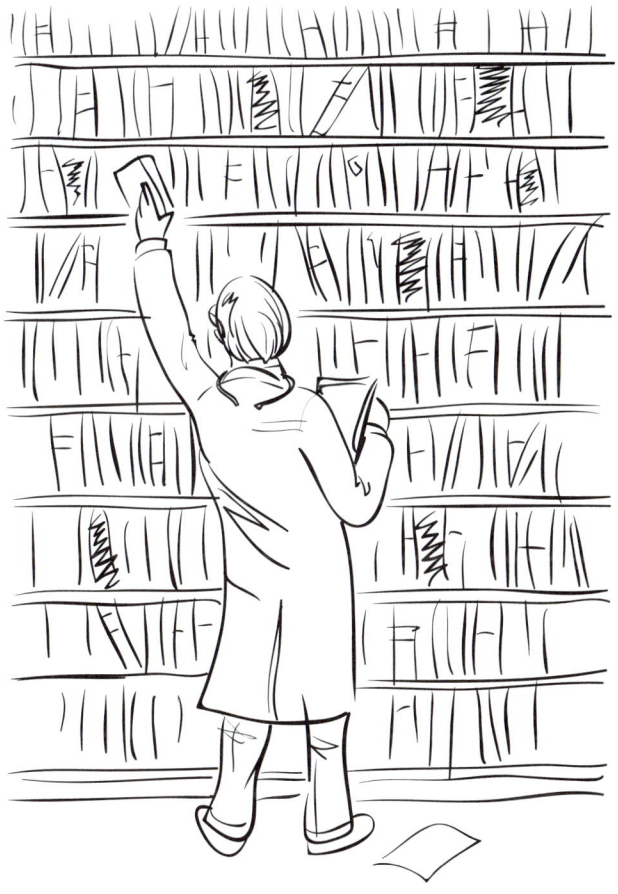

Chapter 27
Blood Chemistries and Body Fluids

Helen K. Hughes, MD, MPH, and Lauren K. Kahl, MD

Determining normal reference ranges of laboratory studies in pediatric patients poses some major challenges. Available literature is often limited because of the small sample sizes of patients in many studies that have been used to derive these suggested normal ranges. **Please use great caution and be aware of this limitation when interpreting pediatric laboratory studies.**

The following values have been compiled from both published literature and the Johns Hopkins Hospital Department of Pathology. Normal values vary with the analytic method used. Consult your laboratory for its analytic method and range of normal values, and for less commonly used parameters which are beyond the scope of this text. Additional normal laboratory values may be found in Chapters 10, 14, and 15.

A special thanks to Lori Sokoll, PhD, and Allison Chambliss, PhD, for their guidance in preparing this chapter.

I. REFERENCE VALUES (Table 27.1)

II. EVALUATION OF BODY FLUIDS

A. Evaluation of Transudate Versus Exudate (Table 27.2)

B. Evaluation of Cerebrospinal Fluid (Table 27.3)

C. Evaluation of Synovial Fluid (Table 27.4)

III. CONVERSION FORMULAS

A. Temperature

1. **To convert degrees Celsius to degrees Fahrenheit:**

$$([9/5] \times \text{Temperature}) + 32$$

2. **To convert degrees Fahrenheit to degrees Celsius:**

$$(\text{Temperature} - 32) \times (5/9)$$

B. Length and Weight

1. **Length:** To convert inches to centimeters, multiply by 2.54
2. **Weight:** To convert pounds to kilograms, divide by 2.2

TABLE 27.1
REFERENCE VALUES

	Conventional Units	SI Units
ALANINE AMINOTRANSFERASE (ALT)[1,2]*		
(Major sources: Liver, skeletal muscle, and myocardium)		
Infant aged <12 mo	13–45 U/L	13–45 U/L
1–3 yr	5–45 U/L	5–45 U/L
4–6 yr	10–25 U/L	10–25 U/L
7–9 yr	10–35 U/L	10–35 U/L
10–11 yr		
Female	10–30 U/L	10–30 U/L
Male	10–35 U/L	10–35 U/L
12–13 yr		
Female	10–30 U/L	10–30 U/L
Male	10–55 U/L	10–55 U/L
14–15 yr		
Female	5–30 U/L	5–30 U/L
Male	10–45 U/L	10–45 U/L
>16 yr		
Female	5–35 U/L	5–35 U/L
Male	10–40 U/L	10–40 U/L
ALBUMIN		
(See Proteins)		
ALDOLASE[3]		
(Major sources: Skeletal muscle and myocardium)		
10–24 mo	3.4–11.8 U/L	3.4–11.8 U/L
2–16 yr	1.2–8.8 U/L	1.2–8.8 U/L
Adult	1.7–4.9 U/L	1.7–4.9 U/L
ALKALINE PHOSPHATASE[4]		
(Major sources: Liver, bone, intestinal mucosa, placenta, and kidney)		
Infant	150–420 U/L	150–420 U/L
2–10 yr	100–320 U/L	100–320 U/L
Adolescent male	100–390 U/L	100–390 U/L
Adolescent female	100–320 U/L	100–320 U/L
Adult	30–120 U/L	30–120 U/L
AMMONIA[2]		
(Heparinized venous specimens on ice, analyzed within 30 min)		
Newborn	90–150 mcg/dL	64–107 µmol/L
0–2 wk	79–129 mcg/dL	56–92 µmol/L
Infant/child	29–70 mcg/dL	21–50 µmol/L
Adult	15–45 mcg/dL	11–32 µmol/L
AMYLASE[5]		
(Major sources: Pancreas, salivary glands, and ovaries)		
0–14 days	3–10 U/L	3–10 U/L
15 days–13 wk	2–22 U/L	2–22 U/L
13 wk–1 yr	3–50 U/L	3–50 U/L
>1 yr	25–101 U/L	25–101 U/L

Continued

TABLE 27.1
REFERENCE VALUES—cont'd

	Conventional Units	SI Units
ANTINUCLEAR ANTIBODY (ANA)[2] IMMUNOFLUORESCENCE ASSAY (IFA)		
Negative	<1:40	
Patterns with clinical correlation:		
Centromere: CREST[†]		
Nucleolar: Scleroderma		
Homogeneous: Systemic lupus erythematosus		
ANTISTREPTOLYSIN O TITER[6]		
(Fourfold rise in paired serial specimens is significant.)		
Newborn	Similar to mother's value	
6–24 mo	≤50 Todd units/mL	
2–4 yr	≤160 Todd units/mL	
≥5 yr	≤330 Todd units/mL	
ASPARTATE AMINOTRANSFERASE (AST)[2]		
(Major sources: Liver, skeletal muscle, kidney, myocardium, and erythrocytes)		
0–10 days	47–150 U/L	47–150 U/L
10 days–24 mo	9–80 U/L	9–80 U/L
>24 mo		
Female	13–35 U/L	13–35 U/L
Male	15–40 U/L	15–40 U/L
BICARBONATE[2,4]		
Newborn	17–24 mEq/L	17–24 mmol/L
Infant	19–24 mEq/L	19–24 mmol/L
2 mo–2 yr	16–24 mEq/L	16–24 mmol/L
>2 yr	22–26 mEq/L	22–26 mmol/L
BILIRUBIN (TOTAL)[4,7]		
Please see Chapter 18 for more complete information about neonatal hyperbilirubinemia and acceptable bilirubin values.		
Cord:		
Term and preterm	<2 mg/dL	<34 µmol/L
0–1 days:		
Term and preterm	<8 mg/dL	<137 µmol/L
1–2 days:		
Preterm	<12 mg/dL	<205 µmol/L
Term	<11.5 mg/dL	<197 µmol/L
3–5 days:		
Preterm	<16 mg/dL	<274 µmol/L
Term	<12 mg/dL	<205 µmol/L
Older infant:		
Preterm	<2 mg/dL	<34 µmol/L
Term	<1.2 mg/dL	<21 µmol/L
Adult	<1.5 mg/dL	<20.5 µmol/L
BILIRUBIN (CONJUGATED)[2,4]		
Neonate	<0.6 mg/dL	<10 µmol/L
Infants/children	<0.2 mg/dL	<3.4 µmol/L

TABLE 27.1
REFERENCE VALUES—cont'd

BLOOD GAS, ARTERIAL (BREATHING ROOM AIR)[2]

	pH	Pao_2 (mmHg)	$Paco_2$ (mmHg)	HCO_3^- (mEq/L)
Cord blood	7.28 ± 0.05	18.0 ± 6.2	49.2 ± 8.4	14–22
Newborn (birth)	7.11–7.36	8–24	27–40	13–22
5–10 min	7.09–7.30	33–75	27–40	13–22
30 min	7.21–7.38	31–85	27–40	13–22
60 min	7.26–7.49	55–80	27–40	13–22
1 day	7.29–7.45	54–95	27–40	13–22
Child/adult	7.35–7.45	83–108	32–48	20–28

NOTE: Venous blood gases can be used to assess acid-base status, not oxygenation. Pco_2 averages 6–8 mm Hg higher than $Paco_2$, and pH is slightly lower. Peripheral venous samples are strongly affected by the local circulatory and metabolic environment. Capillary blood gases correlate best with arterial pH and moderately well with $Paco_2$.

	Conventional Units	SI Units
C-REACTIVE PROTEIN[4]	0–0.5 mg/dL	
CALCIUM (TOTAL)[2]		
Premature neonate	6.2–11 mg/dL	1.55–2.75 mmol/L
0–10 days	7.6–10.4 mg/dL	1.9–2.6 mmol/L
10 days–24 mo	9–11 mg/dL	2.25–2.75 mmol/L
24 mo–12 yr	8.8–10.8 mg/dL	2.2–2.7 mmol/L
12–18 yr	8.4–10.2 mg/dL	2.1–2.55 mmol/L
CALCIUM (IONIZED)[3]		
0–1 mo	3.9–6.0 mg/dL	1.0–1.5 mmol/L
1–6 mo	3.7–5.9 mg/dL	0.95–1.5 mmol/L
1–18 yr	4.9–5.5 mg/dL	1.22–1.37 mmol/L
Adult	4.75–5.3 mg/dL	1.18–1.32 mmol/L
CARBON DIOXIDE (CO_2 CONTENT)[2]		
(See Blood Gas, Arterial)		
CARBON MONOXIDE (CARBOXYHEMOGLOBIN)		
Nonsmoker	0.5%–1.5% of total hemoglobin	
Smoker	4%–9% of total hemoglobin	
Toxic	20%–50% of total hemoglobin	
Lethal	>50% of total hemoglobin	

	Conventional Units	SI Units
CHLORIDE (SERUM)[3]		
0–6 mo	97–108 mEq/L	97–108 mmol/L
6–12 mo	97–106 mEq/L	97–106 mmol/L
Child/adult	97–107 mEq/L	97–107 mmol/L
CHOLESTEROL		
(See Lipids)		
CREATINE KINASE (CREATINE PHOSPHOKINASE)[2]		
(Major sources: Myocardium, skeletal muscle, smooth muscle, and brain)		
Newborn	145–1578 U/L	145–1578 U/L
>6 wk–adult male	20–200 U/L	20–200 U/L
>6 wk–adult female	20–180 U/L	20–180 U/L

Continued

TABLE 27.1
REFERENCE VALUES—cont'd

	Conventional Units	SI Units
CREATININE (SERUM)[2] (ENZYMATIC)		
Cord	0.6–1.2 mg/dL	53–106 μmol/L
Newborn	0.3–1.0 mg/dL	27–88 μmol/L
Infant	0.2–0.4 mg/dL	18–35 μmol/L
Child	0.3–0.7 mg/dL	27–62 μmol/L
Adolescent	0.5–1.0 mg/dL	44–88 μmol/L
Adult male	0.9–1.3 mg/dL	80–115 μmol/L
Adult female	0.6–1.1 mg/dL	53–97 μmol/L
ERYTHROCYTE SEDIMENTATION RATE (ESR)[2]		
Child	0–10 mm/hr	
Adult male	0–15 mm/hr	
Adult female	0–20 mm/hr	
FERRITIN[2]		
Newborn	25–200 ng/mL	56–450 pmol/L
1 mo	200–600 ng/mL	450–1350 pmol/L
2–5 mo	50–200 ng/mL	112–450 pmol/L
6 mo–15 yr	7–140 ng/mL	16–315 pmol/L
Adult male	20–250 ng/mL	45–562 pmol/L
Adult female	10–120 ng/mL	22–270 pmol/L
FIBRINOGEN		
See Chapter 14.		
FOLATE (SERUM)[3]		
Newborn	16–72 ng/mL	16–72 nmol/L
Child	4–20 ng/mL	4–20 nmol/L
Adult	10–63 ng/mL	10–63 nmol/L
FOLATE (RBC)[2]		
Newborn	150–200 ng/mL	340–453 nmol/L
Infant	74–995 ng/mL	168–2254 nmol/L
2–16 yr	>160 ng/mL	>362 nmol/L
>16 yr	140–628 ng/mL	317–1422 nmol/L
GALACTOSE[2]		
Newborn	0–20 mg/dL	0–1.11 mmol/L
Older child	<5 mg/dL	<0.28 mmol/L
GAMMA-GLUTAMYL TRANSFERASE (GGT)[2,6]		
[Major sources: Liver (biliary tree) and kidney]		
Cord	37–193 U/L	37–193 U/L
0–1 mo	13–147 U/L	13–147 U/L
1–2 mo	12–123 U/L	12–123 U/L
2–4 mo	8–90 U/L	8–90 U/L
4 mo–10 yr	5–32 U/L	5–32 U/L
10–15 yr	5–24 U/L	5–24 U/L
Adult male	11–49 U/L	11–49 U/L
Adult female	7–32 U/L	7–32 U/L

TABLE 27.1
REFERENCE VALUES—cont'd

	Conventional Units	SI Units
GLUCOSE (SERUM)[2,6]		
Preterm	20–60 mg/dL	1.1–3.3 mmol/L
Newborn, <1 day	40–60 mg/dL	2.2–3.3 mmol/L
Newborn, >1 day	50–90 mg/dL	2.8–5.0 mmol/L
Child	60–100 mg/dL	3.3–5.5 mmol/L
>16 yr	70–105 mg/dL	3.9–5.8 mmol/L
HAPTOGLOBIN[2]		
Newborn	5–48 mg/dL	50–480 mg/L
>30 days	26–185 mg/dL	260–1850 mg/L
HEMOGLOBIN A_{1c}[8]		
Normal	4.5%–5.6%	
At risk for diabetes	5.7%–6.4%	
Diabetes mellitus	≥6.5%	
HEMOGLOBIN F, % TOTAL HEMOGLOBIN [MEAN (SD)][2]		
1 day	77.0 (7.3)	
5 days	76.8 (5.8)	
3 wk	70.0 (7.3)	
6–9 wk	52.9 (11)	
3–4 mo	23.2 (16)	
6 mo	4.7 (2.2)	
8–11 mo	1.6 (1.0)	
Adult	<2.0	

	Conventional Units	SI Units
IRON[2]		
Newborn	100–250 mcg/dL	17.9–44.8 μmol/L
Infant	40–100 mcg/dL	7.2–17.9 μmol/L
Child	50–120 mcg/dL	9.0–21.5 μmol/L
Adult male	65–175 mcg/dL	11.6–31.3 μmol/L
Adult female	50–170 mcg/dL	9.0–30.4 μmol/L
LACTATE[2,3]		
Capillary blood:		
0–90 days	9–32 mg/dL	1.1–3.5 mmol/L
3–24 mo	9–30 mg/dL	1.0–3.3 mmol/L
2–18 yr	9–22 mg/dL	1.0–2.4 mmol/L
Venous	4.5–19.8 mg/dL	0.5–2.2 mmol/L
Arterial	4.5–14.4 mg/dL	0.5–1.6 mmol/L
LACTATE DEHYDROGENASE (AT 37°C)[2]		
(Major sources: Myocardium, liver, skeletal muscle, erythrocytes, platelets, and lymph nodes)		
0–4 days	290–775 U/L	290–775 U/L
4–10 days	545–2000 U/L	545–2000 U/L
10 days–24 mo	180–430 U/L	180–430 U/L
24 mo–12 yr	110–295 U/L	110–295 U/L
>12 yr	100–190 U/L	100–190 U/L

Continued

TABLE 27.1
REFERENCE VALUES—cont'd

	Conventional Units	SI Units
LEAD[9]		
Child	<5 mcg/dL	<0.24 µmol/L
LIPASE[3]		
0–30 days	6–55 U/L	6–55 U/L
1–6 mo	4–29 U/L	4–29 U/L
6–12 mo	4–23 U/L	4–23 U/L
>1 yr	3–32 U/L	3–32 U/L

	Cholesterol (mg/dL)			LDL (mg/dL)				HDL (mg/dL)
	Desirable	Borderline	High	Optimal	Near/Above Optimal	Borderline	High	Desirable
LIPIDS[10,11]								
Child/adolescent	<170	170–199	>200	<110	-	110–129	≥130	>35
Adult	<200	200–239	≥240	<100	100–129	130–159	≥160	40–60

	Conventional Units	SI Units
MAGNESIUM[2]	1.6–2.4 mg/dL	0.63–1.05 mmol/L
METHEMOGLOBIN[2]	0.78% (±0.37%) of total hemoglobin	
OSMOLALITY[2]	275–295 mOsm/kg (neonates as low as 266)	275–295 mmol/kg
PHENYLALANINE[2]		
Preterm	2.0–7.5 mg/dL	121–454 µmol/L
Newborn	1.2–3.4 mg/dL	73–206 µmol/L
Adult	0.8–1.8 mg/dL	48–109 µmol/L
PHOSPHORUS[2]		
0–9 days	4.5–9.0 mg/dL	1.45–2.91 mmol/L
10 days–24 mo	4–6.5 mg/dL	1.29–2.10 mmol/L
3–9 yr	3.2–5.8 mg/dL	1.03–1.87 mmol/L
10–15 yr	3.3–5.4 mg/dL	1.07–1.74 mmol/L
>15 yr	2.4–4.4 mg/dL	0.78–1.42 mmol/L
PORCELAIN[12]	0.930–6.0 mg/dL	1.2–10.15 mmol/L
POTASSIUM[2]		
Preterm	3.0–6.0 mEq/L	3.0–6.0 mmol/L
Newborn	3.7–5.9 mEq/L	3.7–5.9 mmol/L
Infant	4.1–5.3 mEq/L	4.1–5.3 mmol/L
Child	3.4–4.7 mEq/L	3.4–4.7 mmol/L
Adult	3.5–5.1 mEq/L	3.5–5.1 mmol/L
PREALBUMIN[3]		
Newborn	7–39 mg/dL	
1–6 mo	8–34 mg/dL	
6 mo–4 yr	12–36 mg/dL	
4–6 yr	12–30 mg/dL	
6–19 yr	12–42 mg/dL	

TABLE 27.1
REFERENCE VALUES—cont'd

PROTEIN ELECTROPHORESIS (g/dL)[2]

Age	Total Protein	Albumin	α-1	α-2	β	γ
Cord	4.8–8.0					
Premature	3.6–6.0					
Newborn	4.6–7.0					
0–15 day	4.4–7.6	3.0–3.9	0.1–0.3	0.3–0.6	0.4–0.6	0.7–1.4
15 day–1 yr	5.1–7.3	2.2–4.8	0.1–0.3	0.5–0.9	0.5–0.9	0.5–1.3
1–2 yr	5.6–7.5	3.6–5.2	0.1–0.4	0.5–1.2	0.5–1.1	0.5–1.7
3–16 yr	6.0–8.0	3.6–5.2	0.1–0.4	0.5–1.2	0.5–1.1	0.5–1.7
≥16 yr	6.0–8.3	3.9–5.1	0.2–0.4	0.4–0.8	0.5–1.0	0.6–1.2

	Conventional Units	SI Units
PYRUVATE[3]	0.7–1.32 mg/dL	0.08–0.15 mmol/L
RHEUMATOID FACTOR[2]	<30 U/mL	
SODIUM[1]		
<1 yr	130–145 mEq/L	130–145 mmol/L
>1 yr	135–147 mEq/L	135–147 mmol/L
TOTAL IRON-BINDING CAPACITY (TIBC)[2]		
Infant	100–400 mcg/dL	17.9–71.6 μmol/L
Adult	250–425 mcg/dL	44.8–76.1 μmol/L
TOTAL PROTEIN		
(See Proteins)		
TRANSAMINASE (SGOT)		
[See Aspartate aminotransferase (AST)]		
TRANSAMINASE (SGPT)		
[See Alanine aminotransferase (ALT)]		
TRANSFERRIN[2]		
Newborn	130–275 mg/dL	1.30–2.75 g/L
3 mo–16 yr	203–360 mg/dL	2.03–3.6 g/L
Adult	215–380 mg/dL	2.15–3.8 g/L

TOTAL TRIGLYCERIDE[3]

	Conventional Units (mg/dL)		SI Units (mmol/L)	
	Male	Female	Male	Female
0–7 days	21–182	28–166	0.24–2.06	0.32–1.88
8–30 days	30–184	30–165	0.34–2.08	0.34–1.86
31–90 days	40–175	35–282	0.45–1.98	0.4–3.19
91–180 days	45–291	50–355	0.51–3.29	0.57–4.01
181–365 days	45–501	36–431	0.51–5.66	0.41–4.87
1–3 yr	27–125	27–125	0.31–1.41	0.31–1.41
4–6 yr	32–116	32–116	0.36–1.31	0.36–1.31
7–9 yr	28–129	28–129	0.32–1.46	0.32–1.46
10–19 yr	24–145	37–140	0.27–1.64	0.42–1.58

Continued

TABLE 27.1
REFERENCE VALUES—cont'd

	Conventional Units	SI Units
UREA NITROGEN[1,2]		
Premature (<1 wk)	3–25 mg/dL	1.1–8.9 mmol/L
Newborn	2–19 mg/dL	0.7–6.7 mmol/L
Infant/child	5–18 mg/dL	1.8–6.4 mmol/L
Adult	6–20 mg/dL	2.1–7.1 mmol/L
URIC ACID[3,6]		
0–30 days	1.0–4.6 mg/dL	0.059–0.271 mmol/L
1–12 mo	1.1–5.6 mg/dL	0.065–0.33 mmol/L
1–5 yr	1.7–5.8 mg/dL	0.1–0.35 mmol/L
6–11 yr	2.2–6.6 mg/dL	0.13–0.39 mmol/L
Male 12–19 yr	3.0–7.7 mg/dL	0.18–0.46 mmol/L
Female 12–19 yr	2.7–5.7 mg/dL	0.16–0.34 mmol/L
VITAMIN A (RETINOL)[2,3]		
Preterm	13–46 mcg/dL	0.46–1.61 µmol/L
Full term	18–50 mcg/dL	0.63–1.75 µmol/L
1–6 yr	20–43 mcg/dL	0.7–1.5 µmol/L
7–12 yr	20–49 mcg/dL	0.9–1.7 µmol/L
13–19 yr	26–72 mcg/dL	0.9–2.5 µmol/L
VITAMIN B_1 (THIAMINE)[2]	4.5–10.3 mcg/dL	106–242 µmol/L
VITAMIN B_2 (RIBOFLAVIN)	4–24 mcg/dL	106–638 nmol/L
VITAMIN B_{12} (COBALAMIN)[2]		
Newborn	160–1300 pg/mL	118–959 pmol/L
Child/adult	200–835 pg/mL	148–616 pmol/L
VITAMIN C (ASCORBIC ACID)[2]	0.4–2.0 mg/dL	23–114 µmol/L
VITAMIN D (1,25-DIHYDROXY-VITAMIN D)[2]	16–65 pg/mL	42–169 pmol/L
VITAMIN D (25-HYDROXY-VITAMIN D)[13,14]		
Deficiency‡	<12 ng/mL	<30 mmol/L
Insufficiency‡	12–20 ng/mL	30–50 mmol/L
Sufficient‡	≥20 ng/mL	≥50 mmol/L
VITAMIN E[1-3]		
Preterm	0.5–3.5 mg/L	1–8 µmol/L
Full term	1.0–3.5 mg/L	2–8 µmol/L
1–12 yr	3.0–9.0 mg/L	7–21 µmol/L
13–19 yr	6.0–10.0 mg/L	14–23 µmol/L
ZINC[2]	70–120 mcg/dL	10.7–18.4 mmol/L

*There is evidence to suggest that these cutoffs may not be sensitive enough to detect pediatric chronic liver disease.[15]
†CREST: **C**alcinosis, **R**aynaud syndrome, **E**sophageal dysmotility, **S**clerodactyly, **T**elangiectasia.
‡Controversy exists regarding optimal 25-hydroxyvitamin D level. Some experts recommend a level ≥30 ng/mL as sufficient.[16]

TABLE 27.2
EVALUATION OF TRANSUDATE VS. EXUDATE (PLEURAL, PERICARDIAL, OR PERITONEAL FLUID)

Measurement*	Transudate	Exudate[†]
Protein (g/dL)	<3.0	>3.0
Fluid/serum ratio	<0.5	≥0.5
LDH (IU)	<200	≥200
Fluid/serum ratio (isoenzymes not useful)	<0.6	≥0.6
WBCs[‡]	<10,000/μL	>10,000/μL
RBCs	<5000	>5000
Glucose	>40	<40
pH[§]	>7.2	<7.2

NOTE: Amylase > 5000 U/mL or pleural fluid/serum ratio >1 suggests pancreatitis.
LDH, Lactate dehydrogenase; RBCs, red blood cells; WBCs, white blood cells.
*Always obtain serum for glucose, LDH, protein, amylase, etc.
[†]All of the following criteria do not have to be met for consideration as an exudate.
[‡]In peritoneal fluid, WBC count >800/μL suggests peritonitis.
[§]Collect anaerobically in a heparinized syringe.
Data from Nichols DG, Ackerman AD, Carcillo JA, et al. Rogers Textbook of Pediatric Intensive Care. 4th ed. Baltimore: Williams & Wilkins; 2008.

TABLE 27.3
EVALUATION OF CEREBROSPINAL FLUID

Age[4,17]	WBC Count/μL (median)	95th Percentile
0–28 days	0–12*(3)	19
29–56 days	0–6* (2)	9
Child	0–7	

	Conventional Units	SI Units
GLUCOSE[4,18]		
Preterm	24–63 mg/dL	1.3–3.5 mmol/L
Term	34–119 mg/dL	1.9–6.6 mmol/L
Child	40–80 mg/dL	2.2–4.4 mmol/L
PROTEIN[4,18,19]		
Preterm	65–150 mg/dL	0.65–1.5 g/L
0–14 days	79 (±23) mg/dL[†]	0.79 (±0.23) g/L[†]
15–28 days	69 (±20) mg/dL[†]	0.69 (±0.20) g/L[†]
29–42 days	58 (±17) mg/dL[†]	0.58 (±0.17) g/L[†]
43–56 days	53 (±17) mg/dL[†]	0.53 (±0.17) g/L[†]
Child	5–40 mg/dL	5–40 mg/dL
OPENING PRESSURE (LATERAL RECUMBENT POSITION)[4,20]		
Newborn	8–11 cm H$_2$O	
1–18 yr	11.5–28 cm H$_2$O*	
Respiratory variations	0.5–1 cm H$_2$O	

*Up to 90th percentile.
[†]Mean (±SD).
WBC, White blood cell.

TABLE 27.4
CHARACTERISTICS OF SYNOVIAL FLUID IN THE RHEUMATIC DISEASES

Group	Condition	Synovial Complement	Color/Clarity	Viscosity	Mucin Clot	WBC Count	PMN (%)	Miscellaneous Findings
Noninflammatory	Normal	N	Yellow Clear	↑↑	G	<200	<25	
	Traumatic arthritis	N	Xanthochromic Turbid	↑	F–G	<2000	<25	Debris
	Osteoarthritis	N	Yellow Clear	↑	F–G	1000	<25	
Inflammatory	Systemic lupus erythematosus	↓	Yellow Clear	N	N	5000	10	Lupus cells
	Rheumatic fever	N–↑	Yellow Cloudy	↓	F	5000	10–50	
	Juvenile rheumatoid arthritis	N–↓	Yellow Cloudy	↓	Poor	15,000–20,000	75	
	Reactive arthritis	↑	Yellow Opaque	↓	Poor	20,000	80	
Pyogenic	Tuberculous arthritis	N–↑	Yellow-white Cloudy	↓	Poor	25,000	50–60	Acid-fast bacteria
	Septic arthritis	↑	Serosanguineous Turbid	↓	Poor	50,000–300,000	>75	Low glucose, bacteria

F, Fair; G, good; H, high; N, normal; PMN, polymorphonuclear leukocyte; WBC, white blood cell; ↓, decreased; ↑, increased.
From Cassidy JT, Petty RE. Textbook of Pediatric Rheumatology. 5th ed. Philadelphia: WB Saunders; 2005.

REFERENCES

1. Meites S, ed. *Pediatric Clinical Chemistry*. 3rd ed. Washington, DC: American Association for Clinical Chemistry; 1989.
2. Wu Alan HB. *Tietz Guide to Laboratory Tests*. 4th ed. Philadelphia: WB Saunders; 2006.
3. Soldin SJ, Brugnara C, Wong EC. *Pediatric Reference Intervals*. 6th ed. Washington, DC: Americal Association for Clinical Chemistry Press; 2007.
4. McMillan JA. *Oski's Pediatrics: Principles and Practice*. 4th ed. Philadelphia: JB Lippincott; 2006.
5. Colantonio DA, Kyriakopoulou L, Chan MK, et al. Closing the gaps in pediatric laboratory reference intervals: a CALIPER database of 40 biochemical markers in a healthy and multiethnic population of children. *Clin Chem*. 2012;58:854-868.
6. Kleigman RM, Behrman RE, Jenson HB, et al. *Nelson Textbook of Pediatrics*. 18th ed. Philadelphia: WB Saunders; 2007.
7. Chernecky CC, Berger BJ. *Laboratory Tests and Diagnostic Procedures*. 5th ed. St Louis: Elsevier; 2008.
8. American Diabetes Association. Classification and Diagnosis of Diabetes. *Diabetes Care*. 2016;39:S3-S22.
9. National Center for Environmental Health. Division of Emergency and Environmental Health Services. CDC—Lead—New Blood Lead Level Information. <https://www.cdc.gov/nceh/lead/acclpp/blood_lead_levels.htm>. Accessed November 21, 2016.
10. National Cholesterol Education Program (NCEP). Highlights of the report of the Expert Panel on Blood Cholesterol Levels in Children and Adolescents. NCEP Expert Panel on Blood Cholesterol Levels in Children and Adolescents. *Pediatrics*. 1992;89:495-501.
11. Executive Summary of the Third Report of the National Cholesterol Education Program (NCEP) Expert Panel on Detection, Evaluation, and Treatment of High Blood Cholesterol in Adults (Adult Treatment Panel III). *JAMA*. 2001;285:2486-2497.
12. Hughes HK, Kahl LK. *Mischief managed: until the very end*. Baltimore: Johns Hopkins University Press; 2016-2017.
13. Office of Dietary Supplements—Vitamin D. <https://ods.od.nih.gov/factsheets/VitaminD-HealthProfessional/>. Accessed December 3, 2016.
14. Ross AC, Manson JE, Abrams SA, et al. The 2011 Report on Dietary Reference Intakes for Calcium and Vitamin D from the Institute of Medicine: What Clinicians Need to Know. *J Clin Endocrinol Metab*. 2011;96(1):53-58. doi:10.1210/jc.2010-2704.
15. Schwimmer JB, Dunn W, Norman GJ, et al. SAFETY study: alanine aminotransferase cutoff values are set too high for reliable detection of pediatric chronic liver disease. *Gastroenterology*. 2010;138(4):1357-1364, 1364.e1-e2.
16. Holick MF, Binkley NC, Bischoff-Ferrari HA, et al. Evaluation, treatment, and prevention of vitamin D deficiency: an Endocrine Society clinical practice guideline. *J Clin Endocrinol Metab*. 2011;96(7):1911-1930. doi:10.1210/jc.2011-0385.
17. Kestenbaum LA, Ebberson J, Zorc JJ, et al. Defining cerebrospinal fluid white blood cell count reference values in neonates and young infants. *Pediatrics*. 2010;125:257-264.

18. Sarff LD, Platt LH, McCracken GH. Cerebrospinal fluid evaluation in neonates: comparison of high-risk infants with and without meningitis. *J Pediatr*. 1976;883:473-477.
19. Shah SS, Ebberson J, Kestenbaum LA, et al. Age-specific reference values for cerebrospinal fluid protein concentration in neonates and young infants. *J Hosp Med*. 2011;6:22-27.
20. Avery RA, Shah SS, Licht DJ. Reference range for cerebrospinal fluid opening pressure in children. *N Engl J Med*. 2010;363:891-893.

Chapter 28
Biostatistics and Evidence-Based Medicine
Anirudh Ramesh, MD

See additional content on Expert Consult

I. WEB RESOURCES

A. Evidence-Based Resources
- Centre for Evidence Based Medicine: http://www.cebm.net
- Cochrane Reviews: www.cochranelibrary.com
- National Guideline Clearinghouse: http://guideline.gov/

B. Statistics Resources and Software
- BMJ Statistics at Square One: http://www.bmj.com/collections/statsbk/index.dtl

II. EVIDENCE-BASED MEDICINE

Evidence-based medicine refers to the method of integrating individual clinical expertise with the best available evidence from the literature. Below is a framework on how to evaluate a clinical question and appraise the evidence[1]:

A. Formulate the Clinical Question:
1. **Describe the patient or problem,** deciding whether the evidence you seek is regarding therapy, diagnosis, prognosis, etiology, or cost effectiveness.
2. **Describe the intervention** under consideration.
3. **Compare the intervention** with an alternative or standard of care if applicable.
4. **Formulate a specific outcome** of interest.

B. Search for the Evidence to Answer the Question:
1. **Define search terms** that fit the clinical question.
2. **Develop your search strategy** using PubMed or other primary search sources.
3. **Review your results** and apply methodological filters to target the right type of study.

C. Critically Appraise the Evidence:
1. **Therapy:**
a. Were patient groups randomized for treatment?
b. Were groups comparable and treated equally, aside from the allocated treatment?

c. Were study subjects and investigators blinded?
  d. Were all patients entering the trial accounted for in the groups they were randomized to (intention to treat)?
  e. How large was the treatment effect?
2. **Diagnosis:**
  a. Was the test compared with an independent reference standard?
  b. Was the test evaluated in an appropriate spectrum of patients?
3. **Prognosis:**
  a. Were study patients defined early in their course and followed up over a sufficient time?
  b. How likely is it that the outcomes occur during a defined time period, and how precise are the estimates of prognosis?
4. **Guidelines for judging causality between a variable and outcome**[2]**:**
  a. Is there a temporal relationship?
  b. What is the strength of association?
  c. Is there a dose/response relationship?
  d. Were the findings replicated?
  e. Is there biological plausibility?
  f. What happens with cessation of exposure?
  g. Is this explanation consistent with other knowledge?
5. **Types of bias:** Consider these types of bias that may influence results.[3]
  a. *Selection bias:* A distortion of statistical findings due to a nonrandom or dissimilar sample (between cases and controls) from a population. Mitigated by randomization and selection of participants who are representative of the target population.
  b. *Recall bias:* Cases are more likely to recount an exposure compared to controls.
  c. *Measurement bias:* Collection of information is influenced by interviewers' knowledge of study design and outcomes. Mitigated by blinding interviewers to subject status and standardizing data collection procedures.
  d. *Confounding bias:* Failure to account for factors that influence the desired outcome. Confounders should be controlled for during statistical testing.
  e. *Lead time bias:* Early detection of a disease leads to incorrect conclusions about increased survival.
  f. *Funding bias:* Influence of a financial sponsor on reporting of outcomes or publication bias (bias towards reporting only positive outcomes).

D. Apply the Evidence to the Clinical Question:

If the evidence is valid and important, integrate it with your clinical expertise and decide whether:
1. The patient will benefit from the therapy and be able to tolerate harms.
2. The test is available, affordable, accurate, and precise.

III. BIOSTATISTICS FOR MEDICAL LITERATURE

A. Statistical Tests

The following statistical tests are used to determine whether observed differences are statistically significant (Table 28.1).[4]

1. *Parametric tests* are used when data follow a normal distribution (a bell shaped distribution where the median, mean, and mode are all equal).
2. *Nonparametric tests* are used when a normal distribution cannot be assumed; they rank data rather than taking absolute differences into account.
3. *Paired tests* are performed on paired data; for example, where the same parameter is measured twice on each study subject, often before and after an intervention.
4. *Unpaired tests* compare values from independent samples.
5. *Two-tailed tests* should be used when an intervention could potentially lead to either an increase or decrease of the outcome.
6. *One-tailed tests* should be used when an intervention can have only one plausible effect on the outcome.
7. *Correlation and regression* describe the degree of linear association between two quantitative variables, but they do not imply causation.
a. *Correlation* measures the strength of association between two variables; expressed by the correlation coefficient r, also termed Pearson correlation coefficient.
b. *Regression* constructs an optimal straight line illustrating correlation, and allows for prediction of a dependent variable based on an independent (known) variable.

B. Statistical Terminology

1. **α (Alpha)—Significance level of a statistical test**[5]:
a. **α:** Probability of making a **Type 1 error**, which is a statistical association found by chance alone despite absence of a true association. The null hypothesis is incorrectly rejected in favor of the alternative hypothesis.
b. α is typically set at ≤0.05 (but can be set where a study determines), which allows interpretation with 95% certainty that a detected association is true.
c. **The *p* value** is the probability of a difference occurring by chance, and is judged against α, the preset level of significance. If p is less than the significance level α, the detected association is unlikely to be due to chance alone. For example, if $p < 0.01$, there is less than a 1 in 100 chance of the detected association being due to chance alone.
2. **β (Beta)—Power of a statistical test:**
a. **β:** Probability of making a **Type II error**, which is when no statistical association is found when there truly is one. The null hypothesis is not rejected when in fact it is false.

TABLE 28.1
COMMONLY USED STATISTICAL TESTS

Purpose of Test	Parametric Test	Nonparametric Test	Example
Compares two independent samples	Two-sample (unpaired) t test	Mann-Whitney U test	To compare girls' heights with boys' heights
Compares two sets of observations on a single sample	One-sample (paired) t test	Wilcoxon matched pairs test	To compare weight of infants before and after a feeding
Compares three or more sets of observations made on a single sample	One-way analysis of variance (F test) using total sum of squares (ANOVA)	Kruskal-Wallis analysis of variance by ranks	To determine whether plasma glucose level is higher 1 hour, 2 hours, or 3 hours after a meal
Test the influence (and interaction) of two different variables	Two-way analysis of variance (ANOVA)	Two-way analysis of variance by ranks	In the above example, to determine whether the results differ in male and female subjects
Tests the null hypothesis that the distribution of a variable is the same in two (or more) independent samples	χ^2 (chi square) test	Fisher exact test	To assess whether male or female adolescents are more likely to smoke
Assesses the strength of the straight-line association between two continuous variables	Product moment correlation coefficient (Pearson r)	Spearman rank correlation coefficient ($r\sigma$)	To assess whether and to what extent plasma HbA_{1c} concentration is related to plasma triglyceride concentration in diabetic patients
Describes the numerical relation between two quantitative variables, allowing one value to be predicted from the other	Regression by least squares method	Nonparametric regression (various tests)	To see how peak expiratory flow rate varies with height
Describes the numerical relationship between a dependent variable and several predictor variables (covariates)	Multiple regression by least squares method	Nonparametric regression (various tests)	To determine whether and to what extent a person's age, body fat, and sodium intake determine his or her blood pressure

Data from Greenhalgh T. How to read a paper. Statistics for the non-statistician. I: Different types of data need different statistical tests. BMJ. 1997; 315(7104): 364-366.

Chapter 28 Biostatistics and Evidence-Based Medicine

b. **Power = 1 − β:** the probability of finding a statistical association when there truly is one.
c. **Power** is typically set at a minimum of 0.80, which allows interpretation with 80% certainty that a detected lack of association is true.
3. **Sample size:** The number of subjects required in a study to detect an effect with a sufficiently high power and sufficiently low α.
4. **95% confidence interval:** Describes the values between which there is a 95% chance that the true population value falls within. When confidence intervals for groups overlap, they do not differ in a statistically significant manner.
5. **Confounding:** A variable associated with both the disease and the exposure (risk factor), leading to detection of a false relationship between the disease and exposure. Can be controlled for by matching, blinding, and randomization.
6. **Effect modification (interaction):** A variable that modifies the observed effect of an exposure on disease.
7. **Survival curves:** The most commonly used method is the Kaplan-Meier curve, used to plot time against any well-defined event. The fraction of remaining participants is recalculated each time an event occurs.

C. Types of Study Designs: Table 28.2

D. Measurement of Disease Occurrence and Treatment Effects

1. **Prevalence:** Proportion of study population who has a disease in a defined time period. Often used in cross-sectional studies.

$$Prevalence = \frac{Number\ of\ total\ cases}{Population\ size}$$

2. **Incidence:** Number of new cases in the study population who newly develop a disease in a defined time period. Often used in cohort studies and clinical trials.

$$Incidence = \frac{Number\ of\ new\ cases}{Population\ size}$$

3. **Relative risk (RR):** The ratio of incidence of disease among people with risk factor to incidence of disease among people without risk factor. Used in prospective cohort studies, cross sectional studies, or clinical trials (Table 28.3).

$$RR = \frac{\frac{A}{A+C}}{\frac{B}{B+D}}$$

a. RR =1: No effect of exposure or treatment on outcome
b. RR <1: Exposure or treatment protective against outcome
c. RR >1: Exposure or treatment increases the outcome

TABLE 28.2
STUDY DESIGN COMPARISON

Design Type	Definition	Advantages	Disadvantages
Case-control (often called retrospective)	Define diseased subjects (cases) and nondiseased subjects (controls); compare proportion of cases with exposure (risk factor) with proportion of controls with exposure (risk factor)	Good for rare diseases Small sample size Shorter study times (not followed over time) Less expensive	Highest potential for biases (recall, selection, and others) Weak evidence for causality Unable to determine prevalence, PPV, NPV
Cohort (usually prospective; occasionally retrospective)	In study population, define exposed group (with risk factor) and nonexposed group (without risk factor) Over time, compare proportion of exposed group with outcome (disease) with proportion of nonexposed group with outcome (disease)	Defines incidence Stronger evidence for causality Decreases biases (sampling, measurement, reporting)	Expensive Long study times May not be feasible for rare diseases/outcomes Factors related to exposure and outcome may falsely alter effect of exposure on outcome (confounding)
Cross-sectional	In study population, concurrently measure outcome (disease) and risk factor Compare proportion of diseased group with risk factor with proportion of nondiseased group with risk factor	Defines prevalence Short time to complete	Selection bias Weak evidence for causality
Clinical trial (experiment)	In study population, assign (randomly) subjects to receive treatment or receive no treatment Compare rate of outcome (e.g., disease cure) between treatment and nontreatment groups	Randomized blinded trial is gold standard Randomization reduces confounding Best evidence for causality	Expensive Risks of experimental treatments in humans Longer study time Not suitable for rare outcomes/diseases
Meta-analysis	Collates data from multiple independent studies to maximize precision and power in testing for statistical significance	Higher statistical power Can control for inter-study variation	Possible bias in exclusion of published studies or publication bias

NPV, Negative predictive value; PPV, positive predictive value
Data from Hulley SB, Cummings SR, et al. Study Designs. In: Designing Clinical Research. 4th edition. Philadelphia: Lippincott Williams & Wilkins; 2011:84-207.

Chapter 28 Biostatistics and Evidence-Based Medicine

TABLE 28.3
GRID FOR CALCULATIONS IN CLINICAL STUDIES*

Disease or Outcome	Exposure or Risk Factor or Treatment	
	Positive	Negative
Positive	A	B
Negative	C	D

*Also known as a contingency table

4. **Attributable risk:** Difference in incidence between exposed and unexposed groups.
5. **Odds Ratio (OR):** The ratio of the odds of having the risk factor in people with the disease to the odds of having the risk factor in people without disease. Often used in retrospective case-control studies (see Table 28.3).

$$OR = \frac{\frac{A}{B}}{\frac{C}{D}} = \frac{A \times D}{B \times C}$$

   a. OR approximates RR when the disease is rare (incidence <0.10)
   b. OR =1: No association between risk factor and disease
   c. OR <1: Suggests that risk factor is protective against disease
   d. OR >1: Suggests association between risk factor and disease
6. **Absolute risk reduction (ARR) or absolute benefit increase or absolute risk increase (ARI):** Absolute difference the treatment makes, expressed as difference between the risk of the outcome in control group minus the risk of the outcome in treatment group.
7. **Relative risk reduction or relative benefit increase:** The strength of the impact of the exposure or treatment, expressed as the ARR divided by the risk of the outcome in the control group.
8. **Number needed to treat:** Number of patients who need to be treated to prevent one undesired outcome, expressed as 1 ÷ ARR.
9. **Number needed to harm:** Number of patients who need to be treated to cause one additional patient harm, expressed as 1 ÷ ARI.

E. Measurements of Test Performance: Table 28.4

1. **Sensitivity:** Proportion of all patients with disease who have a positive test. Measures the ability of the test to correctly identify those who have the disease. Use highly sensitive test to help exclude a disease, such as a screening test. Sensitivity is not affected by disease prevalence (see Table 28.4).

$$Sensitivity = \frac{TP}{TP + FN}$$

2. **Specificity:** Proportion of all patients without disease who have a negative test. Measures the ability of the test to correctly identify those

TABLE 28.4
GRID FOR EVALUATING A CLINICAL TEST

Test Result	Disease Status	
	Positive	Negative
Positive	TP (true positive)	FP (false positive)
Negative	FN (false negative)	TN (true negative)

who do not have the disease. Use a highly specific test to help confirm a disease. Specificity is not affected by disease prevalence (see Table 28.4).

$$Specificity = \frac{TN}{FP + TN}$$

3. **Positive predictive value (PPV):** Proportion of those with positive tests who truly have disease. PPV is increased with higher disease prevalence (see Table 28.4).

$$PPV = \frac{TP}{TP + FP}$$

4. **Negative predictive value (NPV):** Proportion of those with negative tests who truly do not have disease. NPV is increased with lower disease prevalence (see Table 28.4).

$$NPV = \frac{TN}{FN + TN}$$

5. **Likelihood ratio (LR):** Used with Bayes nomogram (Fig. EC 28.A available on Expert Consult) to calculate posttest probability of a disease based on a given test result. LR incorporates the performance of the test (sensitivity and specificity) to determine the magnitude of effect of a test on changing the pretest probability of disease. Tests that provide the greatest impetus to changing clinical management are those with an LR ≥10 (or LR ≤0.1 for negative tests). LR is unaffected by disease prevalence.

$$LR \text{ for positive test} = \frac{sensitivity}{1 - specificity}$$

$$LR \text{ for negative test} = \frac{1 - sensitivity}{specificity}$$

REFERENCES

1. Straus SE, Glasziou P, Richardson WS, et al. *Evidence-Based Medicine: How to Practice and Teach It.* 4th ed. Edinburgh: Churchill Livingstone; 2011:1-166.

2. Gordis L. From Association to Causation: Deriving Inferences from Epidemiologic Studies. In: *Epidemiology*. 5th ed. Philadelphia: Elsevier Saunders; 2014:243-261.
3. Gordis L. More on Causal Inferences: Bias, Confounding, and Interactions. In: *Epidemiology*. 5th ed. Philadelphia: Elsevier Saunders; 2014:262-278.
4. Rosner B. Hypothesis Testing: One Sample Inference. In: *Fundamentals of Biostatistics*. 7th ed. Boston: Brooks/Cole; 2011:204-265.
5. Motulsky H. Introduction to P values. In: *Intuitive Biostatistics*. New York: Oxford University Press; 1995:91-152.

PART IV

FORMULARY

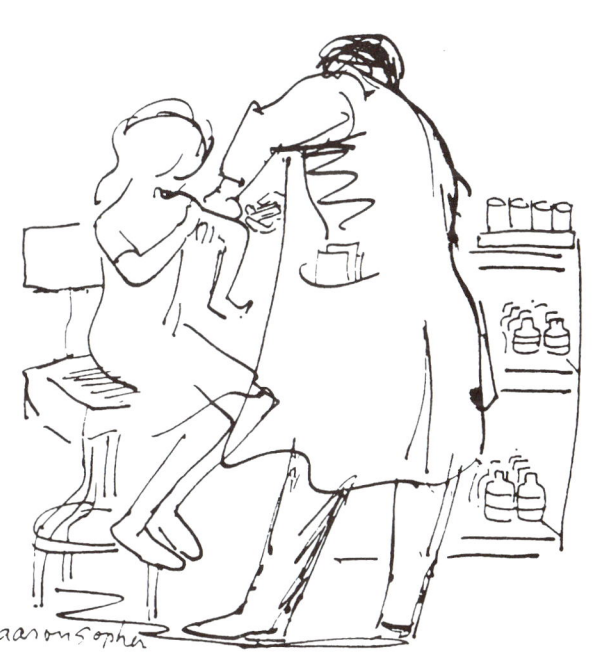

Chapter 29
Drug Dosages
Carlton K.K. Lee, PharmD, MPH

I. NOTE TO READER

The author has made every attempt to check dosages and medical content for accuracy. Because of the incomplete data on pediatric dosing, many drug dosages will be modified after the publication of this text. We recommend that the readers check product information and published literature for changes in dosing, especially for newer medicines. The U.S. Food and Drug Administration (FDA) provides the following pediatric drug information data sources:
- New Pediatric Labeling Information: www.fda.gov/NewPedLabeling
- Drug Safety Reporting Updates: www.fda.gov/PedDrugSafety
- Pediatric Study Characteristics Database: www.fda.gov/PedStudies

To prevent prescribing errors, the use of abbreviations has been greatly discouraged. The following is a list of abbreviations The Joint Commission considers prohibited for use.

THE JOINT COMMISSION

Official "Do Not Use" List*

Do Not Use	Potential Problem	Use Instead
U (unit)	Mistaken for "0" (zero), the number "4" (four) or "cc"	Write "unit"
IU (International Unit)	Mistaken for IV (intravenous) or the number 10 (ten)	Write "International Unit"
Q.D., QD, q.d., qd (daily)	Mistaken for each other	Write "daily"
Q.O.D., QOD, q.o.d, qod (every other day)	Period after the Q mistaken for "I" and the "O" mistaken for "I"	Write "every other day"
Trailing zero (X.0 mg)[†] Lack of leading zero (.X mg)	Decimal point is missed	Write X mg Write 0.X mg
MS	Can mean morphine sulfate or magnesium sulfate	Write "morphine sulfate" Write "magnesium sulfate"
MSO_4 and $MgSO_4$	Confused for one another	

*Applies to all orders and all medication-related documentation that is handwritten (including free-text computer entry) or on preprinted forms.

[†]Exception: A "trailing zero" may be used only where required to demonstrate the level of precision of the value being reported, such as for laboratory results, imaging studies that report size of lesions, or catheter/tube sizes. It may not be used in medication orders or other medication-related documentation.

Additional Abbreviations, Acronyms, and Symbols (For possible future inclusion in the Official "Do Not Use" List)

Do Not Use	Potential Problem	Use Instead
> (greater than) < (less than)	Misinterpreted as the number "7" (seven) or the letter "L" Confused for one another	Write "greater than" Write "less than"
Abbreviations for drug names	Misinterpreted due to similar abbreviations for multiple drugs	Write drug names in full
Apothecary units	Unfamiliar to many practitioners Confused with metric units	Use metric units
@	Mistaken for the number "2" (two)	Write "at"
cc	Mistaken for U (units) when poorly written	Write "mL" or "ml" or "milliliters" ("mL" is preferred)
µg	Mistaken for mg (milligrams), resulting in one thousand-fold overdose	Write "mcg" or "micrograms"

II. SAMPLE ENTRY

Pregnancy: Refer to explanation of pregnancy categories (see p. 735).
Breast: Refer to explanation of breast-feeding categories (see p. 735).
Kidney: Indicates need for caution or need for dose adjustment in renal impairment (see also Chapter 30).
Liver: Indicates need for caution or need for dose adjustment in hepatic impairment.

How supplied

ACETAZOLAMIDE ← Generic name

Diamox and generics ← Trade name and other names
Carbonic anhydrase inhibitor, diuretic ← Drug category

Yes   Yes   1   C

Tabs: 125, 250 mg
Oral suspension: 25 mg/mL ← Mortar and pestle: Indicates need for extemporaneous compounding by a pharmacist
Capsules (sustained release): 500 mg
Injection (sodium): 500 mg
Contains 2.05 mEq Na/500 mg drug

Diuretic (PO, IV)
  Child: 5 mg/kg/dose once daily or every other day
  Adult: 250–375 mg/dose once daily or every other day
Glaucoma
  Child:
    PO: 8–30 mg/kg/24 hr ÷ Q6–8 hr
    IM/IV: 20–40 mg/kg/24 hr ÷ Q6 hr; **max. dose:** 1000 mg/24 hr
  Adult:
    PO (simple chronic; open-angle): 1000 mg/24 hr ÷ Q6 hr
    IV (acute secondary; closed-angle): For rapid decrease in intraocular pressure, administer 500 mg/dose IV
Seizures (extended-release product not recommended):
  Child and adult: 8–30 mg/kg/24 hr ÷ Q6–12 hr PO; **max. dose:** 1 g/24 hr
Urine alkalinization:
  Adult: 5 mg/kg/dose PO repeated BID–TID over 24 hr.
Management of hydrocephalus (see remarks): Start with 20 mg/kg/24 hr ÷ Q8 hr PO/IV; may increase to 100 mg/kg/24 hr up to a **max. dose** of 2 g/24 hr.
Pseudotumor cerebri (PO; see remarks):
  Child: Start with 25 mg/kg/24 hr ÷ once daily–QID, increase by 25 mg/kg/24 hr until clinical response or as tolerated up to a maximum of 100 mg/kg/24 hr.
  Adolescent: Start with 1 g/24 hr ÷ once daily–QID, increase by 250 mg/24 hr until clinical response or as tolerated up to a maximum of 4 g/24 hr.

Drug dosing

Contraindicated in hepatic failure, severe renal failure (GFR <10 mL/min), and hypersensitivity to sulfonamides.

$T_{1/2}$: 2–6 hr; **do not use** sustained release capsules in seizures; IM injection may be painful; bicarbonate replacement therapy may be required during long-term use (see *Citrate or Sodium Bicarbonate*). For use in pseudotumor cerebri, doses of 60 mg/kg/24 hr may be required.

Possible side effects (more likely with long-term therapy) include GI irritation, paresthesias, sedation, hypokalemia, acidosis, reduced urate secretion, aplastic anemia, polyuria, and development of renal calculi.

May increase toxicity of cyclosporine. Aspirin may increase toxicity of acetazolamide. May decrease the effects of salicylates, lithium, and phenobarbital. False-positive urinary protein may occur with several assays. **Adjust dose in renal failure (see Chapter 30).**

Brief remarks about side effects, drug interactions, precautions, therapeutic monitoring, and other relevant information

III. EXPLANATION OF BREASTFEEDING CATEGORIES

See sample entry on page 734.
1 Compatible
2 Use with caution
3 Unknown with concerns
X Contraindicated
? Safety not established

IV. EXPLANATION OF PREGNANCY CATEGORIES

A Adequate studies in pregnant women have not demonstrated a risk to the fetus in the first trimester of pregnancy, and there is no evidence of risk in later trimesters.

B Animal studies have not demonstrated a risk to the fetus, but there are no adequate studies in pregnant women; or animal studies have shown an adverse effect, but adequate studies in pregnant women have not demonstrated a risk to the fetus during the first trimester of pregnancy, and there is no evidence of risk in later trimesters.

C Animal studies have shown an adverse effect on the fetus, but there are no adequate studies in humans; or there are no animal reproduction studies and no adequate studies in humans.

D There is evidence of human fetal risk, but the potential benefits from the use of the drug in pregnant women may be acceptable despite its potential risks.

X Studies in animals or humans demonstrate fetal abnormalities or adverse reaction; reports indicate evidence of fetal risk. The risk of use in pregnant women clearly outweighs any possible benefit.

V. BODY SURFACE NOMOGRAM AND EQUATION

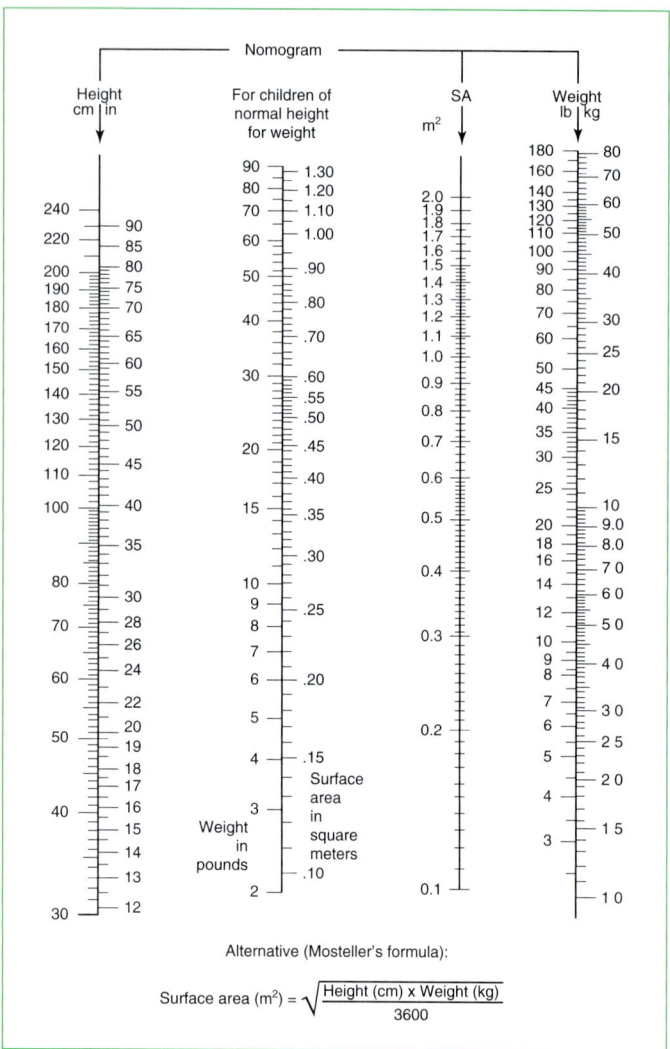

FIGURE 29.1
Body surface area nomogram and equation. (*From Kliegman RM, Stanton BF, Schor NF, et al., eds. Nelson Textbook of Pediatrics. 20th ed. Philadelphia: Elsevier; 2016.*)

VI. DRUG INDEX

Trade Names	Generic Name
1,25-dihydroxycholecalciferol	Calcitriol
2-PAM*	Pralidoxime Chloride
3TC*	Lamivudine
5-aminosalicylic acid	Mesalamine
5-ASA	Mesalamine
5-FC*	Flucytosine
5-Fluorocytosine*	Flucytosine
8-Arginine Vasopressin*	Vasopressin
9-Fluorohydrocortisone*	Fludrocortisone Acetate
27% Elemental Ca	Calcium Chloride
A-200	Pyrethrins
Abelcet	Amphotericin B Lipid Complex
Absorica	Isotretinoin
Abstra	Fentanyl
Accolate	Zafirlukast
AccuNeb (prediluted nebulized solution)	Albuterol
Accutane	Isotretinoin
Acetadote	Acetylcysteine
Acticin	Permethrin
Actigall	Ursodiol
Actiq	Fentanyl
Activase	Alteplase
Acular, Acular LS	Ketorolac
Acuvail	Ketorolac
Aczone	Dapsone
Adalat CC	Nifedipine
Adderall, Adderall XR	Dextroamphetamine + Amphetamine
Adenocard	Adenosine
Adoxa	Doxycycline
Adrenaline	Epinephrine HCl
Advair Diskus, Advair HFA	Fluticasone Propionate and Salmeterol
Advil, Children's Advil	Ibuprofen
Aerospan	Flunisolide
Afrin	Oxymetazoline
AK-Poly-Bac Ophthalmic	Bacitracin + Polymyxin B
AK-Spore H.C. Otic	Polymyxin B Sulfate, Neomycin Sulfate, Hydrocortisone
AK-Sulf	Sulfacetamide Sodium Ophthalmic
AKTob	Tobramycin
AK-Tracin Ophthalmic	Bacitracin
Albuminar	Albumin, Human
Albutein	Albumin, Human
Aldactone	Spironolactone
Aleve [OTC]	Naproxen/Naproxen Sodium
Allegra, Allegra ODT	Fexofenadine
Allegra-D 12 Hour, Allegra-D 24 Hour	Fexofenadine + Pseudoephedrine
Allergen Ear Drops	Antipyrine and Benzocaine

*Common abbreviation or other name (not recommended for use when writing a prescription).

Trade Names	Generic Name
Alloprim	Allopurinol
Almacone, Almacone II Double Strength	Aluminum Hydroxide with Magnesium Hydroxide
Alsuma	Sumatriptan Succinate
AlternaGEL	Aluminum Hydroxide
Alu-Cap	Aluminum Hydroxide
Alvesco	Ciclesonide
AmBisome	Amphotericin B, Liposomal
Amicar	Aminocaproic Acid
Amikin	Amikacin Sulfate
Amnesteem	Isotretinoin
Amoclan	Amoxicillin-Clavulanic Acid
Amoxil	Amoxicillin
Amphadase	Hyaluronidase
Amphocin	Amphotericin B
Amphojel	Aluminum Hydroxide
Anacin	Aspirin
Anaprox	Naproxen/Naproxen Sodium
Ancef	Cefazolin
Ancobon	Flucytosine
Anectine	Succinylcholine
Antilirium	Physostigmine Salicylate
Antipyrine and Benzocaine Otic	Antipyrine and Benzocaine
Antizol	Fomepizole
Anzemet	Dolasetron
Apresoline	Hydralazine Hydrochloride
Apriso	Mesalamine
Aquachloral Supprettes	Chloral Hydrate
Aquasol A	Vitamin A
Aquasol E	Vitamin E
Aquavit-E	Vitamin E
Aralen	Chloroquine HCl/Phosphate
Aranesp	Darbepoetin Alfa
Arbinoxa	Carbinoxamine
Arestin	Minocycline
Aridol	Mannitol
Aristospan	Triamcinolone
ASA*	Aspirin
Asacol, Asacol HD	Mesalamine
Asmanex Twisthaler	Mometasone Furoate
Asprin Free Anacin	Acetaminophen
Astelin	Azelastine
Astepro	Azelastine
Astragraf XL	Tacrolimus
Ativan	Lorazepam
AtroPen	Atropine Sulfate
Atrovent	Ipratropium Bromide
Augmentin, Augmentin ES-600, Augmentin XR	Amoxicillin-Clavulanic Acid

*Common abbreviation or other name (not recommended for use when writing a prescription).

Trade Names	Generic Name
Auralgan (available in Canada)	Antipyrine and Benzocaine
Auro Ear Drops	Carbamide Peroxide
Avinza	Morphine Sulfate
Avita	Tretinoin
Ayr Saline	Sodium Chloride—Inhaled Preparations
Azactam	Aztreonam
Azasan	Azathioprine
Azasite	Azithromycin
Azo-Standard [OTC]	Phenazopyridine HCl
Azulfidine, Azulfidine EN-Tabs	Sulfasalazine
Baciguent Topical	Bacitracin
Bactrim	Sulfamethoxazole and Trimethoprim
Bactroban, Bactroban Nasal	Mupirocin
BAL*	Dimercaprol
Beconase AQ	Beclomethasone Dipropionate
Benadryl	Diphenhydramine
Benzac AC Wash 2½, 5, 10; Benzac 5, 10	Benzoyl Peroxide
Beta-Val	Betamethasone
Bethkis	Tobramycin
Biaxin, Biaxin XL	Clarithromycin
Bicillin C-R, Bicillin C-R 900/300	Penicillin G Preparations—Penicillin G Benzathine and Penicillin G Procaine
Bicillin L-A	Penicillin G Preparations—Benzathine
Bio-Statin	Nystatin
Bioxiverz	Neostigmine
Bleph 10	Sulfacetamide Sodium Ophthalmic
Brevibloc	Esmolol HCl
Brevoxyl Creamy Wash	Benzoyl Peroxide
Brisdelle	Paroxetine
British anti-Lewisite	Dimercaprol
Bufferin	Aspirin
Bumex	Bumetanide
Buminate	Albumin, Human
Cafcit	Caffeine Citrate
Cafergot	Ergotamine Tartrate + Caffeine
Calcidol	Ergocalciferol
Caldolor	Ibuprofen
Calan, Calan SR	Verapamil
Calciferol	Ergocalciferol
Calcijex	Calcitriol
Calcionate	Calcium Glubionate
Calciquid	Calcium Glubionate
Cal-Citrate	Calcium Citrate
Calcium disodium versenate	Edetate (EDTA) Calcium Disodium
Cal-Glu	Calcium Gluconate
Cal-Lac	Calcium Lactate
Calphron	Calcium Acetate
Camphorated opium tincture	Paregoric

*Common abbreviation or other name (not recommended for use when writing a prescription).

Trade Names	Generic Name
Canasa	Mesalamine
Cancidas	Caspofungin
Cankaid	Carbamide Peroxide
Capoten	Captopril
Carafate	Sucralfate
Carbatrol	Carbamazepine
Cardene, Cardene SR	Nicardipine
Cardizem, Cardizem SR, Cardizem CD, Cardizem LA	Diltiazem
Carnitor	Carnitine
Catapres, Catapres TTS	Clonidine
Cathflo Activase	Alteplase
Caysten	Aztreonam
Ceclor, Ceclor CD	Cefaclor
Cecon	Ascorbic Acid
Cedax	Ceftibuten
Cefotan	Cefotetan
Ceftin	Cefuroxime Axetil
Cefzil	Cefprozil
Celestone	Betamethasone
CellCept	Mycophenolate Mofetil
Cephulac	Lactulose
Ceptaz	Ceftazidime
Cerebyx	Fosphenytoin
Chemet	Succimer
Chloromycetin	Chloramphenicol
Chlor-Trimeton	Chlorpheniramine Maleate
Cholestyramine Light	Cholestyramine
Chronulac	Lactulose
Ciloxan ophthalmic	Ciprofloxacin
Cipro, Cipro XR, Ciprodex, Cipro HC Otic	Ciprofloxacin
Citracel	Calcium Citrate
Claforan	Cefotaxime
Claravis	Isotretinoin
Claritin, Claritin Children's Allergy, Claritin RediTabs	Loratadine
Claritin-D 12 Hour, Claritin-D 24 Hour	Loratadine + Pseudoephedrine
Cleocin-T, Cleocin	Clindamycin
Cogentin	Benztropine Mesylate
Colace	Docusate
Colocort	Hydrocortisone
CoLyte	Polyethylene Glycol—Electrolyte Solution
Compazine	Prochlorperazine
Concerta	Methylphenidate HCl
Copegus	Ribavirin
Cordarone	Amiodarone HCl
Cordron-D NR, Cordron-D	Carbinoxamine + Pseudoephedrine
Coreg, Coreg CR	Carvedilol

*Common abbreviation or other name (not recommended for use when writing a prescription).

Trade Names	Generic Name
Cortef	Hydrocortisone
Cortenema	Hydrocortisone
Cortifoam	Hydrocortisone
Cortisporin Otic	Polymyxin B Sulfate, Neomycin Sulfate, Hydrocortisone
Co-Trimoxazole	Sulfamethoxazole and Trimethoprim
Coumadin	Warfarin
Covera-HS	Verapamil
Cozaar	Losartan
Crolom	Cromolyn
Cruex	Clotrimazole
Cuprimine	Penicillamine
Curosurf	Surfactant, Pulmonary/Poractant Alfa
Cutivate	Fluticasone Propionate
Cuvposa	Glycopyrrolate
Cyanoject	Cyanocobalamin/Vitamin B_{12}
Cyclogyl	Cyclopentolate
Cyclomydril	Cyclopentolate with Phenylephrine
Cyomin	Cyanocobalamin/Vitamin B_{12}
Cytovene	Ganciclovir
D-3, D3-5, D3-50	Cholecalciferol
Dantrium	Dantrolene
Daraprim	Pyrimethamine
Daytrana	Methylphenidate HCl
DDAVP*	Desmopressin Acetate
DDS*	Dapsone
D Drops	Cholecalciferol
Debrox	Carbamide Peroxide
Decadron	Dexamethasone
Deltasone	Prednisone
Delzicol	Mesalamine
Deodorized tincture of opium	Opium Tincture
Depacon	Valproic Acid
Depakene	Valproic Acid
Depakote, Depakote ER	Divalproex Sodium
Depen	Penicillamine
Depo-Medrol	Methylprednisolone
Depo-Provera	Medroxyprogesterone
Depo-Sub Q Provera 104	Medroxyprogesterone
Desquam-E 5, Desquam-E 10	Benzoyl Peroxide
Desyrel (previously available as)	Trazodone
Dexedrine Spansules	Dextroamphetamine
DexFerrum	Iron—Injectable Preparations (iron dextran)
Dexpak Taperpak	Dexamethasone
DextroStat	Dextroamphetamine ± Amphetamine
Di-5-ASA*	Olsalazine
Dialume	Aluminum Hydroxide
Diaminodiphenylsulfone	Dapsone

*Common abbreviation or other name (not recommended for use when writing a prescription).

Trade Names	Generic Name
Diamox	Acetazolamide
Diastat, Diastat AcuDial	Diazepam
Diflucan and others	Fluconazole
Digibind, DigiFab	Digoxin Immune Fab (Ovine)
Digitek	Digoxin
Dilacor XR	Diltiazem
Dilantin, Dilantin Infatab	Phenytoin
Dilaudid, Dilaudid-HP	Hydromorphone HCl
Di-mesalazine	Olsalazine
Dimetapp Children's Cold and Allergy	Brompheniramine with Phenylephrine
Diovan	Valsartan
Dipentum	Olsalazine
Diprolene, Diprolene AF	Betamethasone
Diprosone	Betamethasone
DisperMox	Amoxicillin
Ditropan, Ditropan XL	Oxybutynin Chloride
Diuril	Chlorothiazide
DMSA [dimercaptosuccinic acid]*	Succimer
Dobutrex (previously available as)	Dobutamine
Dolophine	Methadone HCl
Dopram	Doxapram HCl
Doryx	Doxycycline
Doxidan	Bisacodyl
Dramamine, Children's Dramamine	Dimenhydrinate
Drisdol	Ergocalciferol
Dulcolax	Bisacodyl
Dulera	Mometasone Furoate + Formoterol Fumarate
Duraclon	Clonidine
Duragesic	Fentanyl
Duramist 12-Hr Nasal	Oxymetazoline
Duricef	Cefadroxil
Dycill	Dicloxacillin Sodium
Dynacin	Minocycline
Dyrenium	Triamterene
EC-Naprosyn	Naproxen
Efidac/24-Pseudoephedrine	Pseudoephedrine
Elavil	Amitriptyline
Elidel	Pimecrolimus
Elimite	Permethrin
Eliphos	Calcium Acetate
Elitek	Rasburicase
Elixophyllin	Theophylline
Elocon	Mometasone Furoate
Emfamil D-Vi-Sol	Cholecalciferol
EMLA, Eutectic mixture of lidocaine and prilocaine	Lidocaine and Prilocaine
E-Mycin	Erythromycin Preparations
Enbrel	Etanercept

*Common abbreviation or other name (not recommended for use when writing a prescription).

Chapter 29 Drug Dosages

Trade Names	Generic Name
Endocet	Oxycodone and Acetaminophen
Endodan	Oxycodone and Aspirin
Enemeez	Docusate
Enlon	Edrophonium Chloride
Entocort EC	Budesonide
Enuloase	Lactulose
Epaned	Enalapril Maleate
EpiPen	Epinephrine HCl
Epitol	Carbamazepine
Epivir, Epivir-HBV	Lamivudine
Epogen	Epoetin Alfa
Epsom salts	Magnesium Sulfate
Ergomar	Ergotamine Tartrate
Ery-Ped	Erythromycin
Erythrocin, Pediamycin, E-Mycin, Ery-Ped	Erythromycin
Erythropoietin	Epoetin Alfa
Eryzole	Erythromycin Ethylsuccinate and Acetylsulfisoxazole
Exalgo	Hydromorphone HCl
Extina	Ketoconazole
Famvir	Famciclovir
Fansidar	Pyrimethamine + Sulfadoxine
Felbatol	Felbamate
Fentora	Fentanyl
Feosol	Iron—Oral Preparations (Ferrous sulfate)
Fergon	Iron—Oral Preparations (Ferrous sulfate)
Fer-In-Sol	Iron—Oral Preparations (Ferrous gluconate)
Ferrlecit	Iron—Injectable Preparations (Ferric gluconate)
Feverall	Acetaminophen
Fiberall	Psyllium
First-Lansoprazole	Lansoprazole
First-Omeprazole	Omeprazole
FK506	Tacrolimus
Flagyl, Flagyl ER	Metronidazole
Flebogamma DIF	Immune Globulin
Fleet Babylax	Glycerin
Fleet Laxative, Fleet Bisacodyl	Bisacodyl
Fleet Mineral Oil	Mineral Oil
Fleet, Fleet Phospho-Soda	Sodium Phosphate
Fletcher's Castoria	Senna/Sennosides
Flonase HFA	Fluticasone Propionate
Florinef Acetate	Fludrocortisone Acetate
Flovent Diskus	Fluticasone Propionate
Floxin, Floxin Otic	Ofloxacin
Flumadine	Rimantadine
Fluohydrisone	Fludrocortisone Acetate
Fluoritab	Fluoride

*Common abbreviation or other name (not recommended for use when writing a prescription).

Trade Names	Generic Name
Focalin, Focalin XR	Dexmethylphenidate
Folvite	Folic Acid
Foradil Aerolizer	Formoterol
Fortamet	Metformin
Fortaz	Ceftazidime
Fortical Nasal Spray	Calcitonin—Salmon
Foscavir	Foscarnet
Fulvicin U/F, Fulvicin P/G	Griseofulvin
Fungizone	Amphotericin B
Furadantin	Nitrofurantoin
Gabitril	Tiagabine
Gablofen	Baclofen
Galzin	Zinc Salts, Systemic
Gamaplex	Immune Globulin
Gamma benzene hexachloride*	Lindane
Gammaked	Immune Globulin
Garamycin	Gentamicin
Gastrocrom	Cromolyn
Gas-X	Simethicone
Gengraf	Cyclosporine Modified
GlucaGen, Glucagon Emergency Kit	Glucagon HCl
Glucophage, Glucophage XR	Metformin
Gly-Oxide	Carbamide Peroxide
Glycate	Glycopyrrolate
GoLYTELY	Polyethylene Glycol—Electrolyte Solution
Gralise	Gabapentin
Granisol	Granisetron
Grifulvin V	Griseofulvin
Grisactin	Griseofulvin
Gris-PEG	Griseofulvin
Gyne-Lotrimin 3, Gyne-Lotrimin	Clotrimazole
H.P. Acthar Gel	Corticotropin
Haldol, Haldol Decanoate 50, Haldol Decanoate 100	Haloperidol
Hecoria	Tacrolimus
Hexadrol	Dexamethasone
Horizant	Gabapentin
Humatin	Paromomycin Sulfate
Hydro-Tussin CBX	Carbinoxamine + Pseudoephedrine
Hylenex	Hyaluronidase
Hypersal	Sodium Chloride—Inhaled Preparations
Imitrex	Sumatriptan Succinate
Imodium, Imodium AD	Loperamide
Imuran	Azathioprine
Inapsine	Droperidol
Inderal, Inderal LA	Propranolol
Indocin, Indocin SR, Indocin IV	Indomethacin
Infasurf	Surfactant, Pulmonary/Calfactant

*Common abbreviation or other name (not recommended for use when writing a prescription).

Trade Names	Generic Name
INFeD	Iron—Injectable Preparations (iron dextran)
INH*	Isoniazid
Intal (previously available as)	Cromolyn
Intropin (previously available as)	Dopamine
Intuniv	Guanfacine
Invanz	Ertapenem
Iosat	Potassium Iodide
Iquix	Levofloxacin
IsonaRif	Isoniazid
Isoptin SR	Verapamil
Isopto Carpine	Pilocarpine HCl
Isopto Hyoscine	Scopolamine Hydrobromide
Isuprel	Isoproterenol
Jantoven	Warfarin
Kadian	Morphine Sulfate
Kantrex	Kanamycin
Kaopectate	Bismuth Subsalicylate
Kao-Tin	Bismuth Subsalicylate
Kapvay	Clonidine
Kayexalate	Sodium Polystyrene Sulfonate
Keflex	Cephalexin
Kemstro	Baclofen
Kenalog	Triamcinolone
Keppra, Keppra XR	Levetiracetam
Ketalar	Ketamine
Kionex	Sodium Polystyrene Sulfonate
Klonopin	Clonazepam
Klout	Pyrethrins with Piperonyl Butoxide
Kondremul	Mineral Oil
Konsyl	Psyllium
K-PHOS Neutral	Phosphorus Supplements
Kristalose	Lactulose
Kytril	Granisetron
Lamictal, Lamictal ODT, Lamictal XR	Lamotrigine
Laniazid	Isoniazid
Lanoxin	Digoxin
Lariam	Mefloquine HCl
Lasix	Furosemide
Lax-Pills	Senna/Sennosides
Lazanda	Fentanyl
L-Carnitine	Carnitine
Levaquin, Quixin, Iquix	Levofloxacin
Levocarnitine	Carnitine
Levophed and others	Norepinephrine Bitartrate
Lialda	Mesalamine
Licide	Pyrethrins with Piperonyl Butoxide
Lidoderm	Lidocaine
Lioresal	Baclofen

*Common abbreviation or other name (not recommended for use when writing a prescription).

Trade Names	Generic Name
Liquid Pred	Prednisone
Lithobid	Lithium
L-M-X	Lidocaine
Loniten (previously available as)	Minoxidil
Lopressor, Toprol-XL	Metoprolol
Lotrimin AF	Clotrimazole
Lotrimin AF	Miconazole
Lovenox	Enoxaparin
Luminal	Phenobarbital
Luride	Fluoride
Luvox CR	Fluvoxamine
Maalox, Maalox Maximum Strength Liquid	Aluminum Hydroxide with Magnesium Hydroxide
Macrobid	Nitrofurantoin
Macrodantin	Nitrofurantoin
Mag-200, Mag-Ox 400, Uro-Mag	Magnesium Oxide
Marinol	Dronabinol
Maxidex	Dexamethasone
Maxipime	Cefepime
Maxivate	Betamethasone
Maxolon	Metoclopramide
Medrol, Medrol Dosepack	Methylprednisolone
Mefoxin	Cefoxitin
Mephyton	Phytonadione/Vitamin K_1
Mepron	Atovaquone
Merrem	Meropenem
Mestinon	Pyridostigmine Bromide
Metadate ER	Methylphenidate HCl
Metamucil	Psyllium
Methadose	Methadone HCl
Methylin, Methylin ER	Methylphenidate HCl
Metozolv	Metoclopramide
MetroCream	Metronidazole
MetroGel, MetroGel-Vaginal	Metronidazole
MetroLotion	Metronidazole
Miacalcin, Miacalcin Nasal Spray	Calcitonin—Salmon
Micatin	Miconazole
Microzide	Hydrochlorothiazide
Milk of Magnesia	Magnesium Hydroxide
Millipred	Prednisolone
Minocin	Minocycline
Mintezol	Thiabendazole
Mintox	Aluminum Hydroxide with Magnesium Hydroxide
MiraLax	Polyethylene Glycol—Electrolyte Solution
Monistat	Miconazole
Motrin, Children's Motrin	Ibuprofen
MS Contin	Morphine Sulfate

*Common abbreviation or other name (not recommended for use when writing a prescription).

Trade Names	Generic Name
Mucomyst	Acetylcysteine
Mucosol	Acetylcysteine
Murine Ear	Carbamide Peroxide
Myambutol	Ethambutol HCl
Mycamine	Micafungin Sodium
Mycelex, Mycelex-7	Clotrimazole
Mycobutin	Rifabutin
Mycostatin	Nystatin
Myfortic	Mycophenolate Sodium
Mylanta Gas	Simethicone
Mylanta, Mylanta Extra Strength	Aluminum Hydroxide with Magnesium Hydroxide
Mylicon	Simethicone
Myorisan	Isotretinoin
Mysoline	Primidone
Nallpen	Nafcillin
Naprelan	Naproxen/Naproxen Sodium
Naprosyn, Naprosen DR	Naproxen/Naproxen Sodium
Narcan	Naloxone
Nasacort AQ	Triamcinolone
Nasalcrom	Cromolyn
Nasarel	Flunisolide
Nascobal	Cyanocobalamin/Vitamin B_{12}
Nasonex	Mometasone Furoate
Nebcin	Tobramycin
NebuPent	Pentamidine Isethionate
Nembutal	Pentobarbital
NeoBenz Micro	Benzoyl Peroxide
Neo-fradin	Neomycin Sulfate
Neo-Polycin	Neomycin/Polymyxin B/Bacitracin
NeoProfen (IV)	Ibuprofen
Neoral	Cyclosporine
Neosporin, Neosporin Ophthalmic, Neo To Go	Neomycin/Polymyxin B/Bacitracin
Neosporin GU Irrigant	Neomycin/Polymyxin B
Neo-Synephrine	Phenylephrine HCl
Neo-Synephrine 12-Hr Nasal	Oxymetazoline
Nephron	Epinephrine, Racemic
Neupogen, G-CSF	Filgrastim
Neurontin	Gabapentin
Neut	Sodium Bicarbonate
Nexiclon XR	Clonidine
Nexium	Esomeprazole
Nexterone	Amiodarone HCl
Niacor	Niacin (Vitamin B_3)
Niaspan	Niacin (Vitamin B_3)
Nicotinic acid	Niacin (Vitamin B_3)
Nifediac CC	Nifedipine
Niferex	Iron—Oral Preparations

*Common abbreviation or other name (not recommended for use when writing a prescription).

Trade Names	Generic Name
Nilstat	Nystatin
Nipride (previously available as)	Nitroprusside
Nitro-Bid	Nitroglycerin
Nitro-Dur	Nitroglycerin
Nitro-Mist	Nitroglycerin
Nitropress	Nitroprusside
Nitrostat	Nitroglycerin
Nitro-Time	Nitroglycerin
Nix	Permethrin
Nizoral, Nizoral A-D	Ketoconazole
Noriate	Metronidazole
Normal Serum Albumin (Human)	Albumin, Human
Normodyne	Labetalol
Noroxin	Norfloxacin
Norvasc	Amlodipine
Nostrilla	Oxymetazoline
NuCort	Hydrocortisone
NuLYTELY	Polyethylene Glycol—Electrolyte Solution
Nutr-E-Sol	Vitamin E/α-Tocopherol
NVP*	Nevirapine
Nydrazid	Isoniazid
OCL*	Polyethylene Glycol—Electrolyte Solution
Ocean	Sodium Chloride—Inhaled Preparations
Ocuflox	Ofloxacin
Ocusulf-10	Sulfacetamide Sodium Ophthalmic
Omnaris	Ciclesonide
Ofirmev	Acetaminophen
Omeprazole and Syrspend SF Alka	Omeprazole
Omnicef	Cefdinir
Omnipaque 140, Omnipaque 180, Omnipaque 240, Omnipaque 300, and Omnipaque 350	Iohexol
Omnipen	Ampicillin
Onfi	Clobazam
Onmel	Itraconazole
Opticrom	Cromolyn
Optivar	Azelastine
Oralone	Corticosteroid
Oramorph SR	Morphine Sulfate
Orapred, Orapred ODT	Prednisolone
Oraqix	Lidocaine and Prilocaine
Orasone	Prednisone
OraVerse	Phentolamine Mesylate
Orazinc	Zinc Salts, Systemic
Os-Cal	Calcium Carbonate
Osmitrol	Mannitol
OsmoPrep	Sodium Phosphate
Oxtellar	Oxcarbazepine
Oxy-5, Oxy-10	Benzoyl Peroxide

*Common abbreviation or other name (not recommended for use when writing a prescription).

Trade Names	Generic Name
OxyContin	Oxycodone
Oxytrol	Oxybutynin Chloride
Pacerone	Amiodarone HCl
Palasbumin	Albumin, Human
Palgic	Carbinoxamine
Pamelor	Nortriptyline Hydrochloride
Pamix	Pyrantel Pamoate
Panadol	Acetaminophen
Paracetamol	Acetaminophen
Pataday	Olopatadine
Patanase	Olopatadine
Patanol	Olopatadine
Pathocil	Dicloxacillin Sodium
Paxil, Paxil CR	Paroxetine
Pediaflor	Fluoride
Pedia-Lax	Glycerin
Pediamycin	Erythromycin Preparations
Pediapred	Prednisolone
Pediazole	Erythromycin Ethylsuccinate and Acetylsulfisoxazole
PediOtic	Polymyxin B Sulfate, Neomycin Sulfate, Hydrocortisone
Pentam 300	Pentamidine Isethionate
Pentasa	Mesalamine
Pepcid, Pepcid AC [OTC], Maximum Strength Pepcid AC [OTC], Pepcid Complete [OTC], Pepcid RPD	Famotidine
Pepto-Bismol	Bismuth Subsalicylate
Percocet	Oxycodone and Acetaminophen
Percodan	Oxycodone and Aspirin
Perforomist	Formoterol
Periactin (previously available as)	Cyproheptadine
Periostat	Doxycycline
Pexeva	Paroxetine
Pfizerpen	Penicillin G Preparations—Aqueous Potassium and Sodium
PGE_1*	Alprostadil
Phazyme	Simethicone
Phenergan	Promethazine
Phenytek	Phenytoin
PhosLo	Calcium Acetate
Phoslyra	Calcium Acetate
Pilopine HS	Pilocarpine HCl
Pima	Potassium Iodide
Pin-Rid	Pyrantel Pamoate
Pin-X	Pyrantel Pamoate
Pipracil	Piperacillin
Pitressin	Vasopressin

*Common abbreviation or other name (not recommended for use when writing a prescription).

Trade Names	Generic Name
Plaquenil	Hydroxychloroquine
Polymox	Amoxicillin
Polysporin Ophthalmic	Bacitracin + Polymyxin B
Polysporin Topical	Bacitracin + Polymyxin B
Polytrim Ophthalmic Solution	Polymyxin B Sulfate and Trimethoprim Sulfate
Posture-D	Calcium Phosphate, Tribasic
Potassium Phosphate	Phosphorus Supplements
Precidex	Dexmedetomidine
Prelone	Prednisolone
Prevacid, Prevacid SoluTab	Lansoprazole
Prevalite	Cholestyramine
Prilosec, Prilosec OTC	Omeprazole
Primacor	Milrinone
Primaxin IV	Imipenem and Cilastatin
Principen	Ampicillin
Prinivil	Lisinopril
Privagen	Immune Globulin
ProAir HFA	Albuterol
Procanbid	Procainamide
Procardia, Procardia XL	Nifedipine
ProCentra	Dextroamphetamine Sulfate
Procrit	Epoetin Alfa
Proglycem	Diazoxide
Prograf	Tacrolimus
Pronestyl	Procainamide
Pronto	Pyrethrins
Prostaglandin E_1	Alprostadil
Prostigmin	Neostigmine
Prostin VR Pediatric	Alprostadil
Protonix	Pantoprazole
Protopam	Pralidoxime Chloride
Protopic	Tacrolimus
Protostat	Metronidazole
Proventil, Proventil HFA (aerosol inhaler)	Albuterol
Provera	Medroxyprogesterone
Prozac, Prozac Weekly	Fluoxetine Hydrochloride
Pseudo Carb Pediatric	Carbinoxamine + Pseudoephedrine
PTU*	Propylthiouracil
Pulmicort Respules, Pulmicort Flexhaler	Budesonide
Pulmozyme	Dornase Alfa/DNase
Pyrazinoic acid amide	Pyrazinamide
Pyridium	Phenazopyridine HCl
Pyrinyl	Pyrethrins
Qnasl	Beclomethasone Dipropionate
Quelicin, Quelicin-1000	Succinylcholine
Questran, Questran Light	Cholestyramine
Quinidex	Quinidine
Quixin	Levofloxacin

*Common abbreviation or other name (not recommended for use when writing a prescription).

Trade Names	Generic Name
QVAR*	Beclomethasone Dipropionate
Raniclor	Cefaclor
Rapamune	Sirolimus
Rayos	Prednisone
Rebetol	Ribavirin
Reese's Pinworm	Pyrantel Pamoate
Regitine	Phentolamine Mesylate
Reglan	Metoclopramide
Regonal	Pyridostigmine Bromide
Renova	Tretinoin
Resectisol	Mannitol
Restasis	Cyclosporine, Cyclosporine Microemulsion, Cyclosporine Modified
Retin-A, Retin-A Micro	Tretinoin
Retrovir, AZT	Zidovudine
Revatio	Sildenafil
Reversol	Edrophonium Chloride
Revonto	Dantrolene
R-Gene 10	Arginine Chloride
Rhinaris	Sodium Chloride—Inhaled Preparations
Rhinocort Aqua Nasal Spray	Budesonide
Ribaspheres	Ribavirin
RID	Pyrethrins
Rifadin	Rifampin
Rifamate	Isoniazid + Rifampin
Rifater	Pyrazinamide + Isoniazid + Rifampin
Rimactane	Rifampin
Riomet	Metformin
Risperdal, Risperdal M-Tab, Risperdal Consta	Risperidone
Ritalin, Ritalin SR, Ritalin LA	Methylphenidate HCl
Robinul	Glycopyrrolate
Rocaltrol	Calcitriol
Rocephin	Ceftriaxone
Rogaine, Men's Rogaine Extra Strength	Minoxidil
Romazicon	Flumazenil
Rowasa, SfRowasa	Mesalamine
Roxanol	Morphine Sulfate
Roxicet	Oxycodone and Acetaminophen
Roxicodone	Oxycodone
Roxilox	Oxycodone and Acetaminophen
RuLox Plus	Aluminum Hydroxide with Magnesium Hydroxide
S-2 Inhalant	Epinephrine, Racemic
Sabril	Vigabatrin
Salagen	Pilocarpine HCl
Salicylazosulfapyridine	Sulfasalazine
Sal-Tropine	Atropine Sulfate
Sancuso	Granisetron

*Common abbreviation or other name (not recommended for use when writing a prescription).

Trade Names	Generic Name
Sandimmune	Cyclosporine
Sandostatin, Sandostatin LAR Depot	Octreotide Acetate
Sani-Supp	Glycerin
Sarafem	Fluoxetine Hydrochloride
SAS*	Sulfasalazine
Scopace	Scopolamine Hydrobromide
Selsun and others	Selenium Sulfide
Senna-Gen	Senna/Sennosides
Senokot	Senna/Sennosides
Septra	Sulfamethoxazole and Trimethoprim
Serevent Diskus	Salmeterol
Sildec	Carbinoxamine + Pseudoephedrine
Silvadene	Silver Sulfadiazine
Simply Saline	Sodium Chloride—Inhaled Preparations
Singulair	Montelukast
Slo-Niacin	Niacin (Vitamin B_3)
Slow FE	Iron—Oral Preparations
Sodium Phosphate	Phosphorus Supplements
Solodyn	Minocycline
Solu-cortef	Hydrocortisone
Solu-Medrol	Methylprednisolone
Soluspan	Betamethasone
Sporanox	Itraconazole
SPS*	Sodium Polystyrene Sulfonate
SSD Cream, SSD AF Cream	Silver Sulfadiazine
SSKI*	Potassium Iodide
Stadol	Butorphanol
Stavzor	Valproic Acid
Stimate	Desmopressin Acetate
Stomach Relief, Stomach Relief Max St, Stomach Relief Plus	Bismuth Subsalicylate
Strattera	Atomoxetine
Streptase	Streptokinase
Sublimaze	Fentanyl
Sudafed	Pseudoephedrine
Sulfatrim	Sulfamethoxazole and Trimethoprim
Sulfazine, Sulfazine EC	Sulfasalazine
Sunkist Vitamin C	Ascorbic Acid
Suprax	Cefixime
Surfak	Docusate
Surfaxin	Surfactant, Pulmonary/Lucinactant
Survanta	Surfactant, Pulmonary/Beractant
Symbicort	Budesonide and Formoterol
Symmetrel	Amantadine Hydrochloride
Synagis	Palivizumab
Synercid	Quinupristin and Dalfopristin
Synthroid	Levothyroxine T_4
Tagamet, Tagamet HB [OTC]	Cimetidine

*Common abbreviation or other name (not recommended for use when writing a prescription).

Trade Names	Generic Name
Tambocor	Flecainide Acetate
Tamiflu	Oseltamivir Phosphate
Tapazole	Methimazole
Tazicef	Ceftazidime
Tazidime	Ceftazidime
Tegretol, Tegretol-XR	Carbamazepine
Tempra	Acetaminophen
Tenex	Guanfacine
Tenormin	Atenolol
Tensilon	Edrophonium Chloride
Tetrahydrocannabinol	Dronabinol
THC*	Dronabinol
Theo-24	Theophylline
Theochron	Theophylline
Thera-Ear	Carbamide Peroxide
Therazene	Silver Sulfadiazine
Thorazine	Chlorpromazine
ThyroSave	Potassium Iodide
ThyroShield	Potassium Iodide
Tiazac	Diltiazem
Tigan	Trimethobenzamide HCl
Timentin	Ticarcillin and Clavulanate
Tinactin	Tolnaftate
Tirosint	Levothyroxine
Tisit	Pyrethrins
TMP-SMX*	Sulfamethoxazole and Trimethoprim
TOBI, TOBI Podhaler	Tobramycin
Tobrex	Tobramycin
Tofranil, Tofranil-PM	Imipramine
Topamax	Topiramate
Topiragen	Topiramate
Toprol-XL	Metoprolol
Totacillin	Ampicillin
tPA*	Alteplase
Trandate	Labetalol
Transderm Scop	Scopolamine Hydrobromide
Trianex	Corticosteroid
Triaz	Benzoyl Peroxide
Triderm	Corticosteroid
Trileptal	Oxcarbazepine
Trilisate and others	Choline Magnesium Trisalicylate
TriLyte	Polyethylene Glycol—Electrolyte Solution
Trimethoprim-Sulfamethoxazole	Sulfamethoxazole and Trimethoprim
Trimox	Amoxicillin
Trokenndi XR	Topiramate
Tums	Calcium Carbonate
Tylenol	Acetaminophen
Tylenol #1, #2, #3, #4	Codeine and Acetaminophen

*Common abbreviation or other name (not recommended for use when writing a prescription).

Trade Names	Generic Name
Tylox	Oxycodone and Acetaminophen
Uceris	Budesonide
Unasyn	Ampicillin/Sulbactam
Unithroid, Unithroid Direct	Levothyroxine
Urecholine	Bethanechol Chloride
Uro-KP-Neutral	Phosphorus Supplements
Urolene Blue	Methylene Blue
Urso 250, Urso Forte	Ursodiol
Vagistat-3	Miconazole
Valcyte	Valganciclovir
Valium	Diazepam
Valtrex	Valacyclovir
Vancocin	Vancomycin
Vantin	Cefpodoxime Proxetil
VariZig	Varicella-Zoster Immune Globulin (Human)
Vasotec	Enalapril Maleate
Vasotec IV	Enalaprilat
Veetids	Penicillin V Potassium
Venofer	Iron—Injectable Preparations (iron sucrose)
Ventolin HFA	Albuterol
Veramyst	Fluticasone Propionate
Verelan, Verelan PM	Verapamil
Veripred	Prednisolone
Vermox	Mebendazole
Versed (previously available as)	Midazolam
VFEND	Voriconazole
Viagra	Sildenafil
Vibramycin	Doxycycline
Vimpat	Lacosamide
Viramune, Viramune XR	Nevirapine
Virazole	Ribavirin
Visicol	Sodium Phosphate
Visine LR	Oxymetazoline
Vistaril	Hydroxyzine
Vistide	Cidofovir
Vitamin B_1	Thiamine
Vitamin B_2	Riboflavin
Vitamin B_{12}	Cyanocobalamin/Vitamin B_{12}
Vitamin B_3	Niacin/Vitamin B_3
Vitamin B_6	Pyridoxine
Vitamin C	Ascorbic Acid
Vitrase	Hyaluronidase
Vitrasert	Ganciclovir
VoSpire ER	Albuterol
Vyvanse	Lisdexamfetamine
VZIG	Varicella-Zoster Immune Globulin (Human)
WinRho-SDF	Rh_0 (D) Immune Globulin Intravenous (Human)
Wycillin	Penicillin G Preparations—Procaine

*Common abbreviation or other name (not recommended for use when writing a prescription).

Trade Names	Generic Name
Wymox	Amoxicillin
Xolegel	Ketoconazole
Xopenex, Xopenex HFA	Levalbuterol
Xylocaine	Lidocaine
Zantac, Zantac 75 [OTC], Zantac 150 Maximum Strength [OTC]	Ranitidine HCl
Zarontin	Ethosuximide
Zaroxolyn	Metolazone
Zegerid	Omeprazole
Zemuron	Rocuronium
Zenatane	Isotretinoin
Zenzedi	Dextroamphetamine Sulfate
Zestril	Lisinopril
Zetonna	Ciclesonide
Zinacef	Cefuroxime
Zirgan	Ganciclovir
Zithromax, Zithromax TRI-PAK, Zithromax Z-PAK, Zmax	Azithromycin
Zoderm	Benzoyl Peroxide
Zofran	Ondansetron
Zolicef	Cefazolin
Zoloft	Sertraline HCl
Zonegran	Zonisamide
ZORprin	Aspirin
Zosyn	Piperacillin with Tazobactam
Zovirax	Acyclovir
Zyloprim	Allopurinol
Zyrtec, Children's Zyrtec	Cetirizine
Zyrtec-D 12 Hour	Cetirizine + Pseudoephedrine
Zyvox	Linezolid

*Common abbreviation or other name (not recommended for use when writing a prescription).

TABLE 29.1
EXAMPLES OF INDUCERS AND INHIBITORS OF CYTOCHROME P450 SYSTEM

Isoenzyme	Substrates (Drugs Metabolized by Isoenzyme)	Inhibitors*	Inducers
CYP1A2	Caffeine, theophylline, estradiol, propranolol	Cimetidine, quinolones, fluvoxamine, ketoconazole, lidocaine	Carbamazepine, smoking, phenobarbital, rifampin
CYP2B6	Cyclophosphamide, efavirenz, propofol	Paroxetine, sertraline	Carbamazepine, (fos)phenytoin, phenobarbital, rifampin
CYP2C9/10	Warfarin, phenytoin, tolbutamide, fluoxetine, sulfamethoxazole, fosphenytoin	Amiodarone, fluconazole, ibuprofen, indomethacin, nicardipine	Carbamazepine, (fos)phenytoin, rifampin, phenobarbital
CYP2C19	Diazepam, PPIs, phenytoin, desogestrel, ifosfamide, phenobarbital, sertraline, voriconazole	Cimetidine fluvoxamine, fluconazole, isoniazid, PPIs, sertraline	Carbamazepine, (fos)phenytoin, rifampin
CYP2D6	Captopril, codeine, haloperidol, dextromethorphan, tricyclic antidepressants, hydrocodone, oxycodone, phenothiazines, metoprolol, propranolol, paroxetine, venlafaxine, risperidone, flecainide, sertraline, aripiprazole, fluoxetine, lidocaine, fosphenytoin, ritonavir	Chlorpromazine, cinacalcet, dexmedetomidine, cocaine, cimetidine, quinidine, ritonavir, fluoxetine, sertraline, amiodarone	None known
CYP2E1	Acetaminophen, alcohol, isoniazid, theophylline, isoflurane	Disulfiram	Alcohol
CYP3A4	Amlodipine, aripiprazole, budesonide, cocaine, clonazepam, diltiazem, efavirenz, erythromycin, estradiol, fentanyl, fluticasone, nifedipine, verapamil, cyclosporine, carbamazepine, cisapride, tacrolimus, midazolam, alfentanil, diazepam, ifosfamide, imatinib, itraconazole, ketoconazole, cyclophosphamide, PPIs, haloperidol, lidocaine, medroxyprogesterone, methadone, methylprednisolone, salmeterol, theophylline, quetiapine, ritonavir, indinavir, sildenafil, ivacaftor	Erythromycin, cimetidine, clarithromycin, isoniazid, ketoconazole, itraconazole, metronidazole, sertraline, ritonavir, indinavir, imatinib, nicardipine, propofol, quinidine	Rifampin, (fos)phenytoin, phenobarbital, carbamazepine, dexamethasone, lumacaftor

NOTE: The cytochrome P450 enzyme system is composed of different isoenzymes. Each isoenzyme metabolizes a unique group of drugs or substrates. When an *inhibitor* of a particular isoenzyme is introduced, the serum concentration of any drug or substrate metabolized by that particular isoenzyme will *increase*. When an *inducer* of a particular isoenzyme is introduced, the serum concentration of drugs or substrates metabolized by that particular isoenzyme will *decrease*.

CYP450, Cytochrome P450; PPI, proton pump inhibitor.

*Only strong and some moderate inhibitors are listed here. Weak inhibitors also exist.

Data from Taketomo CK, Hodding JH, Kraus DM, American Pharmaceutical Association Pediatric Dosage Handbook. 16th ed. Hudson, OH: Lexi-Comp; 2009. Zevin S, Benowitz NL. Drug interactions with tobacco smoking. An update. Clin Pharmacokinet. 1999;36:425-438. Cupp MJ, Tracy TS. Cytochrome P450: new nomenclature and clinical implications. Am Fam Physician. 1998;57:107-116.

ACETAMINOPHEN
Tylenol, Tempra, Panadol, Feverall, Anacin Aspirin Free,
Paracetamol, Ofirmev, and many others
Analgesic, antipyretic

Yes   Yes   1   C

Tabs [OTC]: 325, 500, 650 mg
Chewable tabs [OTC]: 80 mg; some may contain phenylalanine
Infant drops, solution/suspension [OTC]: 80 mg/0.8 mL
Child suspension/syrup [OTC]: 160 mg/5 mL; may contain sodium benzoate
Oral liquid [OTC]: 160 mg/5 mL; may contain sodium benzoate and propylene glycol
Elixir [OTC]: 160 mg/5 mL; may contain sodium benzoate and propylene glycol
Caplet [OTC]: 160, 500, 650 mg
Extended-release caplet [OTC]: 650 mg
Gelcap [OTC]: 325 mg
Capsules [OTC]: 500 mg
Dispersible tabs (Tylenol Children's Meltaways) [OTC]: 80, 160 mg; contains sucralose
Suppositories [OTC]: 80, 120, 325, 650 mg
Injection:
  Ofirmev: 10 mg/mL (100 mL); preservative free

PO/PR:
  Neonate: 10–15 mg/kg/dose PO/PR Q6–8 hr. Some advocate loading doses of 20–25 mg/kg/dose for PO dosing or 30 mg/kg/dose for PR dosing
  Pediatric: 10–15 mg/kg/dose PO/PR Q4–6 hr; **max. dose:** 90 mg/kg/24 hr or 4 g/24 hr. For rectal dosing, some may advocate a 40–45 mg/kg/dose loading dose

Dosing by weight (preferred) or age (PO/PR Q4–6 hr):

Weight (lbs)	Weight (kg)	Age	Dosage (mg)
6–11	2.7–5	0–3 mo	40
12–17	5.1–7.7	4–11 mo	80
18–23	7.8–10.5	1–2 yr	120
24–35	10.6–15.9	2–3 yr	160
36–47	16–21.4	4–5 yr	240
48–59	21.5–26.8	6–8 yr	320
60–71	26.9–32.3	9–10 yr	400
72–95	32.4–43.2	11 yr	480

Adult: 325–650 mg/dose
Max. dose: 4 g/24 hr, 5 doses/24 hr

IV:
  Infant and child < 2 yr: Labeled dosing from the UK and pharmacokinetic studies recommend 7.5–15 mg/kg/dose Q6 hr IV up to a **maximum** of 60 mg/kg/24 hr (see Pediatric Anesthesia 2009;19:329–337). A phase 3 study is currently in progress in children aged <2 yr
  See www.clinicaltrials.gov for updated information.
  Child (≥2 –12 yr) and adolescent/adult < 50 kg: 15 mg/kg/dose Q6 hr, **OR** 12.5 mg/kg/dose Q4 hr IV up to a **maximum** of 75 mg/kg/24 hr up to 3750 mg/24 hr
  Adolescent and adult (≥ 50 kg): 1000 mg Q6 hr, **OR** 650 mg Q4 hr up to a **maximum** of 4000 mg/24 hr

Does not possess antiinflammatory activity. **Use with caution** in patients with known G6PD deficiency.
$T_{1/2}$: 1–3 hr, 2–5 hr in neonates; metabolized in the liver; see Chapter 2 and acetylcysteine for management of drug overdose.

Continued

ACETAMINOPHEN continued

Some preparations contain alcohol (7%–10%) and/or phenylalanine; all suspensions should be shaken before use.

May decrease the activity of lamotrigine and increase the activity/toxicity of busulfan, warfarin, and zidovudine. Barbiturates, phenytoin, rifampin, and anticholinergic agents (e.g., scopolamine) may decrease the effect of acetaminophen. Increased risk for hepatotoxicity may occur with barbiturates, carbamazepine, phenytoin, carmustine (with high acetaminophen doses), and chronic alcohol use. **Adjust dose in renal failure (see Chapter 30).**

FOR IV USE: administer dose undiluted over 15 min. Most common side effects with IV use include nausea, vomiting, constipation, pruritus, agitation, and atelectasis in children and nausea, vomiting, headache, and insomnia in adults. Rare risk of serious skin reactions (e.g., SJS, TEN) has been reported.

ACETAZOLAMIDE
Diamox and generics
Carbonic anhydrase inhibitor, diuretic

Yes Yes 1 C

Tabs: 125, 250 mg
Oral suspension: 25 mg/mL
Capsules (extended release): 500 mg
Injection (sodium): 500 mg
Contains 2.05 mEq Na/500 mg drug

Diuretic (PO, IV)
  Child: 5 mg/kg/dose once daily or every other day
  Adult: 250–375 mg/dose once daily or every other day
Glaucoma
  Child:
    PO: 8–30 mg/kg/24 hr ÷ Q6–8 hr; **max. dose:** 1000 mg/24 hr
    IM/IV: 20–40 mg/kg/24 hr ÷ Q6 hr; **max. dose:** 1000 mg/24 hr
  Adult:
    PO (Simple chronic; open-angle): 1000 mg/24 hr ÷ Q6 hr
    IV (Acute secondary; closed-angle): For rapid decrease in intraocular pressure, administer 500 mg/dose IV
Seizures (extended-release product not recommended):
  Child and adult: 8–30 mg/kg/24 hr ÷ Q6–12 hr PO; **max. dose:** 1 g/24 hr
Urine alkalinization:
  Adult: 5 mg/kg/dose PO repeated BID–TID over 24 hr
Management of hydrocephalus (see remarks): Start with 20 mg/kg/24 hr ÷ Q8 hr PO/IV; may increase to 100 mg/kg/24 hr up to a **max. dose** of 2 g/24 hr
Pseudotumor cerebri (PO; see remarks):
  Child: Start with 25 mg/kg/24 hr ÷ once daily–QID, increase by 25 mg/kg/24 hr until clinical response or as tolerated up to a **maximum** of 100 mg/kg/24 hr
  Adolescent: Start with 1 g/24 hr ÷ once daily–QID, increase by 250 mg/24 hr until clinical response or as tolerated up to a **maximum** of 4 g/24 hr

Contraindicated in hepatic failure, severe renal failure (GFR < 10 mL/min), and hypersensitivity to sulfonamides.

ACETAZOLAMIDE continued

$T_{1/2}$: 2–6 hr; **do not use** sustained-release capsules in seizures; IM injection may be painful; bicarbonate replacement therapy may be required during long-term use (see *Citrate* or *Sodium Bicarbonate*). For use in Pseudotumor cerebri, doses of 60 mg/kg/24 hr may be required.

Possible side effects (more likely with long-term therapy) include GI irritation, paresthesias, sedation, hypokalemia, acidosis, reduced urate secretion, aplastic anemia, polyuria, and development of renal calculi.

May increase toxicity of carbamazepine and cyclosporine. Aspirin may increase toxicity of acetazolamide. May decrease the effects of salicylates, lithium, and phenobarbital. False-positive urinary protein may occur with several assays. **Adjust dose in renal failure (see Chapter 30).**

ACETYLCYSTEINE
Various generics, Acetadote, previously available as Mucomyst
Mucolytic, antidote for acetaminophen toxicity

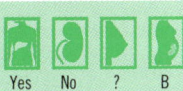
Yes   No   ?   B

Solution for inhalation or oral use: 100 mg/mL (10%) (10, 30 mL) or 200 mg/mL (20%) (4, 10, 30 mL); may contain EDTA.
Injectable (Acetadote): 200 mg/mL (20%) (30 mL); may contain EDTA 0.5 mg/mL
Preservative-free versions of the inhalation and oral solutions and injectable forms exist.

Acetaminophen poisoning (see Chapter 2 for additional information):
  PO: 140 mg/kg × 1, followed by 70 mg/kg/dose Q4 hr for a total of 17 doses. Repeat dose if vomiting occurs within 1 hr of administration
  IV: 150 mg/kg ×1 diluted in D_5W or D_5W ½ NS administered over 60 min, followed by 50 mg/kg diluted in D_5W administered over 4 hr, then 100 mg/kg diluted in D_5W administered over 16 hr.
Recommended weight-based drug dilution volumes:

Weight (kg)	Volume of D_5W or D_5W ½NS for 150 mg/kg Loading Dose Administered Over 60 Minutes	Volume of D_5W for 50 mg/kg Second Dose Administered Over 4 Hours	Volume of D_5W for 100 mg/kg Third Dose Administered Over 16 Hours
≤20	3 mL/kg	7 mL/kg	14 mL/kg
>20–<40	100 mL	250 mL	500 mL
≥40	200 mL	500 mL	1000 mL

Nebulizer:
  Infant: 1–2 mL of 20% solution (diluted with equal volume of H_2O, or sterile saline to equal 10%), or 2–4 mL of 10% solution; administered TID–QID
  Child: 3–5 mL of 20% solution (diluted with equal volume of H_2O, or sterile saline to equal 10%), or 6–10 mL of 10% solution; administer TID–QID
  Adolescent: 5–10 mL of 10% or 20% solution; administer TID–QID
Distal intestinal obstruction syndrome in cystic fibrosis:
  Adolescent and adult: 10 mL of 20% solution (diluted in a sweet drink) PO QID with 100 mL of 10% solution PR as an enema once daily–QID

Use with caution in asthma. For nebulized use, give inhaled bronchodilator 10–15 min before use and follow with postural drainage and/or suctioning after acetylcysteine administration. Prior hydration is essential for distal intestinal obstruction syndrome treatment.

May induce bronchospasm, stomatitis, drowsiness, rhinorrhea, nausea, vomiting, and hemoptysis. Anaphylactoid reactions have been reported with IV use.

Continued

ACETYLCYSTEINE continued

For IV use, elimination $T_{1/2}$ is longer in newborns (11 hr) than in adults (5.6 hr). $T_{1/2}$ is increased by 80% in patients with severe liver damage (Child-Pugh score of 7–13) and biliary cirrhosis (Child-Pugh score of 5–7).

For oral administration, chilling the solution and mixing with carbonated beverages, orange juice, or sweet drinks may enhance palatability.

ACTH

See Corticotropin

ACYCLOVIR
Zovirax and generics
Antiviral

No Yes 1 B

Capsules: 200 mg
Tabs: 400, 800 mg
Oral suspension: 200 mg/5 mL; may contain parabens
Ointment: 5% (5, 15, 30 g)
Cream: 5% (5 g); may contain propylene glycol
Injection in powder (with sodium): 500, 1000 mg
Injection in solution (with sodium): 50 mg/mL (10, 20 mL)
Contains 4.2 mEq Na/1 g drug

IMMUNOCOMPETENT:
Neonatal (HSV and HSV encephalitis; birth–3 mo):
Initial IV therapy (duration of therapy: 14–21 days):
   <30-wk postmenstrual age: 40 mg/kg/24 hr ÷ Q12 hr IV
   ≥30-wk postmenstural age: 60 mg/kg/24 hr ÷ Q8 hr IV; a population pharmacokinetic analysis suggests using 80 mg/kg/24 hr mg/kg/24 hr ÷ Q6 hr IV for neonates 36–41-wk postmenstural age to achieve concentrations > 3 mg/L for ≥ 50% of the dosing interval

Oral therapy for HSV suppression and neurodevelopment following treatment with IV acyclovir for 14–21 days: 300 mg/m²/dose Q8 hr PO × 6 mo

HSV encephalitis (duration of therapy: 14–21 days):
   Birth–3 mo: use above IV dosage
   3 mo–12 yr: 60 mg/kg/24 hr ÷ Q8 hr IV; some experts recommend 45 mg/kg/24 hr ÷ Q8 hr IV to reduce the risk of neurotoxicity and nephrotoxicity
   ≥12 yr: 30 mg/kg/24 hr ÷ Q8 hr IV

Mucocutaneous HSV (including genital, ≥12 yr):
Initial infection:
   IV: 15 mg/kg/24 hr or 750 mg/m²/24 hr ÷ Q8 hr × 5– 7 days
   PO: 1000–1200 mg/24 hr ÷ 3–5 doses per 24 hr × 7–10 days. For pediatric dosing, use 40–80 mg/kg/24 hr ÷ Q6–8 hr × 5–10 days (**max. pediatric dose:** 1000 mg/24 hr)

Recurrence (≥ 12 yr):
   PO: 1000 mg/24 hr ÷ 5 doses per 24 hr × 5 days, or 1600 mg/24 hr ÷ Q12 hr × 5 days, or 2400 mg/24 hr ÷ Q8 hr × 2 days

Chronic suppressive therapy (≥ 12 yr):
   PO: 800 mg/24 hr ÷ Q12 hr for up to 1 year

ACYCLOVIR continued

Zoster:
IV (all ages): 30 mg/kg/24 hr or 1500 mg/m^2/24 hr ÷ Q8 hr × 7–10 days
PO (≥12 yr): 4000 mg/24 hr ÷ 5×/24 hr × 5–7 days

Varicella:
IV (≥2 yr): 30 mg/kg/24 hr or 1500 mg/m^2/24 hr ÷ Q8 hr × 7–10 days
PO (≥2 yr): 80 mg/kg/24 hr ÷ QID × 5 days (begin treatment at earliest signs/symptoms); **max. dose:** 3200 mg/24 hr

Max. dose of oral acyclovir in children = 80 mg/kg/24 hr

IMMUNOCOMPROMISED:

HSV:
IV (all ages): 750–1500 mg/m^2/24 hr ÷ Q8 hr × 7–14 days
PO (≥2 yr): 1000 mg/24 hr ÷ 3–5 times/24 hr × 7–14 days; **max. dose** for child: 80 mg/kg/24 hr

HSV prophylaxis:
IV (all ages): 750 mg/m^2/24 hr ÷ Q8 hr during risk period
PO (≥2 yr): 600–1000 mg/24 hr ÷ 3–5 times/24 hr during risk period; **max. dose** for child: 80 mg/kg/24 hr

Varicella or zoster:
IV (all ages): 1500 mg/m^2/24 hr ÷ Q8 hr × 7–10 days
PO (consider using valacyclovir or famciclovir for better absorption):
    Infant and child: 20 mg/kg/dose (**max.** 800 mg) Q6 hr × 7–10 days
    Adolescent and adult: 20 mg/kg/dose (**max.** 800 mg) 5 times daily × 7–10 days

Max. dose of oral acyclovir in children = 80 mg/kg/24 hr

TOPICAL:

Cream (see remarks):
Herpes labialis (≥12 and adult): Apply to affected areas 5 times a day × 4 days

Ointment:
Immunocompromised genital or mucocutaneous HSV: Apply 0.5-inch ribbon of 5% ointment for 4-inch square surface area 6 times a day × 7 days

---

See most recent edition of the AAP Red Book for further details. Use with **caution** in patients with preexisting neurologic or **renal impairment (adjust dose; see Chapter 30)** or dehydration. Adequate hydration and slow (1 hr) IV administration are essential to prevent crystallization in renal tubules. **Do not use** topical product on the eye or for the prevention of recurrent HSV infections. Oral absorption is unpredictable (15%–30%); consider using valacyclovir or famciclovir for better absorption. Use ideal body weight for obese patients when calculating dosages. Resistant strains of HSV and VZV have been reported in immunocompromised patients (e.g., advanced HIV infection).

Can cause renal impairment; has been infrequently associated with headache, vertigo, insomnia, encephalopathy, GI tract irritation, elevated liver function tests, rash, urticaria, arthralgia, fever, and adverse hematologic effects. Probenecid decreases acyclovir renal clearance. Acyclovir may increase the concentration of tenofovir and of meperidine and its metabolite (normeperidine).

Topical cream acyclovir 5% in combination with hydrocortisone 1% (Xerese) is indicated for herpes labialis (≥ 6 yr and adults) at a dosage of 5 applications per day for 5 days.

ADAPALENE ± BENZOYL PEROXIDE
Differin and generics
In combination with benzoyl peroxide: Epiduo, Epiduo Forte
Synthetic retinoic acid derivative; topical acne product

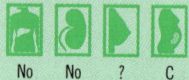
No   No   ?   C

Topical cream: 0.1% (45 g)
Topical gel: 0.1% [OTC], 0.3% (45 g); some preparations may contain methylparabens and propylene glycol
Topical lotion: 0.1% (59 mL); some preparations may contain methylparabens and propylene glycol
Topical solution as a swab: 0.1% (1.2 g per swab; 60 units of swabs per box)
In combination with benzoyl peroxide:
  Epiduo: 0.1% adapalene + 2.5% benzoyl peroxide (45 g)
  Epiduo Forte: 0.3% adapalene + 2.5% benzoyl peroxide (15, 30, 45, 60, 70 g)

Adapalene (≥12 yr and adult): Apply a thin film of cream, gel or lotion to affected areas of cleansed and dried skin QHS
Adapalene and benzoyl peroxide: Apply a thin film to affected areas of cleansed and dried skin once daily
  Epiduo: Indicated for children ≥ 9 yr and adults with limited data in children 7–< 9 yr
  Epiduo Forte: Indicated for children ≥ 12 yr and adults

Avoid contact with eyes, mucous membranes, abraded skin, and open wounds; excessive sun exposure; and use of other irritating topical products. A mild transitory warm or stinging sensation of the skin may occur during the first 4 weeks of use. Clean and dry the skin before each use.

ADAPALENE: Onset of therapeutic benefits seen in 8–12 weeks. Common side effects include dry skin, erythema, and scaly skin. When compared to tretinoin in clinical trials for acne vulgaris, adapalene was as effective and had a more rapid onset of clinical effects with less skin irritation.

ADAPALENE + BENZOYL PEROXIDE: Onset of therapeutic benefits seen in 4–8 weeks. Side effects reported in placebo-controlled studies include dry skin, erythema, skin irritation, and contact dermatitis. When compared to isotretinoin in a clinical trial for nodulocystic acne, adapalene+benzoyl peroxide plus doxycycline was not inferior to isotretinoin and was less effective in reducing the number of total lesions (nodules, papules/pustules, and comedones).

ADDERALL

See Dextroamphetamine ± Amphetamine

ADENOSINE
Adenocard and generics
Antiarrhythmic

No   No   ?   C

Injection: 3 mg/mL (2, 4 mL); preservative free

Supraventricular tachycardia:
  Neonate: 0.05 mg/kg by rapid IV push over 1–2 seconds; may increase dose by 0.05-mg/kg increments every 2 min to **max** of 0.25 mg/kg.
  Child: 0.1–0.2 mg/kg (initial **max. dose:** 6 mg) by rapid IV push over 1–2 seconds; may increase dose by 0.05-mg/kg increments every 2 min to a **max.** of 0.25 mg/kg (up to 12 mg), or until termination of SVT. **Max. subsequent single dose:** 12 mg.

ADENOSINE continued

Adolescent and adults ≥ 50 kg: 6 mg rapid IV push over 1–2 seconds; if no response after 1–2 min, give 12-mg rapid IV push. May repeat a second 12-mg dose after 1–2 min if required.
Max. single dose: 12 mg.

Contraindicated in 2nd- and 3rd-degree AV block or sick-sinus syndrome unless pacemaker placed. **Use with caution** in combination with digoxin (enhanced depressant effects on SA and AV nodes). If necessary, doses may be administered IO.
Follow each dose with NS flush. $T_{1/2}$: <10 seconds.
May precipitate bronchoconstriction, especially in asthmatics. Side effects include transient asystole, facial flushing, headache, shortness of breath, dyspnea, nausea, chest pain, and lightheadedness.
Carbamazepine and dipyridamole may increase the effects/toxicity of adenosine. Methylxanthines (e.g., caffeine and theophylline) may decrease the effects of adenosine.

ALBUMIN, HUMAN
Albuminar, Albutein, Buminate, Plasbumin, Normal Serum
Albumin (human), and many others
Blood product derivative, plasma volume expander

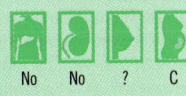

No   No   ?   C

Injection: 5% (50 mg/mL) (50, 100, 250, 500, mL); 25% (250 mg/mL) (20, 50, 100 mL); both concentrations contain 130–160 mEq Na/L

Hypoalbuminemia:
 Child: 0.5–1 g/kg/dose IV over 30–120 min; repeat Q1–2 days PRN
 Adult: 25 g/dose IV over 30–120 min; repeat Q1–2 days PRN
 Max. dose: 2 g/kg/24 hr
Hypovolemia:
 Child: 0.5–1 g/kg/dose IV rapid infusion; may repeat PRN; **max. dose:** 6 g/kg/24 hr
 Adult: 25 g/dose IV rapid infusion; may repeat PRN; **max. dose:** 250 g/48 hr

Contraindicated in cases of CHF or severe anemia; rapid infusion may cause fluid overload; hypersensitivity reactions may occur; may cause rapid increase in serum sodium levels.
Caution: 25% concentration contraindicated in preterm infants due to risk of IVH. For infusion, use 5-micron filter or larger. Both 5% and 25% products are isotonic but differ in oncotic effects. Dilutions of the 25% product should be made with D_5W or NS; **avoid sterile water as a diluent.**

ALBUTEROL
VoSpire ER (sustained-release tabs); ProAir HFA, Proventil
HFA Ventolin HFA (aerosol inhaler); ProAir RespiClick (breath activated aerosol powder inhaler); AccuNeb (prediluted nebulized solution); and many generics
$β_2$-adrenergic agonist

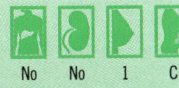

No   No   1   C

Tabs: 2, 4 mg
Sustained-release tabs: 4, 8 mg
Oral solution: 2 mg/5 mL (473 mL)
Aerosol inhaler (HFA): 90 mcg/actuation (60 actuations/inhaler) (8.5 g)
Breath-activated aerosol powder inhaler: 90 mcg/actuation (200 actuations/inhaler) (0.65 g)
Nebulization solution (dilution required): 0.5% (5 mg/mL) (0.5, 20 mL)
Prediluted nebulized solution: 0.63 mg in 3 mL NS, 1.25 mg in 3 mL NS, and 2.5 mg in 3 mL NS (0.083%); some preparations may be preservative free

Continued

ALBUTEROL continued

Inhalations (nonacute use; see remarks):
   Aerosol (HFA): 2 puffs (90 mcg) Q4–6 hr PRN
   Nebulization:
     <1 yr: 0.05–0.15 mg/kg/dose Q4–6 hr
     1–5 yr: 1.25–2.5 mg/dose Q4–6 hr
     5–12 yr: 2.5 mg/dose Q4–6 hr
     >12 yr: 2.5–5 mg/dose Q4–8 hr
For use in acute exacerbations more aggressive dosing may be employed.
Oral (highly discouraged—see remarks):
   2–6 yr: 0.3 mg/kg/24 hr PO ÷ TID; **max. dose:** 12 mg/24 hr
   6–12 yr: 6 mg/24 hr PO ÷ TID; **max. dose:** 24 mg/24 hr
   >12 yr and adult: 2–4 mg/dose PO TID–QID; **max. dose:** 32 mg/24 hr

Inhaled doses may be given more frequently than indicated. In such cases, consider cardiac monitoring and serum potassium (hypokalemia) monitoring. Systemic effects are dose related. Please verify the concentration of the nebulization solution used.

Safety and efficacy of the treatment for symptoms or bronchospasms associated with obstructive airway disease have not been demonstrated for children aged <4 yr (either the dose studied was not optimal in this age or the drug is not effective in this age group).

Use of oral dosage form is discouraged due to increased side effects and decreased efficacy compared to inhaled formulations.

Possible side effects include tachycardia, palpitations, tremors, insomnia, nervousness, nausea, and headache.

The use of tube spacers or chambers may enhance efficacy of the metered dose inhalers and have been proven to be just as effective and sometimes safer than nebulizers.

ALLOPURINOL
Zyloprim, Aloprim, and generics
Uric acid–lowering agent, xanthine oxidase inhibitor

Yes   Yes   2   C

Tabs: 100, 300 mg
Oral suspension: 20 mg/mL
Injection (Aloprim): 500 mg
Contains ~ 1.45 mEq Na/500 mg drug

For use in tumor lysis syndrome, see Chapter 22 for additional information.
Child:
   Oral: 10 mg/kg/24 hr PO ÷ BID–QID; **max. dose:** 800 mg/24 hr
   Injectable: 200 mg/m^2/24 hr IV ÷ Q6–12 hr; **max. dose:** 600 mg/24 hr
Adult:
   Oral: 200–800 mg/24 hr PO ÷ BID–TID
   Injectable: 200–400 mg/m^2/24 hr IV ÷ Q6–12 hr; **max. dose:** 600 mg/24 hr

Adjust dose in renal insufficiency (see Chapter 30). Must maintain adequate urine output and alkaline urine.

Drug interactions: increases serum theophylline level; may increase the incidence of rash with ampicillin and amoxicillin; increased risk of toxicity with azathioprine, didanosine and mercaptopurine; and increased risk of hypersensitivity reactions with ACE inhibitors and thiazide diuretics. Use with didanosine is **contraindicated** due to increased risk for didanosine toxicity. Rhabdomyolysis has been reported with clarithromycin use.

ALLOPURINOL continued

Side effects include rash, neuritis, hepatotoxicity, GI disturbance, bone marrow suppression, and drowsiness.

IV dosage form is very alkaline and must be **diluted to a minimum concentration** of 6 mg/mL and infused over 30 min.

ALMOTRIPTAN MALATE
Axert and generics
Antimigraine agent, selective serotonin agonist

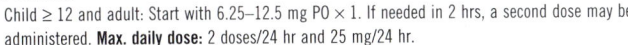

Yes   Yes   3   C

Tabs: 6.25, 12.5 mg

Treatment of acute migraines with or without aura:
Oral (safety of an average of >4 headaches in a 30-day period has not been established; see remarks):
Child ≥ 12 and adult: Start with 6.25–12.5 mg PO × 1. If needed in 2 hrs, a second dose may be administered. **Max. daily dose:** 2 doses/24 hr and 25 mg/24 hr.

Contraindicated in ischemic/vasospastic coronary artery disease, significant underlying cardiovascular disease, cerebrovascular syndromes, peripheral vascular disease, uncontrolled hypertension, or hemiplegic/basilar migrane. **Do not** administer with any ergotamine-containing medication ergot-type medication, any other 5-HT$_1$ agonist (e.g., triptans), methylene blue, or with/within 2 weeks of discontinuing a MAO inhibitor or linezolid.

FDA labeled indication for adolescents is acute migrane treatment in patients with a history of migraine lasting ≥4 hrs when left untreated. Efficacy for the treatment of migrane associated symptoms of nausea, photophobia, and phonophobia were not established for adolescents.

Most common side effects include dizziness, somnolence, headache, paresthesia, nausea and vomiting. Reported serious adverse effects include coronary artery spasm, ischemia (myocardial, gastrointestinal, peripheral vascular), cerebral/subarachnoid hemorrhage, cerebrovascular accident/disease, and vision loss.

Use with **caution** in renal impairment (CrCl ≤ 30 mL/min)or hepatic impairment; use initial dose of 6.25 mg dose with a max. daily dose of 12.5 mg/24 hr.

Alotriptan is a minor substrate for CYP 450 2D6 and 3A4. Use lower initial single dose of 6.25 mg with maximum daily dose of 12.5 mg if receiving a potent CYP 450 3A4 inhibitor (e.g., ritonavir).

Doses may be administered with or without food.

ALPROSTADIL
Prostin VR Pediatric, Prostaglandin E$_1$, PGE$_1$
Prostaglandin E$_1$, vasodilator

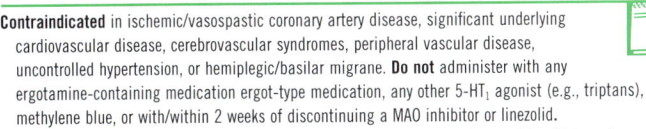

No   No   ?   ?

Injection: 500 mcg/mL (1 mL); contains dehydrated alcohol

Neonate:
Initial: 0.05–0.1 mcg/kg/min. Advance to 0.2 mcg/kg/min if necessary.
Maintenance: When increase in PaO$_2$ is noted, decrease immediately to lowest effective dose. Usual dosage range: 0.01–0.4 mcg/kg/min; doses above 0.4 mcg/kg/min not likely to produce additional benefit.
To prepare infusion: see inside front cover.

Continued

ALPROSTADIL continued

For palliation only. Continuous vital sign monitoring essential. May cause apnea (10%–12%; especially in those weighing < 2 kg at birth), fever, seizures, flushing, bradycardia, hypotension, diarrhea, gastric outlet obstruction, and reversible cortical proliferation of long bones (with prolonged use). May decrease platelet aggregation.

ALTEPLASE
Activase, Cathflo Activase, tPA
Thrombolytic agent, tissue plasminogen activator

Yes   Yes   ?   C

Injection:
  Cathflo Activase: 2 mg
  Activase: 50 mg (29 million units), 100 mg (58 million units)
  Contains: L-arginine and polysorbate 80

Occluded IV catheter:
Aspiration method: Use 1 mg/1 mL concentration as follows:
  Central venous line (dosage per lumen, treating one lumen at a time):
    <30 kg: Instill a volume equal to 110% of internal lumen volume of the catheter **NOT exceeding** 2 mg.
    ≥30 kg: 2 mg each lumen.
  Subcutaneous port: Instill a volume equal to 110% of internal lumen and line volume of the port **NOT exceeding** 2 mg.
Instill into catheter over 1–2 min and leave in place for 2 hr before attempting blood withdrawal. After 2 hr, attempts to withdraw blood may be made every 2 hr for three attempts. Dose may be repeated once in 24 hr using a longer catheter dwell time of 3–4 hr. After 3–4 hr (repeat dose), attempts to withdraw blood may be made every 2 hr for three attempts. **DO NOT** infuse into patient.
Systemic thrombolytic therapy (use in consultation with a hematologist; see remarks): dosage regimens ranging from lower dosages (0.01 mg/kg/hr) to higher dosages (0.1–0.6 mg/kg/hr) have been reported (Chest 2008;133:887–968S). The length of continuous infusion is variable as patients may respond to longer or shorter courses of therapy.

Current use in the pediatric population is limited. May cause bleeding, rash, and increased prothrombin time.
THROMBOLYTIC USE: History of stroke, transient ischemic attacks, other neurologic disease, and hypertension are **contraindications for adults** but considered **relative contraindications for children**. Monitor fibrinogen, thrombin clotting time, PT and aPTT when used as a thrombolytic. For systemic thrombosis therapy, efficacy has been reported at 40%–97%, with the risk for bleeding at 3%–27%. Poor efficacy in VTE in children has been recently reported. **Use with caution** in severe hepatic or renal dysfunction (systemic use only).
Newborns have reduced plasminogen levels (~50% of adult values), which decrease the thrombolytic effects of alteplase. Plasminogen supplementation may be necessary.

ALUMINUM HYDROXIDE
Amphojel and various generics
Antacid, phosphate binder

No Yes ? ?

Oral suspension [OTC]: 320 mg/5 mL (473 mL)
Each 5-mL suspension contains <0.13 mEq Na.

Antacid:
  Child: 320–960 mg PO 1–3 hr PC and HS
  Adult: 640 mg PO 1–3 hr PC and HS; **max. dose:** 3840 mg/24 hr
Hyperphosphatemia (administer all doses between meals and titrate to normal serum phosphorus):
  Child: 50–150 mg/kg/24 hr ÷ Q4–6 hr PO
  Adult: 300–600 mg TID–QID PO between meals and QHS
  Max. dose (all ages): 3000 mg/24 hr

Chronic antacid use is not recommended for children with GERD. **Use with caution** in patients with renal failure and upper GI hemorrhage.
Interferes with the absorption of several orally administered medications, including digoxin, ethambutol, indomethacin, isoniazid, naproxen, mycophenolate, tetracyclines, fluoroquinolones (eg., ciprofloxacin), and iron. In general, **do not** take oral medications within 1–2 hrs of taking aluminum dose, unless specified.
May cause constipation, decreased bowel motility, encephalopathy, and phosphorus depletion.

ALUMINUM HYDROXIDE WITH MAGNESIUM HYDROXIDE
Maalox, Maalox Maximum Strength Liquid, Mylanta, Mylanta Maximum Strength, Mylanta Ultimate Strength, Almacone Antacid Antigas, Almacone Double Strength, RuLox, and many others generics (see remarks)
Antacid

No Yes ? ?

Chewable tabs [OTC]: (Al (OH)$_3$: Mg (OH)$_2$)
  Almacone: 200 mg AlOH, 200 mg MgOH, and 20 mg simethicone
Oral suspension [OTC] (see remarks):
  Maalox, Mylanta, Almacone Antacid Antigas, and RuLox: each 5 mL contains 200 mg AlOH, 200 mg MgOH, and 20 mg simethicone (150, 360, 720 mL)
  Mylanta Maximum Strength, Maalox Maximum Strength liquid, and Almacone Double Strength: each 5 mL contains 400 mg AlOH, 400 mg MgOH, and 40 mg simethicone (360, 480 mL)
  Mylanta Ultimate Strength: each 5 mL contains 500 mg AlOH, 500 mg MgOH (360 mL)
  Many other combinations exist.
  Contains 0.03–0.06 mEq Na/5 mL

Antacid (mL volume dosages are based on the 200 mg AlOH, 200 mg MgOH, and 20 mg simethicone per 5 mL oral suspension concentration):
  Child ≤ 12 yr: 0.5–1 mL/kg/dose (**max. dose:** 20 mL/dose) PO 1–3 hr PC and HS
  >12 yr and adult: 10–20 mL PO 1–3 hr PC and HS; **max. dose:** 80 mL/24 hr

Chronic antacid use is not recommended for children with GERD. May have laxative effect. May cause hypokalemia. **Use with caution** in patients with renal insufficiency (magnesium) and gastric outlet obstruction. **Do not use** for hyperphosphatemia.

Continued

ALUMINUM HYDROXIDE WITH MAGNESIUM HYDROXIDE continued

Interferes with the absorption of the benzodiazepines, chloroquine, digoxin, naproxen, mycophenolate, phenytoin, quinolones (eg. ciprofloxacin), tetracyclines, and iron. In general, do not take oral medications within 1–2 hr of taking an antacid dose, unless specified.

DO NOT use Maalox Total Relief (bismuth subsalicylate), Mylanta Supreme Liquid (calcium carbonate + magnesium hydroxide), Maalox Regular Strength Chewable Tablets and Children's Mylanta Chewable Tablets (calcium carbonate), Maalox Maximum Strength Chewable (calcium carbonate and simethicone), and Mylanta Gas (simethicone) as these products do not contain aluminum hydroxide and magnesium hydroxide.

AMANTADINE HYDROCHLORIDE
Symmetrel and other generics
Antiviral agent

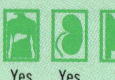
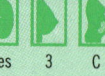

Yes   Yes   3   C

Capsule: 100 mg
Tabs: 100 mg
Oral solution or syrup: 50 mg/5 mL (480 mL); may contain parabens

Influenza A prophylaxis and treatment (for treatment, it is best to initiate therapy immediately after the onset of symptoms; within 2 days; see remarks):
 1–9 yr: 5 mg/kg/24 hr PO ÷ BID; **max. dose:** 150 mg/24 hr
 ≥10 yr:
  <40 kg: 5 mg/kg/24 hr PO ÷ BID; **max. dose** 200 mg/24 hr
  ≥40 kg: 200 mg/24 hr ÷ BID
Duration of therapy:
 Prophylaxis:
  Single exposure: at least 10 days
  Repeated/uncontrolled exposure: up to 90 days
  Use with influenza A vaccine when possible.
 Symptomatic treatment:
  Continue for 24–48 hr after disappearance of symptoms.

Do not use in the first trimester of pregnancy. **Use with caution** in patients with liver disease, seizures, renal disease, congestive heart failure, peripheral edema, orthostatic hypotension, history of recurrent eczematoid rash, and in those receiving CNS stimulants. **Adjust dose in patients with renal insufficiency (see Chapter 30).**

CDC has reported resistance to influenza A and does not recommend its use for treatment and prophylaxis. Check with local microbiology laboratories and the CDC for seasonal susceptibility/resistance. Individuals immunized with live attenuated influenza vaccine should not receive amantadine prophylaxis for 14 days after the vaccine.

May cause dizziness, anxiety, depression, mental status change, rash (livedo reticularis), nausea, orthostatic hypotension, edema, CHF, and urinary retention. Impulse control disorder has been reported. Neuroleptic malignant syndrome has been reported with abrupt dose reduction or discontinuation (especially if patient is receiving neuroleptics).

AMIKACIN SULFATE
Amikin and many generics
Antibiotic, aminoglycoside

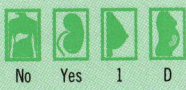
No   Yes   1   D

Injection: 250 mg/mL (2, 4 mL); may contain sodium bisulfite

Initial empirical dosage; patient specific dosage defined by therapeutic drug monitoring (see remarks).

Neonates: See the following table.

Postconceptional Age (wk)	Postnatal Age (days)	Dose (mg/kg/dose)	Interval (hr)
≤29*	0–7	18	48
	8–28	15	36
	>28	15	24
30–34	0–7	18	36
	>7	15	24
≥35	ALL	15	24[†]

*Or significant asphyxia, PDA, indomethacin use, poor cardiac output, reduced renal function.
[†]Use Q36 hr interval for HIE patients receiving whole-body therapeutic cooling.

Infant and child: 15–22.5 mg/kg/24 hr ÷ Q8 hr IV/IM; infants and patients requiring higher doses (eg., cystic fibrosis) may receive initial doses of 30 mg/kg/24 hr ÷ Q8 hr IV/IM
Cystic fibrosis (if available, use patient's previous therapeutic mg/kg dosage):
  Conventional Q8 hr dosing: 30 mg/kg/24 hr ÷ Q8 hr IV
  High-dose extended-interval (once daily) dosing (limited data): 30–35 mg/kg/24 hr Q24 hr IV
Adult: 15 mg/kg/24 hr ÷ Q8–12 hr IV/IM
Initial max. dose: 1.5 g/24 hr, then monitor levels

Use with **caution** in preexisting renal, vestibular, or auditory impairment; concomitant anesthesia or neuromuscular blockers; neurotoxic, concomitant neurotoxic, ototoxic, or nephrotoxic drugs; sulfite sensitivity; and dehydration. **Adjust dose in renal failure (see Chapter 30).** Longer dosing intervals may be necessary for neonates receiving indomethacin for PDAs and for all patients with poor cardiac output. Rapidly eliminated in patients with cystic fibrosis, burns, and in febrile neutropenic patients. CNS penetration is poor beyond early infancy.

Therapeutic levels (using conventional dosing): peak, 20–30 mg/L; trough, 5–10 mg/L. Recommended serum sampling time at steady state: trough within 30 min before the third consecutive dose and peak 30–60 minutes after the administration of the third consecutive dose. Peak levels of 25–30 mg/L have been recommended for CNS, pulmonary, bone, life-threatening, and *Pseudomonas* infections and in febrile neutropenic patients.

Therapeutic levels for cystic fibrosis using high-dose extended-interval (once daily) dosing: peak, 80–120 mg/L; trough, <10 mg/L. Recommended serum sampling time: trough within 30 minutes before the dose and peak 30–60 minutes after administration of dose.

For initial dosing in obese patients, use an adjusted body weight (ABW). ABW = Ideal Body Weight + 0.4 (Total Body Weight − Ideal Body Weight).

May cause ototoxicity, nephrotoxicity, neuromuscular blockade, and rash. Loop diuretics may potentiate the ototoxicity of all aminoglycoside antibiotics.

AMINOCAPROIC ACID
Amicar and other generics
Hemostatic agent

No   Yes   ?   C

Tabs: 500, 1000 mg
Oral liquid/syrup: 250 mg/mL (240, 480 mL); may contain 0.2% methylparaben and 0.05% propylparaben
Injection: 250 mg/mL (20 mL); contains 0.9% benzyl alcohol

Child (IV/PO):
  Loading dose: 100–200 mg/kg
  Maintenance: 100 mg/kg/dose Q4–6 hr; **max. dose:** 30 g/24 hr
Adult (IV/PO): 4–5 g during the first hour, followed by 1 g/hr × 8 hr or until bleeding is controlled.
Max. dose: 30 g/24 hr.

Contraindications: DIC, hematuria. **Use with caution** in patients with cardiac or renal disease. Should not be given with factor IX complex concentrates or antiinhibitor coagulant concentrates because of risk for thrombosis. Dose should be reduced by 75% in oliguria or end stage renal disease. Hypercoagulation may be produced when given in conjunction with oral contraceptives.

May cause nausea, diarrhea, malaise, weakness, headache, decreased platelet function, hypotension, and false increase in urine amino acids. Elevation of serum potassium may occur, especially in patients with renal impairment. Prolonged use may increase risk for skeletal muscle weakness and rhabdomyolysis.

AMINOPHYLLINE
Various generic products
Bronchodilator, methylxanthine

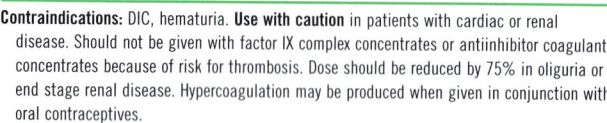
Yes   No   1   C

Injection: 25 mg/mL (79% theophylline) (10, 20 mL)
Note: Pharmacy may dilute IV dosage forms to enhance accuracy of neonatal dosing.

Neonatal apnea:
  Loading dose: 5–6 mg/kg IV
  Maintenance dose: 1–2 mg/kg/dose Q6–8 hr, IV
Asthma exacerbation and reactive airway disease:
  IV loading: 6 mg/kg IV over 20 min (each 1.2 mg/kg dose raises the serum theophylline concentration by 2 mg/L)
  IV maintenance: Continuous IV drip:
    Neonate: 0.2 mg/kg/hr
    6 wk–6 mo: 0.5 mg/kg/hr
    6 mo–1 yr: 0.6–0.7 mg/kg/hr
    1–9 yr: 1–1.2 mg/kg/hr
    9–12 yr and young adult smoker: 0.9 mg/kg/hr
    >12 yr healthy nonsmoker: 0.7 mg/kg/hr
    The above total daily doses may also be administered IV ÷ Q4–6 hr.

Consider milligrams of theophylline available when dosing aminophylline. For oral route of administration, use theophylline.
Monitoring serum levels is essential especially in infants and young children. Intermittent dosing for infants and children 1–5 yr may require Q4 hr dosing regimen due to enhanced

AMINOPHYLLINE continued

metabolism/clearance. Side effects: restlessness, GI upset, headache, tachycardia, seizures (may occur in absence of other side effects with toxic levels).

Therapeutic level (as theophylline): for asthma, 10–20 mg/L; for neonatal apnea, 6–13 mg/L.

Recommended guidelines for obtaining levels:
  IV bolus: 30 min after infusion
  IV continuous; 12–24 hr after initiation of infusion
  PO liquid, immediate-release tab (theophylline product):
    Peak: 1 hr post dose
    Trough: just before dose
  PO sustained release (theophylline product):
    Peak: 4 hr post dose
    Trough: just before dose

Ideally, obtain levels after steady state has been achieved (after at least one day of therapy). Liver impairment, cardiac failure and sustained high fever may increase theophylline levels. See *Theophylline* for drug interactions.

Use while breastfeeding may cause irritability in infant. It is recommended to avoid breastfeeding for 2 hr after IV or 4 hr after immediate-release oral intermittent dose.

AMIODARONE HCL
Cordarone, Pacerone, Nexterone, and various generics
Antiarrhythmic, Class III

Yes   No   3   D

Tabs: 100, 200, 400 mg
Oral suspension: 5 mg/mL
Injection: 50 mg/mL (3, 9, 18 mL) (contains 20.2 mg/mL benzyl alcohol and 100 mg/mL polysorbate 80 or Tween 80)
Premixed injection (Nexterone): 1.5 mg/mL (100 mL) (iso-osmotic solution; each 1 mL contains 15 mg sulfobutylether β-cyclodextrin, 0.362 mg citric acid, 0.183 mg sodium citrate, and 42.1 mg dextrose), 1.8 mg/mL (200 mL) (iso-osmotic solution; each 1 mL contains 18 mg sulfobutylether β-cyclodextrin, 0.362 mg citric acid, 0.183 mg sodium citrate, and 41.4 mg dextrose)
Contains 37.3% iodine by weight.

See algorithms in front cover of book for arrest dosing.
Child PO for tachyarrhythmia:
  <1 yr: 600–800 mg/1.73 m²/24 hr ÷ Q12–24 hr × 4–14 days and/or until adequate control achieved, then reduce to 200–400 mg/1.73 m²/24 hr
  ≥1 yr: 10–15 mg/kg/24 hr ÷ Q12–24 hr × 4–14 days and/or until adequate control achieved, then reduce to 5 mg/kg/24 hr ÷ Q12–24 hr, if effective
Child IV for tachyarrhythmia (limited data):
  5 mg/kg (**max. dose:** 300 mg) over 30 min followed by a continuous infusion starting at 5 micrograms (mcg)/kg/min; infusion may be increased up to a **max. dose** of 15 mcg/kg/min or 20 mg/kg/24 hr or 2200 mg/24 hr.
Adult PO for ventricular arrhythmias:
  Loading dose: 800–1600 mg/24 hr ÷ Q12–24 hr for 1–3 wk
  Maintenance: 600–800 mg/24 hr ÷ Q12–24 hr × 1 mo, then 200 mg Q12–24 hr
  Use lowest effective dose to minimize adverse reactions.

Continued

AMIODARONE HCL continued

Adult IV for ventricular arrhythmias:
Loading dose: 150 mg over 10 min (15 mg/min) followed by 360 mg over 6 hr (1 mg/min); followed by a maintenance dose of 0.5 mg/min. Supplemental boluses of 150 mg over 10 min may be given for breakthrough VF or hemodynamically unstable VT, and the maintenance infusion may be increased to suppress the arrhythmia. **Max. dose:** 2.1 g/24 hr.

Used in the resuscitation algorithm for ventricular fibrillation/pulseless ventricular tachycardia **(see front cover for arrest dosing and back cover for PALS algorithm).** Overall use of this drug may be limited to its potentially life-threatening side effects and the difficulties associated with managing its use.

Contraindicated in severe sinus node dysfunction, marked sinus bradycardia, second- and third-degree AV block. **Use with caution** in hepatic impairment.

Long elimination half-life (40–55 days). Major metabolite is active.

Increases cyclosporine, digoxin, phenytoin, tacrolimus, warfarin, calcium channel blockers, theophylline, and quinidine levels. Amiodarone is a CYP P450 3A3/4 substrate and inhibits CYP 3A3/4, 2C9, and 2D6. Risk of rhabdomyolysis is increased when used with simvastatin at doses greater than 20 mg/24 hr and lovastatin at doses greater than 40 mg/24 hr.

Proposed therapeutic level with chronic oral use: 1–2.5 mg/L.

Asymptomatic corneal microdeposits should appear in all patients. Alters liver enzymes, thyroid function. Pulmonary fibrosis reported in adults. May cause worsening of preexisting arrhythmias with bradycardia and AV block. May also cause hypotension, anorexia, nausea, vomiting, dizziness, paresthesias, ataxia, tremors, SIADH, and hypothyroidism or hyperthyroidism. Drug rash with eosinophilia and systemic symptoms (DRESS) and acute respiratory distress syndrome have been reported.

Correct hypokalemia, hypocalcemia, or hypomagnesemia whenever possible before use, as these conditions may exaggerate QTc prolongation.

Intravenous continuous infusion concentration for peripheral administration should not exceed 2 mg/mL and **must be diluted** with D₅W. The intravenous dosage form can leach out plasticizers, such as DEHP. It is recommended to reduce the potential exposure to plasticizers in pregnant women, toddlers, and younger children by using alternative methods of IV drug administration.

Oral administration should be consistent with regards to meals because food increases the rate and extent of oral absorption.

AMITRIPTYLINE
Elavil and generics
Antidepressant, tricyclic (TCA)

Yes No 2 C

Tabs: 10, 25, 50, 75, 100, 150 mg

Antidepressant:
Child: Start with 1 mg/kg/24 hr ÷ TID PO for 3 days; then increase to 1.5 mg/kg/24 hr. Dose may be gradually increased to a **max. dose** of 5 mg/kg/24 hr, if needed. Monitor ECG, BP, and heart rate for doses > 3 mg/kg/24 hr.

Adolescent: 10 mg TID PO and 20 mg QHS; dose may be gradually increased up to a **max. dose** of 200 mg/24 hr if needed.

Adult: 40–100 mg/24 hr ÷ QHS-BID PO; dose may be gradually increased up to 300 mg/24 hr, if needed; gradually decrease dose to lowest effective dose when symptoms are controlled.

Augment analgesia for chronic pain:
Child: Initial: 0.1 mg/kg/dose QHS PO; increase as needed and tolerated over 2–3 wk to 0.5–2 mg/kg/dose QHS.

AMITRIPTYLINE continued

Migrane prophylaxis (limited data):
  Child: Initial 0.1–0.25 mg/kg/dose QHS PO; increase as needed and tolerated every 2 wk by 0.1–0.25 mg/kg/dose up to a **max. dose** of 2 mg/kg/24 hr or 75 mg/24 hr. For doses > 1 mg/kg/24 hr, divide daily dose BID and monitor ECG.
  Adult: Initial 10–25 mg/dose QHS PO; reported range of 10–400 mg/24 hr.

Contraindicated in narrow-angle glaucoma, seizures, severe cardiac disorders, and patients who received MAO inhibitors within 14 days. See Chapter 2 for management of TCA toxic ingestion.

$T_{1/2}$ = 9–25 hr in adults. **Maximum** antidepressant effects may not occur for 2 wk or more after initiation of therapy. **Do not abruptly discontinue therapy in patients receiving high doses for prolonged periods.**

Therapeutic levels (sum of amitriptyline and nortriptyline): 100–250 ng/mL. Recommended serum sampling time: obtain a single level 8 hr or more after an oral dose (following 4–5 days of continuous dosing). Amitriptyline is a substrate for CYP 450 1A2, 2C9, 2C19, 2D6, and 3A3/4 and inhibitor for CYP 450 1A2, 2C19, 2C9, 2D6, and 2E1. Rifampin can decrease amitriptyline levels. Amitriptyline may increase side effects of tramadol.

Side effects include sedation, urinary retention, constipation, dry mouth, dizziness, drowsiness, liver enzyme elevation, and arrhythmia. May discolor urine (blue/green). QHS dosing during first weeks of therapy will reduce sedation. Monitor ECG, BP, and CBC at start of therapy and with dose changes. Decrease dose if PR interval reaches 0.22 s, QRS reaches 130% of baseline, HR rises above 140/min, or if BP is > 140/90. Tricyclics may cause mania. For antidepressant use, monitor for clinical worsening of depression and suicidal ideation/behavior following the initiation of therapy or after dose changes.

AMLODIPINE
Norvasc and generics
Calcium channel blocker, antihypertensive

Yes   No   3   C

Tabs: 2.5, 5, 10 mg
Oral suspension: 1 mg/mL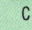

Child:
  Hypertension: Start with 0.1 mg/kg/dose (**max. dose:** 5 mg) PO once daily–BID; dosage may be gradually increased to a **max. dose** of 0.6 mg/kg/24 hr up to 20 mg/24 hr. An effective antihypertensive dose of 2.5–5 mg once daily for those aged 6–17 yr has been reported, and doses > 5 mg have not been evaluated.
Adult:
  Hypertension: 5–10 mg/dose once daily PO; use 2.5 mg/dose once daily PO in patients with hepatic insufficiency. **Max. dose:** 10 mg/24 hr.

Use with caution in combination with other antihypertensive agents. Younger children (<6 yr) may require higher mg/kg doses than older children and adults. A BID dosing regimen may provide better efficacy in children.

Reduce dose in hepatic insufficiency. Allow 5–7 days of continuous initial dose therapy before making dosage adjustments because of the drug's gradual onset of action and lengthy elimination half-life. Amlodipine is a substrate of CYP 450 3A4 and **should be used with caution** with 3A4 inhibitors, such as protease inhibitors and azole antifungals (eg. fluconazole and ketoconazole). May increase levels and toxicity of cyclosporine, tacrolimus, and simvastatin.

Dose-related side effects include edema, dizziness, flushing, fatigue, and palpitations. Other side effects include headache, nausea, abdominal pain, and somnolence.

AMMONIUM CHLORIDE
Various generics
Diuretic, urinary acidifying agent

Yes   Yes   ?   C

Injection: 5 mEq/mL (26.75%) (20 mL); contains EDTA
1 mEq = 53 mg

Urinary acidification:
  Child: 75 mg/kg/24 hr ÷ Q6 hr IV; **max. dose:** 6 g/24 hr
  Adult: 1.5 g/dose Q6 hr IV
Drug administration: Dilute to concentration ≤ 0.4 mEq/mL. Infusion **not to exceed** 50 mg/kg/hr or 1 mEq/kg/hr.

Contraindicated in hepatic or renal insufficiency and primary respiratory acidosis. **Use with caution** in infants.
May produce acidosis, hyperammonemia, and GI irritation. Monitor serum chloride level, acid/base status, and serum ammonia.

AMMONUL

See Sodium Phenylacetate + Sodium Benzoate

AMOXICILLIN
Moxatag and various generics; previously available as Amoxil and Trimox
Antibiotic, aminopenicillin

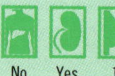
No   Yes   1   B

Oral suspension: 125, 250 mg/5 mL (80, 100, 150 mL); and 200, 400 mg/5 mL (50, 75, 100 mL)
Caps: 250, 500 mg
Tablets: 500, 875 mg
Chewable tabs: 125, 250 mg; may contain phenylalanine
Extended-release tabs (Moxatag; see remarks): 775 mg

Neonate–≤ 3 mo: 20–30 mg/kg/24 hr ÷ Q12 hr PO
Child:
  Standard dose: 25–50 mg/kg/24 hr ÷ Q8–12 hr PO
  High dose (resistant *Streptococcus pneumoniae*; see remarks): 80–90 mg/kg/24 hr ÷ Q8–12 hr PO
  Max. dose: 2–3 g/24 hr; some experts recommend a maximum dosage up to 4 g/24 hr
Adult:
  Mild/moderate infections: 250 mg/dose Q8 hr PO OR 500 mg/dose Q12 hr PO
  Severe infections: 500 mg/dose Q8 hr PO OR 875 mg/dose Q12 hr PO
  Max. dose: 2–3 g/24 hr
Tonsillitis/pharyngitis (S. pyogenes): 50 mg/kg/24 hr ÷ Q12 hr PO × 10 days; **max. dose:** 1 g/24 hr.
  Extended-release tablets (Moxatag): 775 mg once daily PO × 10 days is indicated for children ≥ 12 yr and adults.
SBE prophylaxis: administer dose 1 hour before procedure
  Child: 50 mg/kg PO × 1; max. 2 g/dose
  Adult: 2 g PO × 1
Early lyme disease:
  Child: 50 mg/kg/24 hr ÷ Q8 hr PO × 14–21 days; **max. dose:** 1.5 g/24 hr
  Adult: 500 mg/dose Q8 hr PO × 14–21 days

AMOXICILLIN continued

Renal elimination. **Adjust dose in renal failure (see Chapter 30).** Serum levels about twice those achieved with equal dose of ampicillin. Fewer GI effects, but otherwise similar to ampicillin. Side effects: rash and diarrhea. Rash may develop with concurrent EBV infection. May increase warfarin's effect by increasing INR.

High-dose regimen, increasingly useful, is recommended in respiratory infections (e.g., CAP), acute otitis media, and sinusitis, owing to increasing incidence of penicillin-resistant pneumococci. **Chewable tablets may contain phenylalanine and should not be used by phenylketonurics.**

AMOXICILLIN-CLAVULANIC ACID
Augmentin, Augmentin ES-600, Augmentin XR, and various generic products
Antibiotic, aminopenicillin with β-lactmase inhibitor

No | Yes | 1 | B

Tabs:
  For TID dosing: 250, 500 mg (with 125 mg clavulanate)
  For BID dosing: 875 mg amoxicillin (with 125 mg clavulanate); Augmentin XR: 1g amoxicillin (with 62.5 mg clavulanate)
Chewable tabs:
  For BID dosing: 200, 400 mg amoxicillin (28.5 and 57 mg clavulanate, respectively); contains saccharin and aspartame
Oral suspension:
  For TID dosing: 125, 250 mg amoxicillin/5 mL (31.25 and 62.5 mg clavulanate/5 mL, respectively) (75, 100, 150 mL); contains saccharin
  For BID dosing: 200, 400 mg amoxicillin/5 mL (28.5 and 57 mg clavulanate/ 5 mL, respectively) (50, 75, 100 mL); 600 mg amoxicillin/5 mL (Augmentin ES-600; contains 42.9 mg clavulanate/5 mL) (75, 125, 200 mL); contains saccharin and/or aspartame
Contains 0.63 mEq K^+ per 125 mg clavulanate (Augmentin ES-600 contains 0.23 mEq K^+ per 42.9 mg clavulanate)

Dosage based on amoxicillin component (see remarks for resistant S. pneumoniae).
Infant 1–<3 mo: 30 mg/kg/24 hr ÷ Q12 hr PO (recommended dosage form is 125 mg/5 mL suspension)
Child ≥ 3 mo (for non–high-dose amoxicillin regimens, use adult dosage if ≥ 40 kg):
  TID dosing (see remarks):
    20–40 mg/kg/24 hr ÷ Q8 hr PO
  BID dosing (see remarks):
    25–45 mg/kg/24 hr ÷ Q12 hr PO
  Augmentin ES-600:
    ≥3 mo and <40 kg: 90 mg/kg/24 hr ÷ Q12 hr PO × 10 days
Adult: 250–500 mg/dose Q8 hr PO or 875 mg/dose Q12 hr PO for more severe and respiratory infections
  Augmentin XR:
    ≥16 yr and adult: 2 g Q12 hr PO × 10 days for acute bacterial sinusitis or × 7–10 days for community-acquired pneumonia

See Amoxicillin for additional comments. **Adjust dose in renal failure (see Chapter 30).**
  Contraindicated in patients with a history of cholestatic jaundice/hepatic dysfunction associated with amoxicillin-clavulanic acid. Augmentin XR is **contraindicated** in patients with CrCl < 30 mL/min.

Continued

AMOXICILLIN-CLAVULANIC ACID continued

Clavulanic acid extends the activity of amoxicillin to include β-lactamase–producing strains of *Haemophilus influenzae, Moraxella catarrhalis, Neisseria gonorrhoeae,* and some *Staphylococcus aureus* and may increase the risk for diarrhea.

The BID dosing schedule is associated with less diarrhea. For BID dosing, the 875-mg, 1-g tablets; the 200-mg, 400-mg chewable tablets; or the 200-mg/5 mL, 400-mg/5 mL, 600-mg/5 mL suspensions should be used. These BID dosage forms contain phenylalanine and **should not be used** by phenylketonurics. For TID dosing, the 250-mg, 500-mg tablets; the 125-mg, 250-mg chewable tablets; or the 125-mg/5 mL, 250-mg/5 mL suspensions should be used.

Higher doses of 80–90 mg/kg/24 hr (amoxicillin component) have been recommended for resistant strains of *S. pneumoniae* in acute otitis media and pneumonia (use BID formulations containing 7:1 ratio of amoxicillin to clavulanic acid or Augmentin ES-600).

The 250 or 500 mg tablets **cannot** be substituted for Augmentin XR.

AMPHETAMINE
Evekeo, Adzenys XR-ODT, Dyanavel XR
CNS stimulant

No   No   3   C

Tabs, immediate release:
  Evekeo: 5, 10 mg; both tablets are scored
Extended-release dispersible tabs:
  Adzenys XR-ODT: 3.1, 6.3, 9.4, 12.5, 15.7, 18.8 mg
Extended-release oral suspension:
  Dyanavel XR: 2.5 mg/mL (464 mL); contains parabens and polysorbate 80
DO NOT substitute extended-release formulations for other amphetamine products on a mg per mg basis due to differences in potency and pharmacokinetic profiles. If converting from other amphetamine products, discontinue that treatment first and titrate new dosage forms as indicated in the drug dosage section.

Attention deficit hyperactivity disorder:
  Immediate-release tabs (Evekeo; PO):
    3–5 yr: 2.5 mg/24 hr QAM; increase by 2.5 mg/24 hr at weekly intervals until desired response. Incremental dosages may be administered BID–TID, with the first dose at awakening and subsequent doses spaced at 4–6 hr intervals. Doses rarely exceed 40 mg/24 hr.
    ≥6 yr and adolescent: 5 mg once daily or BID; increase by 5 mg/24 hr at weekly intervals until desired response. Incremental dosages may be administered BID–TID, with the first dose at awakening and subsequent doses spaced at 4–6 hr intervals. Doses rarely exceed 40 mg/24 hr.
  Extended-release suspension (see how supplied section above; Dyanavel XR; PO):
    ≥6 yr and adolescent: 2.5 or 5 mg/24 hr QAM; increase by 2.5–10 mg/24 hr every 4–7 days until desired response up to a **maximum** of 20 mg/24 hr.
  Extended-release dispersible tabs (see how supplied section above; Adzenys XR-ODT; PO):
    6–17 yr: 6.3 mg/24 hr QAM; increase by 3.1 or 6.3 mg/24 hr at weekly intervals until desired response. **Maximum dose:** 6–12 yr: 18.8 mg/24 hr; 13–17 yr: 12.5 mg/24 hr.
    Adult: 12.5 mg/24 hr QAM
Narcolepsy:
  Immediate-release tabs (Evekeo; PO):
    6–12 yr: 5 mg QAM; increase by 5 mg/24 hr at weekly intervals until desired response. Incremental doses may be administered with the first dose at awakening and subsequent doses (5 or 10 mg) spaced at 4–6 hr intervals. Usual daily dosage range: 5–60 mg/24 hr in divided doses.

AMPHETAMINE continued

≥13 yr and adult: 10 mg QAM; increase by 10 mg/24 hr at weekly intervals until desired response. Incremental doses may be administered with the first dose at awakening and subsequent doses (5 or 10 mg) spaced at 4–6 hr intervals. Usual daily dosage range: 5–60 mg/24 hr in divided doses.

Use with caution in presence of hypertension or cardiovascular disease. **Avoid use** in known serious structural cardiac abnormalities, cardiomyopathy, serious heart rhythm abnormalities, coronary artery disease, or other serious cardiac problems that may increase risk of sympathomimetic effects of amphetamines (sudden death, stroke, and MI have been reported). Do not use with MAO inhibitors; hypertensive crisis may occur if used within 14 days of discontinuing MAO inhibitor.

Not recommended for patients aged <3 yr. Medication should generally not be used in children aged <5 yr because diagnosis of ADHD in this age group is extremely difficult (use in consultation with a specialist). Interrupt administration occasionally to determine need for continued therapy.

Common side effects include headache, insomnia, anorexia, abdominal pain, anxiety, mood swings, and agitation. Psychotic disorder, peripheral vascular disease (including Raynaud's phenomenon), and cerebrovascular accidents have been reported.

Evekeo has an additional labeled indication for the treatment of exogenous obesity in those aged ≥12 yr and adults. Doses may be administered with or without food. **Do not** crush or chew the extended-release dispersible tabs (Adzenys XR-ODT).

AMPHOTERICIN B (CONVENTIONAL)
Various generics; previously available as Fungizone
Antifungal, polyene

Yes   Yes   ?   B

Injection: 50-mg vials

IV: mix with D₅W to a concentration 0.1 mg/mL (peripheral administration) or 0.25 mg/mL (central line only). pH > 4.2. Infuse over 2–6 hr.

Optional test dose: 0.1 mg/kg/dose IV up to **max. dose** of 1 mg (followed by remaining initial dose).

Initial dose: 0.5–1 mg/kg/24 hr; if test dose NOT used, infuse first dose over 6 hr and monitor frequently during the first several hours.

Increment: Increase as tolerated by 0.25–0.5 mg/kg/24 hr once daily or every other day. Use larger dosage increments (0.5 mg once daily) for critically ill patients.

Usual maintenance:
  Once-daily dosing: 0.5–1 mg/kg/24 hr once daily
  Every-other-day dosing: 1.5 mg/kg/dose every other day
Max. dose: 1.5 mg/kg/24 hr
Intrathecal: 25–100 mcg Q48–72 hr. Increase to 500 mcg, as tolerated.
Bladder irrigation for urinary tract mycosis: 5–15 mg in 100 mL sterile water for irrigation at 100–300 mL/24 hr. Instill solution into bladder, clamp catheter for 1–2 hr, then drain; repeat TID–QID for 2–5 days.

Monitor renal, hepatic, electrolyte, and hematologic status closely. Hypercalciuria, hypokalemia, hypomagnesemia, RTA, renal failure, acute hepatic failure, hypotension, and phlebitis may occur. **For dosing information in renal failure, see Chapter 30.**

Common infusion-related reactions include fever, chills, headache, hypotension, nausea, vomiting; may premedicate with acetaminophen and diphenhydramine 30 min before and 4 hr after infusion. Meperidine useful for chills. Hydrocortisone, 1 mg/mg ampho (**max.:** 25 mg) added to bottle may

Continued

AMPHOTERICIN B (CONVENTIONAL) continued

help prevent immediate adverse reactions. Use total body weight for obese patients when calculating dosages.

Salt loading with 10–15 mL/kg of NS infused prior to each dose may minimize the risk of nephrotoxicity. Maintaining sodium intake of >4 mEq/kg/24 hr in premature neonates may also reduce risk for nephrotoxicity. Nephrotoxic drugs such as aminoglycosides, chemotherapeutic agents, and cyclosporine may result in synergistic toxicity. Hypokalemia may increase the toxicity of neuromuscular blocking agents and cardiac glycosides.

AMPHOTERICIN B LIPID COMPLEX
Abelcet, ABLC
Antifungal, polyene

Yes Yes ? B

Injection: 5 mg/mL (20 mL)
(formulated as a 1:1 molar ratio of amphotericin B to lipid complex comprised of dimyristoylphosphatidylcholine and dimyristoylphosphatidylglycerol)

IV: 2.5–5 mg/kg/24 hr once daily
For visceral leishmaniasis that failed to respond to or relapsed after treatment with antimony compound, a dosage of 1–3 mg/kg/24 hr once daily × 5 days has been used.

Mix with D_5W to a concentration 1 or 2 mg/mL for fluid restricted patients.
Infusion rate: 2.5 mg/kg/hr; shake the infusion bag every 2 hr if total infusion time exceeds 2 hr.
Do not use an in-line filter.

Monitor renal, hepatic, electrolyte, and hematologic status closely. Thrombocytopenia, anemia, leukopenia, hypokalemia, hypomagnesemia, diarrhea, respiratory failure, skin rash, nephrotoxicity, and increases in liver enzymes and bilirubin may occur. See conventional amphotericin for drug interactions.

Highest concentrations achieved in spleen, lung, and liver from human autopsy data from one heart transplant patient. CNS/CSF levels are lower than amphotericin b, liposomal (AmBisome). In animal models, concentrations are higher in the liver, spleen, and lungs but the same in the kidneys when compared to conventional amphotericin B. Pharmacokinetics in renal and hepatic impairment have not been studied.

Common infusion-related reactions include fever, chills, rigors, nausea, vomiting, hypotension, and headaches; may premedicate with acetaminophen, diphenhydramine and meperidine (see Conventional *Amphotericin B* remarks).

AMPHOTERICIN B, LIPOSOMAL
AmBisome
Antifungal, polyene

Yes Yes ? B

Injection: 50-mg (vials); contains soy, 900-mg sucrose
(formulated in liposomes composed of hydrogenated soy phosphatidylcholine, cholesterol, distearoylphosphatidylglycerol, and α-tocopherol)

Systemic fungal infections: 3–5 mg/kg/24 hr IV once daily; an upper dosage limit of 10 mg/kg/24 hr has been suggested based on pharmacokinetic endpoints and risk for hypokalemia. However, dosages as high as 15 mg/kg/24 hr have been used. Dosages as high as 10 mg/kg/24 hr have been used in patients with Aspergillus.
Empiric therapy for febrile neutropenia: 3 mg/kg/24 hr IV once daily
Cryptococcal meningitis in HIV: 6 mg/kg/24 hr IV once daily

AMPHOTERICIN B, LIPOSOMAL continued

Leishmaniasis (a repeat course may be necessary if infection does not clear):
  Immunocompetent: 3 mg/kg/24 hr IV on days 1 to 5, 14, and 21
  Immunocompromised: 4 mg/kg/24 hr IV on days 1 to 5, 10, 17, 24, 31, and 38
Mix with D₅W to a concentration of 1–2 mg/mL (0.2–0.5 mg/mL may be used for infants and small children).
Infusion rate: Administer dose over 2 hr; infusion may be reduced to 1 hr if well tolerated. A ≥1-micron in-line filter may be used.

Closely monitor renal, hepatic, electrolyte, and hematologic status. Thrombocytopenia, anemia, leukopenia, tachycardia, hypokalemia, hypomagnesemia, hypocalcemia, hyperglycemia, diarrhea, dyspnea, skin rash, low back pain, nephrotoxicity, and increases in liver enzymes and bilirubin may occur. Rhabdomyolysis has been reported. Safety and effectiveness in neonates have not been established. See conventional *amphotericin* for drug interactions.

Compared to conventional amphotericin B, higher concentrations found in the liver and spleen; and similar concentrations found in the lungs and kidney. CNS/CSF concentrations are higher than other *amphotericin* B products. Pharmacokinetics in renal and hepatic impairment have not been studied.

Common infusion-related reactions include fever, chills, rigors, nausea, vomiting, hypotension, and headache; may premedicate with acetaminophen, diphenhydramine, and meperidine (see Conventional *Amphotericin* B remarks).

False elevations of serum phosphate have been reported with the PHOSm assay (used in Beckman Coulter analyzers).

AMPICILLIN
Many generics
Antibiotic, aminopenicillin

No Yes 1 B

Oral suspension: 125 mg/5 mL, 250 mg/5 mL (100, 200 mL)
Caps: 250, 500 mg
Injection: 125, 250, 500 mg; 1, 2, 10 g
Contains 3 mEq Na/1 g IV drug

Neonate (IM/IV):
  <7 days:
    <2 kg: 100 mg/kg/24 hr ÷ Q12 hr
    ≥ 2 kg: 150 mg/kg/24 hr ÷ Q8 hr
    Group B streptococcal meningitis: 200–300 mg/kg/24 hr ÷ Q8 hr
  ≥7 days:
    <1.2 kg: 100 mg/kg/24 hr ÷ Q12 hr
    1.2–2 kg: 150 mg/kg/24 hr ÷ Q8 hr
    >2 kg: 200 mg/kg/24 hr ÷ Q6 hr
    Group B streptococcal meningitis: 300 mg/kg/24 hr ÷ Q4–6 hr
Infant/child (see remarks):
  Mild/moderate infections:
    IM/IV: 100–200 mg/kg/24 hr ÷ Q6 hr
    PO: 50–100 mg/kg/24 hr ÷ Q6 hr; **max. PO dose: 4 g/24 hr**
  Severe infections: 200–400 mg/kg/24 hr ÷ Q4–6 hr IM/IV; max. dose: 12 g/24 hr
  Community-acquired pneumonia in a fully immunized patient (IV/IM):
    S. pneumoniae penicillin MIC ≤ 2.0 or H. influenzae (β-lactamase negative): 150–200 mg/kg/24 hr ÷ Q6 hr
    S. pneumoniae penicillin MIC ≥ 4.0: 300–400 mg/kg/24 hr ÷ Q6 hr
Max. IV/IM dose: 12 g/24 hr

Continued

AMPICILLIN continued

Adult:
  IM/IV: 500–3000 mg Q4–6 hr
  PO: 250–500 mg Q6 hr
Max. IV/IM dose: 14 g/24 hr
SBE prophylaxis:
  Moderate risk patients:
    Child: 50 mg/kg/dose × 1 IV/IM 30 min before procedure; **max. dose:** 2 g/dose
    Adult: 2 g/dose × 1 IV/IM 30 min before procedure
  High-risk patients with GU and GI procedures: Above doses PLUS gentamicin 1.5 mg/kg × 1 (**max. dose:** 120 mg) IV within 30 min of starting procedure. Followed by ampicillin 25 mg/kg/dose IV (or PO amoxicillin) × 1, 6 hr later.

Use higher doses with shorter dosing intervals to treat CNS disease and severe infection. CSF penetration occurs only with inflamed meninges. **Adjust dose in renal failure (see Chapter 30).**

Produces the same side effects as penicillin, with cross-reactivity. Rash commonly seen at 5–10 days and may occur with concurrent EBV infection or allopurinol use. May cause interstitial nephritis, diarrhea, and pseudomembranous enterocolitis. Chloroquine reduces ampicillin's oral absorption.

AMPICILLIN/SULBACTAM
Unasyn and generics
Antibiotic, aminopenicillin with β-lactamase inhibitor

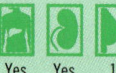

Yes   Yes   1   B

Injection:
  1.5 g = ampicillin 1 g + sulbactam 0.5 g
  3 g = ampicillin 2 g + sulbactam 1 g
  15 g = ampicillin 10 g + sulbactam 5 g
  Contains 5 mEq Na per 1.5 g drug combination

Dosage based on ampicillin component:
Neonate:
  Premature (based on pharmacokinetic data): 100 mg/kg/24 hr ÷ Q12 hr IM/IV
  Full-term: 100 mg/kg/24 hr ÷ Q8 hr IM/IV
Infant ≥ 1 mo:
  Mild/moderate infections: 100–150 mg/kg/24 hr ÷ Q6 hr IM/IV
  Meningitis/severe infections: 200–300 mg/kg/24 hr ÷ Q6 hr IM/IV
Child (see remarks):
  Mild/moderate infections: 100–200 mg/kg/24 hr ÷ Q6 hr IM/IV; **max. dose:** 1 g ampicillin/dose
  Meningitis/severe infections: 200–400 mg/kg/24 hr ÷ Q4–6 hr IM/IV; **max. dose:** 2 g ampicillin/dose
Adult: 1–2 g Q6–8 hr IM/IV
Max. dose: 8 g ampicillin/24 hr

Similar spectrum of antibacterial activity to ampicillin with the added coverage of β-lactamase–producing organisms. Total sulbactam dose should not exceed 4 g/24 hr.

Use higher doses with shorter dosing intervals to treat CNS disease and severe infection. Hepatic dysfunction, including hepatitis and cholestatic jaundice, has been reported. Monitor hepatic function in patients with hepatic impairment.

Adjust dose in renal failure (see Chapter 30). Similar CSF distribution and side effects to ampicillin.

ANTIPYRINE AND BENZOCAINE (OTIC)
Antipyrine and Benzocaine Otic and many generics;
previously available as Auralgan
Otic analgesic, cerumenolytic

No   No   2   C

Otic solution: Antipyrine 5.4%, benzocaine 1.4% (10, 15 mL); may contain oxyquinoline sulfate.

Otic analgesia: Fill external ear canal (2–4 drops) Q1–2 hr PRN. After instillation of the solution, a cotton pledget should be moistened with the solution and inserted into the meatus.
Cerumenolytic: Fill external ear canal (2–4 drops) TID–QID for 2–3 days.

Benzocaine sensitivity may develop and is not intended for prolonged use. **Contraindicated** if tympanic membrane perforated or PE tubes in place. Local reactions (eg., burning, stinging) and hypersensitivity reactions may occur. Risk of benzocaine-induced methemoglobinemia may be increased in infants aged ≤3 mo.

ARGININE CHLORIDE—INJECTABLE PREPARATION
R-Gene 10
Metabolic alkalosis agent, urea cycle disorder treatment agent, growth hormone diagnostic agent

   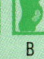
Yes   Yes   ?   B

Injection: 10% (100 mg/mL) arginine hydrochloride, contains 47.5 mEq chloride per 100 mL (300 mL)
Osmolality: 950 mOsmol/L

Used as a secondary alternative agent for patients that are unresponsive or unable to receive sodium chloride and potassium chloride.
Correction of hypochloremia: Arginine chloride dose in milliequivalents (mEq) = $0.2 \times$ patient's weight (kg) $\times$ [103 − patient's serum chloride in mEq/L]. Administer $\frac{1}{2}$ to $\frac{2}{3}$ of the calculated dose and reassess.
Drug administration: Do not exceed an IV infusion rate of 1 g/kg/hr (4.75 mEq/kg/hr). Drug may be administered without further dilution, but should be diluted to reduce risk of tissue irritation.
Hyperammonemia in metabolic disorders: See Chapter 13, Treatment of Metabolic Crisis

Contraindicated in renal or hepatic failure. Use with **extreme caution** as overdose may result in hyperchloremic metabolic acidosis, cerebral edema, and death. Hypersensitivity reactions, including anaphylaxis, and hematuria have been reported.
Arginine hydrochloride is metabolized to nitrogen-containing products for renal excretion. Excess arginine increases the production of nitric oxide (NO) to cause vasodilation/hypotension. Closely monitor acid/base status. Hyperglycemia, hyperkalemia, GI disturbances, IV extravasation, headache, and flushing may occur.
In addition to its use in chloride supplementation, arginine is used in urea cycle disorder therapy (increases arginine levels and prevents breakdown of endogenous proteins) and as a diagnostic agent for growth hormone (stimulates pituitary release of growth hormone).

ARIPIPRAZOLE
Abilify, Abilify Maintena, and generics
Atypical antipsychotic (2nd generation)

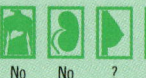

No No ? C

Tabs: 2, 5, 10, 15, 20, 30 mg
Tabs, orally disintegrating (ODT): 10, 15 mg; contains phenylalanine
Oral solution: 1 mg/mL (150, 237 mL); may contain parabens
Intramuscular suspension (extended release):
  Abilify Maintena: 300, 400 mg

Irritability Associated with Autistic Disorder:
  6–17 yr: Start at 2 mg PO once daily × 7 days, then increase to 5 mg PO once daily. If needed, dose may be increased in 5 mg increments ≥ 7 days in duration up to a **maximum** dose of 15 mg/24 hr. Patients should be periodically evaluated to determine the continued need for maintenance treatment.

Schizophrenia:
  13–17 yr: Start at 2 mg PO once daily × 2 days, followed by 5 mg PO once daily × 2 days, then to the recommended target dose of 10 mg PO once daily. If necessary, dose may be increased in 5-mg increments up to a **maximum** of 30 mg/24 hr (30 mg/24 hr was not shown to be more effective than 10 mg/24 hr in clinical trials). Patients should be periodically evaluated to determine the continued need for maintenance treatment.

Bipolar disorder (mono or adjunctive therapy):
  10–17 yr: Start at 2 mg PO once daily × 2 days, followed by 5 mg PO once daily × 2 days, then to the recommended target dose of 10 mg PO once daily. If necessary, dose may be increased in 5-mg increments up to a **maximum** of 30 mg/24 hr.

Tourettes Disorder:
  6–18 yr (Patients should be periodically evaluated to determine the continued need for maintenance treatment):
   50 kg: Start at 2 mg PO once daily × 2 days, then increase to the target dose of 5 mg PO once daily. If necessary after 7 days, dose may be increased to 10 mg PO once daily.
   ≥50 kg: Start at 2 mg PO once daily × 2 days, followed by 5 mg PO once daily × 5 days, and then 10 mg PO once daily. If necessary after 7 days, dose may be increased in 5-mg increments of ≥7 days in duration **up to** a **maximum** of 20 mg/24 hr.

Monitor for clinical worsening of depression and suicidal ideation/behavior after initiation of therapy or after dose changes. **Avoid** use of extended-release IM injection with CYP 450 inducers, including carbamazepine, for > 14 days. Higher cumulative doses and longer treatment duration may increase risk for irreversible tardive dyskinesia.

Weight gain, constipation, GI discomfort, akathisia, dizziness, extrapyramidal symptoms, headaches, insomnia, sedation, blurred vision and fatigue are common. May cause leukopenia, neutropenia, agranulocytosis, hyperthermia, neuroleptic malignant syndrome, hyperglycemia, orthostatic hypotension and prolongation of the QT interval (use considered contraindicated with other medications prolonging the QT interval). Rare impulse-control problems, such as compulsive or uncontrollable urges to gamble, binge eat, shop, and to have sex, have been reported.

Primarily metabolized by the CYP 450 2D6 and 3A4 enzymes. Dosage reduction for using half of the usual dose has been recommended for those who are either known poor metabolizers of CYP 450 2D6; or nonpoor metabolizers of CYP 450 2D6 taking strong CYP 450 2D6 (e.g., quinidine, fluoxetine, paroxetine) or 3A4 inhibitors (e.g., itraconazole, clarithromycin). Use of $\frac{1}{4}$ the usual dose has been recommended for known poor metabolizers of CYP 2D6 taking either a strong 2D6 or 3A4 inhibitor; or nonpoor metabolizers of CYP 450 2D6 taking both strong 2D6 AND 3A4 inhibitors.

ARIPIPRAZOLE continued

Consult with a pediatric psychiatrist for use in ADHD, conduct disorder, and PDD-NOS. Oral doses may be administered with or without meals. Do not split orally-disintegrating tablet dosage form.

ARNUITY ELLIPTA

See Fluticasone preparations

ASCORBIC ACID
Vitamin C, and many others
Water-soluble vitamin

No   No   1   A/C

Tabs [OTC]: 100, 250, 500 mg, 1 g
Chewable tabs (Sunkist Vitamin C and others) [OTC]: 100, 250, 500 mg; some may contain aspartame
Tabs (timed release) [OTC]: 0.5, 1, 1.5 g
Caps [OTC]: 500, 1000 mg
Extended-release caps [OTC]: 500 mg
Injection: 500 mg/mL; may contain sodium hydrosulfite
Oral liquid [OTC]: 500 mg/5 mL (236, 473 mL)
Oral syrup [OTC]: 500 mg/5 mL (118 mL)
Crystals [OTC]: 1 g per ¼ teaspoonful (120 g, 480 g)
Some products may contain approximately 5 mEq Na/1 g ascorbic acid.

Scurvy (PO/IM/IV/SC):
  Child: 100–300 mg/24 hr ÷ once daily–BID for at least 2 wk
  Adult: 100–250 mg once daily–BID for at least 2 wk
U.S. Recommended Daily Allowance (RDA):
  See Chapter 21.

Adverse reactions: Nausea, vomiting, heartburn, flushing, headache, faintness, dizziness, and hyperoxaluria. Use high doses with **caution** in G6PD patients. May cause false-negative and false-positive urine glucose determinations with glucose oxidase and cupric sulfate tests, respectively.
May increase the absorption of aluminum hydroxide and increase the adverse/toxic effects of deferoxamine. May reduce the effects of amphetamines.
Oral dosing is preferred with or without food. IM route is the preferred parenteral route. Protect the injectable dosage form from light.
Pregnancy Category changes to "C" if used in doses above the RDA.

ASPIRIN
ASA, various trade names and generics
Nonsteroidal antiinflammatory agent, antiplatelet agent, analgesic

Yes   Yes   2   D

Tabs/Caplet [OTC]: 325, 500 mg
Tabs, enteric-coated [OTC]: 81, 325, 500, 650 mg
Tabs, time-release [OTC]: 81, 650 mg
Tabs, buffered [OTC]: 325 mg; may contain magnesium, aluminum, and/or calcium

Continued

ASPIRIN continued

Caplet, buffered [OTC]: 500 mg; may contain magnesium, aluminum, and/or calcium
Tabs, chewable [OTC]: 81 mg
Suppository [OTC]: 300, 600 mg (12s)

Analgesic/antipyretic: 10–15 mg/kg/dose PO/PR Q4–6 hr up to total of 60–80 mg/kg/24 hr
Max. dose: 4 g/24 hr
Antiinflammatory: 60–100 mg/kg/24 hr PO ÷ Q6–8 hr
Kawasaki disease: 80–100 mg/kg/24 hr PO ÷ QID during febrile phase until defervesce then decrease to 3–5 mg/kg/24 hr PO QAM. Continue for at least 8 wk or until both platelet count and ESR are normal.

Do not use in children aged <16 yr for treatment of varicella or flu-like symptoms (risk for Reye's Syndrome), in combination with other NSAIDs, or in severe renal failure. **Use with caution** in bleeding disorders, renal dysfunction, gastritis, and gout. May cause GI upset, allergic reactions, liver toxicity, and decreased platelet aggregation.
Drug interactions: may increase effects of methotrexate, valproic acid, and warfarin which may lead to toxicity (protein displacement). Buffered dosage forms may decrease absorption of ketoconazole and tetracycline. GI bleeds have been reported with concurrent use of SSRIs (eg. fluoxetine, paroxetine, sertraline).
Therapeutic levels: antipyretic/analgesic: 30–50 mg/L, antiinflammatory: 150–300 mg/L. Tinnitus may occur at levels of 200–400 mg/L. Recommended serum sampling time at steady state: obtain trough level just prior to dose following 1–2 days of continuous dosing. Peak levels obtained 2 hr (for non-sustained-release dosage forms) after a dose may be useful for monitoring toxicity. **Adjust dose in renal failure (see Chapter 30).**
Breastfeeding considerations:
High-dose aspirin regimens: use of an alternative drug is recommended.
Low-dose (75–162 mg/24 hr) aspirin regimens: avoid breastfeeding for 1–2 hr after a dose.

ATENOLOL
Tenormin and generics
β₁-selective adrenergic blocker

No   Yes   2   D

Tab: 25, 50, 100 mg
Oral suspension: 2 mg/mL

Hypertension:
  Child and adolescent: 0.5–1 mg/kg/dose PO once daily–BID; **max. dose:** 2 mg/kg/24 hr up to 100 mg/24 hr.
  Adult: 25–100 mg/dose PO once daily; **max. dose:** 100 mg/24 hr

Contraindicated in pulmonary edema, cardiogenic shock. May cause bradycardia, hypotension, second- or third-degree AV block, dizziness, fatigue, lethargy, and headache. **Use with caution** in diabetes and asthma. Wheezing and dyspnea have occurred when daily dosage exceeds 100 mg/24 hr. Postmarketing evaluation reports a temporal relationship for causing elevated LFTs and/or bilirubin, hallucinations, psoriatic rash, thrombocytopenia, visual disturbances, and dry mouth. **Avoid** abrupt withdrawal of the drug. Does not cross the blood-brain barrier; lower incidence of CNS side effects compared to propranolol. Neonates born to mothers receiving atenolol during labor or while breastfeeding may be at risk for hypoglycemia.
Use with disopyramide, amiodarone or digoxin may enhance bradycardic effects. **Adjust dose in renal impairment (see Chapter 30).**

ATOMOXETINE
Strattera
Norepinephrine reuptake inhibitor, attention deficit hyperactivity disorder agent

Yes   No   3   C

Capsules: 10, 18, 25, 40, 60, 80, 100 mg

Child ≥ 6 yr and adolescent ≤ 70 kg (see remarks):
Start with 0.5 mg/kg/24 hr PO QAM and increase after a minimum of 3 days to approximately 1.2 mg/kg/24 hr PO ÷ QAM or BID (morning and late afternoon/early evening). **Max. daily dose:** 1.4 mg/kg/24 hr or 100 mg, whichever is less.
If used with a strong CYP 450 2D6 inhibitor (eg., fluoxetine, paroxetine, quinidine) or in patients with reduced CYP 450 2D6 activity: Maintain above initial dose for 4 wk and increase to a **max.** of 1.2 mg/kg/24 hr only if symptoms do not improve and initial dose is tolerated.

Child ≥ 6 yr and adolescent > 70 kg (see remarks):
Start with 40 mg PO QAM and increase after a minimum of 3 days to about 80 mg/24 hr PO ÷ QAM or BID (morning and late afternoon/early evening). After 2–4 wk, dose may be increased to a **max.** of 100 mg/24 hr if needed.
If used with a strong CYP 450 2D6 inhibitor (eg., fluoxetine, paroxetine, quinidine) or in patients with reduced CYP 450 2D6 activity: Maintain above initial dose for 4 wk and increase to 80 mg/24 hr only if symptoms do not improve and initial dose is tolerated.

Contraindicated in patients with narrow angle glaucoma, pheochromocytoma, and severe cardiac disorders. **Do not** administer with or within 2 wk after discontinuing an MAO inhibitor; fatal reactions have been reported. **Use with caution** in hypertension, tachycardia, cardiovascular or cerebrovascular diseases, or with concurrent albuterol therapy. Increased risk of suicidal thinking has been reported; closely monitor for clinical worsening, agitation, aggressive behavior, irritability, suicidal thinking or behaviors and unusual changes in behavior when initiating (first few months) or at times of dose changes (increases or decreases). Atomoxetine is a CYP 450 2D6 substrate; poor 2D6 metabolizers compared to normal and has been reported to have higher rates of adverse effects of insomnia, weight loss, constipation, depression, tremor, and excoriation.

Doses > 1.2 mg/kg/24 hr in patients ≤ 70 kg have not been shown to be of additional benefit. Reduce dose (initial and target doses) by 50% and 75% for patients with moderate (Child-Pugh Class B) and severe (Child-Pugh Class C) hepatic insufficiency, respectively.

Major side effects include GI discomfort, vomiting, fatigue, anorexia, dizziness, and mood swings. Hypersensitivity reactions, aggression, irritability, priapism, allergic reactions and severe liver injury have also been reported. Consider interrupting therapy in patients who are not growing or gaining weight satisfactorily.

Doses may be administered with or without food. Atomoxetine can be discontinued without tapering.

ATOVAQUONE
Mepron and generics
Antiprotozoal

Yes   Yes   3   C

Oral suspension: 750 mg/5 mL (210 mL); contains benzyl alcohol

Pneumocystis jiroveci (carinii) pneumonia (PCP):
  Treatment (21 day course):
    Child: 30–40 mg/kg/24 hr PO ÷ BID with fatty foods; **max. dose:** 1500 mg/24 hr. Infants 3–24 mo may require higher doses of 45 mg/kg/24 hr.
    Adult: 750 mg/dose PO BID

Continued

ATOVAQUONE continued

Prophylaxis (1st episode and recurrence):
   Child 1–3 mo or > 24 mo: 30 mg/kg/24 hr PO once daily; **max. dose:** 1500 mg/24 hr
   Child 4–24 mo: 45 mg/kg/24 hr PO once daily; **max. dose:** 1500 mg/24 hr
   Adult: 1500 mg/dose PO once daily
Toxoplasa gondii:
  Child:
    First-episode prophylaxis and recurrence prophylaxis: use pneumocystis jiroveci prophylaxis dosages ± pyrimethamine 1 mg/kg/dose (max. 25 mg/dose) PO once daily PLUS leucovorin 5 mg PO Q3 days.
  Adult:
    Treatment: 1500 mg/dose PO BID ± (sulfadiazine 1000–1500 mg PO Q6 hr or pyrimethamine PLUS leucovorin).
    First-episode prophylaxis: 1500 mg/dose PO once daily ± pyrimethamine 25 mg PO once daily PLUS leucovorin 10 mg PO once daily.
    Recurrence prophylaxis: 750 mg/dose PO Q6–12 hr ± pyrimethamine 25 mg PO once daily PLUS leucovorin 10 mg PO once daily.

Not recommended in the treatment of severe pneumocystis jiroveci (lack of clinical data). Patients with GI disorders or severe vomiting and who cannot tolerate oral therapy should consider alternative IV therapies. Rash, pruritus, sweating, GI symptoms, LFT elevation, dizziness, headache, insomnia, anxiety, cough, and fever are common. Anemia, Stevens-Johnson syndrome, hepatitis, renal/urinary disorders, and pancreatitis have been reported.

Metoclopramide, rifampin, rifabutin, and tetracycline may decrease atovaquone levels. Shake oral suspension well before dispensing all doses. Take all doses with high fat foods to maximize absorption.

ATROPINE SULFATE
AtroPen, and many generic products
Anticholinergic agent

No   No   2   C

Injection: 0.4, 0.8, 1 mg/mL
Injection (auto-injector for IM use):
  AtroPen 0.25 mg: delivers a single 0.25 mg (0.3 mL) dose (yellow-colored pen)
  AtroPen 0.5 mg: delivers a single 0.5 mg (0.7 mL) dose (blue-colored pen)
  AtroPen 1 mg: delivers a single 1 mg (0.7 mL) dose (dark red–colored pen)
  AtroPen 2 mg: delivers a single 2 mg (0.7 mL) dose (green-colored pen)
Ointment (ophthalmic): 1% (3.5 g)
Solution (ophthalmic): 1% (2, 5, 15 mL)

Preintubation dose (see remarks):
  Neonate: 0.01–0.02 mg/kg/dose IV (over 1 min)/IM prior to other premedications.
  Child: 0.01 mg/kg/dose IV/IM; **max. dose:** 0.4 mg/dose; may repeat Q4–6 hr PRN
  Adult: 0.5 mg/dose IV/IM
Cardiopulmonary resuscitation/Bradycardia (see remarks):
  Neonate: 0.01–0.03 mg/kg/dose IV/IM Q10–15 min PRN up to a total maximum of 0.04 mg/kg. Administer IV over 1 min.
  Child: 0.02 mg/kg/dose IV Q5 min × 2–3 doses PRN; **max. single dose:** 0.5 mg in children, 1 mg in adolescents; **max total dose:** 1 mg children, 2 mg adolescents
  Adult: 0.5–1 mg/dose IV Q5 min; **max. total dose:** 3 mg

ATROPINE SULFATE continued

Bronchospasm: 0.025–0.05 mg/kg/dose (**max. dose:** 2.5 mg/dose) in 2.5 mL NS Q6–8 hr via nebulizer

Nerve agent and insecticide poisoning for muscarinic symptoms (organophosphate or carbamate poisoning) (IV/IM/ET; dilute in 1–2 mL NS for ET administration):
Child: 0.05–0.1 mg/kg Q5–10 min until bronchial or oral secretions terminate.
Adult: 2–5 mg/dose Q5–10 min until bronchial or oral secretions terminate.

AtroPen device (IM route): Inject as soon as exposure is known or suspected. Give one dose for mild symptoms and two additional doses (total 3 doses) in rapid succession 10 min after the first dose for severe symptoms as follows:
Child < 6 mo (<7 kg): 0.25 mg
Child 6 mo–4 yr (7–18 kg): 0.5 mg
Child 4–10 yr (18–41 kg): 1 mg
Child > 10 yr and adult (≥41 kg): 2 mg

Ophthalmic (uveitis):
Child: (0.5% solution; prepared by diluting equal volume of the 1% atropine ophthalmic solution with artificial tears) 1–2 drops in each eye once daily–TID
Adult: (1% solution) 1–2 drops in each eye once daily–QID

Contraindicated in glaucoma, obstructive uropathy, tachycardia, and thyrotoxicosis, except for severe or life-threatening muscarinic symptoms. Use with **caution** in patients sensitive to sulfites.

Recommended minimum dosage of 0.1 mg for neonates for bradycardia is currently recommended by PALS for concerns of paradoxical bradycardia. However, use of this minimum dose could result in an overdose. Additionally, data suggest the minimum 0.1 mg dose may not be warranted for the preintubation indication as well.

Side effects include: dry mouth, blurred vision, fever, tachycardia, constipation, urinary retention, CNS signs (dizziness, hallucinations, restlessness, fatigue, headache).

In case of bradycardia, may give via endotracheal tube (dilute with NS to volume of 1–2 mL and follow each dose with 1 mL NS) or intraosseous (IO) route. Use injectable solution for nebulized use; can be mixed with albuterol for simultaneous administration. AtroPen dosage form is designed for IM administration to the outer thigh.

AURALGAN

See Antipyrine and Benzocaine

AZATHIOPRINE
Imuran, Azasan, and others generics
Immunosuppressant

Yes Yes 3 D

Oral suspension: 50 mg/mL
Tabs:
 Imuran and generic: 50 mg (scored)
 Azasan: 75, 100 mg (scored)
Injection: 100 mg

Immunosuppression (see remarks):
Child and adult:
 Initial: 3–5 mg/kg/24 hr IV/PO once daily
 Maintenance: 1–3 mg/kg/24 hr IV/PO once daily

Continued

AZATHIOPRINE continued

Increased risk for hepatosplenic T-cell lymphoma has been reported in adolescents and young adults. Toxicity: bone marrow suppression, rash, stomatitis, hepatotoxicity, alopecia, arthralgias, and GI disturbances.

Use ¼–⅓ dose when given with allopurinol. Dose reduction or discontinuance is recommended in patients with low or absent thiopurine methyl transferase (TPMT) activity. Individuals with the low functioning alleles for NUDT15 are common among Asian ancestry and Hispanic ethnicity.

Severe anemia has been reported when used in combination with captopril or enalapril. Monitor CBC, platelets, total bilirubin, alkaline phosphatase, BUN, and creatinine. Pancytopenia and bone marrow suppression have been reported with concomitant use of pegylated interferon and ribavirin in patients with hepatitis C. Progressive multifocal leukoencephalopathy (PML) has been reported.
Adjust dose in renal failure (see Chapter 30).

Administer oral doses with food to minimize GI discomfort. To minimize infant exposure via breastmilk, avoid breastfeeding for 4–6 hr after administering a maternal dose.

AZELASTINE
Astelin, Astepro, Opitvar, and generics
Antihistamine

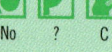
No   No   ?   C

Nasal spray:
 0.1% (Astelin, Astepro): 137 mcg/spray (200 actuations per 30 mL); contains benzalkonium chloride and EDTA
 0.15% (Astepro): 205.5 mcg/spray (200 actuations per 30 mL); contains benzalkonium chloride and EDTA

Ophthalmic drops (Opitvar): 0.05% (0.5 mg/mL) (6 mL); contains benzalkonium chloride

Seasonal allergic rhinitis:
 0.1% strength:
  Child 2–11 yr: 1 spray in each nostril BID
  ≥12 yr and adult: 1–2 sprays in each nostril BID
 0.15% strength:
  Child 6–12 yr: 1 spray in each nostril BID
  ≥12 yr and adult: 1–2 sprays in each nostril BID or 2 sprays in each nostril once daily
Perennial allergic rhinitis:
 0.1% strength:
  ≥6 mo–<12 yr: 1 spray in each nostril BID
 0.15% strength:
  6–<12 yr: 1 spray in each nostril BID
  ≥12 yr and adult: 2 sprays in each nostril BID
Ophthalmic:
  ≥3 yr and adult: Instill 1 drop into each affected eye BID

NASAL USE: Drowsiness may occur despite nasal route of administration (**avoid** concurrent use of alcohol or CNS depressants). Bitter taste, nausea, nasal burning, pharyngitis, weight gain, fatigue, nasal sores, and epistaxis may also occur. Also available in combination with fluticasone as Dymista with labeled dosing information of 1 spray in each nostril BID for seasonal allergic rhinitis (≥6 yr and adult).

OPHTHALMIC USE: Eye burning and stinging have been reported in about 30% of patients receiving the ophthalmic dosage form. **Should not be used** to treat contact lens related irritation. Soft contact lens users should wait at least 10 min after dose instillation before they insert their lenses.

AZITHROMYCIN
Zithromax, Zithromax TRI-PAK, Zithromax Z-PAK, Zmax (extended-release oral suspension), Azasite, and generics
Antibiotic, macrolide

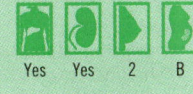
Yes   Yes   2   B

Tablets: 250, 500, 600 mg
  TRI-PAK: 500 mg (3s as unit dose pack)
  Z-PAK: 250 mg (6s as unit dose pack)
Oral suspension: 100 mg/5 mL (15 mL), 200 mg/5 mL (15, 22.5, 30 mL)
Oral Powder (Sachet): 1 g (3s, 10s)
Extended-release oral suspension (microspheres):
  Zmax: 2 g reconstituted with 60 mL of water
Injection: 500 mg; contains 9.92 mEq Na/1 g drug
Ophthalmic solution (Azasite): 1% (2.5 mL)

Infant and child (see remarks):
  Community acquired pneumonia (≥6 mo):
    Tablet or oral suspension: 10 mg/kg PO on day 1 (**max. dose:** 500 mg), followed by 5 mg/kg/24 hr PO once daily (**max. dose:** 250 mg/24 hr) on days 2–5
    Extended-release oral suspension (Zmax): 60 mg/kg (**max. dose:** 1500 mg) PO ×1
  Pharyngitis/tonsillitis (2–15 yr): 12 mg/kg/24 hr PO once daily × 5 days (**max. dose:** 500 mg/24 hr)
  Acute sinusitis (≥ 6 mo): 10 mg/kg/dose (**max. dose:** 500 mg) PO once daily × 3 days
  Pertussis:
    Infant < 6 mo: 10 mg/kg/dose PO once daily × 5 days
    ≥6 mo: 10 mg/kg/dose (**max. dose:** 500 mg) PO × 1, followed by 5 mg/kg/ (**max. dose:** 250 mg) PO once daily on days 2–5.
  Mycobacterium avium complex in HIV (see www.aidsinfo.nih.gov/guidelines for most current recommendations):
    Prophylaxis for first episode: 20 mg/kg/dose PO Q7 days (**max. dose:** 1200 mg/dose); alternatively, 5 mg/kg/24 hr PO once daily (**max. dose:** 250 mg/dose) with or without rifabutin.
    Prophylaxis for recurrence: 5 mg/kg/24 hr PO once daily (**max. dose:** 250 mg/dose), plus ethambutol 15 mg/kg/24 hr (**max. dose:** 900 mg/24 hr) PO once daily with or without rifabutin 5 mg/kg/24 hr (**max. dose:** 300 mg/24 hr).
    Treatment: 10–12 mg/kg/24 hr PO once daily (**max. dose:** 500 mg/24 hr) × 1 month or longer, plus ethambutol 15–25 mg/kg/24 hr (**max. dose:** 1 g/24 hr) PO once daily with or without rifabutin 10–20 mg/kg/24 hr (**max. dose:** 300 mg/24 hr).
  Endocarditis prophylaxis: 15 mg/kg/dose (**max. dose:** 500 mg) PO × 1, 30–60 min before procedure.
  Antiinflammatory agent in Cystic Fibrosis:
    25–39 kg: 250 mg PO every Mondays, Wednesdays and Fridays
    ≥ 40 kg: 500 mg PO every Mondays, Wednesdays and Fridays
Adolescent and adult:
  Pharyngitis, tonsillitis, skin, and soft tissue infection: 500 mg PO day 1, then 250 mg/24 hr PO on days 2–5
  Mild/moderate bacterial COPD exacerbation: above 5 day dosing regimen OR 500 mg PO once daily × 3 days
  Community acquired pneumonia:
    Tablets: 500 mg PO day 1, then 250 mg/24 hr PO on days 2–5
    Extended-release oral suspension (Zmax): Single dose 2 g PO

Continued

AZITHROMYCIN continued

Adolescent and adult:
  Community acquired pneumonia:
    IV and tablet regimen: 500 mg IV once daily × 2 days followed by 500 mg PO once daily to complete a 7–10 day regimen (IV and PO)
  Sinusitis:
    Tablets: 500 mg PO once daily × 3 days
    Extended-release oral suspension (Zmax): Single dose 2 g PO
  Uncomplicated chlamydial cervicitis or urethritis: Single dose 1 g PO
  Gonococcal cervicitis or urethritis: Single 2 g dose PO
  Acute PID (chlamydia): 500 mg IV once daily × 1–2 days followed by 250 mg PO once daily to complete a 7 day regimen (IV and PO).
  Mycobacterium avium complex in HIV (see www.aidsinfo.nih.gov/guidelines for most recent recommendations):
    Prophylaxis for first episode: 1200 mg PO Q7 days with or without rifabutin 300 mg PO once daily
    Prophylaxis for recurrence: 500 mg PO once daily, plus ethambutol 15 mg/kg/dose PO once daily, with or without rifabutin 300 mg PO once daily
    Treatment: 500–600 mg PO once daily with ethambutol 15 mg/kg/dose PO once daily with or without rifabutin 300 mg PO once daily.
  Endocarditis prophylaxis: 500 mg PO × 1, 30–60 min before procedure
  Antiinflammatory agent in Cystic Fibrosis: use same dosing in children.
Ophthalmic:
  ≥1 yr and adult: Instill one drop into the affected eye(s) BID, 8–12 hr apart, × 2 days, followed by one drop once daily for the next 5 days.

No longer recommended for otitis media due to increased resistant pathogens.
Contraindicated in hypersensitivity to macrolides and history of cholestatic jaundice/hepatic dysfunction associated with prior use. **Use with caution** in impaired hepatic function, GFR < 10 mL/min (limited data), hypokalemia, hypomagnesemia, bradycardia, arrhythmias, prolonged QT intervals, and receiving medications that can cause the aforementioned conditions of caution. May cause increase in hepatic enzymes, cholestatic jaundice, GI discomfort, and pain at injection site (IV use). Compared to other macrolides, less risk for drug interactions. Nelfinavir may increase azithromycin levels; monitor for liver enzyme abnormalities and hearing impairment. Vomiting, diarrhea and nausea have been reported at higher frequency in otitis media with 1-day dosing regimen. Exacerbations of myasthenia gravis/syndrome, decreased lymphocytes, and elevated bilirubin, BUN and creatinine have been reported. CNS penetration is poor.

Aluminum- and magnesium-containing antacids decrease absorption. Tablet and oral suspension dosage forms may be administered with or without food. Extended-release oral suspension should be taken on an empty stomach (at least 1 hr before or 2 hr following a meal). Intravenous administration is over 1–3 hr; **do not** give as a bolus or IM injection.
Ophthalmic Use: Do not wear contact lenses. Eye irritation is the most common side effect.

AZTREONAM
Azactam, Cayston, and generic intravenous products
Antibiotic, monobactam

No   Yes   2   B

Injection: 1, 2 g
Frozen injection (Azactam): 1 g/50 mL 3.4% dextrose, 2 g/50 mL 1.4% dextrose (iso-osmotic solutions)
Each 1 g drug contains approximately 780 mg L-Arginine

AZTREONAM continued

Nebulizer solution (Cayston): 75-mg powder to be reconstituted with the supplied diluent of 1 mL 0.17% sodium chloride (28-day course kit contains 84 sterile vials of Cayston and 88 ampules of diluent)

Neonate:
  30 mg/kg/dose IV/IM:
    <1.2 kg and 0–4-wk age: Q12 hr
    1.2–2 kg and 0–7 days: Q12 hr
    1.2–2 kg and >7 days: Q8 hr
    >2 kg and 0–7 days: Q8 hr
    >2 kg and >7 days: Q6 hr
Child: 90–120 mg/kg/24 hr ÷ Q6–8 hr IV/IM
Cystic Fibrosis: 150–200 mg/kg/24 hr ÷ Q6–8 hr IV/IM
Adult:
  Moderate infections: 1–2 g/dose Q8–12 hr IV/IM
  Severe infections: 2 g/dose Q6–8 hr IV/IM
Max. dose: 8 g/24 hr
Inhalation:
  Cystic fibrosis prophylaxis therapy:
    ≥7 yr and adult: 75 mg TID (minimum 4 hr between doses) administered in repeated cycles of 28 days on drug followed by 28 days off drug. Administer each dose with the Altera Nebulizer System.

Typically indicated in multidrug-resistant aerobic gram-negative infections when β-lactam therapy is contraindicated. Well-absorbed IM. **Use with caution** in arginase deficiency. Low cross-allergenicity between aztreonam and other β-lactams. Adverse reactions: thrombophlebitis, eosinophilia, leukopenia, neutropenia, thrombocytopenia, elevation of liver enzymes, hypotension, seizures, and confusion. Good CNS penetration. Probenecid and furosemide increases aztreonam levels. **Adjust dose in renal failure (see Chapter 30).**

INHALATIONAL USE: Cough, nasal congestion, wheezing, pharyngolaryngeal pain, pyrexia, chest discomfort, abdominal pain and vomiting may occur. Bronchospasm has been reported. Use the following order of administration: bronchodilator first, chest physiotherapy, other inhaled medications (if indicated) and aztreonam last.

BACITRACIN ± POLYMYXIN B
Various ophthalmic and topical generic products
In combination with polymyxin b: AK-Poly-Bac Ophthalmic,
Double Antibiotic Topical, Polysporin Topical and others
Antibiotic, topical

No   No   ?   C

BACITRACIN:
  Ophthalmic ointment: 500 units/g (1, 3.5 g)
  Topical ointment (OTC): 500 units/g (15, 30, 113.4, 454 g)
BACITRACIN IN COMBINATION WITH POLYMYXIN B:
  Ophthalmic ointment (AK-Poly-Bac Ophthalmic): 500 units bacitracin + 10,000 units polymyxin B/g (3.5 g)
  Topical ointment: 500 units bacitracin + 10,000 units polymyxin B/g (15, 30 g)

Continued

BACITRACIN ± POLYMYXIN B *continued*

BACITRACIN
Child and adult:
Topical: Apply to affected area once daily to TID
Ophthalmic: Apply 0.25–0.5-inch ribbon into the conjunctival sac of the infected eye(s) Q3–12 hr; frequency depends on severity of infection. Administer Q3–4 hr × 7–10 days for mild/moderate infections.

BACITRACIN + POLYMYXIN B
Child and adult:
Topical: Apply ointment to affected area once daily to TID
Ophthalmic: Apply 0.25–0.5-inch ribbon into the conjunctival sac of the infected eye(s) Q3–12 hr; frequency depends on severity of infection. Administer Q3–4 hr × 7–10 days for mild/moderate infections.

Hypersensitivity reactions to bacitracin and/or polymyxin b can occur. **Do not use** topical ointment for the eyes or for a duration of >7 days. Side effects may include rash, itching, burning, and edema.

Ophthalmic dosage form may cause temporary blurred vision and retard corneal healing. For ophthalmic use, wash hands before use and avoid contact of tube tip with skin or eye.

For neomycin containing products, see Neomycin/Polymyxin B/± Bacitracin.

BACLOFEN
Lioresal, Gablofen, Kemstro, and generic tablets
Centrally acting skeletal muscle relaxant

No | Yes | 2 | C

Tabs: 10, 20 mg
Disintegrating oral tabs (Kemstro): 10, 20 mg; contains phenylalanine
Oral suspension: 5, 10 mg/mL
Intrathecal injection:
   Gablofen: 50 mcg/mL (1 mL), 0.5 mg/mL (20 mL), 1 mg/mL (20 mL), 2 mg/mL (20 mL); preservative-free
   Lioresal: 50 mcg/mL (1 mL), 0.5 mg/mL (20 mL), 2 mg/mL (5, 20 mL); preservative free

---

Oral: Dosage increments, if tolerated, are made at 3-day intervals until desired effect or max. dose is achieved. Initiate first dosage level at QHS, followed by Q12 hr and then Q8 hr. Dosage increments are made by first increasing the QHS dosage, followed by the morning dosage and then the remaining mid-day dosage.

Child (PO, see remarks):
   <20 kg: Start at 2.5 mg QHS, increase in 2.5-mg increments if needed up to the recommended **max. dose** below.
   ≥20–50 kg: Start at 5 mg QHS, increase in 5-mg increments if needed up to the recommended **max. dose** below.
   >50 kg: Start at 10 mg QHS, increase in 10-mg increments if needed up to the recommended **max. dose** below.
   Recommended max. PO dose:
      2 yr–<8 yr: 60 mg/24 hr
      8–16 yr: 80 mg/24 hr
      >16 yr: 120 mg//24 hr
Adult (PO):
   Start at 5 mg TID, increase in 5 mg increments if needed up to a maximum of 80 mg/24 hr.

BACLOFEN continued

Intrathecal continuous-infusion maintenance therapy (not well established):
<12 yr: average dose of 274 mcg/24 hr (range: 24–1199 mcg/24 hr) has been reported.
≥12 yr and adult: most required 300–800 mcg/24 hr (range: 12–2003 mcg/24 hr with limited experience at doses > 1000 mcg/24 hr)

Avoid abrupt withdrawal of drug. **Use with caution** in patients with seizure disorder and impaired renal function. Approximately 70%–80% of the drug is excreted unchanged in the urine. Administer oral dose with food or milk.

Adverse effects: Drowsiness, fatigue, nausea, vertigo, psychiatric disturbances, rash, urinary frequency, and hypotonia. **Avoid** abrupt withdrawal of intrathecal therapy to prevent potential life-threatening events (rhabdomyolysis, multiple organ-system failure and death).

Cases of intrathecal mass at the tip of the implanted catheter leading to withdrawal symptoms have been reported. Inadvertent subcutaneous injection may occur with improper access of the reservoir refill septum and may result in an overdose. Sterile techniques must be employed with intrathecal use accounting for all nonsterile external surfaces.

Usual oral dosage range observed from a single institution retrospective review in 87 patients suggest following:
<2 yr: 10–20 mg/24 hr to a **maximum** of 40 mg/24 hr
2–7 yr: 20–30 mg/24 hr to a **maximum** of 60 mg/24 hr
≥8 yr: 30–40 mg/24 hr to a **maximum** of 200 mg/24 hr

BECLOMETHASONE DIPROPIONATE
QVAR, Beconase AQ, Qnasl Childrens, Qnasl
Corticosteroid

Yes   No   2   C

Inhalation, oral:
QVAR: 40 mcg/inhalation (8.7 g provides 120 inhalations), 80 mcg/inhalation (8.7 g provides 120 inhalations); CFC-free product (HFA)
Inhalation, nasal:
Beconase AQ: 42 mcg/inhalation (25 g provides 180 metered doses); contains benzalkonium chloride
Qnasl Childrens: 40 mcg/inhalation (4.9 g provides 60 metered doses)
Qnasl: 80 mcg/inhalation (8.7 g provides 120 metered doses)

Oral inhalation (QVAR) (see remarks):
5–11 yr: Start at 40 mcg BID; **max. dose:** 80 mcg BID
≥12 yr and adult:
  Corticosteroid naïve: Start at 40–80 mcg BID; **max. dose:** 320 mcg BID
  Previous corticosteroid use: Start at 40–160 mcg BID; **max. dose:** 320 mcg BID
Nasal inhalation:
Beconase AQ:
  6–12 yr: Start with 1 spray (42 mcg) in each nostril BID, may increase to 2 sprays in each nostril BID if needed. Once symptoms are controlled, decrease dose to 1 spray in each nostril BID.
  >12 yr and adult: 1–2 spray(s) (42–84 mcg) in each nostril BID
Qnasl Childrens:
  4–11 yr: 1 spray (40 mcg) each nostril once daily; **max. dose:** 2 sprays (80 mcg)/24 hr
Qnasl:
  12 yr and adult: 2 sprays (160 mcg) in each nostril once daily; **max. dose:** 4 sprays (320 mcg)/24 hr.

Continued

BECLOMETHASONE DIPROPIONATE continued

Not recommended for oral inhalation in children aged <5 yr and for nasal administration in those aged <6 yr (Becnase AQ) or <4 yr (Qnasl Childrens) because of unknown safety and efficacy. Dose should be titrated to lowest effective dose. **Avoid** using higher than recommended doses. **Avoid** use of nasal dosage form in recent nasal ulcers, nasal surgery, or nasal trauma. Nasal septal perforation has been reported with nasal product. Psychiatric and behavioral changes have been reported in children with the oral inhalation product. Routinely monitor growth of pediatric patients with chronic use of all dosage forms.

When converting from fluticasone to beclomethasone for oral inhalation use, consider the following:

Fluticasone MDI (Flovent HFA)	Fluticasone DPI (Flovent Diskus)	Beclomethasone MDI (QVAR)
44 mcg: 2 puffs BID	50 mcg: 2 inhalations BID	40 mcg: 1 puff BID
110 mcg: 2 puffs BID	100 mcg: 2 inhalations BID	40 mcg: 2 puffs BID
220 mcg: 2 puffs BID	250 mcg: 2 inhalations BID	80 mcg: 2 puffs BID

CYP 450 3A4 inhibitors (eg., ketoconazole, erythromycin, and protease inhibitors) or significant hepatic impairment may increase systemic exposure of beclomethasone.

Monitor for hypothalamic, pituitary, adrenal, or growth suppression and hypercorticism. Rinse mouth and gargle with water after oral inhalation; may cause thrush. Use of tube spacers with oral inhalation is recommended.

BENZOYL PEROXIDE
Desquam-DX 5% Wash, Desquam-DX 10% Wash, NeoBenz Micro, Oxy-5, Oxy-10, PanOxyl, and many other products
Topical acne product

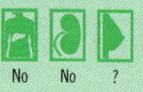

No   No   ?   C

Liquid wash: 5% (120, 150, 200 mL), 10% (120, 150, 240 mL)
Liquid cream wash: 4% (180 g), 8% (180 g)
Bar: 5% [OTC] (113 g), 10% [OTC] (113 g)
Lotion: 4% (297 g), 5% [OTC] (30 mL), 6% (170, 340 g), 8% (297 g), 10% [OTC] (30 mL, 85, 170, 340 g)
Cream: 5% [OTC] (18 g), 10% [OTC] (30 g)
Gel: 2.5% (50 g), 4% (42.5 g), 5% [OTC] (42.5, 60, 90 g), 7% (45 g), 10% (42.5, 60, 90 g)
NOTE: Some preparations may contain alcohol and come in combination packs of cleansers and creams with various strengths.
Combination product with erythromycin (Benzamycin and others):
  Gel: 30 mg erythromycin and 50 mg benzoyl peroxide per g (0.8, 23.3, 46 g); some preparations may contain 20% alcohol
Combination product with clindamycin:
  Gel:
    BenzaClin and generics: 10 mg clindamycin and 50 mg benzoyl peroxide per g (25, 35, 50 g); some preparations may contain methylparaben.
    Duac: 12 mg clindamycin and 50 mg benzoyl peroxide per g (45 g)
    Acanya: 12 mg clindamycin and 25 mg benzoyl peroxide per g (50 g)
Combination product with adapalene: see Adapalene ± Benzoyl Peroxide

Child ≥ 12 yr and adult:
  Cleansers (liquid wash, or bar): Wet affected area prior to application. Apply and wash once daily–BID; rinse thoroughly and pat dry. Modify dose frequency or concentration to control the amount of drying or peeling.

BENZOYL PEROXIDE continued

Lotion, cream, or gel: Cleanse skin and apply small amounts over affected areas once daily initially; increase frequency to BID–TID, if needed. Modify dose frequency or concentration to control drying or peeling.

Combination products:

Benzamycin, BenzaClin and generics: Apply BID (morning and evening) to affected areas after washing and drying skin.

Duac: Apply QHS to affected areas after washing and drying skin.

Acanya: Apply pea-sized amount once daily.

Contraindicated in patients with known history of hypersensitivity to product's components (benzoyl peroxide, clindamycin, or erythromycin). **Avoid** contact with mucous membranes and eyes. May cause skin irritation, stinging, dryness, peeling, erythema, edema, and contact dermatitis. Anaphylaxis has been reported with products containing clindamycin and benzoyl peroxide.

Concurrent use with tretinoin (Retin-A) will increase risk of skin irritation. Products containing clindamycin and erythromycin should not be used in combination.

Any single application resulting in excessive stinging or burning may be removed with mild soap and water. Lotion, cream, and gel dosage forms should be applied to dry skin.

BENZTROPINE MESYLATE
Cogentin and various generics
Anticholinergic agent, drug-induced dystonic reaction antidote, anti-Parkinson's agent

No No ? ?

Injection: 1 mg/mL (2 mL)
Tabs: 0.5, 1, 2 mg

Drug-induced extrapyramidal symptoms (PO/IM/IV):
>**3 yr:** 0.02–0.05 mg/kg/dose once daily–BID
Adult: 1–4 mg/dose once daily–BID
Acute dystonic reaction (phenothiazines) (IM/IV):
Child: 0.02 mg/kg/dose (**max. dose:** 1 mg) × 1
Adult: 1–2 mg/dose ×1

Contraindicated in myasthenia gravis, GI/GU obstruction, untreated narrow-angle glaucoma, and peptic ulcer. Use IV route **only** when PO and IM routes are not feasible. May cause anticholinergic side effects, especially constipation and dry mouth. Drug interactions include: potentiation of CNS-depressant effects when used with CNS depressants, enhanced CNS side effects of amantadine, and inhibition of the response of neuroleptics. This medication has not been formally assigned a pregnancy category by the FDA. The Australian pregnancy ratings have deemed use in pregnancy to a limited number of women without an increase in frequency of malformation or other direct/indirect harmful effects.

Onset of action: 15 min for IV/IM and 1 hr for PO.
Oral doses should be administered with food to decrease GI upset.

BERACTANT

See Surfactant, pulmonary

BETAMETHASONE
AlphaTrex, Celestone Soluspan, Diprolene, Diprolene AF, Luxiq, Sernivo, and many generics
Corticosteroid

No   No   3   C

Na Phosphate and Acetate:
  Injection suspension (Celestone Soluspan and generics): 6 mg/mL (3 mg/mL Na phosphate + 3 mg/mL betamethasone acetate) (5 mL); may contain benzalkonium chloride and EDTA.
Dipropionate:
  Topical cream: 0.05% (15, 45 g)
  Topical emulsion (Sernivo): 0.05% (120 mL); contains parabens
  Topical lotion: 0.05% (60 mL); may contain 46.8% alcohol and propylene glycol
  Topical ointment: 0.05% (15, 45, 50 g)
Valerate:
  Topical cream: 0.1% (15, 45 g)
  Topical foam (Luxiq and generics): 1.2 mg/g (50, 100 g); may contain 60.4% ethanol, cetyl alcohol, stearyl alcohol, and propylene glycol
  Topical lotion: 0.1% (60 mL); may contain 47.5% isopropyl alcohol
  Topical ointment: 0.1% (15, 45 g)
Dipropionate augmented:
  Topical cream (Diprolene AF and generics): 0.05% (15, 50 g); contains propylene glycol
  Topical gel (AlphaTrex and generics): 0.05% (15, 50 g); contains propylene glycol
  Topical lotion (Diprolene and generics): 0.05% (30, 60 mL); contains 30% isopropyl alcohol
  Topical ointment (Diprolene and generics): 0.05% (15, 45, 50 g); contains propylene glycol

All dosages should be adjusted based on patient response and severity of condition (see remarks).
Antiinflammatory:
  Child:
    IM: 0.0175–0.125 mg/kg/24 hr or 0.5–7.5 mg/m^2/24 hr ÷ Q6–12 hr
  Adolescent and adult:
    IM: 0.6–9 mg/24 hr ÷ Q12–24 hr
Topical (use smallest amount for shortest period of time to avoid adrenal suppression and reassess diagnosis if no improvement is achieved after 2 weeks; see remarks):
  Valerate and dipropionate forms:
    Child and adult: Apply to affected areas once daily–BID
  Dipropionate augmented forms:
    ≥13 yr–adult: Apply to affected areas once daily–BID
    Max. dose: 14 days
      Cream and ointment: 45 g/week
      Gel: 50 g/week
      Lotion: 50 mL/week

Use with caution in hypothyroidism, cirrhosis, and ulcerative colitis. See Chapter 8 for relative steroid potencies and doses based on body surface area. Betamethasone is inadequate when used alone for adrenocortical insufficiency because of its minimal mineralocorticoid properties. Like all steroids, it may cause hypertension, pseudotumor cerebri, acne, Cushing syndrome, adrenal axis suppression, GI bleeding, hyperglycemia, and osteoporosis.

Na phosphate and acetate injectable suspension recommended for IM, intraarticular, intrasynovial, intralesional, and soft tissue use only; but **not** for IV use. Topical betamethasone dipropionate

BETAMETHASONE continued

augmented (Diprolene and Diprolene AF) is **not recommended** in children ≤ 12 yr owing to the higher risk of adrenal suppression.

Injectable IM dosage form is used in premature labor to stimulate fetal lung maturation.

BICITRA

See Citrate Mixtures

BISACODYL
Dulcolax, Fleet Laxative, Fleet Bisacodyl, and various other names
Laxative, stimulant

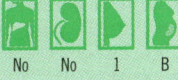
No   No   1   B

Tabs (enteric coated) [OTC]: 5 mg
Suppository [OTC]: 10 mg
Enema (Fleet Bisacodyl) [OTC]: 10 mg/30 mL (37.5 mL)
Delayed-release tabs [OTC]: 5 mg

Oral:
Child (3–12 yr): 0.3 mg/kg/dose or 5–10 mg × 1 administered 6 hr before desired effect; **max. dose:** 30 mg/24 hr
Adolescent and adult (>12 yr): 5–15 mg × 1 administered 6 hr before desired effect; **max. dose:** 30 mg/24 hr
Rectal suppository (as a single dose):
  <2 yr: 5 mg
  2–11 yr: 5–10 mg
  >11 yr and adult: 10 mg
Rectal enema (as a single dose):
  ≥12 yr and adult: 10 mg (30 mL)

Do not use in newborn period. Instruct patient/parent that tablets should be swallowed whole, **not** chewed or crushed; **not** to be given within 1 hr of taking antacids or milk. May cause abdominal cramps, nausea, vomiting, and rectal irritation. Oral dose is usually effective within 6–10 hr; rectal dose is usually effective within 15–60 min.

Antacids may decrease the effect of bisacodyl and may cause the premature release of the delayed-release formulation prior to reaching the large intestine.

BISMUTH SUBSALICYLATE
Pepto-Bismol, Kaopectate, Kaopectate Extra Strength, Kao-Tin, Stomach Relief, Stomach Relief Max St, and many others
(see remarks)
Antidiarrheal, gastrointestinal ulcer agent

No   Yes   3   D

Liquid [OTC]:
  Kaopectate, Pepto-Bismol, Kao-Tin, Stomach Relief, and others: 262 mg/15 mL (240, 360, 480 mL)
  Kaopectate Extra Strength, and Stomach Relief Max St: 525 mg/15 mL (240, 480 mL)
Chewable tabs [OTC]: 262 mg; may contain aspartame
Contains 102 mg salicylate per 262 mg tablet; or 129 mg salicylate per 15 mL of the 262 mg/15 mL liquid.

Continued

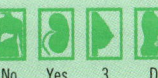

BISMUTH SUBSALICYLATE continued

Diarrhea:
  Child: 100 mg/kg/24 hr ÷ 5 equal doses for 5 days; **max. dose:** 4.19 g/24 hr
  Dosage by age; give following dose Q30 min to 1 hr PRN up to a **max. dose** of 8 doses/24 hrs:
  3–5 yr: 87.3 mg (⅓ tablet or 5 mL of 262 mg/15 mL)
  6–8 yr: 174.7 mg (⅔ tablet or 10 mL of 262 mg/15 mL)
  9–11 yr: 262 mg (1 tablet or 15 mL of 262 mg/15 mL)
  ≥12 yr–adult: 524 mg (2 tablets or 30 mL of 262 mg/15 mL)
H. pylori gastric infection (in combination with ampicillin and metronidazole or with tetracycline and metronidazole for adults; doses not well established for children):
  <10 yr: 262 mg PO QID × 6 wk
  ≥10 yr–adult: 524 mg PO QID /× 6 wk

Generally not recommended in children <16 yr with chicken pox or flu-like symptoms (risk for Reye syndrome), in combination with other nonsteroidal antiinflammatory drugs, anticoagulants, or oral antidiabetic agents, or in severe renal failure. **Use with caution** in bleeding disorders, renal dysfunction, gastritis, and gout. May cause darkening of tongue and/or black stools, GI upset, impaction, and decreased platelet aggregation.

Drug combination appears to have antisecretory and antimicrobial effects with some antiinflammatory effects. Absorption of bismuth is negligible, whereas approximately 80% of the salicylate is absorbed. Decreases absorption of tetracycline.

DO NOT use Children's Pepto (calcium carbonate) since it does not contain bismuth subsalicylate. **Avoid use in renal failure** (see Chapter 30).

BROMPHENIRAMINE WITH PHENYLEPHRINE
Dimetapp Children's Cold and Allergy, and many other products
Antihistamine + decongestant

No   No   3   C

Oral syrup (Dimetapp Children's Cold and Allergy) [OTC]: Brompheniramine 1 mg + phenylephrine 2.5 mg/5 mL (237 mL)
Chewable tab (Dimetapp Children's Cold and Allergy) [OTC]: Brompheniramine 1 mg + phenylephrine 2.5 mg
NOTE: other combination products exist using the Dimetapp name; always check the specific ingredients with each specific product

All doses based on brompheniramine component.
  2–<6 yr: 1 mg Q4 hr PO up to a **max. dose** of 6 mg/24 hr
  6–12 yr: 2 mg Q4 hr PO up to a **max. dose** of 12 mg/24 hr
  ≥12 yr: 4 mg Q4 hr PO up to a **max. dose** of 24 mg/24 hr
Alternatively, dosing based on specific dosage forms/products. CAUTION: These products may be available in different concentrations.
  Oral, elixir (Dimetapp Children's Cold and Allergy):
    6–<12 yr: 10 mL Q4 hr PO up to a **max. dose** of 60 mL/24 hr
    ≥12 yr: 20 mL Q4 hr PO up to a **max. dose** of 120 mL/24 hr
  Oral, chewable tab (Dimetapp Children's Cold and Allergy):
    6–<12 yr: Chew 2 tablets Q4 hr PO; **max. dose:** 6 doses/24 hr
    ≥12 yr: Chew 4 tablets Q4 hr PO; **max. dose:** 6 doses/24 hr

BROMPHENIRAMINE WITH PHENYLEPHRINE continued

Generally not recommended for treating URIs in infants. No proven benefit for infants and young children with URIs. Over-the-counter (OTC or nonprescription) use of this product is **not recommended** for children aged < 6 years due to reports of serious adverse effects (cardiac and respiratory distress, convulsions, and hallucinations) and fatalities (from unintentional overdosages, including combined use of other OTC products containing the same active ingredients).

Contraindicated with use of MAO inhibitors (concurrent use and within 14 days of discontinuing MAO inhibitors). **Use with caution** in narrow-angle glaucoma, bladder neck obstruction, asthma, pyloroduodenal obstruction, symptomatic prostatic hypertrophy, hypertension, coronary artery disease, diabetes mellitus, and thyroid disease. Discontinue use 48 hours prior to allergy skin testing. May cause drowsiness, fatigue, CNS excitation, xerostomia, blurred vision, and wheezing.

BUDESONIDE
Pulmicort Respules, Pulmicort Flexhaler, Rhinocort Aqua Nasal Spray, Entocort EC, Uceris, and generics
Corticosteroid

Yes   No   2/?   B/C

Nasal spray (Rinocort Aqua and generics): 32 mcg/actuation (8.6 g, delivers approx. 120 sprays)
Nebulized inhalation suspension (Pulmicort Respules and generics): 0.25 mg/2 mL, 0.5 mg/2 mL (30s)
Oral inhalation powder:
  Pulmicort Flexhaler: 90 mcg/metered dose (165 mg, delivers 60 doses), 180 mcg/metered dose (225 mg, delivers 120 doses); contains lactose
Enteric-coated caps (Entocort EC and generics): 3 mg
Extended-release tabs (Uceris): 9 mg
Rectal foam (Uceris): 2 mg per metered dose (33.4 g, delivers 14 doses; 2 canisters per kit)

Nebulized inhalation suspension:
  Child 1–8 yr:
    No prior steroid use: 0.5 mg/24 hr ÷ once daily–BID; **max. dose:** 0.5 mg/24 hr
    Prior inhaled steroid use: 0.5 mg/24 hr ÷ once daily–BID; **max. dose:** 1 mg/24 hr
    Prior oral steroid use: 1 mg/24 hr ÷ once daily–BID; **max. dose:** 1 mg/24 hr
    NIH Asthma Guideline 2007 recommendations (divide daily doses once daily–BID):
    Child 0–4 yr:
      Low dose: 0.25–0.5 mg/24 hr
      Medium dose: >0.5–1 mg/24 hr
      High dose: >1 mg/24 hr
    Child 5–11 yr:
      Low dose: 0.5 mg/24 hr
      Medium dose: 1 mg/24 hr
      High dose: 2 mg/24 hr
Oral inhalation:
  Pulmicort Flexhaler:
    Child ≥ 6 yr: Start at 180 mcg BID; **max. dose:** 720 mcg/24 hr.
    Adult: Start at 180–360 mcg BID; **max. dose:** 1440 mcg/24 hr.
Nasal inhalation (≥6 yr and adult):
  Rhinocort Aqua: (initial): 1 spray in each nostril once daily. Increase dose as needed up to **max. dose** (see next page).

Continued

BUDESONIDE continued

Max. nasal dose: 6–11 yr: 128 mcg/24 hr (4 sprays/24 hr); ≥12 yr and adult: 256 mcg/24 hr (8 sprays/24 hr)

Crohn's disease (Encort EC):

Child ≥ 6 yr (see remarks): Data are limited as the following dosages have been reported. Additional studies are needed.

Active disease: 9 mg PO once daily × 7–8 wks

Maintenance of remission: 6 mg PO once daily × 3–4 wks

Additionally, a report in children aged 10–19 years demonstrated higher remission rates, with an induction dose of 12 mg PO once daily × 4 wks, followed by 9 mg PO once daily × 3 wks, and followed by 6 mg PO once daily × 3 wks.

Adult:

Active disease: 9 mg PO QAM × 8 wks; if remission is not achieved, a second 8-week course may be given.

Maintenance of remission: 6 mg PO once daily for up to 3 mo. If symptom control is maintained at 3 mo, taper dosage to compete cessation. Remission therapy beyond 3 mo has not shown to provide substantial clinical benefit.

Ulcerative colitis, induction of remission (Uceris):

Adult:

Oral: 9 mg PO QAM for up to 8 weeks

Rectal: 2 mg PR BID × 2 weeks followed by 2 mg PR once daily × 4 weeks

Reduce maintenance dose to as low as possible to control symptoms. May cause pharyngitis, cough, epistaxis, nasal irritation, and HPA-axis suppression. Rinse mouth after each use via the oral inhalation route. Nebulized budesonide has been shown to be effective in mild to moderate croup at doses of 2 mg × 1. Ref: *N Engl J Med* 331(5):285.

Hypersensitivity reactions, including anaphylaxis, have been reported with the inhaled route. Anaphylactic reactions and benign intracranial hypertension have been reported with oral route of administration.

Safety and effectiveness for mild/moderate Crohn's disease have been established for children aged 8–17 years and weighing ≥ 25 kg. Safety and efficacy has NOT been established in pediatric patients for the maintenance of clinical remission of mild/moderate Crohn's disease. Although the reported safety profile in pediatric Crohn's disease is consistent with adults, there may be increased risk for decreased growth velocity due to higher systemic absorption of corticosteroids in children with Crohn's disease.

CYP 450 3A4 inhibitors (eg., ketoconazole, erythromycin, and protease inhibitors) or significant hepatic impairment may increase systemic exposure of budesonide (inhalation and PO routes)

Onset of action for oral inhalation and nebulized suspension is within 1 day and 2–8 days, respectively, with peak effects at 1–2 wk and 4–6 wk, respectively.

For nasal use, onset of action is seen after 1 day with peak effects after 3–7 days of therapy. Discontinue therapy if no improvement in nasal symptoms after 3 wk of continuous therapy.

Pregnancy category is "B" for inhalation routes of administration and "C" for the oral and rectal routes. **Breast feeding category is "2" for inhalation routes and "?"** for the oral and rectal routes. **Do not** crush or chew the oral capsule dosage form.

BUDESONIDE AND FORMOTEROL
Symbicort
Corticosteroid and long-acting β₂-adrenergic agonist

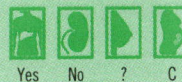
Yes No ? C

Aerosol inhaler:
80 mcg budesonide + 4.5 mcg formoterol fumarate dihydrate (6.9 g delivers 60 inhalations, 10.2 g delivers about 120 inhalations)
160 mcg budesonide + 4.5 mcg formoterol fumarate dihydrate (6 g delivers 60 inhalations, 10.2 g delivers about 120 inhalations)

5–11 yr (NIH Asthma Guideline 2007 recommendations and 6–<12 yr [FDA labeling]): Two inhalations BID of 80 mcg budesonide + 4.5 mcg fomoterol; max. dose: 4 inhalations/24 hr.
≥12 yr and adult:
  No prior inhaled steroid use: Start with two inhalations BID of 80 mcg budesonide + 4.5 mcg fomoterol **OR** 160 mcg budesonide + 4.5 mcg fomoterol, depending on severity.
  Prior low to medium doses of inhaled steroid use: Start with two inhalations BID of 80 mcg budesonide + 4.5 mcg fomoterol.
  Prior medium to high doses of inhaled steroid use: Start with two inhalations BID of 160 mcg budesonide + 4.5 mcg fomoterol.
  Max. dose: 2 inhalations of 160 mcg budesonide + 4.5 mcg fomoterol BID

See *Budesonide* and *Fomoterol* for remarks. Should only be used for patients not adequately controlled on other asthma-controller medications (e.g., low-to-medium–dose inhaled corticosteroids) or whose disease severity requires the use of two maintenance therapies. Titrate to the lowest effective strength after asthma is adequately controlled. Proper patient education including dosage administration technique is essential; see patient package insert for detailed instructions. Rinse mouth after each use.

BUMETANIDE
Generics; previously available as Bumex
Loop diuretic

Yes No ? C

Tabs: 0.5, 1, 2 mg
Injection: 0.25 mg/mL (4, 10 mL); some preparations may contain 1% benzyl alcohol

Neonate and infant (see remarks): PO/IM/IV
  ≤6 mo: 0.01–0.05 mg/kg/dose once daily or every other day
Infant and child: PO/IM/IV
  >6 mo: 0.015–0.1 mg/kg/dose once daily–QID; **max. dose:** 10 mg/24 hr
Adult:
  PO: 0.5–2 mg/dose once daily–BID
  IM/IV: 0.5–1 mg over 1–2 min. May give additional doses Q2–3 hr PRN
Usual max. dose (PO/IM/IV): 10 mg/24 hr

Cross-allergenicity may occur in patients allergic to sulfonamides. Dosage reduction may be necessary in patients with hepatic dysfunction. Administer oral doses with food.
Side effects include cramps, dizziness, hypotension, headache, electrolyte losses (hypokalemia, hypocalcemia, hyponatremia, and hypochloremia), and encephalopathy. May also lead to metabolic alkalosis. Serious skin reactions (eg. Stevens-Johnson syndrome, TEN) have been reported.
Drug elimination has been reported to be slower in neonates with respiratory disorders compared to neonates without. May displace bilirubin in critically ill neonates. **Maximal** diuretic effect for infants ≤ 6 mo has been reported at 0.04 mg/kg/dose, with greater efficacy seen at lower dosages.

BUTORPHANOL
Generics; previously available as Stadol
Narcotic, analgesic

Yes   Yes   3   C

Injection: 1 mg/mL (1 mL), 2 mg/mL (1, 2, 10 mL)
Nasal solution: 10 mg/mL (2.5 mL); 1 mg per spray

Child: 0.03–0.05 mg/kg/dose (**max. dose:** 2 mg/dose) IV Q3–4 hr PRN.
Adult:
  IV: 1 mg/dose Q3–4 hr PRN; usual dosage range: 0.5–2 mg Q3–4 hr PRN
  IM: 2 mg/dose Q3–4 hr PRN; usual dosage range: 1–4 mg Q3–4 hr PRN
Intranasal: 1 spray (1 mg) in one nostril × 1; an additional 1-mg dose may be given at 1–1.5 hr, if needed. This two-dose sequence may be repeated in 3–4 hr, if needed. Alternatively, the patients may receive 2 mg initially (1 mg in each nostril) only if they remain recumbent. If drowsiness or dizziness occurs, an additional dose may be given 3–4 hr later.

A synthetic mixed agonist/antagonist opioid analgesic. **Contraindicated** in patients hypersensitive to benzethonium chloride. **Use with caution** in hypotension, thyroid dysfunction, renal or hepatic impairment, and concomitant CNS depressants. **Suggested dosage reduction** in renal impairment (IV/IM): 75% of usual dose for GFR 10–50 mL/min and 50% of usual dose for GFR < 10 mL/min, with an increase in dosage interval based on duration of clinical effects. A 50% IV/IM dosage reduction with increased dosage interval has been recommended in hepatic dysfunction. Reduced dosage for intranasal administration for both renal and hepatic impairment: initial dose should not exceed 1 mg.

Butorphanol is a P450 3A4 substrate. Cytochrome P450 3A4 inhibitors may increase butorphanol's effects and toxicity (fatal respiratory depression).

Common side effects include drowsiness, dizziness, insomnia (nasal spray), nausea, vomiting, and nasal congestion (nasal spray). Severe respiratory depression has been reported with use of nasal solutions.

Onset of action: 5–10 min (IV); 0.5–1 hr (IM); and within 15 min (intranasal). **Duration:** 3–4 hr (IV/IM) and 4–5 hr (intranasal).

CAFFEINE CITRATE
Cafcit and generics
Methylxanthine, respiratory stimulant

Yes   Yes   2   C

Injection: 20 mg/mL (3 mL)
Oral liquid: 20 mg/mL (3 mL), also available as powder for compounding 10, 20 mg/mL
20 mg/mL caffeine citrate salt = 10 mg/mL caffeine base

Doses expressed in mg of caffeine citrate.
  Neonatal apnea:
    Loading dose: 20–25 mg/kg IV/PO × 1
    Maintenance dose: 5–10 mg/kg/dose PO/IV Q24 hr, to begin 24 hr after loading dose

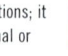

Avoid use in symptomatic cardiac arrhythmias. **Do not use** caffeine benzoate formulations; it has been associated with kernicterus in neonates. **Use with caution** in impaired renal or hepatic function.

CAFFEINE CITRATE continued

Therapeutic levels: 5–25 mg/L. Cardiovascular, neurologic, or gastrointestinal (GI) toxicity reported at serum levels of >50 mg/L. Recommended serum sampling time: obtain trough level within 30 min prior to a dose. Steady state is typically achieved 3 wk after initiation of therapy. Levels obtained prior to steady state are useful for preventing toxicity.
For IV administration, give loading dose over 30 min and maintenance dose over 10 min.

CALCITONIN—SALMON
Miacalcin, Miacalcin Nasal Spray, Fortical Nasal Spray and generic nasal sprays
Hypercalcemia antidote, antiosteoporotic

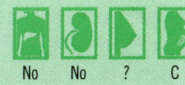
No   No   ?   C

Injection (Miacalcin): 200 U/mL (2 mL); contains phenol
Nasal spray: 200 U/metered dose (2 mL provides at least 14 doses and 3.7 mL provides at least 30 doses); may contain benzyl alcohol

Osteogenesis imperfecta:
>6-mo adolescent: 2 U/kg/dose IM/SC 3 times per week
Hypercalcemia (see remarks):
Adult: Start with 4 U/kg/dose IM/SC Q12 hr; if response is unsatisfactory after 1 or 2 days, increase dose to 8 U/kg/dose Q12 hr. If response remains unsatisfactory after 2 more days, increase to a **max. dose** of 8 U/kg/dose Q6 hr.
Paget's disease (see remarks):
Adult: Start with 100 U IM/SC once daily initially, followed by a usual maintenance dose of 50 U once daily **OR** 50–100 U Q1–3 days.

Contraindicated in patients sensitive to salmon protein or gelatin. Because of hypersensitivity risk (e.g., bronchospasm, airway swelling, anaphylaxis), a skin test is recommended before initiating IM/SC therapy. For skin test, prepare a 10-U/mL dilution with normal saline, administer 0.1 mL intradermally, and observe for 15 min for wheals or significant erythema. Tachyphylaxis has been reported 2–3 days after use for the treatment of hypercalcemia of malignancy.
Nausea, abdominal pain, diarrhea, flushing, and inflammation/urticaria at the injection site have been reported with IM/SC route of administration. May decrease lithium levels via enhanced urinary clearance. Hypocalcemia and increased risk for malignancies have been reported in a meta-analysis.
Intranasal use currently indicated for postmenopausal osteoporosis in adults. Nasal irritation (alternate nostrils to reduce risk), rhinitis, epistaxis may occur with the intranasal product.
Tremors have been reported with both intranasal and injectable routes of administration.
If the injection volume exceeds 2 mL, use IM route and multiple sites of injection.

CALCITRIOL
1,25-dihydroxycholecalciferol, Rocaltrol, Calcijex, and generics
Active form vitamin D, fat soluble

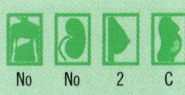
No   No   2   C

Caps: 0.25, 0.5 mcg; may contain parabens
Oral solution: 1 mcg/mL (15 mL)
Injection: (Calcijex and others) 1 mcg/mL (1 mL); contains EDTA

Continued

CALCITRIOL continued

Hypoparathyroidism (evaluate dosage at 2–4 wk intervals):
  Child aged >1 yr and adult: Initial dose of 0.25 mcg/dose PO once daily. May
  increase daily dosage by 0.25 mcg at 2- to 4-wk intervals. Usual maintenance dosage
  as follows:
    <1 yr: 0.02–0.06 mcg/kg/dose PO once daily
    1–5 yr: 0.25–0.75 mcg/dose PO once daily
    >6 yr and adult: 0.5–2 mcg/dose PO once daily
Renal failure: See the National Kidney Foundation guidelines at http://www.kidney.org/professionals/kdoqi/guidelinespedbone/guide9.htm.

Most potent vitamin D metabolite available. Should not be used to treat 25-OH vitamin D deficiency; use cholecalciferol or ergocalciferol. Monitor serum calcium and phosphorus; and parathyroid hormone (PTH) in dialysis patients. **Avoid** concomitant use of Mg^{2+}-containing antacids. IV dosing applies if patient undergoing hemodialysis.

Contraindicated in patients with hypercalcemia, vitamin D toxicity. Side effects include weakness, headache, vomiting, constipation, hypotonia, polydipsia, polyuria, myalgia, metastatic calcification, etc. Allergic reactions, including anaphylaxis, have been reported. May increase serum creatinine in predialysis patients.

CALCIUM ACETATE
PhosLo, Calphron, Eliphos, Phoslyra, and generics;
25% elemental Ca
Calcium supplement, phosphorous-lowering agent

No   Yes   2   C

Tabs (Calphron, Eliphos and generics): 667 mg (169 mg elemental Ca)
Capsules (PhosLo and generics): 667 mg (169 mg elemental Ca)
Oral solution (Phoslyra): 667 mg/5 mL (473 mL) (169 mg elemental Ca per 5 mL); contains methylparabens and propylene glycol
Each 1 g of salt contains 12.7 mEq (250 mg) elemental Ca.

Doses expressed in mg of calcium acetate.
  Hyperphosphatemia (see remarks):
    Child and adolescent: Start with 667–1000 mg PO with each meal. If needed,
    dosage may be titrated every 2–4 wk up to the recommended limits from the KDOQI guidelines:
      Calcium intake as phosphate binders: 1500 mg elemental Ca/24 hr
      Total calcium intake from all sources: 2000 mg elemental Ca/24 hr
    Adult: Start with 1334 mg PO with each meal. Dosage may be increased gradually to bring serum phosphorous levels below 6 mg/dL, as long as hypercalcemia does not occur. Most patients require 2001–2668 mg PO with each meal.

Contraindicated in ventricular fibrillation. **Use with caution** in renal impairment as hypercalcemia may develop in end-stage renal failure. Nausea and hypercalcemia may also occur. Approximately 40% of the dose is systemically absorbed in fasting conditions and up to 30% in nonfasting conditions. May reduce absorption of fluoroquinolones, tetracyclines, iron, and effectiveness of polystyrene sulfonate. May potentiate effects of digoxin.

1 g calcium acetate binds to 45 mg phosphorus.
Administer with meals and plenty of fluids for use as a phosphorus-lowering agent. Calcium is excreted in breast milk and is not expected to harm the infant, provided maternal serum calcium is appropriately monitored.

CALCIUM CARBONATE
Tums, Children's Pepto, and many generics; 40% elemental Ca
Calcium supplement, antacid

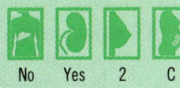

No   Yes   2   C

Tab, chewable [OTC]: 400, 500, 600, 750, 1000, 1250 mg
Children's Pepto [OTC]: 400 mg
Tab [OTC]: 500, 600, 648, 1250, 1500 mg
Oral suspension [OTC]: 1250 mg/5 mL
Powder [OTC]: 800 mg/2 g (480 g)
Each 1 g of salt contains 20 mEq elemental Ca (400 mg elemental Ca).
Some products may be combined with vitamin D; check package labeling.

Hypocalcemia (Doses expressed in mg of elemental Ca. To convert to mg of salt, divide elemental dose by 0.4):
Neonate: 50–150 mg/kg/24 hr ÷ Q4–6 hr PO; **max. dose:** 1 g/24 hr
Child: 45–65 mg/kg/24 hr PO ÷ QID
Adult: 1–2 g/24 hr PO ÷ TID-QID

Antacid (Doses expressed in mg of calcium carbonate; chronic use NOT recommended in gastroesophageal reflux disease [GERD]):
2–5 yr and ≥10.9 kg: 375–400 mg PO as symptoms occur; **max. dose:** 1500 mg/24 hr
>6–11 yr: 750–800 mg PO as symptoms occur; **max. dose:** 3000 mg/24 hr
>11 yr and adult: 500–3000 mg PO as symptoms occur; **max. dose:** 7500 mg/24 hr

See *Calcium acetate* for **contraindications**, **precautions**, and drug interactions. Side effects: constipation, hypercalcemia, hypophosphatemia, hypomagnesemia, nausea, vomiting, headache, and confusion. Some products may contain trace amounts of sodium. Administer with plenty of fluids. For use as a phosphorus-lowering agent, administer with meals. Calcium is excreted in breast milk and is not expected to harm the infant, provided maternal serum calcium is appropriately monitored.

CALCIUM CHLORIDE
Various generics; 27% elemental Ca
Calcium supplement

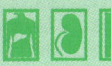

No   Yes   2   C

Injection: 100 mg/mL (10%) (1.36 mEq Ca/mL) (10 mL)
Prefilled syringe for injection: 100 mg/mL (10%) (1.36 mEq Ca/mL) (10 mL)
Each 1 g of salt contains 13.6 mEq (273 mg) elemental Ca.

Doses expressed in mg of calcium chloride.
Cardiac arrest or calcium channel blocker toxicity:
Infant/child: 20 mg/kg/dose (**max. dose:** 2000 mg/dose) IV/IO Q10 min PRN; if effective, an infusion of 20–50 mg/kg/hr may be used.
Adult: 500–1000 mg/dose IV Q10 min PRN or 2–4 mg/kg/dose Q10 min PRN
MAXIMUM IV ADMINISTRATION RATES:
IV push: Do not exceed 100 mg/min (over 10–20 sec in cardiac arrest).
IV infusion: Do not exceed 45–90 mg/kg/hr with a **max. concentration** of 20 mg/mL.

Contraindicated in ventricular fibrillation. **Not recommended** for asystole and electromechanical dissociation. **Use with caution** in renal impairment as hypercalcemia may develop in end-stage renal failure. May potentiate effects of digoxin.

Continued

CALCIUM CHLORIDE continued

Use IV with extreme caution. Extravasation may lead to necrosis. Hyaluronidase may be helpful for extravasation. Central line administration is the preferred IV route of administration. **Do not use scalp veins. Do not administer via IM or SC routes.**

Rapid IV infusion associated with bradycardia, hypotension, and peripheral vasodilation. May cause hyperchloremic acidosis.

Calcium is excreted in breast milk and is not expected to harm the infant, provided maternal serum calcium is appropriately monitored.

CALCIUM CITRATE
Calcitrate, Citracal, and generics; 21% elemental Ca
Calcium supplement

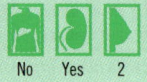
No   Yes   2   C

Tabs [OTC]: 950 mg (200 mg elemental Ca), 1040 mg (218 mg elemental Ca)
Granules [OTC]:
  As elemental Ca: 760 mg/teaspoonful or 3.5 g of granules (480 g)
Each 1 g of salt contains 10.6 mEq (211 mg) elemental Ca.
Some products may be combined with vitamin D; check package labeling.

Doses expressed as mg of elemental Ca. To convert to mg of salt, divide elemental dose by 0.21.
Hypocalcemia:
  Neonate: 50–150 mg/kg/24 hr ÷ Q4–6 hr PO; **max. dose**: 1 g/24 hr
  Child: 45–65 mg/kg/24 hr PO ÷ QID
  Adult: 1–2 g/24 hr PO ÷ TID-QID

See Calcium Acetate for **contraindications, precautions**, and drug interactions. Side effects: constipation, hypercalcemia, hypophosphatemia, hypomagnesemia, nausea, vomiting, headache, and confusion.

Administer with meals for use as a phosphorus-lowering agent or with use of the granule dosage form. For hypocalcemia, do not administer with or before meals/food and take plenty of fluids.

Calcium is excreted in breast milk and is not expected to harm the infant, provided maternal serum calcium is appropriately monitored.

CALCIUM GLUBIONATE
Calcionate and generics; 6.4% elemental Ca
Calcium supplement

No   Yes   2   C

Syrup [OTC]: 1.8 g/5 mL (473 mL) (1.2 mEq Ca/mL)
Each 1 g of salt contains 3.2 mEq (64 mg) elemental Ca.

Doses expressed in mg of calcium glubionate.
Hypocalcemia:
  Neonate: 1200 mg/kg/24 hr PO ÷ Q4–6 hr
  Infant/child: 600–2000 mg/kg/24 hr PO ÷ QID; **max. dose**: 9 g/24 hr
  Adult: 6–18 g/24 hr PO ÷ QID

See *Calcium Acetate* for **contraindications, precautions**, and drug interactions. Side effects include GI irritation, dizziness, and headache. High osmotic load of syrup (20% sucrose) may cause diarrhea.

Best absorbed when administered before meals. Absorption inhibited by high phosphate load.

CALCIUM GLUBIONATE continued

Calcium is excreted in breast milk and is not expected to harm the infant, provided maternal serum calcium is appropriately monitored.

CALCIUM GLUCONATE
Cal-Glu and generics; 9% elemental Ca
Calcium supplement

No   Yes   2   C

Tabs [OTC]: 50, 500 mg
Caps (Cal-Glu) [OTC]: 500 mg
Injection: 100 mg/mL (10%) (0.45 mEq Ca/mL) (10, 50, 100 mL)
Each 1 g of salt contains 4.5 mEq (90 mg) elemental Ca

Doses expressed in mg of calcium gluconate.
Maintenance/hypocalcemia:
  Neonate: IV: 200–800 mg/kg/24 hr ÷ Q6 hr
  Infant:
    IV: 200–500 mg/kg/24 hr ÷ Q6 hr
    PO: 400–800 mg/kg/24 hr ÷ Q6 hr
  Child: 200–500 mg/kg/24 hr IV or PO ÷ Q6 hr
  Adult: 0.5–8 g/24 hr IV or PO ÷ Q6 hr
For cardiac arrest:
  Infant and child: 100 mg/kg/dose IV Q10 min
  Adult: 1.5–3 g/dose IV Q10 min
  Max. dose: 3 g/dose
For tetany:
  Neonate, infant, child: 100–200 mg/kg dose IV over 5–10 min, repeat dose 6 hr later if needed; **max. dose**: 500 mg/kg/24 hr
  Adult: 0.5–2 g IV over 10–30 min, repeat dose 6 hr later if needed.
MAXIMUM IV ADMINISTRATION RATES:
  IV push: **Do not exceed** 100 mg/min (over 10–20 sec in cardiac arrest).
  IV infusion: **Do not exceed** 200 mg/min, with a **maximum** concentration of 50 mg/mL.

Contraindicated in ventricular fibrillation. **Use with caution** in renal impairment as hypercalcemia may develop in end-stage renal failure. **Avoid** peripheral infusion as extravasation may cause tissue necrosis. IV infusion associated with hypotension and bradycardia. Also associated with arrhythmias in digitalized patients. May reduce absorption of fluoroquinolones, tetracyclines, and iron and effectiveness of polystyrene sulfonate with oral route of administration.

May precipitate when used with bicarbonate. **Do not use scalp veins. Do not administer via IM or SC.**
Calcium is excreted in breast milk and is not expected to harm the infant, provided maternal serum calcium is appropriately monitored.

CALCIUM LACTATE
Cal-Lac and various generics; 13% elemental Ca
Calcium supplement

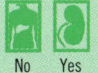

No   Yes   2   C

Tabs [OTC]: 100, 325, 650 mg
Caps (Cal-Lac) [OTC]: 500 mg
Each 1 g salt contains 6.5 mEq (130 mg) elemental Ca.

Continued

CALCIUM LACTATE continued

Doses expressed in mg of calcium lactate.
Hypocalcemia:
  Neonate/Infant: 400–500 mg/kg/24 hr PO ÷ Q4–6 hr
  Child: 500 mg/kg/24 hr PO ÷ Q6–8 hr
  Adult: 1.5–3 g PO Q8 hr
  Max. dose: 9 g/24 hr

See *Calcium Acetate* for **contraindications**, **precautions**, and drug interactions. May cause constipation, headache, and hypercalcemia.
Administer with or following meals and with plenty of fluids. **Do not** dissolve tablets in milk.
Calcium is excreted in breast milk and is not expected to harm the infant, provided maternal serum calcium is appropriately monitored.

CALCIUM PHOSPHATE, TRIBASIC
Posture-D; 39% elemental Ca
Calcium supplement

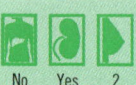
No   Yes   2   C

Tabs [OTC]: 600 mg elemental Ca and 280 mg phosphorus; with 500 IU vitamin D and 50 mg magnesium
Oral suspension: 10 mg elemental Ca/1 mL
NOTE: Pharmacy may crush tablets into a powder to enhance drug delivery for children who are unable to swallow tablets and to accommodate smaller doses.

Doses expressed as mg of elemental Ca.
Hypocalcemia:
  Neonate: 20–80 mg/kg/24 hr ÷ Q4–6 hr PO; **max. dose:** 1 g/24 hr
  Child: 45–65 mg/kg/24 hr PO ÷ Q6 hr
  Adult: 1–2 g/24 hr PO ÷ Q6–8 hr

Contraindicated in ventricular fibrillation. **Use with caution** in renal impairment as hypercalcemia may develop in end-stage renal failure (**avoid use** in dialysis with hypercalcemia), history of kidney stones, and parathyroid disorders. May cause constipation, GI disturbances, and hypercalcemia. See *Calcium Acetate* for drug interactions.
Give with or following meals and with plenty of fluids. Keep in mind the amounts of vitamin D and magnesium your respective dosage may provide.
Calcium is excreted in breast milk and is not expected to harm the infant, provided maternal serum calcium is appropriately monitored.

CALFACTANT

See Surfactant, pulmonary

CAPTOPRIL
Various generics; previously available as Capoten
Angiotensin-converting enzyme inhibitor, antihypertensive

No   Yes   2   D

Tabs: 12.5, 25, 50, 100 mg
Oral suspension: 1 mg/mL

CAPTOPRIL continued

Neonate: 0.01–0.05 mg/kg/dose PO Q8–12 hr.
Infant aged <6 mo: Initially 0.01–0.5 mg/kg/dose PO BID–TID; titrate upward if needed; **max. dose:** 6 mg/kg/24 hr.
Child: Initially, 0.3–0.5 mg/kg/dose PO BID–TID; titrate upward if needed; **max. dose:** 6 mg/kg/24 hr up to 450 mg/24 hr.
Adolescent and adult: Initially, 12.5–25 mg/dose PO BID–TID; increase weekly if necessary by 25 mg/dose to **max. dose:** 450 mg/24 hr. Usual dosage range: 25–100 mg/24 hr ÷ BID.

Onset within 15–30 min of administration. Peak effect within 1–2 hr. **Adjust dose with renal failure (see Chapter 30).** Should be administered on an empty stomach 1 hr before or 2 hr after meals. Titrate to minimal effective dose. Lower doses should be used in patients with sodium and water depletion because of diuretic therapy.

Use with caution in collagen vascular disease and concomitant potassium sparing diuretics. **Avoid use** with dialysis with high-flux membranes as anaphylactoid reactions have been reported. May cause rash, proteinuria, neutropenia, cough, angioedema (head, neck and intestine), hyperkalemia, hypotension, or diminution of taste perception (with long term use). Known to decrease aldosterone and increase renin production. Do not coadminister with angiotensin receptor blockers or aliskiren as use has been associated with increased risks for hypotension, hyperkalemia, and acute renal failure. Captopril is a CYP P450 2D6 substrate. Use with sirolimus, everolimus, or temsirolimus may increase risk for angioedema.

Captopril should be discontinued as soon as possible when pregnancy is detected.

CARBAMAZEPINE
Epitol, Tegretol, Tegretol-XR, Carbatrol, Equetro, Carnexiv, and various generics
Anticonvulsant

Yes   Yes   2   D

Tabs: 200 mg
Chewable tabs: 100 mg
Extended-release tabs (Tegretol-XR and generics): 100, 200, 400 mg
Extended-release caps (Carbatrol, Equetro, and generics): 100, 200, 300 mg
Oral suspension: 100 mg/5 mL (450 mL); may contain propylene glycol
Injection (Carnexiv): 10 mg/mL (20 mL); contains betadex sulfobutyl ether sodium (preservative-free)

See remarks regarding dosing intervals for specific dosage forms:
<6 yr:
  Initial: 10–20 mg/kg/24 hr PO ÷ BID-TID (QID for suspension)
  Increment: Q5–7 days up to **max. dose** of 35 mg/kg/24 hr PO
6–12 yr:
  Initial: 10 mg/kg/24 hr PO ÷ BID up to **max. dose:** 100 mg/dose BID
  Increment: 100 mg/24 hr at 1 wk intervals (÷ TID-QID) until desired response is obtained.
  Maintenance: 20–30 mg/kg/24 hr PO ÷ BID-QID; usual maintenance dose is 400–800 mg/24 hr; **max. dose:** 1000 mg/24 hr.
>12 yr and adult:
  Initial: 200 mg PO BID
  Increment: 200 mg/24 hr at 1 wk intervals (÷ BID-QID) until desired response is obtained.
  Maintenance: 800–1200 mg/24 hr PO ÷ BID-QID (see next page for max. doses)

Continued

CARBAMAZEPINE continued

Max. dose:
Child 12–15 yr: 1000 mg/24 hr
Child >15 yr: 1200 mg/24 hr
Adult: 1.6–2.4 g/24 hr

Intravenous dosage form (Carnexiv; see remarks):
Child: pediatric PK, efficacy, and safety data currently not available
Adult (IV; indicated as replacement therapy for PO carbamazepine when PO route is not feasible): Determine IV daily dose by taking 70% of the established total daily oral dosage and divide into 4 equal doses to be administered Q6 hr. Each dose is further diluted in 100 mL of compatible fluid and infused over 30 min. Use is **NOT recommended** > 7 days.

Contraindicated for patients taking monoamine oxidase (MAO) inhibitors or who are sensitive to tricyclic antidepressants. They should **not** be used in combination with clozapine because of an increased risk for bone marrow suppression and agranulocytosis. Increased risk for severe dermatological reactions (e.g., Stevens-Johnson syndrome [SJS] and toxic epidermal necrolysis [TEN]) has been associated with the HLA-B*1502 (prevalent among Asian descent) and HLA-A*3101 (prevalent among Japanese, Native American, Southern Indians, and some Arabic ancestory) alleles.

Erythromycin, diltiazem, verapamil, cefixime, cimetidine, itraconazole, aprepitant, and INH may increase serum levels. Carbamazepine may decrease activity of warfarin, doxycycline, oral contraceptives, cyclosporine, theophylline, phenytoin, benzodiazepines, ethosuximide, and valproic acid. Carbamazepine is a CYP 450 3A3/4 substrate and inducer of CYP 450 1A2, 2C, and 3A3/4. The enzyme-inducing effects may increase effects/toxicity of cyclophosphamide. CYP 450 3A4 inhibitors may increase carbamazepine levels/toxicity.

Suggested dosing intervals for specific dosage forms: extended-release tabs or caps (BID); chewable and immediate-release tablets (BID–TID); suspension (QID).

Doses may be administered with food. **Do not** crush or chew extended-release dosage forms. Shake bottle well prior to dispensing oral suspension dosage form, and **do not** administer simultaneously with other liquid medicines or diluents.

Drug metabolism typically increases after the first month of therapy initiation because of hepatic autoinduction.

Therapeutic blood levels: 4–12 mg/L. Recommended serum sampling time: obtain trough level within 30 min prior to an oral dose. Steady state is typically achieved 1 mo after initiation of therapy (following enzymatic autoinduction). Levels obtained prior to steady state are useful for preventing toxicity. Blood levels of 7–10 mg/L have been recommended for bipolar disorders.

Side effects include sedation, dizziness, diplopia, aplastic anemia, neutropenia, urinary retention, nausea, SIADH, and SJS. Suicidal behavior or ideation and onychomadesis have been reported. About 1/3 of patients who have hypersensitivity reactions will also experience hypersensitivity to oxcarbazepine. Pretreatment complete blood counts (CBCs) and liver function tests (LFTs) are suggested. Patient should be monitored for hematologic and hepatic toxicity. Most common side effects with the IV route, dizziness, somnolence, blurred vision, diplopia, headache, infusion-related reaction, infusion site pain and anemia.

Adjust dose in renal impairment (see Chapter 30).

Do not use IV dosage form in moderate/severe renal impairment (GFR < 30 mL/min) due to accumulation of betadex sulfobutyl ether sodium which may be nephrotoxic.

CARBAMIDE PEROXIDE
Debrox, Auro Ear Wax Remover, Thera-Ear, Gly-Oxide, and generics
Cerumenolytic, topical oral analgesic

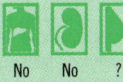
No   No   ?   ?

Otic solution [OTC]: 6.5% (7, 15, 22 mL); may contain propylene glycol or alcohol.
Oral liquid [OTC]: 10% (Gly-Oxide) (15, 60 mL)

Cerumenolytic:
<12 yr: Tilt head sideways and instill 1–5 drops (according to patient size) into affected ear; retain drops in ear for several minutes. Remove wax by gently flushing the ear with warm water using a soft rubber bulb ear syringe. Dose may be repeated BID PRN for up to 4 days.
≥12 yr: Following the abovementioned instructions, instill 5–10 drops into affected ear BID PRN for up to 4 days.
Oral analgesic (see remarks):
≥2 yr (able to follow instructions): Instill several drops of the oral liquid to the affected area and expectorate after 2–3 min **OR** place 10 drops on tongue and mix with saliva, swish for several minutes, and expectorate. Administer up to QID, after meals and QHS, for **up to 7 days**.

Otic solution: Contraindicated if tympanic membrane perforated; following otic surgery; ear discharge, drainage, pain, irritation, or rash; or PE tubes in place. Tip of applicator should not enter ear canal when used as a cerumenolytic.
Oral liquid: Prolonged use may result in fungal overgrowth. **Do not** rinse the mouth or drink for at least 5 min when using oral preparation.
Pregnancy category has not been formally assigned by the FDA.

CARBINOXAMINE
Arbinoxa, Karbinal ER, and generics
Antihistamine

No   No   3   C

Oral liquid: 4 mg/5 mL (473 mL); may contain propylene glycol
Extended-release oral suspension (Karbinal ER): 4 mg/5 mL (480 mL); contains parabens and metasulfite
Tabs: 4 mg

Child (PO; see remarks):
Immediate-release dosage forms: 0.2–0.4 mg/kg/24 hr PO ÷ TID–QID; alternative dosing by age (**do not exceed** 0.4 mg/kg/24 hr):
 2–5 yr: 1–2 mg TID–QID
 6–11 yr: 2–4 mg TID–QID
 ≥12 yr: 4–8 mg TID–QID
Extended-release oral suspension (approximately 0.2–0.4 mg/kg/24 hr):
 2–3 yr: 3–4 mg Q12 hr
 4–5 yr: 3–8 mg Q12 hr
 6–11 yr: 6–12 mg Q12 hr
 ≥12 yr: 6–16 mg Q12 hr
Adult (PO):
 Immediate-release dosage forms: 4–8 mg TID–QID
 Extended-release oral suspension: 6–16 mg Q12 hr

Continued

CARBINOXAMINE continued

Generally not recommended for treating upper respiratory tract infections (URIs) in infants. No proven benefit for infants and young children with URIs. **The FDA does not recommend use for URIs in children aged <2 yr because of reports of increased fatalities.** Karbinal ER use is contraindicated in children aged <2 yr and in nursing mothers.

Contraindicated in acute asthma, hypersensitivity with other ethanolamine antihistamines, MAO inhibitors, severe hypertension, narrow-angle glaucoma, severe coronary artery disease, and urinary retention. Be aware that a combination of decongestant products may exist.

May cause drowsiness, vertigo, dry mucus membranes, and headache. Paradoxical excitation reactions are more likely to occur in younger children. Contact dermatitis and central nervous system (CNS) excitation have been reported.

CARNITINE
Levocarnitine, Carnitor, Carnitor SF, L-Carnitine, and generics
Nutritional supplement, amino acid

No   Yes   ?   B

Tabs: 250, 330 mg
Caps: 250 mg
Oral solution: 100 mg/mL (118 mL); contains methyl- and propylparabens; Carnitor SF is a sugar-free product.
Injection: 200 mg/mL (5, 12.5 mL); preservative free

Primary carnitine deficiency:
Oral:
  Child: 50–100 mg/kg/24 hr PO ÷ Q8–12 hr; increase slowly as needed and tolerated to **max. dose** of 3 g/24 hr
  Adult: 330 mg to 1 g/dose BID–TID PO; **max. dose:** 3 g/24 hr
IV:
  Child and adult: 50 mg/kg as loading dose; may follow with 50 mg/kg/24 hr IV infusion (for severe cases); maintenance: 50 mg/kg/24 hr ÷ Q4–6 hr; increase to **max. dose** of 300 mg/kg/24 hr if needed.

May cause nausea, vomiting, abdominal cramps, diarrhea, and body odor. Seizures have been reported in patients with or without a history of seizures. Safety in end-stage renal disease (ESRD) has not been established. High doses to severely compromised renal function or ESRD on dialysis may result in accumulation of potentially toxic metabolites (trimethylamine and trimethylamine-*N*-oxide).
Give bolus IV infusion over 2–3 min.

CARVEDILOL
Coreg, Coreg CR and generics
Adrenergic antagonist (α and β), antihypertensive

Yes   Yes   ?   C

Tabs: 3.125, 6.25, 12.5, 25 mg
Extended-release caps (Coreg CR): 10, 20, 40, 80 mg
Oral suspension: 0.1, 1.25, 1.67 mg/mL

CARVEDILOL continued

Heart failure:
Immediate-release dosage forms (tablets and oral suspension; see remarks):
  Infant, child, adolescent: Start at 0.05–0.2 mg/kg/24 hr PO ÷ BID. Dose may be titrated at 1- or 2-wk intervals as needed up to a **maximum** of 2 mg/kg/24 hr or 50 mg/24 hr. Reported usual effective dose: 0.2–1 mg/kg/24 hr.
  Adult: Start at 3.125 mg PO BID × 2 wk, if needed and tolerated, may increase to 6.25 mg BID. Dose may be doubled every 2 wk if needed to the following **maximum doses**:
    Mild/moderate heart failure: <85 kg: 25 mg BID; ≥85 kg: 50 mg BID
    Severe heart failure: 25 mg BID
Extended-release capsules:
  Adult: Start at 10 mg PO once daily × 2 wk, if needed and tolerated, double the dose every 2 wk up to a **maximum** of 80 mg once daily.

Hypertension:
Adult:
  Immediate-release dosage forms: Start at 6.25 mg PO BID; dose may be doubled every 1–2 wk up to a maximum of 25 mg PO BID.
  Extended-release capsules: Start at 20 mg PO once daily × 1–2 wk, if needed and tolerated, increase to 40 mg PO once daily. If needed, dose may be further increased in 2-wk intervals up to a **maximum** of 80 mg/24 hr.

Immediate-release and extended-release products are NOT interchangeable on a mg/mg basis.
Contraindicated in asthma or related bronchospastic disease, sick sinus syndrome, 2nd or 3rd degree heart block, severe bradycardia, cardiogenic shock, decompensated cardiac failure requiring IV inotropic therapy, and severe hepatic impairment (Child-Pugh class C)

Use with caution mild/moderate hepatic impairment (Child-Pugh class A or B), renal insufficiency, thyrotoxicosis, ischemic heart disease, diabetes, and cataract surgery. **Avoid abrupt withdrawal** of medication.

Children aged <3.5 years may have faster carvedilol clearance and may require higher dosages or TID dosing. Carvedilol is a CYP 450 2D6 substrate. Digoxin, disopyramide, and dipyridamole may increase bradycardiac effects.

Bradycardia, postural hypotension, peripheral edema, weight gain, hyperglycemia, diarrhea, dizziness, and fatigue are common. Hypersensitivity reactions have been reported. Chest pain, headache, vomiting, edema, and dyspnea have also been reported in children. Administering dose with food can reduce risk for orthostatic hypotension.

CASPOFUNGIN
Cancidas
Antifungal, echinocandin

Yes No ? C

Injection: 50, 70 mg; contains sucrose (39 mg in 50 mg vial and 54 mg in 70 mg vial)

Preterm neonate—<3-mo infant (based on a small pharmacokinetic study, achieving similar plasma exposure as seen in adults receiving 50 mg/24 hr): 25 mg/m^2/dose IV once daily. Alternatively, 1 mg/kg/dose IV once daily × 2 days followed by 2 mg/kg/dose IV once daily has been reported in a case series with excellent microbiological results.

3-mo infant–17 yr (see remarks): 70 mg/m^2/dose IV loading dose on day 1, followed by 50 mg/m^2/dose IV once daily maintenance dose. Increase the maintenance dose to 70 mg/m^2/dose if response is inadequate or if the patient is receiving an enzyme-inducing medication (see remarks).
Maximum loading and maintenance dose: 70 mg/dose.

Continued

CASPOFUNGIN continued

Adolescent and adult (see remarks):
  Loading dose: 70 mg IV × 1
  Maintenance dose:
    Usual: 50 mg IV once daily. If tolerated and response is inadequate or if patient is receiving an enzyme-inducing medication (see remarks), increase to 70 mg IV once daily.
    Hepatic insufficiency (Child-Pugh score 7–9): 35 mg IV once daily.

Use with caution in hepatic impairment and concomitant enzyme-inducing drugs. Higher maintenance doses (70 mg/m^2/dose in children and 70 mg in adults) are recommended for concomitant use of enzyme inducers such as carbamazepime, dexamethasone, phenytoin, nevirapine, efavirenz, or rifampin. Use Mosteller formula for calculating body surface area (BSA).

Most common adverse effects (>10%) in children include fever, diarrhea, rash, elevated aspartate transaminase/alanine transaminase (ALT/AST), hypokalemia, hypotension, and chills. May also cause facial swelling, nausea/vomiting, headache, infusion site phlebitis, and LFT elevation. Anaphylaxis, TEN, SJS, and possible histamine-related reactions (angioedema, bronchospasm, and warm sensation) have been reported. Hepatobiliary adverse effects have been reported in pediatric patients with serious underlying medical conditions.

Reduce daily dose by 30% in moderate hepatic impairment (Child-Pugh score 7–9).

Use with cyclosporine may cause transient increase in LFTs and caspofungin level elevations. May decrease tacrolimus levels.

Administer doses by slow IV infusion over 1 hr. **Do not** mix or coinfuse with other medications and **avoid** using dextrose-containing diluents (e.g., D$_5$W).

CEFACLOR
Generics; previously available as Ceclor
Antibiotic, cephalosporin (second generation)

No Yes 1 B

Caps: 250, 500 mg
Extended-release tabs: 500 mg
Oral suspension: 125 mg/5 mL (150 mL); 250 mg/5 mL (150 mL); 375 mg/5 mL (100 mL)

Child aged >1–mo-old (use regular-release dosage forms): 20–40 mg/kg/24 hr PO ÷ Q8 hr; max. dose: 1 g/24 hr
  Q12 hr dosage interval option for pharyngitis: 20 mg/kg/24 hr; max. dose: 1 g/24 hr
Adult: 250–500 mg/dose PO Q8 hr
  Extended-release tablets: 500 mg/dose PO Q12 hr

Use with caution in penicillin-allergic patients or in the presence of renal impairment. Side effects include elevated LFTs, bone marrow suppression, and moniliasis. Probenecid may increase cefaclor concentrations. May cause positive Coombs test or false-positive test for urinary glucose. Serum sickness reactions have been reported in patients receiving multiple courses of cefaclor.

Do not crush, cut, or chew extended-release tablets. Dose should be given on an empty stomach. **Extended-release tablets not recommended for children. Adjust dose in renal failure (see Chapter 30).**

CEFADROXIL
Duricef and generics
Antibiotic, cephalosporin (first generation)

No　Yes　1　B

Oral suspension: 250 mg/5 mL (50, 100 mL), 500 mg/5 mL (75, 100 mL)
Tabs: 1 g
Caps: 500 mg

Infant and child: 30 mg/kg/24 hr PO ÷ Q12 hr (daily dose may be administered once daily for group A β-hemolytic streptococci pharyngitis/tonsillitis); **max. dose:** 2 g/24 hr
Bacterial endocarditis prophylaxis for dental and upper airway procedures: 50 mg/kg/dose (max. dose: 2 g) × 1 PO 1 hr before procedure.
Adolescent and adult: 1–2 g/24 hr PO ÷ Q12–24 hr (administer Q12 hr for complicated UTIs); **max. dose:** 2 g/24 hr
Bacterial endocarditis prophylaxis for dental and upper airway procedures: 2 g × 1 PO 1 hr before procedure.

See *Cephalexin* for **precautions** and interactions. Rash, nausea, vomiting, and diarrhea are common. Transient neutropenia and vaginitis have been reported. **Adjust dose in renal failure (see Chapter 30).**

CEFAZOLIN
Generics; previously available as Ancef
Antibiotic, cephalosporin (first generation)

Yes　Yes　1　B

Injection: 0.5, 1, 10, 20, 100 g
Frozen injection: 1 g/50 mL (contains 2 g dextrose to make an iso-osmotic solution), 2 g/100 mL (contains 4 g dextrose to make an iso-osmotic solution)
Contains 2.1 mEq Na/g drug

Neonate (IM/IV):
 Postnatal age ≤7 days: 50 mg/kg/24 hr ÷ Q12 hr
 Postnatal age >7 days:
  ≤2000 g: 50 mg/kg/24 hr ÷ Q12 hr
  >2000 g: 75 mg/kg/24 hr ÷ Q8 hr
Infant >1 mo and child (IM/IV):
 Mild/moderate infection: 25–50 mg/kg/24 hr ÷ Q6–8 hr
 Severe infection: 100 mg/kg/24 hr ÷ Q6–8 hr; 150 mg/kg/24 hr ÷ Q6–8 hr has been recommended for community-acquired pneumonia
 Max. dose: 6 g/24 hr
Adult: 2–6 g/24 hr ÷ Q6–8 hr IV/IM; **max. dose:** 12 g/24 hr
Bacterial endocarditis prophylaxis for dental and upper respiratory procedures:
 Infant and child: 50 mg/kg IV/IM (**max. dose:** 1 g) 30 min before procedure
 Adult: 1 g IV/IM 30 min before procedure

Use with caution in the presence of renal impairment or in penicillin-allergic patients. Does not penetrate well into the cerebrospinal fluid (CSF). May cause phlebitis, leukopenia, thrombocytopenia, transient liver enzyme elevation, and false-positive urine–reducing substance (Clinitest) and Coombs test.
For dosing in obese patients, use the higher end of the dosing recommendation. **Adjust dose in renal failure (see Chapter 30).**

CEFDINIR
Generics; previously available as Omnicef
Antibiotic, cephalosporin (third generation)

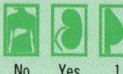
No   Yes   1   B

Caps: 300 mg
Oral suspension: 125 mg/5 mL (60, 100 mL), 250 mg/5 mL (60, 100 mL)

6 mo–12 yr:
  Otitis media, sinusitis, pharyngitis/tonsillitis: 14 mg/kg/24 hr PO ÷ Q12–24 hr; max. dose: 600 mg/24 hr
  Uncomplicated skin infections (see remarks): 14 mg/kg/24 hr PO ÷ Q12 hr; max. dose: 600 mg/24 hr
≥13 yr and adult:
  Bronchitis, sinusitis, pharyngitis/tonsillitis: 600 mg/24 hr PO ÷ Q12–24 hr
  Community-acquired pneumonia, uncomplicated skin infections (see remarks): 600 mg/24 hr PO ÷ Q12 hr

Use with caution in penicillin-allergic patients or in the presence of renal impairment. Good gram-positive cocci activity. May cause diarrhea (especially in children aged <2 yr), headache, vaginitis, and false-positive urine–reducing substance (Clinitest) and Coombs test. Eosinophilia and abnormal LFTs have been reported with higher than usual doses.

Once daily dosing has not been evaluated in pneumonia and skin infections. Probenecid increases serum cefdinir levels. Avoid concomitant administration with iron and iron-containing vitamins and antacids that contain aluminum or magnesium (space 2 hr apart) to reduce the risk for decreasing antibiotic's absorption. Doses may be taken without food. **Adjust dose in renal failure (see Chapter 30).**

CEFEPIME
Maxipime and generics
Antibiotic, cephalosporin (fourth generation)

No   Yes   ?   B

Injection: 1, 2 g
Premixed injection: 1 g/50 mL, 2 g/100 mL (iso-osmotic dextrose solutions)
Each 1 g drug contains 725 mg L-Arginine.

Neonate (IV/IM):
  <14 days old: 60 mg/kg/24 hr ÷ Q12 hr
  ≥14 days old: 100 mg/kg/24 hr ÷ Q12 hr
  Meningitis or Pseudomonas infections:
    <1 kg and 0–14 days old, or 1–2 kg and <0–7 days old: 100 mg/kg/24 hr ÷ Q12 hr
    <1 kg and >14 days old, or 1–2 kg and >7 days old, or >2 kg and 0–30 days old: 150 mg/kg/24 hr ÷ Q8 hr
Child aged ≥2 mo (IV/IM): 100 mg/kg/24 hr ÷ Q12 hr
  Meningitis, fever, and neutropenia, or serious infections: 150 mg/kg/24 hr ÷ Q8 hr
  Max. dose: 2 g/single dose or 6 g/24 hr
Cystic fibrosis: 150 mg/kg/24 hr ÷ Q8 hr IV/IM, up to a **max. dose** of 6 gm/24 hr
Adult: 1–4 g/24 hr ÷ Q12 hr IV/IM
  Severe infections: 6 g/24 hr ÷ Q8 hr IV/IM
  Max. dose: 6 g/24 hr

CEFEPIME continued

Use with caution in penicillin-allergic patients or in the presence of renal impairment. Good activity against *Pseudomonas aeruginosa* and other gram-negative bacteria plus most gram-positive bacteria (methicillin sensitive *Staphylococcus aureus*). May cause thrombophlebitis, GI discomfort, transient increases in liver enzymes, and false-positive urine–reducing substance (Clinitest) and Coombs test. Probenecid increases serum cefepime levels. Encephalopathy, myoclonus, seizures (including nonconvulsive status epilepticus), transient leukopenia, neutropenia, agranulocytosis, and thrombocytopenia have been reported. **Adjust dose in renal failure (see Chapter 30).**

CEFIXIME
Suprax and generics
Antibiotic, cephalosporin (third generation)

No Yes 1 B

Oral suspension: 100 mg/5 mL (50 mL), 200 mg/5 mL (50, 75 mL), 500 mg/5 mL (10, 20 mL)
Chewable tabs: 100, 150, 200 mg; contains aspartame
Caps: 400 mg

Infant (>6 mo) and child: 8 mg/kg/24 hr ÷ Q12–24 hr PO; **max. dose:** 400 mg/24 hr. May be used in infants aged ≥3-mo-old for community-acquired pneumonia.
Alternative dosing for acute UTI: 16 mg/kg/24 hr ÷ Q12 hr on day 1, followed by 8 mg/kg/24 hr Q24 hr PO × 13 days. **Max. dose:** 400 mg/24 hr
Sexual victimization prophylaxis: 8 mg/kg PO × 1 (**max. dose:** 400 mg) PLUS azithromycin 20 mg/kg PO × 1 (**max. dose:** 1 g)

Adolescent and adult: 400 mg/24 hr ÷ Q12–24 hr PO
Uncomplicated cervical, urethral, or rectal infections due to Neisseria gonorrhoeae: 400 mg × 1 PO plus azithromycin 1 g PO × 1 OR doxycycline 100 mg PO BID × 7 days
Sexual victimization prophylaxis: 400 mg PO × 1 PLUS azithromycin 1 g PO × 1 OR doxycycline 100 mg BID PO × 7 days, PLUS metronidazole 2 g PO × 1. PLUS hepatitis B vaccine (if not immunized).

Use with caution in penicillin-allergic patients or in the presence of renal failure. Adverse reactions include diarrhea, abdominal pain, nausea, and headache. Because of reduced bioavailability, do not use tablets for the treatment of otitis media. Probenecid increases serum cefixime levels. Unlike most cephalosporins, drug is excreted unchanged in the bile (5%–10%) and urine (50%). May increase serum carbamazepine concentrations. May cause false-positive urine–reducing substance (Clinitest), Coombs test, and nitroprusside test for ketones. **Adjust dose in renal failure (see Chapter 30).**

CEFOTAXIME
Claforan and generics
Antibiotic, cephalosporin (third generation)

No Yes 1 B

Injection: 0.5, 1, 2, 10 g
Frozen injection: 1 g/50 mL 3.4% dextrose, 2 g/50 mL 1.4% dextrose (iso-osmotic solutions)
Contains 2.2 mEq Na/g drug

Neonate, IV/IM:
  Postnatal age ≤7 days:
    <2000 g: 100 mg/kg/24 hr ÷ Q12 hr
    ≥2000 g: 100–150 mg/kg/24 hr ÷ Q8–12 hr

Continued

CEFOTAXIME continued

Neonate, IV/IM:
  Postnatal age >7 days:
   <1200 g: 100 mg/kg/24 hr ÷ Q12 hr
   1200–2000 g: 150 mg/kg/24 hr ÷ Q8 hr
   >2000 g: 150–200 mg/kg/24 hr ÷ Q6–8 hr
Infant and child (1 mo–12 yr and <50 kg): 100–200 mg/kg/24 hr ÷ Q6–8 hr IV/IM. Higher doses of 150–225 mg/kg/24 hr ÷ Q6–8 hr have been recommended for infections outside the CSF due to penicillin-resistant pneumococci.
  Meningitis: 200 mg/kg/24 hr ÷ Q6 hr IV/IM. Higher doses of 225–300 mg/kg/24 hr ÷ Q6–8 hr, in combination with vancomycin (dosed at CNS target levels), have been recommended for meningitis due to penicillin-resistant pneumococci.
  Max. dose: 12 g/24 hr
Child (>12 yr or ≥50 kg) and adult: 1–2 g/dose Q6–8 hr IV/IM
  Severe infection: 2 g/dose Q4–6 hr IV/IM
  Max. dose: 12 g/24 hr
  Uncomplicated gonorrhea: 0.5–1 g ×1 IM

Use with caution in penicillin-allergic patients and in the presence of renal impairment (reduce dosage). Toxicities similar to other cephalosporins: allergy, neutropenia, thrombocytopenia, eosinophilia, false-positive urine–reducing substance (Clinitest) and Coombs test, elevated blood urine nitrogen (BUN), creatinine, and liver enzymes. Probenecid increases serum cefotaxime levels.
Good CNS penetration. **Adjust dose in renal failure (see Chapter 30).**

CEFOTETAN
Cefotan and generics
Antibiotic, cephalosporin (second generation)

No   Yes   1   B

Injection: 1, 2, 10 g
Frozen injection: 1 g/50 mL 3.8% dextrose, 2 gm/50 mL 2.2% dextrose (iso-osmotic solutions)
Contains 3.5 mEq Na/g drug

Infant and child (IV/IM, limited data):
  Mild/moderate infection: 60 mg/kg/24 hr ÷ Q12 hr; max. single dose: 2 g/dose
  Severe infection: 100 mg/kg/24 hr ÷ Q12 hr; max. single dose: 2–3 g/dose
  Intra-abdominal infection: 40–80 mg/kg/24 hr ÷ Q12 hr
Adolescent and adult: 2–4 g/24 hr ÷ Q12 hr IV/IM; **max. dose:** 6 g/24 hr
  PID: 2 g Q12 hr IV × 24–48 hr after clinical improvement. Doxycycline 100 mg Q12 hr PO/IV × 14 days is also initiated at the same time.
Max. dose (all ages): 6 g/24 hr
Preoperative prophylaxis (30–60 min before procedure):
  Child: 40 mg/kg/dose (**max. dose:** 2 g/dose) IV
  Adult: 1–2 g IV

Use with caution in penicillin-allergic patients or in the presence of renal impairment. May cause disulfiram-like reaction with ethanol, increase effects/toxicities of anticoagulants, false-positive urine–reducing substance (Clinitest), and false elevations of serum and urine creatinine (Jaffe method). Hemolytic anemia has been reported. Good anaerobic activity, but poor CSF penetration. **Adjust dose in renal failure (see Chapter 30).**

CEFOXITIN
Generics; previously available as Mefoxin
Antibiotic, cephalosporin (second generation)

   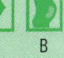
No Yes 1 B

Injection: 1, 2, 10 g
Frozen injection: 1 g/50 mL 4% dextrose, 2 g/50 mL 2.2% dextrose (iso-osmotic solutions)
Contains 2.3 mEq Na/g drug

Neonate: 90–100 mg/kg/24 hr ÷ Q8 hr IM/IV
Infant and child:
  Mild/moderate infections: 80–100 mg/kg/24 hr ÷ Q6–8 hr IM/IV
  Severe infections: 100–160 mg/kg/24 hr ÷ Q4–6 hr IM/IV
Adult: 1–2 g/dose Q6–8 hr IM/IV
  PID: 2 g IV Q6h × 24–48 hr after clinical improvement. Doxycycline 100 mg Q12 hr PO/IV × 14 days is also initiated at the same time.
Max. dose (all ages): 12 g/24 hr

Use with caution in penicillin-allergic patients or in the presence of renal impairment. Has good anaerobic activity, but poor CSF penetration. Probenecid increases serum cefoxitin levels. May cause false-positive urine–reducing substance (Clinitest and other copper reduction method tests), and false elevations of serum and urine creatinine (Jaffe and KDA methods).
Adjust dose in renal failure (see Chapter 30).

CEFPODOXIME PROXETIL
Generics; previously available as Vantin
Antibiotic, cephalosporin (third generation)

No Yes 1 B

Tabs: 100, 200 mg
Oral suspension: 50, 100 mg/5 mL (50, 100 mL)

2 mo–12 yr:
  Otitis media: 10 mg/kg/24 hr PO ÷ Q12 hr × 5 days; **max. dose:** 400 mg/24 hr
  Pharyngitis/tonsillitis: 10 mg/kg/24 hr PO ÷ Q12 hr × 5–10 days; **max. dose:** 200 mg/24 hr
  Acute maxillary sinusitis: 10 mg/kg/24 hr PO ÷ Q12 hr × 10 days; **max. dose:** 400 mg/24 hr
≥13 yr–adult:
  Exacerbation of chronic bronchitis, community-acquired pneumonia, and sinusitis: 400 mg/24 hr PO ÷ Q12 hr × 10 days (14 days for pneumonia)
  Pharyngitis/tonsillitis: 200 mg/24 hr PO ÷ Q12 hr × 5–10 days
  Skin/skin structure infection: 800 mg/24 hr PO ÷ Q12 hr × 7–14 days
  Uncomplicated gonorrhea: 200 mg PO × 1

Use with caution in penicillin-allergic patients or in the presence of renal impairment. May cause diarrhea, nausea, vomiting, vaginal candidiasis, and false-positive Coombs test.
Tablets should be administered with food to enhance absorption. Suspension may be administered without regard to food. High doses of antacids or H₂ blockers may reduce absorption. Probenecid increases serum cefpodoxime levels.
Adjust dose in renal failure (see Chapter 30).

CEFPROZIL
Generics; previously available as Cefzil
Antibiotic, cephalosporin (second generation)

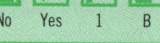

Tabs: 250, 500 mg
Oral suspension: 125 mg/5 mL, 250 mg/5 mL (50, 75, 100 mL); contains aspartame and phenylalanine

Otitis media:
  6 mo–12 yr: 30 mg/kg/24 hr PO ÷ Q12 hr; **max. dose:** 1 g/24 hr
Pharyngitis/tonsillitis:
  2–12 yr: 15 mg/kg/24 hr PO ÷ Q12 hr; **max. dose:** 1 g/24 hr
  ≥13 yr: 500 mg PO Q24 hr
Acute sinusitis:
  6 mo–12 yr: 15–30 mg/kg/24 hr PO ÷ Q12 hr; **max. dose:** 1 g/24 hr
  >13 yr: 250 or 500 mg PO Q12 hr
Uncomplicated skin infections:
  2–12 yr: 20 mg/kg/24 hr PO Q24 hr; **max. dose:** 500 mg/dose
  >12 yr: 250 mg PO Q12 hr or 500 mg PO Q12–24 hr
UTI:
  2–24 mo: 30 mg/kg/24 hr PO ÷ Q12 hr
Other:
  ≥13 yr and adult: 500–1000 mg/24 hr PO ÷ Q12–24 hr

Use with caution in penicillin-allergic patients or in the presence of renal impairment. Oral suspension contains aspartame and phenylalanine and should not be used by patients with phenylketonuria. May cause nausea, vomiting, diarrhea, liver enzyme elevations, and false-positive urine–reducing substance (Clinitest and other copper reduction method tests) and Coombs test. Probenecid increases serum cefprozil levels. Absorption is not affected by food. **Adjust dose in renal failure (see Chapter 30).**

CEFTAROLINE FOSAMIL
Teflaro
Antibiotic, cephalosporin (fifth generation)

Injection: 400, 600 mg; contains L-arginine

Child (2 mo–<18 yr):
Acute bacterial skin and skin structure infection (ABSSSI) and community-acquired bacterial pneumonia (CABP):
  2 mo–<2 yr: 8 mg/kg/dose IV Q8 hr
  ≥2 yr–<18 yr:
    ≤33 kg: 12 mg/kg/dose IV Q8 hr
    >33 kg: 400 mg IV Q8 hr or 600 mg IV Q12 hr
Adult: 600 mg IV Q12 hr
Cystic Fibrosis (limited data):
  Adult: pharmacokinetic simulations in eight patients revealed dosages of 600 mg IV Q8 hr infused over 1 hr or 600 mg IV Q12 hr infused over 3 hr would achieve the targeted serum concentration time above the minimal inhibitory concentration (MIC) of 60%.

CEFTAROLINE FOSAMIL continued

Use with caution in penicillin-allergic patients and in the presence of renal impairment. Common side effects in pediatric trials include diarrhea, rash, vomiting, pyrexia, and nausea. Leukopenia has been reported.

Probenecid increases serum ceftaroline levels. Direct Coombs test seroconversion has been reported with use.

Adjust dose in renal failure (see Chapter 30).

CEFTAZIDIME
Fortaz, Tazicef, and generics
Antibiotic, cephalosporin (third generation)

No   Yes   1   B

Injection: 0.5, 1, 2, 6 g
Frozen injection: 1 g/50 mL 4.4% dextrose, 2 g/50 mL 3.2% dextrose (iso-osmotic solutions)
Contains 2.3 mEq Na/g drug

Neonate (IV/IM):
  Postnatal age ≤7 days:
    <2000 g: 100 mg/kg/24 hr ÷ Q12 hr
    ≥2000 g: 100–150 mg/kg/24 hr ÷ Q8–12 hr
  Postnatal age >7 days:
    <1200 g: 100 mg/kg/24 hr ÷ Q12 hr
    ≥1200 g: 150 mg/kg/24 hr ÷ Q8 hr
Infant (>1 mo) and child (IV/IM): 100–150 mg/kg/24 hr ÷ Q8 hr; max. dose: 6 g/24 hr
  Cystic fibrosis and meningitis (IV/IM): 150–200 mg/kg/24 hr ÷ Q6–8 hr; max. dose: 6 g/24 hr
Adult (IV/IM): 1–2 g/dose Q8–12 hr; **max. dose:** 6 g/24 hr

Use with caution in penicillin-allergic patients or in the presence of renal impairment. Good *Pseudomonas* coverage and CSF penetration. May cause rash, liver enzyme elevations, and false-positive urine–reducing substance (Clinitest and other copper reduction method tests) and Coombs test. Probenecid increases serum ceftazidime levels. **Adjust dose in renal failure (see Chapter 30).**

CEFTIBUTEN
Cedax and generics
Antibiotic, cephalosporin (third generation)

No   Yes   1   B

Oral suspension: 90 mg/5 mL (60, 90, 120 mL), 180 mg/5 mL (60 mL); contains sodium benzoate
Caps: 400 mg

Child (>6 mo):
  Otitis media and pharyngitis/tonsillitis: 9 mg/kg/24 hr (**max. dose:** 400 mg/24 hr) PO once daily × 10 days
≥12 yr and adult:
  Chronic bronchitis exacerbation, otitis media, and pharyngitis/tonsillitis: 400 mg PO once daily × 10 days; max. dose: 400 mg/24 hr

Use with caution in penicillin-allergic patients or in the presence of renal impairment. May cause GI symptoms and elevations in eosinophils and BUN. SJS has been reported. Gastric acid–lowering medications (e.g., ranitidine and omeprazole) may enhance bioavailability of ceftibutin.

Oral suspension should be administered 2 hr before or 1 hr after a meal. **Adjust dose in renal failure (see Chapter 30).**

CEFTRIAXONE
Rocephin and generics
Antibiotic, cephalosporin (third generation)

Yes   Yes   1   B

Injection: 0.25, 0.5, 1, 2, 10 g
Frozen injection: 1 g/50 mL 3.8% dextrose, 2 g/50 mL 2.4% dextrose (iso-osmotic solutions)
Contains 3.6 mEq Na/g drug

Neonate:
  Gonococcal ophthalmia or prophylaxis: 25–50 mg/kg/dose IM/IV × 1; max. dose: 125 mg/dose
Infant (>1 mo) and child:
  Mild/moderate infections: 50–75 mg/kg/24 hr ÷ Q12–24 hr IM/IV; **max. dose**: 2 g/24 hr
  Meningitis (including penicillin-resistant pneumococci): 100 mg/kg/24 hr IM/IV ÷ Q12 hr; **max. dose**: 2 g/dose and 4 g/24 hr
  Penicillin-resistant pneumococci outside the CSF: 80–100 mg/kg/24 hr ÷ Q12–24 hr (**max. dose**: 2 g/dose and 4 g/24 hr)
  Acute otitis media: 50 mg/kg IM/IV (**max. dose**: 1 g) × 1; for persistent or relapse cases use 50 mg/kg IM/IV (**max. dose**: 1 g) Q24 hr × 3 doses.
Adult: 1–2 g/dose Q12–24 hr IV/IM; **max. dose**: 2 g/dose and 4 g/24 hr
  Uncomplicated gonorrhea or chancroid: 250 mg IM × 1
Bacterial endocarditis prophylaxis for dental and upper respiratory procedures:
  Infant and child: 50 mg/kg IV/IM (**max. dose**: 1 g) 30 min before procedure
  Adult: 1 g IV/IM 30 min before procedure

Contraindicated in neonates with hyperbilirubinemia. **Do not** administer with IV calcium-containing solutions or products (mixed or administered simultaneously via different lines) in neonates (<28 days old) because of the risk for precipitation of ceftriaxone–calcium salt. Cases of fatal reactions with calcium–ceftriaxone precipitates in lung and kidneys in preterm and full term neonates have been reported. **Do not** administer simultaneously with IV calcium-containing solutions via a Y-site for any age group. IV calcium-containing products may be administered sequentially only when the infusion lines are thoroughly flushed between infusions with a compatible fluid.

Use with caution in patients with penicillin allergy, gallbladder, biliary tract, liver, or pancreatic disease; in the presence of renal impairment; or in neonates with continuous dosing (risk for hyperbilirubinemia). In neonates, consider using an alternative third-generation cephalosporin with similar activity. Unlike other cephalosporins, ceftriaxone is significantly cleared by the biliary route (35%–45%).

Rash, injection site pain, diarrhea, and transient increase in liver enzymes are common. May cause reversible cholelithiasis, sludging in gallbladder, and jaundice. May interfere with serum and urine creatinine assays (Jaffe method) and cause false-positive urine protein and urine–reducing substances (Clinitest).

For IM injections, dilute drug with either sterile water for injection or 1% lidocaine to a concentration of 250 or 350 mg/mL (250 mg/mL has lower incidence of injection site reactions). Assess the potential risk/benefit for using lidocaine as a diluent; see Lidocaine for additional remarks.

CEFUROXIME (IV, IM)/CEFUROXIME AXETIL (PO)
IV: Zinacef and generics
PO: Ceftin and generics
Antibiotic, cephalosporin (second generation)

No　Yes　1　B

Injection: 0.75, 1.5, 7.5 g
Frozen injection: 1.5 g/50 mL water (iso-osmotic solutions)
Injectable dosage forms contain 2.4 mEq Na/g drug
Tabs: 250, 500 mg
Oral suspension: 125, 250 mg/5 mL (50, 100 mL); may contain aspartame

IM/IV:
  Neonate:
    Postnatal age ≤7 days: 100 mg/kg/24 hr ÷ Q12 hr
    Postnatal age >7 days:
      <1 kg:
        8–≤14 days old: 100 mg/kg/24 hr ÷ Q12 hr
        >15 days old: 150 mg/kg/24 hr ÷ Q8 hr
      ≥1 kg: 150 mg/kg/24 hr ÷ Q8 hr
  Infant (>3 mo)/child:
    Mild/moderate infection: 75–100 mg/kg/24 hr ÷ Q8 hr; **max. dose**: 1500 mg/dose
    Severe infection: 100–200 mg/kg/24 hr ÷ Q6–8 hr; **max. dose**: 1500 mg/dose
  Adult: 750–1500 mg/dose Q8 hr; **max. dose**: 9 g/24 hr
PO (see remarks):
  Child (3 mo–12 yr):
    Pharyngitis and tonsillitis: 20 mg/kg/24 hr ÷ Q12 hr; **max. dose**: 500 mg/24 hr
    Otitis media, impetigo, and maxillary sinusitis: 30 mg/kg/24 hr ÷ Q12 hr; **max. dose**: 1 g/24 hr
    Lyme disease (alternative to doxycycline or amoxicillin):
      Oral suspension: 30 mg/kg/24 hr (**max. dose**: 500 mg/24 hr) ÷ Q12 hr × 14–28 days.
  Child (≥13 yr):
    Sinusitis, otitis media, pharyngitis, and tonsillitis:
      Tab: 250 mg Q12 hr
  Adult: 250–500 mg BID; **max. dose**: 1 g/24 hr

Use with caution in penicillin-allergic patients or in the presence of renal impairment. May cause GI discomfort; thrombophlebitis at the infusion site; and false-positive urine–reducing substance (Clinitest and other copper reduction method tests) and Coombs test; may also interfere with serum and urine creatinine determination by the alkaline picrate method. Not recommended for meningitis.

Tablets and oral suspension are NOT bioequivalent and CANNOT be substituted on a mg/mg basis. Administer the suspension with food. Concurrent use of antacids, H₂ blockers, and proton pump inhibitors may decrease oral absorption. **Adjust dose in renal failure (see Chapter 30).**

CELECOXIB
Celebrex and generics
Nonsteroidal antiinflammatory agent (COX-2 selective)

Yes   Yes   2   C/D

Capsules: 50, 100, 200, 400 mg

JRA (≥2 yr and adolescent; see remarks):
  10–25 kg: 50 mg PO BID
  >25 kg: 100 mg PO BID
Adult (see remarks): 100–200 mg PO BID

Contraindicated for perioperative pain with coronary artery bypass graft (CABG) surgery. Use with caution in patients with systemic onset juvenile rheumatoid arthritis (JRA) because of the risk for serious adverse reactions (e.g., disseminated intravascular coagulation). In adults, serious cardiovascular and GI risks reported include thrombosis, myocardial infarction (MI), stroke, GI bleed, GI ulceration, and GI perforation. Common adverse effects include headache, diarrhea, nausea, and hypertension. TEN, SJS, acute kidney injury, and hyperkalemia have also been reported.

Celecoxib is a substrate of CYP 450 2C9. Poor metabolizers of 2C9 should be used with caution, or alternative therapy should be considered. Angiotensin-converting enzyme (ACE) inhibitors, loop diuretics, and sodium phosphates may increase the risk for renal dysfunction. Celecoxib may reduce the antihypertensive effects of ACE inhibitors and increase the levels/toxicity of lithium, metoprolol, and methotrexate.

Not recommended for use in severe renal dysfunction and severe hepatic impairment (Child-Pugh Class C). Reduce dose by 50%, and monitor patient closely in moderate hepatic impairment (Child-Pugh Class B).

Pregnancy category is "C" for prior to 30 wk of gestation and "D" for 30 wk and greater.

If unable to swallow capsules whole, contents of the capsule may be added to applesauce (stable for up to 6 hr refrigerated) and ingested with water.

CEPHALEXIN
Keflex and generics
Antibiotic, cephalosporin (first generation)

No   Yes   1   B

Caps: 250, 500, 750 mg
Tabs: 250, 500 mg
Oral suspension: 125 mg/5 mL, 250 mg/5 mL (100, 200 mL)

Infant and child:
  Mild/moderate infection: 25–50 mg/kg/24 hr PO ÷ Q6 hr; **max. dose:** 2 g/24 hr. Less frequent dosing (Q8–12 hr) may be used for uncomplicated infections.
  Severe infection: 75–100 mg/kg/24 hr PO ÷ Q6 hr; **max. dose:** 4 g/24 hr
  Streptococcal pharyngitis and skin infections: 25–50 mg/kg/24 hr PO ÷ Q6–12 hr. Total daily dose may be divided Q12 hr for streptococcal pharyngitis (>1 yr).
  UTI: 50–100 mg/kg/24 hr PO ÷ Q6 hr
Adult: 1–4 g/24 hr PO ÷ Q6 hr
Max. dose (all ages): 4 g/24 hr
Bacterial endocarditis prophylaxis for dental and upper respiratory procedures:
  Infant and child: 50 mg/kg PO (**max. dose:** 2 g) 1 hr before procedure
  Adult: 2 g PO 1 hr before procedure

CEPHALEXIN continued

Some cross-reactivity with penicillin. **Use with caution** in the presence of renal insufficiency. May cause GI discomfort and false-positive urine–reducing substance (Clinitest and other copper reduction method tests) and Coombs test; false elevation of serum theophylline levels (high-performance liquid chromatography [HPLC] method); and false urine protein test. Probenecid increases serum cephalexin levels, and concomitant administration with cholestyramine may reduce cephalexin absorption. May increase the effects of metformin.

Administer doses on an empty stomach at 2 hr prior or 1 hr after meals. **Adjust dose in renal failure (see Chapter 30).**

CETIRIZINE ± PSEUDOEPHEDRINE
Zyrtec, Children's Zyrtec, and generics
In combination with pseudoephedrine:
  Zyrtec-D 12 Hour and generics
Antihistamine, less sedating

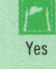
Yes   Yes   ?   B/?

Oral solution or syrup [OTC]: 5 mg/5 mL (120, 473 mL); contains parabens
Tabs [OTC]: 5, 10 mg
Capsule [Liquid filled; OTC]: 10 mg
Chewable tabs [OTC]: 5, 10 mg
Dispersible tabs [OTC]: 10 mg
In combination with pseudoephedrine (PE):
  Extended-release tabs [OTC]: 5 mg cetirizine + 120 mg PE

Cetirizine (see remarks for dosing in hepatic impairment):
  6 mo and <2 yr: 2.5 mg PO once daily; dose may be increased for children 12–23 mo to a **max. dose** of 2.5 mg PO Q12 hr.
  ***2–5 yr:* Initial dose:** 2.5 mg PO once daily; if needed, may increase dose to a **max. dose** of 5 mg/24 hr once daily or divided BID.
  ≥6 yr–adult: 5–10 mg PO once daily
Cetirizine in combination with pseudoephedrine (PE) (see remarks for dosing in hepatic impairment):
  ≥12 yr and adult:
    Zyrtec-D 12 Hour: 1 tablet PO BID

Generally not recommended for treating URIs in infants. No proven benefits in infants and young children with URIs. The FDA does not recommend use for URIs in children aged <2 yr because of reports of increased fatalities.

May cause headache, pharyngitis, GI symptoms, dry mouth, and sedation. Aggressive reactions and convulsions have been reported. Has NOT been implicated in causing cardiac arrhythmias when used with other drugs that are metabolized by hepatic microsomal enzymes (e.g., ketoconazole and erythromycin).

In hepatic impairment, the following doses have been recommended:
  Cetirizine:
    <6 yr: use not recommended
    6–11 yr: <2.5 mg PO once daily
    ≥12 yr–adult: 5 mg PO once daily
  Cetirizine in combination with pseudoephedrine:
    ≥12 yr–adult: 1 tablet PO once daily

Continued

CETIRIZINE ± PSEUDOEPHEDRINE continued

Doses may be administered regardless of food. For Zyrtec-D 12 Hour, see Pseudoephedrine for additional remarks. Pregnancy category is "B" for cetirizine and "?" or unknown when combined with pseudoephedrine. **Dosage adjustment is recommended in renal impairment (see Chapter 30).**

CHARCOAL, ACTIVATED

See Chapter 2

CHLORAMPHENICOL
Generics
Antibiotic

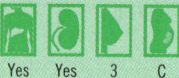
Yes   Yes   3   C

Injection: 1 g
Contains 2.25 mEq Na/g drug

Neonate IV:
  Loading dose: 20 mg/kg
  Maintenance dose (first dose should be given 12 hr after loading dose):
    ≤7 days: 25 mg/kg/24 hr Q24 hr
    >7 days:
      ≤2 kg: 25 mg/kg/24 hr Q24 hr
      >2 kg: 50 mg/kg/24 hr ÷ Q12 hr
Infant/child/adult: 50–75 mg/kg/24 hr IV ÷ Q6 hr
  Meningitis: 75–100 mg/kg/24 hr IV ÷ Q6 hr
Max. dose (all ages): 4 g/24 hr

Dose recommendations are just guidelines for therapy; monitoring of blood levels is essential. Follow hematologic status for dose-related or idiosyncratic marrow suppression. "Gray baby" syndrome may be seen with levels of >50 mg/L. **Use with caution** in G6PD deficiency, renal or hepatic dysfunction, and in neonates.

Concomitant use of phenobarbital and rifampin may lower serum chloramphenicol levels. Phenytoin may increase serum chloramphenicol levels. Chloramphenicol may increase the effects/toxicity of phenytoin, chlorpropamide, cyclosporine, tacrolimus, and oral anticoagulants and decrease the absorption of vitamin B_{12}. Chloramphenicol is an inhibitor of CYP 450 2C9.

Therapeutic levels: Peak: 15–25 mg/L for meningitis and 10–20 mg/L for other infections. Trough: 5–15 mg/L for meningitis and 5–10 mg/L for other infections. Recommended serum sampling time: trough within 30 min prior to next dose; peak 30 min after the end of infusion. Time to achieve steady state: 2–3 days for newborns; 12–24 hr for children and adults.

CHLOROQUINE PHOSPHATE
Aralen and generics
Amebicide, antimalarial

Yes   Yes   2   C

Tabs: 250, 500 mg as phosphate (150, 300 mg base, respectively)
Oral suspension: 16.67 mg/mL as phosphate (10 mg/mL base), 15 mg/mL as phosphate (9 mg/mL base)

CHLOROQUINE PHOSPHATE continued

Doses expressed in mg of chloroquine base.
Malaria prophylaxis (start 1 wk prior to exposure and continue for 4 wk after leaving endemic area):
  Infant and child: 5 mg/kg/dose PO every week; **max. dose**: 300 mg/dose
  Adult: 300 mg/dose PO every week
Malaria treatment (chloroquine sensitive strains):
  For treatment of malaria, consult the infectious disease (ID) specialist or see the latest edition of the AAP Red Book.
  Infant and child: 10 mg/kg/dose (**max. dose**: 600 mg/dose) PO × 1; followed by 5 mg/kg/dose (**max. dose**: 300 mg/dose) 6, 24, and 48 hr after the initial dose.
  Adult: 600 mg/dose PO × 1; followed by 300 mg/dose 6, 24, and 48 hr after the initial dose.

Use with caution in liver disease, preexisting auditory damage or seizures, G6PD deficiency, psoriasis, porphyria, or concomitant hepatotoxic drugs. May cause nausea, vomiting, electrocardiogram (ECG) abnormalities, prolonged QT interval, blurred vision, retinal and corneal changes (reversible corneal opacities), headache, confusion, skeletal muscle weakness, increased liver enzymes, and hair depigmentation. SJS, TEN, anaphylactic reactions, and maculopathy and macular degeneration have been reported.

Antacids, ampicillin, and kaolin may decrease the absorption of chloroquine (allow 4-hr interval between these drugs and chloroquine). Cimetidine may increase effects/toxicity of chloroquine. May increase serum cyclosporine levels. Coadministration with mefloquine may increase the risk for convulsions. May reduce the antibody response to intradermal human diploid cell rabies vaccine.
Adjust dose in renal failure (see Chapter 30).

CHLOROTHIAZIDE
Diuril and generics
Thiazide diuretic

Yes   Yes   2   C/D

Tabs: 250, 500 mg
Oral suspension: 250 mg/5 mL (237 mL); contains 0.5% alcohol, 0.12% methylparaben, 0.02% propylparaben, and 0.1% benzoic acid
Injection: 500 mg; contains 5 mEq Na/1 g drug

<6 mo:
  PO: 20–40 mg/kg/24 hr ÷ Q12 hr
  IV: Start at 5–10 mg/kg/24 hr ÷ Q12 hr, may increase to 20–40 mg/kg/24 hr ÷ Q12 hr if needed.
≥6 mo:
  PO: 10–20 mg/kg/24 hr ÷ Q12 hr; **maximum PO dose** by age:
    6 mo–2 yr: 375 mg/24 hr
    2–12 yr: 1 g/24 hr
    >12 yr: 2 g/24 hr
  IV: Start at 5–10 mg/kg/24 hr ÷ Q12–24 hr, may increase to 20 mg/kg/24 hr ÷ Q12 hr, if needed.
Adult: 500–2000 mg/24 hr ÷ Q12–24 hr PO/IV; alternative IV dosing, some may respond to intermittent dosing on alternate days or on 3–5 days each week.

Contraindicated in anuria. **Use with caution** in liver and severe renal disease and sulfonamide hypersensitivity. May increase serum calcium, bilirubin, glucose, and uric acid. May cause alkalosis, pancreatitis, dizziness, hypokalemia, and hypomagnesemia.

Continued

CHLOROTHIAZIDE continued
Avoid IM or subcutaneous administration.
Pregnancy category changes to "D" if used in pregnancy-induced hypertension.

CHLORPHENIRAMINE MALEATE
Chlor-Trimeton and generics
Antihistamine

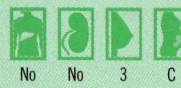
No   No   3   C

Tabs [OTC]: 4 mg
Sustained-release tabs [OTC]: 12 mg
Syrup [OTC]: 2 mg/5 mL (473 mL); may contain 5% alcohol and/or parabens

Child aged <12 yr: 0.35 mg/kg/24 hr PO ÷ Q4–6 hr or dose based on age as follows:
  2–5 yr: 1 mg/dose PO Q4–6 hr; **max. dose:** 6 mg/24 hr
  6–11 yr: 2 mg/dose PO Q4–6 hr; **max. dose** 12 mg/24 hr
≥*12 yr–adult:* 4 mg/dose Q4–6 hr PO; **max. dose**: 24 mg/24 hr
  Sustained release: 12 mg PO Q 12 hr

Use with caution in asthma. May cause sedation, dry mouth, blurred vision, urinary retention, polyuria, and disturbed coordination. Paradoxically, young children may be excited.
Found in many combination over-the-counter (OTC or nonprescription) cough and cold products and are **not recommended** for children aged <6 yr because of reports of serious adverse effects (cardiac and respiratory distress, convulsions, and hallucinations) and fatalities (from unintentional overdosages, including combined use of other OTC products containing the same active ingredients).
Doses may be administered PRN. Administer doses with food. Sustained-release forms are **NOT recommended** in children aged <6 yr and should **NOT** be crushed, chewed, or dissolved.

CHLORPROMAZINE
Thorazine and generics
Antiemetic, antipsychotic, phenothiazine derivative

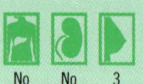
No   No   3   C

Tabs: 10, 25, 50, 100, 200 mg
Injection: 25 mg/mL (1, 2 mL); contains 2% benzyl alcohol

Psychosis:
  Child >6 mo:
    PO: 2.5–6 mg/kg/24 hr ÷ Q4–6 hr; **max. PO dose:** 500 mg/24 hr
    IM/IV: 2.5–4 mg/kg/24 hr ÷ Q6–8 hr
    Max. IM/IV dose:
      <5 yr: 40 mg/24 hr
      5–12 yr: 75 mg/24 hr
  Adult:
    PO: 10–25 mg/dose Q4–6 hr; **max. dose:** 2 g/24 hr
    IM/IV: Initial: 25 mg; repeat with 25–50 mg/dose, if needed, Q1–4 hr up to a **max. dose** of 400 mg/dose Q4–6 hr
Antiemetic:
  Child (≥6 mo):
    IV/IM/PO: 0.5–1 mg/kg/dose Q6–8 hr PRN
    Max. IM/IV/PO dose:
      <5 yr: 40 mg/24 hr
      5–12 yr: 75 mg/24 hr

CHLORPROMAZINE continued

Adult:
  IV/IM: 25–50 mg/dose Q4–6 hr PRN
  PO: 10–25 mg/dose Q4–6 hr PRN

Adverse effects include drowsiness, jaundice, lowered seizure threshold, extrapyramidal/anticholinergic symptoms, hypotension (more with IV), arrhythmias, agranulocytosis, and neuroleptic malignant syndrome. May potentiate effect of narcotics, sedatives, and other drugs. Monitor BP closely. ECG changes include prolonged PR interval, flattened T waves, and ST depression; do not use in combination with fluoxetine, haloperidol, citalopram, and other drugs that can prolong the QT interval. **Do not administer oral liquid dosage form simultaneously with carbamazepine oral suspension**; an orange rubbery precipitate may form.

CHOLECALCIFEROL
D-3, D3-5, D3-50, Decara, D Drops, Emfamil D-Vi-Sol, and many others
Vitamin D₃

No   No   2   A/D

Tablet [OTC]: 400; 1000; 2000; 3000; 5000; 50,000 IU
Caps [OTC]: 1000; 2000; 5000; 10,000; 25,000; 50,000 IU
  D3-5: 5000 IU
  Decra: 25,000 IU
  D3-50, Decara: 50,000 IU
Oral drops (D Drops) [OTC]: 400, 1000, 2000 IU/drop (10 mL)
Oral liquid: (Emfamil D-Vi-Sol and generics): 400 IU/mL (50 mL)

Dietary supplementation (see Chapter 21 for additional information):
  Preterm: 200–400 IU/24 hr PO
  Infant (<1 yr): 400 IU/24 hr PO
  Breast-fed neonate and infant: 400 IU/24 hr PO
  Child (≥1 yr) and adolescent: 600 IU/24 hr PO
Vitamin D deficiency and/or rickets (with calcium and phosphorus supplementation; decrease dose maintenance dosage when radiologically proven healing is achieved):
  <1 mo: 1000 IU/24 hr PO × 2–3 mo; maintenance dose: 400 IU/24 hr
  1–12 mo: 1000–5000 IU/24 hr PO × 2–3 mo; maintenance dose: 400–1000 IU/24 hr
  >12 mo: 5000–10,000 IU/24 hr PO × 2–3 mo; maintenance dose: 600–1000 IU/24 hr
Renal failure (CKD stages 2–5) and 25-OH vitamin D levels of ≤30 ng/mL (monitor serum 25-OH vitamin D and corrected calcium/phosphorus 1 mo after initiation and Q3 mo thereafter):
  Child (PO):
    25-OH vitamin D < 5 ng/mL: 8000 IU/24 hr × 4 wk followed by 4000 IU/24 hr × 2 mo; OR 50,000 IU weekly × 4 wk followed by 50,000 IU twice monthly for 3 mo
    25-OH vitamin D 5–15 ng/mL: 4000 IU/24 hr × 12 wk; OR 50,000 IU every other week × 12 wk
    25-OH vitamin D 16–30 ng/mL: 2000 IU/24 hr × 3 mo; OR 50,000 IU monthly × 3 mo
    Maintenance dose (after repletion): 200–1000 IU once daily

Biological potency and oral absorption may be greater than ergocalciferol (vitamin D₂). Requires activation by the liver (25-hydroxylation) and kidney (1-hydroxylation) to the active form, calcitriol.
Monitor serum Ca^{2+}, PO$_4$, 25-OH vitamin D (goal level for infant and child: ≥20 ng/mL) and alkaline phosphate. Serum Ca^{2+}, PO$_4$ product should be <70 mg/dL to avoid ectopic calcification. Serum

Continued

CHOLECALCIFEROL continued

25-OH vitamin D level of ≥35 ng/mL has been used in Cystic Fibrosis patients to decrease the risk for hyperparathyroidism and bone loss.

Toxic effects in infants may result in nausea, vomiting, constipation, abdominal pain, loss of appetite, polydipsia, polyuria, muscle weakness, muscle/joint pain, confusion, and fatigue; renal damage may also occur.

Pregnancy category changes to "D" if used in doses above the US RDA.

CHOLESTYRAMINE
Questran, Cholestyramine Light, Prevalite, and generics
Antilipemic, binding resin

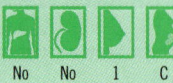
No   No   1   C

Powder for oral suspension:
    Questran and generics: 4 g anhydrous resin per 9 g powder (9, 378 g)
    Cholestyramine Light: 4 g anhydrous resin per 5.7 g powder with aspartame (210, 239 g)
    Prevalite: 4 g anhydrous resin per 5.5 g powder with aspartame (5.5, 231 g)

All doses based in terms of anhydrous resin. Titrate dose based on response and tolerance.
Child: 240 mg/kg/24 hr ÷ TID; doses normally do not exceed 8 g/24 hr (higher doses do not provide additional benefit). Give PO as slurry in water, juice, or milk before meals.
Adult: 3–4 g of cholestyramine BID-QID; **max. dose**: 24 g/hr

In addition to the use for managing hypercholesterolemia, drug may be used for itching associated with elevated bile acids and diarrheal disorders associated with excess fecal bile acids or *Clostridium difficile* (pseudomembranous colitis). May also be applied topically for diaper dermatitis by preparing a 5% or 10% topical product with hydrophilic topical ointment (Aquaphor); other compounded topical formulations exist (e.g., Butt paste: Cholestyramine, sucralfate, zinc oxide, and Eucerin).

May cause constipation, abdominal distention, vomiting, vitamin deficiencies (A, D, E, K), and rash. Hyperchloremic acidosis may occur with prolonged use.

Give other oral medications 4–6 hr after cholestyramine or 1 hr before dose to avoid decreased absorption.

CHOLINE MAGNESIUM TRISALICYLATE
Generic; previously available as Trilisate
Nonsteroidal antiinflammatory agent

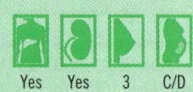
Yes   Yes   3   C/D

Combination of choline salicylate and magnesium salicylate (1:1.24 ratio, respectively); strengths expressed in terms of mg salicylate:
Oral liquid: 500 mg/5 mL (240 mL)

Dose based on total salicylate content.
Child: 30–60 mg/kg/24 hr PO ÷ TID-QID
Adult: 500 mg–1.5 g/dose PO once daily–TID

Avoid use in patients with suspected varicella or influenza due to concerns of Reye's Syndrome. **Use with caution** in severe hepatic or renal (hypermagnesemia risk) failure, asthma, or peptic ulcer disease. Less GI irritation than aspirin and other NSAIDs. No antiplatelet effects.

Pregnancy category changes to "D" if used during the third trimester.

CHOLINE MAGNESIUM TRISALICYLATE continued

Therapeutic salicylate levels, see *Aspirin*. 500 mg choline magnesium trisalicylate is equivalent to 650 mg aspirin.

CICLESONIDE
Alvesco, Omnaris, Zetonna
Corticosteroid

Yes   No   2   C

Aerosol inhaler (Alvesco): 80 mcg/actuation (6.1 g = 60 doses), 160 mcg/actuation (6.1 g = 60 doses)
Nasal spray:
  Omnaris (nasal suspension): 50 mcg/actuation (12.5 g = 120 doses)
  Zetonna (nasal aerosol solution): 37 mcg/actuation (6.1 g = 60 doses)

Intranasal (allergic rhinitis):
  Omnaris:
   2–11 yr (limited data): 1–2 sprays (50–100 mcg) per nostril once daily. **Max. dose**: 200 mcg/24 hr. 2 sprays (100 mcg) per nostril once daily is approved for use in children aged ≥6 yr for seasonal allergic rhinitis.
   ≥12 yr and adult: 2 sprays (100 mcg) per nostril once daily. **Max. dose**: 200 mcg/24 hr.
  Zetonna:
   ≥12 yr and adult: 1 spray (37 mcg) per nostril once daily. **Max. dose**: 74 mcg/24 hr.
Oral inhalation (asthma; Alvesco):
  Dosage suggested by the Global Strategy for Asthma Management and Prevention (see later for current FDA labeled dosage information for ≥12 yr):

Age	Low Dose (mcg/24 hr)	Medium Dose (mcg/24 hr)	High Dose (mcg/24 hr)
<5 yr	160	ND	ND
6–11 yr	80	>80–160	>160–640 mcg/24 hr
≥12 yr and adult	80–160	>160–320	>320–640 mcg/24 hr

ND, Not defined

  ≥12 yr and adult (FDA labeling):
   Prior use with bronchodilator only: 80 mcg/dose BID; max. dose: 320 mcg/24 hr
   Prior use with inhaled corticosteroid: 80 mcg/dose BID; max. dose: 640 mcg/24 hr
   Prior use with oral corticosteroid: 320 mcg/dose BID; max. dose: 640 mcg/24 hr

Ciclesonide is a prodrug hydrolyzed to an active metabolite, des-ciclesonide via esterases in nasal mucosa and lungs; further metabolism via hepatic CYP3A4 and 2D6. Concurrent use with ketoconazole and other CYP 450 3A4 inhibitors may increase systemic des-ciclesonide levels. **Use with caution** and monitor in hepatic impairment.

Oral inhalation (asthma): Rinse mouth after each use. May cause headache, arthralgia, nasal congestion, nasopharyngitis, and URIs. Maximum benefit may not be achieved until 4 wk after initiation; consider dose increase if response is inadequate after 4 wk after initial dosage.

Intranasal (allergic rhinitis): Clear nasal passages prior to use. May cause otalgia, epistaxis, nasopharyngitis, and headache. Nasal septal perforation has also been reported. Patients should be free of nasal disease, except for allergic rhinitis, before starting therapy. Monitor linear growth of pediatric patients routinely. Onset of action: 24–48 hr; further improvement observed over 1–2 wk in seasonal allergic rhinitis or 5 wk in perennial allergic rhinitis. Discontinue use if nasal erosion, ulceration, or perforation occurs.

CIDOFOVIR
Vistide and generics
Antiviral

No   Yes   3   C

Injection: 75 mg/mL (5 mL); preservative-free

Safety and efficacy has not been established in children.
CMV retinitis:
  Adult:
   Induction: 5 mg/kg IV once weekly × 2 with probenecid and hydration
   Maintenance: 5 mg/kg IV Q2 weeks with probenecid and hydration
Adenovirus infection in immunocompromised oncology patients (limited data and other regimens exist; see remarks):
  Child: 5 mg/kg/dose IV once weekly until PCR negative. Administer oral probenecid 1–1.25 g/m^2/dose (rounded to the nearest 250 mg interval) 3 hr before and 1 hr and 8 hr after each dose of cidofovir. Also, give normal saline (NS) via IV at maintenance fluid concentration, 3 times, 1 hr before and 1 hr after cidofovir, followed by 2 times maintenance fluid for an additional 2 hr. For patients with renal dysfunction (see remarks), give 1 mg/kg/dose IV three times weekly until PCR negative.
BK virus hemorrhagic cystitis (limited data and other regimens exist): 1 mg/kg/dose IV once weekly without probenecid.

Contraindicated in hypersensitivity to probenecid or sulfa-containing drugs; sCr > 1.5 mg/dL, CrCl ≤ 55 mL/min, urine protein ≥ 100 mg/dL (2+ proteinuria), direct intraocular injection of cidofovir, and concomitant nephrotoxic drugs. **Renal impairment is the major dose-limiting toxicity.** IV NS prehydration and probenecid must be used (unless not indicated) to reduce risk for nephrotoxicity. May also cause nausea, vomiting, headache, rash, metabolic acidosis, uveitis, decreased intraocular pressure, and neutropenia.
Reported criteria for defining renal dysfunction in children include a sCr > 1.5 mg/dL, GFR < 90 mL/min/1.73 m^2 and >2+ proteinuria. For adults, reduce dose to 3 mg/kg if sCr increases 0.3–0.4 mg/dL from baseline. Discontinue therapy if sCr increases to ≥0.5 mg/dL from baseline or development of ≥3+ proteinuria.
Administer doses via IV infusion over 1 hr at a concentration of ≤8 mg/mL.

CIMETIDINE
Tagamet, Tagamet HB [OTC] and generics
Histamine-2-antagonist

Yes   Yes   2   B

Tabs: 200 [OTC], 300, 400, 800 mg
Oral solution: 300 mg/5 mL (240 mL); may contain 2.8% alcohol

Neonate: 5–20 mg/kg/24 hr PO ÷ Q6–12 hr
Infant: 10–20 mg/kg/24 hr PO ÷ Q6–12 hr
Child: 20–40 mg/kg/24 hr PO ÷ Q6 hr
Adult: 300 mg/dose PO QID **OR** 400 mg/dose PO BID **OR** 800 mg/dose PO QHS
  Ulcer prophylaxis: 400–800 mg PO QHS

Diarrhea, rash, myalgia, confusion, neutropenia, gynecomastia, elevated LFTs, or dizziness may occur. **Use with caution** in hepatic and renal impairment **(adjust dose in renal failure; see Chapter 30).**

CIMETIDINE continued

Inhibits CYP 450 1A2, 2C9, 2C19, 2D6, 2E1, and 3A4 isoenzymes, therefore increases levels and effects of many hepatically metabolized drugs (i.e., theophylline, phenytoin, lidocaine, nicardipine, diazepam, warfarin). Cimetidine may decrease the absorption of iron, ketoconazole, and tetracyclines.

CIPROFLOXACIN
Cipro, Cipro XR, Ciloxan ophthalmic, Cetraxal, Ciprodex,
Cipro HC Otic, Otovel Otic, and generics
Antibiotic, quinolone

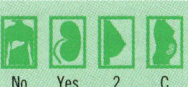

No   Yes   2   C

Tabs: 100, 250, 500, 750 mg
Extended-release tabs (Cipro XR and generics): 500, 1000 mg
Oral suspension: 250 mg/5 mL (100 mL), 500 mg/5 mL (100 mL)
Injection: 10 mg/mL (20, 40 mL)
Premixed injection: 200 mg/100 mL 5% dextrose, 400 mg/200 mL 5% dextrose (iso-osmotic solutions)
Ophthalmic solution (Ciloxan and generics): 3.5 mg/mL (2.5, 5, 10 mL); may contain benzalkonium chloride
Ophthalmic ointment (Ciloxan): 3.3 mg/g (3.5 g)
Otic suspension:
  Cetraxal and generics: 0.5 mg/0.25 mL (14s)
  With dexamethasone (Ciprodex): 3 mg/mL ciprofloxacin + 1 mg/mL dexamethasone (7.5 mL); contains benzalkonium chloride
  With hydrocortisone (Cipro HC Otic): 2 mg/mL ciprofloxacin + 10 mg/mL hydrocortisone (10 mL); contains benzyl alcohol
  With fluocinolone (Otovel Otic): 3 mg/mL ciprofloxacin + 0.25 mg/mL fluocinolone acetonide (0.25 mL; carton of 14s)

Child:
  PO:
    Mild/moderate infection: 20 mg/kg/24 hr ÷ Q12 hr; **max. dose:** 1 g/24 hr
    Severe Infection: 30–40 mg/kg/24 hr ÷ Q12 hr; **max. dose:** 1.5 g/24 hr
  IV:
    Severe infection: 10 mg/kg/dose Q8–12 hr; **max. dose:** 400 mg/dose
  Complicated UTI or pyelonephritis (× 10–21 days):
    PO: 20–40 mg/kg/24 hr ÷ Q12 hr; **max. dose:** 1.5 g/24 hr
    IV: 18–30 mg/kg/24 hr ÷ Q8 hr; **max. dose:** 1.2 g/24 hr
  Cystic fibrosis:
    PO: 40 mg/kg/24 hr ÷ Q12 hr; **max. dose:** 2 g/24 hr
    IV: 30 mg/kg/24 hr ÷ Q8 hr; **max. dose:** 1.2 g/24 hr
  Anthrax (see remarks):
    Inhalational/systemic/cutaneous: Start with 20–30 mg/kg/24 hr ÷ Q12 hr IV (**max. dose:** 800 mg/24 hr) and convert to oral dosing with clinical improvement at 20–30 mg/kg/24 hr ÷ Q12 hr PO (**max. dose:** 1 g/24 hr). Duration of therapy: 60 days (IV and PO combined)
    Post exposure prophylaxis: 20–30 mg/kg/24 hr ÷ Q12 hr PO × 60 days; **max. dose:** 1 g/24 hr
Adult:
  PO:
    Immediate release: 250–750 mg/dose Q12 hr
    Extended release (Cipro XR):
      Uncomplicated UTI/Cystitis: 500 mg/dose Q24 hr
      Complicated UTI/Uncomplicated pyelonephritis: 1000 mg/dose Q24 hr

Continued

CIPROFLOXACIN continued

Adult:
> **IV:** 200–400 mg/dose Q12 hr; 400 mg/dose Q8 hr for more severe/complicated infections
> **Anthrax (see remarks):**
>> **Inhalational/systemic/cutaneous:** Start with 400 mg/dose Q12 hr IV and convert to oral dosing with clinical improvement at 500 mg/dose Q12 hr PO. Duration of therapy: 60 days (IV and PO combined).
>> **Post exposure prophylaxis:** 500 mg/dose Q12 hr PO × 60 days.
> **Ophthalmic solution:**
>> **≥1 yr and adult:** 1–2 drops Q2 hr while awake × 2 days, then 1–2 drops Q4 hr while awake × 5 days
> **Ophthalmic ointment:**
>> **≥2 yr and adult:** Apply 0.5 inch ribbon TID × 2 days, then BID × 5 days
> **Otic:**
>> **Cetraxal and generics:**
>>> **Acute otitis externa (≥1 yr and adult):** 0.25 mL to affected ear(s) BID × 7 days
>> **Ciprodex:**
>>> **Acute otitis media with tympanostomy tubes or acute otitis externa (≥6 mo and adult):** 4 drops to affected ear(s) BID × 7 days
>> **Cipro HC Otic:**
>>> **Otitis externa (>1 yr and adult):** 3 drops to affected ear(s) BID × 7 days
>> **Otovel Otic:**
>>> **Acute otitis media with tympanostomy tubes (≥6 mo):** 0.25 mL to affected ear(s) BID × 7 days

Systemic fluoroquinolones are associated with disabling and potentially permanent side effects of the tendons, muscles, joints, nerves and CNS.

Can cause GI upset, renal failure, and seizures. GI symptoms, headache, restlessness, and rash are common side effects. Peripheral neuropathy has been reported. **Use with caution** in children aged <18 yr (like other quinolones, tendon rupture can occur during or after therapy, especially with concomitant corticosteroid use), alkalinized urine (crystalluria), seizures, excessive sunlight (photosensitivity), and renal dysfunction **(adjust systemic dose in renal failure; see Chapter 30). Do not use otic suspension with perforated tympanic membranes and with viral infections of the external ear canal.**

For dosing in obese patients, use an adjusted body weight (ABW). ABW = Ideal Body Weight + 0.45 (Total Body Weight − Ideal Body Weight).

Combinational antimicrobial therapy is recommended for anthrax. For penicillin susceptible strains, consider changing to high dose amoxicillin (25–35 mg/kg/dose TID PO). See www.bt.cdc.gov for the latest information.

Inhibits CYP 450 1A2. Ciprofloxacin can increase effects and/or toxicity of caffeine, methotrexate, theophylline, warfarin, tizanidine (excessive sedation and dangerous hypotension), and cyclosporine. Probenecid increases ciprofloxacin levels.

Do not administer antacids or other divalent salts with or within 2–4 hr of oral ciprofloxacin dose.
  Do not administer oral suspension through feeding tubes as this dosage form adheres to the tube.

CITRATE MIXTURES
Alkalinizing agent, electrolyte supplement

No Yes ? ?

Oral liquid:
Each mL of oral solution contains the following mEq of electrolyte:

	Na	K	Citrate or HCO₃
Tricitrates*, Virtrate-3*, or Sodium Citrate/Potassium Citrate/Citric Acid (480 mL)	1	1	2
Cytra-K*, Vitrate-K*, or Potassium Citrate/Citric Acid (480 mL)	0	2	2
Cytra-2*, Virtrate-2*, or Sodium Citrate/Citric Acid* (480 mL)	1	0	1
Oracit (15, 30, 500 mL)	1	0	1

*Sugar free

Oral powder for oral solution:
Cytra-K: each packet of powder contains 30 mEq each of potassium and citrate/HCO₃ (100 packets per box) and must be diluted in at least 6 ounces of cold water or juice.

Dilute dose in water or juice.
All mEq doses based on citrate.
Infant and child (PO): 2–3 mEq/kg/24 hr ÷ Q6–8 hr or 5–15 mL/dose Q6–8 hr (after meals and before bedtime)
Adult (PO): 100–200 mEq/24 hr ÷ Q6–8 hr or 15–30 mL/dose Q6–8 hr (after meals and before bedtime)

Contraindicated in severe renal impairment and acute dehydration. **Use with caution** in patients already receiving potassium supplements or who are sodium-restricted. May have laxative effect and cause hypocalcemia and metabolic alkalosis.

Adjust dose to maintain desired pH. 1 mEq of citrate is equivalent to 1 mEq HCO₃ in patients with normal hepatic function.

Potassium citrate has a pregnancy category of "C"; otherwise the pregnancy category is not known for the other components in this medication.

CLARITHROMYCIN
Biaxin, Biaxin XL, and generics
Antibiotic, macrolide

Yes Yes 2 C

Film tablets: 250, 500 mg
Extended-release tablets (Biaxin XL and generics): 500 mg
Granules for oral suspension: 125, 250 mg/5 mL (50, 100 mL)

Infant and child:
Acute otitis media, pharyngitis/tonsillitis, pneumonia, acute maxillary sinusitis, or uncomplicated skin infections: 15 mg/kg/24 hr PO ÷ Q12 hr; max. dose: 1 g/24 hr
Pertussis (≥1 mo): 15 mg/kg/24 hr PO ÷ Q12 hr × 7 days; max. dose: 1 g/24 hr
Bacterial endocarditis prophylaxis: 15 mg/kg (max. dose: 500 mg) PO 1 hr before procedure
Helicobacter pylori: 20 mg/kg/24 hr PO ÷ Q12 hr × 7–14 days; max. dose: 1 g/24 hr with amoxicillin and proton pump inhibitor with/without metronidazole

Continued

CLARITHROMYCIN continued

Infant and child (cont.):
- ***Mycobacterium avium complex (MAC):***
  - ***Prophylaxis (1st episode and recurrence):*** 15 mg/kg/24 hr PO ÷ Q12 hr
  - ***Treatment:*** 15 mg/kg/24 hr PO ÷ Q12 hr with other antimycobacterial drugs
  - ***Max. dose (prophylaxis and treatment):*** 1 g/24 hr

Adolescent and adult:
- ***Pharyngitis/tonsillitis, acute maxillary sinusitis, bronchitis, pneumonia, or uncomplicated skin infections:***
  - ***Immediate release:*** 250–500 mg/dose Q12 hr PO
  - ***Extended release (Biaxin XL):*** 1000 mg Q24 hr PO (currently not indicated for pharyngitis/tonsillitis or uncomplicated skin infections)

Adult:
- ***Pertussis:*** 500 mg (immediate release)/dose Q12 hr PO × 7 days
- ***Bacterial endocarditis prophylaxis:*** 500 mg PO 1 hr before procedure
- ***MAC:***
  - ***Prophylaxis (1st episode and recurrence):*** 500 mg/dose Q12 hr PO
  - ***Treatment:*** 500 mg Q12 hr PO with other antimycobacterial drugs
- ***Helicobacter pylori GI infection:*** 500 mg Q12 hr PO with proton pump inhibitor (lansoprazole or omeprazole) and amoxicillin

Contraindicated in patients allergic to erythromycin and history of cholestatic jaundice/hepatic dysfunction with prior use. As with other macrolides, clarithromycin has been associated with QT prolongation and ventricular arrhythmias, including ventricular tachycardia and torsades de pointes. May cause cardiac arrhythmias in patients also receiving cisapride. Side effects: diarrhea, nausea, abnormal taste, dyspepsia, abdominal discomfort (less than erythromycin but greater than azithromycin), and headache. Anaphylaxis, angioedema, hepatic dysfunction, rhabdomyolysis, SJS, and TEN have been reported.

May increase effects/toxicity of carbamazepine, theophylline, cyclosporine, digoxin, ergot alkaloids, fluconazole, midazolam, selected oral hypoglycemic agents, tacrolimus, triazolam, quetiapine, and warfarin. Substrate and inhibitor of CYP 450 3A4, and inhibits CYP 1A2.

Adjust dose in renal failure (see Chapter 30). Doses, regardless of dosage form, may be administered with food.

CLINDAMYCIN
Cleocin-T, Cleocin, ClindaMax, Evoclin, and generics
Antibiotic, lincomycin derivative

Yes   Yes   2   B

Caps: 75, 150, 300 mg
Oral solution: 75 mg/5 mL (100 mL); may contain ethyl parabens
Injection: 150 mg/mL; contains 9.45 mg/mL benzyl alcohol
Premixed injection in 5% dextrose: 300 mg/50 mL, 600 mg/50 mL, 900 mg/50 mL; contains edetate disodium and may contain benzyl alcohol
Solution, topical (Cleocin-T): 1% (30, 60 mL); may contain 50% isopropyl alcohol
Gel, topical (Cleocin-T, ClindaMax, and generics): 1% (30, 60 g); may contain methylparaben
Lotion, topical (Cleocin-T and generics): 1% (60 mL); may contain methylparaben
Foam, topical (Evoclin and generics): 1% (50, 100 g); contains 58% ethanol
See benzoyl peroxide for combination topical product (clindamycin and benzoyl peroxide)
See tretinoin for combination topical product (clindamycin and tretinoin)
Vaginal cream: 2% (40 g); may contain benzyl alcohol
Vaginal suppository: 100 mg (3s)

CLINDAMYCIN continued

Neonate:
   IV/IM: 5 mg/kg/dose with the following dosage intervals:
     ≤7 days:
       ≤2 kg: Q12 hr
       >2 kg: Q8 hr
     >7 days:
       <1 kg: Q12 hr for 8–14 days old and Q8 hr for ≥15 days old
       1–2 kg: Q8 hr
       >2 kg: Q6 hr

Child and adolescent:
   PO: 10–40 mg/kg/24 hr ÷ Q6–8 hr; **max. dose:** 1.8 g/24 hr
   IM/IV: 25–40 mg/kg/24 hr ÷ Q6–8 hr; **max. dose:** 2.7 g/24 hr
   Bacterial endocarditis prophylaxis: 20 mg/kg (**max. dose:** 600 mg) × 1 PO or IV; 1 hr before procedure with PO route and 30 min before procedure with IV route.

Adult:
   PO: 150–450 mg/dose Q6–8 hr; **max. dose:** 1.8 g/24 hr
   IM/IV: 1200–2700 mg/24 hr IM/IV ÷ Q6–12 hr; **max. dose:** 4.8 g/24 hr. Max. IM dose: 600 mg/dose
   Bacterial endocarditis prophylaxis: 600 mg ×1 PO or IV; 1 hr before procedure with PO route and 30 min before procedure with IV route.

Topical (≥12 yr and adult; administer after washing and fully dry the affected skin): apply to affected area BID.
   Evoclin foam: apply to affected area once daily.

Bacterial vaginosis (adolescent and adult):
   Suppositories: 100 mg/dose QHS × 3 days
   Vaginal cream (2%): 1 applicator dose (5 g) QHS for 3 or 7 days in non-pregnant patients and for 7 days in pregnant patients in the second and third trimesters.

Not indicated in meningitis; CSF penetration is poor.

Pseudomembranous colitis may occur up to several weeks after cessation of therapy. May cause diarrhea, rash, granulocytopenia, thrombocytopenia, or sterile abscess at injection site. Anaphylaxis, DRESS, SJS, severe taste alterations including metallic taste (with high IV doses), and TEN have been reported.

Clindamycin may increase the neuromuscular blocking effects of tubocurarine and pancuronium. **Do not exceed** IV infusion rate of 30 mg/min because hypotension, cardiac arrest has been reported with rapid infusions. May diminish the effects of erythromycin when administered together.

Dosage reduction may be required in severe renal or hepatic disease but not necessary in mild/moderate conditions. Oral liquid preparation may not be palatable; consider sprinkling oral capsules onto applesauce or pudding.

CLOBAZAM
Onfi
Benzodiazepine, anticonvulsant

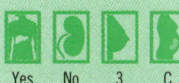
Yes   No   3   C

Tabs: 10, 20 mg
Oral suspension: 2.5 mg/mL (120 mL); contains parabens, polysorbate 80, and propylene glycol

Lennox-Gastaut (adjunctive therapy; see remarks):
   Child (≥2 yr) and adult (PO): Dosage increments (if needed), should not be more rapid than every 7 days. See next page for dose titration.

Continued

CLOBAZAM continued

Weight (kg)	Initial Dose	Dose at Day 8, if Needed	Dose at Day15, if Needed
≤30 kg	5 mg once daily	5 mg BID	10 mg BID (**max. dose**)
>30 kg	5 mg BID	10 mg BID	20 mg BID (**max. dose**)

Dosage adjustment for mild/moderate hepatic impairment (Child-Pugh score 5–9) and individuals with poor CYP 450 2C19 activity (PO):

Weight (kg)	Initial Dose	First Dose Increment, if Needed	Second Dose Increment, if Needed	Third Dose Increment, if Needed
≤30 kg	5 mg once daily × ≥14 days	5 mg BID × ≥7 days	10 mg BID (**max. dose**)	N/A
>30 kg	5 mg once daily × ≥7 days	5 mg BID × ≥7 days	10 mg BID × ≥7 days	20 mg BID (**max. dose**)

N/A = Not applicable

Seizures (generalized or partial, as monotherapy or adjunctive therapy; limited data and prescribing information from Canada and the UK):
  Infant and child (<2 yr): Start at 0.5–1 mg/kg/24 hr (**max. dose:** 5 mg/24 hr) PO ÷ BID, if needed and tolerated, slowly increase dosage at 5–7 day intervals up to the **maximum** of 10 mg/kg/24 hr.
  2–16 yr: Start at 5 mg PO once daily, if needed and tolerated, slowly increase dosage at 5–7 day intervals up to the **maximum** of 40 mg/kg/24 hr. Usual dosage range: 10–20 mg/24 hr or 0.3–1 mg/kg/24 hr ÷ BID.

Use with caution in hepatic impairment (dose adjustment may be needed). **Do not discontinue use abruptly** as seizures/withdrawal symptoms may occur. Common side effects include constipation, drooling, ataxia, drowsiness, insomnia, aggressive behavior, cough and fever. SJS, TEN, urinary retention, hypothermia, leukopenia, and thrombocytopenia have been reported.

Do not use in combination with azelastine, olanzapine, sodium oxybate, and thioridazine; increased risk for adverse events. Proton pump inhibitors, azole antifungal agents (e.g., itraconazole and ketoconazole), St. Johns Wort, grapefruit juice, CNS depressants, cimetidine, and calcium channel blockers may increase the effects/toxicity of clobazam. Carbamazepine, rifamycin derivatives (e.g., rifampin), and theophylline may decrease the effects of clobazam. Clobazam is a major substrate for CYP 450 2C19 and P-glycoprotein, minor substrate for CYP 450 2B6 and 3A4, inhibitor of CYP 450 2D6 and inducer of CYP 3A4. Carefully review the patient's medication profile for other drug interactions each time clobazam is initiated or when a new drug is added to a regimen containing clobazam.

Doses may be taken with or without food. Tablets may be crushed and mixed with applesauce.

CLONAZEPAM
Klonopin and generics
Benzodiazepine, anticonvulsant

Yes   Yes   3   D

Tabs: 0.5, 1, 2 mg
Disintegrating oral tabs: 0.125, 0.25, 0.5, 1, 2 mg; contains phenylalanine
Oral suspension: 100 mcg/mL

CLONAZEPAM continued

Infant and child: <10 yr or <30 kg:
 Initial: 0.01–0.03 mg/kg/24 hr PO ÷ BID–TID; **maximum initial dose:** 0.05 mg/kg/24 hr.
 Increment: 0.25–0.5 mg/24 hr Q3 days, up to **maximum maintenance dose** of 0.1–0.2 mg/kg/24 hr ÷ TID
Child ≥10 yr or ≥30 kg and adult:
 Initial: 1.5 mg/24 hr PO ÷ TID
 Increment: 0.5–1 mg/24 hr Q3 days; **max. dose:** 20 mg/24 hr

Contraindicated in severe liver disease and acute narrow-angle glaucoma. Drowsiness, behavior changes, increased bronchial secretions, GI, CV, GU, and hematopoietic toxicity (thrombocytopenia, leukopenia) may occur. Monitor for depression, suicidal behavior/ideation, and unusual changes in behavior/mood. **Use with caution** in patients with compromised respiratory function, porphyria and renal impairment. **Do not discontinue abruptly.** $T_{1/2}$ = 24–36 hr.

Proposed therapeutic levels (not well established): 20–80 ng/mL. Recommended serum sampling time: Obtain trough level within 30 min prior to an oral dose. Steady state is typically achieved after 5–8 days continuous therapy using the same dose.

Carbamazepine, phenytoin, and phenobarbital may decrease clonazepam levels and effect. Drugs that inhibit CYP-450 3A4 isoenzymes (e.g., erythromycin) may increase clonazepam levels and effects/toxicity.

CLONIDINE
Catapres, Kapvay, Catapres TTS, Duraclon, Nexiclon XR, and generics
Central α-adrenergic agonist, antihypertensive

| No | No | 3 | C |

Tabs: 0.1, 0.2, 0.3 mg
Oral suspension: 20, 100, 1000 mcg/mL
Transdermal patch (Catapres TTS and generics): 0.1, 0.2, 0.3 mg/24 hr (7 day patch); contains metallic components (see remarks)
Injection, epidural (Duraclon and generics): 100, 500 mcg/mL (10 mL); preservative free
Extended-release oral preparations:
 Extended-release oral tab:
  Kapvay and generics: 0.1, 0.2 mg; also available as dose pack blister cards 60 tablets each of 0.1 and 0.2 mg tablets
  Nexiclon XR: 0.17, 0.26 mg; for Q24 hr dosing
 Extended-release oral liquid (Nexiclon XR): 0.09 mg/mL (118 mL); for Q24 hr dosing

Hypertension (use immediate-release products unless noted):
 Child (PO): 5–10 mcg/kg/24 hr ÷ Q8–12 hr initially; if needed, increase at 5–7 day intervals to 5–25 mcg/kg/24 hr ÷ Q6 hr; **max. dose:** 25 mcg/kg/24 hr up to 0.9 mg/24 hr.
 ≥12 yr and adult (PO): 0.1 mg BID initially; increase in 0.1 mg/24 hr increments at weekly intervals until desired response is achieved (usual range: adolescent: 0.2–0.6 mg/24 hr ÷ BID; adult: 0.1–0.8 mg/24 hr ÷ BID), **max. dose:** 2.4 mg/24 hr
Transdermal patch:
 Child: conversion to patch only after establishing an optimal oral dose first. Use a transdermal dosage closest to the established total oral daily dose.
 Adult: Initial 0.1 mg/24 hr patch for first wk. May increase dose by 0.1 mg/24 hr at 1–2 wk intervals PRN. Usual range: 0.1–0.3 mg/24 hr. Each patch last for 7 days. Doses of >0.6 mg/24 hr do not provide additional benefit.

Continued

CLONIDINE continued

ADHD (Child ≥6 yr and adolescent):
Immediate-release product (PO): Start with 0.05 mg QHS; if needed, increase by 0.05 mg every 3–7 days up to a **max. dose** of 0.4 mg/24 hr. Titrated doses may be divided TID-QID.
Extended-release product (Kapvay and generics, PO): Start with 0.1 mg QHS; if needed increase by 0.1 mg every 7 days by administering the dose BID up to a **maximum** of 0.4 mg/24 hr. Depending on dosage level, BID dosing should be either the same amount or with the higher dosage given at bedtime. If therapy is to be discontinued, slowly reduce dosage at ≤0.1 mg every 3–7 days to avoid withdrawal.
Neonatal abstinence syndrome, adjunctive therapy (use immediate-release product; limited data):
0.5–1 mcg/kg/dose Q4–6 hr PO; use Q6 hr interval for preterm neonates.

Side effects: Dry mouth, dizziness, drowsiness, fatigue, constipation, anorexia, arrhythmias, and local skin reactions with patch. Somnolence, fatigue, URI irritability, throat pain, insomnia, nightmares, and emotional disorder were reported as common side effects in ADHD clinical trials. May worsen sinus node dysfunction and AV block especially for patients taking other sympatholytic drugs. **Do not abruptly discontinue**; signs of sympathetic overactivity may occur; taper gradually over >1 wk.

β-Blockers may exacerbate rebound hypertension during and following the withdrawal of clonidine. If patient is receiving both clonidine and a β-blocker and clonidine is to be discontinued, the β-blocker should be withdrawn several days prior to tapering the clonidine. If converting from clonidine over to a β-blocker, introduce the β-blocker several days after discontinuing clonidine (after taper).

Monitor heart rate when used with digitalis, calcium channel blockers and β-blockers. Use with diltiazem or verapamil may result in sinus bradycardia. Use with neuroleptics may induce/exacerbate orthostatic hypotension, dizziness and fatigue.

$T_{1/2}$: 44–72 hr (neonate), 6–20 hr (adult). Onset of action (antihypertensive): 0.5–1 hr for oral route, 2–3 days for transdermal route. **Do not** use transdermal route while patient is undergoing a magnetic resonance imaging (MRI) procedure; transdermal patches contains metals and may result in serious patient burns when undergoing MRI.

CLOTRIMAZOLE
Alevazol, Lotrimin AF, Gyne-Lotrimin 3, Gyne-Lotrimin 7, and generics
Antifungal, imidazole

Yes   No   ?   B/C

Oral troche: 10 mg
Cream, topical (Lotrimin AF and generics; OTC): 1% (15, 30, 45 g); may contain benzyl alcohol
Ointment, topical (Alevazol; OTC): 1% (56.7 g)
Solution, topical [OTC]: 1% (10, 30 mL)
Vaginal cream [OTC]:
 Gyne-Lotrimin 7 and generics: 1% (45 g)
 Gyne-Lotrimin 3 and generics: 2% (21 g)

Topical (cream, ointment or solution): Apply to affected skin areas BID × 4–8 wk
Vaginal cream (>12 yr and adult; may be used in combination with other antifungal vaginal suppository):
 1 applicator dose (5 g) of 1% cream intravaginally QHS × 7–14 days, or
 1 applicator dose of 2% cream intravaginally QHS × 3 days

CLOTRIMAZOLE continued

Thrush:
>**3 yr–adult:** Dissolve slowly (15–30 min) one troche in the mouth 5 times/24 hr × 14 days

May cause erythema, blistering, or urticaria with topical use. Liver enzyme elevation, nausea and vomiting may occur with troches. **Avoid use** of condoms and diaphragms with vaginal cream as latex can be weakened. **Do not use** troches for systemic infections.
Pregnancy code is a "B" for topical and vaginal dosage forms and "C" for troches.

CORTICOTROPIN
HP Acthar, ACTH
Adrenocorticotropic hormone

No   No   ?   C

Injection, repository gel: 80 U/mL (5 mL); contains phenol
1 unit = 1 mg

Infantile spasms (many regimens exist):
20–40 U/24 hr IM once daily × 6 wk or 150 U/m^2/24 hr ÷ BID for 2 wk; followed by a gradual 2-wk taper of 30 U/m^2/dose QAM × 3 days, followed by 15 U/m^2/dose QAM × 3 days, followed by 10 U/m^2/dose QAM × 3 days and 10 U/m^2/dose every other morning ×6 days.

Antiinflammatory:
≥**2 yr and adolescent:** 0.8 U/kg/24 hr ÷ Q12–24 hr IM

Contraindicated in acute psychoses, CHF, Cushing's disease, TB, peptic ulcer, ocular herpes, fungal infections, recent surgery, and sensitivity to porcine products. **Use with caution** in osteoporosis. Repository gel dosage form is only for IM route.
Hypersensitivity reactions may occur. Similar adverse effects as corticosteroids.

CORTISONE ACETATE
Various generics
Corticosteroid

No   No   ?   C/D

Tabs: 25 mg

Antiinflammatory/immunosuppressive:
Child: 2.5–10 mg/kg/24 hr ÷ Q6–8 hr PO
Adult: 25–300 mg/24 hr ÷ Q12–24 hr PO

May produce glucose intolerance, Cushing's syndrome, edema, hypertension, adrenal suppression, cataracts, hypokalemia, skin atrophy, peptic ulcer, osteoporosis, and growth suppression.
Pregnancy category changes to "D" if used in the first trimester.

CO-TRIMOXAZOLE

See SULFAMETHOXAZOLE AND TRIMETHOPRIM

CROMOLYN
Nasalcrom, Gastrocrom, and generics; previously available as Intal
Antiallergic agent, mast cell stabilizer

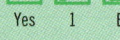

Yes   Yes   1   B

Nebulized solution: 10 mg/mL (2 mL)
Oral concentrate (Gastrocrom and generics): 100 mg/5 mL (5 mL)
Ophthalmic solution: 4% (10 mL)
Nasal spray (Nasalcrom and generics) [OTC]: 4% (5.2 mg/spray) (100 sprays, 13 mL; 200 sprays, 26 mL); contains benzalkonium chloride and EDTA

Nebulization:
   Child aged ≥2 yr and adult: 20 mg Q6–8 hr
      Exercise-induced asthma: 20 mg × 1, 10–15 min prior to and no longer than 1 hr before exercise.
Nasal:
   Child aged ≥2 yr and adult: 1 spray each nostril TID-QID; **max. dose:** 1 spray 6 times/24 hr.
Ophthalmic:
   Child aged >4 yr and adult: 1–2 gtts 4–6 times/24 hr
Food allergy/inflammatory bowel disease:
   2–12 yr: 100 mg PO QID; give 15–20 min AC and QHS; **max. dose:** 40 mg/kg/24 hr
   >12 yr and adult: 200–400 mg PO QID; give 15–20 min AC and QHS
Systemic mastocytosis (taper to lowest effective maintenance dose once desired effect is achieved):
   Infant and child aged <2 yr: 20 mg/kg/24 hr ÷ QID PO; **max. dose:** <6 mo: 20 mg/kg/24 hr, ≥6 mo–<2 yr: 40 mg/kg/24 hr
   2–12 yr: 100 mg PO QID; give 30 min AC and QHS; **max. dose:** 40 mg/kg/24 hr
   >12 yr and adult: 200 mg PO QID; give 30 min AC and QHS; **max. dose:** 40 mg/kg/24 hr

May cause rash, cough, bronchospasm, and nasal congestion. May cause headache, diarrhea with oral use. **Use with caution** in patients with renal or hepatic dysfunction.
Therapeutic response often occurs within 2 wk; however, a 4- to 6-wk trial may be needed to determine maximum benefit. Oral concentrate can only be diluted in water. Nebulized solution can be mixed with albuterol nebs.

CYANOCOBALAMIN/VITAMIN B₁₂
B-12 Compliance, Physicians EZ Use B-12, Nascobal, Vitamin B₁₂ and generics
Vitamin (synthetic), water soluble

No   No   1   A/C

Tabs [OTC]: 100, 250, 500, 1000 mcg
Extended-release tabs: 1000 mcg
Sublingual tabs: 2500 mcg
Sublingual liquid: 3000 mcg/mL (52 mL)
Lozenges [OTC]: 50, 100, 250, 500 mcg
Nasal spray (Nascobal): 500 mcg/spray (1.3 mL delivers 4 doses); contains benzalkonium chloride
Injection: 1000 mcg/mL (1, 10, 30 mL); may contain benzyl alcohol
Injection kit (B-12 Compliance, Physicians EZ Use B-12, and generics): 1000 mcg/mL (1 mL); may contain benzyl alcohol
Contains cobalt (4.35%)

CYANOCOBALAMIN/VITAMIN B₁₂ continued

US RDA: See Chapter 21.
Vitamin B₁₂ deficiency, treatment:
  Child (IM or deep SC): 100 mcg/24 hr × 10–15 days followed by 100 mcg once or twice weekly for several months
    Maintenance: At least 60 mcg/mo
  Adult (IM or deep SC): 30–100 mcg/24 hr × 5–10 days
    Maintenance: 100–200 mcg/mo
Pernicious anemia:
  Child (IM or deep SC): 30–50 mcg/24 hr for at least 14 days to a total dose of 1000–5000 mcg
    Maintenance: 100 mcg/mo
  Adult (IM or deep SC): 100 mcg/24 hr × 7 days, followed by 100 mcg/dose every other day × 14 days, then 100 mcg/dose Q3–4 days until remission is complete.
    Maintenance:
      IM/deep SC: 100–1000 mcg/mo
      Intranasal: 500 mcg in one nostril once weekly
      Sublingual: 1000–2000 mcg/24 hr

Contraindicated in optic nerve atrophy. May cause hypokalemia, hypersensitivity, pruritus, and vascular thrombosis. Pregnancy category changes to "C" if used in doses above the RDA or if administered by the intranasal route.

Prolonged use of acid-suppressing medications may reduce cyanocobalamin oral absorption. Protect product from light. Oral route of administration is generally **not recommended** for pernicious anemia and B₁₂ deficiency because of poor absorption. IV route of administration is **NOT recommended** because of a more rapid elimination. See Chapter 21 for multivitamin preparations.

CYCLOPENTOLATE
Cyclogyl and generics
Anticholinergic, mydriatic agent

No   No   ?   C

Ophthalmic solution: 0.5% (15 mL), 1% (2, 5, 15 mL), 2% (2, 5, 15 mL); may contain benzalkonium chloride

Administer dose approximately 40–50 min prior to examination/procedure.
Infant: Use of cyclopentolate/phenylephrine (Cyclomydril) due to lower cyclopentolate concentration and reduced risk for systemic side effects.
Child: 1 drop of 0.5%–1% solution OU, followed by repeat drop, if necessary, in 5 min. Use 2% solution for heavily pigmented iris.
Adult: 1 drop of 1% solution OU followed by another drop OU in 5 min. Use 2% solution for heavily pigmented iris.

Do not use in narrow-angle glaucoma. May cause a burning sensation, behavioral disturbance, tachycardia, and loss of visual accommodation. Psychotic reactions and behavioral disturbances have been reported in children. To minimize absorption, apply pressure over nasolacrimal sac for at least 2 min. CNS and cardiovascular side effects are common with the 2% solution in children. **Avoid** feeding infants within 4 hr of dosing to prevent potential feeding intolerance.
Onset of action: 15–60 min. Duration of action: 6–24 hr; complete recovery of accommodation may take several days for some patients. Observe patient closely for at least 30 min after dose.

CYCLOPENTOLATE WITH PHENYLEPHRINE
Cyclomydril
Anticholinergic/sympathomimetic, mydriatic agent

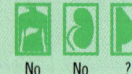
No   No   ?   C

Ophthalmic solution: 0.2% cyclopentolate and 1% phenylephrine (2, 5 mL); contains 0.1% benzalkonium chloride, EDTA and boric acid

Administer dose approximately 40–50 min prior to examination/procedure.
Neonate–adult: 1 drop OU Q5–10 min; **max. dose:** 3 drops per eye

Used to induce mydriasis. See *cyclopentolate* for additional remarks.
Onset of action: 15–60 min. Duration of action: 4–12 hr.

CYCLOSPORINE, CYCLOSPORINE MICROEMULSION, CYCLOSPORINE MODIFIED
Sandimmune, Gengraf, Neoral, Restasis, and generics
Immunosuppressant

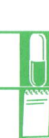
Yes   Yes   X   C

CYCLOSPORINE (Sandimmune and generics):
　Injection: 50 mg/mL (5 mL); contains 32.9% alcohol and 650 mg/mL polyoxyethylated castor oil
　Oral solution: 100 mg/mL (50 mL); contains 12.5% alcohol
　Caps: 25, 50, 100 mg; contains 12.8% alcohol
CYCLOSPORINE MICROEMULSION (Neoral):
　Caps: 25, 100 mg
　Oral solution: 100 mg/mL (50 mL)
　Neoral products contain 11.9% alcohol
CYCLOSPORINE MODIFIED (Gengraf):
　Caps: 25, 50, 100 mg; contains 12.8% alcohol
　Oral solution: 100 mg/mL (50 mL): contains propylene glycol
Ophthalmic emulsion (Restasis): 0.05% (0.4 mL as 30 single-use vials/box); preservative free

Neoral manufacturer recommends a 1:1 conversion ratio with Sandimmune. Because of its better absorption, lower doses of Neoral and Gengraf may be required. Exact dosing will vary depending on transplant type.
Oral: 15 mg/kg/24 hr as a single dose given 4–12 hr pretransplantation; give same daily dose ÷ Q12–24 hr for 1–2 wk posttransplantation, then reduce by 5% per wk to 3–10 mg/kg/24 hr ÷ Q12–24 hr
IV: 5–6 mg/kg/24 hr as a single dose given 4–12 hr pretransplantation; administer over 2–6 hr; give same daily dose posttransplantation until patient able to tolerate oral form
Ophthalmic:
　≥16 yr and adult: Instill one drop onto affected eye(s) Q12 hr.

May cause nephrotoxicity, hepatotoxicity, hypomagnesemia, hyperkalemia, hyperuricemia, hypertension, hirsutism, acne, GI symptoms, tremor, leukopenia, sinusitis, gingival hyperplasia, and headache. Encephalopathy, convulsions, lower extremity pain, vision and movement disturbances, and impaired consciousness have been reported, especially in liver transplant patients. Psoriasis patients previously treated with PUVA and, to a lesser extent, methotrexate or other immunosuppressive agents, UVB, coal tar, or radiation therapy, are at increased risk for skin malignancies when taking Neoral or Gengraf.
Opportunistic infections and activation of latent viral infections have been reported.
BK virus-associated nephropathy has been observed in renal transplant patients.

CYCLOSPORINE, CYCLOSPORINE MICROEMULSION, CYCLOSPORINE MODIFIED continued

Use caution with concomitant use of other nephrotoxic drugs (e.g., amphotericin B, aminoglycosides, non-steroidal anti-inflammatory drugs, and tacrolimus).

Plasma concentrations increased with the use of boceprevir, telaprevir, fluconazole, ketoconazole, itraconazole, erythromycin, clarithromycin, voriconazole, nefazodone, diltiazem, verapamil, nicardipine, carvedilol, and corticosteroids. Plasma concentrations decreased with the use of carbamazepine, nafcillin, rifampin, oxcarbazepine, bosentin, phenobarbital, octreotide, and phenytoin. May increase bosentan, dabigatran, methotrexate, repaglinide, and anthracycline antibiotics (e.g., doxorubicin, mitoxantrone, daunorubicin) levels/effects/toxicity. Use with nifedipine may result in gingival hyperplasia. Cyclosporine is a substrate and inhibitor for CYP 450 3A4 and P-glycoprotein.

Children may require dosages 2–3 times higher than adults. Plasma half-life 6–24 hr.

Monitor trough levels (just prior to a dose at steady state). Steady state is generally achieved after 3–5 days of continuous dosing. Interpretation will vary based on treatment protocol and assay methodology (RIA monoclonal vs. RIA polyclonal vs. HPLC) as well as whole blood vs. serum sample. Additional monitoring and dosage adjustments may be necessary in renal and hepatic impairment or when changing dosage forms.

For ophthalmic use: Remove contact lens prior to use; lens may be inserted 15 min after dose administration. May be used with artificial tears but need to be separated by 15 min for one another.

CYPROHEPTADINE
Various generics; previously available as Periactin
Antihistamine

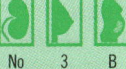
Yes   No   3   B

Tabs: 4 mg
Syrup: 2 mg/5 ml (473 mL); may contain alcohol

Antihistaminic uses:
  Child: 0.25 mg/kg/24 hr or 8 mg/m^2/24 hr ÷ Q8–12 hr PO or by age:
   2–6 yr: 2 mg Q8–12 hr PO; **max. dose:** 12 mg/24 hr
   7–14 yr: 4 mg Q8–12 hr PO; **max. dose:** 16 mg/24 hr
  Adult: Start with 12 mg/24 hr ÷ TID PO; dosage range: 12–32 mg/24 hr ÷ TID PO; **max. dose:** 0.5 mg/kg/24 hr
Migraine prophylaxis: 0.25–0.4 mg/kg/24 hr ÷ BID–TID PO up to following **max. dose**s:
  2–6 yr: 12 mg/24 hr
  7–14 yr: 16 mg/24 hr
  Adult: 0.5 mg/kg/24 hr or 32 mg/24 hr
Appetite stimulation (see remarks):
  ≥2 yr and adolescent: 0.25 mg/kg/24 hr ÷ Q12 hr PO up to the following maximum dose by age: 2–6 yr: 12 mg/24 hr, 7–14 yr: 16 mg/24 hr, ≥15 yr: 32 mg/24 hr.
  Alternative dosing by age:
   4–8 yr (limited data): 2 mg Q8 hr PO
   >13 yr and adult: Start with 2 mg Q6 hr PO; dose may be gradually increased to 8 mg Q6 hr over a 3 wk period.

Contraindicated in neonates, patients currently on MAO inhibitors, and patients suffering from asthma, glaucoma, or GI/GU obstruction. May produce anticholinergic side effects including sedation and appetite stimulation. Consider reducing dosage with hepatic insufficiency.

Continued

CYPROHEPTADINE continued

Allow 4–8 wk of continuous therapy for assessing efficacy in migraine prophylaxis. For use as an appetite stimulant, a dosing cycle of 3 weeks on therapy followed by 1 wk off of therapy may enhance efficacy.

DANTROLENE
Dantrium, Revonto, Ryanodex, and generics
Skeletal muscle relaxant

Yes   No   ?   C

Cap: 25, 50, 100 mg
Oral suspension: 5 mg/mL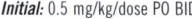
Injection:
  Dantrium and Revonto: 20 mg; injectable solution containing 3 g mannitol per 20 mg drug
  Ryanodex: 250 mg; injectable suspension containing 125 mg mannitol, 25 mg polysorbate 80, 4 mg povidone K12 per 250 mg drug

Chronic spasticity:
  Child: (<5 yr)
    Initial: 0.5 mg/kg/dose PO BID
    Increment: Increase frequency to TID-QID at 4- to 7-day intervals, then increase doses by 0.5 mg/kg/dose
    Max. dose: 3 mg/kg/dose PO BID-QID, up to 400 mg/24 hr
Malignant hyperthermia:
  Prevention:
    PO: 4–8 mg/kg/24 hr ÷ Q6 hr × 1–2 days before surgery with last dose administered 3–4 hr prior to surgery.
    IV (see remarks for specific dosage form administration rates): 2.5 mg/kg beginning 1.25 hr before anesthesia, additional doses PRN
  Treatment (see remarks for specific dosage form administration rates): 1 mg/kg IV, repeat PRN to **maximum cumulative dose** of 10 mg/kg, followed by a postcrisis regimen of 4–8 mg/kg/24 hr PO ÷ Q6 hr for 1–3 days

Contraindicated in active hepatic disease. Monitor transaminase levels for hepatotoxicity. **Use with caution** with cardiac or pulmonary impairment. May cause change in sensorium, drowsiness, weakness, diarrhea, constipation, incontinence, and enuresis. Rare cardiovascular collapse has been reported in patients receiving concomitant verapamil. May potentiate vecuronium-induced neuromuscular block.
Avoid unnecessary exposure of medication to sunlight. **Avoid** extravasation into tissues. A decrease in spasticity sufficient to allow daily function should be therapeutic goal. Discontinue if benefits are not evident in 45 days.

IV administration rates for malignant hyperthermia:

Dosage Form	Prevention Use	Treatment Use
Injectable solution	Over 1 hr	IV push
Injectable suspension	Over at least 1 min	IV push

DAPSONE
Aczone, Diaminodiphenylsulfone, DDS, and generics
Antibiotic, sulfone derivative

Yes | Yes | 2 | C

Tabs: 25, 100 mg
Oral suspension: 2 mg/mL
Topical gel (Aczone): 5% (60, 90 g), 7.5% (60, 90 g)

Pneumocystis jirovecii (formerly carinii) treatment:
  Child and adult: 2 mg/kg/24 hr PO once daily (**max. dose**: 100 mg/24 hr) with trimethoprim 15 mg/kg/24 hr PO ÷ TID × 21 days

Pneumocystis jirovecii (formerly carinii) prophylaxis (first episode and recurrence):
  Child ≥1 mo: 2 mg/kg/24 hr PO once daily; **max. dose**: 100 mg/24 hr. Alternative weekly dosing, 4 mg/kg/dose PO Q7 days; **max. dose**: 200 mg/dose
  Adult: 100 mg/24 hr PO ÷ once daily–BID with or without pyrimethamine 50 mg PO Q7 days and leucovorin 25 mg PO Q7 days; other combination regimens with pyrimethamine and leucovorin may be used (see http://www.aidsinfo.gov).

Toxoplasma gondii prophylaxis (prevent first episode):
  Child ≥1 mo: 2 mg/kg/24 hr (**max. dose**: 25 mg/24 hr) PO once daily with pyrimethamine 1 mg/kg/24 hr (max. 25 mg/dose) PO once daily and leucovorin 5 mg PO Q3 days.
  Adult: 50 mg PO once daily with pyrimethamine 50 mg PO Q7 days and leucovorin 25 mg PO Q7 days; other combination regimens with pyrimethamine and leucovorin may be used (see http://www.aidsinfo.gov).

Leprosy (See www.who.int/en/ for the WHO latest recommendations, including combination regimens such as rifampin ± clofazimine):
  Child: 1–2 mg/kg/24 hr PO once daily; **max. dose**: 100 mg/24 hr
  Adult: 100 mg PO once daily

Acne vulgaris (topical gel, Aczone):
  ≥12 yr:
    5% gel: Apply small amount (pea size) of topical gel onto clean, acne affected areas BID.
    7.5% gel: Apply small amount (pea size) of topical gel onto clean, acne affected areas once daily

Patients with HIV, glutathione deficiency, or G6PD deficiency may be at increased risk for developing methemoglobinemia. Side effects include hemolytic anemia (dose related), agranulocytosis, methemoglobinemia, aplastic anemia, nausea, vomiting, hyperbilirubinemia, headache, nephrotic syndrome, and hypersensitivity reaction (sulfone syndrome). Cholestatic jaundice, hepatitis, peripheral neuropathy, and suicidal intent have been reported with systemic use.

Didanosine, rifabutin, and rifampin decrease dapsone levels. Trimethoprim increases dapsone levels. Pyrimethamine, nitrofurantoin, primaquine, and zidovudine increase risk for hematological side effects.

Oral suspension may not be absorbed as well as tablets.

TOPICAL USE: Dry skin, erythema, and peeling of the skin may occur. Use of topical gel, followed by benzoyl peroxide for acne, has resulted in temporary local discoloration (yellow/orange) of the skin and facial hair. **Avoid use** of topical gel in G6PD deficiency or congenital/idiopathic methemoglobinemia.

DARBEPOETIN ALFA
Aranesp
Erythropoiesis stimulating protein

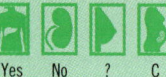
Yes   No   ?   C

Injection: 25, 40, 60, 100, 200, 300 mcg/1 mL (1 mL); 10 mcg/0.4 mL (0.4 mL)
Single dose prefilled injection syringe (27 gauge 1/2-inch needle): 25 mcg/0.42 mL (0.42 mL), 40 mcg/0.4 mL (0.4 mL), 60 mcg/0.3 mL (0.3 mL), 100 mcg/0.5 mL (0.5 mL), 150 mcg/0.3 mL (0.3 mL), 200 mcg/0.4 mL (0.4 mL), 300 mcg/0.6 mL (0.6 mL), 500 mcg/1 mL (1 mL)
Both dosage forms contain polysorbate (0.05 mg/mL).

Anemia in chronic renal failure (see remarks):
  Child (>1 yr) and adult:
    Receiving dialysis: Start with 0.45 mcg/kg/dose IV/SC once weekly **OR** 0.75 mcg/kg/dose IV/SC once every 2 wk; IV route is recommended for patients on hemodialysis. Adjust dose according to the table that follows.
    Not receiving dialysis: Start with 0.45 mcg/kg/dose IV/SC once every 4 wk and adjust dose according to the table that follows:

Darbepoetin Alfa Dose Adjustment in Anemia Associated with Chronic Renal Failure

Response to Dose	Dose Adjustment
<1 g/dL increase in hemoglobin and below target range after 4 wk of therapy	Increase dose by 25% not more frequently than once monthly. Further increases, if needed, may be done at 4-wk intervals.
>1 g/dL increase in hemoglobin in any 2-wk period, or if hemoglobin exceeds and approaches 11 g/dL	Decrease dose by 25%
Hemoglobin continues to increase despite dosage reduction	Discontinue therapy; reinitiate therapy at a 25% lower dose than that of the previous dose after hemoglobin starts to decrease

Anemia associated with chemotherapy (patients with nonmyeloid malignancies):
  Child (limited data) and adult (see remarks): Start with 2.25 mcg/kg/dose SC once weekly and adjust dose according to the table that follows:

Darbepoetin Alfa Dose Adjustment in Anemia Associated with Chemotherapy

Response to Dose	Dose Adjustment
<1 g/dL increase in hemoglobin and remains below 10 g/dL after 6 wk of therapy	Increase dose to 4.5 mcg/kg/dose once weekly SC/IV
>1 g/dL increase in hemoglobin in any 2-wk period, or when hemoglobin reaches a level needed to avoid transfusion	Decrease dose by 40%
If hemoglobin exceeds a level needed to avoid transfusion	Hold therapy until hemoglobin approaches a level where transfusions may be required and reinitiate at a reduced dose by 40%
Lack or response after 8 wk or completion of chemotherapy	Discontinue therapy

DARBEPOETIN ALFA continued
Conversion from epoetin alfa to darbepoetin alfa (see table below):

Previous Weekly Epoetin Alfa Dose (units/wk)*	Pediatric Weekly Darbepoetin Alfa Dose (mcg/wk) Administered Sc/Iv Once Weekly†	Adult Weekly Darbepoetin Alfa Dose (mcg/wk) Administered Sc/Iv Once Weekly†	Adult Once Every 2 wk Darbepoetin Alfa Dose (mcg Every 2 wk) Administered Sc/Iv Once Every 2 wk‡
<1500	Insufficient data	6.25	12.5
1500–2499	6.25	6.25	12.5
2500–4999	10	12.5	25
5000–10,999	20	25	50
11,000–17,999	40	40	80
18,000–33,999	60	60	120
34,000–89,000	100	100	200
≥90,000	200	200	400

*200 units of epoetin alfa is equivalent to 1 mcg darbepoetin alfa.
†If patient was receiving epoetin alfa 2–3 times weekly, darbepoetin alfa should be administered once weekly.

‡If patient was receiving epoetin alfa once weekly, darbepoetin alfa should be administered once every 2 wk.**Contraindicated** in patients with uncontrolled hypertension and those who are hypersensitive to albumin/polysorbate 80 or epoetin alfa. Darbepoetin alfa is not intended for patients requiring acute correction of anemia. **Use with caution** in seizures and liver disease. Evaluate serum iron, ferritin, and TIBC; concurrent iron supplementation may be necessary. Red cell aplasia and severe anemia associated with neutralizing antibodies to erythropoietin have been reported.

USE IN CHRONIC RENAL FAILURE: Higher doses may be needed for pediatric patients being switched from epoetin alfa than those for naïve patients. May cause edema, fatigue, gastrointestinal (GI) disturbances, headache, blood pressure changes, fever, cardiac arrhythmia/arrest, infections, and myalgia. Higher risk for mortality and serious cardiovascular events have been reported with higher targeted hemoglobin levels (>11 g/dL). If hemoglobin levels do not increase or reach targeted levels despite appropriate dose titrations over 12 wk, (1) **do not** administer higher doses and use the lowest dose that will maintain hemoglobin levels to avoid the need for recurrent blood transfusions; (2) evaluate and treat other causes of anemia; (3) always follow the dose adjustment instructions; and (4) discontinue use if the patient remains transfusion dependent.

USE IN CANCER: Use only for anemia that is a result of myelosuppressive chemotherapy; not effective in reducing the need for transfusions in patients with anemia that is not a result of chemotherapy. Shortened survival and time to tumor progression have been reported in patients with various cancers. May cause fatigue, fever, edema, dizziness, headache, GI disturbances, arthralgia/myalgia, and rash. Use lowest dose to avoid transfusions and **do not exceed hemoglobin levels of >12 g/dL**; increased frequency of adverse events, including mortality and thrombotic vascular events, have been reported. **Prescribers and hospitals must enroll in and comply with the ESA APPRISE Oncology Program to prescribe and/or dispense this drug to patients with cancer.**

Monitor hemoglobin, blood pressure (BP), serum chemistries, and reticulocyte count. Increases in dose should not be made more frequently than once a month. For IV administration, infuse over 1–3 min.

DEFEROXAMINE MESYLATE
Desferal and generics
Chelating agent

Yes   Yes   2   C

Injection: 500, 2000 mg

Acute iron poisoning (if using IV route, convert to IM as soon as the patient's clinical condition permits; see remarks):
  Child:
   IV: 15 mg/kg/hr
   IM: 50 mg/kg/dose Q6 hr
   Max. dose: 6 g/24 hr
  Adult:
   IV: 15 mg/kg/hr
   IM: 1 g × 1, then 0.5 g Q4 hr × 2; may repeat 0.5 g Q4–12 hr
   Max. dose: 6 g/24 hr
Chronic iron overload (see remarks):
  Child and adolescent:
   IV: 20–40 mg/kg/dose over 8–12 hr once daily × 5–7 days per week; usual **max. dose:** 40 mg/kg/24 hr (child) or 60 mg/kg/24 hr (adolescent)
   SC: 20–40 mg/kg/dose once daily as infusion over 8–12 hr; **max. dose:** 2 g/24 hr
  Adult:
   IV: 40–50 mg/kg/dose over 8–12 hr once daily × 5–7 days per week; **max. dose:** 6 g/24 hr
   IM: 0.5–1 g/dose once daily; **max. dose:** 1 g/24 hr
   SC: 1–2 g/dose once daily as infusion over 8–24 hr

Contraindicated in severe renal disease or anuria. **Not approved** for use in primary hemochromatosis. May cause flushing, erythema, urticaria, hypotension, tachycardia, diarrhea, leg cramps, fever, cataracts, hearing loss, nausea, and vomiting. Iron mobilization may be poor in children aged <3 yr. Serum creatinine elevation, acute renal failure, renal tubular disorders, and hepatic dysfunction have been reported.

Avoid use if GFR of <10 mL/min and administer 25%–50% of usual dose if GFR is 10–50 mL/min or patient is receiving continuous renal replacement therapy (CRRT).

High doses and concomitant low ferritin levels have also been associated with growth retardation. Growth velocity may resume to pretreatment levels by reducing the dosage. Acute respiratory distress syndrome (ARDS) has been reported following treatment with excessively high IV doses in patients with acute iron intoxication or thalassemia. Toxicity risk has been reported with infusions of >8 mg/kg/hr for >4 days for thalassemia and with infusions of 15 mg/kg/hr for >1 day for acute iron toxicity. Pulmonary toxicity was not seen in 193 courses.

For IV infusion, **maximum rate:** 15 mg/kg/hr. Infuse IV infusion over 6–12 hr for mild/moderate iron intoxication and over 24 hr for severe cases and then reassess. SC route is via a portable controlled–infusion device and is **not recommended** in acute iron poisoning.

DESMOPRESSIN ACETATE
DDAVP, Stimate, and generics
Vasopressin analog, synthetic; hemostatic agent

No   No   2   B

Tabs: 0.1, 0.2 mg
Nasal solution (with rhinal tube): DDAVP, 100 mcg/mL (2.5, 5 mL); contains 9 mg NaCl/mL

DESMOPRESSIN ACETATE continued

Injection: 4 mcg/mL (1, 10 mL); contains 9 mg NaCl/mL
Nasal spray:
  100 mcg/mL, 10 mcg/spray (50 sprays, 5 mL); contains 7.5 mg NaCl/mL
  Stimate: 1500 mcg/mL, 150 mcg/spray (25 sprays, 2.5 mL); contains 9 mg NaCl/mL
Conversion: 100 mcg = 400 IU arginine vasopressin

Diabetes insipidus (see remarks):
  Oral:
    Child aged ≤12 yr: Start with 0.05 mg/dose BID; titrate to effect; usual dose range: 0.1–0.8 mg/24 hr.
    Child aged >12 yr and adult: Start with 0.05 mg/dose BID; titrate dose to effect; usual dose range: 0.1–1.2 mg/24 hr ÷ BID–TID.
  Intranasal (titrate dose to achieve control of excessive thirst and urination. Morning and evening doses should be adjusted separately for diurnal rhythm of water turnover):
    3 mo–12 yr: 5–30 mcg/24 hr ÷ once daily–BID
    >12 yr and adult: 10–40 mcg/24 hr ÷ once daily–TID
  IV/SC:
    <12 yr (limited data): 0.1–1 mcg/24 hr ÷ once daily–BID; start with lower dose and increase as needed.
    ≥12 yr and adult: 2–4 mcg/24 hr ÷ BID
Hemophilia A and von Willebrand disease:
  Intranasal: 2–4 mcg/kg/dose 2 hr before procedure
  IV: 0.2–0.4 mcg/kg/dose over 15–30 min, administered 30 min before procedure
Nocturnal enuresis (≥6 yr; see remarks):
  Oral: 0.2 mg at bedtime, titrated to a **max. dose** of 0.6 mg to achieve desired effect.

Use with caution in hypertension, patients at risk for water intoxication with hyponatremia, and coronary artery disease. May cause headache, nausea, seizures, BP changes, hyponatremia, nasal congestion, abdominal cramps, and hypertension.

NOCTURNAL ENURESIS: Intranasal formulations are no longer indicated by the FDA for primary nocturnal enuresis (children are susceptible for severe hyponatremia and seizures) or in patients with a history of hyponatremia. Patients using tablets should reduce their fluid intake to prevent potential water intoxication and hyponatremia and should have their therapy interrupted during acute illnesses that may lead to fluid and/or electrolyte imbalance.

Injection may be used SC or IV at approximately 10% of intranasal dose. Adjust fluid intake to decrease risk for water intoxication and monitor serum sodium.

If switching from intranasal route to IV/SC route stabilized the patient, use 10% of intranasal dose. Peak effects: 1–5 hr with intranasal route; 1.5–3 hr with IV route; and 2–7 hr with PO route.

DEXAMETHASONE
Dexpak Taperpak, Maxidex, and generics; previously available as Decadron and Hexadrol
Corticosteroid

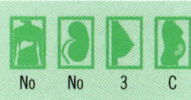

Tabs (Decadron and other generics): 0.5, 0.75, 1, 1.5, 2, 4, 6 mg
  Dexpak Taperpak: 1.5 mg [21 tabs (6 day), 35 tabs (10 day), 51 tabs (13 day)]
Injection (sodium phosphate salt): 4, 10 mg/mL (some preparations contain benzyl alcohol or methyl/propyl parabens)
Elixir: 0.5 mg/5 mL; some preparations contain 5% alcohol

Continued

DEXAMETHASONE continued

Oral solution: 0.1, 1 mg/mL; some preparations contain 30% alcohol
Ophthalmic solution: 0.1% (5 mL)
Ophthalmic suspension (Maxidex): 0.1% (5 mL)

Airway edema: 0.5–2 mg/kg/24 hr IV/IM ÷ Q6 hr (begin 24 hr before extubation and continue for 4–6 doses after extubation)
Asthma exacerbation: 0.6 mg/kg/dose (max. 16 mg/dose) PO/IV/IM Q24 hr × 1 or 2 doses; use beyond 2 days increases risk for metabolic adverse effects
Croup: 0.6 mg/kg/dose PO/IV/IM × 1
Antiemetic (chemotherapy induced):
 Initial: 10 mg/m^2/dose IV; **max. dose**: 20 mg
 Subsequent: 5 mg/m^2/dose Q6 hr IV
Antiinflammatory:
 Child: 0.08–0.3 mg/kg/24 hr PO, IV, IM ÷ Q6–12 hr
 Adult: 0.75–9 mg/24 hr PO, IV, IM ÷ Q6–12 hr
Brain tumor–associated cerebral edema:
 Loading dose: 1–2 mg/kg/dose IV/IM × 1
 Maintenance: 1–1.5 mg/kg/24 hr ÷ Q4–6 hr; **max. dose**: 16 mg/24 hr
Ophthalmic use (child and adult):
 Solution: Instill 1–2 drops into the conjunctival sac(s) of the affected eye(s) Q1 hr during the day and Q2 hr during the night as initial therapy. When a favorable response is achieved, reduce dosage to Q3–4 hr. Further dose reduction to 1 drop TID–QID may be sufficient to control symptoms.
 Suspension: Shake well before using. Instill 1–2 drops in the conjunctival sac(s) of the affected eye(s) up to 4–6 times/24 hr. For severe disease, drops may be Q1 hr, which is tapered to discontinuation as inflammation subsides. For mild disease, drops may be used ≤4–6 times/24 hr.

Not recommended for systemic therapy in the prevention or treatment of chronic lung disease in infants with very low birth weight because of increased risk for adverse events. Dexamethasone is a substrate of CYP450 3A3/4 and P-glycoprotein.
Compared with prednisone, dexamethasone has no mineralocorticoid effects with greater glucocorticoid effects. Consider use of alternative low glucocorticoid systemic steroid for patients with hyperglycemia. **Contraindicated** in active untreated infections and fungal, viral, and mycobacterial ocular infections.
Oral peak serum levels occur 1–2 hr and within 8 hr following IM administration. **For other uses, doses based on body surface area, and dose equivalence to other steroids, see Chapter 10.**
OPHTHALMIC USE: Use ophthalmic preparation only in consultation with an ophthalmologist. **Use with caution** in corneal/scleral thinning and glaucoma. Consider the possibility of persistent fungal infections of the cornea after prolonged use. Ophthalmic solution/suspension may be used in otitis externa.

DEXMEDETOMIDINE
Precedex and generics
α-Adrenergic agonist, sedative

Yes No ? C

Injection (Precedex and generics): 200 mcg/2 mL (2 mL); preservative free
Premixed injection in NS (Precedex): 80 mcg/20 mL (20 mL), 200 mcg/50 mL (50 mL), 400 mcg/100 mL (100 mL); preservative free

DEXMEDETOMIDINE continued

NOTE: Maintenance infusion rate dosing metric is mcg/kg/HR
ICU sedation:
  Child (limited data): 0.5–1 mcg/kg/dose IV × 1 over 10 min followed by 0.2–1 mcg/kg/hr infusion titrated to effect. Children <1 yr of age may require higher dosages.
  Adult: 1 mcg/kg/dose IV × 1 over 10 min, followed by 0.2–0.7 mcg/kg/hr infusion and titrated to effect.
Procedural sedation:
  Child (limited data):
    IV: 2 mcg/kg/dose × 1 IV followed by 1.5 mcg/kg/hr was administered to children with autism/pervasive developmental disorders for sedation for electroencephalography (EEG).
    IM: 1–4.5 mcg/kg/dose × 1 IM was administered to children for sedation for EEG. Extremely anxious, inconsolable, aggressive, and noncompliant children received doses of >2.5 mcg/kg and calm and relatively compliant children received doses of ≤2.5 mcg/kg. A second lower repeat dose (~2 mcg/kg/dose IM) was administered because adequate sedation was not achieved after 10 min of the first dose.
    Intranasal route (limited data): 1–2 mcg/kg/dose × 1 for premedication anesthesia induction.
  Adult: 1 mcg/kg/dose IV × 1 over 10 min, followed by 0.6 mcg/kg/hr titrated to effect; dosage has ranged from 0.2–1 mcg/kg/hr.

Use with caution with other vasodilating or negative chronotropic agents (additive pharmacodynamic effects), hepatic impairment (decrease drug clearance; consider dose reduction), advanced heart block, hypovolemia, diabetes mellitus, chronic hypertension, and severe ventricular dysfunction. Prolonged use >24 hr may be associated with tolerance and tachyphylaxis and dose-related side effects (ARDS, respiratory failure, and agitation).

Hypotension and bradycardia are common side effects; may be more pronounced in hypovolemia, diabetes, or chronic hypertension. Transient hypertension has been observed during loading doses. QT prolongation, hypernatremia, sinus arrest, and polyuria have been reported. **Do not** abruptly withdraw therapy as withdrawal symptoms (nausea, vomiting, and agitation) are possible; taper the dose when discontinuing use.

Use with anesthetics, sedatives, hypnotics, and opioids may lead to enhanced effects; consider dosage reduction of dexmedetomidine. Dexmedetomidine is a CYP450 2A6 substrate and a weak inhibitor of CYP450 1A2, 2C9, and 3A4.

Onset of action for procedural sedation: IV or IM: 15 min, intranasal: 15–30 min. Duration of action for procedural sedation: IM: 1 hr, intranasal: 1–1.5 hr.

This drug should be administered by individuals skilled in the management of patients in the ICU and OR. Concentrated IV solution (200 mcg/2 mL) must be diluted with normal saline (NS) to a concentration of 4 mcg/mL prior to administration. See Chapter 6 for additional information.

DEXMETHYLPHENIDATE
Focalin, Focalin XR, and generics
CNS stimulant

| No | No | 3 | C |

Immediate-release tab (Focalin and generics): 2.5, 5, 10 mg
Extended-release caps (Focalin XR and generics): 5, 10, 15, 20, 25, 30, 35, 40 mg

Continued

DEXMETHYLPHENIDATE continued

Attention deficit/hyperactivity disorder:
METHYLPHENIDATE NAIVE:

Age/Dosage Form	Initial Dose	Dosage Increase at Weekly Intervals, if Needed	Daily Maximum Dose
≥6 YR AND ADOLESCENT			
Immediate-release tabs*	2.5 mg PO BID	2.5–5 mg/24 hr	20 mg/24 hr (10 mg BID)
Extended-release caps**	5 mg PO once daily	5 mg/24 hr	30 mg/24 hr
ADULT			
Immediate-release tabs*	2.5 mg PO BID	2.5–5 mg/24 hr	20 mg/24 hr (10 mg BID)
Extended-release caps**	10 mg PO once daily	10 mg/24 hr	40 mg/24 hr

*BID dosing (at least 4 hr apart), **Once-daily dosing

CONVERTING FROM METHYLPHENIDATE:
  ≥6 yr and adult: Start at 50% of the total daily dose of racemic methylphenidate with the following maximum doses:
    Immediate-release tabs (BID dosing): 20 mg/24 hr
    Extended-release caps (once-daily dosing): 30 mg/24 hr for ≥6 yr–adolescents; 40 mg/24 hr for adults.
CONVERTING FROM IMMEDIATE-RELEASE TABS (BID) TO EXTENDED-RELEASE CAPS (once daily)
DEXMETHYLPHENIDATE: Use the equivalent mg dosage amount.

Dexmethylphenidate is the d-enantiomer of methylphenidate and accounts for the majority of clinical effects for methylphenidate. **Contraindicated** in glaucoma, anxiety disorders, motor tics, and Tourette syndrome. **Do not** use with monoamine oxidase (MAO) inhibitor; hypertensive crisis may occur if used within 14 days of discontinuance of MAO inhibitor. See *methylphendate* for additional warnings and drug interactions.

Common side effects include abdominal pain, indigestion, appetite suppression, nausea, headache, insomnia, and anxiety. Peripheral vasculopathy, including Raynaud phenomenon, and priapism have been reported.

Immediate-release tablets are dosed BID (minimum 4 hr between doses), and extended-release capsules are dosed once daily. Contents of the extended-release capsule may be sprinkled on a spoonful of applesauce and consumed immediately for those who are unable to swallow capsules.

DEXTROAMPHETAMINE ± AMPHETAMINE
Dexedrine, ProCentra, Zenzedi, and many generics
In combination with amphetamine: Adderall, Adderall XR, and generics
CNS stimulant, amphetamine

No   No   X   C

Immediate-release tabs:
  Dexedrine and generics: 5, 10 mg
  Zenzedi: 2.5, 5, 7.5, 10, 15, 20, and 30 mg
Sustained-release caps (Dexedrine and generics): 5, 10, 15 mg
Oral solution (ProCentra and generics): 1 mg/mL (473 mL)

DEXTROAMPHETAMINE ± AMPHETAMINE continued

In combination with amphetamine (Adderall): Available as 1:1:1:1 mixture of dextroamphetamine sulfate, dextroamphetamine saccharate, amphetamine aspartate, and amphetamine sulfate salts (e.g., 5 mg tablet contains 1.25 mg dextroamphetamine sulfate, 1.25 mg dextroamphetamine saccharate, 1.25 mg amphetamine aspartate, and 1.25 mg amphetamine sulfate; 5 mg of the mixture is equivalent to 3.1 mg amphetamine base):

Tabs: 5, 7.5, 10, 12.5, 15, 20, 30 mg
Caps, extended-release (Adderall XR and generics): 5, 10, 15, 20, 25, 30 mg
Oral suspension: 1 mg/mL

Dosages are in terms of mg of dextroamphetamine when using dextroamphetamine alone OR in terms of mg of the total dextroamphetamine and amphetamine salts when using Adderall. Nonextended-release dosage forms are usually given BID–TID (first dose on awakening and subsequent doses at intervals of 4–6 hr later). Extended/sustained-released dosage forms are usually given PO once daily, sometimes BID.

Attention deficit/hyperactivity disorder:
3–5 yr: 2.5 mg/24 hr QAM; increase by 2.5 mg/24 hr at weekly intervals to a **max. dose** of 40 mg/24 hr ÷ once daily–BID (some may require TID dosing).
≥6 yr: 5 mg/24 hr QAM; increase by 5 mg/24 hr at weekly intervals to a **max. dose** of 40 mg/24 hr ÷ once daily–BID (some may require TID dosing). **Max. dose** of 60 mg/24 hr has been used patients >50 kg.

Narcolepsy:
6–12 yr: 5 mg/24 hr ÷ once daily–TID; increase by 5 mg/24 hr at weekly intervals to a **max. dose** of 60 mg/24 hr
>12 yr and adult: 10 mg/24 hr ÷ once daily–TID; increase by 10 mg/24 hr at weekly intervals to a **max. dose** of 60 mg/24 hr

Use with caution in the presence of hypertension or cardiovascular disease. **Avoid** use in known serious structural cardiac abnormalities, cardiomyopathy, serious heart rhythm abnormalities, coronary artery disease, or other serious cardiac problems that may increase risk for sympathomimetic effects of amphetamines (sudden death, stroke, and MI have been reported). **Do not** administer with MAO inhibitors (also within 14 days of discontinuance) or general anesthetics. Use with proton pump inhibitors (PPIs) may reduce the effectiveness of either dextroamphetamine or the combination with amphetamine.

Not recommended for <3 yr. Medication should generally **not** be used in children aged <5 yr as diagnosis of ADHD in this age group is extremely difficult (use in consultation with a specialist). Interrupt administration occasionally to determine need for continued therapy. Many side effects, including insomnia (**avoid** dose administration within 6 hr of bedtime), restlessness/irritability, anorexia, psychosis, visual disturbances, headache, vomiting, abdominal cramps, dry mouth, and growth failure. Paranoia, mania, peripheral vasculopathy (including Raynaud phenomenon), priapism, bruxism, and auditory hallucination have been reported. Tolerance develops. Same guidelines as for methylphenidate apply. See Amphetamine for amphetamine-only–containing product.

DIAZEPAM
Valium, Diastat, Diastat AcuDial, and generics
Benzodiazepine; anxiolytic, anticonvulsant

Yes | Yes | X | D

Tabs: 2, 5, 10 mg
Oral solution: 1 mg/mL, 5 mg/mL; contains 19% alcohol

Continued

DIAZEPAM continued

Injection: 5 mg/mL; contains 40% propylene glycol, 10% alcohol, 5% sodium benzoate, and 1.5% benzyl alcohol

Intramuscular auto-injector: 5 mg/mL (2 mL); contains 40% propylene glycol, 10% alcohol, 5% sodium benzoate, and 1.5% benzyl alcohol

Rectal gel:

   Pediatric rectal gel (Diastat and generics): 2.5 mg (5 mg/mL concentration with 4.4-cm rectal tip delivery system; contains 10% alcohol, 1.5% benzyl alcohol, and propylene glycol); in twin packs.

   Pediatric/Adult rectal gel (Diastat AcuDial and generics):

     4.4-cm rectal tip delivery system (Pediatric/Adult): 10 mg (5 mg/mL, delivers set doses of either 5, 7.5, or 10 mg); contains 10% alcohol, and 1.5% benzyl alcohol; in twin packs.

     6-cm rectal tip delivery system (Adult): 20 mg (5 mg/mL, delivers set doses of either 10, 12.5, 15, 17.5, 20 mg); contains 10% alcohol, and 1.5% benzyl alcohol; in twin packs.

Sedative/muscle relaxant:

   Child:

     IM or IV: 0.04–0.2 mg/kg/dose Q2–4 hr; **max. dose**: 0.6 mg/kg within an 8-hr period.

     PO: 0.12–0.8 mg/kg/24 hr ÷ Q6–8 hr

   Adult:

     IM or IV: 2–10 mg/dose Q3–4 hr PRN

     PO: 2–10 mg/dose Q6–12 hr PRN

Status epilepticus:

   Neonate: 0.3–0.75 mg/kg/dose IV Q15–30 min × 2–3 doses; max. total dose: 2 mg.

   Child >1 mo: 0.2–0.5 mg/kg/dose IV Q15–30 min; max. total dose: <5 yr: 5 mg; ≥5 yr: 10 mg. May repeat dosing in 2–4 hr, as needed.

   Adult: 5–10 mg/dose IV Q10–15 min; max. total dose: 30 mg in an 8-hr period. May repeat dosing in 2–4 hr, as needed.

   Rectal dose (using IV dosage form): 0.5 mg/kg/dose followed by 0.25 mg/kg/dose in 10 min PRN; max. dose: 20 mg/dose.

   Rectal gel: all doses rounded to the nearest available dosage strength; repeat dose in 4–12 hr PRN. Do not use >5 times per month or more than once every 5 days.

     2–5 yr: 0.5 mg/kg/dose

     6–11 yr: 0.3 mg/kg/dose

     ≥12 yr: and adult: 0.2 mg/kg/dose

       Max. dose (all ages): 20 mg/dose

Contraindicated in myasthenia gravis, severe respiratory insufficiency, severe hepatic failure, and sleep apnea syndrome. Hypotension and respiratory depression may occur. **Use with caution** in hepatic and renal dysfunction, glaucoma, shock, and depression. **Do not** use in combination with protease inhibitors. Concurrent use with CNS depressants, cimetidine, erythromycin, itraconazole, and valproic acid may enhance the effects of diazepam. Diazepam is a substrate for CYP450 2B6, 2C8, 2C9, and 3A5–7 and is a minor substrate and inhibitor for CYP450 2C19 and 3A3/4. The active desmethyldiazepam metabolite is a CYP450 2C19 substrate.

Administer the conventional IV product undiluted no faster than 2 mg/min. **Do not** mix with IV fluids. In status epilepticus, diazepam must be followed by long-acting anticonvulsants. Onset of anticonvulsant effect: 1–3 min with IV route; 2–10 min with rectal route. **For management of status epilepticus, see Chapter 1.**

DIAZOXIDE
Proglycem
Antihypoglycemic agent, antihypertensive agent

No Yes ? C

Oral suspension: 50 mg/mL (30 mL); contains 7.25% alcohol

Hyperinsulinemic hypoglycemia (because of insulin-producing tumors; start at the lowest dose):
  Newborn and infant: 8–15 mg/kg/24 hr ÷ Q8–12 hr PO; usual range: 5–20 mg/kg/24 hr ÷ Q8 hr
  Child and adult: 3–8 mg/kg/24 hr ÷ Q8–12 hr PO

Hypoglycemia should be treated initially with IV glucose; diazoxide should be introduced only if refractory to glucose infusion. Should **not** be used in patients who are hypersensitive to thiazides unless benefit outweighs risk. Thiazides may enhance diazoxide's hyperglycemic effects. **Use with caution** in renal impairment (clearance of drug is reduced); consider dosage reduction.

Sodium and fluid retention is common in young infants and adults and may precipitate CHF in patients with compromised cardiac reserve (usually responsive to diuretics). Hirsutism (reversible), GI disturbances, transient loss of taste, tachycardia, ketoacidosis, palpitations, rash, headache, weakness, and hyperuricemia may occur. Pulmonary hypertension in newborns/infant treated for hypoglycemia has been reported as resolution/improvement of the condition was achieved after discontinuing diazoxide. Monitor BP closely for hypotension.

Hyperglycemic effect with PO administration occurs within 1 hr, with a duration of 8 hr.

DICLOXACILLIN SODIUM
Various generics; previously available as Dycill and Pathocil
Antibiotic, penicillin (penicillinase resistant)

No No 1 B

Caps: 250, 500 mg; contains 0.6 mEq Na/250 mg

Child (<40 kg) (see remarks):
  Mild/moderate infections: 25–50 mg/kg/24 hr PO ÷ Q6 hr
  Severe infections: 50–100 mg/kg/24 hr PO ÷ Q6 hr
  Max. dose: 2 g/24 hr
Child (≥40 kg) and adult: 125–500 mg/dose PO Q6 hr; **max. dose:** 2 g/24 hr

Contraindicated in patients with a history of penicillin allergy. **Use with caution** in cephalosporin hypersensitivity. May cause nausea, vomiting, and diarrhea. Immune hypersensitivity has been reported.

Limited experience in neonates and very young infants. Higher doses (50–100 mg/kg/24 hr) are indicated following IV therapy for osteomyelitis.

May decrease the effects of oral contraceptives and warfarin. Administer 1 hr before meals or 2 hr after meals.

DIGOXIN
Lanoxin, Lanoxin Pediatric, and generics
Antiarrhythmic agent, inotrope

No Yes 2 C

Tabs: 125, 250 mcg
Oral solution: 50 mcg/mL (60 mL); may contain 10% alcohol

Continued

DIGOXIN continued

Injection:
Lanoxin Pediatric: 100 mcg/mL (1 mL); may contain propylene glycol and alcohol
Lanoxin and generics: 250 mcg/mL (2 mL); may contain propylene glycol and alcohol

Digitalizing: Total digitalizing dose (TDD) and maintenance doses in mcg/kg/24 hr (see the table that follows):

DIGOXIN DIGITALIZING AND MAINTENANCE DOSES

Age	TDD		Daily Maintenance	
	PO	IV/IM	PO	IV/IM
Premature neonate	20	15	5	3–4
Full-term neonate	30	20	8–10	6–8
1 mo–<2 yr	40–50	30–40	10–12	7.5–9
2–10 yr	30–40	20–30	8–10	6–8
>10 yr and <100 kg	10–15	8–12	2.5–5	2–3

Initial: 1/2 TDD, then 1/4 TDD Q8–18 hr × 2 doses; obtain electrocardiogram (ECG) 6 hr after dose to assess for toxicity

Maintenance:
<10 yr: Give maintenance dose ÷ BID
≥10 yr: Give maintenance dose once daily

Contraindicated in patients with ventricular dysrhythmias. Use should be **avoided** in patients with preserved left ventricular systolic function. **Use with caution** in renal failure, calcium channel blockers (may result in heart block), and adenosine [enhanced depressant effects on sinoatrial (SA) and atrioventricular (AV) nodes]. May cause AV block or dysrhythmias. In patients treated with digoxin, cardioversion or calcium infusion may lead to ventricular fibrillation (pretreatment with lidocaine may prevent this). Patients with beriberi heart disease may not respond to digoxin if underlying thiamine deficiency is not treated concomitantly. Decreased serum potassium and magnesium or increased magnesium and calcium may increase risk for digoxin toxicity. For signs and symptoms of toxicity, see Chapter 2.

Excreted via the kidney; **adjust dose in renal failure (see Chapter 30).** Therapeutic concentration: 0.8–2 ng/mL. Higher doses may be required for supraventricular tachycardia. Neonates, pregnant women, and patients with renal, hepatic, or heart failure may have falsely elevated digoxin levels because of the presence of digoxin-like substances.

Digoxin is a CYP450 3A4 and P-glycoprotein substrate. Calcium channel blockers, captopril, carvedilol, amiodarone, quinidine, cyclosporine, itraconazole, tetracycline, and macrolide antibiotics may increase digoxin levels. Use with β-blockers may increase risk for bradycardia. Succinylcholine may cause arrhythmias in digitalized patients.

$T_{1/2}$: Premature infants, 61–170 hr; full-term neonates, 35–45 hr; infants, 18–25 hr; and children, 35 hr.

Recommended serum sampling at steady state: Obtain a single level from 6 hr postdose to just before the next scheduled dose following 5–8 days of continuous dosing. Levels obtained prior to steady state may be useful in preventing toxicity.

DIGOXIN IMMUNE FAB (OVINE)
DigiFab
Antidigoxin antibody

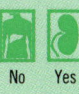

No Yes ? C

Injection: 40 mg

Dosing based on known amounts of digoxin acutely ingested:
 First determine total body digoxin load (TBL):
  TBL (mg) = mg digoxin ingested × 0.8
 Then, calculate digoxin immune Fab dose:
  Dose in number of digoxin immune Fab vials (DigiFab):
 vials = TBL ÷ 0.5

Dosing based on steady-state serum digoxin levels:

DigiFab Dose (mg) from Steady-State Digoxin Levels

Patient Weight (kg)	Serum Digoxin Concentration (ng/mL)						
	1	2	4	8	12	16	20
1	0.4 mg*	1 mg*	1.5 mg*	3 mg*	5 mg	6.5 mg	8 mg
3	1 mg*	2.5 mg*	5 mg	10 mg	14 mg	19 mg	24 mg
5	2 mg*	4 mg	8 mg	16 mg	24 mg	32 mg	40 mg
10	4 mg	8 mg	16 mg	32 mg	48 mg	64 mg	80 mg
20	8 mg	16 mg	32 mg	64 mg	96 mg	128 mg	160 mg
40	20 mg	40 mg	80 mg	120 mg	200 mg	280 mg	320 mg
60	20 mg	40 mg	120 mg	200 mg	280 mg	400 mg	480 mg
70	40 mg	80 mg	120 mg	240 mg	360 mg	440 mg	560 mg
80	40 mg	80 mg	120 mg	280 mg	400 mg	520 mg	640 mg
100	40 mg	80 mg	160 mg	320 mg	480 mg	640 mg	800 mg

*Use 1 mg/mL DigiFab concentration for dose accuracy

Dosage Administration:
Reconstitute each vial with 4 mL NS for a 10 mg/mL concentration and infuse IV dose over 30 min. If an infusion rate reaction occurs, stop infusion and restart at a slower rate. In situations of cardiac arrest, DigiFab can be administered as a bolus injection but has an increased risk for infusion-related reactions. For smaller doses, vials may be reconstituted with 36 mL NS for a 1 mg/mL concentration.

Contraindicated if hypersensitive to sheep products. **Use with caution** in renal or cardiac failure. May cause rapidly developing severe hypokalemia, decreased cardiac output (from withdrawal of digoxin's inotropic effects), rash, edema, and phlebitis. Digoxin therapy may be reinstituted in 3–7 days when toxicity has been corrected. Digoxin immune FAB will interfere with digitalis immunoassay measurements to result in misleading concentrations.

DILTIAZEM
Cardizem, Cardizem CD, Cardizem LA, Cartia XT, Matzim LA, Taztia XT, Tiazac, and many others, including generics
Calcium channel blocker, antihypertensive

Yes Yes 1 C

Tabs: 30, 60, 90, 120 mg
Extended-release tabs (for Q24 hr dosing):
 Various generics: 180, 240, 300, 360, 420 mg
 Cardizem LA: 120, 180, 240, 300, 360, 420 mg
 Matzim LA: 180, 240, 300, 360, 420 mg

Continued

DILTIAZEM continued

Extended-release caps (for Q12 hr dosing): 60, 90, 120 mg
Extended-release caps (for Q24 hr dosing):
  Various generics: 120, 180, 240, 300, 360, 420 mg
  Cardizem CD, Taztia XT: 120, 180, 240, 300, 360 mg
  Cartia XT: 120, 180, 240, 300 mg
  Tiazac: 120, 180, 240, 300, 360, 420 mg
Oral liquid: 12 mg/mL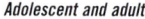
Injection: 5 mg/mL (5, 10, 25 mL)

Child: 1.5–2 mg/kg/24 hr PO ÷ TID-QID; max. dose: 3.5 mg/kg/24 hr, alternative max. dose of 6 mg/kg/24 hr up to 360 mg/24 hr have been recommended.
Adolescent and adult:
  Immediate release: 30–120 mg/dose PO TID-QID; usual range 180–360 mg/24 hr.
  Extended release: 120–360 mg/24 hr PO ÷ once daily–BID (BID dosing with Q12 hr extended-release generic capsule; once-daily dosing with extended-release tabs, Cardizem CD, Cartia XT, Cardizem LA, Matzim LA, Taztia XT, Tiazac and Q24 hr generic extended-release capsule or tab); max. dose: 540 mg/24 hr.

Contraindicated in acute MI with pulmonary congestion, second- or third-degree heart block, and sick sinus syndrome. **Use with caution** in congestive heart failure (CHF) or renal and hepatic impairment. Dizziness, headache, edema, nausea, vomiting, heart block, and arrhythmias may occur. Acute hepatic injury and severe skin reactions have been reported. Monitor heart rate with concurrent clonidine use (sinus bradycardia has been reported).

Diltiazem is a substrate and inhibitor of the CYP450 3A4 enzyme system. May increase levels and effects/toxicity of buspirone, cyclosporine, carbamazepine, fentanyl, digoxin, quinidine, tacrolimus, benzodiazepines, and β-blockers. Cimetidine and statins may increase serum diltiazem levels. Rifampin may decrease serum diltiazem levels.

Maximal antihypertensive effect seen within 2 wk. Extended-release dosage forms should be swallowed whole and NOT crushed or chewed. Cardizem immediate-release tablets should be swallowed whole because crushing or chewing may alter its pharmacokinetics.

DIMENHYDRINATE
Dramamine, Driminate, and generics
Antiemetic, antihistamine

No   No   3   B

Tabs [OTC]: 50 mg
Chewable tabs [OTC]: 50 mg; contains 1.5 mg phenylalanine
Injection: 50 mg/mL; contains benzyl alcohol and propylene glycol

Child (<12 yr): 5 mg/kg/24 hr ÷ Q6 hr PO/IM/IV; alternative oral dosing by age:
  2–5 yr: 12.5–25 mg/dose Q6–8 hr PRN PO with the max. dosage in the subsequent list
  6–12 yr: 25–50 mg/dose Q6–8 hr PRN PO with the max. dosage in the subsequent list
≥12 yr and adult: 50–100 mg/dose Q4–6 hr PRN PO/IM/IV
MAXIMUM PO DOSE:
  2–5 yr: 75 mg/24 hr
  6–12 yr: 150 mg/24 hr
  ≥12 yr and adult: 400 mg/24 hr
MAXIMUM IM DOSE:
  Child: 300 mg/24 hr

DIMENHYDRINATE continued

Causes drowsiness and anticholinergic side effects. May mask vestibular symptoms and cause CNS excitation in young children. **Caution** when taken with ototoxic agents or history of seizures. **Use should be limited to management of prolonged vomiting of known etiology. Not recommended** in children aged <2 yr. Toxicity resembles anticholinergic poisoning.

DIMERCAPROL
Bal in Oil, BAL (British Anti-Lewisite), and generics
Heavy metal chelator (arsenic, gold, mercury, lead)

Yes Yes ? C

Injection (in oil): 100 mg/mL (3 mL); contains 20% benzyl benzoate and peanut oil

Give all injections deep IM.
Lead poisoning:
  Acute severe encephalopathy (lead level > 70 mcg/dL): 4 mg/kg/dose Q4 hr × 2–7 days with the addition of Ca-EDTA (given at a separate site) at the time of the second dose.
  Less severe poisoning: 4 mg/kg × 1, then 3 mg/kg/dose Q4 hr × 2–7 days.
Arsenic or gold poisoning (see table as follows):

	Mild Cases	Severe Cases
Days 1 and 2	2.5 mg/kg/dose Q6 hr	3 mg/kg/dose Q4 hr
Day 3	2.5 mg/kg/dose Q12 hr	3 mg/kg/dose Q6 hr
Days 4–13	2.5 mg/kg/dose Q24 hr	3 mg/kg/dose Q12 hr

Mercury poisoning: 5 mg/kg × 1, then 2.5 mg/kg/dose once daily–BID × 10 days

Contraindicated in hepatic or renal insufficiency. May cause hypertension, tachycardia, GI disturbance, headache, fever (30% of children), nephrotoxicity, and transient neutropenia. Symptoms are usually relieved by antihistamines. Urine should be kept alkaline to protect the kidneys. **Use with caution** with G6PD deficiency and peanut-sensitive patients. **Do not** use concomitantly with iron.

DIPHENHYDRAMINE
Benadryl, many other brand names, and generics
Antihistamine

No Yes 3 B

Elixir [OTC]: 12.5 mg/5 mL; may contain 5.6% alcohol
Syrup [OTC]: 12.5 mg/5 mL; some may contain 5% alcohol
Oral liquid/solution [OTC]: 12.5 mg/5 mL
Caps/Tabs [OTC]: 25, 50 mg
Tabs, orally disintegrating [OTC]: 12.5 mg; contains aspartame, phenylalanine
Strips, orally disintegrating [OTC]: 12.5 mg; may contain <5% alcohol
Chewable tabs [OTC]: 12.5 mg; contains aspartame, phenylalanine
Injection: 50 mg/mL
Cream [OTC]: 1, 2% (30 g)
Topical gel [OTC]: 2% (118 mL); contains parabens
Topical solution [OTC]: 2% (60 mL); contains alcohol
Topical stick [OTC]: 2% (14 mL); contains alcohol

Continued

DIPHENHYDRAMINE continued

Severe allergic reaction (anaphylaxis) and dystonic reactions (including phenothiazine toxicity) (PO/IM/IV):
Child: 1–2 mg/kg/dose Q6 hr; usual dose: 5 mg/kg/24 hr ÷ Q6 hr. Max. dose: 50 mg/dose and 300 mg/24 hr.
Adult: 25–50 mg/dose Q4–8 hr; max. dose: 400 mg/24 hr
Sleep aid (PO/IM/IV): Administer dose 30 min before bedtime.
2–11 yr: 1 mg/kg/dose; max. dose: 50 mg/dose
≥12 yr: 50 mg
Topical (cream, gel, solution, stick):
≥2 yr–adult: Apply 1% or 2% to affected area no more than TID–QID.

Contraindicated with concurrent MAO inhibitor use, acute attacks of asthma, and GI or urinary obstruction. **Use with caution** in infants and young children, and **do not** use in neonates because of potential CNS effects. Side effects include sedation, nausea, vomiting, xerostoma, blurred vision, and other reactions common to antihistamines. CNS side effects more common than GI disturbances. May cause paradoxical excitement in children. **Adjust dose in renal failure (see Chapter 30).**
TOPICAL USE: side effects include rash, urticaria, and photosensitivity.

DIVALPROEX SODIUM
Depakote, Depakote ER, and generics
Anticonvulsant

Yes   No   2   D/X

Delayed-release tabs: 125, 250, 500 mg
Extended-release tabs (Depakote ER and generics): 250, 500 mg
Sprinkle caps: 125 mg

Dose: see Valproic Acid

See *Valproic Acid*. Preferred over valproic acid for patients on ketogenic diet. Depakote ER is prescribed by a once-daily interval, whereas Depakote is typically prescribed BID.
Depakote and Depakote ER are not bioequivalent; see package insert for dose conversion.
Efficacy was not established in separate randomized double-blinded, placebo-controlled trials for the treatment of pediatric bipolar disorder (age, 10–17 yr) and migraine prophylaxis (ages, 12–17 yr).
Pregnancy category is "X" when used for migraine prophylaxis and is a "D" for all other indications.

DOBUTAMINE
Various generics; previously available as Dobutrex
Sympathomimetic agent

No   No   ?   B

Injection: 12.5 mg/mL (20, 40 mL); contains sulfites
Prediluted injection in D₅W: 1 mg/mL (250 mL), 2 mg/mL (250 mL), 4 mg/mL (250 mL)

Continuous IV infusion (all ages): 2.5–15 mcg/kg/min;
  Max. dose: 40 mcg/kg/min
To prepare infusion: see IV infusions on page i.

DOBUTAMINE continued

Contraindicated in idiopathic hypertrophic subaortic stenosis (IHSS). Tachycardia, arrhythmias (PVCs), and hypertension may occasionally occur (especially at higher infusion rates). Correct hypovolemic states before use. Increases AV conduction, may precipitate ventricular ectopic activity.

Dobutamine has been shown to increase cardiac output and systemic pressure in pediatric patients of every age group. However, in premature neonates, dobutamine is less effective than dopamine in increasing raising systemic BP without causing undue tachycardia, and dobutamine has not been shown to provide any added benefit when given to such infants already receiving optimal infusions of dopamine.

Monitor BP and vital signs. $T_{1/2}$: 2 min. Peak effects in 10–20 min. Use with linezolid may potentially increase BP.

DOCUSATE
Colace, DocuSol Kids, DocuSol, Kao-Tin, Sur-Q-Lax, Enemeez Mini, and many other brands
Stool softener, laxative

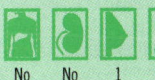

No No 1 C/?

Available as docusate sodium:
  Caps [OTC]: 50, 100, 250 mg; sodium content (50 mg cap: 3 mg; 100 mg cap: ~5 mg)
  Tabs [OTC]: 100 mg
  Syrup [OTC]: 20 mg/5 mL (473 mL); may contain alcohol
  Oral liquid [OTC]: 10 mg/mL (118, 473 mL); contains 1 mg/mL sodium
  Rectal enema:
    DocuSol Kids [OTC]: 100 mg/5 mL (5 mL); contains polyethylene glycol
    Enemeez Mini, and DocuSol [OTC]: 283 mg/5 mL (5 mL); DocuSol Plus product contains benzocaine
Available as docusate calcium:
  Caps [Kao-Tin, Sur-Q-Lax; OTC]: 240 mg

PO (take with liquids; see remarks):
  <3 yr: 10–40 mg/24 hr ÷ once daily–QID
  3–6 yr: 20–60 mg/24 hr ÷ once daily–QID
  6–12 yr: 40–150 mg/24 hr ÷ once daily–QID
  >12 yr and adult: 50–400 mg/24 hr ÷ once daily–QID
Rectal (see remarks):
  2–<12 yr: 100 mg/5 mL or 283 mg/5 mL PR once daily
  ≥12 yr and adult: 283 mg/5 mL PR once daily–TID. Alternatively, 50–100 mg of oral liquid (not syrup) mixed in enema fluid (saline or oil retention enemas) may be used.

Oral dosage effective only after 1–3 days of therapy, whereas the enema has an onset of action in 2–15 min. Reassess therapy if no response seen after 7 days of continuous use.
Incidence of side effects is exceedingly low. Rash, nausea, and throat irritation have been reported. Oral liquid is bitter; give with milk, fruit juice, or formula to mask the taste.
A few drops of the 10 mg/mL oral liquid may be used in the ear as a cerumenolytic. Effect is usually seen within 15 min.
Pregnancy category has not been formally assigned by the FDA but is considered a "C."

DOLASETRON
Anzemet
Antiemetic agent, 5-HT₃ antagonist

No   Yes   ?   B

Injection: 20 mg/mL (0.625, 5, 25 mL)
Tabs: 50, 100 mg
Oral suspension: 10 mg/mL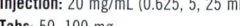

Chemotherapy-induced nausea and vomiting prevention:
2 yr–adult: 1.8 mg/kg/dose PO up to a max. dose of 100 mg. Administer PO dose 60 min prior to chemotherapy. IV route of administration is considered contraindicated for this indication because of increased risk for QTc prolongation.

Postoperative nausea and vomiting prevention: Administer IV doses 15 min prior to cessation of anesthesia and PO doses 2 hr prior to surgery.
2–16 yr:
  IV: 0.35 mg/kg/dose (max. dose: 12.5 mg) × 1
  PO: 1.2 mg/kg/dose × 1 (max. dose: 100 mg) × 1
Adult:
  IV: 12.5 mg/dose ×1

Postoperative nausea and vomiting treatment: Administer IV at onset of nausea and vomiting.
2–16 yr: 0.35 mg/kg/dose (max. dose: 12.5 mg) IV
>16 yr–adult: 12.5 mg/dose IV

May cause hypotension and prolongation of cardiac conduction intervals, particularly QTc interval (dose dependent effect). Common side effects include dizziness, headache, sedation, blurred vision, fever, chills, and sleep disorders. Rare cases of sustained supraventricular and ventricular arrhythmias, fatal cardiac arrest, and MI have been reported in children and adolescents.

Avoid use in patients with congenital long QTc syndrome, hypomagnesemia, hypokalemia, or with concurrent use with other drugs that increase QTc interval (e.g., erythromycin, cisapride). Drug's active metabolite (hydrodolasetron) is a substrate for CYP450 2D6 and 3A3/4 isoenzymes; concomitant use of enzyme inhibitors (e.g., cimetidine) may increase risk for side effects and use of enzyme inducers (e.g., rifampin) may decrease dolasetron's efficacy. Serotonin syndrome has been associated with concurrent use of selective serotonin reuptake inhibitors (SSRIs; e.g., fluoxetine, sertraline), serotonin and norepinephrine reuptake inhibitors (SNRIs; e.g., duloxetine, venlafaxine), MAO inhibitors, mirtazapine, fentanyl, lithium, tramadol, and IV methylene blue.

Although no dosage adjustments are necessary, hydrodolasetron's clearance decreases by 42% with severe hepatic impairment and 44% with severe renal impairment.

ECG monitoring is recommended in patients with electrolyte abnormalities, CHF, bradyarrhythmias, or renal impairment.

IV doses may be administered undiluted over 30 sec.

DOPAMINE
Various generics; previously available as Intropin
Sympathomimetic agent

No   No   ?   C

Injection: 40 mg/mL (5, 10 mL), 80 mg/mL (5 mL), 160 mg/mL (5 mL)
Prediluted injection in D₅W: 0.8, 1.6, 3.2 mg/mL (250, 500 mL)

DOPAMINE continued

All ages:
Low dose: 2–5 mcg/kg/min IV; increases renal blood flow; minimal effect on heart rate and cardiac output
Intermediate dose: 5–15 mcg/kg/min IV; increases heart rate, cardiac contractility, cardiac output, and to a lesser extent, renal blood flow.
High dose: >20 mcg/kg/min IV; α-adrenergic effects are prominent; decreases renal perfusion.
Max. dose recommended: 20–50 mcg/kg/min IV
To prepare infusion: see IV infusions on page i.

Do not use in pheochromocytoma, tachyarrhythmia, or hypovolemia. Monitor vital signs and BP continuously. Correct hypovolemic states. Tachyarrhythmias, ectopic beats, hypertension, vasoconstriction, and vomiting may occur. **Use with caution** with phenytoin because hypotension and bradycardia may be exacerbated. Use with linezolid potentially increases BP.
Newborn infants may be more sensitive to vasoconstrictive effects of dopamine. Children aged <2 yr clear dopamine faster and exhibit high variability in neonates.
Should be administered through a central line or large vein. Extravasation may cause tissue necrosis; treat with phentolamine. **Do not** administer into an umbilical arterial catheter.

DORNASE ALFA/DNASE
Pulmozyme
Inhaled mucolytic

No / No / ? / B

Inhalation solution: 1 mg/mL (2.5 mL)

Cystic fibrosis:
Child aged >5 yr and adult: 2.5 mg via nebulizer once daily. Some patients may benefit from 2.5 mg BID.

Contraindicated in patients with hypersensitivity to epoetin alfa. Voice alteration, pharyngitis, laryngitis may result. These are generally reversible without dose adjustment. Safety and efficacy has not been demonstrated in patients >1 yr of continuous use.
Do not mix with other nebulized drugs. A β-agonist may be useful before administration to enhance drug distribution. Chest physiotherapy should be incorporated into treatment regimen. The following nebulizer compressor systems have been recommended for use: Pulmo-Aide, Pari-Proneb, Mobilaire, Porta-Neb, or PariBaby. Use of the "Sidestream" nebulizer cup can significantly reduce the medication administration time.

DOXAPRAM HCL
Dopram and generics
CNS stimulant

No / No / ? / B

Injection: 20 mg/mL (20 mL); may contain 0.9% benzyl alcohol

Methylxanthine-refractory neonatal apnea (see remarks): Load with 2.5–3 mg/kg IV over 15 min, followed by a continuous IV infusion of 1 mg/kg/hr titrated to the lowest effective dose; **max. dose**: 2.5 mg/kg/hr

Contraindicated in seizures, proven or suspected pulmonary embolism, head injuries, cerebral vascular accident, cerebral edema, cardiovascular or coronary artery disease, severe hypertension, pheochromocytoma, hyperthyroidism, and in patients with mechanical

Continued

DOXAPRAM HCL continued

disorders of ventilation. **Do not** use with general anesthetic agents that can sensitize the heart to catecholamines (e.g., halothane, cyclopropane, and enflurane) to reduce the risk for cardiac arrhythmias, including ventricular tachycardia and ventricular fibrillation. **Do not** initiate doxapram until the general anesthetic agent has been completely excreted.

Hypertension occurs with higher doses (>1.5 mg/kg/hr). May also cause tachycardia, arrhythmia, seizure, hyperreflexia, hyperpyrexia, abdominal distension, bloody stools, and sweating. **Avoid** extravasation into tissues.

DOXYCYCLINE
Adoxa, Vibramycin, Doryx, Monodox, Oracea, many others, and generics
Antibiotic, tetracycline derivative

Yes   Yes   2   D

Caps: 50, 75, 100, 150 mg
Tabs: 20, 50, 75, 100, 150 mg
Delayed-release caps (Oracea and generics): 40 mg
Delayed-release tabs (Doryx and generics): 50, 75, 100, 150, 200 mg
Syrup: 50 mg/5 mL (473 mL); contains parabens
Oral suspension: 25 mg/5 mL (60 mL)
Injection: 100 mg

Initial:
  ≤45 kg: 2.2 mg/kg/dose BID PO/IV × 1 day to max. dose: of 200 mg/24 hr
  >45 kg: 100 mg/dose BID PO/IV × 1 day
Maintenance:
  ≤45 kg: 2.2–4.4 mg/kg/24 hr once daily–BID PO/IV
  >45 kg: 100–200 mg/24 hr ÷ once daily–BID PO/IV
  Max. dose: 200 mg/24 hr
PID:
  Inpatient: 100 mg Q12 hr with cefotetan or cefoxitin or ampicillin/sulbactam. Convert to oral therapy 24 hr after patient improves on IV to complete a 14-day total course (IV and PO).
  Outpatient: 100 mg PO Q12 hr × 14 days with ceftriaxone, cefoxitin + probenecid, or other parenteral third–generation cephalosporin with or without metronidazole
Anthrax (inhalation/systemic/cutaneous; see remarks): Initiate therapy with IV route and convert to PO route when clinically appropriate. Duration of therapy is 60 days (IV and PO combined):
  ≤8 yr or ≤45 kg: 2.2 mg/kg/dose BID IV/PO; max. dose: 200 mg/24 hr
  >8 yr and >45 kg: 100 mg/dose BID IV/PO
Malaria prophylaxis (start 1–2 days prior to exposure and continue for 4 wk after leaving endemic area):
  >8 yr: 2.2 mg/kg/24 hr PO once daily; max. dose: 100 mg/24 hr; and max. duration of 4 mo.
  Adult: 100 mg PO once daily
Periodontitis:
  Adult: 20 mg BID PO × ≤9 mo

Use with caution in hepatic and renal disease. Generally **not recommended** for use in children aged <8 yr because of risk for tooth enamel hypoplasia and discoloration. However, the AAP Redbook recommends doxycycline as the drug of choice for rickettsial disease regardless of age. May cause GI symptoms, photosensitivity, hemolytic anemia, rash, and hypersensitivity reactions. Increased intracranial pressure (pseudotumor cerebri), toxic epidermal necrolysis (TEN), drug rash with eosinophilia and systemic symptom (DRESS), erythema multiforme, and Stevens-Johnson syndrome have been reported.

DOXYCYCLINE continued

Doxycycline is approved for the treatment of anthrax *(Bacillus anthracis)* in combination with one or two other antimicrobials. If meningitis is suspected, consider using an alternative agent because of poor CNS penetration. Consider changing to high-dose amoxicillin (25–35 mg/kg/dose TID PO) for penicillin-susceptible strains. See www.bt.cdc.gov for the latest information.

Rifampin, barbiturates, phenytoin, and carbamazepine may increase clearance of doxycycline. Doxycycline may enhance the hypoprothrombinemic effect of warfarin. See *Tetracycline* for additional drug/food interactions and remarks.

Infuse IV over 1–4 hr. **Avoid** prolonged exposure to direct sunlight.

For periodontitis, take tablets ≥1 hr prior or 2 hr after meals.

DRONABINOL
Marinol, Tetrahydrocannabinol, THC, and generics
Antiemetic

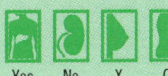
Yes   No   X   C

Caps: 2.5, 5, 10 mg; may contain sesame oil

Antiemetic:
  Child & adult (PO): 5 mg/m^2/dose 1–3 hr prior to chemotherapy, then Q2–4 hr up to a max. dose of 6 doses/24 hr; doses may be gradually increased by 2.5 mg/m^2/dose increments up to a max. dose of 15 mg/m^2/dose if needed and tolerated.

Appetite stimulant:
  Adult (PO): 2.5 mg BID 1 hr before lunch and dinner; if not tolerated, reduce dose to 2.5 mg QHS.
  Max. dose: 20 mg/24 hr (use caution when increasing doses because of increased risk for dose-related adverse reactions at higher dosages)

Contraindicated in patients with history of substance abuse and mental illness, and allergy to sesame oil. **Use with caution** in heart disease, seizures, and hepatic disease (reduce dose if severe). Side effects: euphoria, dizziness, difficulty concentrating, anxiety, mood change, sedation, hallucinations, ataxia, paresthesia, hypotension, excessively increased appetite, and habit-forming potential.

Onset of action: 0.5–1 hr; duration of psychoactive effects 4–6 hr, appetite stimulation 24 hr.

DROPERIDOL
Inapsine and generics
Sedative, antiemetic

Yes   Yes   3   C

Injection: 2.5 mg/mL (2 mL)

Antiemetic/sedation:
  Child: 0.03–0.07 mg/kg/dose IM or IV over 2–5 min; if needed, may give 0.1–0.15 mg/kg/dose; initial max. dose: 0.1 mg/kg/dose and subsequent max. dose: 2.5 mg/dose.
    Dosage interval:
      Antiemetic: PRN Q4–6 hr
      Sedation: Repeat dose in 15–30 min, if necessary
  Adult: 2.5–5 mg IM or IV over 2–5 min; initial max. dose is 2.5 mg.
    Dosage interval:
      Antiemetic: PRN Q3–4 hr
      Sedation: Repeat dose in 15–30 min if necessary.

Continued

DROPERIDOL continued

Use with caution in renal and hepatic impairment; 75% of metabolites are excreted renally, and drug is extensively metabolized in the liver. Side effects include hypotension, tachycardia, extrapyramidal side effects such as dystonia, feeling of motor restlessness, laryngospasm, and bronchospasm. May lower seizure threshold. **Fatal arrhythmias and QT interval prolongation has been associated with use.**

Onset in 3–10 min. Peak effects within 10–30 min. Duration of 2–4 hr. Often given as adjunct to other agents.

EDETATE (EDTA) CALCIUM DISODIUM
Calcium disodium versenate and generics
Chelating agent, antidote for lead toxicity

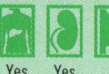
Yes Yes 3 B

Injection: 200 mg/mL (5 mL)

Lead poisoning:
  Lead level > 70 mcg/dL (use with dimercaprol): Initiate at the time of the 2nd dimercaprol dose and treat for 3–5 days. May repeat a course as needed after 2–4 days of no EDTA.
    IM: 1000–1500 mg/m^2/24 hr ÷ Q4 hr.
    IV: 1000–1500 mg/m^2/24 hr as an 8–24 hour infusion or divided Q12 hr.
    Use 1500 mg/m^2/24 hr for 5 days in the presence of encephalopathy.
  Lead level 20–70 mcg/dL: 1000 mg/m^2/24 hr IV as an 8–24 hr infusion OR intermittent dosing divided Q12 hr × 5 days. May repeat course as needed after 2–4 days of no EDTA.
  Max. daily dose: 75 mg/kg/24 hr.

Edetate (EDTA) calcium disodium is not interchangeable with edetate disodium (Na$_2$EDTA); erroneous substitutions have led to fatalities. Prescribe this product by its full name and **avoid** the EDTA abbreviation to prevent dispensing errors.

May cause renal tubular necrosis. **Do not use** in the presence of anuria, hepatitis, and active renal disease. Dosage reduction is recommended with mild renal disease. Follow urinalysis and renal function. Monitor ECG continuously for arrhythmia when giving IV. Rapid IV infusion may cause sudden increase in intracranial pressure in patients with cerebral edema. May cause zinc and copper deficiency. Monitor Ca^{2+} and PO$_4$.

IM route preferred. Give IM with 0.5% procaine.

EDROPHONIUM CHLORIDE
Enlon
Anticholinesterase agent, antidote for neuromuscular blockade

No Yes ? ?

Injection: 10 mg/mL (15 mL) (contains 0.45% phenol and 0.2% sulfite)

Diagnosis for myasthenia gravis (IV; see remarks):
  Neonate: 0.1 mg single dose
  Infant and child:
    Initial: 0.04 mg/kg/dose × 1
    Max. dose: 1 mg for <34 kg, 2 mg for ≥34 kg
    If no response after 1 min, may give 0.16 mg/kg/dose for a total of 0.2 mg/kg
    Total **max. dose:** 5 mg for <34 kg, 10 mg for ≥34 kg
  Adult: 2-mg test dose IV; if no reaction, give 8 mg after 45 sec

EDROPHONIUM CHLORIDE continued

May precipitate cholinergic crisis, arrhythmias, and bronchospasm. Keep atropine available in a syringe and have resuscitation equipment ready. Hypersensitivity to test dose (fasciculations or intestinal cramping) is an indication to stop giving drug. Contraindicated in GI or GU obstruction or arrhythmias. Dose may need to be reduced in chronic renal failure.

Reported doses for reversing neuromuscular blockade in children have ranged from 0.1–1.43 mg/kg/dose. Antagonism of nondepolarizing neuromuscular blocking drugs is more rapid in children than in adults.

Short duration of action with IV route (5–10 min). Antidote: atropine 0.01–0.04 mg/kg/dose. Pregnancy category has not been established.

EMLA

See Lidocaine and Prilocaine

ENALAPRIL MALEATE (PO), ENALAPRILAT (IV)
Enalapril: Vasotec, Epaned, and generics
Enalaprilat: generics; previously available as Vasotec IV
Angiotensin converting enzyme inhibitor, antihypertensive

No   Yes   2   D

Enalapril:
Tabs: 2.5, 5, 10, 20 mg (scored)
Oral solution (Epaned): 1 mg/mL (150 mL); contains parabens and saccharin
Oral suspension: 0.1, 1 mg/mL

Enalaprilat:
Injection: 1.25 mg/mL (1, 2 mL); contains benzyl alcohol

Hypertension:
Infant and child:
PO: 0.08 mg/kg/24 hr up to 5 mg/24 hr once daily; increase PRN over 2 wk
Max. dose (higher doses have not been evaluated): 0.58 mg/kg/24 hr up to 40 mg/24 hr
IV: 0.005–0.01 mg/kg/dose Q8–24 hr; **max. dose:** 1.25 mg/dose
Adolescent and adult:
PO: 2.5–5 mg/24 hr once daily initially to **max. dose** of 40 mg/24 hr ÷ once daily–BID
IV: 0.625–1.25 mg/dose IV Q6 hr; doses as high as 5 mg Q6 hr is reported to be tolerated for up to 36 hr

Use with caution in bilateral renal artery stenosis. **Avoid use** in dialysis with high-flux membranes because anaphylactoid reactions have been reported. Side effects: nausea, diarrhea, headache, dizziness, hyperkalemia, hypoglycemia, hypotension, and hypersensitivity. Cough is a reported side effect of ACE inhibitors.

Enalapril (PO) is converted to its active form (Enalaprilat) by the liver. Administer IV over 5 min. **Adjust dose in renal impairment (see Chapter 30).**

Nitritoid reactions have been observed in patients receiving concomitant IV gold therapy. Enalapril/enalaprilat should be discontinued as soon as possible when pregnancy is confirmed. If oliguria or hypotension occurs in a neonate with in utero exposure to enalapril/enalaprilat, exchange transfusions or dialysis may be needed to reverse hypotension and/or support renal function.

ENOXAPARIN
Lovenox and generics
Anticoagulant, low molecular weight heparin

Yes   Yes   1   B

Injection: 100 mg/mL (3 mL); contains 15 mg/mL benzyl alcohol
Injection (prefilled syringes with 27-gauge × ½-inch needle): 30 mg/0.3 mL, 40 mg/0.4 mL, 60 mg/0.6 mL, 80 mg/0.8 mL, 100 mg/1 mL, 120 mg/0.8 mL, 150 mg/1 mL; preservative free and may contain pork proteins
Approximate anti–factor Xa activity: 100 IU per 1 mg

Initial empiric dosage; patient specific dosage defined by therapeutic drug monitoring when indicated (see remarks).

DVT treatment:
<2 mo: 1.5 mg/kg/dose Q12 hr SC; higher doses of 1.7–2 mg/kg/dose Q12 hr SC have been recommended for neonates
≥2 mo–adult: 1 mg/kg/dose Q12 hr SC; alternatively, 1.5 mg/kg/dose Q24 hr SC can be used in adults

Dosage adjustment for DVT treatment to achieve target anti–factor Xa low-molecular-weight heparin (LMWH) levels of 0.5–1 units/mL (see the following table).

Anti–factor Xa Level LMWH (units/mL)	Hold Next Dose?	Dose Change	Repeat Anti–factor Xa Level LMWH?
<0.4	No	Increase by 25%	4 hr post next new AM dose
0.4	No	Increase by 10%	4 hr post next new AM dose
0.5	No	No	4 hr post next AM dose; if within therapeutic range recheck 1 wk later at 4 hr post dose
0.6–0.7	No	No	1 wk later at 4 hr post dose
0.8–1	No	No	4 hr post next AM dose; if within therapeutic range, recheck 1 wk later at 4 hr post dose
1.1–1.5	No	Decrease by 20%	4 hr post next new AM dose
1.6–2	3 hr	Decrease by 30%	Trough level (goal: <0.5) prior to next new dose and 4 hr post next new dose
>2	Until anti–factor Xa LMWH reaches 0.5 units/mL (levels can be measured Q12 hr until it reaches ≤0.5 units/mL).	When anti–factor Xa LMWH reaches 0.5 units/mL, dose may be restarted at a dose 40% less than originally prescribed.	4 hr post next new AM dose

DVT prophylaxis:
Infant < 2 mo: 0.75 mg/kg/dose Q12 hr SC.
Infant ≥ 2 mo–child 18 yr: 0.5 mg/kg/dose Q12 hr SC; **max. dose**: 30 mg/dose.

ENOXAPARIN continued

DVT prophylaxis:
  Patients with indwelling epidural catheters/neuraxial anesthesia (≥2 mo–child 18 yr): 1 mg/kg/dose Q24 hr SC; **max. dose**: 40 mg/dose. Twice daily dosing is **contraindicated** for these patients. See remarks.
  Adjust dosage for DVT prophylaxis to achieve target anti–factor Xa levels of 0.1–0.3 units/mL for all children.
  Adult:
    Knee or hip replacement surgery: 30 mg BID SC × 7–14 days; initiate therapy 12–24 hr after surgery provided hemostasis is established. Alternatively, for hip replacement surgery, 40 mg once daily SC × 7–14 days initially up to 3 wk thereafter; initiate therapy 9–15 hr prior to surgery.
    Abdominal surgery: 40 mg once daily SC × 7–12 days initiated 2 hr prior to surgery.
    Patients at risk due to severe restricted mobility during an acute illness: 40 mg once daily SC × 6–14 days.

Inhibits thrombosis by inactivating factor Xa without significantly affecting bleeding time, platelet function, PT, or aPTT at recommended doses. Dosages of enoxaparin, heparin, or other LMWHs **CANNOT** be used interchangeably on a unit-for-unit (or mg-for-mg) basis because of differences in pharmacokinetics and activity. Peak anti–factor Xa LMWH activity is achieved 4 hr after a dose. **Anti–factor Xa LMWH is NOT THE SAME as unfractionated heparin anti–Xa level (used for monitoring heparin therapy).**

Contraindicated in major bleeding and drug-induced thrombocytopenia. Use with caution in uncontrolled arterial hypertension, bleeding diathesis, history of recurrent GI ulcers, diabetic retinopathy, and severe renal dysfunction (reduce dose by increasing the dosage interval from Q12 hr to Q24 hr if GFR is <30 mL/min). Prophylactic use is not recommended in patients with prosthetic heart valves (especially in pregnant women) due to reports of fatalities in patients and fetuses. **Concurrent use with spinal or epidural anesthesia, or spinal puncture has resulted in long-term or permanent paralysis; potential benefits must be weighed against the risks.** May cause fever, confusion, edema, nausea, hemorrhage, thrombocytopenia, hypochromic anemia, and pain/erythema at injection site. Allergic reactions, headache, eosinophilia, alopecia, hepatocellular and cholestatic liver injury, and osteoporosis (long-term use) have been reported. **Protamine sulfate is the antidote;** 1 mg protamine sulfate neutralizes 1 mg enoxaparin.

DVT prophylaxis for patients with epidural catheters/neuraxial anesthesia: If placing needle, hold anticoagulation for 12 hr and restart dosing no sooner than 4 hr after needle insertion. If removing catheter, hold anticoagulation for 12 hr and restart dosing no sooner than 2 hr after catheter removal.

Recommended anti–factor Xa LMWH levels obtained 4 hr after subcutaneous dose after the third consecutive dose:
  DVT treatment: 0.5–1 units/mL
  DVT prophylaxis: 0.1–0.3 units/mL

Administer by deep SC injection by having the patient lie down. Alternate administration between the left and right anterolateral and left and right posterolateral abdominal wall. See package insert for detailed SC administration recommendations. To minimize bruising, do not rub the injection site. IV or IM route of administration is not recommended.

For additional information, see *Chest* 2008;133:887–968 and *Regional Anesthesia and Pain Medicine* 2003;28(3):172–197.

EPINEPHRINE HCL
Adrenalin, EpiPen, other brand names and generics
Sympathomimetic agent

No   No   2   C

Injection:
  1:1000 (aqueous): 1 mg/mL (1, 30 mL); may contain chlorobutanol and metabisulfite
  1:10,000 (aqueous): 0.1 mg/mL (10 mL prefilled syringes with either 18-G 3.5 inch or 21-G 1.5 inch needles or 10 mL vials)
Autoinjector:
  EpiPen and others: Delivers a single 0.3 mg (0.3 mL) dose (1 or 2 pack)
  EpiPen Jr and others: Delivers a single 0.15 mg (0.3 mL) dose (1 or 2 pack)
Some preparations may contain sulfites.

Cardiac uses:
  Neonate:
    Asystole and bradycardia: 0.01–0.03 mg/kg of 1:10,000 solution (0.1–0.3 mL/kg) IV/ET Q3–5 min PRN.
  Infant and child:
    Bradycardia/asystole and pulseless arrest: See page ii and PALS algorithms in the back of the book.
    Bradycardia, asystole, and pulseless arrest (see remarks):
      First dose: 0.01 mg/kg of 1:10,000 solution (0.1 mL/kg) IO/IV; **max. dose:** 1 mg (10 mL). Subsequent doses Q3–5 min PRN should be the same. High-dose epinephrine after the failure of standard dose has not been shown to be effective (see remarks). Must circulate drug with CPR. For ET route see below.
      All ET doses: 0.1 mg/kg of 1:1000 solution (0.1 mL/kg) ET Q3–5 min.
  Adult:
    Asystole: 1 mg IV or 2–2.5 mg ET Q3–5 min.
IV drip (all ages): 0.1–1 mcg/kg/min; titrate to effect; to prepare infusion, see inside front cover.
Respiratory uses:
  Bronchodilator:
    1:1000 (aqueous):
      Infant and child: 0.01 mL/kg/dose SC (**max. single dose** 0.5 mL); repeat Q15 min × 3–4 doses or Q4 hr PRN.
      Adult: 0.3–0.5 mg (0.3–0.5 mL)/dose SC Q20 min × 3 doses.
    Nebulization (alternative to racemic epinephrine): 0.5 mL/kg of 1:1000 solution diluted in 3 mL NS; **max. doses:** ≤4 yr: 2.5 mL/dose; >4 yr: 5 mL/dose.
Hypersensitivity reactions (see remarks for IV dosing):
  Child: 0.01 mg/kg/dose IM up to a **max. dose** of 0.5 mg/dose Q20 min–4 hr PRN. If using EpiPen or EpiPen Jr, administer the following dosage IM × 1 (an additional dose may be repeated in 5–15 min):
    <30 kg: 0.15 mg.
    ≥30 kg: 0.3 mg.
  Adult: Start with 0.1–0.5 mg IM/SC Q20 min–4 hr PRN; doses may be increased if necessary to a single **max. dose** of 1 mg. If using EpiPen, use 0.3 mg IM × 1; an additional dose may be repeated in 5–15 min.

High-dose rescue therapy for in-hospital cardiac arrest in children after the failure of an initial standard dose has been reported to be of no benefit compared to standard dose (*N Engl J Med* 2004;350:1722–1730).

EPINEPHRINE HCL continued

Hypersensitivity reactions: For bronchial asthma and certain allergic manifestations (e.g., angioedema, urticaria, serum sickness, anaphylactic shock) use epinephrine SC. Patients with anaphylaxis may benefit from IM administration. The adult IV dose for hypersensitivity reactions or to relieve bronchospasm usually ranges from 0.1 to 0.25 mg injected slowly over 5–10 min Q5–15 min as needed. Neonates may be given a dose of 0.01 mg/kg body weight; for infants, 0.05 mg is an adequate initial dose and this may be repeated at 20–30 min intervals in the management of asthma attacks.

May produce arrhythmias, tachycardia, hypertension, headaches, nervousness, nausea, and vomiting. Necrosis may occur at site of repeated local injection. Rare cases of serious skin and soft tissue infections, including necrotizing fasciitis and myonecrosis, have been reported with IM or deep SC injections.

Concomitant use of noncardiac selective β-blockers or tricyclic antidepressants may enhance epinephrine's pressor response. Chlorpromazine may reverse the pressor response.

ETT doses should be diluted with NS to a volume of 3–5 mL before administration. Follow with several positive pressure ventilations.

EpiPen and EpiPen Jr should be administered IM into the anterolateral aspect of the thigh. See EpiPen product information for proper use of the device and to prevent injury and/or inadvertent dose administration to the individual administering the dose. Accidental injection into the digits, hands, or feet may result in the loss of blood flow to the affected area. Do not inject into the buttock area.

EPINEPHRINE, RACEMIC
Asthmanefrin and S-2
Sympathomimetic agent

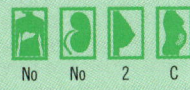
No   No   2   C

Solution for inhalation (OTC): 2.25% (1.25% epinephrine base) (0.5 mL)
Contains edetate disodium and may contain sulfites.

<4 yr:
Croup (using 2.25% solution): 0.05 mL/kg/dose up to a **max. dose** of 0.5 mL/dose diluted to 3 mL with NS. Given via nebulizer over 15 min PRN but **not** more frequently than Q1–2 hr.
≥4 yr: 0.5 mL/dose diluted to 3 mL with NS via a nebulizer over 15 min Q3–4 hr PRN.

Tachyarrhythmias, headache, nausea, and palpitations have been reported. Rebound symptoms may occur. Cardiorespiratory monitoring should be considered if administered more frequently than Q1–2 hr.

EPOETIN ALFA
Epogen, Procrit, and Erythropoietin
Recombinant human erythropoietin

No   No   2   C

Injection (single-dose, preservative-free vials): 2000, 3000, 4000, 10,000, 40,000 U/mL (1 mL).
Injection (multidose vials): 10,000 U/mL (2 mL), 20,000 U/mL (1 mL); contains 1% benzyl alcohol. All dosage forms contains 2.5 mg albumin per 1 mL.

Anemia in chronic renal failure (see remarks for dosage adjustment and withholding therapy): SC/IV (IV preferred for hemodialysis patients).
Initial dose:
Child and adolescent: Start at 50 U/kg/dose 3 times per week. Reported dosage range for children (3 mo–20 yr) not requiring dialysis, 50–250 U/kg/dose 3 times per week.

Continued

EPOETIN ALFA continued

Reported dosage range for children receiving hemodialysis, 50–450 U/kg/dose 2–3 times a week.

Adult: Start at 50–100 U/kg/dose 3 times per week.

Maintenance dose: Dose is individualized to achieve and maintain the lowest Hgb level sufficient to avoid transfusions and **not to exceed** 11 g/dL.

Anemia in cancer (use until chemotherapy is completed; see remarks for dosage reduction and withholding therapy):

Initial dose:

Child (5–18 yr): Start at 600 U/kg (**max. dose:** 40,000 U) IV once weekly.

Adult: Start at 150 U/kg/dose SC 3 times per week or 40,000 U SC once every week.

Increasing doses (if needed):

Three-times-a-week dosing regimen (adult): If no increase in Hgb > 1 g/dL and Hgb remains < 10 g/dL after initial 4 wk of therapy, increase dosage to 300 U/kg/dose 3 times per week.

Weekly dosing regimen: If no increase in Hgb > 1 g/dL and Hgb remains < 10 g/dL after initial 4 wk of therapy:

Child: increase dose to 900 U/kg/dose IV (**max. dose:** 60,000 U) once weekly.

Adult: 60,000 U SC once weekly.

For all ages, discontinue use after 8 wk of therapy if transfusions are still required or no hemoglobin response is observed.

AZT-treated HIV patients (Hgb should not exceed 12 g/dL): SC/IV.

Child: Reported dosage range in children (8 mo–17 yr), 50–400 U/kg/dose 2–3 times per wk.

Adult (with serum erythropoietin ≤ 500 milliunits/mL and receiving ≤ 4200 mg AZT per week): Start at 100 U/kg/dose 3 times per wk × 8 wk. If response is NOT satisfactory in reducing transfusion requirements or increasing Hgb levels after 8 wk of therapy, dose may be increased by 50–100 U/kg/dose given 3 times per wk and reevaluate every 4–8 wk thereafter. Patients are unlikely to respond to doses > 300 U/kg/dose 3 times a week.

For all ages, withhold therapy if Hgb > 12 g/dL and resume therapy by decreasing dosage by 25% once Hgb falls below 11 g/dL. For adults, discontinue therapy if Hgb does not increase after 8 wk of the 300 U/kg/dose 3 times per wk dosage.

Anemia of prematurity (many regimens exist):

250 U/kg/dose SC 3 times per wk × 10 doses; alternatively, 200–400 U/kg/dose IV/SC 3–5 times per wk for 2–6 wk (total dose per wk is 600–1400 U/kg). Administer with supplemental iron at 3–6 mg elemental iron/kg/24 hr.

Use the lowest dose to avoid transfusions. Increased risk for death, serious cardiovascular events, and thrombosis/stroke have been reported in patients treated with chronic kidney disease and hemoglobin levels > 11 g/dL. Increased risk for death, shorten survival and/or shorten time to tumor progression/regression, serious cardiovascular events, and thrombosis in various cancer patients, especially with Hgb levels > 12 g/dL have been reported with epoetin alfa and other erythropoiesis-stimulating agents.

Evaluate serum iron, ferritin, TIBC before therapy. Iron supplementation recommended during therapy unless iron stores are already in excess. Monitor Hct, BP, clotting times, platelets, BUN, serum creatinine. Peak effect in 2–3 wk.

DOSAGE ADJUSTMENT FOR ANEMIA IN CHRONIC RENAL FAILURE:

Reduce dose by ≥25%: when Hgb increases >1 g/dL in any 2-wk period. Dose reductions can be made more frequently than once every 4 wk if needed.

Increase dose by 25%: when Hgb does not increase by 1 g/dL after 4 wk of therapy. Dosage increments should not be made more frequently than once every 4 wk.

Withholding therapy: when Hgb > 11 g/dL; restart therapy at a 25% lower dose after Hgb decreases to target levels or < 11 g/dL.

EPOETIN ALFA continued

Inadequate response after a 12-wk dose escalation: Use minimum effective dosage that will maintain hemoglobin levels to avoid the need for recurrent blood transfusions and evaluate other causes of anemia. Discontinue use if patient remains transfusion dependent.

DOSAGE REDUCTION ADJUSTMENT/WITHHOLDING THERAPY FOR ANEMIA IN CANCER:

If Hgb exceeds a level needed to avoid blood transfusion: Withhold dose and resume therapy at a reduced dosage by 25% when Hgb approaches a level where blood transfusions may be needed.

If Hgb increases >1 g/dL in any 2-wk period or Hgb reaches a level to avoid blood transfusion: Reduce dose by 25%.

May cause hypertension, seizure, hypersensitivity reactions, headache, edema, dizziness. SC route provides sustained serum levels compared to IV route. For IV administration, infuse over 1–3 min.

Do not use multidose vial preparation for breastfeeding mothers because of concerns for benzyl alcohol.

ERGOCALCIFEROL
Calciferol, Calcidiol, and generics
Vitamin D$_2$

No　No　2　A/C

Caps: 50,000 IU (1.25 mg)
Tabs: 400, 2000 IU
Drops (OTC): 8000 IU/mL (200 mcg/mL) (60 mL); contains propylene glycol
1 mg = 40,000 IU vitamin D activity

Dietary supplementation (see Chapter 21 for additional information):
  Preterm: 400–800 IU/24 hr PO
  Infant (<1 yr): 400 IU/24 hr PO
  Child (≥1 yr) and adolescent: 600 IU/24 hr PO

Renal failure (CKD stages 2–5) and 25-OH vitamin D levels < 30 ng/mL (monitor serum 25-OH vitamin D and corrected calcium/phosphorus 1 mo after initiation and Q3 mo thereafter):
  25-OH vitamin D < 5 ng/mL:
    Child: 8000 IU/24 hr × 4 wk followed by 4000 IU/24 hr × 2 mo; or 50,000 IU weekly × 4 wk followed by 50,000 IU twice monthly for 2 mo
  25-OH vitamin D 5–15 ng/mL:
    Child: 4000 IU/24 hr PO × 12 wk or 50,000 IU every other wk × 12 wk
  25-OH vitamin D 16–30 ng/mL:
    Child: 2000 IU/24 hr PO × 3 mo or 50,000 IU every mo × 3 mo

Vitamin D–dependent rickets:
  Child: 3000–5000 IU/24 hr PO; **max. dose**: 60,000 IU/24 hr

Nutritional rickets:
  Child and adult with normal GI absorption: 2000–5000 IU/24 hr PO × 6–12 wk
  Malabsorption:
    Child: 10,000–25,000 IU/24 hr PO
    Adult: 10,000–300,000 IU/24 hr PO

Vitamin D–resistant rickets (with phosphate supplementation):
  Child: initial dose 40,000–80,000 IU/24 hr PO; increase daily dose by 10,000–20,000 IU PO Q3–4 mo if needed
  Adult: 10,000–60,000 IU/24 hr PO

Hypoparathyroidism (with calcium supplementation):
  Child: 50,000–200,000 IU/24 hr PO
  Adult: 25,000–200,000 IU/24 hr PO

Continued

ERGOCALCIFEROL continued

Monitor serum Ca^{2+}, PO_4, 25-OH vitamin D (goal level for infant and child: ≥20 ng/mL) and alkaline phosphate. Serum Ca^{2+}, PO_4 product should be <70 mg/dL to avoid ectopic calcification. Titrate dosage to patient response. Watch for symptoms of hypercalcemia: weakness, diarrhea, polyuria, metastatic calcification, nephrocalcinosis. Vitamin D_2 is activated by 25-hydroxylation in liver and 1-hydroxylation in kidney.

Serum 25-OH vitamin D level of ≥35 ng/mL has been suggested in Cystic Fibrosis patients to decrease the risk of hyperparathyroidism and bone loss.

Pregnancy category changes to "C" if used in doses above the U.S. RDA.

ERGOTAMINE TARTRATE ± CAFFEINE
Ergomar
In combination with caffeine: Cafergot, Migergot, and generics
Ergot alkaloid

Yes   Yes   X   X

Sublingual tabs (Ergomar): 2 mg
In combination with caffeine:
  Tabs: 1 and 100 mg caffeine
  Suppository: 2 and 100 mg caffeine (12s)

ERGOTAMINE:
Adolescent and adult:
SL: 1 mg at the onset of migraine attack, then 1 mg Q30 min PRN up to **max. dose** of 3 mg per 24 hr; **do not exceed** 5 mg per wk.

ERGOTAMINE PLUS CAFFEINE
Doses based on mg of ergotamine.
Adolescent and adult:
PO: 2 mg at the onset of migraine attack, then 1–2 mg Q30 min up to 6 mg per attack; **do not exceed** 10 mg per wk.
Suppository: 2 mg at first sign of attack; follow with second 2 mg dose after 1 hr if needed; **max. dose** 4 mg per attack, **not to exceed** 10 mg/wk.

Use with caution in renal or hepatic disease. May cause paresthesias, GI disturbance, angina-like pain, rebound headache with abrupt withdrawal, or muscle cramps. **Contraindicated** in pregnancy and has **not been recommended** in breast-feeding. Concurrent administration with protease inhibitors, clarithromycin, erythromycin, other CYP450 3A4 inhibitors, and nitroglycerin are **contraindicated** owing to risk of ergotism (nausea, vomiting, and vasospastic ischemia leading to cerebral and peripheral ischemia).

For sublingual administration, place tablet under the tongue and do not crush.

ERTAPENEM
Invanz
Antibiotic, carbapenem

No   Yes   2   B

Injection: 1 g
Contains ~6 mEq Na/g drug

Infant < 3 mo: 15 mg/kg/dose IV/IM Q12 hr
3 mo–12 yr: 15 mg/kg/dose IV/IM Q12 hr; **max. dose:** 1 g/24 hr

ERTAPENEM continued

Adolescent and adult: 1 g IV/IM Q24 hr
  Recommended duration of therapy (all ages):
    Complicated intraabdominal infection: 5–14 days
    Complicated skin/subcutaneous tissue infections: 7–14 days
    Diabetic foot infection without osteomyelitis: up to 28 days
    Community acquired pneumonia, complicated UTI/pyelonephritis: 10–14 days
    Acute pelvic infection: 3–10 days
Surgical prophylaxis:
  Child and adolescent: 15 mg/kg (**max. dose**: 1 g/dose) IV 1 hr before procedure
  Adult (colorectal surgery): 1 g IV 1 hr before procedure

Ertapenem has poor activity against *Pseudomonas aeruginosa*, *Acinetobacter*, MRSA, and *Enterococcus*. **Do not use** in meningitis due to poor CSF penetration. **Use with caution** in CNS disorders, including seizures. **Adjust dosage in renal impairment; see Chapter 30.**

Diarrhea, infusion complications, nausea, headache, vaginitis, phlebitis/thrombophlebitis, and vomiting are common. Seizures (primarily with renal insufficiency and/or CNS disorders such as brain lesions and seizures), decreased consciousness, muscle weakness, gait disturbance, abnormal coordination, teeth staining, and DRESS syndrome have been reported. Increased ALT, AST, and neutropenia have been reported in pediatric clinical trials. Decreases valproic acid levels. Probenecid may increase ertapenem levels.

IM route requires reconstitution with 1% lidocaine and **should not** be administer IV. **Do not** reconstitute or co-infuse with dextrose containing solutions.

ERYTHROMYCIN PREPARATIONS
Erythrocin, Pediamycin, EES, E-Mycin, EryPed, Ery-Tab, PCE, Erygel, and generics
Ophthalmic ointment: Ilotycin and generics
Antibiotic, macrolide

Yes Yes 2 B

Erythromycin base:
  Tabs: 250, 500 mg
  Delayed-release tabs (Ery-Tab, PCE): 250, 333, 500 mg
  Delayed-release caps: 250 mg
  Topical gel (Erygel and generics): 2% (30, 60 g); contains alcohol 92%
  Topical solution: 2% (60 mL); may contain 44%–66% alcohol
  Topical pad/swab: 2% (60s); may contain propylene glycol
  Ophthalmic ointment: 0.5% (1, 3.5 g)
Erythromycin ethyl succinate (EES):
  Oral suspension (EES and EryPed): 200 mg/5 mL (100, 200 mL), 400 mg/5 mL (100 mL)
  Tabs (EES and generics): 400 mg
Erythromycin stearate:
  Tabs: 250 mg
Erythromycin lactobionate:
  Injection: 500 mg; may contain benzyl alcohol

Oral:
  Neonate (use EES preparation):
    <1.2 kg: 20 mg/kg/24 hr ÷ Q12 hr PO

Continued

ERYTHROMYCIN PREPARATIONS continued

Neonate (use EES preparation):
≥1.2 kg:
0–7 days: 20 mg/kg/24 hr ÷ Q12 hr PO
>7 days:
1.2–2 kg: 30 mg/kg/24 hr ÷ Q8 hr PO
≥2 kg: 30–40 mg/kg/24 hr ÷ Q6–8 hr PO
Chlamydial conjunctivitis and pneumonia: 50 mg/kg/24 hr ÷ Q6 hr PO × 14 days; **max. dose:** 2 g/24 hr
Child (use base, EES, or stearate preparation): 30–50 mg/kg/24 hr ÷ Q6–8 hr; max. dose: 4 g/24 hr
Pertussis: 40–50 mg/kg/24 hr ÷ Q6 hr PO × 14 days (**max. dose:** 2 g/24 hr); use azithromycin for infants <1 mo old
Adult: 2 g/24 hr ÷ Q6 hr PO × 14 days
Parenteral:
Child and adult: 15–20 mg/kg/24 hr ÷ Q6 hr IV; **max. dose:** 4 g/24 hr
Ophthalmic:
Neonatal gonococcal ophthalmia prophylaxis: Apply 1-inch ribbon to both eyes × 1
Conjunctivitis: Apply 1-inch ribbon to affected eye(s) several times a day up to 6 times daily
Preoperative bowel prep: 20 mg/kg/dose PO erythromycin base × 3 doses, with neomycin, 1 day before surgery
Prokinetic agent:
Infant and child: 10–20 mg/kg/24 hr PO ÷ TID-QID (QAC or QAC and QHS)

Avoid use in patients with known QT prolongation, proarrhythmic conditions (e.g., hypokalemia, hypomagnesemia, and significant bradycardia), and receiving class IA or class III antiarrhythmic agents, astemizole, cisapride, pimozide, or terfenadine. Hypertrophic pyloric stenosis in neonates receiving prophylactic therapy for pertussis; life-threatening episodes of ventricular tachycardia associated with prolonged QTc interval; and exacerbation of myasthenia gravis have been reported. May produce false positive urinary catecholamines, 17-hydroxycorticosteroids, and 17-ketosteroids.

GI side effects are common (nausea, vomiting, abdominal cramps). Cardiac dysrhythmia, anaphylaxis, interstitial nephritis, and hearing loss have been reported. Use with **caution** in liver disease. Estolate formulation may cause cholestatic jaundice, although hepatotoxicity is uncommon (2% of reported cases). Inhibits CYP450 1A2, 3A3/4 isoenzymes. May produce elevated digoxin, theophylline, carbamazepine, clozapine, cyclosporine, and methylprednisolone levels. **Adjust dose in renal failure (see Chapter 30).** Use ideal body weight for obese patients when calculating doses.

Oral therapy should replace IV as soon as possible. Give oral doses after meals. Because of different absorption characteristics, higher oral doses of EES are needed to achieve therapeutic effects. **Avoid** IM route (pain and necrosis). For ophthalmic use, avoid contact of ointment tip with eye or skin.

ERYTHROPOIETIN

See Epoetin Alfa

ESCITALOPRAM
Lexapro and generics
Antidepressant, selective serotonin reuptake inhibitor

Yes   Yes   3   C

Tabs: 5, 10, 20 mg.
Oral solution: 1 mg/mL (240 mL); contains parabens and propylene glycol.

ESCITALOPRAM continued

Depression:
<12 yr: Limited data, only one placebo-controlled RCT did not demonstrate efficacy.
≥12 yr and adolescent: Start with 10 mg PO once daily. If needed after 3 weeks, dose may be increased to 20 mg once daily.
Adult: Start with 10 mg PO once daily. If needed after 1 week, dose may be increased to 20 mg once daily.

Autism and Pervasive Developmental Disorders (PDD; limited data):
6–17 yr: In a 10-wk, open-label trial, 28 subjects were given a weekly increasing PO dosage regimen of 2.5, 5, 10, 15, and 20 mg/24 hr. Mean dosage of responders with significant improvement at 11.1 ± 6.5 mg/24 hr; 25% of subjects responded at doses < 10 mg/24 hr and 36% responded at doses ≥ 10 mg/24 hr. Seven of the 17 (41%) responders and 25% of all treated subjects could not tolerate the 10 mg/24 hr dose.

Social Anxiety Disorder (limited data):
10–17 yr: In a 12-week, open-label trial, 20 subjects were given an initial PO dosage of 5 mg once daily × 7 days followed by 10 mg once daily. If needed and tolerated, it was increased by 5 mg/24 hr at weekly intervals up to a maximum of 20 mg/24 hr. Two subjects did not complete the trial due to a lack of efficacy and tolerability; 65% of the remaining subjects met the response criteria with a mean final dose of 13 ± 4.1 mg/24 hr. Common adverse events included somnolence (25%), insomnia (20%), flu symptoms (15%), increased appetite (15%), and decreased appetite (15%).

Increased risk for serotonin syndrome when used with MAO inhibitors (or within 14 days of discontinuance), linezolid, or methylene blue; concurrent use considered contraindicated. **Do not** use with pimozide because of increased QTc interval risk. **Use with caution** in hepatic or severe renal impairment; dosage adjustment may be needed. **Avoid** abrupt discontinuation to prevent withdrawal symptoms.

Diaphoresis, GI discomfort, xerostomia, dizziness, headache, insomnia, somnolence, sexual dysfunction, and fatigue are common side effects. Abnormal bleeding, depression, QTc prolongation, and suicidal ideation have been reported.

Primarily metabolized by the CYP450 2C19 and 3A4 enzymes and is a weak inhibitor for CYP450 2D6 enzyme. Taking with other medications with QTc prolongation may further increase that risk. Omeprazole may increase the toxicity of escitalopram. Doses may be administered with or without food.

ESMOLOL HCL
Brevibloc and generics
β₁-selective adrenergic blocking agent, antihypertensive agent, class II antiarrhythmic

No | No | ? | C

Injection: 10 mg/mL (10 mL).
Injection, premixed infusion in iso-osmotic sodium chloride: 2000 mg/100 mL (100 mL), 2500 mg/250 mL (250 mL).

Postopertaive hypertension: Titrate to response (limited information):
   Loading dose: 500 mcg/kg IV over 1 min.
   Maintenance dose: 50–250 mcg/kg/min IV as infusion. Titrate doses upward 50–100 mcg/kg/min Q5–10 min as needed. Heart surgery patients may require higher doses (~700 mcg/kg/min). Dosages as high as 1000 mcg/kg/min have been administered to children 1–12 yr.

Continued

ESMOLOL HCL continued

SVT: Titrate to response (limited information).
  Loading dose: 100–500 mcg/kg IV over 1 min.
  Maintenance dose: 25–100 mcg/kg/min IV as infusion. Titrate doses upward 50–100 mcg/kg/min Q5–10 min as needed. Dosages as high as 1000 mcg/kg/min have been administered.

Contraindicated in sinus bradycardia, >first-degree heart block, and cardiogenic shock or heart failure. Short duration of action; $T_{1/2}$ = 2.9–4.7 min for children and 9 min for adults. May cause bronchospasm, congestive heart failure, hypotension (at doses > 200 mcg/kg/min), nausea, and vomiting. May increase digoxin (by 10%–20%) and theophylline levels. Morphine may increase esmolol level by 46%. Theophylline may decrease esmolol's effects.
Administer only in a monitored setting. Concentration for administration is typically ≤10 mg/mL, but 20 mg/mL has been administered in pediatric patients.

ESOMEPRAZOLE
Nexium and generics
Gastric acid proton pump inhibitor

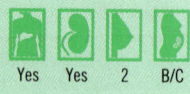
Yes   Yes   2   B/C

Caps, delayed release: 20, 40 mg; contains magnesium
Tab, delayed release: 20 mg; contains magnesium
Powder for oral suspension: 2.5, 5, 10, 20, 40 mg packets (30s); contains magnesium
Injection: 20, 40 mg; contains EDTA

Child (PO):
  GERD (use for up to 8 weeks):
    1–11 yr: 10 mg once daily
    ≥12 yr: 20–40 mg once daily
  Erosive esophagitis in GERD (use up to 6 weeks):
    Infant (1 mo–< 1 yr):
      3–5 kg: 2.5 mg once daily
      >5–7.5 kg: 5 mg once daily
      >7.5–12 kg: 10 mg once daily
    1–11 yr:
      <20 kg: 10 mg once daily
      ≥20 kg: 10 or 20 mg once daily
Child (IV):
  GERD with erosive esophagitis:
    Infant: 0.5–1 mg/kg/dose once daily
    Child 1–17 yr:
      <55 kg: 10 mg once daily
      ≥55 kg: 20–40 mg once daily
Adult (PO/IV):
  GERD: 20 or 40 mg once daily × 4–8 wk
  Prevention of NSAID-induced gastric ulcers: 20 or 40 mg once daily for up to 6 mo
  Pathological hypersecretory conditions (e.g., Zollinger-Ellison Syndrome): 40 mg BID; doses up to 240 mg/24 hr have been used
  Hepatic impairment: Patients with severe hepatic function impairment (Child-Pugh class C) should not exceed 20 mg/24 hr

---

Cross-allergic reactions with other proton pump inhibitors (e.g., lansoprazole, pantoprazole, and rabeprazole). **Use with caution** in liver impairment (see dosage adjustment recommendation in dosing section). GI disturbances and headache are common.

ESOMEPRAZOLE continued

Hypomagnesemia may occur with continuous use. Anaphylaxis; angioedema; bronchospasm; acute interstitial nephritis; erythema multiforme; urticaria; Stevens–Johnson syndrome; TEN; pancreatitis; and fractures of the hip, wrist, and spine (in adults > 50 yr old receiving high doses or prolonged therapy for >1 yr) have been reported. Drug is a substrate and inhibitor of CYP450 2C19 and substrate of CYP450 3A4. May decrease the absorption or effects of atazanavir, clopidogrel, ketoconazole, itraconazole, mycophenolate mofetil, and iron salts. May increase the effect/toxicity of diazepam, midazolam, digoxin, carbamazepine, and warfarin. Voriconazole may increase the effects of esomeprazole. May be used in combination with clarithromycin and amoxicillin for Helicobacter pylori infections.

Pregnancy category is a "B" for the magnesium containing product and a "C" for the strontium containing product.

Administer all oral doses before meals and 30 min before sucralfate (if receiving). **Do not** crush or chew capsules. IV doses may be given as fast as 3 min or infused over 10–30 min.

ETANERCEPT
Enbrel and Enbrel SureClick
Antirheumatic, immunomodulatory agent, tumor necrosis factor receptor p75 Fc fusion protein

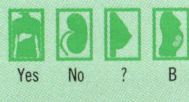

Yes   No   ?   B

Prefilled injection (single use): 25 mg (0.51 mL of 50 mg/mL solution), 50 mg (0.98 mL of 50 mg/mL solution); contains sucrose, L-arginine (preservative free) (carton of 4 prefilled syringes).
Injection (powder; multidose vial): 25 mg with diluent (1 mL bacteriostatic water containing 0.9% benzyl alcohol); contains mannitol, sucrose, tromethamine.
Autoinjector:
   Enbrel SureClick (single use): 50 mg (0.98 mL of 50 mg/mL solution); contains sucrose, L-arginine (preservative free) (carton of four auto-injectors).

Juvenile idiopathic arthritis:
   Child 2–17 yr: 0.4 mg/kg/dose SC twice weekly administered 72–96 hr apart; **max. dose:** 25 mg. Alternatively, once weekly dose of 0.8 mg/kg/dose SC (**max. dose:** 50 mg/wk and **max. single injection site dose** of 25 mg) may be used.
Rheumatoid arthritis, psoriatic arthritis, ankylosing spondylitis:
   Adult: 25 mg SC twice weekly administered 72–96 hr apart. Alternatively, once weekly dose of 50 mg SC (**max. single injection site dose** of 25 mg) may be used.
Plaque psoriasis:
   Child and adolescent (4–17 yr): 0.8 mg/kg/dose (max. dose: 50 mg) SC once weekly.
   Adult: Start with 50 mg SC twice weekly administered 72–96 hr apart × 3 mo, followed by a reduced maintenance dose of 50 mg SC per wk. Starting doses of 25 mg or 50 mg per wk have also been shown to be effective.
   Max. single injection site dose: 25 mg.

Contraindicated in serious infections, sepsis, or hypersensitivity to any of medication components. **Use with caution** in patients with history of recurrent infections (including hepatitis B) or underlying conditions that may predispose them to infections (including concomitant immunosuppressive therapy), CNS demyelinating disorders, malignancies, immune-related diseases, and latex allergy. Common adverse effects in children include headache, abdominal pain, vomiting, and nausea. Injection site reactions (e.g., discomfort, itching, and swelling), rhinitis, dizziness, rash, depression, infections (varicella, aseptic meningitis, rare cases of TB, and fatal/serious infections and sepsis), bone marrow

Continued

ETANERCEPT continued

suppression (e.g., aplastic anemia), sarcoidosis, vertigo, and CNS demyelinating disorder have also been reported. Malignancies (some were fatal and ~50% were lymphomas) have been reported in children and adolescents.

Do not administer live vaccines concurrently with this drug. In JRA, it is recommended that before initiating therapy, the patient be brought up to date with all immunizations in agreement with current immunization guidelines.

Onset of action is 1–4 wk, with peak effects usually within 3 mo.

Patients must be properly instructed on preparing and administering the medication. For multi-dose vial, reconstitute vial by gently swirling its contents with the supplied diluent (**do not** shake or vigorously agitate) as some foaming will occur. Reconstituted solutions should be clear and colorless as unused portions must be stored in the refrigerator and used within 14 days.

Drug is administered subcutaneously by rotating injection sites (thigh, abdomen, or upper arm) with a **max. single injection site dose** of 25 mg. Administer new injections ≥1 inch from an old site and never where the skin is tender, bruised, red, or hard.

ETHAMBUTOL HCL
Myambutol and generics
Antituberculosis drug

No   Yes   2   C

Tabs: 100, 400 mg
400 mg tabs may be scored

Tuberculosis:
  Infant, child, adolescent, and adult: 15–25 mg/kg/dose PO once daily or 50 mg/kg/dose PO twice weekly
  Max. dose: 2.5 g/24 hr
Nontuberculous mycobacterial infection and Mycobacterium avium complex in AIDS (recurrence prophylaxis or treatment; use in combination with other medications):
  Infant, child, adolescent, and adult: 15–25 mg/kg/24 hr PO once daily; **max. dose:** 2.5 g/24 hr

May cause reversible optic neuritis, especially with larger doses. Obtain baseline ophthalmologic studies before beginning therapy and then monthly. Follow visual acuity, visual fields, and (red-green) color vision. **Do not use** in optic neuritis and in children in whom visual acuity cannot be assessed. **Discontinue** if any visual deterioration occurs. Monitor uric acid, liver function, heme status, and renal function. Hyperuricemia, GI disturbances and mania are common. Erythema multiforme has been reported. Coadministration with aluminum hydroxide can reduce ethambutol's absorption; space administration by 4 hr. Give with food. **Adjust dose with renal failure (see Chapter 30).**

ETHOSUXIMIDE
Zarontin and generics
Anticonvulsant

Yes   Yes   2   D

Caps: 250 mg
Oral solution: 250 mg/5 mL (473 mL)

ETHOSUXIMIDE continued

Oral:
≤6 yr:
  Initial: 15 mg/kg/24 hr ÷ BID; *max. dose:* 500 mg/24 hr; increase as needed Q4–7 days
  Usual maintenance dose: 15–40 mg/kg/24 hr ÷ BID
>6 yr and adult: 250 mg BID; increase by 250 mg/24 hr as needed Q4–7 days.
  Usual maintenance dose: 20–40 mg/kg/24 hr ÷ BID
Max. dose (all ages): 1500 mg/24 hr

Use with caution in hepatic and renal disease. Ataxia, anorexia, drowsiness, sleep disturbances, rashes, and blood dyscrasias are rare idiosyncratic reactions. May cause lupus-like syndrome; may increase frequency of grand mal seizures in patients with mixed type seizures. Serious dermatological reactions (e.g., Stevens Johnson and DRESS) has been reported. May increase risk of suicidal thoughts/behavior. Cases of birth defects have been reported; ethosuximide crosses the placenta. Drug of choice for absence seizures.

Carbamazepine, phenytoin, primidone, phenobarbital, valproic acid, nevirapine, and ritonavir may decrease ethosuximide levels.

Therapeutic levels: 40–100 mg/L. $T_{1/2}$ = 24–42 hr. Recommended serum sampling time at steady state: obtain trough level within 30 min prior to the next scheduled dose after 5–10 days of continuous dosing.

To minimize GI distress, may administer with food or milk. Abrupt withdrawal of drug may precipitate absence status.

FAMCICLOVIR
Famvir and generics
Antiviral

Yes   Yes   ?   B

Tabs: 125, 250, 500 mg

Adult:
  Herpes zoster: 500 mg Q8 hr PO × 7 days; initiate therapy promptly as soon as diagnosis is made (initiation within 48 hr after rash onset is ideal; currently no data for starting treatment > 72 hr after rash onset).
  Genital herpes (first episode): 250 mg Q8 hr PO × 7–10 days.
  Recurrent genital herpes:
    Immunocompetent: 1000 mg Q12 hr PO × 1 day or 125 mg Q12 hr PO × 5 days; initiate therapy at first sign or symptom. Efficacy has not been established when treatment is initiated >6 hr after onset of symptoms or lesions.
    Immunocompromised: 500 mg Q8 hr PO × 7 days.
  Suppression of recurrent genital herpes (immunocompetent): 250 mg Q12 hr PO up to 1 yr, then reassess for HSV infection recurrence.
  Recurrent herpes labialis:
    Immunocompetent: 1500 mg PO × 1.
    Immunocompromised: 500 mg Q8 hr PO × 7 days.
  Recurrent mucocutaneous herpes in HIV: 500 mg Q12 hr PO × 7 days.

Drug is converted to its active form (penciclovir). Hepatic impairment may impair/reduce the conversion of famciclovir to penciclovir. Better absorption than PO acyclovir.

May cause headache, diarrhea, nausea, and abdominal pain. Serious skin reactions (e.g., TEN and Stevens–Johnson syndrome), angioedema, leukocytoclastic vasculitis, palpitations, cholestatic

Continued

FAMCICLOVIR continued

jaundice, and abnormal LFTs have been reported. Concomitant use with probenecid and other drugs eliminated by active tubular secretion may result in decreased penciclovir clearance. **Reduce dose in renal impairment (see Chapter 30).**

Safety and efficacy in suppression of recurrent genital herpes have not been established beyond 1 yr. No efficacy data is available for children 1–<12 yr to support its use for genital herpes, recurrent herpes labialis, and varicella. Furthermore, efficacy has not been established for recurrent herpes labialis for children 12–<18 yr. May be administered with or without food.

FAMOTIDINE
Pepcid, Pepcid AC [OTC], Pepcid AC EZ Chews [OTC], Pepcid AC Maximum Strength [OTC], Pepcid Complete [OTC], and generics
Histamine-2-receptor antagonist

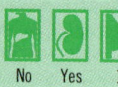

No Yes 1 B

Injection: 10 mg/mL (2, 4, 20, 50 mL); multidose vials contain 0.9% benzyl alcohol
Premixed injection: 20 mg/50 mL in iso-osmotic sodium chloride
Oral suspension: 40 mg/5 mL (contains parabens) (50 mL)
Tabs: 10 (OTC), 20 (OTC), 40 mg
Chewable tabs:
 Pepcid Complete: 10 mg famotidine with 800 mg calcium carbonate and 165 mg magnesium hydroxide (25s, 50s); may contain aspartame
 Pepcid AC EZChews (OTC): 20 mg (25s)

Neonate and <3 mo:
 IV: 0.25–0.5 mg/kg/dose Q24 hr
 PO: 0.5–1 mg/kg/dose Q24 hr
≥3 mo–1 yr (GERD): 0.5 mg/kg/dose PO Q12 hr
Child (1–12 yr):
 IV: initial: 0.6–0.8 mg/kg/24 hr ÷ Q12 hr up to a **max.** of 40 mg/24 hr
 PO: initial: 1–1.2 mg/kg/24 hr ÷ Q12 hr up to a **max.** of 40 mg/24 hr
 Peptic ulcer: 0.5–1 mg/kg/24 hr PO QHS or ÷ Q12 hr up to a **max. dose** of 40 mg/24 hr
 GERD: 1–2 mg/kg/24 hr PO ÷ Q 12 hr up to a **max. dose** of 80 mg/24 hr
Adolescent and adult:
 Duodenal ulcer:
  PO: 20 mg BID or 40 mg QHS × 4–8 wk; then, maintenance therapy at 20 mg QHS
  IV: 20 mg BID
 GERD: 20 mg BID PO × 6 wk
 Esophagitis: 20–40 mg BID PO × 12 wk

A Q12-hr dosage interval is generally recommended; however, infants and young children may require a Q8-hr interval because of enhanced drug clearance. Headaches, dizziness, constipation, diarrhea, and drowsiness have occurred. **Dosage adjustment is required in severe renal failure (see Chapter 30);** prolonged QT interval has been reported very rarely in patients with renal impairment whose dosage had not been adjusted appropriately. Rhabdomyolysis has been reported.

Shake oral suspension well prior to each use. Disintegrating oral tablets should be placed on the tongue to be disintegrated and subsequently swallowed. Doses may be administered with or without food.

FELBAMATE
Felbatol and generics
Anticonvulsant

Yes   Yes   3   C

Tabs: 400, 600 mg
Oral suspension: 600 mg/5 mL (240, 473 mL)

Lennox-Gastaut for child 2–14 yr (adjunctive therapy):
  Start at 15 mg/kg/24 hr PO ÷ TID–QID; increase dosage by 15 mg/kg/24 hr increments at weekly intervals up to a **max. dose** of 45 mg/kg/24 hr or 3600 mg/24 hr (whichever is less). See remarks for adjusting concurrent anticonvulsants.

Child ≥ 14 yr–adult:
  Adjunctive therapy: Start at 1200 mg/24 hr PO ÷ TID–QID; increase dosage by 1200 mg/24 hr at weekly intervals up to a **max. dose** of 3600 mg/day. See remarks for adjusting concurrent anticonvulsants.
  Monotherapy (as initial therapy): Start at 1200 mg/24 hr PO ÷ TID–QID. Increase dose under close clinical supervision at 600 mg increments Q2 wk to 2400 mg/24 hr. **Max. dose:** 3600 mg/24 hr.
  Conversion to monotherapy: Start at 1200 mg/24 hr ÷ PO TID–QID for 2 wk; then increase to 2400 mg/24 hr for 1 wk. At wk 3, increase to 3600 mg/24 hr. Reduce dose of other anticonvulsants by 33% at the initiation of felbamate, then an additional 33% of original dose at week 2, and continue to reduce other anticonvulsants as clinical indicated at week 3 and beyond.

Drug should be prescribed under strict supervision by a specialist. **Contraindicated** in blood dyscrasias or hepatic dysfunction (prior or current); and hypersensitivity to meprobamate. Aplastic anemia and hepatic failure leading to death have been associated with drug. May cause headache, fatigue, anxiety, GI disturbances, gingival hyperplasia, increased liver enzymes, and bone marrow suppression. Suicidal behavior or ideation have been reported. **Obtain serum levels of concurrent anticonvulsants.** Monitor liver enzymes, bilirubin, CBC with differential, platelets at baseline and every 1–2 wk. Doses should be decreased by 50% in renally impaired patients.

When initiating adjunctive therapy (all ages), doses of other antiepileptic drugs (AEDs) are reduced by 20% to control plasma levels of concurrent phenytoin, valproic acid, phenobarbital, and carbamazepine. Further reductions of concomitant AED dosage may be necessary to minimize side effects caused by drug interactions.

When converting to monotherapy, reduce other AEDs by one third at start of felbamate therapy. Then after 2 wk and at the start of increasing the felbamate dosage, reduce other AEDs by an additional one third. At wk 3, continue to reduce other AEDs as clinically indicated.

Carbamazepine levels may be decreased; however, phenytoin and valproic acid levels may be increased. Phenytoin and carbamazepine may increase felbamate clearance; valproic acid may decrease its clearance.

Doses can be administered with or without food.

FENTANYL
Sublimaze, Durasegic, Fentora, Actiq, Lanzanda, and generics
Narcotic; analgesic, sedative

No   Yes   2   C/D

Injection: 50 mcg/mL
SR patch (Duragesic and generics): 12.5, 25, 50, 75, 100 mcg/hr (5s)

Continued

FENTANYL continued

Tabs for buccal administration:
  Fentora: 100, 200, 400, 600, 800 mcg (28s)
Lozenge on a stick:
  Actiq and generics: 200, 400, 600, 800, 1200, 1600 mcg (30s)
Nasal solution:
  Lazanda: 100 mcg/spray, 300 mcg/spray, 400 mcg/spray (5 mL; delivers 8 sprays)

Titrate dose to effect.
Neonate and younger infant:
  Sedation/analgesia: 1–4 mcg/kg/dose IV Q2–4 hr PRN
  Continuous IV infusion: 1–5 mcg/kg/hr; tolerance may develop
Older infant and child:
  Sedation/analgesia: 1–2 mcg/kg/dose IV/IM Q30–60 min PRN
  Continuous IV infusion: 1 mcg/kg/hr; titrate to effect; usual infusion range 1–3 mcg/kg/hr
To prepare infusion, use the following formula:

$$50 \times \frac{\text{Desired dose (mcg/kg/hr)}}{\text{Desired infusion rate (mL/hr)}} \times \text{Wt (kg)} = \frac{\text{mcg Fentanyl}}{50 \text{ mL fluid}}$$

Oral, breakthrough cancer pain for opioid-intolerant patients (see remarks):
  Buccal tabs (Fentora; ≥18 yr): Start with 100 mcg by placing tablet in the buccal cavity (above a rear molar between the upper cheek and gum) and letting the tablet dissolve for 15–25 min. A second 100 mcg dose, if needed, may be administered 30 min after the start of the first dose. If needed, increase dose initially in multiples of 100 mcg tablet when patients require > 1 dose per breakthrough pain episode for several consecutive episodes. If titration requires > 400 mcg/dose, use 200 mcg tabs.
  Lozenges (≥16 yr): Start with 200 mcg by placing lozenge in the mouth between the cheek and lower gum. If needed, may repeat dose 15 min after the completion of the first dose (30 min after start of prior dose). If therapy requires >1 lozenge per episode, consider increasing the dose to the next higher strength. **Do not** give more than 2 doses for each episode of breakthrough pain and re-evaluate long-acting opioid therapy if patient requires >4 doses/24 hr.
Transdermal (see remarks): Safety has not been established in children <2 yr and should be administered in children ≥2 yr who are opioid tolerant. Use is **contraindicated** in acute or postoperative pain in opiate-naïve patients.
  Opioid-tolerant child receiving at least 60 mg morphine equivalents/24 hr: Use 25 mcg/hr patch Q72 hr. Patch titration should not occur before 3 days of administration of the initial dose or more frequently than every 6 days thereafter.
See Chapter 6 for equianalgesic dosing and PCA dosing.
Intranasal route for acute and preprocedure analgesia (see remarks):
  ≥1 yr–adolescent: 1–2 mcg/kg/dose intranasally (max. dose: 50 mcg) Q1 hr PRN

Use with caution in bradycardia, respiratory depression, and increased intracranial pressure. **Adjust dose in renal failure (see Chapter 30).** Fatalities and life-threatening respiratory depression have been reported with inappropriate use (overdoses, use in opioid-naïve patients, changing the patch too frequently and exposing the patch to a heat source) of the transdermal route.

Highly lipophilic and may deposit into fat tissue. IV onset of action 1–2 min with peak effects in 10 min. IV duration of action 30–60 min. Give IV dose over 3–5 min. Rapid infusion may cause respiratory depression and chest wall rigidity. Respiratory depression may persist beyond the period of analgesia. Transdermal onset of action 6–8 hr with a 72-hr duration of action. See Chapter 6 for pharmacodynamic information with transmucosal and transdermal routes.

FENTANYL continued

Buccal tabs and oral lozenges are indicated only for the management of breakthrough cancer pain in patients who are already receiving and who are tolerant to opioid therapy. Buccal tabs (Fentora) and lozenge (Actiq) dosage forms are available through a restricted distribution program (REMS) and are NOT bioequivalent (see package insert for conversion).

Intranasal route of administration for analgesia has an onset of action at 10–30 min. Pediatric studies have demonstrated that the intranasal fentanyl is equivalent to and better than morphine (PO/IV/IM) and equivalent to intravenous fentanyl for providing analgesia.

Fentanyl is a substrate for the CYP450 3A4 enzyme. Be aware of medications that inhibit or induce this enzyme, for it may increase or decrease the effects of fentanyl, respectively.

Pregnancy category changes to "D" if drug is used for prolonged periods or in high doses at term.

FERRIC GLUCONATE

See Iron—Injectable Preparations

FERROUS SULFATE

See Iron—Oral Preparations

FEXOFENADINE ± PSEUDOEPHEDRINE
Allegra, Allegra ODT, Allegra-D 12 Hour, Allegra-D 24 Hour, and generics
Antihistamine, less-sedating ± decongestant

No Yes 2 C

Tabs: 30 mg, 60 mg [OTC], 180 mg [OTC]
Tabs, orally disintegrating (Allegra Allergy Children's**; ODT) [OTC]:** 30 mg; contains phenylalanine
Oral suspension [OTC]: 6 mg/mL (120 mL)
Extended-release tab in combination with pseudoephedrine (PE):
   Allegra-D 12 Hour [OTC]: 60 mg fexofenadine + 120 mg PE
   Allegra-D 24 Hour [OTC]: 180 mg fexofenadine + 240 mg PE

Fexofenadine:
   6 mo–<2 yr: 15–30 mg PO BID
   2–11 yr: 30 mg PO BID
   ≥12 yr–adult: 60 mg PO BID; 180 mg PO once daily may be used in seasonal rhinitis
Extended-release tabs of fexofenadine and pseudoephedrine:
   ≥12 yr–adult:
      Allegra-D 12 Hour: 1 tablet PO BID
      Allegra-D 24 Hour: 1 tablet PO once daily

May cause drowsiness, fatigue, headache, dyspepsia, nausea, and dysmenorrhea. Has not been implicated in causing cardiac arrhythmias when used with other drugs that are metabolized by hepatic microsomal enzymes (e.g., ketoconazole and erythromycin). **Reduce dose to 30 mg PO once daily for child 6–11 yr old and 60 mg PO once daily for ≥ 12 yr old if CrCl < 40 mL/min.** For use of Allegra-D 12 Hour and decreased renal function, an initial dose of 1 tablet PO once daily is recommended. **Avoid use** of Allegra-D 24 Hour in renal impairment. See pseudoephedrine for additional remarks if using the combination product.

Continued

FEXOFENADINE ± PSEUDOEPHEDRINE continued

Medication as a single agent may be administered with or without food. Do not administer antacids with or within 2 hr of fexofenadine dose. The extended-release combination product should be swallowed whole without food.

FILGRASTIM
Neupogen, Granix, Zarxio, G-CSF
Colony stimulating factor

No   Yes   ?   C

Injection: 300 mcg/mL (1, 1.6 mL vials)
Injection, prefilled syringes with 27-gauge 1/2-inch needles: 600 mcg/mL (300 mcg per 0.5 mL and 480 mcg per 0.8 mL) (10s)
All dosage forms contain polysorbate 80 and are preservative free.

Individual protocols may direct dosing.
IV/SC: 5–10 mcg/kg/dose once daily × 14 days or until ANC > 10,000/mm³. Dosage may be increased by 5 mcg/kg/24 hr if desired effect is not achieved within 7 days. Discontinue therapy when ANC > 10,000/mm³.

May cause bone pain, fever, and rash. Monitor CBC, uric acid, and LFTs. Glomerulonephritis and thrombocytopenia have been reported. Decreased bone density/osteoporosis has been reported in pediatric patients with severe chronic neutropenia. **Use with caution** in patients with malignancies with myeloid characteristics. **Contraindicated** for patients sensitive to E. coli-derived proteins. Do not administer 24 hr before or after administration of chemotherapy.

SC routes of administration are preferred because of prolonged serum levels over IV route. If used via IV route and G-CSF final concentration < 15 mcg/mL, add 2 mg albumin/1 mL of IV fluid to prevent drug adsorption to the IV administration set.

FLECAINIDE ACETATE
Generics; previously available as Tambocor
Antiarrhythmic, class Ic

Yes   Yes   2   C

Tabs: 50, 100, 150 mg
Oral suspension: 20 mg/mL

Child: Initial: 1–3 mg/kg/24 hr ÷ Q8 hr PO; usual range: 3–6 mg/kg/24 hr ÷ Q8 hr PO, monitor serum levels to adjust dose if needed.
Adult:
  Sustained V tach: 100 mg PO Q12 hr; may increase by 50 mg Q12 hr (100 mg/24 hr) every 4 days to **max. dose** of 600 mg/24 hr.
  Paroxysmal SVT/paroxysmal AF: 50 mg PO Q12 hr; may increase dose by 50 mg Q12 hr every 4 days to **max. dose** of 300–400 mg/24 hr.

May aggravate LV failure, sinus bradycardia, preexisting ventricular arrhythmias. May cause AV block, dizziness, blurred vision, dyspnea, nausea, headache, and increased PR or QRS intervals. **Reserve for life-threatening cases. Use with caution** in renal and/or hepatic impairment.

Flecainide is a substrate for the CYP450 2D6 enzyme. Be aware of medications that inhibit (e.g., certain SSRIs) or induce this enzyme for it may increase or decrease the effects of flecainide, respectively.

FLECAINIDE ACETATE continued

Therapeutic trough level: 0.2–1 mg/L. Recommended serum sampling time at steady-state: Obtain trough level within 30 min prior to the next scheduled dose after 2–3 days of continuous dosing for children; after 3–5 days for adults. **Adjust dose in renal failure (see Chapter 30).**

FLUCONAZOLE
Diflucan and generics
Antifungal agent

Yes   Yes   2   C/D

Tabs: 50, 100, 150, 200 mg
Injection: 2 mg/mL (50, 100, 200 mL); contains 9 mEq Na/2 mg drug
Oral suspension: 10 mg/mL (35 mL), 40 mg/mL (35 mL)

Neonate (IV/PO):
  Loading dose: 12–25 mg/kg
  Maintenance dose: 6–12 mg/kg with the following dosing intervals (see following table); use higher doses for severe infections of Candida strains with MICs > 4–8 mcg/mL

Postconceptional Age (wk)	Postnatal Age (days)	Dosing Interval (hr) & Time (hr) to Start First Maintenance Dose After Load
≤29	0–14	48
	>14	24
≥30	0–7	48
	>7	24

Child (IV/PO):

Indication	Loading Dose	Maintenance Dose (Q24 hr) to Begin 24 hr After Loading Dose
Oropharyngeal Candidiasis	6 mg/kg	3 mg/kg
Esophageal Candidiasis	12 mg/kg	6 mg/kg
Invasive Systemic Candidiasis and Cryptococcal meningitis	12 mg/kg	6–12 mg/kg
Suppressive therapy for HIV infected with Cryptococcal meningitis	6 mg/kg	6 mg/kg

Max. dose: 12 mg/kg/24 hr
Adult:
  Oropharyngeal and esophageal candidiasis: Loading dose of 200 mg PO/IV followed by 100 mg Q24 hr (24 hr after load); doses up to **max. dose** of 400 mg/24 hr should be used for esophageal candidiasis
  Systemic candidiasis and cryptococcal meningitis: Loading dose of 400 mg PO/IV, followed by 200–800 mg Q24 hr (24 hr after load)
  Bone marrow transplant prophylaxis: 400 mg PO/IV Q24 hr
  Suppressive therapy for HIV infected patients with cryptococcal meningitis: 200 mg PO/IV Q24 hr
  Vaginal candidiasis: 150 mg PO × 1

Use with other medications that are known to prolong the QT interval and are metabolized via the CYP450 3A4 enzyme (e.g., erythromycin) is considered **contraindicated**. May cause nausea, headache, rash, vomiting, abdominal pain, hepatitis, cholestasis, and diarrhea. Neutropenia, agranulocytosis, and thrombocytopenia have been reported. **Use with caution** in hepatic or renal dysfunction and in patients with proarrhythmic conditions.

Continued

FLUCONAZOLE continued

Inhibits CYP450 2C9/10 and CYP450 3A3/4 (weak inhibitor). May increase effects, toxicity, or levels of cyclosporine, midazolam, phenytoin, rifabutin, tacrolimus, theophylline, warfarin, oral hypoglycemics, and AZT. Rifampin increases fluconazole metabolism.

Pediatric to adult dose equivalency: every 3 mg/kg pediatric dosage is equal to 100 mg adult dosage. Consider using higher doses in morbidly obese patients. **Adjust dose in renal failure (see Chapter 30).**

Pregnancy category is "C" for single 150-mg use for vaginal candidiasis but a recent Danish study reports a higher risk of miscarriages during weeks 7–22 of gestation. The FDA is currently evaluating this and additional data. Pregnancy category is "D" for all other indications (high-dose use during first trimester of pregnancy may result in birth defects).

FLUCYTOSINE
Ancobon, 5-FC, 5-Fluorocytosine, and generics
Antifungal agent

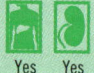

Yes   Yes   3   C

Caps: 250, 500 mg
Oral suspension: 10, 50 mg/mL

Neonate (monitor serum concentrations):
<1 kg:
  ≤14 days old: 75 mg/kg/24 hr ÷ Q8 hr PO
  15–28 days old: 75 mg/kg/24 hr ÷ Q6 hr PO
1–2 kg:
  ≤7 days old: 75 mg/kg/24 hr ÷ Q8 hr PO
  8–28 days old: 75 mg/kg/24 hr ÷ Q6 hr PO
>2 kg and ≤60 days old: 75 mg/kg/24 hr ÷ Q6 hr PO

Dosages of 75–100 mg/kg/24 hr have been used in neonates (preterm and term) for candidal meningitis.
Child and adult (monitor serum concentrations): 50–150 mg/kg/24 hr ÷ Q6 hr PO

Monitor CBC, BUN, serum creatinine, alkaline phosphatase, AST, and ALT. Common side effects: nausea, vomiting, diarrhea, rash, CNS disturbance, anemia, leukopenia, and thrombocytopenia. **Use with caution** in hepatic and renal impairment and hematologic disorders. Use is **contraindicated** in the first trimester of pregnancy.

Therapeutic levels: 25–100 mg/L. Recommended serum sampling time at steady-state: Obtain peak level 2–4 hr after oral dose following 4 days of continuous dosing. Peak levels of 40–60 mg/L have been recommended for systemic candidiasis. Maintain trough levels above 25 mg/L. Prolonged levels above 100 mg/L can increase risk for bone marrow suppression. Bone marrow suppression in immunosuppressed patients can be irreversible and fatal.

Flucytosine interferes with creatinine assay tests using the dry-slide enzymatic method (Kodak Ektachem analyzer). **Adjust dose in renal failure (see Chapter 30).**

FLUDROCORTISONE ACETATE
Generics (previously available as Florinef); 9-fluorohydrocortisone
Corticosteroid

No   Yes   3   C

Tabs: 0.1 mg

Infant and child: 0.05–0.1 mg/24 hr once daily PO
  Congenital adrenal hyperplasia: 0.05–0.3 mg/24 hr once daily PO
Adult: 0.05–0.2 mg/24 hr once daily PO

FLUDROCORTISONE ACETATE continued

Contraindicated in CHF and systemic fungal infections. Has primarily mineralocorticoid activity. **Use with caution** in hypertension, edema, or renal dysfunction. May cause hypertension, hypokalemia, acne, rash, bruising, headaches, GI ulcers, and growth suppression.

Monitor BP and serum electrolytes. See Chapter 10 for steroid potency comparison.

Drug interactions: Drug's hypokalemic effects may induce digoxin toxicity; phenytoin and rifampin may increase fludrocortisone metabolism.

Doses 0.2–2 mg/24 hr has been used in the management of severe orthostatic hypotension in adults. Use a gradual dosage; taper when discontinuing therapy.

FLUMAZENIL
Generics; previously available as Romazicon
Benzodiazepine antidote

Yes   No   ?   C

Injection: 0.1 mg/mL (5, 10 mL); contains parabens

Benzodiazepine overdose (IV, see remarks):
  Child (limited data): 0.01 mg/kg (**max. dose**: 0.2 mg) Q1 min PRN to a max. total cumulative dose of 1 mg. As an alternative for repeat bolus doses, a continuous infusion of 0.005–0.01 mg/kg/hr has been used.
  Adult: Initial dose: 0.2 mg over 30 sec; if needed, give 0.3 mg 30 sec later over 30 sec. Additional doses of 0.5 mg given over 30 sec Q1 min PRN up to a cumulative dose of 3 mg (usual cumulative dose: 1–3 mg). Patients with only a partial response to 3 mg may require additional slow titration to a total of 5 mg.

Reversal of benzodiazepine sedation (IV):
  Child: Initial dose: 0.01 mg/kg (**max. dose**: 0.2 mg) given over 15 sec; if needed, after 45 sec, give 0.01 mg/kg (**max. dose**: 0.2 mg) Q1 min to a max. total cumulative dose of 0.05 mg/kg or 1 mg, whichever is lower. Usual total dose: 0.08–1 mg (average 0.65 mg).
  Adult: Initial dose: 0.2 mg over 15 sec; if needed, after 45 sec, give 0.2 mg Q1 min to a max. total cumulative dose of 1 mg. Doses may be repeated at 20 min interval (**max. dose** of 1 mg per 20 min interval) up to a **max. dose** of 3 mg in 1 hr.

Does not reverse narcotics. Onset of benzodiazepine reversal occurs in 1–3 min. Reversal effects of flumazenil ($T_{1/2}$ approximately 1 hr) may wear off sooner than benzodiazepine effects. If patient does not respond after cumulative 1–3-mg dose, suspect agent other than benzodiazepines.

May precipitate seizures, especially in patients taking benzodiazepines for seizure control or in patients with tricyclic antidepressant overdose. Fear, panic attacks in patients with history of panic disorders have been reported.

Use with caution in liver dysfunction; flumazenil's clearance is significantly reduced. Use normal dose for initial dose and decrease the dosage and frequency for subsequent doses.

See Chapter 2 for complete management of suspected ingestions.

FLUNISOLIDE
Nasal solution: generics; previously available as Nasarel or Nasalide
Oral inhaler: Aerospan
Corticosteroid

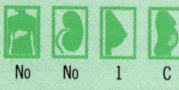
No   No   1   C

Nasal solution: 25 mcg/spray (200 sprays/bottle) (25 mL)
Oral aerosol inhaler:
  Aerospan: 80 mcg/dose (60 doses/5.1 g, 120 doses/8.9 g); CFC-free (HFA)

For all dosage forms, after symptoms are controlled, reduce to lowest effective maintenance dose (e.g., 1 spray each nostril once daily) to control symptoms.
Nasal solution:
  Child (6–14 yr):
    Initial: 1 spray per nostril TID or 2 sprays per nostril BID; **max. dose**: 4 sprays per nostril/24 hr.
  ≥15 yr and adult:
    Initial: 2 sprays per nostril BID; if needed in 4–7 days, increase to 2 sprays per nostril TID; **max. dose**: 8 sprays per nostril/24 hr.
Oral inhaler (see remarks):
  Aerospan:
    Child 6–11 yr: 1 puff BID; **max. dose**: 4 puffs/24 hr
    ≥12 yr–adult: 2 puffs BID; **max. dose**: 8 puffs/24 hr

May cause a reduction in growth velocity. Shake inhaler or nasal solution well before use. Patients using nasal solution should clear nasal passages before use. Flunisolide is a minor substrate of CYP450 3A4.

Do not use a spacer with Aerospan because the product has a self-contained spacer. Rinse mouth after administering drug by inhaler to prevent thrush.

FLUORIDE
Fluorabon, Fluor-A-Day, Fluoritab, Lozi-Flur, many others, and generics
Mineral

No   No   2   B

Concentrations and strengths based on fluoride ion:
Oral drops: 0.125 mg/drop (30 mL), 0.25 mg/drop (24 mL)
  Fluorabon: 0.42 mg/mL (60 mL)
Chewable tabs (Fluor-A-Day, Fluoritab, and generics): 0.25, 0.5, 1 mg
Lozenges (Lozi-Flur): 1 mg
See Chapter 21 for fluoride-containing multivitamins.

All doses/24 hr (see table below):
Recommendations from American Academy of Pediatrics and American Dental Association.

Age	Concentration of fluoride in drinking water (ppm)		
	<0.3	0.3–0.6	>0.6
Birth–6 mo	0	0	0
6 mo–3 yr	0.25 mg	0	0
3–6 yr	0.5 mg	0.25 mg	0
6–16 yr	1 mg	0.5 mg	0

FLUORIDE continued

Contraindicated in areas where drinking water fluoridation is > 0.7 ppm. **Acute overdose:** GI distress, salivation, CNS irritability, tetany, seizures, hypocalcemia, hypoglycemia, and cardiorespiratory failure. Chronic excess use may result in mottled teeth or bone changes.
Take with food, but **not** milk, to minimize GI upset. The doses have been decreased owing to concerns over dental fluorosis.

FLUOXETINE HYDROCHLORIDE
Prozac, Sarafem, Prozac Weekly, and generics
Antidepressant, selective serotonin reuptake inhibitor

Yes   Yes   X   C

Oral solution: 20 mg/5 mL; may contain alcohol
Caps: 10, 20, 40 mg
Delayed-released caps (Prozac Weekly and generics): 90 mg
Tabs: 10, 20, 60 mg

Depression:
  Child, 8–18 yr: Start at 10–20 mg once daily PO. If started with 10 mg/24 hr, may increase dose to 20 mg/24 hr after 1 wk. Use lower 10 mg/24 hr initial dose for lower-weight children; if needed, increase to 20 mg/24 hr after several weeks.
  Adult: Start at 20 mg once daily PO. May increase after several weeks by 20 mg/24 hr increments to **max. dose** of 80 mg/24 hr. Doses > 20 mg/24 hr should be divided BID.

Obsessive-compulsive disorder:
  Child, 7–18 yr:
    Lower-weight child: Start at 10 mg once daily PO. May increase after several weeks. Usual dose range: 20–30 mg/24 hr. There is very minimal experience with doses > 20 mg/24 hr and no experience with doses > 60 mg/24 hr.
    Higher-weight child and adolescent: Start at 10 mg daily PO and increase dose to 20 mg/24 hr after 2 wk. May further increase dose after several weeks. Usual dose range: 20–60 mg/24 hr.

Bulimia:
  Adolescent (PO; limited data): 20 mg QAM × 3 days, then 40 mg QAM × 3 days, then 60 mg QAM.
  Adult: 60 mg QAM PO; it is recommended to titrate up to this dose over several days.

Premenstrual dysphoric disorder:
  Adult: Start at 20 mg once daily PO using the Sarafem product. **Max. dose:** 80 mg/24 hr. Systematic evaluation has shown that efficacy is maintained for periods of 6 mo at a dose of 20 mg/day. Reassess patients periodically to determine the need for continued treatment.

Contraindicated in patients taking MAO inhibitors (e.g., linezolid) due to possibility of seizures, hyperpyrexia, and coma. **Use with caution** in patients with angle-closure glaucoma, receiving diuretics, or with liver (reduce dose with cirrhosis) or renal impairment. May increase the effects of tricyclic antidepressants. May cause headache, insomnia, nervousness, drowsiness, GI disturbance, and weight loss. Increased bleeding diathesis with unaltered prothrombin time may occur with warfarin. Hyponatremia has been reported. Monitor for clinical worsening of depression and suicidal ideation/behavior following the initiation of therapy or after dose changes.

May displace other highly protein-bound drugs. Inhibits CYP450 2C19, 2D6, and 3A3/4 drug metabolism isoenzymes, which may increase the effects or toxicity of drugs metabolized by these

Continued

FLUOXETINE HYDROCHLORIDE continued

enzymes. Use with serotonergic drugs (e.g., triptans and methylene blue) and drugs that impair serotonin metabolism (MAOIs) may increase the risk for serotonin syndrome. Carefully review the patients' medication profile for potential interactions.

Delayed-release capsule is currently indicated for depression and is dosed at 90 mg Q7 days. It is unknown if weekly dosing provides the same protection from relapse as does daily dosing.

Breast-feeding is not recommended by the manufacturer as adverse events in nursing infants have been reported. Fluoxetine and metabolite are variable and are higher when compared to other SSRIs. Maternal use of SSRIs during pregnancy and postpartum may result in more difficult breastfeeding. Infants exposed to SSRIs during pregnancy may also have an increased risk for persistent pulmonary hypertension of the newborn.

FLUTICASONE FUROATE + VILANTEROL
Breo Ellipta
Corticosteroid and long-acting β_2-adrenergic agonist

Yes   No   2   C

Aerosol powder for inhalation (Breo Ellipta):
100 mcg fluticasone furoate + 25 mcg vilanterol per inhalation (28, 60 inhalations)
200 mcg fluticasone furoate + 25 mcg vilanterol per inhalation (28, 60 inhalations)
For Fluticasone Furoate (Arnuity Ellipta) as a single agent, see Fluticasone Preparations.

Asthma:
Adult: one inhalation of 100 mcg fluticasone furoate + 25 mcg vilanterol OR 200 mcg fluticasone furoate + 25 mcg vilanterol once daily.
Max. dose: one inhalation/24 hr for either dosage strength (25 mcg vilanterol/24 hr).

See Fluticasone Preparations for remarks. Vilanterol is a long-acting β_2-adrenergic agonist with a faster onset and longer duration of action compared to salmeterol.
Hypersensitivity reactions, muscle spasms, and tremor have been reported.
Titrate to the lowest effective strength after asthma is adequately controlled. Proper patient education including dosage administration technique is essential; see patient package insert for detailed instructions. Rinse mouth after each use.

FLUTICASONE PREPARATIONS
Fluticasone propionate: Flonase, Cutivate, Flovent Diskus, Flovent HFA, and generics
Fluticasone furoate: Veramyst, Flonase Sensimist, and Arnuity Ellipta
Corticosteroid

Yes   No   2   C

FLUTICASONE PROPIONATE
Nasal spray (Flonase and generics; OTC): 50 mcg/actuation (9.9 mL = 60 doses, 15.8 mL = 120 doses)
Topical cream (Cutivate and generics): 0.05% (15, 30, 60 g)
Topical ointment (Cutivate and generics): 0.005% (15, 30, 60 g)
Topical lotion (Cutivate and generics): 0.05% (60, 120 mL)
Aerosol inhaler (MDI) (Flovent HFA): 44 mcg/actuation (10.6 g), 110 mcg/actuation (12 g), 220 mcg/actuation (12 g); each inhaler provides 120 metered inhalations

FLUTICASONE PREPARATIONS continued

Dry-powder inhalation (DPI) (Flovent Diskus): 50 mcg/dose, 100 mcg/dose, 250 mcg/dose; all strengths come in a package of 15 Rotadisks; each Rotadisk provides 4 doses for a total of 60 doses per package

FLUTICASONE FUROATE

Nasal spray (Veramyst, Flonase Sensimist [OTC]): 27.5 mcg/actuation (10 g = 120 doses)
Oral inhalation powder (Arnuity Ellipta): 100 mcg/metered dose (14, 30), 200 mcg/metered dose (14, 30)

Intranasal (allergic rhinitis):
  Fluticasone propionate (Flonase and generics):
    ≥4 yr and adolescent: 1 spray (50 mcg) per nostril once daily. Dose may be increased to 2 sprays (100 mcg) per nostril once daily if inadequate response or severe symptoms. Reduce to 1 spray per nostril once daily when symptoms are controlled.
    Adult: Initial 200 mcg/24 hr [2 sprays (100 mcg) per nostril once daily; OR 1 spray (50 mcg) per nostril BID]. Reduce to 1 spray per nostril once daily when symptoms are controlled.
    Max. dose (4 yr–adult): 2 sprays (100 mcg) per nostril/24 hr
  Fluticasone furoate (Veramyst):
    2–11 yr: 1 spray (27.5 mcg) per nostril once daily. If needed, dose may be increased to 2 sprays each nostril once daily. Reduce to 1 spray per nostril once daily when symptoms are controlled.
    ≥11 yr and adult: 2 sprays (55 mcg) each nostril once daily. Reduce to 1 spray per nostril once daily when symptoms are controlled.
    Max. dose (2 yr–adult): 2 sprays (55 mcg) per nostril/24 hr

Oral inhalation (asthma):
  Fluticasone propionate (Flovent HFA and Diskus): **Divide all 24-hr doses BID.** If desired response is not seen after 2 wk of starting therapy, increase dosage. Then reduce to the lowest effective dose when asthma symptoms are controlled. Administration of MDI (HFA) with aerochamber enhances drug delivery.
  Recommended dosages for asthma (see following table).

Age	Previous Use of Bronchodilators Only: (Max. Dose)	Previous Use of Inhaled Corticosteroid: (Max. Dose)	Previous Use of Oral Corticosteroid: (Max. Dose)
Child (4–11 yr)	MDI: 88 mcg/24 hr (176 mcg/24 hr) DPI: 100 mcg/24 hr (200 mcg/24 hr)	MDI: 88 mcg/24 hr (176 mcg/24 hr) DPI: 100 mcg/24 hr (200 mcg/24 hr)	Dose not available
≥12 yr and adult	MDI: 176 mcg/24 hr (880 mcg/24 hr) DPI: 200 mcg/24 hr (1000 mcg/24 hr)	MDI: 176–440 mcg/24 hr (880 mcg/24 hr) DPI: 200–500 mcg/24 hr (1000 mcg/24 hr)	MDI: 880 mcg/24 hr (1760 mcg/24 hr) DPI: 1000–2000 mcg/24 hr (2000 mcg/24 hr)

DPI, Dry powder inhaler; MDI, metered dose inhaler

  Fluticasone furoate (Arnuity Ellipta):
    ≥12 yr and adult: Inhale 100–200 mcg once daily; **max. dose**: 200 mcg/24 hr.
  Eosinophillic esophagitis (limited data; use oral fluticasone propionate HFA dosage form without spacer for PO administration as doses are swallowed):
    Child (1–10 yr): 220 mcg QID × 4 wk, then 220 mcg TID × 3 wk, then 220 mcg BID × 3 wk, and 220 mcg once daily × 2 wk.
    Child ≥11 yr and adult: 440 mcg QID × 4 wk, then 440 mcg TID × 3 wk, then 440 mcg BID × 3 wk, and 440 mcg once daily × 2 wk.

Continued

FLUTICASONE PREPARATIONS continued

Topical (reassess diagnosis if no improvement in 2 wk):
  Cream (see Chaper 10 for topical steroid comparisons):
    ≥3 mo and adult: Apply thin film to affected areas once daily–BID; then reduce to a less potent topical agent when symptoms are controlled.
  Lotion (see remarks):
    ≥1 yr and adult: Apply thin film to affected areas once daily. Safety of use has not been evaluated longer than 4 weeks.
  Ointment:
    Adult: Apply thin film to affected areas BID.

Fluticasone propionate and fluticasone furoate do not have equivalent potencies; follow specific dosing regimens for the respective products.

Concurrent administration with ritonavir and other CYP450 3A4 inhibitors may increase fluticasone levels resulting in Cushing syndrome and adrenal suppression. **Use with caution** and monitor closely in hepatic impairment.

Intranasal: Clear nasal passages prior to use. May cause epistaxis and nasal irritation, which are usually transient. Taste and smell alterations, rare hypersensitivity reactions (angioedema, pruritus, urticaria, wheezing, dyspnea), and nasal septal perforation have been reported in postmarketing studies.

Oral inhalation: Rinse mouth after each use. May cause dysphonia, oral thrush, and dermatitis. Esophageal candidiasis and hypersensitivity reactions have been reported. Compared to beclomethasone, it has shown to have less of an effect on suppressing linear growth in asthmatic children. Eosinophilic conditions may occur with the withdrawal or decrease of oral corticosteroids after the initiation of inhaled fluticasone.

Topical use: **Avoid** application/contact to face, eyes, and open skin. Occlusive dressings are not recommended because they may increase local side effects (irritation, folliculitis, acneiform eruptions, hypopigmentation, perioral dermatitis, contact dermatitis, secondary infection, skin atrophy, striae, hypertrichosis, and miliaria). **Do not use** lotion dosage form with formaldehyde hypersensitivity.

FLUTICASONE PROPIONATE AND SALMETEROL
Advair Diskus, Advair HFA
Corticosteroid and long-acting β_2-adrenergic agonist

Yes   No   2   C

Dry powder inhalation (DPI) (Advair Diskus; contains lactose):
  100 mcg fluticasone propionate + 50 mcg salmeterol per inhalation (14, 60 inhalations).
  250 mcg fluticasone propionate + 50 mcg salmeterol per inhalation (60 inhalations).
  500 mcg fluticasone propionate + 50 mcg salmeterol per inhalation (60 inhalations).
Aerosol inhaler (MDI) (Advair HFA):
  45 mcg fluticasone propionate + 21 mcg salmeterol per inhalation (8 g delivers 60 doses, 12 g delivers 120 doses).
  115 mcg fluticasone propionate + 21 mcg salmeterol per inhalation (8 g delivers 60 doses, 12 g delivers 120 doses).
  230 mcg fluticasone propionate + 21 mcg salmeterol per inhalation (8 g delivers 60 doses, 12 g delivers 120 doses).

Asthma:
  Without prior inhaled steroid use:
    Dry powder inhalation (DPI):
      4–11 yr: Start with one inhalation BID of 100 mcg fluticasone propionate + 50 mcg salmeterol.

FLUTICASONE PROPIONATE AND SALMETEROL continued

≥12 yr and adult: Start with one inhalation BID of 100 mcg fluticasone propionate + 50 mcg salmeterol, OR 250 mcg fluticasone propionate + 50 mcg salmeterol; **max. dose:** one inhalation BID of 500 mcg fluticasone propionate + 50 mcg salmeterol.

Aerosol inhaler (MDI):
≥12 yr and adult: 2 inhalations BID of 45 mcg fluticasone + 21 mcg salmeterol, OR 115 mcg fluticasone + 21 mcg salmeterol; **max. dose:** 2 inhalations BID of 230 mcg fluticasone + 21 mcg salmeterol.

With prior inhaled steroid use (conversion from other inhaled steroids; see following table):

Inhaled Corticosteroid	Current Daily Dose	Recommended Strength of Fluticasone Propionate + Salmeterol Diskus (DPI) (Advair Diskus) Administered at One Inhalation BID	Recommended Strength of Fluticasone Propionate + Salmeterol Aerosol Inhaler (MDI) (Advair HFA) Administered at Two Inhalations BID
Beclomethasone dipropionate (Qvar; CFC-free, HFA)	160 mcg	100 mcg + 50 mcg	45 mcg + 21 mcg
	320 mcg	250 mcg + 50 mcg	115 mcg + 21 mcg
	640 mcg	500 mcg + 50 mcg	230 mcg + 21 mcg
Budesonide	≤400 mcg	100 mcg + 50 mcg	45 mcg + 21 mcg
	800–1200 mcg	250 mcg + 50 mcg	115 mcg + 21 mcg
	1600 mcg	500 mcg + 50 mcg	230 mcg + 21 mcg
Flunisolide (Aerospan; CFC-free, HFA)	≤320 mcg	100 mcg + 50 mcg	45 mcg + 21 mcg
	640 mcg	250 mcg + 50 mcg	115 mcg + 21 mcg
Fluticasone propionate aerosol (HFA)	≤176 mcg	100 mcg + 50 mcg	45 mcg + 21 mcg
	440 mcg	250 mcg + 50 mcg	115 mcg + 21 mcg
	660–880 mcg	500 mcg + 50 mcg	230 mcg + 21 mcg
Fluticasone propionate dry powder (DPI)	≤200 mcg	100 mcg + 50 mcg	45 mcg + 21 mcg
	500 mcg	250 mcg + 50 mcg	115 mcg + 21 mcg
	1000 mcg	500 mcg + 50 mcg	230 mcg + 21 mcg
Mometasone furoate	220 mcg	100 mcg + 50 mcg	45 mcg + 21 mcg
	440 mcg	250 mcg + 50 mcg	115 mcg + 21 mcg
	880 mcg	500 mcg + 50 mcg	230 mcg + 21 mcg

Max. doses:
Dry powder inhalation (DPI): one inhalation BID of 500 mcg fluticasone propionate + 50 mcg salmeterol.
Aerosol inhaler (MDI): two inhalations BID of 230 mcg fluticasone propionate + 21 mcg salmeterol.

See *Fluticasone Preparations* and *Salmeterol* for remarks. Titrate to the lowest effective strength after asthma is adequately controlled. Proper patient education, including dosage administration technique, is essential; see patient package insert for detailed instructions. Rinse mouth after each use.

FLUVOXAMINE
Generics; previously available as Luvox and Luvox CR
Antidepressant, selective serotonin reuptake inhibitor

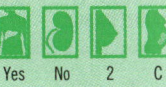

Yes   No   2   C

Tabs: 25, 50, 100 mg
Extended-release capsules: 100, 150 mg

Continued

FLUVOXAMINE continued

Obsessive-compulsive disorder (use immediate-release tablets unless noted otherwise):
8–17 yr: Start at 25 mg PO QHS. Dose may be increased by 25 mg/24 hr Q7–14 days (slower titration for minimizing behavioral side effects). Total daily doses >50 mg/24 hr should be divided BID. Female patients may require lower dosages compared to males.
   Max. dose: Child: 8–11 yr: 200 mg/24 hr; and child ≥12–17 yr: 300 mg/24 hr.
Adult: Start at 50 mg PO QHS. Dose may be increased by 50 mg/24 hr Q4–7 days up to a **max. dose** of 300 mg/24 hr. Total daily doses >100 mg/24 hr should be divided BID.
   Extended-release capsule (adult): Start at 100 mg PO QHS. Dose may be increased by 50 mg/24 hr Q7 days up to a **max. dose** of 300 mg/24 hr.

Contraindicated with the coadministration of cisapride, pimozide, thioridazine, tizanidine, or MAO inhibitors. **Use with caution** in hepatic disease (dosage reduction may be necessary); drug is extensively metabolized by the liver. Monitor for clinical worsening of depression and suicidal ideation/behavior following the initiation of therapy or after dose changes.

Inhibits CYP450 1A2, 2C19, 2D6, and 3A3/4, which may increase the effects or toxicity of drugs metabolized by these enzymes. Dose-related use of thioridazine with fluvoxamine may cause the prolongation of QT interval and serious arrhythmias. May increase warfarin plasma levels by 98% and prolong PT. May increase toxicity and/or levels of theophylline, caffeine, and tricyclic antidepressants. Side effects include: headache, insomnia, somnolence, nausea, diarrhea, dyspepsia, and dry mouth.

Titrate to lowest effective dose. Use a gradual taper when discontinuing therapy to prevent withdrawal symptoms.

Consider the benefits to potential risk for maternal use in breast feeding. Maternal use during pregnancy and postpartum may result in breastfeeding difficulties.

FOLIC ACID
Folvite and many other generics
Water-soluble vitamin

| No | No | 1 | A/C |

Tabs [OTC]: 0.4, 0.8, 1 mg
Caps: 0.4 mg [OTC], 0.8 mg [OTC], 5 mg, 20 mg
Oral solution: 50 mcg/mL
Injection: 5 mg/mL; contains 1.5% benzyl alcohol

For U.S. RDA, see Chapter 21.
Folic acid deficiency PO, IM, IV, SC (see following table)

Infant	Child 1–10 yr	Child ≥ 11 yr and Adult
INITIAL DOSE		
15 mcg/kg/dose; **max. dose** 50 mcg/24 hr	1 mg/dose	1 mg/dose
MAINTENANCE		
30–45 mcg/24 hr once daily	0.1–0.4 mg/24 hr once daily	0.4 mg/24 hr once daily; Pregnant/lactating women: 0.8 mg/24 hr once daily

Normal levels: **see Chapter 21.** May mask hematologic effects of vitamin B$_{12}$ deficiency but will not prevent the progression of neurologic abnormalities. High dose folic acid may decrease the absorption of phenytoin.

FOLIC ACID continued

Women of child-bearing age considering pregnancy should take at least 0.4 mg once daily before and during pregnancy to reduce the risk of neural tube defects in the fetus. Pregnancy category changes to "C" if used in doses above the RDA.

FOMEPIZOLE
Antizol and generics
Antidote for ethylene glycol or methanol toxicity

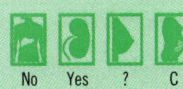
No   Yes   ?   C

Injection: 1 g/mL (1.5 mL); preservative free

Child and adult not requiring hemodialysis (IV, all doses administered over 30 min):
  Load: 15 mg/kg/dose × 1
  Maintenance: 10 mg/kg/dose Q12 hr × 4 doses, then 15 mg/kg/dose Q12 hr until ethylene glycol or methanol level decreases to <20 mg/dL and the patient is asymptomatic with normal pH.
Child and adult requiring hemodialysis (IV following the recommended doses at the intervals indicated here. Fomepizole is removed by dialysis. All doses administered IV over 30 min):
  Dosing at the beginning of hemodialysis:
    If < 6 hr since last fomepizole dose: **DO NOT** administer dose.
    If ≥ 6 hr since last fomepizole dose: Administer next scheduled dose.
  Dosing during hemodialysis: Administer Q4 hr or as continuous infusion of 1–1.5 mg/kg/hr.
  Dosing at the time hemodialysis is completed (based on the time between last dose and end of hemodialysis):
    <1 hr: **DO NOT** administer dose at end of hemodialysis.
    1–3 hr: Administer 1/2 of next scheduled dose.
    >3 hr: Administer next scheduled dose.
  Maintenance dose off hemodialysis: Give next scheduled dose 12 hr from last dose administered.

Works by competitively inhibiting alcohol dehydrogenase. Safety and efficacy in pediatrics have not been established. **Contraindicated** in hypersensitivity to any components or other pyrazole compounds. Most frequent side effects include headache, nausea, and dizziness. Fomepizole is extensively eliminated by the kidneys (**use with caution** in renal failure) and removed by hemodialysis.

Drug may solidify at temperatures <25°C (77°F); vial can be liquefied by running it under warm water (efficacy, safety, and stability are not affected). All doses must be diluted with at least 100 mL of D_5W or NS to prevent vein irritation.

FORMOTEROL
Foradil Aerolizer, Perforomist
β₂-adrenergic agonist (long acting)

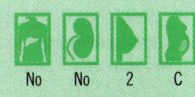
No   No   2   C

Inhalation powder in capsules (Foradil Aerolizer): 12 mcg (12s and 60s); contains lactose and milk proteins. Use with Aerolizer inhaler.
Inhalation solution (Perforomist): 20 mcg/2 mL (60s)

≥5 yr and adult:
  Asthma/Bronchodilation (should be used with an inhaled corticosteroid):
    Foradil Aerolizer: 12 mcg Q12 hr; **max. dose:** 24 mcg/24 hr (12 mcg spaced 12 hr apart)

Continued

FORMOTEROL continued

Prevention of exercise-induced asthma for patients NOT receiving maintenance long-acting β₂-agonists (e.g., formoterol or salmeterol):
    Foradil Aerolizer: 12 mcg 15 min prior to exercise. If needed, an additional dose may be given only AFTER 12 hr. **Max. dose:** 24 mcg/24 hr (12 mcg spaced 12 hr apart). Consider alternative therapy if maximum dosage is not effective.

Fast onset of action (1–3 min) with peak effects in 0.5–1 hr and long duration (up to 12 hr). Although long-acting β₂-adrenergic agonists may decrease the frequency of asthma episodes, they may make asthma episodes more severe when they occur. **Use with caution** in seizures, thyrotoxicosis, diabetes, ketoacidosis, aneurysm, and pheochromocytoma. Abdominal pain, dyspepsia, nausea, and tremor may occur.

Inhalation solution product (Perforomist) is indicated for COPD in adults [20 mcg Q12 hr; **max. dose:** 40 mcg/24 hr (20 mcg spaced 12 hr apart)].

WARNING: Long-acting β₂-agonists may increase the risk of asthma-related death. Only use formoterol as additional therapy for patients not adequately controlled on other asthma-controller medications (e.g., low- to medium-dose inhaled corticosteroids) or whose disease severity clearly requires initiation of treatment with 2 maintenance therapies. Should **not** be used in conjunction with an inhaled, long-acting β₂-agonist and is **not** a substitute for inhaled or systemic corticosteroids. See Chapter 24 for recommendations for asthma controller therapy.

FOSCARNET
Foscavir and generics
Antiviral agent

No   Yes   3   C

Injection: 24 mg/mL (250, 500 mL)
Contains 10 mEq Na/g drug

HIV positive or exposed with the following infection (IV):
  CMV disease:
    Infant and child:
      Induction: 180 mg/kg/24 hr ÷ Q8 hr in combination with ganciclovir, continue until symptom improvement and convert to maintenance therapy
      Maintenance: 90–120 mg/kg/dose Q24 hr
  CMV retinitis (disseminated disease):
    Infant and child:
      Induction: 180 mg/kg/24 hr ÷ Q8 hr × 14–21 days with or without ganciclovir,
      Maintenance: 90–120 mg/kg/24 hr once daily
    Adolescent and adult:
      Induction: 180 mg/kg/24 hr ÷ Q8–12 hr × 14–21 days
      Maintenance: 90–120 mg/kg/24 hr once daily
  Acyclovir-resistant herpes simplex:
    Infant and child: 40 mg/kg/dose Q8 hr or 60 mg/kg/dose Q12 hr for up to 3 wk or until lesions heal
    Adolescent and adult: 40 mg/kg/dose Q8–12 hr × 14–21 days or until lesions heal
  Varicella zoster unresponsive to acyclovir:
    Infant and child: 40–60 mg/kg/dose Q8 hr × 7–10 days
    Adolescent: 90 mg/kg/dose Q12 hr
  Varicella zoster, progressive outer retinal necrosis:
    Infant and child: 90 mg/kg/dose Q12 hr in combination with ganciclovir IV and intravitreal foscarnet with or without ganciclovir
    Adolescent: 90 mg/kg/dose every 12 hr in combination with IV ganciclovir and intravitreal foscarnet and/or ganciclovir

FOSCARNET continued

Intravitreal route for progressive outer retinal necrosis (HIV positive or exposed):
  Child and adolescent: 1.2 mg/0.05 mL per dose twice weekly in combination with IV foscarnet and ganciclovir and/or intravitreal ganciclovir

Use with caution in patients with renal insufficiency and hypernatremia (large sodium content). **Discontinue** use in adults if serum Cr ≥ 2.9 mg/dL. **Adjust dose in renal failure (see Chapter 30).**

May cause peripheral neuropathy, seizures, neutropenia, esophageal ulceration, hallucinations, GI disturbance, increased LFTs, hypertension, chest pain, ECG abnormalities, coughing, dyspnea, bronchospasm, and renal failure (adequate hydration and avoiding nephrotoxic medications may reduce risk). Hypocalcemia (increased risk if given with pentamidine), hypokalemia, and hypomagnesemia may also occur. Use with ciprofloxacin may increase risk for seizures.

Correction of dehydration and adequate hydration reduces the risk for nephrotoxicity; 10–20 mL/kg IV (**max. dose:** 1000 mL) of NS or D₅W should be administer prior to the first dose and concurrently with subsequent doses. For lower foscarnet dosage regimens of 40–60 mg/kg, use 50% of the aforementioned hydration recommendations. Actual hydration may need to be reduced when clinically indicated. Oral hydration methods may also be considered in patients who are able to tolerate.

For peripheral line IV administration, the concentration must be diluted to 12 mg/mL in NS or D₅W.

FOSPHENYTOIN
Cerebyx and generics
Anticonvulsant

Yes Yes 3 D

Injection: 50 mg phenytoin equivalent (75 mg fosphenytoin)/1 mL (2, 10 mL)
1 mg phenytoin equivalent provides 0.0037 mmol phosphate.

All doses are expressed as phenytoin sodium equivalents (PE) (see remarks for dose administration information):
Child: See Phenytoin and use the conversion of 1 mg phenytoin = 1 mg PE
Adult:
  Loading dose:
    Status epilepticus: 15–20 mg PE/kg IV
    Nonemergent loading: 10–20 mg PE/kg IV/IM
  Nonemergent initial maintenance dose: 4–6 mg PE/kg/24 hr IV/IM ÷ Q12–24 hr

All doses should be prescribed and dispensed in terms of mg phenytoin sodium equivalents (PE) to avoid medication errors. Safety in pediatrics has not been fully established.

Use with caution in patients with renal or hepatic impairment and porphyria (consider amount of phosphate delivered by fosphenytoin in patients with phosphate restrictions). Drug is also metabolized to liberate small amounts of formaldehyde, which is considered clinically insignificant with short-term use (e.g., 1 wk). Side effects: hypokalemia (with rapid IV administration), slurred speech, dizziness, ataxia, rash, exfoliative dermatitis, nystagmus, diplopia, and tinnitus. Increased unbound phenytoin concentrations may occur in patients with renal disease or hypoalbuminemia; measure "free" or "unbound" phenytoin levels in these patients.

Abrupt withdrawal may cause status epilepticus. BP and ECG monitoring should be present during IV loading dose administration. **Max. IV infusion rate:** 3 mg PE/kg/min up to a **max.** of 150 mg PE/min. Administer IM via 1 or 2 injection sites and IM route is **not recommended** in status epilepticus.

Continued

FOSPHENYTOIN continued

Therapeutic levels: 10–20 mg/L (free and bound phenytoin) *OR* 1–2 mg/L (free only). Recommended peak serum sampling times: 4 hr following an IM dose or 2 hr following an IV dose.

See *Phenytoin* remarks for drug interactions and additional side effects. Drug is more safely administered via peripheral IV than phenytoin.

FUROSEMIDE
Lasix and generics
Loop diuretic

Yes   Yes   3   C/D

Tabs: 20, 40, 80 mg
Injection: 10 mg/mL (2, 4, 10 mL)
Oral solution: 10 mg/mL (60, 120 mL), 40 mg/5 mL (5, 500 mL)

IM, IV:
 Neonate (see remarks): 0.5–1 mg/kg/dose Q8–24 hr; **max. dose:** 2 mg/kg/dose
 Infant and child: 1–2 mg/kg/dose Q6–12 hr
 Adult: 20–40 mg/24 hr ÷ Q6–12 hr; **max. dose:** 200 mg/dose

PO:
 Neonate: Bioavailability by this route is poor; doses of 1–3 mg/kg/dose once daily to BID have been used
 Infant and child: Start at 2 mg/kg/dose; may increase by 1–2 mg/kg/dose no sooner than 6–8 hr following the previous dose. **Max. dose:** 6 mg/kg/dose. Dosages have ranged from 1–6 mg/kg/dose Q12–24 hr
 Adult: 20–80 mg/dose Q6–12 hr; **max. dose:** 600 mg/24 hr

Continuous IV infusion:
 Infant and child: Start at 0.05 mg/kg/hr and titrate to effect
 Adult: Start at 0.1 mg/kg/hr and titrate to effect; **max. dose:** 0.4 mg/kg/hr

Contraindicated in anuria and hepatic coma. **Use with caution** in hepatic disease (hepatic encephalopathy has been reported); cirrhotic patients may require higher than usual doses. Ototoxicity may occur in presence of renal disease (especially when used with aminoglycosides), with rapid IV injection (do not infuse > 4 mg/min in adults), or with hypoproteinemia. May cause hypokalemia, alkalosis, dehydration, hyperuricemia, and increased calcium excretion. Rash with eosinophilia and systemic symptoms and acute generalized exanthematous pustulosis have been reported. Prolonged use in premature infants and in children <4 yr may result in nephrocalcinosis. May increase risk for PDA in premature infants during the first week of life.

Furosemide-resistant edema in pediatric patients may benefit with the addition of metolazone. Some of these patients may have an exaggerated response leading to hypovolemia, tachycardia, and orthostatic hypotension requiring fluid replacement. Severe hypokalemia has been reported with a tendency for diuresis persisting for up to 24 hr after discontinuing metolazone.

Max. rate of intermittent IV dose: 0.5 mg/kg/min. For patients receiving ECMO, **do not** administer IV doses directly into the ECMO circuit as the medication is absorbed in the circuit, which may result in diminished effects and the need for higher doses.

Pregnancy category changes to "D" if used in pregnancy-induced hypertension.

GABAPENTIN
Neurontin, Fanatrex FusePaq, Gralise, Horizant, and other generics
Anticonvulsant

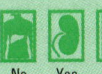
No   Yes   2   C

Caps: 100, 300, 400 mg
Tabs: 300, 600, 800 mg
Slow-release/extended-release tabs (these dosage forms are **not** interchangeable with other gabapentin products due to different pharmacokinetic profiles affecting the dosing interval; see specific product information for specific indications for use and dosage):
  Gralise: 300, 600 mg
  Horizant (Gabapentin Enacarbil): 300, 600 mg
Oral solution: 250 mg/5 mL (470 mL)
Oral suspension (Fanatrex FusePaq): 25 mg/mL (420 mL); contains saccharin and sodium benzoate

Seizures, *adjunctive therapy (maximum time between doses should not exceed 12 hr):*
  3–<12 yr (PO, see remarks):
    Day 1: 10–15 mg/kg/24 hr ÷ TID, then gradually titrate dose upward to the following dosages over a 3-day period:
      3–4 yr: 40 mg/kg/24 hr ÷ TID
      ≥5–12 yr: 25–35 mg/kg/24 hr ÷ TID
    Dosages up to 50 mg/kg/24 hr have been well tolerated.
  ≥12 yr and adult (PO, see remarks): Start with 300 mg TID; if needed, increase dose up to 1800 mg/24 hr ÷ TID. Usual effective doses: 900–1800 mg/24 hr ÷ TID. Doses as high as 3.6 g/24 hr have been tolerated.
Neuropathic pain:
  Child (PO; limited data):
    Day 1: 5 mg/kg/dose (max. 300 mg/dose) at bedtime
    Day 2: 5 mg/kg/dose (max. 300 mg/dose) BID
    Day 3: 5 mg/kg/dose (max. 300 mg/dose) TID; then titrate dose to effect. Usual dosage range: 8–35 mg/kg/24 hr
    Maximum daily dose of 3600 mg/24 hr has been suggested but not formally evaluated.
  Adult (PO):
    Day 1: 300 mg at bedtime
    Day 2: 300 mg BID
    Day 3: 300 mg TID; then titrate dose to effect. Usual dosage range: 1800–2400 mg/24 hr; max. dose: 3600 mg/24 hr
    Postherpetic neuralgia: The above dosage regimen may be titrated up PRN for pain relief to a daily dose of 1800 mg/24 hr ÷ TID (efficacy has been shown from 1800 to 3600 mg/24 hr; however, no additional benefit has been shown for doses >1800 mg/24 hr). The Gralise dosage form is designed for once daily administration with evening meals, whereas the Horizant dosage form is dosed once daily-BID. See specific product information for details.

Generally used as adjunctive therapy for partial and secondary generalized seizures and neuropathic pain.
Somnolence, dizziness, ataxia, fatigue, and nystagmus were common when used for seizures (≥12 yr). Viral infections, fever, nausea and/or vomiting, somnolence, and hostility have been reported in patients aged 3–12 yr receiving other antiepiletics. Dizziness, somnolence, and peripheral edema are common side effects in adults with postherpetic neuralgia. Suicidal behavior

Continued

GABAPENTIN continued

or ideation and multiorgan hypersensitivity (e.g., anaphylaxis, angioedema, or DRESS) have been reported.

Do not withdraw medication abruptly (withdraw gradually over a minimum of 1 wk). Drug is not metabolized by the liver and is primarily excreted unchanged in the urine. Higher doses may be required for children aged <5 yr because of faster clearance in this age group.

May be taken with or without food. In TID dosing schedule, **interval between doses should not exceed 12 hr. Adjust dose in renal impairment (see Chapter 30).**

GANCICLOVIR
Cytovene, Zirgan, and generics
Antiviral agent

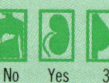

No　Yes　3　C

Injection (Cytovene and generics): 500 mg; contains 4 mEq Na per 1 g drug
Ophthalmic gel (drops):
　Zirgan: 0.15% (5 g); contains benzalkonium chloride

Cytomegalovirus (CMV) infections:
　Neonate (congenital CMV): 12 mg/kg/24 hr ÷ Q12 hr IV × 6 wk
　Child >3 mo and adult:
　　Induction therapy (duration 14–21 days): 10 mg/kg/24 hr ÷ Q12 hr IV
　　IV maintenance therapy: 5 mg/kg/dose once daily IV for 7 days/wk or 6 mg/kg/dose once daily IV for 5 days/wk
Prevention of CMV in transplant recipients:
　Child and adult:
　　Induction therapy (duration 7–14 days): 10 mg/kg/24 hr ÷ Q12 hr IV
　　IV maintenance therapy: 5 mg/kg/dose once daily IV for 7 days/wk or 6 mg/kg/dose once daily IV for 5 days/wk for 100–120 days posttransplant
Prevention of CMV in HIV-infected individuals (see www.aidsinfo.nih.gov for latest recommendations and guidelines for CMV treatment as well):
　Recurrence prophylaxis:
　　Infant, child, adolescent, and adult: 5 mg/kg/dose IV once daily. Consider valganciclovir as an oral alternative
Herpetic keratitis (ophthalmic gel/drops):
　≥2 yr and adult: Apply 1 drop on affected eye(s) 5 times a day (~Q3 hr while awake) until corneal ulcer is healed, then 1 drop TID × 7 days

Limited experience with use in children aged <12 yr. **Contraindicated** in severe neutropenia (ANC < 500/microliter) or severe thrombocytopenia (platelets < 25,000/microliter). **Use with extreme caution. Reduce dose in renal failure (see Chapter 30).** For oral route of administration, see *Valganciclovir*.

Common side effects include neutropenia, thrombocytopenia, retinal detachment, and confusion. Drug reactions alleviated with dose reduction or temporary interruption. Ganciclovir may increase didanosine and zidovudine levels, whereas didanosine and zidovudine may decrease ganciclovir levels. Immunosuppressive agents may increase hematologic toxicities. Amphotericin B, cyclosporine, and tacrolimus increase risk for nephrotoxicity. Imipenem/cilastatin may increase risk for seizures.

Minimum dilution is 10 mg/mL and should be infused IV over ≥ 1 hr. IM and SC administration is **contraindicated** because of a high pH of 11.

GATIFLOXACIN
Zymaxid, Zymar, and generics
Antibiotic, quinolone

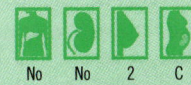
No　No　2　C

Ophthalmic solution:
  Zymaxid and generics: 0.5% (2.5 mL); may contain benzalkonium chloride
  Zymar: 0.3% (5 mL); contains benzalkonium chloride

Conjunctivitis:
  Zymaxid and generics (0.5%):
    ≥1 yr–adult: Instill 1 drop to affected eye(s) Q2 hr while awake (up to 8 times/24 hr) for the first day, then 1 drop BID–QID while awake on days 2–7.
  Zymar (0.3%):
    ≥1 yr–adult: Instill 1 drop to affected eye(s) Q2 hr while awake (up to 8 times/24 hr) for the first 2 days, then 1 drop QID while awake on days 3–7.

Worsening of conjunctivitis, decreased visual acuity, excessive tear production, and keratitis are common side effects. Conjunctival hemorrhage has been reported.

Avoid touching the applicator tip to eyes, fingers, or other surfaces, and do not wear contact lenses during treatment of ocular infections. Apply pressure to the lacrimal sac during and for 1–2 min after dose administration to reduce risk of systemic absorption.

GCSF
See Filgrastim

GENTAMICIN
Garamycin and generics
Antibiotic, aminoglycoside

No　Yes　2　C/D

Injection: 10 mg/mL (2 mL), 40 mg/mL (2, 20 mL); some products may contain sodium metabisulfite
Premixed injection in NS: 40 mg (50 mL), 60 mg (50 mL), 70 mg (50 mL), 80 mg (50, 100 mL), 90 mg (100 mL), 100 mg (50, 100 mL), 120 mg (50, 100 mL)
Ophthalmic ointment: 0.3% (3.5 g); may contain parabens
Ophthalmic drops: 0.3% (5, 15 mL)
Topical ointment: 0.1% (15, 30 g)
Topical cream: 0.1% (15, 30 g)

Initial empiric dosage; patient-specific dosage defined by therapeutic drug monitoring (see remarks).
Parenteral (IM or IV):
  Neonate/Infant (see table below):

Postconceptional Age (wk)	Postnatal Age (days)	Dose (mg/kg/dose)	Interval (hr)
≤29*	0–7	5	48
	8–28	4	36
	>28	4	24
30–34	0–7	4.5	36
	>7	4	24
≥35	ALL	4	24[†]

*Or significant asphyxia, PDA, indomethicin use, poor cardiac output, reduced renal function
[†]Use Q36 hr interval for HIE patients receiving whole-body therapeutic cooling.

Continued

GENTAMICIN continued

Child: 7.5 mg/kg/24 hr ÷ Q8 hr
Adult: 3–6 mg/kg/24 hr ÷ Q8 hr
Cystic Fibrosis: 7.5–10.5 mg/kg/24 hr ÷ Q8 hr
Intrathecal/intraventricular (use preservative-free product only):
  Newborn: 1 mg once daily
  >3 mo: 1–2 mg once daily
  Adult: 4–8 mg once daily
Ophthalmic ointment: Apply Q8–12 hr
Ophthalmic drops: Instill 1–2 drops Q2–4 hr
Topical cream or ointment:
  >1 yr and adult: Apply to affected area TID–QID

Use with caution in patients receiving anesthetics or neuromuscular blocking agents and in patients with neuromuscular disorders. May cause nephrotoxicity and ototoxicity. Ototoxicity may be potentiated with the use of loop diuretics. Eliminated more quickly in patients with cystic fibrosis, neutropenia, and burns. **Adjust dose in renal failure (see Chapter 30).** Monitor peak and trough levels.

Therapeutic peak levels are 6–10 mg/L in general and 8–10 mg/L in pulmonary infections, cystic fibrosis, neutropenia, osteomyelitis, and severe sepsis.

To maximize bactericidal effects, an individualized peak concentration to target a peak/MIC ratio of 8–10:1 may be applied.

Therapeutic trough levels: <2 mg/L. Recommended serum sampling time at steady state: trough within 30 min prior to the 3rd consecutive dose and peak 30–60 min after the administration of the 3rd consecutive dose.

For initial dosing in obese patients, use an adjusted body weight (ABW). ABW = Ideal Body Weight + 0.4 (Total Body Weight − Ideal Body Weight).

Pregnancy category is a "C" for ophthalmic use, a "D" for IV use, and not classified for topical use.

GLUCAGON HCL
GlucaGen, Glucagon Emergency Kit, and generics
Antihypoglycemic agent

No   No   ?   B

Injection: 1-mg vial (requires reconstitution)
1 unit = 1 mg

Hypoglycemia (IM, IV, SC; see remarks):
  Neonate, infant, and child < 20 kg: 0.5 mg/dose (or 0.02–0.03 mg/kg/dose) Q20 min PRN
  Child ≥ 20 kg and adult: 1 mg/dose Q20 min PRN
β-blocker and calcium channel blocker overdose: Load with 0.05–0.15 mg/kg (usually about 10 mg in adults) IV over 1 min followed by an IV infusion of 0.05–0.1 mg/kg/hr.
Alternatively, 5-mg IV bolus Q5–10 min PRN up to 4 doses. If patient is responsive at a particular bolus dose, initiate an hourly IV infusion at that same responsive dose. For example, if the patient responded at 10 mg, start an infusion of 10 mg/hr.

Use with caution in insulinoma and/or pheochromocytoma. Drug product is genetically engineered and identical to human glucagon. High doses have a cardiac stimulatory effect and have been used with some success in β-blocker and calcium channel blocker overdose. May cause nausea, vomiting, urticaria, and respiratory distress. **Do not delay** glucose infusion; dose for hypoglycemia is 2–4 mL/kg of 25% dextrose.

Onset of action: IM: 8–10 min; IV: 1 min. Duration of action: IM: 12–27 min; IV: 9–17 min.

GLYCERIN
Pedia-Lax, Sani-Supp, Fleet Liquid Glycerin Supp, and others including generics
Osmotic Laxative

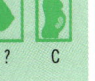

| No | No | ? | C |

Rectal solution (Fleet Liquid Glycerin Supp and generics; OTC): each dose contains 7.5 mL to deliver 5.4 mL of glycerin on average (box of 4)
Suppository (OTC):
Infant/pediatric: 1, 1.2 g (10s, 12s, 25s)
Adult: 2 g (10s, 12s, 24s, 25s, 50s)

Constipation:
Neonate: 0.5 mL/kg/dose rectal solution PR as an enema once daily PRN or sliver/chip of infant/pediatric suppository PR once daily PRN
Child < 6 yr: 2–5-mL rectal solution PR as an enema or 1 infant/pediatric suppository PR once daily PRN
>6 yr–adult: 5–15-mL rectal solution PR as an enema or 1 adult suppository PR once daily PRN

Onset of action: 15–30 min. May cause rectal irritation, abdominal pain, bloating, and dizziness. Insert suppository high into rectum and retain for 15 min.

GLYCOPYRROLATE
Robinul, Cuvposa, and generics
Anticholinergic agent

| Yes | Yes | ? | B/C |

Tabs: 1, 2 mg
Oral solution (Cuvposa): 1 mg/5 mL; contains propylene glycol and parabens
Injection: 0.2 mg/mL (1, 2, 5, 20 mL); some multidose vials contain 0.9% benzyl alcohol.

Respiratory antisecretory:
IM/IV:
Child: 0.004–0.01 mg/kg/dose TID–QID
Adult: 0.1–0.2 mg/dose TID–QID
Max. dose 0.2 mg/dose or 0.8 mg/24 hr
Oral:
Child: 0.04–0.1 mg/kg/dose TID–QID
Alternative dosage for those aged 3–16 yr with chronic severe drooling secondary to neurological conditions: Start with 0.02 mg/kg/dose PO TID and titrate in increments of 0.02 mg/kg/dose every 5–7 days as needed and tolerated up to a **max. dose** of 0.1 mcg/kg/dose TID not exceeding 1.5–3 mg/dose.
Adult: 1–2 mg/dose BID–TID
Reverse neuromuscular blockade:
Child and adult: 0.2 mg IV for every 1-mg neostigmine or 5-mg pyridostigmine

Use with caution in hepatic and renal disease, ulcerative colitis, asthma, glaucoma, ileus, or urinary retention. Atropine-like side effects: tachycardia, nausea, constipation, confusion, blurred vision, and dry mouth. These may be potentiated if given with other drugs having anticholinergic properties.
Onset of action: PO: within 1 hr; IM/SC: 15–30 min; IV: 1 min. Duration of antisialogogue effect: PO: 8–12 hr; IM/SC/IV: 7 hr. Oral doses should be administered 1 hr before and 2 hr after meals.
Pregnancy category is "B" for the injection and tablet dosage forms and "C" for the oral solution.

GRANISETRON
Sancuso, Sustol, and generics; previously available as Kytril
Antiemetic agent, 5-HT₃ antagonist

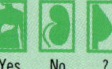

Yes No ? B

Injection: 0.1 mg/mL (1 mL), 1 mg/mL (1, 4 mL); 4-mL multidose vials contain benzyl alcohol
Prefilled syringe for subcutaneous extended-release injection (Sustol): 10 mg/0.4 mL (0.4 mL); contains propylene glycol
Tabs: 1 mg
Oral suspension: 0.2 mg/mL, 50 mcg/mL
Transdermal patch (Sancuso): 3.1 mg/24 hr

Chemotherapy-induced nausea and vomiting:
  IV:
    Child ≥ 2 yr and adult: 10–20 mcg/kg/dose 15–60 min before chemotherapy; the same dose may be repeated 2–3 times at ≥10-min intervals following chemotherapy (within 24 hr after chemotherapy) as a treatment regimen. **Max. dose:** 3 mg/dose or 9 mg/24 hr. Alternatively, a single 40-mcg/kg/dose 15–60 min before chemotherapy has been used.
  SC (Sustol): 10 mg at least 30 min prior to first dose of moderately emetogenic chemotherapy used in combination with dexamethasone. Do not administer more frequently than Q7 days.
  PO:
    Infant, child, and adolescent: 40-mcg/kg/dose BID is recommended for moderately emetogenic chemotherapy; initiate first dose 1 hr prior to chemotherapy
    Adult: 2 mg/24 hr ÷ once daily–BID; initiate first dose 1 hr prior to chemotherapy
Postoperative nausea and vomiting prevention (dosed prior to anesthesia or immediately before anesthesia reversal) and treatment (IV; see remarks):
  Adult: 1 mg × 1
Radiation-induced nausea and vomiting prevention:
  Adult: 2 mg once daily PO administered within 1 hr of radiation
Transdermal patch (see remarks):
  Prophylaxis for chemotherapy-induced nausea and vomiting (adult): Apply 1 patch 24–48 hr prior to chemotherapy. Patch may be worn for up to 7 days, depending on the chemotherapy regimen duration.

Use with caution in liver disease and preexisting cardiac conduction disorders and arrhythmias. May cause hypertension, hypotension, arrhythmias, agitation, and insomnia. Inducers or inhibitors of the CYP450 3A3/4 drug metabolizing enzymes may increase or decrease, respectively, the drug's clearance. QT prolongation has been reported.
Safety and efficacy in pediatric patients for the prevention of postoperative nausea and vomiting has not been established due to lack of efficacy and QT prolongation in a prospective, multicenter, randomized double-blinded trial in 157 patients aged 2–16 yr.
Avoid external heat sources (e.g., heating pads) on and around the transdermal patch dosage form as heat may increase the rate of drug release. Application site reactions of pain, pruritus, rash, irritation, vesicles, and discoloration have been reported with transdermal patch use.
Onset of action: IV: 4–10 min. Duration of action: IV: ≤24 hr.

GRISEOFULVIN
Microsize: Generics; previously available as Grifulvin V, Griseofulvin Microsize
Ultramicrosize: Gris-PEG and generics
Antifungal agent

Yes   No   3   X

Microsize:
  Tabs: 125, 250, 500 mg
  Oral suspension: 125 mg/5 mL (120 mL); contains 0.2% alcohol, parabens, and propylene glycol
Ultramicrosize:
  Tabs (Gris-PEG and generics): 125, 250 mg
250 mg ultramicrosize is approximately 500 mg microsize

Microsize:
  Child > 2 yr and adolescent: 10–20 mg/kg/24 hr PO ÷ once daily–BID; give with milk, eggs, or fatty foods. Use higher dose of 20–25 mg/kg/24 hr PO for tinea capitis to improve efficacy due to relative resistance of the organism.
  Adult: 500–1000 mg/24 hr PO ÷ once daily–BID
  Max. dose (all ages): 1 g/24 hr
Ultramicrosize:
  Child > 2 yr and adolescent: 10–15 mg/kg/24 hr PO ÷ once daily–BID
  Adult: 375–750 mg/24 hr PO ÷ once daily–BID
  Max. dose (all ages): 750 mg/24 hr

Contraindicated in porphyria, pregnancy, and hepatic disease. Monitor hematologic, renal, and hepatic function. May cause leukopenia, rash, headache, paresthesias, and GI symptoms. Severe skin reactions (e.g., Stevens-Johnson, TEN), erythema multiforme, LFT elevations (AST, ALT, bilirubin), and jaundice have been reported. Possible cross-reactivity in penicillin-allergic patients. Usual treatment period is 8 wk for tinea capitis and 4–6 mo for tinea unguium. Photosensitivity reactions may occur. May reduce effectiveness or decrease level of oral contraceptives, warfarin, and cyclosporine. Induces CYP450 1A2 isoenzyme. Phenobarbital may enhance clearance of griseofulvin. Coadministration with fatty meals will increase the drug's absorption.

GUANFACINE
Intuniv, Tenex, and generics
α_2-*Adrenergic agonist*

Yes   Yes   3   B

Tabs: 1, 2 mg
Extended-release tabs: 1, 2, 3, 4 mg

Attention-deficit hyperactivity disorder (see remarks):
  Immediate-release tab:
    ≥6 yr and adolescent:
      ≤45 kg: Start at 0.5 mg QHS, if needed and tolerated; increase dose every 3–4 days at 0.5 mg/24 hr increments by increasing the dosing frequency to BID, TID, QID. **Max. dose:** 27–40.5 kg: 2 mg/24 hr and 40.5–45 kg: 3 mg/24 hr.
      >45 kg: Start at 1 mg QHS, if needed and tolerated; increase dose every 3–4 days at 1 mg/24 hr increments by increasing the dosing frequency to BID, TID, QID. **Max. dose:** 4 mg/24 hr.

Continued

GUANFACINE continued

Attention-deficit hyperactivity disorder (see remarks):
Extended-release tab:
6–17 yr: Start at 1 mg Q24 hr, if needed and tolerated, and increase dose no more than 1 mg per week up to the **maximum dose** of 4 mg/24 hr for 6–12 yr and 7 mg/24 hr for 13–17 yr.
Use with strong CYP450 3A4 inhibitors or inducers:

CYP450 3A4 Characteristic	Adding Guanfacine With Respective CYP450 3A4 Inducer/Inhibitor Already on Board	Adding Respective CYP450 3A4 Inducer/Inhibitor With Guanfacine Already on Board
Strong inducer (e.g., carbamazepine, phenytoin, rifampin, St. John's Wort)	Guanfacine may be titrated up to double the recommended target dose.	Consider increasing guanfacine dose to double the recommended target dose over 1–2 wk as tolerated. If the strong inducer is discontinued, decrease guanfacine dose to target dose over 1–2 wk.
Strong inhibitor (e.g., clarithromycin, azole antifungals)	Decrease guanfacine dose to 50% of recommended target dose.	Decrease guanfacine dose to 50% of recommended target dose. If the strong inhibitor is discontinued, increase guanfacine dose to recommended target dose.

Use with caution in patients at risk for hypotension, bradycardia, heart block, and syncope. A dose-dependent hypotension and bradycardia may occur. Somnolence, fatigue, insomnia, dizziness, and abdominal pain are the common side effects. Orthostatic hypotension, hallucinations, and syncope have been reported.

Drug is a substrate for CYP450 3A4. See dosing section for dosage adjustment with inhibitors and inducers.

Do not abruptly discontinue therapy. Dose reductions may be required with clinically significant renal or hepatic impairment. When converting from an immediate-release tab to the extended-release tab, **do not** covert on an mg-per-mg basis (due to differences in pharmacokinetic profiles) but discontinue the immediate release and titrate with the extended-release product using the recommended dosing schedules.

HALOPERIDOL
Haldol, Haldol Decanoate, and generics
Antipsychotic agent

Yes   Yes   3   C

Injection (IM use only):
Lactate: 5 mg/mL (1, 10 mL); may contain parabens
Decanoate (long acting): 50, 100 mg/mL (1, 5 mL); in sesame oil with 1.2% benzyl alcohol
Tabs: 0.5, 1, 2, 5, 10, 20 mg
Oral solution: 2 mg/mL (15, 120 mL)

Child 3–12 yr:
PO: Initial dose at 0.5 mg/24 hr ÷ BID–TID. If necessary, increase daily dosage by 0.25–0.5 mg/24 hr Q5–7 days PRN. Benefits are not to be expected for doses beyond 6 mg/24 hr. Usual maintenance doses for specific indications include the following:
Agitation: 0.01–0.03 mg/24 hr once daily PO
Psychosis: 0.05–0.15 mg/kg/24 hr ÷ BID–TID PO

HALOPERIDOL continued

Tourette's syndrome: 0.05–0.075 mg/kg/24 hr ÷ BID–TID PO; may increase daily dose by 0.5 mg Q5–7 days
IM, as lactate, for 6–12 yr: 1–3 mg/dose Q4–8 hr; **max. dose**: 0.15 mg/kg/24 hr
>12 yr:
  Acute agitation: 2–5 mg/dose IM as lactate or 1–15 mg/dose PO; repeat in 1 hr PRN
  Psychosis: 2–5 mg/dose Q4–8 hr IM PRN or 1–15 mg/24 hr ÷ BID–TID PO
  Tourette's syndrome: 0.5–2 mg/dose BID–TID PO; 3–5 mg/dose BID–TID PO may be used for severe symptoms

Use with caution in patients with cardiac disease (risk of hypotension), renal or hepatic dysfunction, thyrotoxicosis, and epilepsy because the drug lowers the seizure threshold. Extrapyramidal symptoms, drowsiness, headache, tachycardia, ECG changes, nausea, and vomiting can occur. Higher than recommended doses are associated with a higher risk of QT prolongation and torsades de pointes. Leukopenia/neutropenia, including agranulocytosis, and rhabdomyolysis (IM route) have been reported.

Drug is metabolized by CYP450 1A2, 2D6, and 3A3/4 isoenzymes. May also inhibit CYP450 2D6 and 3A3/4 isoenzymes. Serotonin-specific reuptake inhibitors (e.g., fluoxetine) may increase levels and effects of haloperidol. Carbamazepine and phenobarbital may decrease levels and effects of haloperidol. Monitor for encephalopathy syndrome when used in combination with lithium.

Acutely aggravated patients may require doses as often as Q60 min. **Decanoate salt is given every 3–4 wk in doses that are 10–15 times the individual patient's stabilized oral dose.**

HEPARIN SODIUM
Various generics
Anticoagulant

No   No   1   C

Injection:
  Porcine intestinal mucosa: 1000, 2500, 5000, 10,000, 20,000 U/mL (some products may be preservative free; multidose vials contain benzyl alcohol)
Lock flush solution (porcine based): 1, 10, 100 U/mL (some products may be preservative free or contain benzyl alcohol)
Injection for IV infusion (porcine based):
  D_5W: 40 U/mL (500 mL), 50 U/mL (500 mL), 100 U/mL (100, 250 mL); contains bisulfite
  NS (0.9% NaCl): 2 U/mL (500, 1000 mL)
  0.45% NaCl: 50 U/mL (250, 500 mL), 100 U/mL (250 mL); contains EDTA
120 U = approximately 1 mg

Anticoagulation empiric dosage (see Chapter 14, Table 14.9 for dosage adjustments):
Continuous IV infusion [initial doses for goal unfractionated heparin (UFH) anti-Xa level of 0.3–0.7 units/mL]:

Age	Loading Dose (IV)*	Initial IV Infusion Rate (units/kg/hr)
Neonate and infant < 1 yr	75 U/kg IV	28
Child ≥ 1–16 yr	75 U/kg IV (max. dose: 7700 U)	20 (max. initial rate: 1650 U/hr)
>16 yr	70 U/kg IV (max. dose: 7700 U)	15 (max. initial rate: 1650 U/hr)

*Do not give a loading dose for stroke patients and obtain aPPT 4 hr after the loading dose.

DVT or PE prophylaxis:
  Adult: 5000 U/dose SC Q8–12 hr until ambulatory

Continued

HEPARIN SODIUM continued

Heparin flush (doses should be less than heparinizing dose):
  Younger child: lower doses should be used to avoid systemic heparinization
  Older child and adult:
    Peripheral IV: 1–2 mL of 10 U/mL solution Q4 hr
    Central lines: 2–3 mL of 100 U/mL solution Q24 hr
    TPN (central line) and arterial line: add heparin to make a final concentration of 0.5–1 U/mL

Contraindicated in active major bleeding, known or suspected HIT, and concurrent epidural therapy. **Use with caution** if platelets < 50,000/mm³. **Avoid** IM injections and other medications affecting platelet function (e.g., NSAIDS and ASA). Toxicities include bleeding, allergy, alopecia, and thrombocytopenia.
Adjust dose with one of the following laboratory goals:
  Unfractionated heparin (UFH) anti-Xa level: 0.3–0.7 units/mL
  aPTT level (reagent specific to reflect anti-Xa level of 0.3–0.7 units/mL): 50–80 seconds.
  These laboratory measurements are best measured 4–6 hr after initiation or changes in infusion rate. **Do not** collect blood from the heparinized line or same extremity as site of heparin infusion. If *unfractionated* heparin anti-Xa or aPTT levels are not available, a ratio of aPPT 1.5–2.5 times the control value has been used in the past. *Unfractionated* heparin anti-Xa level is NOT THE SAME *as low-molecular-weight* heparin anti-Xa (used for monitoring low-molecular-weight heparin products such as enoxaparin).
Use preservative-free heparin in neonates. **Note:** heparin flush doses may alter aPTT in small patients; consider using more dilute heparin in these cases.
Use actual body weight when dosing obese patients. Due to recent regulatory changes to the manufacturing process, heparin products may exhibit decreased potency.
Antidote: Protamine sulfate (1 mg per 100 U heparin in previous 4 hr). For *low-molecular-weight* heparin (LMWH), see Enoxaparin.

HYALURONIDASE
Amphadase, Hydase, Hylenex, and Vitrase
Antidote, extravasation

No   No   ?   C

Injection:
  Amphadase and Hydase: 150 U/mL (1 mL); bovine source; may contain edetate disodium and thimerosal
  Hylenex: 150 U/mL (1 mL); recombinant human source; contains 1 mg albumin per 150 U
  Vitrase: 200 U/mL (1.2 mL); ovine source, preservative free
  Pharmacy can make a 15 U/mL dilution.

Extravasation:
  Infant and child: Give 1 mL (150 U) by injecting five separate injections of 0.2 mL (30 U) at borders of extravasation site SC or intradermal using a 25- or 26-gauge needle. Alternatively, a diluted 15-U/mL concentration has been used with the same dosing instructions.

Contraindicated in dopamine and α-agonist extravasation and hypersensitivity to the respective product sources (bovine or ovine). May cause urticaria. Patients receiving large amounts of salicylates, cortisone, ACTH, estrogens, or antihistamines may decrease the effects of hyaluronidase (larger doses may be necessary). Administer as early as possible (minutes to 1 hr) after IV extravasation.
Hylenex is chemically incompatible with sodium metabisulfite, furosemide, benzodiazepines, and phenytoin.

HYDRALAZINE HYDROCHLORIDE
Generics; previously available as Apresoline
Antihypertensive, vasodilator

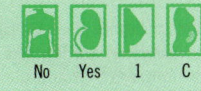

No Yes 1 C

Tabs: 10, 25, 50, 100 mg
Injection: 20 mg/mL (1 mL)
Oral liquid: 2, 4 mg/mL
Some dosage forms may contain tartrazines or sulfites.

Hypertensive crisis (may result in severe and prolonged hypotension; see Chapter 4, Table 4.7 for alternatives):
  Child: 0.1–0.2 mg/kg/dose IM or IV Q4–6 hr PRN; **max. dose:** 20 mg/dose. Usual IV/IM dosage range is 1.7–3.5 mg/kg/24 hr.
  Adult: 10–40 mg IM or IV Q4–6 hr PRN
Chronic hypertension:
  Infant and child: Start at 0.75–1 mg/kg/24 hr PO ÷ Q6–12 hr (**max. dose:** 25 mg/dose). If necessary, increase dose over 3–4 wk up to a **max. dose** of 5 mg/kg/24 hr for infants and 7.5 mg/kg/24 hr for children; or 200 mg/24 hr
  Adult: 10–50 mg/dose PO QID; **max. dose:** 300 mg/24 hr

Use with caution in severe renal and cardiac disease. Slow acetylators, patients receiving high-dose chronic therapy and those with renal insufficiency are at highest risk for lupus-like syndrome (generally reversible). May cause reflex tachycardia, palpitations, dizziness, headaches, and GI discomfort. MAO inhibitors and β-blockers may increase hypotensive effects. Indomethacin may decrease hypotensive effects.
Drug undergoes first-pass metabolism. Onset of action: PO: 20–30 min; IV: 5–20 min. Duration of action: PO: 2–4 hr; IV: 2–6 hr. **Adjust dose in renal failure (see Chapter 30).**

HYDROCHLOROTHIAZIDE
Microzide and generics; previously available as Hydrodiuril
Diuretic, thiazide

No Yes 2 B/D

Tabs: 12.5, 25, 50 mg
Caps (Microzide and generics): 12.5 mg

Edema:
  Neonate and infant < 6 mo: 1–3 mg/kg/24 hr ÷ once daily–BID PO; **max. dose:** 37.5 mg/24 hr
  ≥6 mo, child, and adolescent: 1–2 mg/kg/24 hr ÷ once daily–BID PO; **max. dose:** <2 yr: 37.5 mg/24 hr, child 2–12 yr: 100 mg/24 hr, and adolescent: 200 mg/24 hr
  Adult: 25–100 mg/24 hr ÷ once daily–BID PO; **max. dose:** 200 mg/24 hr
Hypertension:
  Infant and child: Start at 0.5–1 mg/kg/24 hr once daily PO; dose may be increased to a **max. dose** of 3 mg/kg/24 hr up to 50 mg/24 hr.
  Adult: 12.5–25 mg/dose once daily–BID PO; doses > 50 mg/24 hr often results in hypokalemia.

See *Chlorothiazide*. May cause fluid and electrolyte imbalances and hyperuricemia. Drug may not be effective when creatinine clearance is less than 25–50 mL/min. Use with carbamazepine may result in symptomatic hyponatremia.

Continued

HYDROCHLOROTHIAZIDE continued

Hydrochlorothiazide is also available in combination with potassium-sparing diuretics (e.g., spironolactone), ACE inhibitors, angiotensin II receptor antagonists, hydralazine, methyldopa, reserpine, and β-blockers.

Pregnancy category is "D" if used in pregnancy-induced hypertension.

HYDROCORTISONE
Systemic dosage forms: Solu-Cortef, Cortef, and generics
Topical: Cortifoam, Colocort, Cortenema, NuCort, and many others including generics
Corticosteroid

No   No   3   C

Hydrocortisone base:
  Tabs (Cortef and generics): 5, 10, 20 mg
  Oral suspension: 2 mg/mL
  Rectal cream: 1% (30 g), 2.5% (30 g)
  Rectal suspension as an enema (Colocort, Cortenema): 100 mg/60 mL
  Topical ointment: 0.5% [OTC], 1% [OTC], 2.5%
  Topical cream: 0.5% [OTC], 1% [OTC], 2.5%
  Topical gel [OTC]: 1%
  Topical lotion: 1% [OTC], 2%, 2.5%
Na Succinate (Solu-Cortef):
  Injection: 100, 250, 500, 1000 mg/vial; contains benzyl alcohol
Acetate:
  Topical cream [OTC]: 1%
  Topical lotion (NuCort): 2% (60 g); contains benzyl alcohol
  Suppository: 25, 30 mg
  Rectal foam aerosol (Cortifoam): 10% (90 mg/dose) (15 g)

Status asthmaticus:
  Child:
    Load (optional): 4–8 mg/kg/dose IV; **max. dose**: 250 mg
    Maintenance: 8 mg/kg/24 hr ÷ Q6 hr IV
  Adult: 100–500 mg/dose Q6 hr IV
Physiologic replacement: see Chapter 30 for dosing
Anti-inflammatory/immunosuppressive:
  Child:
    PO: 2.5–10 mg/kg/24 hr ÷ Q6–8 hr
    IM/IV: 1–5 mg/kg/24 hr ÷ Q12–24 hr
  Adolescent and adult:
    PO/IM/IV: 15–240 mg/dose Q12 hr
Acute adrenal insufficiency: see Chapter 10 for dosing
Topical use:
  Child and adult: Apply to affected areas BID–QID, depending on severity
Ulcerative colitis, induction for mild/moderate case:
  Adolescent and adult: Insert 1 application of 100 mg rectal enema once daily–BID × 2–3 weeks
Hemorrhoids:
  Adult: 25 or 30 mg suppository PR BID × 2 weeks

Use with caution in immunocompromised patients as they should avoid exposure to chicken pox or measles.
For potency comparisons of topical preparations, see Chapter 8. For doses based on body surface area, see Chapter 10.

HYDROMORPHONE HCL
Dilaudid, Dilaudid-HP, Exalgo, and generics
Narcotic, analgesic

Yes   Yes   3   C/D

Tabs: 2, 4, 8 mg
Extended-release tabs (Exalgo and generics): 8, 12, 16, 32 mg
Injection: 1, 2, 4, 10 mg/mL (may contain parabens)
Prefilled injectable syringes: 10 mg/50 mL (50 mL), 15 mg/30 mL (30 mL)
  Preservative free: 12 mg/60 mL (60 mL)
Powder for injection (Dilaudid-HP): 250 mg
Suppository: 3 mg (6s)
Oral solution: 1 mg/mL; may contain parabens

Analgesia, initial doses with immediate-release dosage forms (titrate to effect):
  Child (<50 kg):
    IV: 0.015 mg/kg/dose Q3–6 hr PRN
    PO: 0.03–0.08 mg/kg/dose Q3–4 hr PRN; **max. dose:** 5 mg/dose
  Child and adolescent (≥50 kg; NOTE: doses are NOT weight-based):
    IV: 0.2–0.6 mg/dose Q2–4 hr PRN
    IM, SC: 0.8–1 mg/dose Q4–6 hr PRN
    PO: 1–2 mg/dose Q3–4 hr PRN
    PR: 3 mg Q4–8 hr PRN
  Adult:
    IV: 0.2–1 mg/dose Q2–3 hr PRN
    IM, SC: 0.8–1 mg/dose Q3–4 hr PRN
    PO: 2–4 mg/dose Q4–6 hr PRN
    PR: 3 mg Q6–8 hr PRN

Refer to Chapter 6 for equianalgesic doses and for patient-controlled analgesia dosing.
  Less pruritus than morphine. Similar profile of side effects to other narcotics. **Use with caution** in infants and young children, and **do not use** in neonates due to potential CNS effects. Dose reduction recommended in renal insufficiency or severe hepatic impairment. Pregnancy category changes to "D" if used for prolonged periods or in high doses at term.
Extended-release tab use requires Risk Evaluation and Mitigation Strategies (REMS)-based provision of safety information and postmarketing safety studies.

HYDROXYCHLOROQUINE
Plaquenil and generics
Antimalarial, antirheumatic agent

Yes   Yes   2   ?

Tabs: 200 mg (155 mg base)
Oral suspension: 25 mg/mL (19.375 mg/mL base)

All doses expressed in mg of hydroxychloroquine base.
Malaria prophylaxis (start 2 wk prior to exposure and continue for 4 wk after leaving endemic area):
  Child: 5 mg/kg/dose PO once weekly; **max. dose:** 310 mg
  Adult: 310 mg PO once weekly

Continued

HYDROXYCHLOROQUINE continued

Malaria treatment (acute uncomplicated cases):
For treatment of malaria, consult with ID specialist or see the latest edition of the AAP Red Book.
Child: 10 mg/kg/dose (**max. dose:** 620 mg) PO × 1 followed by 5 mg/kg/dose (**max. dose:** 310 mg) 6 hr later. Then 5 mg/kg/dose (**max. dose:** 310 mg) Q24 hr × 2 doses starting 24 hr after the first dose.
Adult: 620 mg PO × 1 followed by 310 mg 6 hr later. Then 310 mg Q24 hr × 2 doses starting 24 hr after the first dose.

Juvenile rheumatoid arthritis or systemic lupus erythematosus:
Child: 2.325–3.875 mg/kg/24 hr (base) PO ÷ once daily–BID; **max. dose:** 310 mg/24 hr not to exceed 5.425 mg/kg/24 hr.

Contraindicated in psoriasis, porphyria, retinal or visual field changes, and 4-aminoquinoline hypersensitivity. **Use with caution** in liver disease, G6PD deficiency, concomitant hepatic toxic drugs, renal impairment, metabolic acidosis, or hematologic disorders.

Long-term use in children is **not recommended**. May cause headaches, myopathy, GI disturbances, skin and mucosal pigmentation, agranulocytosis, visual disturbances, and increased digoxin serum levels. Use with aurothioglucose may increase risk for blood dyscrasias.

When used in combination with other immunosuppressive agents for SLE and JRA, lower doses of hydroxychloroquine can be used.

Pregnancy category has not been formally assigned by the FDA. The only situation where use is recommended during pregnancy is during the suppression or treatment of malaria, when the benefits outweigh the risks.

HYDROXYZINE
Vistaril and generics
Antihistamine, anxiolytic, antiemetic

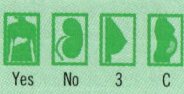

Yes   No   3   C

Tabs (HCl salt): 10, 25, 50 mg
Caps (pamoate salt): 25, 50, 100 mg
Oral syrup, solution (HCl salt): 10 mg/5 mL (120, 473 mL); may contain alcohol
Injection for IM use (HCl salt): 25, 50 mg/mL; may contain benzyl alcohol
Note: pamoate and HCl salts are equivalent in regards to mg of hydroxyzine.

Pruritus and anxiety:
Oral:
  Child and adolescent: 2 mg/kg/24 hr ÷ Q6–8 hr PRN, **max. single dose:** <6 yr: 12.5 mg, 6–12 yr: 25 mg, and >12 yr: 100 mg.
  Alternative dosing by age:
   <6 yr: 50 mg/24 hr ÷ Q6–8 hr PRN
   ≥6 yr: 50–100 mg/24 hr ÷ Q6–8 hr PRN
  Adult: 25 mg/dose TID–QID PRN; **max. dose:** 600 mg/24 hr
IM:
  Child and adolescent: 0.5–1 mg/kg/dose Q4–6 hr PRN; **max. single dose:** 100 mg
  Adult: 25–100 mg/dose Q4–6 hr PRN; **max. dose:** 600 mg/24 hr
Antiemetic (excluding use during pregnancy):
  Child and adolescent: 1.1 mg/kg/dose IM, **max. single dose:** 100 mg
  Adult: 25–100 mg IM

Contraindicated in prolonged QT interval. May potentiate barbiturates, meperidine, and other CNS depressants. **Use with caution** with concomitant use of other medications known to prolong the QT interval. May cause dry mouth, drowsiness, tremor, convulsions, blurred

HYDROXYZINE continued

vision, and hypotension. May cause pain at injection site. Fixed drug eruptions have been reported with use of the oral dosage form.

Increase dosage interval to Q24 hr or longer in the presence of liver disease (e.g., Primary biliary cirrhosis).

Onset of action within 15–30 min. Duration of action: 4–6 hr. IV administration is **NOT recommended.**

IBUPROFEN
PO: Motrin, Advil, Children's Advil, Children's Motrin, and generics
IV: NeoProfen, Caldolor
Nonsteroidal antiinflammatory agent

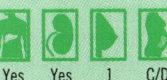

Yes   Yes   1   C/D

Oral suspension [OTC]: 100 mg/5 mL (60, 120, 480 mL)
Oral drops [OTC]: 40 mg/mL (15, 30 mL)
Chewable tabs [OTC]: 50, 100 mg
Caplets [OTC]: 100, 200 mg
Tabs: 100 [OTC], 200 [OTC], 400, 600, 800 mg
Capsules [OTC]: 200 mg
Injection:
   NeoProfen (lysine salt): 10 mg ibuprofen base/1 mL (2 mL)
   Caldolor: 100 mg/mL (4, 8 mL); contains 78 mg/mL arginine

PO:
  Infant and child (≥6 mo):
    Analgesic/antipyretic: 5–10 mg/kg/dose Q6–8 hr PO; **max. dose**: 40 mg/kg/24 hr
    JRA (6 mo–12 yr): 30–50 mg/kg/24 hr ÷ Q6 hr PO; **max. dose**: 2400 mg/24 hr
  Adult:
    Inflammatory disease: 400–800 mg/dose Q6–8 hr PO; **max. dose**: 800 mg/dose or 3.2 g/24 hr
    Pain/fever/dysmenorrhea: 200–400 mg/dose Q4–6 hr PRN PO; **max. dose**: 1.2 g/24 hr

IV:
  6 mo–<12 yr:
    Analgesic and antipyretic: 10 mg/kg/dose up to 400 mg/dose Q4–6 hr PRN; **max. dose**: the lesser of 40 mg/kg/24 hr or 2400 mg/24 hr
  12–17 yr:
    Analgesic and antipyretic: 400 mg/dose Q4–6 hr PRN; **max. dose**: 2400 mg/24 hr
  ≥18 yr and adult:
    Analgesic (see remarks): 400–800 mg/dose Q6 hr PRN; **max. dose**: 3200 mg/24 hr
    Antipyretic (see remarks): 400 mg/dose Q4–6 hr or 100–200 mg/dose Q4 hr PRN; **max. dose**: 3200 mg/24 hr

Closure of ductus arteriosus:
<32 wk of gestation and 0.5–1.5 kg (use birth weight to calculate all doses and infuse all doses over 15 min; see remarks): 10 mg/kg/dose IV × 1 followed by two doses of 5 mg/kg/dose each, 24 and 48 hr after the initial dose. Hold second or third dose if urinary output is <0.6 mL/kg/hr; dosing should resume when laboratory studies indicate the return of normal renal function. If the ductus arteriosus fails to close or reopens, a second course of ibuprofen, use of IV indomethacin, or surgery may be necessary.

Contraindicated in active GI bleeding and ulcer disease. **Use caution** in aspirin hypersensitivity, hepatic/renal insufficiency, heart disease (risk for MI and stroke with prolonged use), dehydration, and in patients receiving anticoagulants. GI distress (lessened with milk), rashes, ocular problems, hypertension, granulocytopenia, and anemia may occur.

Continued

IBUPROFEN continued

Inhibits platelet aggregation. Consumption of more than three alcoholic beverages per day or use with corticosteroids or anticoagulants may increase the risk for GI bleeding.

May increase serum levels and effects of digoxin, methotrexate, and lithium. May decrease the effects of antihypertensives, aspirin (antiplatelet effects), furosemide, and thiazide diuretics. Pregnancy category changes to "D" if used in the 3rd trimester or near delivery.

IV USE for analgesia/antipyretic: Hydrate patient well before use. Doses must be diluted to a concentration of ≤4 mg/mL with NS, D$_5$W, or LR and infused over ≥30 min for adults and ≥10 min for children. Most common reported side effects in clinical trials include nausea, flatulence, vomiting, and headache.

IV USE for PDA: Contraindicated in untreated infections, congenital heart diseases requiring a patent ductus arteriosus to facilitate satisfactory pulmonary and systemic blood flow, active intracranial or gastrointestinal bleeds, thrombocytopenia, coagulation defects, suspected/active NEC, and significant renal impairment. **Use with caution** in hyperbilirubinemia. Not indicated for IVH prophylaxis. Renal side effects are generally less frequent and severe when compared with IV indomethacin. NEC, GI perforation, and pulmonary hypertension have been reported. Neoprofen doses must be administered within 30 min of preparation and infused intravenously over 15 min.

IMIPENEM AND CILASTATIN
Primaxin IV and generics
Antibiotic, carbapenem

No   Yes   2   C

Injection: 250, 500 mg; contains 3.2 mEq Na/g drug
Each 1 mg drug contains 1 mg imipenem and 1 mg cilastatin

Dosages based on imipenem component.
Neonate (see remarks):
<1 kg:
    ≤14 days old: 40 mg/kg/24 hr ÷ Q12 hr IV
    15–28 days old: 50 mg/kg/24 hr ÷ Q12 hr IV
1–2 kg:
    ≤7 days old: 40 mg/kg/24 hr ÷ Q12 hr IV
    8–28 days old: 50 mg/kg/24 hr ÷ Q12 hr IV
>2 kg:
    ≤7 days old: 50 mg/kg/24 hr ÷ Q12 hr IV
    8–28 days old: 75 mg/kg/24 hr ÷ Q8 hr IV
Child (4 wk–3 mo): 100 mg/kg/24 hr ÷ Q6 hr IV
Child (>3 mo): 60–100 mg/kg/24 hr ÷ Q6 hr IV; **max. dose**: 4 g/24 hr
Cystic fibrosis: 90 mg/kg/24 hr ÷ Q6 hr IV; **max. dose**: 4 g/24 hr
Adult: 1–4 g/24 hr ÷ Q6–8 hr IV; **max. dose**: 4 g/24 hr or 50 mg/kg/24 hr, whichever is less.

For IV use, give slowly over 30–60 min at a concentration of ≤5 mg/mL to reduce risk for nausea (lowering the rate may reduce severity). Adverse effects: thrombophlebitis, pruritus, urticaria, GI symptoms, seizures, dizziness, hypotension, elevated LFTs, blood dyscrasias, and penicillin allergy. Greater risk for seizures may occur with CNS infections, concomitant use with ganciclovir, higher doses, and renal impairment. CSF penetration is variable but best with inflamed meninges. Not recommended in CNS infections for neonates due to cilastatin accumulation and seizure risk.

Do not administer with probenecid (increases imipenem/cilastatin levels) and ganciclovir (increased risk for seizures). May significantly reduce valproic acid levels.

Adjust dose in renal insufficiency (see Chapter 30).

IMIPRAMINE
Tofranil and generics
Antidepressant, tricyclic

Yes   Yes   3   ?

Tabs (HCl): 10, 25, 50 mg
Caps (pamoate): 75, 100, 125, 150 mg; strengths are expressed as imipramine HCl equivalent

Antidepressant:
  Child:
    Initial: 1.5 mg/kg/24 hr ÷ TID PO; increase 1–1.5 mg/kg/24 hr Q3–4 days to a **max. dose** of 5 mg/kg/24 hr
  Adolescent:
    Initial: 25–50 mg/24 hr ÷ once daily–TID PO; **max. dose**: 200 mg/24 hr. Dosages exceeding 100 mg/24 hr are generally not necessary
  Adult:
    Initial: 75–100 mg/24 hr ÷ TID PO
    Maintenance: 50–300 mg/24 hr QHS PO; **max. dose**: 300 mg/24 hr
Enuresis (≥6 yr):
  Initial: 10–25 mg QHS PO
  Increment: 10–25 mg/dose at 1- to 2-wk intervals until **max. dose** for age or desired effect is achieved. Continue × 2–3 mo, then taper slowly
  Max. dose:
    6–12 yr: the lesser of 2.5 mg/kg/24 hr or 50 mg/24 hr
    ≥12 yr: 75 mg/24 hr
Augment analgesia for chronic pain:
Initial: 0.2–0.4 mg/kg/dose QHS PO; increase 50% every 2–3 days to a **max. dose** of 1–3 mg/kg/dose QHS PO

Contraindicated in narrow-angle glaucoma and patients who used MAO inhibitors within 14 days. See Chapter 2 for management of toxic ingestion. Monitor for clinical worsening of depression and suicidal ideation/behavior following the initiation of therapy or after dose changes. **Use with caution** in renal or hepatic impairment. Side effects include sedation, urinary retention, constipation, dry mouth, dizziness, drowsiness, and arrhythmia. QHS dosing during first weeks of therapy will reduce sedation. Monitor ECG, BP, and CBC at start of therapy and with dose changes. Tricyclics may cause mania.

Therapeutic reference range (sum of imipramine and desipramine) = 150–250 ng/mL. Levels > 1000 ng/mL are toxic; however, toxicity may occur at >300 ng/mL.

Recommended serum sampling time at steady state: Obtain trough level within 30 min prior to the next scheduled dose after 5–7 days of continuous therapy. Carbamazepine may reduce imipramine levels, and cimetidine, fluoxetine, fluvoxamine, labetolol, and quinidine may increase imipramine levels.

Onset of antidepressant effects: 1–3 wk. **Do not discontinue** abruptly in patients receiving long-term high dose therapy.

Pregnancy category has not been officially assigned by the FDA as congenital abnormalities have been reported in humans with the causal relationship not being established.

IMMUNE GLOBULIN
Immune globulins

No   Yes   ?   C

IM preparations:
   GamaSTAN S/D: 150–180 mg/mL (2, 10 mL); contains 0.21–0.32 M glycine; preservative free

IV preparations in solution (preservative free):
   Bivigam: 10% (100 mg/mL) (50, 100 mL); contains polysorbate 80; sucrose free
   Flebogamma DIF: 5% (50 mg/mL) (10, 50, 100, 200, 400 mL) 10% (100 mg/mL) (50, 100, 200 mL); contains 50 mg/mL sorbitol and ≤6 mg/mL polyethylene glycol; sucrose free
   Gamunex-C: 10% (100 mg/mL) (10, 25, 50, 100, 200, 400 mL); contains 0.16–0.24 M glycine; sucrose free
   Gammagard liquid: 10% (100 mg/mL) (10, 25, 50, 100, 200, 300 mL); contains 0.25 M glycine; sucrose free
   Gammaked: 10% (100 mg/mL) (10, 25, 50, 100, 200 mL); contains 0.16–0.24 M glycine; sucrose free
   Octagam: 5% (50 mg/mL) (20, 50, 100, 200, 500 mL), 10% (100 mg/mL) (20, 50, 100, 200); contains 100 mg/mL maltose; sucrose free
   Privagen 10% (100 mg/mL) (50, 100, 200, 400 mL); contains 210–290 mmol/L L-proline; sucrose free

IV preparations in powder for reconstitution:
   Carimune NF: 3, 6, 12 g (contains 1.67 g sucrose and <20 mg NaCl per 1 g Ig); dilute to 3%, 6%, 9% or 12%
   Gammagard S/D: 5, 10 g (when diluted at 5% or 50 mg/mL, contains <1 mcg/mL of IgA, 3 mg/mL albumin, 22.5 mg/mL glycine, 20 mg/mL glucose, 2 mg/mL polyethylene glycol, 1 mcg/mL tri-n-butyl phosphate, 1 mcg/mL octoxynol 9, and 100 mcg/mL polysorbate 80); may be diluted to 5% or 10%

Subcutaneous (SC) preparations (sucrose and preservative free):
   Hizentra: 20% (200 mg/mL) (5, 10, 20, 50 mL); contains 210–290 mmol/L L-proline and 10–30 mg/L polysorbate 80

Intravenous (IV) preparations:
   Kawasaki disease (should be initiated within first 10 days of symptoms): 2 g/kg × 1 dose over 8–12-hr infusion. If signs and symptoms persist, consider a second 2 g/kg dose. Some recommend using a different drug brand or lot number for the second dose.
   Immune thrombocytopenia (ITP) [see RH$_o$(D) immune globulin intravenous for Rh-positive patients]:
     Acute therapy: 400–1000 mg/kg/dose once daily for 2–5 days for a total cumulative dose of 2000 mg/kg
     Maintenance therapy: 400–1000 mg/kg/dose Q3–6 wk based on clinical response
   Replacement therapy for antibody-deficient disorders: Start at 400–500 mg/kg/dose Q4 wk and adjust dose based on clinical response and maintain a trough IgG level ≥ 500 mg/dL. For severe hypogammaglobulinemia (<100 mg/dL), patients may benefit with a loading dose of 400 mg/kg/dose once daily × 2, followed by 400–500 mg/kg/dose Q4 wk.
   Pediatric HIV with IgG <400 mg/dL: see replacement therapy for antibody-deficient disorder from above.
   Bone marrow transplantation (may decrease risk for infection and death but not acute graft-versus host disease): Start at 400–500 mg/kg/dose to maintain IgG levels at ≥400 mg/dL, resulting in dosage intervals ranging from once weekly to Q3–4 wk.
General guidelines for administration (see package insert of specific products):

IMMUNE GLOBULIN continued

IV: Begin infusion at 0.01 mL/kg/min, double the rate every 15–30 min up to max. of 0.08 mL/kg/min. If adverse reactions occur, stop infusion until side effects subside and may restart at rate that was previously tolerated.

IM: Administer in the anterolateral aspects of the upper thigh or deltoid muscle of the upper arm. Avoid gluteal region because of risk of injury to sciatic nerve. Consider splitting doses for multiple injection sites to address age specific maximum IM injection volumes.

Subcutaneous (SC) preparation:
Converting to SC route from previous IV dosage for patients receiving IV immune globulin (IVIG) infusions at regular intervals for at least 3 mo (≥2 yr):
  Initial weekly dose (start 1 wk after last IV dose):
    Dose (g) = 1.53 × Previous IVIG dose in grams (g) ÷ number of weeks between IVIG doses
    To convert the above dose in grams to milliliters of drug, multiply dose (g) by 5.
    Adjust dose over time by clinical response and serum IgG trough levels. Obtain a previous trough level from IVIG therapy prior to SC conversion, and repeat trough level 2–3 mo after initiating the SC route. A goal trough with the SC route of ~290 mg/dL higher than a trough with the IV route has been recommended.

SC administration: Injection sites include the abdomen, thigh, upper arm, and/or lateral hip. Doses may be administered into multiple sites (spaced ≥ 2 inches apart) simultaneously. See following table.

SC Product	Max. Simultaneous Injection Sites	Max. Infusion Rate	Max. Infusion Volume
Hizentra	4	First infusion: 15 mL/hr per infusion site Subsequent infusions: 25 mL/hr per infusion site (max. 50 mL/hr for all simultaneous sites combined)	First four infusions: 15 mL per infusion site Subsequent infusions: 20–25 mL per infusion site

Use with caution in patients with an increased risk of thrombosis (e.g., hypercoagulable states, prolonged immobilization, in-dwelling catheters, estrogen use, thrombosis history, cardiovascular risks, and hyperviscosity) or hemolysis (e.g., non-O blood type, associated inflammatory conditions, and receiving high cumulative doses of immune globulins over several days).

May cause flushing, chills, fever, headache, and hypotension. Hypersensitivity reaction may occur when IV form is administered rapidly. Maltose containing products may cause an osmotic diuresis. May cause **anaphylaxis** in IgA-deficient patients due to varied amounts of IgA. Some products are IgA depleted; consult a pharmacist.

To decrease risk of renal dysfunction, including acute renal failure, IV preparations containing sucrose should not be infused at a rate such that the amount of sucrose exceeds 3 mg/kg/min.

SC route provides higher serum trough levels, lower rate of adverse reactions, and shorter administration time when compared with the IV route. Use an adjusted body weight [ABW = Ideal Body Weight + 0.5 (Actual Body Weight – Ideal Body Weight)] for dosing in obese patients has been recommended.

Delay immunizations after immune globulin administration (see latest AAP *Red Book* for details).

INDOMETHACIN
Indocin, Tivorbex, and generics
Nonsteroidal antiinflammatory agent

Yes   Yes   1   C/D

Caps: 25, 50 mg
  Tivorbex: 20, 40 mg
Sustained-release caps: 75 mg
Oral suspension: 25 mg/5 mL (237 mL); contains 1% alcohol
Suppositories: 50 mg (30s)
Injection: 1 mg

Antiinflammatory/rheumatoid arthritis:
  Child (≥2 yr): Start at 1–2 mg/kg/24 hr ÷ BID-QID PO; **max. dose:** the lesser of 4 mg/kg/24 hr or 200 mg/24 hr
  Adult: 50–150 mg/24 hr ÷ BID-QID PO; **max. dose:** 200 mg/24 hr
  Tivorbex: 20 mg TID PO or 40 mg BID–TID PO
Closure of ductus arteriosus:
  Infuse intravenously over 20–30 min:

Postnatal Age	Dose (mg/kg/dose Q12–24 hr)*		
	1	2	3
<48 hr	0.2	0.1	0.1
2–7 days	0.2	0.2	0.2
>7 days	0.2	0.25	0.25

*Do not administer if urine output is < 0.6 mL/kg/hr or anuric.

For infants <1500 g, 0.1–0.2 mg/kg/dose IV Q24 hr may be given for an additional 3–5 days.
Intraventricular hemorrhage prophylaxis: 0.1 mg/kg/dose IV Q24 hr × 3 doses initiated at 6–12 hr of age (give in consultation with a neonatologist).

Contraindicated in active bleeding, coagulation defects, necrotizing enterocolitis, and renal insufficiency (urine output < 0.6 mL/kg/hr). **Use with caution** in cardiac dysfunction, hypertension, heart disease (risk for MI and stroke with prolonged use), and renal or hepatic impairment. May cause (especially in neonates) decreased urine output, thrombocytopenia, and decreased GI blood flow and may reduce the antihypertensive effects of β-blockers, hydralazine, and ACE inhibitors. **Fatal hepatitis has been reported in JRA treatment.** Thrombotic events have been observed in adults receiving high doses or prolonged therapy. Monitor renal and hepatic function before and during use.
Reduction in cerebral blood flow associated with rapid IV infusion; infuse all IV doses over 20–30 min.
Sustained-release capsules are dosed once daily–BID. Pregnancy category changes to "D" if used for >48 hr or after 34 wk of gestation or close to delivery.

INSULIN PREPARATIONS
Pancreatic hormone

   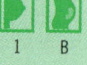
Yes   Yes   1   B

Many preparations at concentrations of 100, 500 U/mL. See Chapter 10, Table 10.3.
  Diluted concentrations of 1 U/mL or 10 U/mL may be necessary for smaller doses in neonates and infants.

INSULIN PREPARATIONS *continued*

Hyperkalemia: See Chapter 11, Fig. 11.3.
DKA: See Chapter 10, Fig. 10.1.

When using insulin drip with new IV tubing, fill the tubing with the insulin infusion solution and wait for 30 min (before connecting tubing to the patient). Flush the line and connect the IV line to the patient to start the infusion. This will ensure proper drug delivery. **Adjust dose in renal failure (see Chapter 30). Use with caution** and monitor closely in hepatic impairment.

IODIDE

See Potassium Iodide

IOHEXOL
Omnipaque 140, Omnipaque 180, Omnipaque 240,
Omnipaque 300, and Omnipaque 350
Radiopaque agent, contrast media

Yes   Yes   3   B

Injection:
  Omnipaque 140: 302 mg iohexol equivalent to 140 mg iodine/mL (50 mL)
  Omnipaque 180: 388 mg iohexol equivalent to 180 mg iodine/mL (10, 20 mL)
  Omnipaque 240: 518 mg iohexol equivalent to 240 mg iodine/mL (10, 20, 50, 100, 150, 200 mL)
  Omnipaque 300: 647 mg iohexol equivalent to 300 mg iodine/mL (10, 30, 50, 75, 100, 125, 150 mL)
  Omnipaque 350: 755 mg iohexol equivalent to 350 mg iodine/mL (50, 75, 100, 125, 150, 200, 250 mL)

Contrast-enhanced CT scan of the abdomen:
  Oral (administered prior to IV dose):
    Child: Mix 20 mL of Omnipaque 350 with 500 mL of noncarbonated beverage of patient's choice (apple juice works well for younger patients). Administer diluted contrast media PO 30–60 min prior to the IV dose and image acquisition using the following dosage:
      <6 mo: 40–60 mL
      6–18 mo: 120–160 mL
      18 mo–3 yr: 165–240 mL
      3 yr–12 yr: 250–360 mL
      >12 yr: 480–520 mL
    Adult: Mix 50 mL of Omnipaque 350 with 1/2 gallon of noncarbonated beverage of patient's choice. Give 2–4 cups containing 480 mL (16 oz) of the diluted contrast media PO 20–40 min prior to the IV dose and image acquisition.
  IV (administered after PO dose):
    Child: 1–2 mL/kg IV of Omnipaque 240 or Omipaque 300 given 30–60 min after the oral dose.
    Max. dose: 3 mL/kg.
    Adult: 100–150 mL IV of Omnipaque 300 given 20–40 min after the oral dose.

Use with caution in dehydration, previous allergic reaction to a contrast medium, iodine sensitivity, asthma, hay fever, food allergy, congestive heart failure, severe liver or renal impairment, diabetic nephropathy, multiple myeloma, pheochromocytoma, hyperthyroidism, and sickle cell disease. Allergic reactions, arrhythmias, hypothyroidism, transient thyroid suppression, and nephrotoxicity have been rarely reported.

Continued

IOHEXOL *continued*

Children at higher risk for adverse events with contrast medium administration may include those having asthma, sensitivity to medication and/or allergens, congestive heart failure, or serum creatinine > 1.5 mg/dL or those aged <12 mo.

Use **NOT** recommended with drugs that lower seizure threshold (e.g., phenothiazines), amiodarone (increased risk of cardiotoxicity), and metformin (lactic acidosis and acute renal failure).

Many other uses exist; see package insert for additional information. Iohexol is particularly useful when barium sulfate is **contraindicated** in patients with suspected bowel perforation or those where aspiration of contrast medium is of concern. Oral dose is poorly absorbed from the normal GI tract (0.1%–0.5%); absorption increases with bowel perforation or bowel obstruction. Concentrations of 302–755 mg iohexol/mL have osmolalities 1.1–3 times that of plasma (285 mOsm/kg) and CSF (301 mOsm/kg) and may be hypertonic.

IPRATROPIUM BROMIDE ± ALBUTEROL
Atrovent and generics
In combination with albuterol: Combivent Respimat and generics; previously available as DuoNeb
Anticholinergic agent

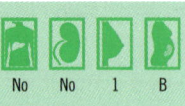

No   No   1   B

Aerosol (HFA): 17 mcg/dose (200 actuations per canister, 12.9 g); contains alcohol
Nebulized solution: 0.02% (500 mcg/2.5 mL) (25s, 30s, 60s)
Nasal spray: 0.03% (21 mcg per actuation, 30 mL provides 345 sprays); 0.06% (42 mcg per actuation, 15 mL provides 165 sprays)
In combination with albuterol:
  Nebulized solution (generic; previously available as DuoNeb): 0.5 mg ipratropium bromide and 2.5 mg albuterol in 3 mL (30s, 60s)
  Inhalation spray (Combivent Respimat): 20 mcg ipratropium and 100 mcg albuterol per actuation (120 actuations per canister, 4 g)

Ipratropium:
Acute use in ED or ICU:
  Nebulizer treatments:
    <12 yr: 250–500 mcg/dose Q20 min × 3, then Q2–4 hr PRN
    ≥12 yr: 500 mcg/dose Q20 min × 3, then Q2–4 hr PRN
  Inhaler:
    <12 yr: 4–8 puffs Q20 min PRN up to 3 hr
    ≥12 yr: 8 puffs Q20 min PRN up to 3 hr
Nonacute use:
  Inhaler:
    <12 yr: 1–2 puffs Q6 hr; **max. dose:** 12 puffs/24 hr
    ≥12 yr: 2–3 puffs Q6 hr; **max. dose:** 12 puffs/24 hr
  Nebulized treatments:
    Infant: 125–250 mcg/dose Q8 hr
    Child ≤ 12 yr: 250 mcg/dose Q6–8 hr
    >12 yr and adult: 250–500 mcg/dose Q6–8 hr
Nasal spray:
  0.03% strength (21 mcg/spray):
    Allergic and nonallergic rhinitis (≥6 yr and adult): 2 sprays (42 mcg) per nostril BID–TID
  0.06% strength (42 mcg/spray):
    Rhinitis associated with common cold (use up to a total of 4 days; safety and efficacy have not been evaluated for >4 days):
      5–11 yr: 2 sprays (84 mcg) per nostril TID
      12 yr–adult: 2 sprays (84 mcg) per nostril TID–QID

IPRATROPIUM BROMIDE ± ALBUTEROL continued

Rhinitis associated with seasonal allergies (use up to a total of 3 weeks; safety and efficacy have not been evaluated for >3 weeks):
≥5 yr–adult: 2 sprays (84 mcg) per nostril QID

Ipratropium in combination with albuterol:
Acute use in the ED or ICU:
Nebulizer treatments:
<12 yr: 1.5 or 3 mL (0.25 mg ipratropium and 1.25 mg albuterol or 0.5 mg ipratropium and 2.5 mg albuterol) Q 20 min × 3 then Q2–4 hr PRN
≥12 yr: 3 mL (0.5 mg ipratropium and 2.5 mg albuterol) Q 20 min × 3 then Q2–4 hr PRN
Inhaler:
<12 yr: 4–8 puffs Q20 min PRN up to 3 hr
≥12 yr: 8 puffs Q20 min PRN up to 3 hr

Contraindicated in soy or peanut allergy (for aerosol inhaler) and atropine hypersensitivity.
Use with caution in narrow-angle glaucoma or bladder neck obstruction, although ipratropium has fewer anticholinergic systemic effects than atropine. May cause anxiety, dizziness, headache, GI discomfort, and cough with inhaler or nebulized use. Epistaxis, nasal congestion, and dry mouth/throat have been reported with the nasal spray. Reversible anisocoria may occur with unintentional aerosolization of drug to the eyes, particularly with mask nebulizers. Proven efficacy of nebulized solution in pediatrics is currently limited to reactive airway disease management in the emergency room and intensive care unit areas.

Combination ipratropium and albuterol products are currently approved for use only in adults and have not been officially studied in children. See albuterol for additional remarks if using the combination product.

Bronchodilation: Onset of action is 1–3 min; peak effects within 1.5–2 hr, and duration of action is 4–6 hr.

Shake inhaler well prior to use with spacer. Nebulized solution may be mixed with albuterol (or use the combination product).

Breastfeeding safety **extrapolated** from safety of atropine.

IRON DEXTRAN

See Iron—Injectable Preparations

IRON SUCROSE

See Iron—Injectable Preparations

IRON—INJECTABLE PREPARATIONS
Ferric gluconate: Ferrlecit and generics
Iron dextran: INFeD, DexFerrum
Iron sucrose: Venofer
Parenteral iron

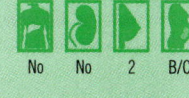

No   No   2   B/C

Injection:
Ferric gluconate (Ferrlecit and generics): 62.5 mg/mL (12.5 mg elemental Fe/mL) (5 mL); contains 9 mg/mL benzyl alcohol and 20% sucrose
Iron dextran (INFeD, DexFerrum): 50 mg/mL (50 mg elemental Fe/mL) (2 mL); products containing 0.5% phenol are only for IM administration; products containing 0.9% sodium chloride can be administered via the IM or IV route.

Continued

IRON—INJECTABLE PREPARATIONS continued

Iron sucrose (Venofer): 20 mg/mL (20 mg elemental Fe/mL) (2.5, 5, 10 mL); contains 300 mg/mL sucrose; preservative free

FERRIC GLUCONATE (IV):
Iron deficiency anemia in patients undergoing chronic hemodialysis who are receiving supplemental erythropoietin therapy (most require 8 doses at 8 sequential dialysis treatments to achieve a favorable response):

Child ≥ 6 yr: 1.5 mg/kg elemental Fe (0.12 mL/kg) IV; **max. dose:** 125 mg elemental Fe/dose. Dilute dose in 25 mL NS and infuse over 1 hr.

Adult: 125 mg elemental Fe in 100 mL NS IV; infuse over 1 hr. Most require a minimum cumulative dose of 1 g elemental Fe administered over 8 sessions.

IRON DEXTRAN (IV or IM):
Iron deficiency anemia (≥4 mo, child, adolescent):

Test dose: 25 mg (12.5 mg for infants) IV (over 5 min) or IM. May initiate treatment dose 1 hr after test dose.

Total replacement dose of iron dextran (mL) = 0.0476 × lean body wt (kg) × [desired Hb (g/dL) − measured Hb (g/dL)] + 1 mL per 5 kg lean body weight (up to **max.** of 14 mL). Total replacement dose is divided into smaller daily doses if it exceeds respective IV or IM daily maximum doses (see below).

Acute blood loss: Total replacement dose of iron dextran (mL) = 0.02 × blood loss (mL) × hematocrit expressed as decimal fraction. Assumes 1 mL of RBC = 1 mg elemental iron.

If no reaction to test dose, give remainder of replacement dose ÷ over 2–3 daily doses.

Max. daily IV dose: 100 mg

Max. daily IM dose:
- **<5 kg:** 0.5 mL (25 mg)
- **5–10 kg:** 1 mL (50 mg)
- **>10 kg:** 2 mL (100 mg)

IM administration: Use "Z-track" technique.

IV administration: Dilute in NS at a max. concentration of 50 mg/mL, and infuse over 1–6 hr at a max. rate of 50 mg/min.

IRON SUCROSE (IV):
Test dose (optional): Infuse 25% of first day dose up to a max. of 25 mg undiluted over 30 min.

Iron deficiency anemia in patients with chronic kidney disease:

Child:

ESRD on hemodialysis: (limited data from 14 children): 1 mg/kg/dialysis was adequate for correcting ferritin levels, and 0.3 mg/kg/dialysis was successful in maintaining ferritin levels between 193–250 mcg/L. Doses were administered during the last hr of each dialysis and are recommended at a frequency of 3 times a week. A 10-mg test dose was administered.

Nonrenal iron deficiency, refractory to PO therapy (limited data):
Total iron replacement dose (mg) = 0.6 × wt (kg) × [100 − (measured Hb ÷ desired Hb × 100)]. Replacement dose is administered by giving an initial dose of 5–7 mg/kg (**max. dose:** 100 mg/24 hr) followed by a maintenance dose of 5–7 mg/kg/dose (**max. dose:** 300 mg/24 hr) Q3–7 days until total iron replacement dose is achieved.

Adult:

Hemodialysis dependent: 100 mg elemental Fe 1–3 times a wk during dialysis up to a total cumulative dose of 1000 mg. May continue to administer at lowest dose to maintain target Hb, Hct, and iron levels.

Nonhemodialysis dependent: 200 mg elemental Fe on 5 different days over a 2-wk period (total cumulative dose: 1000 mg).

IRON—INJECTABLE PREPARATIONS continued

IV administration: May administer undiluted over 2–5 min. For an infusion, dilute each 100 mg with a **max.** of 100-mL NS and infuse over at least 15 min.

Oral therapy with iron salts is preferred; injectable routes are painful. Gluconate and sucrose salts may be better tolerated than iron dextran. Adverse effects include hypotension, GI disturbances, fever, rash, myalgia, arthralgias, cramps, and headaches. Hypersensitivity reactions have been reported for iron dextran and sucrose products; use of test dose prior to first therapeutic dose is recommended.

IM administration is only possible with iron dextran salt. Follow infusion recommendations for specific product. Monitor vital signs during IV infusion. TIBC levels may not be meaningful within 3 wk after dosing.

Efficacy and safety of iron sucrose for maintenance therapy have been evaluated in children aged 2 yr and above with CKD and receiving erythropoietin therapy. Common side effects include headache, respiratory tract viral infection, peritonitis, vomiting, pyrexia, dizziness, and cough.

Pregnancy category is "B" for ferric gluconate and iron sucrose and "C" for iron dextran.

IRON—ORAL PREPARATIONS
Ferrous sulfate: Fer-In-Sol, FeroSul, Slow FE, Slow Iron, and many generics
Ferrous gluconate: Ferate and generics
Ferrous fumarate: Ferretts and generics
Polysaccharide-iron complex: Myferon 150, PIC 200, Poly-Iron 150, NovaFerrum, NovaFerrum Pediatric Drops, and many other brands; previously available as Niferex
Oral iron supplements

No No 2 A

Ferrous sulfate (20% elemental Fe):
Drops and oral solution (Fer-In-Sol and generics; OTC): 75 mg (15 mg Fe)/1 mL (50 mL); contains 0.2% alcohol and sodium bisulfite
Oral elixir and liquid (FeroSul and generics; OTC): 220 mg (44 mg Fe)/5 mL; may contain 5% alcohol
Oral syrup (OTC): 300 mg (60 mg Fe)/5 mL
Tabs (OTC): 325 mg (65 mg Fe)
Extended-release tabs (Slow FE and generics, OTC): 140 mg (45 mg Fe), 160 mg (50 mg Fe), 324 mg (65 mg Fe), and 325 mg (65 mg Fe)

Ferrous gluconate (12% elemental Fe):
Tabs (Ferate and generics; OTC): 240 mg (27 mg Fe), 325 mg (36 mg Fe)

Ferrous fumarate (33% elemental Fe):
Tabs (OTC): 90 mg (29.5 mg Fe), 324 mg (106 mg Fe), 325 mg (106 mg Fe), 456 mg (150 mg Fe)

Polysaccharide-iron complex and ferrous bis-glycinate chelate (expressed in mg elemental Fe):
Caps (OTC): 50 mg (NovaFerrum 50), 150 mg (Myferon 150, Poly-Iron 150, and others), 200 mg (PIC 200); 150 mg strength may contain 50 mg vitamin C
Oral liquid (NovaFerrum 125; OTC): 125 mg/5 mL (180 mL); contains sodium benzoate and 100 units cholecalciferol/5 mL
Oral drops (NovaFerrum Pediatric Drops; OTC): 15 mg/mL (120 mL); contains sodium benzoate

Iron deficiency anemia:
Premature infant: 2–4 mg elemental Fe/kg/24 hr ÷ once daily–BID PO; **max. dose**: 15 mg elemental Fe/24 hr
Child: 3–6 mg elemental Fe/kg/24 hr ÷ once daily–TID PO
Adult: 60–100 mg elemental Fe BID PO up to 60 mg elemental Fe QID

Continued

IRON—ORAL PREPARATIONS continued

Prophylaxis:
Child: Give dose below PO ÷ once daily–TID
  Premature infant: 2 mg elemental Fe/kg/24 hr; **max. dose**: 15 mg elemental Fe/24 hr
  Full-term infant: 1–2 mg elemental Fe/kg/24 hr; **max. dose**: 15 mg elemental Fe/24 hr
  Child 2–12 yr: 2 mg elemental Fe/kg/24 hr; **max. dose**: 30 mg elemental Fe/24 hr
Adolescent and adult: 60 mg elemental Fe/24 hr PO once daily

Contraindicated in hemolytic anemia and hemochromatosis. **Avoid** use in GI tract inflammation. May cause constipation, dark stools (false positive guaiac is controversial), nausea, and epigastric pain. Iron and tetracycline inhibit each other's absorption. Antacids may decrease iron absorption.

Iron preparations are variably absorbed. Less GI irritation when given with or after meals. Vitamin C, 200 mg per 30 mg iron, may enhance absorption. Liquid iron preparations may stain teeth. Give with dropper or drink through straw.

ISONIAZID
INH, Nydrazid, Laniazid, and other generics
In combination with rifampin: Rifamate and IsonaRif
In combination with rifampin and pyrazinamide: Rifater
Antituberculous agent

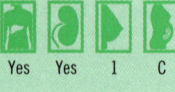
Yes   Yes   1   C

Tabs: 100, 300 mg
Syrup: 50 mg/5 mL (473 mL)
Injection: 100 mg/mL (10 mL); contains 0.25% chlorobutanol
In combination with rifampin:
  Caps (Rifamate, IsonaRif): 150 mg isoniazid + 300 mg rifampin
In combination with rifampin and pyrazinamide:
  Caps (Rifater): 50 mg isoniazid + 120 mg rifampin + 300 mg pyrazinamide

See most recent edition of the AAP Red Book for details and length of therapy.
Prophylaxis:
  Infant and child: 10–15 mg/kg (**max. dose**: 300 mg) PO once daily. After 1 mo of daily therapy and in cases where daily compliance cannot be assured, may change to 20–30 mg/kg (**max. dose**: 900 mg) per dose PO given twice weekly.
  Adult: 300 mg PO once daily
Treatment:
  Infant and child:
  10–15 mg/kg (**max. dose**: 300 mg) PO once daily or 20–30 mg/kg (**max. dose**: 900 mg) per dose twice weekly with rifampin for uncomplicated pulmonary tuberculosis in compliant patients. Additional drugs are necessary in complicated diseases.
  Adult:
  5 mg/kg (**max. dose**: 300 mg) PO once daily or 15 mg/kg (**max. dose**: 900 mg) per dose twice weekly with rifampin. Additional drugs are necessary in complicated diseases.
For INH-resistant TB: Discuss with Health Department or consult ID specialist.

Should not be used alone for treatment. Contraindicated in acute liver disease and previous isoniazid-associated hepatitis. Peripheral neuropathy, optic neuritis, seizures, encephalopathy, psychosis, and hepatic side effects may occur with higher doses, especially in combination with rifampin. Severe liver injury has been reported in children and adults treated for latent TB. Follow LFTs monthly. Supplemental pyridoxine (1–2 mg/kg/24 hr) is recommended for prevention of neurological side effects. Toxic epidermal necrolysis and DRESS have been reported. May cause false-positive urine glucose test.

ISONIAZID continued

Inhibits CYP450 1A2, 2C9, 2C19, and 3A3/4 microsomal enzymes; decrease dose of carbamazepine, diazepam, phenytoin, and prednisone. Prednisone may decrease isoniazid's effects. Also a substrate and inducer of CYP450 2E1 and may potentiate acetaminophen hepatotoxicity. **Avoid** daily alcohol use to reduce risk of isoniazid-induced hepatitis.

May be given IM (same as oral doses) when oral therapy is not possible. Administer oral doses 1 hr prior to and 2 hr after meals. Aluminum salts may decrease absorption. **Adjust dose in renal failure (see Chapter 30).**

ISOPROTERENOL
Isuprel
Adrenergic agonist

No Yes ? C

Injection: 0.2 mg/mL (5, 10 mL); contains disodium EDTA

NOTE: The dosage units for adults are in mcg/min compared to mcg/kg/min for children.
IV infusion:
  Neonate–child: 0.05–2 mcg/kg/min; start at minimum dose and increase every 5–10 min by 0.1 mcg/kg/min until desired effect or onset of toxicity; **max. dose**: 2 mcg/kg/min.
  Adult: 2–20 mcg/min; titrate to desired effect.

Use with caution in diabetes, hyperthyroidism, renal disease, CHF, ischemia, and aortic stenosis. May cause flushing, ventricular arrhythmias, profound hypotension, anxiety, and myocardial ischemia. Monitor heart rate, respiratory rate, and blood pressure. **Not** for treatment of asystole or for use in cardiac arrests, unless bradycardia is due to heart block.

Continuous infusion for bronchodilatation must be gradually tapered over a 24–48-hr period to prevent rebound bronchospasm. Tolerance may occur with prolonged use. Clinical deterioration, myocardial necrosis, congestive heart failure, and **death** have been reported with continuous infusion use in refractory asthmatic children.

ISOTRETINOIN
Absorica, Claravis, Myorisan, Zenatane; previously available as Accutane
Retinoic acid, vitamin A derivative

Yes No 3 X

Caps: 10, 20, 25, 30, 35, 40 mg; may contain soybean oil, EDTA, and parabens

Cystic acne/Severe Recalcitrant Nodular acne (see remarks):
  Child (>12 yr) and adult: 0.5–2 mg/kg/24 hr ÷ BID PO × 15–20 wk or until the total cyst count decreases by 70%, whichever comes first. Dosages as low as 0.05 mg/kg/24 hr have been reported to be beneficial.

Contraindicated during pregnancy; known teratogen. Use with caution in females of childbearing age. May cause conjunctivitis, xerosis, pruritus, photosensitivity reactions (avoid exposure to sunlight and use sunscreen), epistaxis, anemia, hyperlipidemia, pseudotumor cerebri (especially in combination with tetracyclines; avoid this combination), cheilitis, bone pain, muscle aches, skeletal changes, lethargy, nausea, vomiting, elevated ESR, mental depression, aggressive/violent behavior, and psychosis. Serious skin reactions (e.g., Stevens Johnson syndrome and TEN) have been reported.

Elevation of liver enzymes may occur during treatment; a dosage reduction or continued treatment may result in normalization. Discontinue use if liver enzymes do not normalize or if hepatitis is suspected.

Continued

ISOTRETINOIN continued

To avoid additive toxic effects, **do not** take vitamin A concomitantly. Increases clearance of carbamazepine. Hormonal birth control (oral, injectable, and implantable) failures have been reported with concurrent use. Monitor CBC, ESR, triglycerides, and LFTs.

Prescribers, site pharmacists, patients, and wholesalers must register with the iPLEDGE system (a risk minimization program) at www.ipledgeprogram.com or 1–866–495–0654 before doses are dispensed. Prescriptions may not be written for more than a 1-mo supply.

ITRACONAZOLE
Sporanox, Onmel, and generics
Antifungal agent

   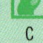

Yes   Yes   3   C

Caps (Sporanox and generics): 100 mg
Tabs (Onmel): 200 mg
Oral solution (Sporanox): 10 mg/mL (150 mL); contains propylene glycol and saccharin

Neonate (limited data in full-term neonates treated for tinea capitis): 5 mg/kg/24 hr PO once daily × 6 wk
Child (limited data): 3–5 mg/kg/24 hr PO ÷ once daily–BID; dosages as high as 5–10 mg/kg/24 hr have been used for Aspergillus prophylaxis in chronic granulomatous disease. Population pharmacokinetic data in pediatric cystic fibrosis and bone marrow transplant patients suggest an oral liquid dosage of 10 mg/kg/24 hr PO ÷ BID or oral capsule dosage of 20 mg/kg/24 hr PO ÷ BID to be more reliable in achieving trough plasma levels between 500 and 2000 ng/mL.
  Prophylaxis for recurrence of opportunistic disease in HIV:
    Coccidioides spp.: 2–5 mg/kg/dose PO Q12 hr; **max. dose**: 400 mg/24 hr
    Cryptococcus neoformans: 5 mg/kg/dose PO Q24 hr; **max. dose**: 200 mg/24 hr
    Histoplasma capsulatum: 5 mg/kg/dose PO Q12 hr; **max. dose**: 400 mg/24 hr
  Treatment of opportunistic disease in HIV:
    Candidiasis: 5 mg/kg/24 hr PO ÷ Q12–24 hr; **max. dose**: 400 mg/24 hr
    Coccidioides spp.: 5–10 mg/kg/dose PO BID × 3 days, followed by 2–5 mg/kg/dose PO BID; **max. dose**: 400 mg/24 hr
    Cryptococcus neoformans: 2.5–5 mg/kg/dose (**max. dose**: 200 mg/dose) PO TID × 3 days, followed by 5–10 mg/kg/24 hr (**max. dose**: 400 mg/24 hr) ÷ once to twice daily for a minimum of 8 wk.
    Histoplasma capsulatum: 2–5 mg/kg/dose (**max. dose**: 200 mg/dose) PO TID × 3 days, followed by 2–5 mg/kg/dose (**max. dose**: 200 mg/dose) PO BID × 12 mo.
Adult:
  Blastomycosis and nonmeningeal histoplasmosis: 200 mg PO once daily up to a **max. dose** of 400 mg/24 hr ÷ BID (**max. dose**: 200 mg/dose)
  Aspergillosis and severe infections: 600 mg/24 hr PO ÷ TID × 3–4 days, followed by 200–400 mg/24 hr ÷ BID; **max. dose**: 600 mg/24 hr ÷ TID.

Oral solution and capsule dosage form should NOT be used interchangeably; oral solution is more bioavailable. Only the oral solution has been demonstrated as effective for oral and/or esophageal candidiasis. **Contraindicated** in CHF and certain interacting drugs (see below). **Use with caution** in hepatic and/or renal impairment, cardiac dysrhythmias, and azole hypersensitivity. May cause GI symptoms, headaches, rash, liver enzyme elevation, hepatitis, and hypokalemia. Double/blurred vision, dizziness, and tremor have been reported.

Like ketoconazole, it inhibits the activity of the CYP450 3A4 drug metabolizing isoenzyme. Thus, the coadministration of cisapride, dofetilide, felodipine, methadone, nisoldipine, pimozide, quinidine,

ITRACONAZOLE continued

triazolam, lovastatin, simvastatin, ergot derivatives, and oral midazolam is **contraindicated.** See remarks in Ketoconazole for additional drug interaction information.

Steady-state serum concentrations of >0.25 mg/L itraconazole and >1 mg/L hydroxyitraconazole (metabolite) have been recommended. Recommended serum sampling time at steady state: any time after 2 wk of continuous dosing. Itraconazole has 34–42-hr $T_{1/2}$.

Administer oral solution on an empty stomach, but administer capsules with food. Achlorhydria reduces absorption of the drug. **Do not** use oral liquid dosage form in patients with GFR <30 mL/min because the hydroxypropyl-β-cyclodextrin excipient has reduced clearance with renal failure.

KETAMINE
Ketalar and generics
General anesthetic

No / No / 3 / B

Injection: 10 mg/mL (20 mL), 50 mg/mL (10 mL), 100 mg/mL (5, 10 mL); contains benzethonium chloride

Child (see remarks):
  Sedation:
    PO: 5 mg/kg × 1
    IV: 0.25–1 mg/kg
    IM: 2–5 mg/kg × 1
Adult:
  Analgesia with sedation:
    IV (see remarks): 0.2–1 mg/kg
    IM: 0.5–4 mg/kg

Contraindicated in elevated ICP, hypertension, aneurysms, thyrotoxicosis, CHF, angina, and psychotic disorders. May cause hypertension, hypotension, emergence reactions, tachycardia, laryngospasm, respiratory depression, and stimulation of salivary secretions. Cystitis has been reported with chronic use/abuse. Intravenous use may induce general anesthesia. Coadministration of an anticholinergic agent may be added in situations of clinically significant hypersalivation in patients with impaired ability to mobilize secretions. Benzodiazepine may be used in the presence of a ketamine-associated recovery reaction (prophylaxis use in adults may be beneficial). Ondansetron prophylaxis can slightly reduce vomiting. See Ann Emerg Med. 2001;57:449–461 for additional use information in the emergency department.

Drug is a substrate for CYP450 2B6, 2C9 and 3A4 isoenzymes. Consider potential drug interactions with respective enzyme inhibitors and inducers, especially with prolonged use.

Rate of IV infusion should **not** exceed 0.5 mg/kg/min and **should not** be administered over less than 60 s. For additional information including onset and duration of action, see Chapter 6.

Pregnancy category is considered by many as a "B" despite no formal designation by the FDA.

KETOCONAZOLE
Nizoral, Nizoral A-D, Xolegel, Extina, Ketodan, and generics
Antifungal agent, imidazole

Yes / No / 2 / C

Tabs: 200 mg
Oral suspension: 100 mg/5 mL

Continued

KETOCONAZOLE continued

Cream: 2% (15, 30, 60 g); contains sulfites
Gel: 2% [Xolegel] (45 g); contains 34% alcohol
Shampoo: 1% [Nizoral A-D, OTC] (125, 200 mL), 2% [Nizoral and generics] (120 mL)
Foam: 2% [Extina, Ketodan and generics] (50, 100 g); contains alcohol and propylene glycol

Oral:
 Child ≥ 2 yr: 3.3–6.6 mg/kg/24 hr once daily
 Adult: 200–400 mg/24 hr once daily
 Max. dose (all ages): 800 mg/24 hr ÷ BID
Topical (see remarks):
 Cream: 1–2 applications/24 hr
 Gel (Xolegel): 1 application once daily
Shampoo (dandruff): Twice weekly with at least 3 days between applications for up to 8 weeks PRN. Thereafter, intermittently as needed to maintain control.

The systemic dosage form should NOT be first-line treatment for any fungal infection due to concerns of hepatotoxicity and adrenal gland effects (per the FDA).

Monitor LFTs in long-term use and adrenal function for patients at risk. Drugs that decrease gastric acidity will decrease absorption. May cause nausea, vomiting, rash, headache, pruritus, and fever. Hepatotoxicity (including fatal cases) has been reported; use in hepatic impairment is **contraindicated**. High doses may decrease adrenocortical function and serum testosterone levels. Hypersensitivity reactions (including anaphylaxis) have been reported with all dosage forms.

Safety and efficacy with topical use in seborrheic dermatitis for patients aged >12 yr has been established. **Avoid** topical use on breast or nipples in nursing mothers.

Inhibits CYP450 3A4. **Contraindicated** when used with cisapride, disopyramide, methadone, mefloquine, quinidine, terfinadine, pimozide, or any drug that can prolong the QT interval (because of risk for cardiac arrhythmias) and HMG-CoA reductase inhibitors (e.g., simvastatin and lovastatin). Excessive sedation and prolonged hypnotic effects with triazolam use (also **contraindicated**). May increase levels/effects of phenytoin, digoxin, cyclosporine, corticosteroids, nevirapine, protease inhibitors, and warfarin. Achlorhydria, phenobarbital, rifampin, isoniazid, H_2 blockers, antacids, and omeprazole can decrease levels of oral ketoconazole.

Administering oral doses with food or acidic beverages and 2 hr prior to antacids will increase absorption.

To use shampoo, wet hair and scalp with water; apply sufficient amount to the scalp and gently massage for about 1 min. Rinse hair thoroughly, reapply shampoo, leave on the scalp for an additional 3 min, and rinse.

KETOROLAC
Many generics (previously available as Toradol), Acular, Acular LS, Acuvail
Nonsteroidal antiinflammatory agent

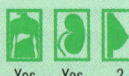 Yes   Yes   2   C/D

Injection: 15 mg/mL (1 mL), 30 mg/mL (1, 2, 10 mL); contains 10% alcohol and tromethamine
Tabs: 10 mg; contains tromethamine
Ophthalmic solution (all containing tromethamine):
 Acular: 0.5% (5 mL); contains benzalkonium chloride
 Acular LS and generics: 0.4% (3, 5, 10 mL); contains benzalkonium chloride
 Acuvail: 0.45% (0.4 mL; 30s); preservative free

KETOROLAC continued

Systemic use is not to exceed 3–5 days; regardless of administration route (IM, IV, PO)
IM/IV:
  Child: 0.5 mg/kg/dose IM/IV Q6–8 hr. **Max. dose**: 30 mg Q6 hr or 120 mg/24 hr. Alternatively, the manufacturer has recommended the following doses for children aged 2–16 yr with moderate/severe acute pain:
    IV: 0.5 mg/kg × 1; **max. dose**: 15 mg
    IM: 1 mg/kg × 1; **max. dose**: 30 mg
  Adult: 30 mg IM/IV Q6 hr. **Max. dose**: 120 mg/24 hr
PO:
  Child > 16 yr (>50 kg) and adult: 10 mg PRN Q6 hr; max. dose: 40 mg/24 hr
Ophthalmic (see remarks):
  ≥3 yr–adult: 1 drop in each affected eye QID

May cause GI bleeding, nausea, dyspepsia, drowsiness, decreased platelet function, and interstitial nephritis. **Not recommended** in patients at increased risk of bleeding. **Do not use** in hepatic or renal failure. **Use with caution** in heart disease (risk for MI and stroke with prolonged use).

Duration of therapy for ophthalmic use: 14 days after cataract surgery and up to 4 days after corneal refractive surgery. Also indicated for ocular itching associated with seasonal allergic conjunctivitis. Bronchospasm or asthma exacerbations, corneal erosion/perforation/thinning/melt, and epithelial breakdown have been reported with ophthalmic use.

Pregnancy category changes to a "D" if used in the third trimester.

LABETALOL
Generics; previously available as Normodyne and Trandate
Adrenergic antagonist (α and β), antihypertensive

Yes   No   2   C/D

Tabs: 100, 200, 300 mg
Injection: 5 mg/mL (4, 20, 40 mL); contains parabens
Oral suspension: 10, 40 mg/mL

Child (see remarks):
  PO: Initial: 1–3 mg/kg/24 hr ÷ BID. May increase up to a **maximum** of 12 mg/kg/24 hr up to 1200 mg/24 hr
  IV: Hypertensive emergency (start at lowest dose and titrate to effect; see Chapter 4 for additional information)
    Intermittent dose: 0.2–1 mg/kg/dose Q10 min PRN; **max. dose:** 40 mg/dose
    Infusion (hypertensive emergencies): 0.4–1 mg/kg/hr, to a **max. dose** of 3 mg/kg/hr; may initiate with a 0.2–1 mg/kg bolus; **max. bolus:** 40 mg
Adult (see remarks):
  PO: 100 mg BID, increase by 100 mg/dose Q2–3 days PRN to a **max. dose** of 2.4 g/24 hr. Usual range: 200–800 mg/24 hr ÷ BID
  IV: Hypertensive emergency (start at lowest dose and titrate to effect with a **max. total dose** of 300 mg for both methods of administration):
    Intermittent dose: 20–80 mg/dose (begin with 20 mg) Q10 min PRN
    Infusion: 2 mg/min, increase to titrate to response

Contraindicated in asthma, pulmonary edema, cardiogenic shock, and heart block. May cause orthostatic hypotension, edema, CHF, bradycardia, AV conduction disturbances,

Continued

LABETALOL continued

bronchospasm, urinary retention, and skin tingling. **Use with caution** in hepatic disease (dose reduction may be necessary), diabetes, liver function test elevation, hepatic necrosis, and hepatitis. Cholestatic jaundice has been reported. Use with digitalis glycosides may increase risk for bradycardia.

Patient should remain supine for up to 3 hr after IV administration. Pregnancy category changes to "D" if used in second or third trimesters.

Onset of action: PO: 1–4 hr; IV: 5–15 min.

LACOSAMIDE
Vimpat
Anticonvulsant

Yes   Yes   ?   C

Oral solution: 10 mg/mL (200, 465 mL); contains aspartame, parabens, and propylene glycol
Tabs: 50, 100, 200 mg
Injection: 10 mg/mL (20 mL)

Child (3–18 yr; limited data in 18 patients with refractory partial seizures as adjunctive therapy with moderate response): Start at 1 mg/kg/24 hr (initial max. 100 mg/24 hr) PO ÷ BID. If needed, dose may be increased at weekly intervals by 1 mg/kg/24 hr administered BID up to 10 mg/kg/24 hr. The final doses range from 2 to 10 mg/kg/24 hr. A retrospective trial in 16 patients aged 8–21 yr with focal seizures as adjunctive therapy received an average dose of 4.7 mg/kg/24 hr PO with moderate response.

Phase III trials for lacosamide as an add-on therapy for patients with partial-onset seizures (1 mo–≤18 yr) and tonic clonic seizures are evaluating the following dosage (see www.clinicaltrials.gov for updates):
  <30 kg: 10 mg/kg/24 hr PO ÷ BID
  ≥30–<50 kg: 6–8 mg/kg/24 hr PO ÷ BID
  ≥50 kg: 150–200 mg PO BID

≥17 yr and adult:
  Partial-onset seizures, adjunctive therapy: Start at 50 mg BID IV/PO. If needed, dose may be increased at weekly intervals by 100 mg/24 day administered BID up to the usual maintenance dose of 200–400 mg/24 hr ÷ BID. Use same dose when converting from IV to PO and vice versa. IV use should be considered for temporary use.

Use with caution with known cardiac conduction problems (e.g., second-degree AV block), severe cardiac disease (e.g., MI or heart failure), concomitant use with drugs known to prolong PR interval, and renal (see Chaper 30) and hepatic impairment. Lacosamide undergoes 95% renal excretion, and a **maximum** dosage of 300 mg/24 hr is recommended in adults with GFR < 30 mL/min and ESRD. Dose reduction may be necessary with hepatic or renal impairment and concurrent strong inhibitor of CYP450 3A4 or 2C9 medication. Use is **not recommended** in severe hepatic impairment, and an adult **max. dose** of 300 mg/24 hr is recommended for mild/moderate hepatic impairment. Oral bioavailability is approximately 100%.

Most common side effects in adults include diplopia, headache, dizziness, and nausea. Somnolence and irritability were frequently reported in pediatric studies. Patients should be informed about potential dizziness, ataxia, and syncope with use. Multiorgan hypersensitivity reactions (affecting the skin, kidney, and liver), agranulocytosis, and euphoria (high doses) have been reported. As with other AEDs, monitor for suicidal behavior and ideation.

Oral doses may be administered with or without food. IV doses should be administered over 30–60 min. **Do not** abruptly withdraw therapy (gradually taper) to prevent potential seizures.

LACTULOSE
Cephulac, Chronulac, Enulose, Kristalose, and generics
Ammonium detoxicant, hyperosmotic laxative

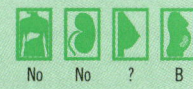

No   No   ?   B

Oral syrup: 10 g/15 mL (15, 30, 237, 473, 960, 1893 mL); contains galactose, lactose, and other sugars
Crystals for reconstitution (Kristalose): 10 g (30s), 20 g (30s)

Constipation:
  Child: 1.5–3 mL/kg/24 hr PO ÷ BID; **max. dose:** 60 mL/24 hr
  Adult: 15–30 mL/24 hr PO once daily to a **max. dose** of 60 mL/24 hr
Portal systemic encephalopathy (adjust dose to produce 2–3 soft stools/day):
  Infant: 2.5–10 mL/24 hr PO ÷ TID–QID
  Child and adolescent: 40–90 mL/24 hr PO ÷ TID–QID
  Adult: 30–45 mL/dose PO TID–QID; acute episodes 30–45 mL Q1–2 hr until 2–3 soft stools/day
  Rectal (adult): 300 mL diluted in 700 mL water or NS in 30–60 min retention enema; may give Q4–6 hr

Contraindicated in galactosemia. **Use with caution** in diabetes mellitus. GI discomfort and diarrhea may occur. For portal systemic encephalopathy, monitor serum ammonia, serum potassium, and fluid status.
Adjust dose to achieve 2–3 soft stools per day. **Do not use** with antacids. Dissolve crystal dosage form with 4 ounces of water or juice. All doses may be administered with juice, milk, or water.

LAMIVUDINE
Epivir, Epivir-HBV, 3TC, and generics
Antiviral agent, nucleoside analogue reverse transcriptase inhibitor

Yes   Yes   3   C

Tabs: 100 mg (Epivir-HBV and generics), 150, 300 mg
Oral solution: 5 mg/mL (Epivir-HBV) (240 mL), 10 mg/mL (Epivir and generics) (240 mL); contains parabens

HIV: See www.aidsinfo.nih.gov/guidelines
Prevention of maternal–fetal transmission to reduce nevirapine resistance (for infants born to mothers with no antiretroviral therapy before or during labor, infants born to mothers with only intrapartum antiretroviral therapy, infants born to mothers with suboptimal viral suppression at delivery, or infants born to mothers with known antiretroviral drug resistance):
  Neonate: 2 mg/kg/dose PO BID × 7–14 days from birth
Chronic hepatitis B (see remarks):
  2–17 yr: 3 mg/kg/dose PO once daily up to a **max. dose** of 100 mg/dose
  ≥18 and adult: 100 mg/dose PO once daily

See aidsinfo.nih.gov/guidelines for remarks for use in HIV. Oral tablet dosage form is preferred over oral solution for children ≥ 14 kg because subjects in the ARROW clinical trial receiving oral solution had lower rates of HIV viral suppression, lower plasma lamivudine exposure, and developed viral resistance more frequently.
May cause headache, fatigue, GI disturbances, rash, and myalgia/arthralgia. Lactic acidosis, severe hepatomegaly with steatosis, posttreatment exacerbations of hepatitis B and ALT elevations,

Continued

LAMIVUDINE continued

pancreatitis, and emergence of resistant viral strains have been reported. Concomitant use with co-trimoxazole (TMP/SMX) may result in increased lamivudine levels.

Use Epivir-HBV product for chronic hepatitis B indication. Safety and effectiveness beyond 1 yr have not been determined. Patients with both HIV and hepatitis B should use the higher HIV doses along with an appropriate combination regimen.

May be administered with food. **Adjust dose in renal impairment (see Chapter 30).**

LAMOTRIGINE
Lamictal, Lamictal ODT, Lamictal XR, and generics
Anticonvulsant

Yes   Yes   2   C

Tabs: 25, 100, 150, 200 mg
Extended-release tabs (Lamictal XR and generics): 25, 50, 100, 200, 250, 300 mg
Chewable tabs: 5, 25 mg
Orally disintegrated tabs (Lamictal ODT and generics): 25, 50, 100, 200 mg
Oral suspension: 1 mg/mL

Child 2–12 yr adjunctive seizure therapy (see remarks):
  WITH antiepileptic drugs (AEDs) other than carbamazepine, phenytoin, phenobarbital, primidone, or valproic acid (use immediate-release dosage forms):
  Wk 1 and 2: 0.3 mg/kg/24 hr PO ÷ once daily–BID; rounded down to the nearest whole tablet.
  Wk 3 and 4: 0.6 mg/kg/24 hr PO ÷ BID; rounded down to the nearest whole tablet.
  Usual maintenance dose: 4.5–7.5 mg/kg/24 hr PO ÷ BID titrate to effect. To achieve the usual maintenance dose, increase doses Q1–2 wk by 0.6 mg/kg/24 hr (rounded down to the nearest whole tablet) as needed.
  Max. dose: 300 mg/24 hr ÷ BID.
  WITH enzyme inducing AEDs WITHOUT valproic acid (use immediate-release dosage forms):
  Wk 1 and 2: 0.6 mg/kg/24 hr PO ÷ BID; rounded down to the nearest whole tablet.
  Wk 3 and 4: 1.2 mg/kg/24 hr PO ÷ BID; rounded down to the nearest whole tablet.
  Usual maintenance dose: 5–15 mg/kg/24 hr PO ÷ BID titrate to effect. To achieve the usual maintenance dose, increase doses Q1–2 wk by 1.2 mg/kg/24 hr (rounded down to the nearest whole tablet) as needed.
  Max. dose: 400 mg/24 hr ÷ BID.
  WITH AEDs WITH valproic acid (use immediate-release dosage forms):
  Wk 1 and 2: 0.15 mg/kg/24 hr PO ÷ once daily–BID; rounded down to the nearest whole tablet (see following table)
  Wk 3 and 4: 0.3 mg/kg/24 hr PO ÷ once daily–BID; rounded down to the nearest whole tablet (see following table)

Weight (kg)	Weeks 1 & 2	Weeks 3 & 4
6.7–14	2 mg every other day	2 mg once daily
14.1–27	2 mg once daily	4 mg/24 hr ÷ once daily–BID
27.1–34	4 mg/24 hr ÷ once daily–BID	8 mg/24 hr ÷ once daily–BID
34.1–40	5 mg once daily	10 mg/24 hr ÷ once daily–BID

  Usual maintenance dose: 1–5 mg/kg/24 hr PO ÷ once daily–BID titrate to effect. To achieve the usual maintenance dose, increase doses Q1–2 wk by 0.3 mg/kg/24 hr (rounded down to the nearest whole tablet) as needed. If adding lamotrigine with valproic acid alone, usual maintenance dose is 1–3 mg/kg/24 hr.
  Max. dose: 200 mg/24 hr.

LAMOTRIGINE continued

>12 yr and adult adjunctive therapy:
  WITH AEDs other than carbamazepine, phenytoin, phenobarbital, primidone, or valproic acid (use immediate-release dosage forms):
    Wk 1 and 2: 25 mg once daily PO.
    Wk 3 and 4: 50 mg once daily PO.
    Usual maintenance dose: 225–375 mg/24 hr ÷ BID PO titrate to effect. To achieve the usual maintenance dose, increase doses Q1–2 wk by 50 mg/24 hr as needed.
  WITH enzyme-inducing AEDs WITHOUT valproic acid (use immediate-release dosage forms):
    Wk 1 and 2: 50 mg once daily PO.
    Wk 3 and 4: 50 mg BID PO.
    Usual maintenance dose: 300–500 mg/24 hr ÷ BID PO titrate to effect. To achieve the usual maintenance dose, increase doses Q1–2 wk by 100 mg/24 hr as needed. Doses as high as 700 mg/24 hr ÷ BID have been used.
  WITH AEDs WITH valproic acid: (use immediate-release dosage forms)
    Wk 1 and 2: 25 mg every other day PO.
    Wk 3 and 4: 25 mg once daily PO.
    Usual maintenance dose: 100–400 mg/24 hr ÷ once daily–BID PO titrate to effect. To achieve the usual maintenance dose, increase doses Q1–2 wk by 25–50 mg/24 hr as needed. If adding lamotrigene to valproic acid alone, usual maintenance dose is 100–200 mg/24 hr.

Extended-release dosage form (Lamictal XR):
  ≥13 yr and adult adjunctive therapy (dose increases at week 8 or later should not exceed 100 mg/24 hr at weekly intervals; see remarks):

	Weeks 1 & 2	Weeks 3 & 4	Week 5	Week 6	Week 7	Maintenance Dose
Patient NOT receiving enzyme-inducing drugs (e.g., carbamazepine) OR valproic acid	25 mg once daily	50 mg once daily	100 mg once daily	150 mg once daily	200 mg once daily	300–400 mg once daily
Patients receiving enzyme-inducing drugs (e.g., carbamazepine) WITHOUT valproic acid	50 mg once daily	100 mg once daily	200 mg once daily	300 mg once daily	400 mg once daily	400–600 mg once daily
Patients receiving valproic acid	25 mg every other day	25 mg once daily	50 mg once daily	100 mg once daily	150 mg once daily	200–250 mg once daily

Converting from a single enzyme-inducing AED to lamotrigine monotherapy for a child ≥ 16 yr and adult (titrate lamotrigine to maintenance dose; then gradually withdraw enzyme-inducing AED by 20% decrements over a 4-wk period; use immediate-release dosage forms):
  Wk 1 and 2: 50 mg once daily PO.
  Wk 3 and 4: 50 mg BID PO.
  Usual maintenance dose: 500 mg/24 hr ÷ BID PO titrate to effect; to achieve the usual maintenance dose, increase doses Q1–2 wk by 100 mg/24 hr as needed.

Continued

LAMOTRIGINE continued

Bipolar disease (use immediate-release dosage forms; see remarks):
≥18 yr and adult (PO; see table below):

	Weeks 1 & 2	Weeks 3 & 4	Week 5	Weeks 6 and Thereafter
Patient NOT receiving enzyme-inducing drugs (e.g., carbamazepine) OR valproic acid	25 mg/24 hr	50 mg/24 hr	100 mg/24 hr	200 mg/24 hr (target dose)
Patients receiving enzyme-inducing drugs (e.g., carbamazepine) WITHOUT valproic acid	50 mg/24 hr	100 mg/24 hr ÷ once daily–BID	200 mg/24 hr ÷ once daily–BID	Week 6: 300 mg/24 hr ÷ once daily–BID. Week 7 and thereafter: may increase to 400 mg/24 hr ÷ once daily–BID (target dose)*
Patients receiving valproic acid	25 mg every other day	25 mg/24 hr	50 mg/24 hr	100 mg/24 hr (target dose)†

*If carbamazepine or other enzyme-inducing drug is discontinued, maintain current lamotrigine dose for 1 week, then decrease daily lamotrigine dose in 100-mg increments at weekly intervals until 200 mg/24 hr.
†If valproic acid is discontinued, increase by 50 mg weekly intervals up to 200 mg/24 hr.

Enzyme-inducing antiepileptic drugs (AEDs) include carbamazepine, phenytoin, and phenobarbital. Stevens–Johnson syndrome, toxic epidermal necrolysis, and other potentially life-threatening rashes have been reported in children (0.3%–0.8%) and adults (0.08%–0.3%) for adjunctive therapy in seizures. Reported rates for adults treated for bipolar/mood disorders as monotherapy and adjunctive therapy are 0.08% and 0.13%, respectively. May cause fatigue, drowsiness, ataxia, rash (especially with valproic acid), headache, nausea, vomiting, and abdominal pain. Diplopia, nystagmus, aseptic meningitis, aggression, and alopecia have also been reported. Use during the first 3 mo of pregnancy may result in a higher chance for cleft lip or cleft palate in the newborn. Suicidal behavior or ideation has been reported.

If converting from immediate- to extended-release dosage form, initial dose of extended release should match the total daily dose of the immediate-release dosage and be administered once daily. Adjust dose as needed with the recommended dosage guidelines.

Reduce maintenance dose in renal failure. Reduce all doses (initial, escalation, and maintenance) in liver dysfunction defined by the Child-Pugh grading system as follows:
Grade B: moderate dysfunction, decrease dose by ~50%
Grade C: severe dysfunction, decrease dose by ~75%

Withdrawal symptoms may occur if discontinued suddenly. A stepwise dose reduction over ≥2 wk (~50% per week) is recommended unless safety concerns require a more rapid withdrawal.

Acetaminophen, carbamazepine, oral contraceptives (ethinylestradiol), phenobarbital, primidone, phenytoin, and rifampin may decrease levels of lamotrigine. Valproic acid may increase levels. False positive urine drug screen for phencyclidine (PCP) has been reported.

Safety and efficacy of maintenance therapy for bipolar disorder in 10–17 yr old were not established in an RCT of 301 subjects.

LANSOPRAZOLE
Prevacid, Prevacid SoluTab, First-Lansoprazole, and generics
Gastric acid pump inhibitor

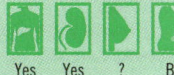
Yes Yes ? B

Caps, delayed release: 15, 30 mg
Tabs, disintegrating delayed release (Prevacid SoluTab): 15, 30 mg; contains aspartame
Oral suspension (First-Lansoprazole): 3 mg/mL (90, 150, 300 mL); contains benzyl alcohol

1–11 yr (short-term treatment of GERD and erosive esophagitis, for up to 12 wk):
  Initial dose using fixed dosing:
    ≤30 kg: 15 mg PO once daily
    >30 kg: 30 mg PO once daily–BID
  Subsequent dosage increase (if needed): May be increased up to 30 mg PO BID after ≥2 wk of therapy without response at initial dose level.
  Alternative weight-based dosing:
    Infant: 1–2 mg/kg/24 hr PO once daily
    Child: 0.7–3 mg/kg/24 hr PO ÷ once daily–BID
12 yr–adult:
  GERD: 15 mg PO once daily for up to 8 wk
  Erosive esophagitis: 30 mg PO once daily × 8–16 wk; maintenance dose: 15 mg PO once daily
  Duodenal ulcer: 15 mg PO once daily × 4 wk; maintenance dose: 15 mg PO once daily
  Gastric ulcer and NSAID induced ulcer: 30 mg PO once daily for up to 8 wk
  Hypersecretory conditions: 60 mg PO once daily; dosage may be increased up to 90 mg PO BID, where doses > 120 mg/24 hr are divided BID

- Common side effects include GI discomfort, headache, fatigue, rash, and taste perversion. Hypersensitivity reactions may result in anaphylaxis, angioedema, bronchospasm, interstitial nephritis, and urticaria. Prolonged use may result in vitamin B_{12} deficiency (≥2 yr) or hypomagnesemia (>1 yr). Microscopic colitis resulting in watery diarrhea has been reported, and switching to an alternative proton-pump inhibitor may be beneficial in resolving diarrhea.
- Drug is a substrate for CYP450 2C19 and 3A3/4. May decrease levels of itraconazole, ketoconazole, iron salts, mycophenolate, nelfinavir, and ampicillin esters and increase the levels/effects of methotrexate, tacrolimus, and warfarin. Theophylline clearance may be enhanced. **Reduce dose in severe hepatic impairment.** May be used in combination with clarithromycin and amoxicillin for *Helicobacter pylori* infections.
- A multicenter, double blind, parallel-group study in infants (1 mo–1 yr) with GERD was no more effective than placebo.
- Administer all oral doses before meals and 30 min prior to sucralfate. **Do not** crush or chew the granules (all dosage forms). Capsule may be opened and intact granules may be administered in an acidic beverage or food (e.g., apple or cranberry juice or apple sauce). **Do not** break or cut the orally disintegrating tablets. Use of oral disintegrating tablets dissolved in water has been reported to clog and block oral syringes and feeding tubes (gastric and jejunostomy). For IV use, use a 1.2-micron inline filter.

LEVALBUTEROL
Xopenex, Xopenex HFA, and generics
β₂-Adrenergic agonist

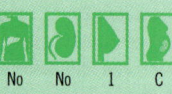
No   No   1   C

Prediluted nebulized solution: 0.31 mg in 3 mL, 0.63 mg in 3 mL, 1.25 mg in 3 mL (30s)
Concentrated nebulized solution: 1.25 mg/0.5 mL (0.5 mL) (30s)
Aerosol inhaler (MDI; Xopenex HFA): 45 mcg/actuation (15 g delivers 200 doses)

Nebulizer:
  ≤*4 yr:* Start at 0.31 mg inhaled Q4–6 hr PRN; dose may be increased up to 1.25 mg Q4–6 hr PRN
  5–11 yr: Start at 0.31 mg inhaled Q8 hr PRN; dose may be increased to 0.63 mg Q8 hr PRN
  ≥*12 yr and adult:* Start at 0.63 mg inhaled Q6–8 hr PRN; dose may be increased to 1.25 mg inhaled Q8 hr PRN
Aerosol inhaler (MDI):
  ≥*4 yr and adult:* 2 puffs Q4–6 hr PRN
For use in acute exacerbations, more aggressive dosing may be employed.

R-isomer of racemic albuterol. Side effects include tachycardia, palpitations, tremor, insomnia, nervousness, nausea, and headache.
Clinical data in children demonstrate levalbuterol is as effective as albuterol with fewer cardiac side effects at equipotent doses (0.31–0.63 mg levalbuterol ~ 2.5 mg albuterol). However, when higher doses of levalbuerol (1.25 mg) were compared to 2.5 mg albuterol changes in heart rate were similar.
More frequent dosing may be necessary in asthma exacerbation.

LEVETIRACETAM
Keppra, Keppra XR, Roweepra, Spritam, and generics
Anticonvulsant

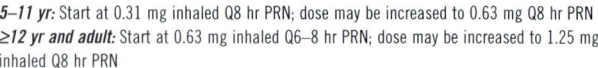
No   Yes   2   C

Tabs: 250, 500, 750, 1000 mg
Extended-release tabs (Keprra XR and generics; see remarks): 500, 750 mg
Tabs, disintegrating (Spritam; see remarks): 250, 500, 750, 1000 mg
Oral solution: 100 mg/mL (480 mL); dye free and contains parabens
Injection: 100 mg/mL (5 mL); contains 45 mg sodium chloride and 8.2 mg sodium acetate trihydrate per 100 mg drug
Premixed injection: 500 mg/100 mL in 0.82% sodium chloride, 1000 mg/100 mL in 0.75% sodium chloride, 1500 mg/100 mL in 0.54% sodium chloride

Partial seizures (adjunctive therapy; using immediate-release dosage forms):
  Infant (1–5 mo): Start at 7 mg/kg/dose PO BID; increase by 7 mg/kg/dose BID every 2 wk as tolerated to the recommended dose of 21 mg/kg/dose BID. An average daily dose of 35 mg/kg/24 hr was reported in clinical trials.
  Infant ≥6 mo–child 3 yr (>20 kg): Start at 10 mg/kg/dose PO BID; increase by 10 mg/kg/dose BID every 2 wk as tolerated to the recommended dose of 25 mg/kg/dose BID. An average daily dose of 47 mg/kg/24 hr was reported in clinical trials.
  Child 4–15 yr: Start at 10 mg/kg/dose PO BID; increase by 10 mg/kg/dose BID every 2 wk as tolerated up to a **max. dose** of 30 mg/kg/dose BID or 3000 mg/24 hr. An average daily dose of 44 mg/kg/24 hr was reported in clinical trials.

LEVETIRACETAM continued

Alternative dosing with oral tablets:
   20–40 kg: Start at 250 mg PO BID; increase by 250 mg BID every 2 wk as tolerated up to a **maximum** of 750 mg BID.
   >40 kg: Start at 500 mg PO BID; increase by 500 mg BID every 2 wk as tolerated up to a **maximum** of 1500 mg BID.
16 yr–adult: Start at 500 mg PO BID; may increase by 500 mg/dose BID every 2 wk as tolerated up to a **max. dose** of 1500 mg BID.

Myoclonic seizure (adjunctive therapy; using immediate-release dosage forms):
   ≥12 yr and adult: Start at 500 mg PO BID; then increase dosage by 500 mg/dose BID every 2 wk as tolerated to reach the target dosage of 1500 mg BID.

Tonic-clonic seizure (primary generalized, adjunctive therapy; use immediate-release dosage forms):
   Child 6–15 yr: Start at 10 mg/kg/dose PO BID; increase by 10 mg/kg/dose BID every 2 wk as tolerated to reach the target dosage of 30 mg/kg/dose BID.

   Alternative fixed dosing with disintegrating tabs (Spritam):
      20–40 kg: Start at 250 mg PO BID; increase by 250 mg BID every 2 wk as tolerated up to a **maximum** of 750 mg BID.
      >40 kg: Start at 500 mg PO BID; increase by 500 mg BID every 2 wk as tolerated up to a **maximum** of 1500 mg BID.
   16 yr–adult: Start at 500 mg PO BID; then increase dosage by 500 mg/dose BID every 2 wk as tolerated to reach the target dosage of 1500 mg BID.

Refractory seizures (add-on therapy to various seizure types; data limited to 6 mo–4 yr): Start at 5–10 mg/kg/24 hr PO ÷ BID–TID, if needed and tolerated, increase dose by 10 mg/kg/24 hr at weekly intervals up to a **max. dose** of 60 mg/kg/24 hr.

Do not abruptly withdraw therapy to reduce risk for seizures. **Use with caution** in renal impairment **(reduce dose; see Chapter 30)**, hemodialysis, and neuropsychiatric conditions.

May cause loss of appetite, vomiting, dizziness, headaches, somnolence, agitation, depression, and mood swings. Drowsiness, fatigue, nervousness, and aggressive behavior have been reported in children. Nonpsychotic behavioral symptoms reported in children are approximately 3 times higher than in adults (37.6% vs 13.3%). Suicidal behavior or ideation, serious dermatological reactions (e.g., Stevens–Johnson syndrome and TEN), hematologic abnormalities (e.g., anemia and leukopenia), hyponatremia, and hypertension have been reported. Levetiracetam may decrease carbamazepine's effects. Ginkgo may decrease levetriacetam's effects.

Drug has excellent PO absorption. For IV use, use similar immediate-release PO dosages only when the oral route of administration is not feasible. Extended-release tablet is designed for once daily administration at similar daily dosage of the immediate-release forms (e.g., 1000 mg once daily of the extended-release tablet is equivalent to 500 mg BID of the immediate-release tablet). Disintegrating tabs (Spritam) may be administered by allowing the tablet to disintegrate in the mouth when taken with a sip of liquid or made into a suspension (see package insert); **do not** swallow this dosage form whole.

LEVOCARNITINE

See Carnitine

LEVOFLOXACIN
Levaquin, Quixin, Iquix, and generics
Antibiotic, quinolone

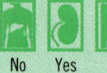

No Yes 2 C

Tabs: 250, 500, 750 mg
Oral solution: 25 mg/mL (100, 200, 480 mL)
Injection: 25 mg/mL (20, 30 mL)
Premixed injection in D$_5$W: 250 mg/50 mL, 500 mg/100 mL, 750 mg/150 mL
Ophthalmic drops:
  Quixin: 0.5% (5 mL)
  Iquix: 1.5% (5 mL)

Child:
  <5 yr: 10 mg/kg/dose IV/PO Q12 hr; **max. dose:** 500 mg/24 hr
  ≥5 yr: 10 mg/kg/dose IV/PO Q24 hr; **max. dose:** 750 mg/24 hr
  Recurrent or persistent acute otitis media (6 mo–<5 yr): 10 mg/kg/dose PO Q12 hr ×10 days; **max. dose:** 500 mg/24 hr
  Community acquired pneumonia (IDSA/Pediatric Infectious Disease Society):
    6 mo–<5 yr: 8–10 mg/kg/dose PO/IV Q12 hr; **max. dose:** 750 mg/24 hr
    5–16 yr: 8–10 mg/kg/dose PO/IV Q24 hr; **max. dose:** 750 mg/24 hr
  Inhalational anthrax (postexposure) and plague:
    ≥6 mo and <50 kg: 8 mg/kg/dose PO/IV Q12 hr; **max. dose:** 500 mg/24 hr
    >50 kg: 500 mg PO/IV once daily
      Duration of therapy:
        Inhalational anthrax (postexposure): 60 days
        Plague: 10–14 days
Adult:
  Community acquired pneumonia: 500 mg PO/IV Q24 hr × 7–14 days; OR 750 mg PO/IV Q24 hr × 5 days
  Complicated UTI/acute pyelonephritis: 250 PO/IV Q24 hr × 10 days; OR 750 mg PO/IV Q24 hr × 5 days
  Uncomplicated UTI: 250 mg PO/IV Q24 hr × 3 days
  Uncomplicated skin/skin structure infection: 500 mg PO/IV Q24 hr × 7–10 days
  Acute bacterial sinusitis: 500 mg PO/IV Q24 hr × 10–14 days; OR 750 mg PO/IV Q24 hr × 5 days
  Inhalational anthrax (postexposure) and plague: 500 mg PO/IV Q24 hr.
    Duration of therapy:
      Inhalational anthrax: 60 days
      Plague: 10–14 days
  Conjunctivitis:
    ≥1 yr and adult: Instill 1–2 drops of the 0.5% solution to affected eye(s) Q2 hr up to 8 times/24 hr while awake for the first 2 days, then Q4 hr up to 4 times/24 hr while awake for the next 5 days.
  Corneal ulcer:
    ≥6 yr and adult: Instill 1–2 drops of the 1.5% solution to affected eye(s) Q30 min–2 hr while awake and 4 and 6 hr after retiring for the first 3 days, then Q1–4 hr while awake.

Contraindicated in hypersensitivity to other quinolones. **Avoid** in patients with history of QTc prolongation or taking QTc prolonging drugs and excessive sunlight exposure. **Use with caution** in diabetes, seizures, myasthenia gravis, children < 18 yr, and renal impairment **(adjust dose, see Chapter 30).** May cause GI disturbances, headache, and blurred vision with the ophthalmic solution. Musculoskeletal disorders (e.g., arthralgia, arthritis,

LEVOFLOXACIN continued

tendinopathy, and gait abnormality) may occur. Peripheral neuropathy and uveitis have been reported. Safety in pediatric patients treated for more than 14 days has not been evaluated. Like other quinolones, tendon rupture can occur during or after therapy (risk increases with concurrent corticosteroids). Use with NSAIDs may increase risk for CNS stimulation and seizures.

Infuse IV over 1–1.5 hr; **avoid** IV push or rapid infusion because of risk for hypotension. **Do not** administer antacids or other divalent salts with or within 2 hr of oral levofloxacin dose; otherwise may be administered with or without food.

LEVOTHYROXINE (T₄)
Synthroid, Levoxyl, Tirosint, Unithroid, Unithroid Direct, and generics
Thyroid product

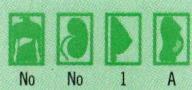

No   No   1   A

Tabs: 25, 50, 75, 88, 100, 112, 125, 137, 150, 175, 200, 300 mcg
Caps (Tirosint): 13, 25, 50, 75, 88, 100, 112, 125, 137, 150 mcg
Injection: 100, 200, 500 mcg; preservative free
Oral suspension: 25 mcg/mL

Child PO dosing:
  1–3 mo: 10–15 mcg/kg/dose once daily. If patient is at risk for developing cardiac failure, start with lower dose of 25 mcg/24 hr, and if patient has very low T₄ (<5 mcg/dL), use higher dose of 12–17 mcg/kg/24 hr.
  3–6 mo: 8–10 mcg/kg/dose once daily
  6–12 mo: 6–8 mcg/kg/dose once daily
  1–5 yr: 5–6 mcg/kg/dose once daily
  6–12 yr: 4–5 mcg/kg/dose once daily
  >12 yr:
    Incomplete growth and prepuberty: 2–3 mcg/kg/dose once daily
    Complete growth and puberty: 1.7 mcg/kg/dose once daily
Child IM/IV dose: 50%–75% of oral dose once daily
Adult:
  PO: Start with 12.5–25 mcg/dose once daily. Increase by 25–50 mcg/24 hr at intervals of Q2–4 wk until euthyroid. Usual adult dose: 100–200 mcg/24 hr
  IM/IV dose: 50% of oral dose once daily
  Myxedema coma or stupor: 200–500 mcg IV × 1, then 100–300 mcg IV once daily; convert to oral therapy once patient is stabilized

Contraindications include acute MI, thyrotoxicosis, and uncorrected adrenal insufficiency. May cause hyperthyroidism, rash, growth disturbances, hypertension, arrhythmias, diarrhea, and weight loss. Pseudotumor cerebri has been reported in children. Overtreatment may cause craniosynostosis in infants and premature closure of the epiphyses in children.

Total replacement dose may be used in children unless there is evidence of cardiac disease; in that case, begin with one-fourth of maintenance dose and increase weekly. Titrate dosage with clinical status and serum T₄ and TSH. Increases the effects of warfarin. Phenytoin, rifampin, carbamazepine, iron and calcium supplements, antacids, and orlistat may decrease levothyroxine levels. Tricyclic antidepressants and SSRIs may enhance toxic effects.

100 mcg levothyroxine = 65 mg thyroid USP. Administer oral doses on an empty stomach and tablets with a full glass of water. Iron and calcium supplements and antacids may decrease absorption; do not administer within 4 hr of these agents. Excreted in low levels in breast milk; preponderance of evidence suggests no clinically significant effect in infants.

LIDOCAINE
Xylocaine, L-M-X, Lidoderm, and generics
Antiarrhythmic class Ib, local anesthetic

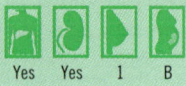

Yes   Yes   1   B

Injection: 0.5%, 1%, 1.5%, 2%, 4%, 5% (1% sol = 10 mg/mL)
IV infusion (in D₅W): 0.4% (4 mg/mL) (250, 500 mL); 0.8% (8 mg/mL) (250 mL)
Injection with epinephrine (some preparations may contain metasulfite or are preservative free):
  Injection with 1:50,000 epi: 2%
  Injection with 1:100,000 epi: 1%, 2%
  Injection with 1:200,000 epi: 0.5%, 1%, 1.5%, 2%
Ointment: 5% (30, 50 g)
Cream, topical: 3% (30, 85 g), 4% (L-M-X-4 and generics)[OTC] (5, 15, 30, 45 g), 5% (L-M-X-5 and generics) (15, 30 g); may contain benzyl alcohol
Cream, rectal: 5% (L-M-X-5 and others; 15, 30 g); contains benzyl alcohol
Gel (external): 2% (5, 10, 20, 30 mL), 3% (10, 30 mL), 4% (10, 30, 113 g), 5% (10, 30, 113 g); may contain benzyl alcohol and EDTA
Lotion: 3% (118, 177 mL)
Solution (external): 4% (50 mL); may contain parabens
Oral solution (mouth/throat): 2% (15, 100 mL), 4% (4 mL)
Transdermal patch (Lidoderm and generics): 5% (1s, 15s, 30s)
Topical 2.5% (with 2.5% prilocaine): See Lidocaine and Prilocaine

Anesthetic:
  Injection:
    Without epinephrine: **max. dose** of 4.5 mg/kg/dose (up to 300 mg); do not repeat within 2 hr.
    With epinephrine: **max. dose** of 7 mg/kg/dose (up to 500 mg); do not repeat within 2 hr.
  Topical:
    Cream (child ≥ 2 yr and adult): Apply to affected intact skin areas BID–QID.
    Gel or ointment (child ≥ 2 yr and adult): Apply to affected intact skin areas once daily–QID; **max. dose:** 4.5 mg/kg up to 300 mg.
    Patch (adult): Apply to most painful area with up to 3 patches at a time. Patch(es) may be applied for up to 12 hr in any 24-hr period.
Antiarrhythmic (infant, child, adolescent):
  Bolus: 1 mg/kg/dose (**max. dose:** 100 mg) slowly IV; may repeat in 10–15 min × 2; **max. total dose** 3–5 mg/kg within the first hr. ETT dose = 2–3 × IV dose.
  Continuous infusion: 20–50 mcg/kg/min IV/IO (**do not exceed** 20 mcg/kg/min for patients with shock, CHF, hepatic disease, or cardiac arrest); see inside cover for infusion preparation. Administer a 1 mg/kg bolus when infusion is initiated if bolus has not been given within previous 15 min.
Oral use (viscous liquid):
  Child (≥3 yr): up to the lesser of 4.5 mg/kg/dose or 300 mg/dose swish and spit Q3 hr PRN up to a **max. dose** of 4 doses per 12 hr period
  Adult: 15 mL swish and spit Q3 hr PRN up to a **max. dose** of 8 doses/24 hr

For cardiac arrest, amiodarone is the preferred agent over lidocaine; lidocaine may be used only when amiodarone is not available.
Contraindicated in Stokes-Adams or Wolff-Parkinson-White syndromes and SA, AV, or intraventricular heart block without a pacemaker. Solutions containing dextrose may be contraindicated in patients with known allergy to corn or corn products. Side effects include hypotension, asystole, seizures, and respiratory arrest. Anaphylactic reactions have been reported.

LIDOCAINE continued

CYP450 2D6 and 3A3/4 substrate. **Use with caution** in severe liver or renal disease. Decrease dose in hepatic failure or decreased cardiac output. **Do not use** topically for teething. Prolonged infusion may result in toxic accumulation of lidocaine, especially in infants. **Do not use** epinephrine-containing solutions for treatment of arrhythmias.

Therapeutic levels 1.5–5 mg/L. Toxicity occurs at >7 mg/L. Toxicity in neonates may occur at >5 mg/L due to reduced protein binding of drug. Elimination $T_{1/2}$: premature infant, 3.2 hr; adult, 1.5–2 hr.

When using the topical patch, avoid exposing the application site to external heat sources as it may increase the risk for toxicity.

LIDOCAINE AND PRILOCAINE
Many brand names, Oraqix, Eutectic mixture of lidocaine and prilocaine; previously available as EMLA
Topical analgesic

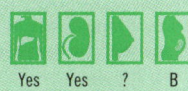

Yes Yes ? B

Cream: Lidocaine 2.5% + prilocaine 2.5% (5, 30 g)
Peridontal gel (Oraqix): Lidocaine 2.5% + prilocaine 2.5% (1.7 g in dental cartridges; 20s)

See Chapter 6, for general use information.

Neonate:
  <37-wk gestation (limited data):
    Painful procedures (e.g., IM injections): 0.5 g/site for 60 min.
  ≥37-wk gestation:
    Painful procedures (e.g., IM injections): 1 g/site for 60 min. **Max. dose**: 1 g for all sites combined with a **max**. application area of 10 cm² and **max**. application time of 1 hr.
    Circumcision: 1–2 g and cover with occlusive dressing for 60–90 min.
Infant and child: The following are the recommended **max. doses** based on the child's age and weight.

Age and Weight	Maximum Total EMLA Dose (g)	Maximum Application Area (cm²)	Maximum Application Time
Birth–<3 mo or <5 kg	1	10	1 hr
3–12 mo and >5 kg*	2	20	4 hr
1–6 yr and >10 kg	10	100	4 hr
7–12 yr and >20 kg	20	200	4 hr

*If patient is > 3 months and not >5 kg, use the **maximum** total dose that corresponds to the patient's weight.
EMLA, Eutectic mixture of local anesthetics.

Adult:
  Minor procedures: 2.5 g/site for at least 60 min.
  Painful procedures: 2 g/10 cm² of skin for at least 2 hr

Should not be used in neonates < 37 wk of gestation or in infants aged <12 mo receiving treatment with methemoglobin-inducing agents (e.g., sulfa drugs, acetaminophen, nitrofurantoin, nitroglycerin, nitroprusside, phenobarbital, and phenytoin). **Use with caution** in patients with G6PD deficiency, patients treated with class I or III antiarrhythmic drugs (additive or toxic cardiac effects), and in patients with renal and hepatic impairment. Prilocaine has been associated with methemoglobinemia. Long duration of application, large treatment area, small patients, or impaired elimination may result in high blood levels.

Apply topically to intact skin and cover with occlusive dressing; **avoid** mucous membranes or the eyes. Wipe cream off before procedure.

LINDANE
Gamma-benzene hexachloride and various generics
Scabicidal agent, pediculocide

No   No   3   C

Shampoo: 1% (60 mL)
Lotion: 1% (60 mL)

Child and adult (see remarks):
  Scabies: Apply thin layer of lotion to skin. Bathe and rinse off medication in adults after 8–12 hr; children 6–8 hr. May repeat × 1 in 7 days PRN.
  Pediculosis capitis: Apply 15–30 mL of shampoo, lather for 4–5 min, rinse hair, and comb with fine comb to remove nits. May repeat × 1 in 7 days PRN.
  Pediculosis pubis: May use lotion or shampoo (applied locally) as for scabies and pediculosis capitis (see above).

Contraindicated in premature infants and seizure disorders. **Use with caution** with drugs that lower seizure threshold. Systemically absorbed. Risk of toxic effects is greater in young children; use other agents (permethrin) in infants, young children (<2 yr), and during pregnancy. Lindane is considered second-line therapy owing to side-effect risk and reports of resistance.

May cause a rash; rarely may cause seizures or aplastic anemia. For scabies, change clothing and bed sheets after starting treatment and treat family members. For pediculosis pubis, treat sexual contacts.

Avoid contact with face, urethral meatus, damaged skin, or mucous membranes. **Do not** use any covering that does not breathe (e.g., plastic lining or clothing) over the applied lindane.

LINEZOLID
Zyvox and generics
Antibiotic, oxazolidinone

No   No   2   C

Tabs: 600 mg; contains ~0.45 mEq Na per 200 mg drug
Oral suspension: 100 mg/5 mL (150 mL); contains phenylalanine and sodium benzoate and 0.8 mEq Na per 200 mg drug
Injection, premixed: 200 mg in 100 mL, 600 mg in 300 mL; contains 1.7 mEq Na per 200 mg drug

Neonate:
  <1 kg:
    <14 days old: 10 mg/kg/dose IV Q12 hr
    ≥14 days old: 10 mg/kg/dose IV Q8 hr
  ≥1–2 kg:
    <7 days old: 10 mg/kg/dose IV/PO Q12 hr
    ≥7 days old: 10 mg/kg/dose IV/PO Q8 hr
  >2 kg: 10 mg/kg/dose IV/PO Q8 hr
  Alternate dosing by gestational age:
    <34-wk gestation:
      <7 days old: 10 mg/kg/dose IV/PO Q12 hr
      ≥7 days old: 10 mg/kg/dose IV/PO Q8 hr
    ≥34-wk gestation and 0–28 days old: 10 mg/kg/dose IV/PO Q8 hr
Infant and child aged <12 yr:
  Pneumonia, bacteremia, bone/joint infections, septic thrombosis (MRSA), complicated skin/skin structure infections, vancomycin-resistant Enterococcus. faecium (VRE) infections (including endocarditis): 10 mg/kg/dose IV/PO Q8 hr.

LINEZOLID continued

Uncomplicated skin/skin structure infections:
<5 yr: 10 mg/kg/dose IV/PO Q8 hr
5–11 yr: 10 mg/kg/dose IV/PO Q12 hr
Max. dose for all indications <12 yr: 600 mg/dose
≥12 yr and adult: 600 mg Q12 hr IV/PO; 400 mg Q12 hr IV/PO may be used for adults with uncomplicated infection.

Duration of therapy:
MRSA infections: variable based on response
Pneumonia: 10–14 days for non-MRSA and 7–21 days (per clinical response) for MRSA
Bacteremia: 10–28 days
Bone/joint infections: 3–6 weeks
Skin/skin structure infections: 10–14 days; longer for complicated cases
Septic thrombosis (MRSA): 4–6 weeks
VRE infections: 14–28 days, minimum of 8 wk for endocarditis

Most common side effects include diarrhea, headache, and nausea. Anemia, leukopenia, pancytopenia, and thrombocytopenia may occur in patients who are at a risk for myelosuppression and who receive regimens > 2 wk. Complete blood count monitoring is recommended in these individuals. Pseudomembranous colitis and neuropathy (peripheral and optic) have also been reported. CSF penetration is variable in patients with VP shunts.

Do not use with SSRIs (e.g., fluoxetine and paroxetine), tricyclic antidepressants, venlafaxine, and trazodone; may cause serotonin syndrome. **Avoid** use with monoamine oxidase inhibitors (e.g., phenelzine) and in patients with uncontrolled hypertension, pheochromocytoma, thyrotoxicosis, and those taking sympathomimetics or vasopressive agents (may elevate blood pressure). **Use with caution** when consuming large amounts of foods and beverages containing tyramine; may increase blood pressure. Dosing information in severe hepatic failure and renal impairment with multidoses have not been established.

Protect all dosage forms from light and moisture. Oral suspension product must be gently mixed by inverting the bottle 3–5 times prior to each use (**do not shake**). All oral doses may be administered with or without food.

LISDEXAMFETAMINE
Vyvanse
CNS stimulant

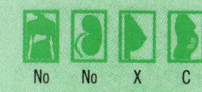

No No X C

Capsules: 10, 20, 30, 40, 50, 60, 70 mg

Attention-deficit hyperactivity disorder:
Child ≥ 6 yr and adult: Start with 30 mg PO QAM. May increase dose by 10–20 mg/24 hr at weekly intervals if needed up to a **max. dose** of 70 mg/24 hr.

Lisdexamfetamine is a prodrug of dextroamphetamine that requires activation by intestinal/hepatic metabolism.

Contraindicated in amphetamine or sympathomimetic hypersensitivity, symptomatic cardiovascular disease, moderate/severe hypertension, hyperthyroidism, glaucoma, agitated states, drug/alcohol abuse history, and MAO inhibitors (concurrent or use within 14 days). As with other CNS simulant medications, serious cardiovascular events, including **death**, have been reported in patients with preexisting structural cardiac abnormalities or other serious heart problems. **Use with caution** in patients with hypertension, psychiatric conditions, and epilepsy. May cause insomnia, irritability, rash, appetite suppression/weight

Continued

LISDEXAMFETAMINE continued

loss, dizziness, xerostomia, and GI disturbances. Dermatillomania, bruxism, Stevens–Johnson syndrome, and TEN have been reported.

Urinary acidifying agents may reduce levels of amphetamines, and urinary alkalinizing agents may increase levels. May increase the effects of TCAs; increase or decrease the effects of guanfacine, phenytoin, and phenobarbital and decrease the effects of adrenergic blockers, antihistamines, and antihypertensives. Norepinephrine may increase the effects of amphetamines.

See *Dextroamphetamine ± Amphetamine* for additional remarks.

LISINOPRIL
Prinivil, Qbrelis, Zestril, and generics
Angiotensin converting enzyme inhibitor, antihypertensive

Yes   Yes   3   D

Tabs: 2.5, 5, 10, 20, 30, 40 mg
Oral solution (Qbrelis): 1 mg/mL (150 mL); contains sodium benzoate
Oral suspension: 1, 2 mg/mL

Hypertension (see remarks):
Child (<6 yr; limited data): Use 6–16 yr dosing below.
6–16 yr: Start with 0.07–0.1 mg/kg/dose PO once daily; max. initial dose: 5 mg/dose. If needed, titrate dose upward at 1–2-week intervals to doses up to 0.61 mg/kg/24 hr or 40 mg/24 hr (higher doses have not been evaluated).
Adult: Start with 10 mg PO once daily. If needed, increase dose by 5–10 mg/24 hr at 1–2 week intervals. Usual dosage range: 10–40 mg/24 hr. Max. dose: 80 mg/24 hr.

Use lower initial dose (50% of recommended dose) if using with a diuretic or in the presence of hyponatremia, hypovolemia, severe CHF, or decreased renal function.

Contraindicated in hypersensitivity and history of angioedema with other ACE inhibitors. **Do not** use with aliskiren in patients with diabetes. **Avoid** use with dialysis with high-flux membranes because anaphylactoid reactions have been reported. **Use with caution** in aortic or bilateral renal artery stenosis and hepatic impairment. Side effects include cough, dizziness, headache, hyperkalemia, hypotension (especially with concurrent diuretic or antihypertensive agent use), rash, and GI disturbances. Mood alterations, including depressive symptoms, have been reported.

Dual blockade of the renin–angiotensin system with lisinopril and angiotensin receptor antagonist (e.g., losartan) or aliskiren is associated with increased risk for hypotension, syncope, hyperkalemia, and renal impairment. Use in diabetic patients treated with oral antidiabetic agents should be monitored for hypoglycemia, especially during the first month of use. NSAIDs (e.g., indomethacin) may decrease linsinopril's effects. Use with mTOR inhibitors (e.g., sirolimus and everolimus) may increase risk for angioedema. **Adjust dose in renal impairment (see Chapter 30).**

Onset of action: 1 hr with maximal effect in 6–8 hr. Lisinopril should be discontinued as soon as possible when pregnancy is detected.

Additional indications with limited data in children include proteinuria associated with mild IgA nephropathy and renal protection for diabetes or renal parenchymal disease.

LITHIUM
Lithobid and many generics; previously available as Eskalith
Antimanic agent

No   Yes   X   D

Carbonate:
300 mg carbonate = 8.12 mEq lithium
Caps: 150, 300, 600 mg

LITHIUM continued

Tabs: 300 mg
Extended-release tabs: 300 mg (Lithobid), 450 mg
Citrate:
Syrup: 8 mEq/5 mL (5, 500 mL); 5 mL is equivalent to 300 mg lithium carbonate.

Child:
Initial (immediate-release dosage forms): 15–60 mg/kg/24 hr ÷ TID–QID PO. Adjust as needed (weekly) to achieve therapeutic levels.
Adolescent: 600–1800 mg/24 hr ÷ TID–QID PO (divided BID using controlled-/slow-release tablets).
Adult:
Initial: 300 mg TID PO. Adjust as needed to achieve therapeutic levels. Usual dose is about 300 mg TID–QID with immediate-release dosage form. For controlled-/slow-release tablets, 900–1800 mg/24 hr PO ÷ BID.
Max. dose: 2400 mg/24 hr.

Contraindicated in severe cardiovascular (including Brugada syndrome) or renal disease. Decreased sodium intake or increased sodium wasting and significant renal or cardiovascular disease may increase lithium levels, resulting in toxicity. May cause goiter, nephrogenic diabetes insipidus, hypothyroidism, arrhythmias, or sedation at therapeutic doses. Nephrotic syndrome has been reported.

Co-administration with diuretics, metronidazole, ACE inhibitors, angiotensin receptor antagonists (e.g., losartan), or nonsteroidal antiinflammatory drugs may increase risk for lithium toxicity. Use with iodine may increase risk for hypothyroidism. If used in combination with haloperidol, closely monitor neurologic toxicities because an encephalopathic syndrome followed by irreversible brain damage has been reported.

Therapeutic levels: 0.6–1.5 mEq/L. In either acute or chronic toxicity, confusion and somnolence may be seen at levels of 2–2.5 mEq/L. **Seizures or death** may occur at levels > 2.5 mEq/L. Recommended serum sampling: trough level within 30 min prior to the next scheduled dose. Steady state is achieved within 4–6 days of continuous dosing. **Adjust dose in renal failure (see Chapter 30).**

LODOXAMIDE
Alomide
Antiallergic agent, mast cell stabilizer

No   No   ?   B

Ophthalmic solution: 0.1% (10 mL); contains benzalkonium chloride

≥2 yr and adult: Instill 1–2 drops to affected eye(s) QID for up to 3 months.

Transient burning, stinging, or discomfort of the eye and headache are common side effects. Itching/pruritus, blurred vision, dry eye, tearing, hyperemia, crystalline deposits, and foreign body sensation may also occur.

Do not wear soft contact lenses during treatment because medication contains benzalkonium chloride.

LOPERAMIDE
Imodium, Imodium A-D, and generics
Antidiarrheal

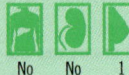

No   No   1   C

Caps (OTC): 2 mg
Tabs (OTC): 2 mg
Chewable tabs (OTC): 2 mg
Caplets (OTC): 2 mg
Oral liquid (OTC): 1 mg/5 mL (120 mL); contains 0.5% alcohol
Oral suspension (OTC): 1 mg/7.5 mL (120 mL); each 30 mL contains 16 mg of sodium

Acute diarrhea (see remarks):
  Child (initial doses within the first 24 hr):
   2–5 yr (13–<21 kg): 1 mg PO TID
   6–8 yr (21–27 kg): 2 mg PO BID
   9–11 yr (>27–43 kg): 2 mg PO TID
   Max. single dose 2 mg
   Follow initial day's dose with 0.1 mg/kg/dose after each loose stool (not to exceed the aforementioned initial doses).
  ≥12 yr and adult: 4 mg/dose × 1, followed by 2 mg/dose after each stool up to **max. dose** of 16 mg/24 hr.
Chronic diarrhea (see remarks):
  Infant–child (limited data): 0.08–0.24 mg/kg/24 hr ÷ BID–TID; **max. dose**: 2 mg/dose

Contraindicated in acute dysentery; acute ulcerative colitis; bacterial enterocolitis caused by *Salmonella, Shigella, Campylobacter,* and *Clostridium difficile*; and abdominal pain in the absence of diarrhea. **Avoid** use in children < 2 yr due to reports of paralytic ileus associated with abdominal distention. Rare hypersensitivity reactions including anaphylactic shock have been reported. May cause nausea, rash, vomiting, constipation, cramps, dry mouth, and CNS depression. Use of higher than recommended dosages via abuse or misuse can cause serious cardiac events (e.g., Torsades de Pointes, arrhythmias, cardiac arrest, and QT prolongation).
Discontinue use if no clinical improvement is observed within 48 hr. Naloxone may be administered for CNS depression.

LORATADINE ± PSEUDOEPHEDRINE
Alavert, Claritin, Claritin Children's Allergy, Claritin RediTabs,
Claritin-D 12 Hour, Claritin-D 24 Hour, many others, and generics
Antihistamine, less sedating ± decongestant

Yes   Yes   2   B

Tabs [OTC]: 10 mg
Chewable tabs (Claritin Children's Allergy) [OTC]: 5 mg; contains aspartame
Disintegrating tabs (RediTabs) [OTC]: 5, 10 mg; contains aspartame
Oral solution or syrup [OTC]: 1 mg/mL (120 mL); contains propylene glycol and sodium benzoate; some preparations may contain metasulfite
Time-release tabs in combination with pseudoephedrine (PE):
  Claritin-D 12 Hour [OTC]: 5 mg loratadine + 120 mg PE
  Claritin-D 24 Hour [OTC]: 10 mg loratadine + 240 mg PE

Loratadine:
  2–5 yr: 5 mg PO once daily
  ≥6 yr and adult: 10 mg PO once daily

LORATADINE ± PSEUDOEPHEDRINE continued

Time-release tabs of loratidine and pseudoephedrine:
≥12 yr and adult (see remarks):
  Claritin-D 12 Hour and generics: 1 tablet PO BID
  Claritin-D 24 Hour and generics: 1 tablet PO once daily

May cause drowsiness, fatigue, dry mouth, headache, bronchospasms, palpitations, dermatitis, and dizziness. Has **not** been implicated in causing cardiac arrhythmias when used with other drugs that are metabolized by hepatic microsomal enzymes (e.g., ketoconazole and erythromycin). May be administered safely in patients who have allergic rhinitis and asthma.

In hepatic and renal function impairment (GFR < 30 mL/min), prolong loratadine (single agent) dosage interval to every other day. **Adjust dose in renal failure (see Chapter 30).**

For time-release tablets of the combination product (loratadine and pseudoephedrine), prolong dosage interval in renal impairment (GFR < 30 mL/min) as follows: Claritin-D 12 Hour: 1 tablet PO once daily; Claritin-D 24 Hour: 1 tablet PO every other day. **Do not** use the combination product in hepatic impairment because drugs cannot be individually titrated.

Administer doses on an empty stomach. For use of RediTabs, place tablet on tongue and allow it to disintegrate in the mouth with or without water. For Claritin-D products, also see remarks in Pseudoephedrine.

LORAZEPAM
Ativan and many generics
Benzodiazepine anticonvulsant

Yes Yes 2 D

Tabs: 0.5, 1, 2 mg
Injection: 2, 4 mg/mL (each contains 2% benzyl alcohol and propylene glycol)
Oral solution: 2 mg/mL (30 mL); some dosage forms may be alcohol and dye free

Status epilepticus (IV route is preferred but may use IM route if IV is not available):
  Neonate, infant, child, and adolescent: 0.05–0.1 mg/kg/dose IV over 2–5 min. May repeat dose in 10–15 min. **Max. dose:** 4 mg/dose.
  Adult: 4 mg/dose IV given slowly over 2–5 min. May repeat in 10–15 min. Usual total **max. dose** in 12-hr period is 8 mg.
Antiemetic adjunct therapy:
  Child: 0.02–0.05 mg/kg/dose IV Q6 hr PRN; **max. single dose:** 2 mg.
Anxiolytic/sedation:
  Infant and child: 0.05 mg/kg/dose Q4–8 hr PO/IV; **max. dose:** 2 mg/dose.
    May also give IM for preprocedure sedation.
  Adult: 1–10 mg/24 hr PO ÷ BID–TID

Contraindicated in narrow-angle glaucoma and severe hypotension. **Use with caution** in renal insufficiency (glucoronide metabolite clearance is reduced), hepatic insufficiency (may worsen hepatic encephalopathy; decrease dose with severe hepatic impairment), compromised pulmonary function, and use of CNS depressant medications. May cause respiratory depression, especially in combination with other sedatives. May also cause sedation, dizziness, mild ataxia, mood changes, rash, and GI symptoms. Paradoxical excitation has been reported in children (10%–30% of patients aged <8 yr).

When compared to diazepam for status epilepticus (3 mo–17 yr), lorazepam was found to be more sedating with a longer time to return to baseline mental status.

Continued

LORAZEPAM continued

Significant respiratory depression and/or hypotension has been reported when used in combination with loxapine. Probenecid and valproic acid may increase the effects/toxicity of lorazepam, and oral contraceptive steroids may decrease lorazepam's effects.

Injectable product may be rectally administered. Benzyl alcohol and propylene glycol may be toxic to newborns at higher doses.

Onset of action for sedation: PO, 20–30 min; IM, 30–60 min; IV, 1–5 min. Duration of action: 6–8 hr. **Flumazenil is the antidote.**

LOSARTAN
Cozaar and generics
Angiotensin II receptor antagonist

Yes   Yes   ?   C/D

Tabs: 25, 50, 100 mg
Oral suspension: 2.5 mg/mL
Contains 2.12 mg potassium per 25 mg drug

Hypertension (see remarks):
  6–16 yr: Start with 0.7 mg/kg/dose (**max. dose:** 50 mg/dose) PO once daily. Adjust dose to desired blood pressure response. **Max. dose** (higher doses have not been evaluated): 1.4 mg/kg/24 hr or 100 mg/24 hr.
  ≥17 yr and adult: Start with 50 mg PO once daily (use lower initial dose of 25 mg PO once daily if patient is receiving diuretics, experiencing intravascular volume depletion, or has hepatic impairment). Usual maintenance dose is 25–100 mg/24 hr PO ÷ once daily–BID.

Use with caution in angioedema (current or past), excessive hypotension (volume depletion), hepatic (use lower starting dose) or renal (contains potassium) impairment, hyperkalemia, renal artery stenosis, and severe CHF. Not recommended in patients < 6 yr or in children with GFR < 30 mL/min/1.73 m^2, owing to lack of data.

Discontinue use as soon as possible when pregnancy is detected because injury and death to developing fetus may occur. Pregnancy category is "C" during the first trimester but changes to "D" for the second and third trimesters.

Diarrhea, asthenia, dizziness, fatigue, and hypotension are common. Thrombocytopenia, rhabdomyolysis, hallucinations, and angioedema have been rarely reported.

Losartan is a substrate for CYP450 2C9 (major) and 3A4. Fluconazole and cimetidine may increase losartan effects/toxicity. Rifampin, phenobarbital, and indomethacin may decrease its effects. Losartan may increase the risk of lithium toxicity. **Do not use** with aliskiren in patients with diabetes or with renal impairment (GFR < 60 mL/min). Dual blockade of the renin–angiotensin system with losartan and ACE inhibitors (e.g., captopril) or aliskiren is associated with increased risk for hypotension, syncope, hyperkalemia, and renal impairment.

LOW MOLECULAR WEIGHT HEPARIN

See Enoxaparin

LUCINACTANT

See Surfactant, pulmonary

MAGNESIUM CITRATE
Various generics
16.17% Elemental Magnesium
Laxative/cathartic

No Yes 1 D

Oral solution (OTC): 1.75 g/30 mL (300 mL); 5 mL = 3.9–4.7 mEq Mg
Tabs: 100 mg

Cathartic:
  <6 yr: 2–4 mL/kg/24 hr PO ÷ once daily–BID
  6–12 yr: 100–150 mL/24 hr PO ÷ once daily–BID
  >12 yr–adult: 150–300 mL/24 hr PO ÷ once daily–BID

Use with caution in renal insufficiency (monitor magnesium level) and patients receiving digoxin. May cause hypermagnesemia, diarrhea, muscle weakness, hypotension, and respiratory depression. Up to about 30% of dose is absorbed. May decrease absorption of H_2 antagonists, phenytoin, iron salts, tetracycline, steroids, benzodiazepines, and quinolone antibiotics.

MAGNESIUM HYDROXIDE
Milk of Magnesia and various generics
41.69% Elemental Magnesium
Antacid, laxative

No Yes 1 D

Oral liquid (OTC): 400 mg/5 mL (Milk of Magnesia and others) (355, 473 mL)
Concentrated oral liquid (OTC): 2400 mg/10 mL (Milk of Magnesia concentrate) (100, 400 mL)
Chewable tabs (OTC): 400 mg
400 mg magnesium hydroxide is equivalent to 166.76 mg elemental magnesium
Combination product with aluminum hydroxide: See Aluminum Hydroxide

Laxative (all liquid mL doses based on 400 mg/5 mL magnesium hydroxide, unless noted otherwise):
Dose/24 hr ÷ once daily–QID PO
  <2 yr: 0.5 mL/kg
  2–5 yr: 5–15 mL ***OR*** 400–1200 mg (1–3 chewable tabs)
  6–11 yr: 15–30 mL ***OR*** 1200–2400 mg (3–6 chewable tabs)
  ≥12 yr and adult: 30–60 mL ***OR*** 2400–4800 mg (6–12 chewable tabs)
Antacid:
Child:
  Liquid: 2.5–5 mL/dose once daily–QID PO
  Tabs: 400 mg once daily–QID PO
Adult:
  Liquid: 5–15 mL/dose once daily–QID PO
  Concentrated liquid (800 mg/5 mL): 2.5–7.5 mL/dose once daily–QID PO
  Tabs: 400–1200 mg/dose once daily–QID PO

See Magnesium Citrate. **Use with caution** in renal insufficiency (monitor magnesium level) and patients receiving digoxin. Drink a full 8 oz. of liquid with each dose of the chewable tablets.

MAGNESIUM OXIDE
Mag-200, Mag-Ox 400, Uro-Mag, and other generics
60.32% Elemental Magnesium
Oral magnesium salt

No   Yes   1   D

Tabs (OTC): 200, 400, 420, 500 mg
Caps (Uro-Mag; OTC): 140 mg
400 mg magnesium oxide is equivalent to 241.3 mg elemental Mg or 20 mEq Mg

Doses expressed in magnesium oxide salt.
Magnesium supplementation:
  Child: 5–10 mg/kg/24 hr ÷ TID–QID PO
  Adult: 400–800 mg/24 hr ÷ BID–QID PO
Hypomagnesemia:
  Child: 65–130 mg/kg/24 hr ÷ QID PO
  Adult: 2000 mg/24 hr ÷ QID PO

See *Magnesium Citrate*. **Use with caution** in renal insufficiency (monitor magnesium level) and patients receiving digoxin. **For dietary recommended intake (U.S. RDA) for magnesium, see Chapter 21.**

MAGNESIUM SULFATE
Epsom salts, many others, and generics
9.9% Elemental Magnesium
Magnesium salt

No   Yes   1   D

Injection: 500 mg/mL (4 mEq/mL) (2, 10, 20, 50 mL)
Injection, prediluted in sterile water for injection; ready to use: 40 mg/mL (0.325 mEq/mL) (50, 100, 500, 1000 mL); 80 mg/mL (0.65 mEq/mL) (50 mL)
Injection, prediluted in D$_5$W; ready to use: 10 mg/mL (0.081 mEq/mL) (100 mL); 20 mg/mL (0.163 mEq/mL) (500 mL)
Granules: Approx. 40 mEq Mg per 5 g (454, 1810 g)
500 mg magnesium sulfate is equivalent to 49.3 mg elemental Mg or 4.1 mEq Mg

All doses expressed in magnesium sulfate salt.
Cathartic:
  Child: 0.25 g/kg/dose PO Q4–6 hr
  Adult: 10–30 g/dose PO Q4–6 hr
Hypomagnesemia or hypocalcemia:
  IV/IM: 25–50 mg/kg/dose Q4–6 hr × 3–4 doses; repeat PRN. Max. single dose: 2 g
  PO: 100–200 mg/kg/dose QID PO
Daily maintenance:
  30–60 mg/kg/24 hr or 0.25–0.5 mEq/kg/24 hr IV
  Max. dose: 1 g/24 hr
Adjunctive therapy for moderate to severe reactive airway disease exacerbation (bronchodilation):
  Child: 25–75 mg/kg/dose (**max. dose:** 2 g) × 1 IV over 20 min.
  Adult: 2 g/dose × 1 IV over 20 min.

When giving IV, **beware** of hypotension, respiratory depression, complete heart block, and/or hypermagnesemia. Calcium gluconate (IV) should be available as **antidote**. **Use with caution** in patients with renal insufficiency (monitor magnesium levels) and with patients on digoxin. **Serum level dependent toxicity** includes the following: >3 mg/dL, CNS

Chapter 29 Drug Dosages **955**

MAGNESIUM SULFATE continued
depression; >5 mg/dL, decreased deep tendon reflexes, flushing, and somnolence; and >12 mg/dL, respiratory paralysis and heart block.
Max. IV intermittent infusion rate: 1 mEq/kg/hr or 125 mg $MgSO_4$ salt/kg/hr.
Pregnancy category is "D" because hypocalcemia, osteopenia, and fractures in the developing baby or fetus have been reported in pregnant women receiving magnesium > 5–7 days of preterm labor.

MANNITOL
Osmitrol, Resectisol, and generics
Osmotic diuretic

No   Yes   ?   C

Injection: 50, 100, 150, 200, 250 mg/mL (5%, 10%, 15%, 20%, 25%, respectively)
Irrigation solution (Resectisol): 50 mg/mL (5%) (2000 mL)

Anuria/oliguria (Child and adult):
  Test dose to assess renal function: 0.2 g/kg/dose (**max. dose**: 12.5 g) IV over 3–5 min. If there is no diuresis within 2 hr, discontinue mannitol.
  Initial: 0.5–1 g/kg/dose IV over 2–6 hr
  Maintenance: 0.25–0.5 g/kg/dose Q4–6 hr IV over 2–6 hr

Contraindicated in severe renal disease, active intracranial bleed, dehydration, and pulmonary edema. May cause circulatory overload and electrolyte disturbances. For hyperosmolar therapy, keep serum osmolality at 310–320 mOsm/kg.
Caution: Drug may crystallize at low temperatures with concentrations ≥ 15%; redissolve crystals by warming solution up to 70°C with agitation. Use an in-line filter. May cause hypovolemia, headache, and polydipsia. Reduction in ICP occurs in 15 min and lasts 3–6 hr.

MEBENDAZOLE
Emverm; previously available as Vermox
Anthelmintic

Yes   No   1   C

Chewable tabs: 100 mg (may be swallowed whole or chewed) (boxes of 12s)

Child (>2 yr) and adult:
  Pinworms (Enterobius): 100 mg PO × 1, repeat in 2 wk if not cured.
  Hookworms, roundworms (Ascaris), and whipworm (Trichuris): 100 mg PO BID × 3 days. Repeat in 3–4 wk if not cured. Alternatively, may administer 500 mg PO × 1 and repeat in 3–4 wk if not cured.
  Capillariasis: 200 mg PO BID × 20 days
  Visceral larva migrans (Toxocariasis): 100–200 mg PO BID × 5 days
  Trichinellosis (Trichinella spiralis): 200–400 mg PO TID × 3 days, then 400–500 mg PO TID × 10 days; use with steroids for severe symptoms
  Ancylostoma caninum (Eosinophilic enterocolitis): 100 mg PO BID × 3 days
See latest edition of the AAP *Red Book* for additional information.

Experience in children aged <2 yr and pregnancy is limited. May cause rash, headache, diarrhea, and abdominal cramping in cases of massive infection. Liver function test elevations and hepatitis have been reported with prolonged courses; monitor hepatic function with prolonged therapy. Family may need to be treated as a group. Therapeutic effect may decrease if administered to patients receiving aminoquinolones, carbamazepine, or phenytoin. Cimetidine may increase the effects/toxicity of mebendazole. Administer with food. Tablets may be crushed and mixed with food, swallowed whole, or chewed.

MEDROXYPROGESTERONE
Depo-Provera, Provera, and various generics; Depo-Sub Q Provera 104
Contraceptive, progestin

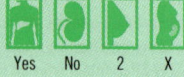
Yes No 2 X

Tabs (Provera and generics): 2.5, 5, 10 mg
Injection, suspension as acetate:
  Depo-Provera and generics, for IM use only: 150 mg/mL (1 mL), 400 mg/mL (2.5 mL); may contain parabens and polyethylene glycol
Injection, prefilled syringe as acetate:
  Depo-Sub Q Provera 104, for SC use only: 104 mg (0.65 mL of 160 mg/mL); contains parabens

Adolescent and adult:
  Contraception: Initiate therapy during the first 5 days after onset of a normal menstrual period; within 5 days postpartum if not breastfeeding, or if breastfeeding, at 6 wk postpartum. When converting contraceptive method to Depo-Sub Q Provera, dose should be administered within 7 days after the last day of using the previous method (pill, ring, or patch).
    IM (Depo-Provera and generics): 150 mg Q3 mo
    SC (Depo-Sub Q Provera 104): 104 mg Q3 mo (every 12–14 wk)
  Amenorrhea: 5–10 mg PO once daily × 5–10 days
  Abnormal uterine bleeding: 5–10 mg PO once daily × 5–10 days initiated on the 16th or 21st day of the menstrual cycle
  Endometriosis-associated pain (Depo-Sub Q Provera 104): 104 mg SC Q3 mo. Do not use for more than 2 yr due to its impact on bone mineral density

Consider patient's risk for osteoporosis because of the potential for decrease in bone mineral density with long-term use. **Contraindicated** in pregnancy, breast and genital cancer, liver disease, missed abortion, thrombophlebitis, thromboembolic disorders, cerebral vascular disease, and undiagnosed vaginal bleeding. **Use with caution** in patients with family history of breast cancer, depression, diabetes, and fluid retention. May cause dizziness, headache, insomnia, fatigue, nausea, weight increase, appetite changes, amenorrhea, and breakthrough bleeding. Cholestatic jaundice, adrenal suppression, and increased intracranial pressure have been reported. Injection site reactions may include pain/tenderness, persistent atrophy/indentation/dimpling, lipodystrophy, sterile abscess, skin color change, and node/lump.

Drug is a substrate to CYP450 3A4 isoenzyme. Aminoglutethimide may decrease medroxyprogesterone levels. May alter thyroid and liver function tests; prothrombin time; factors VII, VIII, IX and X; and metyrapone test.

Do not inject IM or SC product intravenously. Shake IM injection vial well before use and administer in the upper arm or buttock. Administer SC injection product into the anterior thigh or abdomen. Administer oral doses with food.

MEFLOQUINE HCL
Generics; previously available as Lariam
Antimalarial

Yes No 2 B

Tabs: 250 mg (228 mg base)

Doses expressed in mg mefloquine HCl salt
Malaria prophylaxis (start 2 wk prior to exposure and continue for 4 wk after leaving edemic area; see remarks):
  Child (PO, administered Q weekly):
    <10 kg: 5 mg/kg
    10–19 kg: 62.5 mg (1/4 tablet)

MEFLOQUINE HCL continued

20–30 kg: 125 mg (1/2 tablet)
31–45 kg: 187.5 mg (3/4 tablet)
>45 kg: 250 mg (1 tablet)
Adult: 250 mg PO Q weekly

Malaria treatment (uncomplicated/mild infection, chloroquine-resistant Plasmodium vivax):
Child ≥6 mo and >5 kg: 15 mg/kg (**max. dose:** 750 mg) ×1 PO followed by 10 mg/kg (**max. dose:** 500 mg) × 1 PO 12 hr later
Adult: 750 mg × 1 PO followed by 500 mg × 1 PO 12 hr later
See latest edition of the Red Book for additional information.

Contraindicated in active or recent history of depression, anxiety disorders, psychosis or schizophrenia, seizures, or hypersensitivity to quinine or quinidine. **Use with caution** in cardiac dysrhythmias and neurologic disease. May cause dizziness, ringing of the ears, headache, syncope, psychiatric symptoms (e.g., anxiety, paranoia, depression, hallucinations, and psychotic behavior), seizures, ocular abnormalities, GI symptoms, leukopenia, and thrombocytopenia. If neurological or psychiatric side effects occur, discontinue therapy and use an alternative medication. Most adverse events occur within 3 doses of prophylaxis use. Monitor liver enzymes and ocular exams for therapies > 1 yr.

Mefloquine is a substrate and inhibitor of P-glycoprotein and may reduce valproic acid levels. ECG abnormalities may occur when used in combination with quinine, quinidine, chloroquine, halofantrine, and β-blockers. If any of the aforementioned antimalarial drugs is used in the initial treatment of severe malaria, initiate mefloquine at least 12 hours after the last dose of any of these drugs. **Do not** initiate halofantrine or ketoconazole within 15 days of the last dose of mefloquine. Use with chloroquine may increase risk for seizures. Rifampin may decrease mefloquine levels.

Do not take on an empty stomach. Administer with at least 240-mL (8 oz) water. Treatment failures in children may be related to vomiting of administered dose. If vomiting occurs in less than 30 min after the dose, administer a second full dose. If vomiting occurs 30–60 min after the dose, administer an additional half-dose. If vomiting continues, monitor patient closely and consider alternative therapy.

MEROPENEM
Merrem and generics
Carbapenem antibiotic

No   Yes   2   B

Injection: 0.5, 1 g
Contains 3.92 mEq Na/g drug

Neonate and infant < 3 mo (IV):
  Non-CNS general dosing (meropenem MIC < 4):
   ≤2 kg:
    ≤14 days old: 20 mg/kg/dose Q12 hr
    15–28 days old: 20 mg/kg/dose Q8 hr
    29–60 days old: 30 mg/kg/dose Q8 hr
   >2 kg:
    ≤14 days old: 20 mg/kg/dose Q8 hr
    15–60 days old: 30 mg/kg/dose Q8 hr
  Non-CNS infection with moderately resistant meropenem isolate (MIC 4–8 mcg/mL; from a single-dose PK simulation study):
   >30-wk gestation and >7 days old: 40 mg/kg/dose IV Q8 hr

Continued

MEROPENEM continued

Neonate and infant < 3 mo (IV):
  Intraabdominal infection (meropenem MIC < 4 mcg/mL):
    <32-wk gestation:
      <14 days old: 20 mg/kg/dose Q12 hr
      ≥14 days old: 20 mg/kg/dose Q8 hr
    ≥32-wk gestation:
      <14 days old: 20 mg/kg/dose Q8 hr
      ≥14 days old: 30 mg/kg/dose Q8 hr
  Meningitis (1–3 mo, IV; recommendation from 2004 IDSA meningitis practice guidelines): 40 mg/kg/dose Q8 hr
Infant (≥3 mo), child, and adolescent (IV):
  Meningitis, severe infections, cystic fibrosis pulmonary exacerbations: 40 mg/kg/dose (max. 2 g/dose) Q8 hr
  Complicated skin and skin structure infection: 10 mg/kg/dose (max. dose: 500 mg/dose) Q8 hr. If *Pseudomonas aeruginosa* is suspected or confirmed, use 20 mg/kg/dose (max. dose: 1 g/dose) Q8 hr.
  Intraabdominal and mild/moderate infections and fever/neutropenia empiric therapy: 20 mg/kg/dose (max. dose: 1 g/dose) Q8 hr
Adult (IV):
  Skin and subcutaneous tissue infections: 500 mg Q8 hr; use 1 g Q8 hr for suspected or confirmed *P. aeruginosa*
  Intraabdominal and mild/moderate infections; fever/neutropenia empiric therapy: 1 g Q8 hr
  Meningitis and severe infections: 2 g Q8 hr

Contraindicated in patients sensitive to carbapenems or with a history of anaphylaxis to β-lactam antibiotics. **Use with caution** in meningitis and CNS disorders (may cause seizures) and renal impairment **(adjust dose; see Chapter 30).** Drug penetrates well into the CSF.
May cause diarrhea, rash, nausea, vomiting, oral moniliasis, glossitis, pain and irritation at the IV injection site, and headache. Hepatic enzyme and bilirubin elevation, dermatological reactions (including Stevens–Johnson, DRESS, and TEN), leukopenia, thrombocytopenia (in renal dysfunction), and neutropenia have been reported. Probenecid may increase serum meropenem levels. May reduce valproic acid levels.
Increasing the IV drug administration time to 4 hr will improve the meropenem concentration time above the MIC and may be useful in conditions with resistant organisms.

MESALAMINE
Apriso, Asacol, Asacol HD, Canasa, Delzicol, Lialda, Pentasa, Rowasa, SfRowasa, and generics; 5-aminosalicylic acid, 5-ASA
Salicylate, GI antiinflammatory agent

Yes   Yes   2   B/C

Caps, controlled release:
  Pentasa: 250, 500 mg
  Delzicol: 400 mg
  Apriso (for Q24 hr dosing): 375 mg; contains aspartame
Tabs, delayed release: 400 mg (Asacol), 800 mg (Asacol HD and generics), 1200 mg (Lialda)
Suppository (Canasa): 1000 mg (30s, 42s)
Rectal suspension (Rowasa, SfRowasa, and generics): 4 g/60 mL; contains sulfites (SfRowasa is sulfite free) and sodium benzoate

Child and adolescent:
  Caps, controlled release: 50–100 mg/kg/24 hr ÷ Q6–12 hr PO; **max. dose**: 1 g/dose

MESALAMINE continued

Child and adolescent:
   Delzicol (mild/moderate ulcerative colitis; ≥5–18 yr; see remarks):
      17–32 kg: 800 mg QAM and 400 mg Q afternoon PO
      33–53 kg: 1200 mg QAM and 800 mg Q afternoon PO
      54–90 kg: 1200 mg QAM and Q afternoon PO
   Tabs, delayed release: 50–100 mg/kg/24 hr ÷ Q8–12 hr PO; **max. dose:** 4.8 g/24 hr.
Adolescent:
   Enema (Rowasa; for ulcerative colitis): 4 g QHS
   Suppository (Canasa; for ulcerative colitis): 500 mg QHS–BID
Adult (Ulcerative colitis):
   Caps, controlled release:
      Initial therapy: 1 g QID PO × 3–8 wk
      Maintenance therapy for remission:
         Apriso: 1.5 g QAM PO
         Pentasa: 1 g QID PO
   Tabs, delayed release:
      Initial therapy:
         Asacol: 800 mg TID PO × 6 wk
         Asacol HD: 1.6 g TID PO × 6 wk
         Lialda: 2.4–4.8 g once daily PO up to 8 wk
      Maintenance therapy for remission:
         Asacol: 1.6 g/24 hr PO in divided doses
         Lialda: 2.4 g PO once daily
   Suppository: 1000 mg QHS PR × 3–6 wk; retain each dose in the rectum for 1–3 hr or longer, if possible
   Rectal suspension: 60 mL (4 g) QHS × 3–6 wk, retaining each dose for about 8 hr; lie on left side during administration to improve delivery to the sigmoid colon.

Generally **not recommended** in children < 16 yr with chicken pox or flu-like symptoms (risk of Reye's syndrome). **Contraindicated** in active peptic ulcer disease, severe renal failure, and salicylate hypersensitivity. Rectal suspension should not be used in patients with history of sulfite allergy. **Use with caution** in sulfasalazine hypersensitivity, impaired hepatic, or renal function, pyloric stenosis, and with concurrent thrombolytics. May cause headache, GI discomfort, pancreatitis, pericarditis, and rash. Angioedema, Stevens–Johnson syndrome, DRESS, and fatal infections (e.g., sepsis and pneumonia; discontinue use) have been reported.

Safety and efficacy of Asacol in children 5–17 yr for mild/moderate acute ulcerative colitis have been established over a 6-wk period. However, efficacy for maintenance of remission was not established in a 26-wk RCT (potential factors affecting outcome included improper dosage used and premature termination of trial). Safety and efficacy of Canasa suppositories have not been demonstrated for mild/moderate active ulcerative proctitis in a 6-wk open-label study in 49 patients aged 5–17 yr.

Two Delzicol 400 mg capsules have not been shown to be interchangeable or substitutable with one mesalamine 800 delayed-release tablet.

Do not administer with lactulose or other medications that can lower intestinal pH. Oral capsules are designed to release medication throughout the GI tract and oral tablets release medication at the terminal ileus and beyond; 400 mg PO mesalamine is equivalent to 1 g sulfasalazine PO. Tablets should be swallowed whole.

May cause a false-positive urinary normetanephrine test. All products have a pregnancy category "B" except for Asacol HD, which has a pregnancy category "C."

METFORMIN
Glucophage, Glucophage XR, Glumetza, Fortamet, Riomet, and generics
Antidiabetic, biguanide

Yes   Yes   2   B

Tabs: 500, 850, 1000 mg
Tabs, extended release:
  Glucophage XR and generics: 500, 750 mg
  Fortamet, Glumetza, and generics: 500, 1000 mg
Oral suspension (Riomet): 100 mg/mL (120, 480 mL); contains saccharin

Administer all doses with meals (e.g., BID: morning and evening meals).
Child (10–16 yr) (see remarks): Start with 500 mg BID; may increase dose weekly by 500 mg/24 hr in two divided doses up to a **max. dose** of 2000 mg/24 hr.
Child ≥17 yr and adult (see remarks):
  500 mg tabs: Start with 500 mg PO BID; may increase dose weekly by 500 mg/24 hr in two divided doses up to a **max. dose** of 2500 mg/24 hr. Administer 2500 mg/24 hr doses by dividing daily dose TID with meals.
  850 mg tabs: Start with 850 mg PO once daily with morning meal; may increase by 850 mg every 2 wk up to a **max. dose** of 2550 mg/24 hr (first dosage increment: 850 mg PO BID; second dosage increment: 850 mg PO TID).
  Extended-release tabs: Start with 500 mg PO once daily with evening meal; may increase by 500 mg every wk up to a **max. dose** of 2000 mg/24 hr (if glycemic control is not achieved at **max. dose**, divide dose to 1000 mg PO BID). If using Fortamet, **max. dose** is 2500 mg/24 hr. If a dose > 2000 mg is needed, consider switching to nonextended-release tablets in divided doses and increase dose to a **max. dose** of 2550 mg/24 hr.

Assess patient's eGFR prior to initiating therapy. **Contraindicated** in severe renal impairment (<30 mL/min/1.73 m^2), hepatic impairment (increased risk for lactic acidosis), CHF, metabolic acidosis, and during radiology studies using iodinated contrast media. **Use with caution** when transferring patients from chlorpropamide therapy (potential hypoglycemia risk), excessive alcohol intake, hypoxemia, dehydration, surgical procedures, mild/moderate renal impairment, hepatic disease, anemia, and thyroid disease.

Fatal lactic acidosis (diarrhea; severe muscle pain, cramping; shallow and fast breathing; and unusual weakness and sleepiness) and decrease in vitamin B$_{12}$ levels have been reported. May cause GI discomfort (~50% incidence), anorexia, and vomiting. Transient abdominal discomfort or diarrhea have been reported in 40% of pediatric patients. Cimetidine, furosemide, and nifedipine may increase the effects/toxicity of metformin. In addition to monitoring serum glucose and glycosylated hemoglobin, monitor renal function and hematologic parameters (baseline and annual).

Adult patients initiated on 500 mg PO BID may also have their dose increased to 850 mg PO BID after 2 wk.

COMBINATION THERAPY WITH SULFONYLUREAS: If patient has not responded to 4 wk of **maximum** doses of metformin monotherapy, consider gradual addition of an oral sulfonylurea with continued **maximum** metformin dosing (even if failure with sulfonylurea has occurred). Attempt to identify the minimum effective dosage for each drug (metformin and sulfonylurea) because the combination can increase risk for sulfonylurea-induced hypoglycemia. If patient does not respond to 1–3 mo of combination therapy with **maximum** metformin doses, consider discontinuing combination therapy and initiating insulin therapy.

Administer all doses with food.

METHADONE HCL
Dolophine, Methadose, and generics
Narcotic, analgesic

Yes   Yes   2   C

Tabs: 5, 10 mg
Tabs (dispersible): 40 mg
Oral solution: 5 mg/5 mL, 10 mg/5 mL; contains 8% alcohol
Concentrated. solution: 10 mg/mL
Injection: 10 mg/mL (20 mL), contains 0.5% chlorobutanol

Analgesia:
  Child: 0.7 mg/kg/24 hr ÷ Q4–6 hr PO, SC, IM, or IV PRN pain; **max. dose**: 10 mg/dose.
  Adult: 2.5–10 mg/dose Q3–4 hr PO, SC, IM, or IV PRN pain.
Detoxification or maintenance: See package insert.

Unintentional overdoses have resulted in fatalities and severe adverse events such as respiratory depression and cardiac arrhythmias. Use with caution in hepatic (avoid in severe cases) and biliary tract impairment. May cause respiratory depression, sedation, increased intracranial pressure, hypotension, and bradycardia. Average $T_{1/2}$: children, 19 hr and adults, 35 hr. Duration of action PO is 6–8 hr initially and 22–48 hr after repeated doses. Respiratory effects last longer than analgesia. Accumulation may occur with continuous use, making it necessary to adjust dose. Nevirapine may decrease serum levels of methadone. Fatalities have been reported with abuse in combination with benzodiazepines. Methadone is a substrate for CYP450 3A3/4, 2D6, and 1A2 and inhibitor of 2D6.
See Chapter 6 for equianalgesic dosing and onset of action. **Adjust dose in renal failure (see Chapter 30).**

METHIMAZOLE
Tapazole and generics
Antithyroid agent

No   No   2   D

Tabs: 5, 10 mg

Hyperthyroidism:
  Child:
    Initial: 0.4–0.7 mg/kg/24 hr or 15–20 mg/m²/24 hr PO ÷ Q8 hr
    Maintenance: 1/3–2/3 of initial dose PO ÷ Q8 hr
    Max. dose: 30 mg/24 hr
  Adult:
    Initial: 15–60 mg/24 hr PO ÷ TID
    Maintenance: 5–15 mg/24 hr PO ÷ TID

Readily crosses placental membranes and distributes into breast milk (maternal dose ≤ 20 mg/24 hr is considered safe, but there is insufficient data to support safe use with maternal dose > 20 mg/24 hr). Blood dyscrasias, dermatitis, hepatitis, arthralgia, CNS reactions, pruritus, nephritis, hypoprothrombinemia, agranulocytosis, headache, fever, and hypothyroidism may occur.
May increase the effects of oral anticoagulants. When correcting hyperthyroidism, existing β-blocker, digoxin, and theophylline doses may need to be reduced to avoid potential toxicities.
Switch to maintenance dose when patient is euthyroid. Administer all doses with food.

METHYLDOPA
Various generics
Central α-adrenergic blocker, antihypertensive

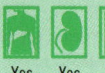

Yes | Yes | 1 | B/C

Tabs: 250, 500 mg
Injection: 50 mg/mL (5 mL); may contain sulfites
Oral suspension: 50 mg/mL

Hypertension:
  Child: 10 mg/kg/24 hr ÷ Q6–12 hr PO; increase PRN Q2 days. **Max. dose**: 65 mg/kg/24 hr or 3 g/24 hr, whichever is less
  Adult: 250 mg/dose BID-TID PO. Increase PRN Q2 days to **max. dose** of 3 g/24 hr
Hypertensive crisis:
  Child: 2–4 mg/kg/dose IV, if no response within 4–6 hr, may increase dose to 5–10 mg/kg/dose IV; give doses Q6–8 hr. **Max. dose** (whichever is less): 65 mg/kg/24 hr or 3 g/24 hr
  Adult: 250–1000 mg IV Q6–8 hr; **max. dose**: 4 g/24 hr

Contraindicated in pheochromocytoma and active liver disease. **Use with caution** if patient is receiving haloperidol, propranolol, lithium, or sympathomimetics. Positive Coombs' test is rarely associated with hemolytic anemia. Fever, leukopenia, sedation, memory impairment, hepatitis, GI disturbances, orthostatic hypotension, black tongue, and gynecomastia may occur. May interfere with lab tests for creatinine, urinary catecholamines, uric acid, and AST.
May increase AV blocking effects of β-blockers and antihypertensive effects of other antihypertensives. $α_2$-antagonist antidepressants, serotonin/norepinephrine reuptake inhibitors, and methylphenidate may reduce the antihypertensive effects of methyldopa. **Do not use** in combination with MAO inhibitors (may enhance adverse effects of methyldopa). **Do not co-administer** oral doses with iron; decreases methyldopa absorption. **Adjust dose in renal failure (see Chapter 30).**
Pregnancy category is "C" for the injectable dosage form and "B" for the oral dosage forms.

METHYLENE BLUE
ProvayBlue and generics
Antidote, drug-induced methemoglobinemia and cyanide toxicity

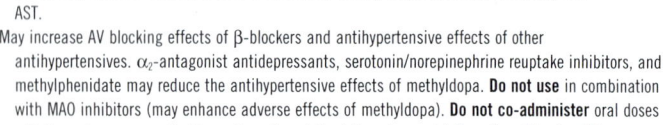

No | Yes | ? | X

Injection: 10 mg/mL (1%) (1, 10 mL)
Intravenous solution (ProvayBlue): 50 mg/10 mL (10 mL)

Methemoglobinemia:
  Child and adult: 1–2 mg/kg/dose or 25–50 mg/m^2/dose IV over 5 min. May repeat in 1 hr if needed

At high doses, may cause methemoglobinemia. **Avoid** subcutaneous or intrathecal routes of administration. **Use with caution** in G6PD deficiency or renal insufficiency. May cause nausea, vomiting, dizziness, headache, diaphoresis, stained skin, and abdominal pain. Causes blue-green discoloration of urine and feces.
Serotonin syndrome has been reported with the co-administration of selective serotonin reuptake inhibitors (SSRI), serotonin norepinephrine reuptake inhibitor (SNRI), or clomipramine. Use with bupropion, paroxetine, sertraline, duloxetine, vilazodone, venlafaxine, fluoxetine, or desipramine is considered contraindicated.

METHYLPHENIDATE HCL
Ritalin, Aptensio XR, Methylin, Metadate ER, Methylin ER, Concerta, Ritalin SR, QuilliChew ER, Quillivant XR, Metadate CD, Ritalin LA, Daytrana, and generics
CNS stimulant

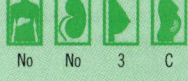
No   No   3   C

Tabs (Ritalin and generics): 5, 10, 20 mg
Chewable tabs (Methylin and generics): 2.5, 5, 10 mg; contains phenylalanine
Extended-release chewable tabs (QuilliChew ER): 20, 30, 40 mg; contains phenylalanine
Oral solution (Methylin and generics): 1 mg/mL, 2 mg/mL; may contain propylene glycol
Oral suspension (Quillivant XR): 25 mg/5 mL (60, 120, 150, 180 mL); contains sodium benzoate
Extended-release tabs:
 8-hr duration (Metadate ER): 20 mg
 24-hr duration (Concerta and generics): 18, 27, 36, 54 mg
Sustained-release tabs:
 8-hr duration (Ritalin SR): 20 mg
Extended-release caps
 24-hr duration:
  Metadate CD, Ritalin LA, and generics: 10, 20, 30, 40, 50, 60 mg
  Aptensio XR: 10, 15, 20, 30, 40, 50, 60 mg
Transdermal patch (Daytrana): 10 mg/9 hr (each 12.5 cm^2 patch contains 27.5 mg), 15 mg/9 hr (each 18.75 cm^2 patch contains 41.3 mg), 20 mg/9 hr (each 25 cm^2 patch contains 55 mg), 30 mg/9 hr (each 37.5 cm^2 patch contains 82.5 mg) (30s)

Attention-deficit hyperactivity disorder:
 Immediate-release oral dosage forms (Methylin, Ritalin; ≥6 yr):
  Initial: 0.3 mg/kg/dose (or 2.5–5 mg/dose) given before breakfast and lunch. May increase by 0.1 mg/kg/dose PO (or 5–10 mg/24 hr) weekly until maintenance dose achieved. May give extra afternoon dose if needed
  Maintenance dose range: 0.3–1 mg/kg/24 hr
  Max. dose: 2 mg/kg/24 hr or 60 mg/24 hr for those weighing ≤50 kg and 100 mg/24 hr >50 kg
 Extended-release once daily oral dosage form (Concerta; ≥6 yr):
  Methylphenidate naive patients: Start with 18 mg PO QAM for children and adolescents and 18–36 mg PO QAM for adults, dosage may be increased at weekly intervals with 18 mg increments up to the following **max. dose**:
   6–12 yr: 54 mg/24 hr
   13–17 yr: 72 mg/24 hr **not to exceed** 2 mg/kg/24 hr
   Patients weighing >50 kg: higher **max. dose** of 108 mg/24 hr may be used
  Patients currently receiving methylphenidate: See following table.

RECOMMENDED DOSE CONVERSION FROM METHYLPHENIDATE REGIMENS TO CONCERTA:

Previous Methylphenidate Daily Dose	Recommended Concerta Dose
5 mg PO BID–TID or 20 mg SR PO once daily	18 mg PO QAM
10 mg PO BID–TID or 40 mg SR PO once daily	36 mg PO QAM
15 mg PO BID–TID or 60 mg SR PO once daily	54 mg PO QAM
20 mg PO BID–TID	72 mg PO QAM

After a week of receiving the above-recommended Concerta dose, dose may be increased in 18-mg increments at weekly intervals PRN up to a **maximum** of 54 mg/24 hr for 6–12 yr and 72 mg/24 hr (not to exceed 2 mg/kg/24 hr) for 13–17 yr.

Continued

METHYLPHENIDATE HCL *continued*

Other extended-release oral dosage forms (see specific product information if converting from another product or dosage form):

Product (Dosage Form)	Initial Dose (≥6 Yr)*	Dosage Adjustment	Max. Dose
Metadate CD (extended-release caps)	20 mg PO once daily	Increase at 20 mg increments Q7 days PRN	≤50 kg: 60 mg/24 hr >50 kg: 100 mg/24 hr
Ritalin LA (extended-release caps)	20 mg PO once daily	Increase at 10 mg increments Q7 days PRN	≤50 kg: 60 mg/24 hr >50 kg: 100 mg/24 hr
Quillivant XR (extended-release oral suspension)*	20 mg PO once daily	Increase at 10–20 mg increments Q7 days PRN	60 mg/24 hr
QuilliChew (extended-release chewable tabs)	20 mg PO once daily	Increase or decrease by 10, 15, or 20 mg Q7 days PRN	Doses > 60 mg/24 hr have not been studied

*Quillivant XR dosing recommendations for children 6–12 yr

Transdermal patch (Daytrana): Apply to the hip 2 hr before the effect is needed and remove 9 hr later. Patch may be removed before 9 hr if a shorter duration of effect is desired or if late-day adverse effects appear.

6–17 yr: Start with 10 mg/9 hr patch once daily. Increase dose PRN Q7 days by increasing to the next dosage strength. Higher starting doses have been reported in patients converting from oral dosage forms > 20 mg/24 hr.

Contraindicated in glaucoma, anxiety disorders, motor tics, and Tourette's syndrome. Medication should generally **not** be used in children aged <5 yr; diagnosis of ADHD in this age group is extremely difficult and should only be done in consultation with a specialist. Sudden death (children, adolescents, and adults), stroke (adults), and MI (adults) have been reported in patients with preexisting structural cardiac abnormalities or other serious heart problems. **Use with caution** in patients with hypertension, psychiatric conditions, and epilepsy. Insomnia, weight loss, anorexia, rash, nausea, emesis, abdominal pain, hyper- or hypotension, tachycardia, arrhythmias, palpitations, restlessness, headaches, fever, tremor, visual disturbances, and thrombocytopenia may occur. Abnormal liver function, cerebral arteritis and/or occlusion, peripheral vasculopathy (including Raynaud's phenomenon), leukopenia and/or anemia, hypersensitivity reactions, transient depressed mood, paranoia, mania, auditory hallucination, priapism, and scalp hair loss have been reported. Skin irritation, chemical leukoderma, and contact dermatitis has been reported with transdermal route. High doses may slow growth by appetite suppression. GI obstruction has been reported with Concerta.

May increase serum concentrations/effects of tricyclic antidepressants, dopamine agonists (e.g., haloperidol), phenytoin, phenobarbital, and warfarin. May decrease the effects of antihypertensive drugs. Effect of methylphenidate may be potentiated by MAO inhibitors; hypertensive crisis may also occur if used within 14 days of discontinuance of the MAO inhibitor.

Extended/sustained-release dosage forms have either an 8- or 24-hour dosage interval (as stipulated previously). Concerta dosage form delivers 22.2% of its dose as an immediate-release product with the remaining amounts as an extended-release product (e.g., 18-mg strength: 4 mg as immediate release and 14 mg as extended release). **Do not** consume alcohol with Ritalin LA or Metadate CD dosage forms as it may result in a more rapid release of the drug. **Do not** expose transdermal application site to external heat sources (e.g., electric blankets, heating pads); this may increase drug release.

METHYLPREDNISOLONE
Medrol, Medrol Dosepack, Solu-Medrol, Depo-Medrol, and generics
Corticosteroid

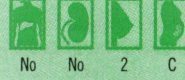
No No 2 C

Tabs: 2, 4, 8, 16, 32 mg
Tabs, dose pack (Medrol Dosepack and generics): 4 mg (21s)
Injection, Na succinate (Solu-Medrol and generics): 40, 125, 500, 1000, 2000 mg (IV or IM use); may contain benzyl alcohol
Injection, Acetate (Depo-Medrol and generics): 20, 40, 80 mg/mL (IM repository); may contain polyethylene glycol (1, 5 mL)

Antiinflammatory/immunosuppressive:
  PO/IM/IV: 0.5–1.7 mg/kg/24 hr ÷ Q6–12 hr
Asthma exacerbations (2007 National Heart, Lung, and Blood Institute Guideline Recommendations; dose until peak expiratory flow reaches 70% of predicted or personal best):
  Child ≤ 12 yr (IM/IV/PO): 1–2 mg/kg/24 hr ÷ Q12 hr (**max. dose:** 60 mg/24 hr). Higher alternative regimen of 1 mg/kg/dose Q6 hr × 48 hr followed by 1–2 mg/kg/24 hr (**max. dose:** 60 mg/24 hr) ÷ Q12 hr has been suggested
  >12 yr and adult (IV/IM/PO): 40–80 mg/24 hr ÷ Q12–24 hr
Outpatient asthma exacerbation burst therapy (longer durations may be necessary):
  PO:
    Child ≤ 12 yr: 1–2 mg/kg/24 hr ÷ Q12–24 hr (**max. dose:** 60 mg/24 hr) × 3–10 days
    Child > 12 yr and adult: 40–60 mg/24 hr ÷ Q12–24 hr × 3–10 days
  IM (use methylprednisolone acetate product) for patients vomiting or with adherence issues:
    Child ≤ 12 yr: 7.5 mg/kg (**max. dose:** 240 mg) IM × 1
    Child > 12 yr and adult: 240 mg IM × 1
Acute spinal cord injury:
  30 mg/kg IV over 15 min followed in 45 min by a continuous infusion of 5.4 mg/kg/hr × 23 hr.

See Chapter 10 for relative steroid potencies. Acetate form may also be used for intraarticular and intralesional injection and has longer times to max. effect and duration of action; it should **NOT** be given IV. Like all steroids, may cause hypertension, pseudotumor cerebri, acne, Cushing syndrome, adrenal axis suppression, GI bleeding, hyperglycemia, and osteoporosis.
Barbiturates, phenytoin, and rifampin may enhance methylprednisolone clearance. Erythromycin, itraconazole, and ketoconazole may increase methylprednisone levels. Methylprednisolone may increase cyclosporine and tacrolimus levels.

METOCLOPRAMIDE
Reglan, Metozolv, and generics
Antiemetic, prokinetic agent

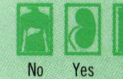
No Yes 2 B

Tabs: 5, 10 mg
Tabs, orally disintegrating (ODT) (Metozolv and generics): 5, 10 mg
Injection: 5 mg/mL (2 mL)
Oral solution: 5 mg/5 mL (473 mL)

Gastroesophageal reflux (GER) or GI dysmotility:
  Infant and child: 0.1–0.2 mg/kg/dose up to QID IV/IM/PO; **max. dose:** 0.8 mg/kg/24 hr or 10 mg/dose
  Adult: 10–15 mg/dose QAC and QHS IV/IM/PO

Continued

METOCLOPRAMIDE continued

Antiemetic (all ages): Premedicate with diphenydramine to reduce EPS
1–2 mg/kg/dose Q2–6 hr IV/IM/PO

Postoperative nausea and vomiting:
Child: 0.1–0.2 mg/kg/dose Q6–8 hr PRN IV; **max. dose**: 10 mg/dose
>14 yr and adult: 10 mg Q6–8 hr PRN IV

Contraindicated in GI obstruction, seizure disorder, pheochromocytoma, or in patients receiving drugs likely to cause extrapyramidal symptoms (EPS). May cause EPS, especially at higher doses. Sedation, headache, anxiety, depression, leukopenia, and diarrhea may occur. Neuroleptic malignant syndrome and tardive dyskinesia (increased risk with prolong duration of therapy; avoid use for >12 wk) have been reported.

For GER, give 30 min before meals and at bedtime. **Reduce dose in renal impairment (see Chapter 30).**

METOLAZONE
Generics; previously available as Zaroxolyn
Diuretic, thiazide-like

Yes   Yes   2   B

Tabs: 2.5, 5, 10 mg
Oral suspension: 0.25, 1 mg/mL

Dosage based on Zaroxolyn (for oral suspension, see remarks):
Child: 0.2–0.4 mg/kg/24 hr ÷ once daily–BID PO
Adult:
  Hypertension: 2.5–5 mg once daily PO
  Edema: 2.5–20 mg once daily PO

Contraindicated in patients with anuria, hepatic coma, or hypersensitivity to sulfonamides or thiazides. **Use with caution** in severe renal disease, impaired hepatic function, gout, lupus erythematosus, diabetes mellitus, and elevated cholesterol and triglycerides. Electrolyte imbalance, GI disturbance, hyperglycemia, marrow suppression, chills, hyperuricemia, chest pain, hepatitis, and rash may occur.

Oral suspensions have increased bioavailability; therefore, lower doses may be necessary when using these dosage forms. More effective than thiazide diuretics in impaired renal function; may be effective in GFRs as low as 20 mL/min. Furosemide-resistant edema in pediatric patients may benefit with the addition of metolazone.

Pregnancy category changes to "D" if used for pregnancy-induced hypertension.

METOPROLOL
Lopressor, Toprol-XL, and generics
Adrenergic blocking agent (β$_1$-selective), class II antiarrhythmic

Yes   No   1   C

Tabs: 25, 37.5, 50, 75, 100 mg
Extended-release tabs (Toprol-XL and generics): 25, 50, 100, 200 mg
Oral liquid: 10 mg/mL
Injection: 1 mg/mL (5 mL)

Hypertension:
Child ≥ 1 yr and adolescent:
  Nonextended-release oral dosage forms: Start at 1–2 mg/kg/24 hr PO ÷ BID; **max. dose:** 6 mg/kg/24 hr **up to** 200 mg/24 hr.

METOPROLOL continued

Extended-release tabs (≥6 yr and adolescent): Start at 1 mg/kg/dose (**max. dose**: 50 mg) PO once daily; if needed, adjust dose **up to** a **max. dose** of 2 mg/kg/24 hr or 200 mg/24 hr once daily (higher doses have not been evaluated).

Adult:

Nonextended-release tabs: Start at 50–100 mg/24 hr PO ÷ once daily–BID; if needed, increase dosage at weekly intervals to desired blood pressure. Usual effective dosage range is 100–450 mg/24 hr. Doses > 450 mg/24 hr have not been studied. Patients with bronchospastic diseases should receive the lowest possible daily dose divided TID.

Extended-release tabs: Start at 25–100 mg/24 hr PO once daily; if needed, increase dosage at weekly intervals to desired blood pressure. Usual dosage range is 50–100 mg/24 hr. Doses > 400 mg/24 hr have not been studied.

Contraindicated in sinus bradycardia, heart block > 1st degree, sick sinus syndrome (except with functioning pacemaker), cardiogenic shock, and uncompensated CHF. **Use with caution** in hepatic dysfunction; peripheral vascular disease; history of severe anaphylactic hypersensitivity drug reactions; pheochromocytoma; and concurrent use with verapamil, diltiazem, or anesthetic agents that may decrease myocardial function. Should not be used with bronchospastic diseases. Reserpine and other drugs that deplete catecholamines (e.g., MAO inhibitors) may increase the effects of metoprolol. Metoprolol is a CYP450 2D6 substrate.

Avoid abrupt cessation of therapy in ischemic heart disease; angina, ventricular arrhythmias, and MI have occurred. Common side effects include bradyarrhythmia, heart block, heart failure, pruritus, rash, GI disturbances, dizziness, fatigue, and depression. Bronchospasm; dyspnea; and elevations in transaminase, alkaline phosphatase, and LDH have all been reported.

METRONIDAZOLE
Flagyl, Flagyl ER, First-Metronidazole, MetroGel, MetroLotion, MetroCream, Rosadan, Noritate, MetroGel-Vaginal, Vandazole, Nuvessa, and generics
Antibiotic, antiprotozoal

Yes   Yes   3   B

Tabs: 250, 500 mg
Tabs, extended release (Flagyl ER): 750 mg
Caps: 375 mg
Oral suspension: 50 mg/mL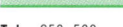
 First-Metronidazole: 50 mg/mL (150 mL), 100 mg/mL (150 mL); contains sodium benzoate and saccharin
Ready-to-use injection: 5 mg/mL (100 mL); contains 28 mEq Na/g drug
Gel, topical:
 Rosadan and generics: 0.75% (45 g)
 MetroGel and generics: 1% (55, 60 g)
Lotion (MetroLotion and generics): 0.75% (59 mL); contains benzyl alcohol
Cream, topical:
 MetroCream, Rosadan, and generics: 0.75% (45 g); contains benzyl alcohol
 Noritate: 1% (30 g); contains parabens
Gel, vaginal:
 MetroGel-Vaginal, Vandazole, and generics: 0.75% (70 g with 5 applicators); contains parabens
 Nuvessa: 1.3% (5 g containing ~65 mg metronidazole); contains parabens

Continued

METRONIDAZOLE continued

Amebiasis:
  Child: 35–50 mg/kg/24 hr PO ÷ TID × 10 days
  Adult: 500–750 mg/dose PO TID × 10 days
Anaerobic infection (see remarks):
  Neonate: PO/IV:
    <1 kg:
      ≤14 days old: 15 mg/kg × 1 loading dose followed by 7.5 mg/kg/dose Q48 hr
      15–28 days old: 15 mg/kg/dose Q24 hr
    1–2 kg:
      ≤7 days old: 15 mg/kg × 1 loading dose followed by 7.5 mg/kg/dose Q24–48 hr
      8–28 days old: 15 mg/kg/dose Q24 hr
    > 2 kg:
      ≤7 days old: 15 mg/kg/dose Q24 hr
      8–28 days old: 15 mg/kg/dose Q12 hr
  Infant/child/adolescent:
    PO: 30–50 mg/kg/24 hr ÷ Q8 hr; **max. dose:** 2250 mg/24 hr
    IV: 22.5–40 mg/kg/24 hr ÷ Q8 hr; **max. dose:** 1500 mg/24 hr
  Adult:
    PO/IV: 30 mg/kg/24 hr ÷ Q6 hr; **max. dose:** 4 g/24 hr
Other parasitic infections:
  Infant/child: 15–30 mg/kg/24 hr PO ÷ Q8 hr
  Adult: 250 mg PO Q8 hr or 2 g PO × 1
Bacterial vaginosis:
  Adolescent and adult:
    PO:
      Immediate-release tabs: 500 mg BID × 7 days
      Extended-release tabs: 750 mg once daily × 7 days
    Vaginal: 5 g (1 applicator full) QHS–BID × 5 days
Giardiasis:
  Child: 15 mg/kg/24 hr PO ÷ TID × 5–7 days; **max. dose:** 750 mg/24 hr
  Adult: 250 mg PO TID × 5 days
Trichomoniasis: Treat sexual contacts
  Child: 15 mg/kg/24 hr PO ÷ TID × 7 days; **max. dose:** 2000 mg/24 hr
  Adolescent/adult: 2 g PO × 1, or 250 mg PO TID, or 375 mg PO BID × 7 days
Clostridium difficile infection (IV may be less efficacious):
  Child: 30 mg/kg/24 hr ÷ Q6 hr PO/IV × 7–14 days; **max. dose:** 2000 mg/24 hr
  Adult: 500 mg TID PO/IV × 10–14 days
Helicobacter pylori infection (use in combination with amoxicillin and acid suppressing agent with/without clarithromycin):
  Child: 20 mg/kg/24 hr (**max. dose:** 1000 mg/24 hr) ÷ BID PO × 10–14 days
  Adult: 250–500 mg QID (QAC and QHS) PO × 10–14 days
Topical use: Apply and rub a thin film to affected areas at the following frequencies specific to product concentration.
  0.75% cream: BID
  1% cream: once daily

Avoid use in the first-trimester of pregnancy. **Use with caution** in patients with CNS disease, blood dyscrasias, severe liver, or **renal disease (GFR < 10 mL/min; see Chapter 30).** If using single 2-g dose in a breastfeeding mother, discontinue breastfeeding for 12–24 hr to allow excretion of the drug.

METRONIDAZOLE continued

Nausea, diarrhea, urticaria, dry mouth, leukopenia, vertigo, metallic taste, and peripheral neuropathy may occur. Candidiasis may worsen. May discolor urine. Patients **should not** ingest alcohol for 24–48 hr after dose (disulfuram-type reaction).

Single-dose oral regimen no longer recommended in bacterial vaginosis due to poor efficacy. May increase levels or toxicity of phenytoin, lithium, and warfarin. Phenobarbital and rifampin may increase metronidazole metabolism.

IV infusion must be given slowly over 1 hr. For intravenous use in all ages, some references recommend a 15 mg/kg loading dose. Use of an adjusted body weight (ABW) for dosing [ABW = IBW + (actual or total BW − IBW)] has been recommended for obese patients.

MICAFUNGIN SODIUM
Mycamine
Antifungal, echinocandin

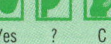
Yes   Yes   ?   C

Injection: 50, 100 mg; contains lactose

Invasive candidiasis (see remarks):
  Neonate and infant (based on a multidose pharmacokinetic and safety trial in 13 neonates/infants aged >48 hr and <120 days with suspected or invasive candidiasis; minimum of 4–5 days of therapy):
    <1 kg: 10 mg/kg/dose IV once daily; additional data from another multidose trial in 12 preterm neonates (median birth weight: 775 g, 27 wk gestation) suggest 15 mg/kg/dose IV once daily will provide similar AUC drug exposure of approximately 5 mg/kg/dose in adults.
    ≥1 kg: 7–10 mg/kg/dose IV once daily; 10–12 mg/kg/dose IV once daily may be needed for HIV-exposed/infected neonates.
  Child and adolescent: 3–4 mg/kg/dose IV once daily; **max. dose**: 200 mg/dose
  Adult: 100–150 mg IV once daily
Esophageal candidiasis (see remarks):
  Child and adult:
    <50 kg: 3–4 mg/kg/dose IV once daily; **max. dose**: 200 mg/dose.
    ≥50 kg: 150 mg IV once daily; mean duration for successful therapy was 15 days (range: 10–30 days).
Candida prophylaxis in hematopoietic stem cell transplant:
  Child and adult:
    <50 kg: 1.5 mg/kg/dose IV once daily; **max. dose**: 50 mg/dose.
    ≥50 kg: 50 mg IV once daily.
Invasive aspergillosis (limited data; see remarks):
  Child and adult:
    <50 kg: 3–4 mg/kg/dose IV once daily; dosages as high as 7.5 mg/kg/24 hr have been tolerated.
    ≥50 kg: 150 mg IV once daily.

Prior hypersensitivity to other echinocandins (anidulafungin, casopofungin) increases risk; anaphylaxis with shock has been reported. **Use with caution** in hepatic and renal impairment.

No dosing adjustments are required based on race or gender or in patients with severe renal dysfunction or mild to moderate hepatic function impairment. Effect of severe hepatic function impairment on micafungin pharmacokinetics has not been evaluated. Higher dosage requirements in premature and young infants may be attributed to faster drug clearance due to lower protein

Continued

MICAFUNGIN SODIUM continued

binding. Higher treatment doses in infants and children have been reported at 8.6–12 mg/kg/dose IV once daily.

May cause GI disturbances, phlebitis, rash, hyperbilirubinemia, liver function test elevation, headache, fever, and rigor. Anemia, leukopenia, neutropenia, thrombocytopenia, TEN, Stevens–Johnson syndrome, and hemolysis have been reported. Micafungin is CYP450 3A isoenzyme substrate and weak inhibitor. May increase the effects/toxicity of nifedipine and sirolimus.

Safety and efficacy in children ≥ 4 mo have been demonstrated based on well-controlled studies and pharmacokinetic/safety studies.

MICONAZOLE
Topical products: Micatin, Lotrimin AF, and other brands
Vaginal products: Monistat, Vagistat-3, and other brands
Antifungal agent

No   No   2   C

Cream (OTC): 2% (15, 30, 57, 141 g)
Ointment (OTC): 2% (56, 71, 141 g)
Solution (OTC): 2% with alcohol (29.57 mL)
Gel (OTC): 2% with alcohol (24 g)
Topical solution (OTC): 2% with alcohol (30.3 mL)
Powder (OTC): 2% (70, 85, 90 g)
Spray, liquid (OTC): 2% (150 g); contains alcohol
Spray, powder (OTC): 2% (85, 113, 133 g); contains alcohol
Vaginal cream (OTC): 2% (45 g)
Vaginal suppository (OTC): 100 mg (7s), 200 mg (3s)
Vaginal combination packs:
  Monistat 1 Combination Pack (OTC): 1200 mg suppository (1) and 2% cream (9 g)
  Monistat 3, Vagistat-3 (OTC): 200 mg suppository (3s) and 2% cream (9 g)
  Monistat 7 (OTC): 100 mg suppository (7s) and 2% cream (9 g)

Topical: Apply BID × 2–4 wk
Vaginal:
  7-day regimen: 1 applicator full of 2% cream or 100 mg suppository QHS × 7 days
  3-day regimen: 1 applicator full of 4% cream or 200 mg suppository QHS × 3 days
  1-day regimen (Monistat 1): 1200 mg suppository × 1 at bedtime or during the day

Use with caution in hypersensitivity to other imidazole antifungal agents (e.g., clotrimazole, ketoconazole). Side effects include pruritis, rash, burning, phlebitts, headaches, and pelvic cramps.

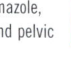

Drug is a substrate and inhibitor of CYP450 3A3/4 isoenzymes. Vaginal use with concomitant warfarin use has also been reported to increase warfarin's effect. Vegetable oil base in vaginal suppositories may interact with latex products (e.g., condoms and diaphragms); consider switching to the vaginal cream.

Avoid contact with eyes.

MIDAZOLAM
Various generics; previously available as Versed
Benzodiazepine

Yes Yes 2 D

Injection: 1 mg/mL (2, 5, 10 mL), 5 mg/mL (1, 2, 5, 10 mL); some preparations may contain 1% benzyl alcohol
Oral syrup: 2 mg/mL (118 mL); contains sodium benzoate

Titrate to effect under controlled conditions (see remarks).
See Chapter 6 for additional routes of administration.
Sedation for procedures:
  Child and adolescent:
    IM: 0.1–0.15 mg/kg/dose 30–60 min prior to procedure. Higher dose of 0.5 mg/kg/dose has been used for anxious patients. **Max. dose:** 10 mg.
    IV:
      6 mo–5 yr: 0.05–0.1 mg/kg/dose over 2–3 min. May repeat dose PRN in 2–3 min intervals up to a max. total dose of 6 mg. A total dose up to 0.6 mg/kg may be necessary for desired effect.
      6–12 yr: 0.025–0.05 mg/kg/dose over 2–3 min. May repeat dose PRN in 2–3 min intervals up to a max. total dose of 10 mg. A total dose up to 0.4 mg/kg may be necessary for desired effect.
      >12–16 yr: Use adult dose; up to max. total dose of 10 mg.
    PO:
      ≥6 mo: 0.25–0.5 mg/kg/dose × 1; **max. dose:** 20 mg. Younger patients (6 mo–5 yr) may require higher doses of 1 mg/kg/dose, whereas older patients (6–15 yr) may require only 0.25 mg/kg/dose. Use 0.25 mg/kg/dose for patients with cardiac or respiratory compromise, concurrent CNS depressive drug, or high-risk surgery.
  Adult:
    IM: 0.07–0.08 mg/kg/dose 30–60 min prior to procedure; usual dose is 5 mg.
    IV: 0.5–2 mg/dose over 2 min. May repeat PRN in 2–3 min intervals until desired effect. Usual total dose: 2.5–5 mg. **Max. total dose:** 10 mg.
Sedation with mechanical ventilation:
  Intermittent:
    Infant and child: 0.05–0.15 mg/kg/dose IV Q1–2 hr PRN
  Continuous IV infusion (initial doses, titrate to effect):
    Neonate:
      <32-wk gestation: 0.5 mcg/kg/min
      ≥32-wk gestation: 1 mcg/kg/min
    Infant and child: 1–2 mcg/kg/min
Refractory status epilepticus:
  ≥2 mo and child: Load with 0.15 mg/kg IV × 1 followed by a continuous infusion of 1 mcg/kg/min; titrate dose upward Q5 min to effect (mean dose of 2.3 mcg/kg/min with a range of 1–18 mcg/kg/min has been reported).

Contraindicated in patients with narrow angle glaucoma and shock. **Use with caution** in CHF, **renal impairment (adjust dose; see Chapter 30)**, pulmonary disease, hepatic dysfunction, and in neonates. Causes respiratory depression, hypotension, and bradycardia. Cardiovascular monitoring is recommended. Use lower doses or reduce dose when given in combination with narcotics or in patients with respiratory compromise.
Higher recommended dosage for younger patients (6 mo–5 yr) is attributed to the water soluble properties of midazolam and the higher percent body water for younger patients.

Continued

MIDAZOLAM continued

Drug is a substrate for CYP450 3A4. Serum concentrations may be increased by cimetidine, clarithromycin, diltiazem, erythromycin, itraconazole, ketoconazole, ranitidine, and protease inhibitors (use contraindicated). Sedative effects may be antagonized by theophylline. **Effects can be reversed by flumazenil.** For pharmacodynamic information, see Chapter 6.

MILRINONE
Generics; previously available as Primacor
Inotrope

No   Yes   ?   C

Injection: 1 mg/mL (10, 20, 50 mL)
Premixed injection in D$_5$W: 200 mcg/mL (100, 200 mL)

Child (limited data): 50 mcg/kg IV bolus over 15 min, followed by a continuous infusion of 0.25–0.75 mcg/kg/min and titrate to effect.
Adult: 50 mcg/kg IV bolus over 10 min, followed by a continuous infusion of 0.375–0.75 mcg/kg/min and titrate to effect. **Max. dose:** 1.13 mg/kg/24 hr.

Contraindicated in severe aortic stenosis, severe pulmonic stenosis, and acute MI. May cause headache, dysrhythmias, hypotension, hypokalemia, nausea, vomiting, anorexia, abdominal pain, hepatotoxicity, and thrombocytopenia. Pediatric patients may require higher mcg/kg/min doses because of a faster elimination T$_{1/2}$ and larger volume of distribution when compared to adults. Hemodynamic effects can last up to 3–5 hr after discontinuation of infusion in children. **Reduce dose in renal impairment.**

MINERAL OIL
Kondremul, Fleet Mineral Oil, and generics
Laxative, lubricant

No   No   2   ?

Liquid, oral (OTC): 30, 472, 500, 1000 mL
Emulsion, oral (Kondremul; OTC): 480 mL; each 5 mL Kondremul contains 2.5 mL mineral oil
Rectal liquid (Fleet Mineral Oil, OTC): 133 mL

Constipation:
  Child 5–11 yr (see remarks):
    Oral liquid: 5–15 mL/24 hr ÷ once daily–TID PO
    Oral emulsion (Kondremul): 10–30 mL/24 hr ÷ once daily–TID PO
    Rectal (2–11 yr): 66.5 mL as single dose
  Child ≥ 12 yr and adult (see remarks):
    Oral liquid: 15–45 mL/24 hr ÷ once daily–TID PO
    Oral emulsion (Kondremul): 30–90 mL/24 hr ÷ once daily–TID PO
    Rectal: 133 mL as single dose

May cause diarrhea, cramps, and lipid pneumonitis via aspiration. Use as a laxative **should not exceed > 1 wk.** Onset of action is approximately 6–8 hr. Higher doses may be necessary to achieve desired effect. **Do not** give QHS dose and **use with caution** in children aged <5 yr to minimize risk of aspiration. May impair the absorption of fat-soluble vitamins, calcium, phosphorus, oral contraceptives, and warfarin. Emulsified preparations are more palatable and are dosed differently than the oral liquid preparation.
For disimpaction, doses up to 1 ounce (30 mL) per yr of age (**max. dose** of 240 mL) BID can be given. Pregnancy category has not been officially assigned by the FDA.

MINOCYCLINE
Minocin, Solodyn, Arestin, and generics
Antibiotic, tetracycline derivative

Yes Yes X D

Tabs: 50, 75, 100 mg
Caps: 50, 75, 100 mg
Extended-release tabs (Q24 hr dosing):
 Generics: 45, 90, 135 mg
 Solodyn: 55, 65, 80, 105, 115 mg
Caps (pellet filled): 50, 100 mg
Sustained-release microspheres (Arestin): 1 mg (12s)
Injection (Minocin): 100 mg

General infections:
 Child (8–12 yr): 4 mg/kg/dose × 1 IV/PO, then 2 mg/kg/dose Q12 hr IV/PO; **max. dose**: 200 mg/24 hr
 Adolescent and adult: 200 mg/dose × 1 IV/PO, then 100 mg Q12 hr IV/PO
Chlamydia trachomatis/Ureaplasma urealyticum:
 Adolescent and adult: 100 mg IV/PO Q12 hr × 7 days
Acne (≥12 yr–adult):
 Immediate-release dosage forms: 50–100 mg PO once daily–BID
 Extended-release tabs:
  45–49 kg: 45 mg PO once daily
  50–59 kg: 55 mg PO once daily
  60–71 kg: 65 mg PO once daily
  72–84 kg: 80 mg PO once daily
  85–96 kg: 90 mg PO once daily
  97–110 kg: 105 PO once daily
  111–125 kg: 115 mg PO once daily
  126–136 kg: 135 mg PO once daily

Not recommended for children <8 yr and during the last half of pregnancy due to risk for permanent tooth discoloration. **Use with caution** in renal failure; lower dosage may be necessary. High incidence of vestibular dysfunction (30%–90%). Nausea, vomiting, allergy, increased intracranial pressure (e.g., pseudotumor cerebri), photophobia, and injury to developing teeth may occur. Hepatitis, including autoimmune hepatitis, liver failure, hypersensitivity reactions (e.g., anaphylaxis, Stevens–Johnson syndrome, erythema multiforme), and lupus-like syndrome have been reported.

May increase effects/toxicity of warfarin and decrease the efficacy of live attenuated oral typhoid vaccine. May be administered with food but **NOT** with milk or dairy products. See Tetracycline for additional drug/food interactions and comments.

MINOXIDIL
Tabs: Generics; previously available as Loniten
Topical: Minoxidil form Men, Hair Regrowth Treatment Men, Men's Rogaine Extra Strength
Antihypertensive agent, hair growth stimulant

   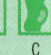
No   Yes   2   C

Tabs: 2.5, 10 mg
Topical solution:
  Minoxidil for Men (OTC): 2% (60 mL)
  Hair Regrowth Treatment for Men, Men's Rogaine Extra Strength, and Minoxidil for Men (OTC): 5% (60, 120 mL); contains 30% alcohol

Child < 12 yr:
  Start with 0.1–0.2 mg/kg/24 hr PO once daily; **max. dose**: 5 mg/24 hr. Dose may be increased in increments of 0.1–0.2 mg/kg/24 hr at 3-day intervals. Usual effective range: 0.25–1 mg/kg/24 hr PO ÷ once daily–BID; **max. dose**: 50 mg/24 hr.
≥12 yr and adult:
  Oral: Start with 5 mg once daily. Dose may be gradually increased at 3-day intervals. Usual effective range: 10–40 mg/24 hr ÷ once daily–BID; **max. dose**: 100 mg/24 hr.
Topical (alopecia; see remarks):
  Adult: Apply solution topically to the affected areas of the scalp BID (QAM and QHS).

Contraindicated in acute MI, dissecting aortic aneurysm, and pheochromocytoma. Concurrent use with a β-blocker and diuretic is recommended to prevent reflex tachycardia and reduce water retention, respectively. May cause drowsiness, dizziness, CHF, pulmonary edema, pericardial effusion, pericarditis, thrombocytopenia, leukopenia, Stevens–Johnson syndrome, TEN, and hypertrichosis (reversible) with systemic use. Neonatal hypertrichosis has been reported following use during pregnancy.

Concurrent use of guanethidine may cause profound orthostatic hypotension; use with other antihypertensive agents may cause additive hypotension. Patients with renal failure or those receiving dialysis may require a dosage reduction. Antihypertensive onset of action within 30 min and peak effects within 2–8 hr.

TOPICAL USE: Local irritation, contact dermatitis may occur. **Do not use** in conjunction with other topical agents including topical corticosteroids, retinoids, petrolatum, or agents that are known to enhance cutaneous drug absorption. Onset of hair growth is 4 mo. Wash hands thoroughly after each application. The 5% solution is flammable.

MOMETASONE FUROATE ± FOMOTEROL FUMARATE
Asmanex, Nasonex, Elocon, and other generic nasal and topical products
In combination with fomoterol: Dulera
Corticosteroid

Yes   No   2   C

Nasal spray (Nasonex and generics): 0.05%, 50 mcg per actuation (17 g, provides 120 doses)
Aerosol for inhalation (Asmanex HFA): 100 mcg per actuation (13 g, provides 120 actuations), 200 mcg per actuation (13 g; provides 120 actuations)
Powder for inhalation, breath activated (Asmanex Twisthaler; see remarks): 110 mcg per actuation (7, 30 units), 220 mcg per actuation (14, 60, 120 units); contains lactose and milk proteins
Topical cream and ointment (Elocon and other generics): 0.1% (15, 45 g)
Topical lotion and solution (Elocon and generics): 0.1% (30, 60 mL); contains isopropyl alcohol

MOMETASONE FUROATE ± FOMOTEROL FUMARATE *continued*

In combination with fomoterol:
  Aerosol inhaler (Dulera):
    100 mcg mometasone furoate + 5 mcg fomoterol fumarate dihydrate per inhalation (8.8 g delivers 60 inhalations; 13 g delivers 120 inhalations)
    200 mcg mometasone furoate + 5 mcg fomoterol fumarate dihydrate per inhalation (8.8 g delivers 60 inhalations; 13 g delivers 120 inhalations)

MOMETASONE FUROATE:
Intranasal (allergic rhinitis): Patients with known seasonal allergic rhinitis should initiate therapy 2–4 wk prior to anticipated pollen season.
  2–11 yr: 50 mcg (1 spray) each nostril once daily.
  ≥12 yr and adult: 100 mcg (2 sprays) each nostril once daily.
Oral inhalation:
  4–11 yr: Start with 110 mcg (1 inhalation) QHS of the 110 mcg inhaler regardless of prior therapy. **Max. dose:** 110 mcg/24 hr.
  ≥12 yr and adult: Max. effects may not be achieved until 1–2 wk or longer. Titrate doses to the lowest effective dose once asthma stabilized.
    Previously treated with bronchodilators alone or with inhaled corticosteroids: Start with 220 mcg (1 inhalation) QHS. Dose may be increased up to a **max. dose** of 440 mcg/24 hr ÷ QHS or BID.
    Previously treated with oral corticosteroids: Start with 440 mcg BID; **max. dose:** 880 mcg/24 hr.
Topical (see Chapter 8 for topical steroid comparisons):
  Cream and ointment:
    ≥2 yr and adult: Apply a thin film to the affected area once daily. Safety and efficacy for >3 wk has not been established for pediatric patients.
  Lotion:
    ≥12 yr and adult: Apply a few drops to the affected area and massage lightly into the skin once daily until it disappears.

MOMETASONE FUROATE + FOMOTEROL FUMARATE (Dulera):
≥12 yr and adult: Two inhalations BID of either 100 mcg mometasone + 5 mcg formoterol or 200 mcg mometasone + 5 mcg formoterol based on prior asthma therapy (see table below). **Max. dose:** Two inhalations BID of 200 mcg mometasone + 5 mcg formoterol.

Previous Therapy	Recommended Starting Dose	Recommended Maximum Daily Dose
Medium-dose Inhaled corticosteroids	100 mcg mometasone + 5 mcg formoterol: 2 inhalations BID	400 mcg mometasone + 20 mcg fomoterol
High-dose inhaled corticosteroids	200 mcg mometasone + 5 mcg formoterol: 2 inhalations BID	800 mcg mometasone + 20 mcg fomoterol

Concurrent administration with ketoconazole and other CYP450 3A4 inhibitors (e.g., protease inhibitors) may increase mometasone levels, resulting in Cushing syndrome and adrenal suppression. **Use with caution** in hepatic impairment; increased drug exposure is possible.

INTRANASAL: Clear nasal passages and shake nasal spray well before each use. Onset of action for nasal symptoms of allergic rhinitis has been shown to occur within 11 hr after the first dose. Nasal burning and irritation may occur. Nasal septal perforation, taste, and smell disturbances have been rarely reported. A clinical trial in children aged 6–17 yr was not able to demonstrate effectiveness for treating nasal polyps.

Continued

MOMETASONE FUROATE ± FOMOTEROL FUMARATE continued

ORAL INHALATION (all forms): Rinse mouth after each use. Fever, allergic rhinitis, URI, UTI, GI discomfort, and sore throat have been reported in children. Musculoskeletal pain, oral candidiasis, arthralgia, and fatigue may occur. May potentially worsen tuberculosis; fungal, bacterial, viral, or parasitic infections; or ocular herpes simplex. Do not use Asmanex Twisthaler if allergic to milk proteins. Breastfeeding information is currently unknown, but most experts consider use of inhaled corticosteroids acceptable.

MOMETASONE + FOMOTEROL (Dulera): Common side effects include nasopharyngitis, sinusitis, and headache. Angioedema, anaphylaxis, and arrhythmias have been reported. See *Formoterol* for additional remarks.

TOPICAL USE: HPA axis suppression and skin atrophy have been reported with cream and ointment use in infants 6–23 mo. Avoid application/contact to face, eyes, underarms, groin, and mucous membranes. Occlusive dressings and use in diaper dermatitis are not recommended.

MONTELUKAST
Singulair and generics
Antiasthmatic, antiallergic, leukotriene receptor antagonist

Yes   No   ?   B

Chewable tabs: 4, 5 mg; contains phenylalanine
Tabs: 10 mg
Oral granules: 4 mg per packet (30s)

Asthma and seasonal allergic rhinitis:
  Child (6 mo–5 yr): 4 mg (oral granules or chewable tablet) PO QHS; minimum age for use in asthma (per product label) is 12 mo.
  Child (6–14 yr): 5 mg (chewable tablet) PO QHS
  ≥15 yr and adult: 10 mg PO QHS
Prevention of exercise-induced bronchospasm (administer dose at least 2 hr prior to exercise; additional doses should not be administered within 24 hr):
  Child (6–14 yr): 5 mg (chewable tablet) PO
  ≥15 yr and adult: 10 mg PO

Chewable tablet dosage form is **contraindicated** in phenylketonuric patients. Side effects include headache, abdominal pain, dyspepsia, fatigue, dizziness, cough, and elevated liver enzymes. Diarrhea, enuresis, epistaxis, pulmonary eosinophilia, thrombocytopenia, hypersensitivity reactions (including Stevens–Johnson and TEN), pharyngitis, nausea, otitis, sinusitis, and viral infections have been reported in children. Neuropsychiatric events, including aggression, anxiety, dream abnormalities, hallucinations, depression, suicidal behavior, and insomnia, have been reported.

Drug is a substrate for CYP450 3A4 and 2C9. Phenobarbital and rifampin may induce hepatic metabolism to increase the clearance of montelukast.

Doses may be administered with or without food.

MORPHINE SULFATE
Roxanol, MS Contin, Oramorph SR, Avinza, Kadian, and many generics
Narcotic, analgesic

Yes   Yes   2   C/D

Oral solution: 10 mg/5 mL, 20 mg/5 mL
Concentrated oral solution: 100 mg/5 mL
Tabs: 15, 30 mg

MORPHINE SULFATE continued

Controlled-release tabs (MS Contin, Oramorph SR): 15, 30, 60, 100, 200 mg
Extended-release tabs: 15, 30, 60, 100, 200 mg
Extended-release caps:
  Avinza (10% of dose as immediate release): 30, 60, 90, 120 mg
  Kadian: 10, 20, 30, 40, 50, 60, 70, 80, 100, 130, 150, 200 mg
  Generics: 10, 20, 30, 45, 50, 60, 75, 80, 90, 100, 120 mg
Rectal suppository: 5, 10, 20, 30 mg
Injection: 0.5, 1, 2, 4, 5, 8, 10, 15, 25, 50 mg/mL

Titrate to effect.
Neonate:
  Analgesia/tetralogy (cyanotic) spells: 0.05–0.2 mg/kg/dose IM, slow IV, SC Q4 hr
  Opiate withdrawal: 0.08–0.2 mg/kg/dose PO Q3–4 hr PRN
Infant 1–6 mo:
  PO: 0.08–0.1 mg/kg/dose Q3–4 hr PRN
  IV: 0.025–0.03 mg/kg/dose Q2–4 hr PRN
Infant > 6 mo and child:
  PO: 0.2–0.5 mg/kg/dose (**initial max. dose:** 15–20 mg/dose) Q4–6 hr PRN (immediate release) or 0.3–0.6 mg/kg/dose Q12 hr PRN (controlled release)
  IM/IV/SC: 0.1–0.2 mg/kg/dose Q2–4 hr PRN; **max. initial dose:** infant: 2 mg/dose, 1–6 yr: 4 mg/dose, 7–12 yr: 8 mg/dose, and adolescent: 10 mg/dose.
Adult:
  PO: 10–30 mg Q4 hr PRN (immediate release) or 15–30 mg Q8–12 hr PRN (controlled release)
  IM/IV/SC: 2–15 mg/dose Q2–6 hr PRN
Continuous IV infusion and SC infusion: Dosing ranges, titrate to effect.
  Neonate (IV route only): 0.01–0.02 mg/kg/hr
  Infant and child:
    Postoperative pain: 0.01–0.04 mg/kg/hr
    Sickle cell and cancer: 0.04–0.07 mg/kg/hr
  Adult: 0.8–10 mg/hr
To prepare infusion for neonates, infants, and children, use the following formula:

$$50 \times \frac{\text{Desired dose (mg/kg/hr)}}{\text{Desired infusion rate (mL/hr)}} \times \text{Wt (kg)} = \frac{\text{mg morphine}}{50 \text{ mL fluid}}$$

Dependence, CNS and respiratory depression, nausea, vomiting, urinary retention, constipation, hypotension, bradycardia, increased ICP, miosis, biliary spasm, and allergy may occur. **Naloxone may be used to reverse effects, especially respiratory depression.** Causes histamine release resulting in itching and possible bronchospasm. Low-dose naloxone infusion may be used for itching. Inflammatory masses (e.g., granulomas) have been reported with continuous infusions via indwelling intrathecal catheters.

Dosage reduction may be necessary with liver cirrhosis. See Chapter 6 for equianalgesic dosing. Pregnancy category changes to "D" if used for prolonged periods or in higher doses at term. Rectal dosing is same as oral dosing but is not recommended due to poor absorption.

The FDA has recently announced safety labeling changes and postmarket study requirements for extended-release/long-acting opioid analgesics; see www.fda.gov/drugs/drugsafety for updated information. Controlled/sustained-release oral tablets must be administered whole. Controlled-release oral capsules may be opened and the entire contents sprinkled on applesauce immediately prior to ingestion. Be aware of the various oral solution concentrations; the concentrated oral

Continued

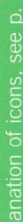

MORPHINE SULFATE *continued*
solution (100 mg/5 mL) has been associated with accidental overdoses. **Adjust dose in renal failure (see Chapter 30).**

MUPIROCIN
Bactroban, Bactroban Nasal, and generics
Topical antibiotic

No / No / 2 / B

Ointment: 2% (22, 30 g); contains polyethylene glycol
Cream: 2% (15, 30 g); may contain benzyl alcohol
Nasal ointment (Bactroban Nasal): 2% (1 g), as calcium salt

Topical (see remarks):

  ≥3 mo–adult: Apply small amount TID to affected area × 5–14 days. Topical ointment may be used in infants aged ≥2 mo for impetigo.
Intranasal for elimination of nasal colonization of Staphylococcus aureus, including MRSA (all ages): Apply small amount intranasally BID × 5–10 days.

Avoid contact with the eyes. Topical cream is **not** intended for use in lesions > 10 cm in length or 100 cm^2 in surface area. **Do not use** topical ointment preparation on open wounds because of concerns about systemic absorption of polyethylene glycol. May cause minor local irritation and dry skin. Intranasal route may cause nasal stinging, taste disorder, headache, rhinits, and pharyngitis.
If clinical response is not apparent in 3–5 days with topical use, reevaluate infection.

MYCOPHENOLATE
Mycophenolate mofetil: CellCept and generics
Mycophenolic acid: Myfortic and generics
Immunosuppressant agent

No / Yes / 3 / D

Mycophenolate mofetil:
  Caps: 250 mg
  Tabs: 500 mg
  Oral suspension: 200 mg/mL (160 mL); contains phenylalanine (0.56 mg/mL) and methylparabens
  Injection: 500 mg
Mycophenolic acid:
  Delayed-release tabs (Myfortic and generics): 180, 360 mg

Child and adolescent (see remarks):
Renal transplant:
  Caps, tabs, or suspension: 600 mg/m^2/dose PO/IV BID up to a **max. dose** of 2000 mg/24 hr; alternatively, patients with body surface areas (BSAs) ≥1.25 m^2 may be dosed as follows:
    1.25–1.5 m^2: 750 mg PO BID
    >1.5 m^2: 1000 mg PO BID
  Delayed-release tabs (Myfortic): 400 mg/m^2/dose PO BID; **max. dose:** 720 mg BID; this dosage form is not recommended in patients with BSAs < 1.19 m^2. Alternatively, patients with body surface areas ≥ 1.19 m^2 may be dosed as follows:
    1.19–1.58 m^2: 540 mg PO BID
    >1.58 m^2: 720 mg PO BID
Nephrotic syndrome:
  Frequently relapsing: 12.5–18 mg/kg/dose or 600 mg/m^2/dose PO BID up to a **max. dose** of 2000 mg/24 hr for 1–2 yr and taper prednisone regimen

MYCOPHENOLATE continued

Steroid dependent: 12–18 mg/kg/dose or 600 mg/m^2/dose PO BID up to a **max. dose** of 2000 mg/24 hr

Adult (in combination with corticosteroids and cyclosporine; check specific transplantation protocol for specific dosage):

IV: 2000–3000 mg/24 hr ÷ BID

Oral:
   Caps, tabs, or suspension: 2000–3000 mg/24 hr PO ÷ BID
   Delayed-release tabs (Myfortic): 720–1080 mg PO BID

Check specific transplantation protocol for specific dosage. Mycophenolate mofetil is a prodrug for mycophenolic acid. Owing to differences in absorption, the delayed-release tablets should **not** be interchanged with other oral dosage forms on an equivalent mg-to-mg basis. Increases risk of first trimester pregnancy loss and increased risk of congenital malformations (especially external ear and facial abnormalities, including cleft lip and palate, and anomalies of the distal limbs, heart, and esophagus).

Common side effects may include headache, hypertension, diarrhea, vomiting, bone marrow suppression, anemia, fever, opportunistic infections, and sepsis. May increase the risk for bacterial, fungal, protozoal, and viral infections and lymphomas or other malignancies. GI bleeds and increased risk of rejection in heart transplant patients switched from calcineurin inhibitors (e.g., cyclosporine and tacrolimus) and CellCept to sirolimus and CellCept have been reported. Cases of progressive multifocal leukoencephalopathy (PML), pure red cell aplasia (PRCA), and hypogammaglobulinemia have also been reported.

Use with caution in patients with active GI disease or renal impairment (GFR < 25 mL/min/1.73 m^2) outside of the immediate posttransplant period. In adults with renal impairment, **avoid** doses > 2 g/24 hr and observe carefully. Dose should be interrupted or reduced in the presence of neutropenia (ANC < 1.3 × 10^3/μL). No dose adjustment is needed for patients experiencing delayed graft function postoperatively.

Drug interactions: (1) Displacement of phenytoin or theophylline from protein-binding sites will decrease total serum levels and increase free serum levels of these drugs. Salicylates displace mycophenolate to increase free levels of mycophenolate. (2) Competition for renal tubular secretion results in increased serum levels of acyclovir, ganciclovir, probenecid, and mycophenolate (when any of these are used together). (3) **Avoid** live and live attenuated vaccines (including influenza); decreases vaccine effectiveness. (4) Proton-pump inhibitors, antacids, cholestyramine, cyclosporine, and telmisartan may reduce mycophenolate levels.

Administer oral doses on an empty stomach. Infuse intravenous doses over 2 hr. Oral suspension may be administered via NG tube with a minimum size of 8 French.

NAFCILLIN
Generics; previously available as Nallpen
Antibiotic, penicillin (penicillinase resistant)

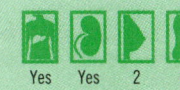

Yes   Yes   2   B

Injection: 1, 2, 10 g; contains 2.9 mEq Na/g drug
Injection, premixed in iso-osmotic dextrose: 1 g in 50 mL, 2 g in 100 mL

Neonate (IM/IV):
   <1 kg:
      ≤14 days old: 50 mg/kg/24 hr ÷ Q12 hr
      15–28 days old: 75 mg/kg/24 hr ÷ Q8 hr

Continued

NAFCILLIN continued

Neonate (IM/IV):
  1–2 kg:
    ≤7 days old: 50 mg/kg/24 hr ÷ Q12 hr
    8–28 days old: 75 mg/kg/24 hr ÷ Q8 hr
  >2 kg:
    ≤7 days old: 75 mg/kg/24 hr ÷ Q8 hr
    8–28 days old: 100 mg/kg/24 hr ÷ Q6 hr

Infant and child (IM/IV):
  Mild to moderate infections: 100–150 mg/kg/24 hr ÷ Q6 hr
  Severe infections: 150–200 mg/kg/24 hr ÷ Q4–6 hr; give 200 mg/kg/24 hr ÷ Q4–6 hr for staphylococcal endocarditis or meningitis.
  Max. dose: 12 g/24 hr

Adult:
  IV: 1000–2000 mg Q4–6 hr
  IM: 500–1000 mg Q4–6 hr
  Max. dose: 12 g/24 hr

Allergic cross-sensitivity with penicillin. Solutions containing dextrose may be **contraindicated** in patients with known allergy to corn or corn products. High incidence of phlebitis with IV dosing. CSF penetration is poor unless meninges are inflamed. **Use with caution** in patients with combined renal and hepatic impairment (reduce dose by 33%–50%). Nafcillin may increase elimination of cyclosporine and warfarin. Acute interstitial nephritis is rare. May cause rash and bone marrow suppression and false-positive urinary and serum proteins. Hypokalemia has been reported.

NALOXONE
Narcan, Evzio, and generics
Narcotic antagonist

No   No   ?   C

Injection: 0.4 mg/mL (1, 10 mL); some preparations may contain parabens
Injection, in syringe: 2 mg/2 mL (2 mL)
Autoinjector (Evzio): 0.4 mg/0.4 mL (0.4 mL)
Nasal liquid (Narcan): 4 mg/0.1 mL (1 ea); contains benzalkonium chloride

Opiate intoxication (IM/IV/SC, use 2–10 times IV dose for ETT route; see remarks):
  Neonate, infant, child ≤ 20 kg or ≤ 5 yr: 0.1 mg/kg/dose. May repeat PRN Q2–3 min.
  Child > 20 kg or > 5 yr: 2 mg/dose. May repeat PRN Q2–3 min.
  Continuous infusion (child and adult): 0.005 mg/kg loading dose followed by infusion of 0.0025 mg/kg/hr has been recommended. A range of 0.0025–0.16 mg/kg/hr has been reported. Taper gradually to avoid relapse.
  Adult: 0.4–2 mg/dose. May repeat PRN Q2–3 min. Use 0.1- to 0.2-mg increments in opiate-dependent patients.

Intranasal route for opiate intoxication:
  Child, adolescent, and adult: 4 mg (0.1 mL) of nasal liquid (Narcan) into one nostril, PRN Q2–3 min in alternate nostrils. Alternatively for adolescents and adults, the 2 mg/2 mL intravenous syringe dosage form with nasal adaptor may be used by administering 1 mg (1 mL) per nostril.
  Opiate induced pruritis (limited data): 0.25–2 mcg/kg/hr IV; a dose finding study in 59 children suggests a minimum dose of 1 mcg/kg/hr when used as prophylactic therapy. Doses ≥ 3 mcg/kg/hr increases the risk for reduced pain control.

Short duration of action may necessitate multiple doses. For severe intoxication, doses of 0.2 mg/kg may be required. If no response is achieved after a cumulative dose of 10 mg,

NALOXONE continued

reevaluate diagnosis. **In the nonarrest situation, use the lowest effective dose (may start at 0.001 mg/kg/dose). See** Chapter 6 **for additional information.**

Will produce narcotic withdrawal syndrome in patients with chronic dependence. **Use with caution** in patients with chronic cardiac disease. Abrupt reversal of narcotic depression may result in nausea, vomiting, diaphoresis, tachycardia, hypertension, and tremulousness.

IV administration is preferred. Onset of action may be delayed with other routes of administration.

NAPROXEN/NAPROXEN SODIUM
Naprosyn, Anaprox, EC-Naprosyn, Naprosyn DR, Naprelan,
Aleve [OTC], and many others including generics
Nonsteroidal antiinflammatory agent

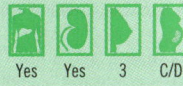
Yes   Yes   3   C/D

Naproxen:
  Tabs (Naprosyn and generics): 250, 375, 500 mg
  Delayed-release tabs (EC-Naprosyn, Naprosyn DR): 375, 500 mg
  Oral suspension (Naprosyn and generics): 125 mg/5 mL; contains 0.34 mEq Na/1 mL and parabens
Naproxen Sodium:
  Tabs:
  Aleve and generics (OTC): 220 mg (200 mg base); contains 0.87 mEq Na
  Anaprox and generics: 275 mg (250 mg base), 550 mg (500 mg base); contains 1 mEq, 2 mEq Na, respectively
  Controlled-release tabs (Naprelan and generics): 412.5 mg (375 mg base), 550 mg (500 mg base), 825 mg (750 mg base)

All doses based on naproxen base
Child >2 yr:
  Analgesia: 5–7 mg/kg/dose Q8–12 hr PO
  JRA: 10–20 mg/kg/24 hr ÷ Q12 hr PO
  Usual max. dose: 1000 mg/24 hr
Adolescent and adult:
  Analgesia:
    Over the counter dosage forms: 200 mg Q8–12 hr PRN PO; 400 mg initial dose may be needed.
    Max. dose: 600 mg/24 hr
    Prescription strength dosage forms: 250 mg Q8–12 hr PRN (500 mg initial dose may be needed) **or** 500 mg Q12 hr PRN PO. **Max. dose:** 1250 mg/24 hr for first day then 1000 mg/24 hr
  Rheumatoid arthritis, ankylosing spondylitis:
    Immediate-release forms: 250–500 mg BID PO
    Delayed-release tabs (EC-Naprosyn, Naprosyn DR): 375–500 mg BID PO
    Controlled-release tabs (Naprelan): 750–1000 mg once daily PO. For patients converting from immediate- and delayed-release forms, calculate daily dose and administer Naprelan as a single daily dose
    Max. dose (all dosage forms): 1500 mg/24 hr
  Dysmenorrhea:
    500 mg × 1, then 250 mg Q6–8 hr PRN PO or 500 mg Q12 hr PRN PO; **max. dose:** 1250 mg/24 hr for first day then 1000 mg/24 hr.

Contraindicated in treating perioperative pain for coronary artery bypass graft surgery. May cause GI bleeding, thrombocytopenia, heartburn, headache, drowsiness, vertigo, and tinnitus. **Use with caution** in patients with GI disease, cardiac disease (risk for thrombotic

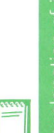

Continued

NAPROXEN/NAPROXEN SODIUM continued

events, MI, stroke), renal or hepatic impairment, and those receiving anticoagulants. Use is **NOT** recommended for moderate/severe renal impairment (CrCl < 30 mL/min). See *Ibuprofen* for other side effects.

Pregnancy category changes to "D" if used in the third trimester or near delivery. Administer doses with food or milk to reduce GI discomfort.

NEO-POLYMYCIN OPHTHALMIC OINTMENT

See Neomycin/polymyxin B ophthalmic products

NEO-POLYCIN HC

See Neomycin/polymyxin B ophthalmic products

NEOMYCIN SULFATE
Neo-fradin and generics
Antibiotic, aminoglycoside; ammonium detoxicant

No Yes 2 D

Tabs: 500 mg
Oral solution (Neo-Fradin): 125 mg/5 mL (480 mL); contains parabens
125 mg neomycin sulfate is equivalent to 87.5 mg neomycin base

Diarrhea:
  Preterm and newborn: 50 mg/kg/24 hr ÷ Q6 hr PO
Hepatic encephalopathy:
  Infant and child: 50–100 mg/kg/24 hr ÷ Q6–8 hr PO × 5–6 days. **Max. dose:** 12 g/24 hr
  Adult: 4–12 g/24 hr ÷ Q4–6 hr PO × 5–6 days
Bowel prep (in combination with erythromycin base):
  Child: 90 mg/kg/24 hr PO ÷ Q4 hr × 2–3 days
  Adult: 1 g Q1 hr PO × 4 doses, then 1 g Q4 hr PO × 5 doses; many other regimens exist

Contraindicated in ulcerative bowel disease, intestinal obstruction, or aminoglycoside hypersensitivity. Monitor for nephrotoxicity and ototoxicity. Oral absorption is limited but levels may accumulate. Consider dosage reduction in the presence of renal failure. May cause itching, redness, edema, colitis, candidiasis, or poor wound healing if applied topically. Prevalence of neomycin hypersensitivity has increased. May decrease absorption of penicillin V, vitamin B_{12}, digoxin, and methotrexate. May potentiate oral anticoagulants and the adverse effects of other neurotoxic, ototoxic, or nephrotoxic drugs.

NEOMYCIN/POLYMYXIN B OPHTHALMIC PRODUCTS
Neomycin/Polymyxin B + Bacitracin:
  Neo Polycin and generics
Neomycin/Polymyxin B + Gramicidin:
  Neosporin Ophthalmic Solution and generics
Neomycin/Polymyxin B + Hydrocortisone:
  Generics
Neomycin/Polymyxin B + Bacitracin + Hydrocortisone:
  Neo-Polycin HC and generics
Ophthalmic antibiotic ± corticosteroid

No No 2 C

Neomycin/Polymyxin B + Bacitracin:
  Ophthalmic ointment (Neo-Polycin Ophthalmic Ointment and generics): 3.5 g neomycin, 10,000 U polymyxin B, and 400 U bacitracin per g ointment (3.5 g)
Neomycin/Polymyxin B + Gramicidin:
  Ophthalmic solution (Neosporin Ophthalmic Solution and generics): 1.75 neomycin, 10,000 U polymyxin B, and 0.025 mg gramicidin per 1 mL (10 mL)
Neomycin/Polymyxin B + Hydrocortisone:
  Ophthalmic suspension: 3.5 mg neomycin, 10,000 U polymyxin B, and 10 mg hydrocortisone per 1 mL (7.5 mL)
Neomycin/Polymyxin B + Bacitracin + Hydrocortisone:
  Ophthalmic ointment (Neo-Polycin HC and generics): 3.5 mg neomycin, 10,000 U polymyxin B, 400 U bacitracin, and 10 mg hydrocortisone per 1 g (3.5 g)

Neomycin/Polymyxin B + Bacitracin:
  Child and adult: Apply 0.5-inch ribbon to affected eye(s) Q3–4 hr for acute infections or BID–TID for mild/moderate infections × 7–10 days
Neomycin/Polymyxin B + Gramicidin:
  Child and adult: Instill 1–2 drops to affected eye(s) Q4 hr or 2 drops every hour for severe infections × 7–10 days
Neomycin/Polymyxin B + Hydrocortisone:
  Child and adult: Instill 1–2 drops to affected eye(s) Q3–4 hr. More frequent dosing has been used for severe infection in adults
Neomycin/Polymyxin B + Bacitracin + Hydrocortisone:
  Child and adult: Apply to inside of lower lid of affected eye(s) Q3–4 hr

Contraindicated if hypersensitive to specific medications (e.g., neomycin, polymyxin b, gramicidin, bacitracin, or hydrocortisone) of respective product. **Use with caution** in glaucoma. Blurred vision, burning, and stinging may occur. Increased intraocular pressure and mycosis may occur with prolonged use. Avoid prolonged use with products containing corticosteroids.
Ophthalmic solution/suspension: Shake well before use and **avoid** contamination of tip of eye dropper. Apply finger pressure to lacrimal sac during and 1–2 min after dose application.
Ophthalmic ointment: Do not touch tube tip to eyelids or other surfaces to prevent contamination.

NEOMYCIN/POLYMYXIN B ± BACITRACIN
Neomycin/Polymyxin B:
  Neosporin GU irrigant and generics
Neomycin/Polymyxin B + Bacitracin:
  Neosporin, Neo To Go, Neo-Polycin, Triple Antibiotic, and generics
Topical antibiotic

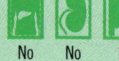
No   No   ?   C/D

NEOMYCIN/POLYMYXIN B:
  Solution, genitourinary irrigant: 40 mg neomycin sulfate, 200,000 U polymyxin B/ mL (1, 20 mL); multidose vial contains methylparabens
NEOMYCIN/POLYMYXIN B + BACITRACIN:
  Ointment, topical (Neosporin, Neo To Go, Triple Antibiotics and generics) (OTC): 3.5 mg neomycin sulfate, 400 U bacitracin, 5000 U polymyxin B/g (0.9, 15, 30, 454 g)
For ophthalmic products, see Neomycin/Polymyxin B Ophthalmic Products

NEOMYCIN/POLYMYXIN B + BACITRACIN:
Child and adult:
  Topical: Apply to minor wounds and burns once daily–TID
NEOMYCIN/POLYMYXIN B:
Bladder irrigation:
  Child and adult: Mix 1 mL in 1000 mL NS and administer via a three-way catheter at a rate adjusted to the patient's urine output. Do not exceed 10 days of continuous use.

Do not use for extended periods. May cause superinfection, delayed healing. See *Neomycin* for additional remarks. **Avoid** use of bladder irrigant in patients with defects in the bladder mucosa or wall. Prevalence of neomycin hypersensitivity has increased.
Pregnancy category is "C" for neomycin/polymyxin B/bacitracin and "D" for neomycin/polymyxin B.

NEOSPORIN OPHTHALMIC SOLUTION

See Neomycin/polymyxin B ophthalmic products

NEOSTIGMINE
Prostigmin, Bioxiverz, and generics
Anticholinesterase (cholinergic) agent

No   Yes   2   C

Injection: 0.5, 1 mg/mL (10 mL) (as methylsulfate); may contain parabens or phenol

Myasthenia gravis diagnosis: Use with atropine (see remarks)
  Child: 0.025–0.04 mg/kg IM × 1
  Adult: 0.02 mg/kg IM × 1
Treatment:
  Child: 0.01–0.04 mg/kg/dose IM/IV/SC Q2–4 hr PRN
  Adult: 0.5–2.5 mg/dose IM/IV/SC Q1–3 hr PRN up to **max. dose** of 10 mg/24 hr
Reversal of nondepolarizing neuromuscular blocking agents: Administer with atropine or glycopyrrolate
  Infant: 0.025–0.1 mg/kg/dose IV
  Child: 0.025–0.08 mg/kg/dose IV
  Adult: 0.5–2 mg/dose IV
  Max. dose (all ages): 5 mg/dose

NEOSTIGMINE continued

Contraindicated in GI and urinary obstruction. **Caution** in asthmatics. May cause cholinergic crisis, bronchospasm, salivation, nausea, vomiting, diarrhea, miosis, diaphoresis, lacrimation, bradycardia, hypotension, fatigue, confusion, respiratory depression, and seizures. Titrate for each patient, but **avoid** excessive cholinergic effects.

For reversal of neuromuscular blockade, infants and small children may be at greater risk of complications from incomplete reversal of neuromuscular blockade due to decreased respiratory reserve.

For diagnosis of myasthenia gravis (MG), administer atropine 0.011 mg/kg/dose IV immediately before or IM (0.011 mg/kg/dose) 30 min before neostigmine. For treatment of MG, patients may need higher doses of neostigmine at times of greatest fatigue.

Antidote: Atropine 0.01–0.04 mg/kg/dose. Atropine and epinephrine should be available in the event of a hypersensitivity reaction.

Adjust dose in renal failure (see Chapter 30).

NEVIRAPINE
Viramune, Viramune XR, NVP, and generics
Antiviral, nonnucleoside reverse transcriptase inhibitor

Yes Yes 3 B

Tabs: 200 mg
Extended-release tabs (Viramune XR and generics): 100, 400 mg
Oral suspension: 10 mg/mL (240 mL); contains parabens

HIV: See www.aidsinfo.nih.gov/guidelines
Prevention of vertical transmission during high-risk situations (women who received no antepartum antiretroviral prophylaxis, women with suboptimal viral suppression at delivery, or women with known antiretroviral drug-resistant virus) and in combination with other antiretroviral medications (see Chapter 17 for additional information):
Newborn: 3 doses (based on birth weight) in the first week of life; Dose 1: within 0–48 hr of birth; Dose 2: 48 hr after Dose 1; Dose 3: 96 hr after Dose 2
  Birth weight: 1.5–2 kg: 8 mg/dose PO
  Birth weight: >2 kg: 12 mg/dose PO

See www.aidsinfo.nih.gov/guidelines for additional remarks.

Use with caution in patients with hepatic or renal dysfunction. **Contraindicated** in moderate/severe hepatic impairment (Child-Pugh Class B or C) and postexposure (occupational or nonoccupational) prophylactic regimens. Most frequent side effects include skin rash (may be life-threatening, including Stevens–Johnson Syndrome and DRESS; permanently discontinue and never restart), fever, abnormal liver function tests, headache, and nausea. **Discontinue therapy** if any of the following occurs: severe rash and rash with fever, blistering, oral lesions, conjunctivitis, or muscle aches. Permanently discontinue and do not restart therapy if symptomatic hepatitis, severe transaminase elevations, or hypersensitivity reactions occur.

Life-threatening hepatotoxicity has been reported primarily during the first 12 wk of therapy. Patients with increased serum transaminase or a history of hepatitis B or C infection prior to nevirapine are at greater risk for hepatotoxicity. Women, including pregnant women, with CD_4 counts > 250 cells/mm^3 or men with CD_4 counts > 400 cells/mm^3 are at risk for hepatotoxicity. Monitor liver function tests (obtain transaminases immediately after development of hepatitis signs/symptoms, hypersensitivity reactions, or rash) and CBCs. Hypophosphatemia has been reported.

Continued

NEVIRAPINE continued

Nevirapine induces the drug metabolizing isoenzyme CYP450 3A4 to cause an autoinduction of its own metabolism within the first 2–4 wk of therapy and has the potential to interact with many drugs. **Carefully review the patient's drug profile for other drug interactions each time nevirapine is initiated or when a new drug is added to a regimen containing nevirapine.**
Doses can be administered with food and concurrently with didanosine.

NIACIN/VITAMIN B₃
Niacor, Niaspan, Slo-Niacin, Nicotinic acid, Vitamin B₃, and many generics
Vitamin, water soluble

Yes   Yes   2   A/C

Tabs (OTC): 50, 100, 250, 500 mg
Timed or extended-release tabs (all OTC except 1000 mg): 250, 500, 750, 1000 mg
Timed or extended-release caps (OTC): 250, 500 mg

US RDA: See Chapter 21.
Pellagra (PO):
  Child: 50–100 mg/dose TID
  Adult: 50–100 mg/dose TID–QID
  Max. dose: 500 mg/24 hr

Contraindicated in hepatic dysfunction, active peptic ulcer, and severe hypotension. **Use with caution** in unstable angina; acute MI (especially if receiving vasoactive drugs); renal dysfunction; and patients with history of jaundice, hepatobiliary disease, or peptic ulcer. Adverse reactions of flushing, pruritis, or GI distress may occur with PO administration. May cause hyperglycemia, hyperuricemia, blurred vision, abnormal liver function tests, dizziness, and headaches. Burning sensation of the skin, skin discoloration, hepatitis, and elevated creatine kinase have been reported. May cause false-positive urine catecholamines (fluorometric methods) and urine glucose (Benedict's reagent).
Pregnancy category changes to "C" if used in doses above the RDA or for typical doses used for lipid disorders. **See Chapter 21 for multivitamin preparations.**

NICARDIPINE
Cardene IV, Cardene SR, and generics
Calcium channel blocker, antihypertensive

Yes   Yes   2   C

Caps (immediate release): 20, 30 mg
Sustained-release caps (Cardene SR): 30, 45, 60 mg
Injection (Cardene IV): 0.1 mg/mL (200 mL), 0.2 mg/mL (200 mL), 2.5 mg/mL (10 mL); also available in generic)

Child (see remarks):
  Hypertension:
    Continuous IV infusion for severe hypertension: Start at 0.5–1 mcg/kg/min, dose may be increased as needed every 15–30 min up to a **max.** of 4–5 mcg/kg/min.
Adult (see remarks):
  Hypertension:
    Oral:
      Immediate release: 20 mg PO TID, dose may be increased after 3 days to 40 mg PO TID if needed.

NICARDIPINE continued
Adult:
> *Sustained release:* 30 mg PO BID, dose may be increased after 3 days to 60 mg PO BID if needed.
> *Continuous IV infusion:* Start at 5 mg/hr, increase dose as needed by 2.5 mg/hr Q5–15 min up to a **max. dose** of 15 mg/hr. Following attainment of desired BP, decrease infusion to 3 mg/hr and adjust rate as needed to maintain desired response.

Reported use in children has been limited to a small number preterm infants, infants, and children. **Contraindicated** in advanced aortic stenosis. **Avoid** systemic hypotension in patients following an acute cerebral infarct or hemorrhage. **Use with caution** in hepatic or renal dysfunction by carefully titrating dose. The drug undergoes significant first-pass metabolism through the liver and is excreted in the urine (60%). Use caution when converting to another dosage form; they are NOT equivalent on a mg per mg basis.

May cause headache, dizziness, asthenia, peripheral edema, and GI symptoms. Nicardipine is a substrate for CYP450 3A and inhibitor of CYP450 2 C9/19. Cimetidine increases the effects/toxicity of nicardipine. **See** *Nifedipine* **for additional drug and food interactions.**

Onset of action for PO administration is 20 min, with peak effects in 0.5–2 hr. IV onset of action is 1 min. Duration of action following a single IV or PO dose is 3 hr. To reduce the risk for venous thrombosis, phlebitis, and vascular impairment with IV administration, do not use small veins (e.g., dorsum of hand or wrist). Avoid intraarterial administration or extravasation. For additional information, **see Chapter 4.**

NIFEDIPINE
Adalat CC, Nifediac CC, Procardia, Procardia XL, and many generics
Calcium channel blocker, antihypertensive

Yes   No   2   C

Caps: (Procardia and generics): 10 mg (0.34 mL), 20 mg (0.45 mL)
Sustained-release tabs: (Adalat CC, Afeditab CR, Nifediac CC, Procardia XL, and others): 30, 60, 90 mg
Oral suspension: 1, 4 mg/mL

Child (see remarks for precautions):
> *Hypertensive urgency:* 0.1–0.25 mg/kg/dose Q4–6 hr PRN PO/SL. **Max. dose**: 10 mg/dose or 1–2 mg/kg/24 hr
> *Hypertension:*
> > *Sustained-release tabs:* Start with 0.25–0.5 mg/kg/24 hr (initial **max. dose**: 30–60 mg/24 hr) ÷ Q12–24 hr. May increase to **max. dose**: 3 mg/kg/24 hr up to 120 mg/24 hr
> *Hypertrophic cardiomyopathy (infant):* 0.6–0.9 mg/kg/24 hr ÷ Q6–8 hr PO/SL

Adult:
> *Hypertension or Angina:*
> > *Sustained-release tabs:* Start with 30 or 60 mg PO once daily. May increase to **max. dose** of 90 mg/24 hr for Adalat CC, Afeditab CR, and Nifediac CC, and 120 mg/24 hr for Procardia XL

Use of immediate-release dosage form in children is controversial and has been abandoned by some. **Use with caution** in children with acute CNS injury due to increased risk for stroke, seizure, hepatic impairment, and altered level of consciousness. To prevent rapid decrease in blood pressure in children, an initial dose of ≤0.25 mg/kg is recommended.

Use with caution in patients with CHF, aortic stenosis, GI obstruction/narrowing (bezoar formation), and cirrhosis (reduced drug clearance). May cause severe hypotension, peripheral edema, flushing,

Continued

NIFEDIPINE continued

tachycardia, headaches, dizziness, nausea, palpitations, and syncope. Acute generalized exanthematous pustulosis has been reported.

Although overall use in adults has been abandoned, the immediate-release dosage form is **contraindicated** in adults with severe obstructive coronary artery disease or recent MI, and hypertensive emergencies.

Nifedipine is a substrate for CYP450 3A3/4 and 3A5–7. **Do not administer** with grapefruit juice; may increase bioavailability and effects. Itraconazole and ketoconazole may increase nifedipine levels/effects. CYP3A inducers (e.g., rifampin, rifabutin, phenobarbital, phenytoin, carbamazepine) may reduce nifedipine's effects. Nifedipine may increase phenytoin, cyclosporine, and digoxin levels. For hypertensive emergencies, **see Chapter 4**.

For sublingual administration, capsule must be punctured and liquid expressed into mouth. A small amount is absorbed via the SL route. Most effects are due to swallowing and oral absorption. **Do not** crush or chew sustained-release tablet dosage form.

NITROFURANTOIN
Furadantin, Macrodantin, Macrobid, and generics
Antibiotic

Yes   Yes   2   B/X

Caps (macrocrystals; Macrodantin and generics): 25, 50, 100 mg
Caps (dual release; Macrobid and generics): 100 mg (25 mg macrocrystal/75 mg monohydrate)
Oral suspension (Furadantin and generics): 25 mg/5 mL (230 mL); contains parabens and saccharin

Child (>1 mo; oral suspension or macrocrystals):
 Treatment: 5–7 mg/kg/24 hr ÷ Q6 hr PO; **max. dose:** 400 mg/24 hr
 UTI prophylaxis: 1–2 mg/kg/dose QHS PO; **max. dose:** 100 mg/24 hr
≥12 yr and adult:
 Macrocrystals: 50–100 mg/dose Q6 hr PO
 Dual release (Macrobid): 100 mg/dose Q12 hr PO
 UTI prophylaxis (macrocrystals): 50–100 mg/dose PO QHS

Contraindicated in severe renal disease, infants aged <1 mo, GFR < 60 mL/min (reduced drug distribution in the urine), active/previous cholestatic jaundice/hepatic dysfunction, and pregnant women at term. **Use with caution** in G6PD deficiency, anemia, lung disease, and peripheral neuropathy. May cause nausea, hypersensitivity reactions (including vasculitis), vomiting, cholestatic jaundice, headache, hepatotoxicity, polyneuropathy, and hemolytic anemia.

Anticholinergic drugs and high-dose probenecid may increase nitrofurantoin toxicity. Magnesium salts may decrease nitrofurantoin absorption. Causes false-positive urine glucose with Clinitest. Administer doses with food or milk.

Pregnancy category changes to "X" at term (38–42 wk gestation). Breastfeeding in mothers receiving nitrofurantoin is not recommended for infants <1 mo and those with G6PD deficiency; use in infants ≥1 mo without G6PD deficiency is compatible.

NITROGLYCERIN
Nitro-Bid, Nitrostat, Nitro-Time, Nitro-Dur, Nitrolingual, Minitran, and generics
Vasodilator, antihypertensive

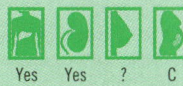
Yes   Yes   ?   C

Injection: 5 mg/mL (10 mL); may contain alcohol or propylene glycol
Prediluted injection in D$_5$W: 100 mcg/mL (250, 500 mL), 200 mcg/mL (250 mL), 400 mcg/mL (250, 500 mL)
Sublingual tabs (Nitrostat and generics): 0.3, 0.4, 0.6 mg
Sustained-release caps (Nitro-Time and generics): 2.5, 6.5, 9 mg
Ointment, topical (Nitro-Bid): 2% (1, 30, 60 g)
Patch (Nitro-Dur, Minitran, and generics): 2.5 mg/24 hr (0.1 mg/hr), 5 mg/24 hr (0.2 mg/hr), 7.5 mg/24 hr (0.3 mg/hr), 10 mg/24 hr (0.4 mg/hr), 15 mg/24 hr (0.6 mg/hr), 20 mg/24 hr (0.8 mg/hr) (30s, 100s)
Spray, translingual (Nitrolingual and generics): 0.4 mg per metered spray (4.9, 12 g; delivers 60 and 200 doses, respectively); contains 20% alcohol (flammable)

NOTE: The IV dosage units for children are in mcg/kg/min, compared to mcg/min for adults.

Infant/child:
 Continuous IV infusion: Begin with 0.25–0.5 mcg/kg/min; may increase by 0.5–1 mcg/kg/min Q3–5 min PRN. Usual dose: 1–5 mcg/kg/min. **Max. dose**: 20 mcg/kg/min.
Adult:
 Continuous IV infusion: 5 mcg/min IV, then increase Q3–5 min PRN by 5 mcg/min up to 20 mcg/min. If no response, increase by 10 mcg/min Q3–5 min PRN up to a **max.** of 400 mcg/min.
 Sublingual: 0.2–0.6 mg Q5 min. Max. of three doses in 15 min
 Oral: 2.5–9 mg BID–TID; up to 26 mg QID
 Ointment: Apply 1–2 inches Q8 hr, up to 4–5 inches Q4 hr
 Patch: 0.2–0.4 mg/hr initially, then titrate to 0.4–0.8 mg/hr; apply new patch daily (tolerance is minimized by removing patch for 10–12 hr/24 hr)

Contraindicated in glaucoma, severe anemia, concurrent phosphodiesterase-5 inhibitor (e.g., sildenafil), and concurrent guanylate cyclase stimulator (e.g., riociguat). In small doses (1–2 mcg/kg/min), acts mainly on systemic veins and decreases preload. At 3–5 mcg/kg/min, acts on systemic arterioles to decrease resistance. May cause headache, flushing, GI upset, blurred vision, and methemoglobinemia. **Use with caution** in severe renal impairment, increased ICP, and hepatic failure. IV nitroglycerin may antagonize anticoagulant effect of heparin.

Decrease dose gradually in patients receiving drug for prolonged periods to **avoid** withdrawal reaction. Must use polypropylene infusion sets to **avoid** adsorption of drug to plastic tubing. Use in heparinized patients may result in a decrease of PTT with subsequent rebound effect upon discontinuation of nitroglycerin.

Onset (duration) of action: IV, 1–2 min (3–5 min); sublingual, 1–3 min (30–60 min); PO sustained release, 40 min (4–8 hr); topical ointment, 20–60 min (2–12 hr); and transdermal patch, 40–60 min (18–24 hr).

NITROPRUSSIDE
Nitropress (previously available as Nipride)
Vasodilator, antihypertensive

Yes   Yes   3   C

Injection: 25 mg/mL (2 mL)

Child, adolescent, and adult: IV, continuous infusion
  Dose: Start at 0.3–0.5 mcg/kg/min, titrate to effect. Usual dose is 3–4 mcg/kg/min. **Max. dose:** 10 mcg/kg/min.

Contraindicated in patients with decreased cerebral perfusion and in situations of compensatory hypertension (increased ICP). Monitor for hypotension and acidosis. Dilute with D$_5$W and protect from light.

Nitroprusside is nonenzymatically converted to cyanide, which is converted to thiocyanate. Cyanide may produce metabolic acidosis and methemoglobinemia; thiocyanate may produce psychosis and seizures. Monitor thiocyanate levels if used for >48 hr or if dose ≥ 4 mcg/kg/min. **Thiocyanate levels should be <50 mg/L. Monitor cyanide levels (toxic levels > 2 mcg/mL)** in patients with hepatic dysfunction and thiocyanate levels in patients with renal dysfunction.
Onset of action is 2 min with a 1- to 10-min duration of effect.

NOREPINEPHRINE BITARTRATE
Levophed and generics
Adrenergic agonist

No   No   ?   C

Injection: 1 mg/mL as norepinephrine base (4 mL); contains sulfites

NOTE: *The dosage units for children are in mcg/kg/min; compared to mcg/min for adults.*
Child: Continuous IV infusion doses as norepinephrine base. Start at 0.05–0.1 mcg/kg/min. Titrate to effect. **Max. dose:** 2.5 mcg/kg/min.
Adult: Continuous IV infusion **doses as norepinephrine base.** Start at 8–12 mcg/min and titrate to effect. Usual maintenance dosage range: 2–4 mcg/min.

May cause cardiac arrhythmias, hypertension, hypersensitivity, headaches, vomiting, uterine contractions, and organ ischemia. May cause decreased renal blood flow and urine output. Avoid extravasation into tissues; may cause severe tissue necrosis. If this occurs, treat locally with phentolamine.

NORTRIPTYLINE HYDROCHLORIDE
Pamelor and generics
Antidepressant, tricyclic

Yes   No   2   D

Caps: 10, 25, 50, 75 mg; may contain benzyl alcohol, EDTA
Oral solution: 10 mg/5 mL (473 mL); contains up to 4% alcohol

Depression:
  Child 6–12 yr: 1–3 mg/kg/24 hr ÷ TID–QID PO or 10–20 mg/24 hr ÷ TID–QID PO
  Adolescent: 1–3 mg/kg/24 hr ÷ TID–QID PO or 30–50 mg/24 hr ÷ TID–QID PO
  Adult: 75–100 mg/24 hr ÷ TID–QID PO
  Max. dose (all ages): 150 mg/24 hr
Nocturnal enuresis:
  6–7 yr (20–25 kg): 10 mg PO QHS
  8–11 yr (26–35 kg): 10–20 mg PO QHS
  >11 yr (36–54 kg): 25–35 mg PO QHS

NORTRIPTYLINE HYDROCHLORIDE continued

See Imipramine for **contraindications** and common side effects. Also **contraindicated** with linezolid or IV methylene blue due to increased risk for serotonin syndrome. Fewer CNS and anticholinergic side effects than amitriptyline. May cause mild pupillary dilation, which may lead to narrow angle glaucoma.

Lower doses and slower dose titration is recommended in hepatic impairment. Therapeutic antidepressant effects occur in 7–21 days. Monitor for clinical worsening of depression and suicidal ideation/behavior following the initiation of therapy or after dose changes. **Do not** discontinue abruptly. Nortriptyline is a substrate for CYP450 1A2 and 2D6 drug metabolizing enzymes. Rifampin may increase the metabolism of nortriptyline.

Therapeutic nortriptyline levels for depression: 50–150 ng/mL. Recommended serum sampling time: obtain a single level 8 or more hr after an oral dose (following 4 days of continuous dosing for children and after 9–10 days for adults).

Administer with food to decrease GI upset.

NYSTATIN
Bio-Statin and generics; previously available as Mycostatin and Nilstat
Antifungal agent

No | No | 1 | C

Tabs: 500,000 U
Caps (Bio-Statin): 500,000, 1,000,000 U
Oral suspension: 100,000 U/mL (5, 60, 480 mL)
Topical cream and ointment: 100,000 U/g (15, 30 g)
Topical powder: 100,000 U/g (15, 30, 60 g)

Oropharyngeal candidiasis:
  Preterm infant: 0.5 mL (50,000 U) to each side of mouth QID
  Term infant: 1–4 mL (100,000–400,000 U) to each side of mouth QID
  Child/adult:
    Oral suspension: 4–6 mL (400,000–600,000 U) swish and swallow QID
  Topical: Apply to affected areas BID–QID.

May produce diarrhea and GI side effects. Local irritation, contact dermatitis, and Stevens–Johnson syndrome have been reported. Treat until 48–72 hr after resolution of symptoms. Drug is poorly absorbed through the GI tract. **Do not** swallow troches whole (allow to dissolve slowly). Oral suspension should be swished about the mouth and retained in the mouth as long as possible before swallowing.

OCTREOTIDE ACETATE
Sandostatin, Sandostatin LAR Depot, and generics
Somatostatin analog, antisecretory agent

No | Yes | ? | B

Injection (amps): 0.05, 0.1, 0.5 mg/mL (1 mL)
Injection (multidose vials): 0.2, 1 mg/mL (5 mL); contains phenol
Injection, microspheres for suspension (Sandostatin LAR Depot; see remarks): 10, 20, 30 mg (in kits with 2 mL diluent and 1.5-inch, 20-gauge needles)

Infant and child (limited data):
  Intractable diarrhea:
    IV/SC: 1–10 mcg/kg/24 hr ÷ Q12–24 hr. Dose may be increased within the recommended range by 0.3 mcg/kg/dose every 3 days as needed. **Max. dose:** 1500 mcg/24 hr.

Continued

OCTREOTIDE ACETATE continued

Infant and child (limited data) for Intractable diarrhea:
IV continuous infusion: 1 mcg/kg/dose bolus followed by 1 mcg/kg/hr has been used in diarrhea associated with graft versus host disease.

Cholelithiasis, hyperglycemia, hypoglycemia, hypothyroidism, nausea, diarrhea, abdominal discomfort, headache, dizziness, and pain at injection site may occur. Growth hormone suppression may occur with long-term use. Bradycardia, thrombocytopenia, and increased risk for pregnancy in patients with acromegaly and pancreatitis have been reported. Cyclosporine levels may be reduced in patients receiving this drug. May increase the effects/toxicity of bromocriptine.

Patients with severe renal failure requiring dialysis may require dosage adjustments due to an increase in half-life. Effects of hepatic dysfunction on octreotide have not been evaluated.

Sandostatin LAR Depot is administered once every 4 wk **only** by the IM route and is currently indicated for use in adults who have been stabilized on IV/SC therapy. See package insert for details.

OFLOXACIN
Floxin Otic, Ocuflox, and generics; previously available as Floxin
Antibiotic, quinolone

Yes Yes 2 C

Otic solution (Floxin Otic and generics): 0.3% (5 mL)
Ophthalmic solution (Ocuflox and generics): 0.3% (5, 10 mL); may contain benzalkonium chloride
Tabs: 200, 300, 400 mg

Otic use:

Otitis externa:
  6 mo–12 yr: 5 drops to affected ear(s) once daily × 7 days
  ≥13 yr–adult: 10 drops to affected ear(s) once daily × 7 days
Chronic suppurative otitis media:
  ≥12 yr–adult: 10 drops to affected ear(s) BID × 14 days
Acute otitis media with tympanostomy tubes:
  1–12 yr: 5 drops to affected ear(s) BID × 10 days
Ophthalmic use (>1 yr–adult):
Conjunctivitis: 1–2 drops to affected eye(s) Q2–4 hr while awake × 2 days, then QID × 5 additional days
Corneal ulcer: 1–2 drops to affected eye(s) Q30 min while awake and Q4–6 hr while asleep at night × 2 days, followed by Q1 hr while awake × 5 days, and then QID until treatment is completed

Pruritus, local irritation, taste perversion, dizziness, and earache have been reported with otic use. Ocular burning/discomfort is frequent with ophthalmic use. Consult with ophthalmologist in corneal ulcers.

When using otic solution, warm solution by holding the bottle in the hand for 1–2 min. Cold solutions may result in dizziness. For otitis externa, patient should lie with affected ear upward before instillation and remain in the same position after dose administration for 5 min to enhance drug delivery. For acute otitis media with tympanostomy tubes, patient should lie in the same position prior to instillation, and the tragus should be pumped four times after the dose to assist in drug delivery to the middle ear.

Systemic use of ofloxacin is typically replaced by its S-isomer, levofloxacin, which has a more favorable side effect profile than ofloxacin. See **Levofloxacin**.

OLANZAPINE
Zyprexa, Zyprexa Zydis, Zyprexa Relprevv, and generics
Antipsychotic, atypical second generation

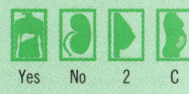
Yes   No   2   C

Tabs: 2.5, 5, 7.5, 10, 15, 20 mg
Orally disintegrating tabs (Zyprexa Zydis and generics): 5, 10, 15, 20 mg
IM injection:
  Short acting: 10 mg; contains tartaric acid
  Long acting (Zyprexa Relprevv):
    Every 2 wk dosing: 210, 300 mg; contains polysorbate 80
    Every 4 wk dosing: 405 mg; contains polysorbate 80

PO DOSING:
Bipolar I disorder (manic or mixed episodes):
  Child 4–<6 yr (limited data, based on an open label trial in 15 subjects): Start at 1.25 mg PO once daily × 7 days, then increase dose Q7 days PRN and tolerated to a target dose of 10 mg once daily.
  Child 6–12 yr (limited data): Start at 2.5 mg PO once daily × 7 days, then increase dose in 2.5 or 5 mg increments Q7 days to a target dose of 10 mg once daily. Suggested **max. dose**: 20 mg/24 hr.
  Adolescent (see remarks): Start at 2.5 or 5 mg PO once daily × 7 days, then increase dose in 2.5 or 5 mg increments Q7 days to a target dose of 10 mg once daily. Doses >20 mg/24 hr have not been evaluated.
  Adult: Start at 10 or 15 mg PO once daily (use 10 mg if used with lithium or valproate). If needed, increase or decrease dose by 5 mg daily at intervals not < 24 hr. Maintenance dosage range: 5–20 mg/24 hr. Doses >20 mg/24 hr have not been evaluated.

Schizophrenia:
  Adolescent (see remarks): Start with 2.5 or 5 mg PO once daily, increase dose in 2.5 or 5 mg increments Q7 days to the target dose of 10 mg once daily. Doses >20 mg/24 hr have not been evaluated.
  Adult: Start with 5 or 10 mg PO once daily (use 5 mg for individuals who are debilitated, predisposed to hypotension, or may exhibit slower metabolism) with a target dose of 10 mg once daily within 5–7 days. If needed, increase or decrease dose by 5 mg daily at weekly intervals. Usual dosage range: 10–15 mg once daily. Additional clinical assessment is recommended for doses >10 mg/24 hr. Doses >20 mg/24 hr have not been evaluated.

IM DOSING:
Short acting for acute agitation associated with bipolar I or schizophrenia:
  Child and adolescent (limited retrospective data in 15 children and 35 adolescents): ≤12 yr: 5 mg and adolescent (13–17 yr): 10 mg. Dosing frequencies and max. doses were not reported.
  Adult: 10 mg (5 or 7.5 mg may be for individuals who are debilitated, predisposed to hypotension, or may exhibit slower metabolism). If needed, additional doses × 2 may be given in 2–4 hr intervals. Recommended **max. dose** is 30 mg/24 hr (10 mg × 3 separated 2–4-hr apart); safety of doses >30 mg/24 hr have not been evaluated.

Long-acting (Zyprexa Relprevv) for schizophrenia (adult): see remarks and package insert for specific dosage based on established oral dosage.

Use with caution in cardiovascular or cerebrovascular disease, hypotensive conditions, diabetes/hyperglycemia, elevated serum lipids and cholesterol, paralytic ileus, hepatic impairment, seizure disorders, narrow angle glaucoma, and prostatic hypertrophy. Medication exhibits anticholinergic effects.

Continued

OLANZAPINE continued

Common side effects include orthostatic hypotension, peripheral edema, hypercholesterolemia, hyperprolactinemia, appetite simulation, weight gain (greater in adolescents than in adults; monitoring is recommended), hypertriglyceridemia, constipation, xerostomia, akathisia, asthenia, dizziness, somnolence, tremor, and personality disorder. Neuroleptic malignant syndrome, dystonia, cognitive and motor impairment, tardive dyskinesia (irreversible with cumulative high doses), neutropenia, leukopenia, agranulocytosis, suicidal intent, acute pancreatitis, pulmonary embolism, increases in LFTs (ALT, AST, GGT), and hyperthermia have been reported.

Olanzapine is a major substrate for CYP450 1A2 and minor substrate for 2D6. It also is a weak inhibitor to CYP450 1A2, 2C9/19. Do not use in combination with benzodiazepines or opiates due to increased risk for sedation and cardiopulmonary depression and with anticholinergic agents (e.g., azelastine, glycopyrrolate) as olanzapine may enhance anticholinergic effects. Use with QTc prolonging medications may further increase the risk for QTc prolongation. Metoclopramide may enhance neurological side effects of olanzapine. $T_{1/2}$: 37 hr for children and 21–54 hr for adults via PO route. Short-acting IM $T_{1/2}$ in adults is similar to PO route but long-acting IM $T_{1/2}$ is ~30 days in adults.

Maintenance treatment for bipolar I disorder and schizophrenia has not been systematically evaluated in adolescents. Therefore, it is recommended to utilize the lowest dose to maintain efficacy and periodically reassess the need for maintenance treatment for this age group.

All oral dosages may be taken with or without food. For orally disintegrating tabs, place tablet in mouth immediately after removing from foil pack (peel off foil and do not push tablet through foil) and allow the tablet to dissolve in saliva and swallow with or without liquids.

Zyrexa Relprevv (long acting IM injection): postinjection delirium and sedation syndrome have been reported with this dosage form. Patients must be observed at a health care provider at a health care facility for at least 3 hr after administration. The FDA REMS program requires prescribers, healthcare facilities, and pharmacies to register with the Zyprexa Relprevv Patient Care Program at 1-877-772-9390 for use of this product.

OLOPATADINE
Patanol, Pataday, Pazeo, Patanase, and generics
Antihistamine

No   No   ?   C

Ophthalmic solution (products may contain benzalkonium chloride):
  Patanol and generics: 0.1% (5 mL)
  Pataday: 0.2% (2.5 mL)
  Pazeo: 0.7% (2.5 mL)
Nasal spray (Patanase and generics): 0.6% (30.5 g provides 240 metered spray doses); contains benzalkonium chloride

Ophthalmic use for allergic conjunctivitis:
  0.1% solution (Patanol and generics):
    ≥3 yr and adult: 1 drop in affected eye(s) BID (spaced 6–8 hr apart)
  0.2% solution (Pataday) or 0.7% (Pazeo):
    ≥2 yr and adult: 1 drop in affected eye(s) once daily
Intranasal use of allergic rhinitis:
  6–11 yr: Inhale 1 spray into each nostril BID
  ≥12 yr and adult: Inhale 2 sprays into each nostril BID

Ocular use: DO NOT use while wearing contact lenses; wait at least 10 min after instilling drops before inserting lenses. Ocular side effects include burning or stinging, dry eye,

OLOPATADINE continued

foreign body sensation, hyperemia, keratitis, lid edema, and pruritus. May also cause headaches, asthenia, pharyngitis, rhinitis, and taste perversion.

Nasal use: Common side effects include bitter taste and headaches. Nasal ulceration, epistaxis, nasal septal perforation, throat pain, and postnasal drip have been reported.

OMEPRAZOLE
Prilosec, Prilosec OTC, First-Omeprazole, Omeprazole and Syrspend SF Alka, and generics
In combination with sodium bicarbonate: Zegerid and generics
Gastric acid pump inhibitor

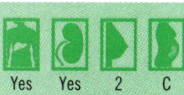
Yes Yes 2 C

Caps, sustained release: 10, 20, 40 mg; may contain magnesium
Tabs, delayed release (Prilosec OTC and generics; OTC): 20 mg; may contain magnesium
Oral suspension:
  First-Omeprazole: 2 mg/mL (90, 150, 300 mL); contains benzyl alcohol
  Omeprazole and Syrspend SF Alka: 2 mg/mL (100 mL); sugar free and preservative free
  Compounded formulation: 2 mg/mL; contains ~ 0.5 mEq sodium bicarbonate per 1 mg drug
Granules for oral suspension (Prilosec): 2.5, 10 mg packets (30s); contains magnesium
In combination with sodium bicarbonate:
  Powder for oral suspension (Zegerid and generics): 20-, 40-mg packets (30s); each packet (regardless of strength) contains 1680 mg (20 mEq) sodium bicarbonate
  Caps, immediate release (Zegerid and generics): 20, 40 mg; each capsule (regardless of strength) contains 1100 mg (13.1 mEq) sodium bicarbonate
  Chewable tabs (Zegerid): 20, 40 mg; each tab (regardless of strength) contains 600 mg (7.1 mEq) sodium bicarbonate and 700 mg magnesium hydroxide

Infant and child:
  Esophagitis, GERD, or ulcers: Start at 1 mg/kg/24 hr PO ÷ once daily–BID (**max. dose:** 20 mg/24 hr). Reported effective range: 0.2–3.5 mg/kg/24 hr. Children 1–6 yr may require higher doses due to enhanced drug clearance. Alternative dosing by weight category:
  3–<5 kg: 2.5 mg PO once daily
  5–<10 kg: 5 mg PO once daily
  10–<20 kg: 10 mg PO once daily
  ≥20 kg: 20 mg PO once daily

Adult:
  Duodenal ulcer or GERD: 20 mg/dose PO once daily × 4–8 wk; may give up to 12 wk for erosive esophagitis.
  Gastric ulcer: 40 mg/24 hr PO ÷ once daily–BID × 4–8 wk.
  Pathological hypersecretory conditions: Start with 60 mg/24 hr PO once daily. If needed, dose may be increased up to 120 mg/24 hr PO ÷ TID. Daily doses >80 mg should be administered in divided doses.

Common side effects: headache, diarrhea, nausea, and vomiting. Allergic reactions including anaphylaxis, acute interstitial nephritis, and vitamin B_{12} deficiency (with prolonged use) have been reported. Has been associated with increased risk for *Clostridium Difficile*–associated diarrhea.

Drug induces CYP450 1A2 (decreases theophylline levels) and is also a substrate and inhibitor of CYP2C19. Increases $T_{1/2}$ of citalopram, diazepam, phenytoin, and warfarin. May decrease the effects of itraconazole, ketoconazole, clopidogrel, iron salts, and ampicillin esters. St. Johns's Wort and

Continued

OMEPRAZOLE continued

rifampin may decrease omeprazole effects. May be used in combination with clarithromycin and amoxicillin for *Helicobacter pylori* infections. Omeprazole may interfere with diagnostic tests for neuroendocrine tumors; discontinue use at least 14 days prior to testing.

Bioavailability may be increased with hepatic dysfunction or in patients of Asian descent. Safety and efficacy for GERD in children <1 mo have not been established.

Administer all doses before meals. Administer 30 min prior to sucralfate. Capsules contain enteric-coated granules to ensure bioavailability. Do **not** chew or crush capsule. For doses unable to be divided by 10 mg, capsule may be opened and intact pellets may be administered in an acidic beverage (e.g., apple juice, cranberry juice) or apple sauce. The extemporaneously compounded oral suspension product may be less bioavailable due to the loss of the enteric coating.

OMNIPAQUE

See Iohexol

ONDANSETRON
Zofran, Zofran ODT, Zuplenz, and generics
Antiemetic agent, 5-HT₃ antagonist

Yes No ? B

Injection: 2 mg/mL (2, 20 mL); may contain parabens and some preparations are preservative free
Tabs: 4, 8. 24 mg
Tabs, orally disintegrating (ODT): 4, 8 mg; contains aspartame
Oral solution: 4 mg/5 mL (50 mL); contains sodium benzoate
Oral film: 4, 8 mg (1, 10s)

Preventing nausea and vomiting associated with chemotherapy:
　Oral (give initial dose 30 min before chemotherapy):
　　Child (≥2 yr and adolescent), dose based on body surface area:
　　　<0.3 m²: 1 mg TID PRN nausea
　　　0.3–0.6 m²: 2 mg TID PRN nausea
　　　0.6–1 m²: 3 mg TID PRN nausea
　　　>1 m²: 4–8 mg TID PRN nausea
　　Dose based on age:
　　　<4 yr: Use dose based on body surface area from preceding dosages
　　　4–11 yr: 4 mg TID PRN nausea
　　　>11 yr and adult: 8 mg TID or 24 mg once daily PRN nausea
　IV (child and adult):
　　Moderately emetogenic drugs: 0.15 mg/kg/dose (**max. dose:** 8 mg/dose for child and 16 mg/dose adult) at 30 min before, 4 and 8 hr after emetogenic drugs. Then same dose Q4 hr PRN.
　　Highly emetogenic drugs: 0.15 mg/kg/dose (**max. dose:** 16 mg/dose) 30 min before, 4 and 8 hr after emetogenic drugs. Then 0.15 mg/kg/dose (**max. dose:** 16 mg/dose) Q4 hr PRN.
Preventing nausea and vomiting associated with surgery (additional doses for controlling nausea and vomiting may not provide any benefits):
　IV/IM (administered prior to anesthesia over 2–5 min):
　　Child (2–12 yr):
　　　<40 kg: 0.1 mg/kg/dose × 1
　　　≥40 kg: 4 mg × 1
　　Adult: 4 mg × 1

ONDANSETRON continued

PO:
  Adult: 16 mg × 1, 1 hr prior to induction of anesthesia
Preventing nausea and vomiting associated with radiation therapy:
  Child: use above dosage for preventing nausea and vomiting associated with chemotherapy and give initial dose 1–2 hr prior to radiation
  Adult:
    Total body irradiation: 8 mg PO 1–2 hr prior to radiation once daily
    Single high-dose fraction radiation to abdomen: 8 mg PO 1–2 hr prior to radiation with subsequent doses Q8 hr after first dose × 1–2 days after completion of radiation
    Daily fractionated radiation to abdomen: 8 mg PO 1–2 hr prior to radiation with subsequent doses Q8 hr after first dose for each day radiation is given
Vomiting in acute gastroenteritis (PO route is preferred, use IV when PO is not possible):
  PO (6 mo–10 yr and ≥8 kg; use oral disintegrating tablet):
    8–15 kg: 2 mg × 1
    >15 and ≤30 kg: 4 mg × 1
    >30 kg: 8 mg × 1
  IV (≥1 mo): 0.15–0.3 mg/kg/dose × 1; **max. dose:** 4 mg/dose

Avoid use in congenital long QTc syndrome. Bronchospasm; tachycardia; hypokalemia; seizures; headaches; lightheadedness; constipation; diarrhea; and transient increases in AST, ALT, and bilirubin may occur. Transient blindness (resolution within a few min up to 48 hr), arthralgia, Stevens–Johnson syndrome, TEN, hepatic dysfunction, and rare/transient ECG changes (including QTc interval prolongation) have been reported. Data limited for use in children <3 yr.

ECG monitoring is recommended in patients with electrolyte abnormalities, CHF, or bradyarrhythmias. Drug clearance is higher for surgical and cancer patients <18 yr when compared to adults. Clearance is slower in children aged 1–4 mo than in those aged >4–24 mo.

Ondansetron is a substrate for CYP450 1A2, 2D6, 2E1, and 3A3/4 drug-metabolizing enzymes. It is likely that the inhibition/loss of one of the previously listed enzymes will be compensated by others and may result in insignificant changes to ondansetron's elimination. Ondansetron's elimination may be affected by CYP450 enzyme inducers. Follow theophylline, phenytoin, or warfarin levels closely if used in combination. Use with apomorphine may result in profound hypotension and loss of consciousness and is **contraindicated**.

To administer the oral film dosage form, place film on top of tongue, allow it to dissolve completely in 4–20 s, and swallow with or without liquid.

OSELTAMIVIR PHOSPHATE
Tamiflu and generics
Antiviral

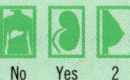

No   Yes   2   C

Caps: 30, 45, 75 mg
Oral suspension: 6 mg/mL (60 mL,); may contain saccharin and sodium benzoate

Treatment of influenza (initiate therapy within 2 days of onset of symptoms):
  Preterm neonate (24–37-wk gestation; based on pharmacokinetic data from 20 neonates):
  1 mg/kg/dose PO BID
  Full-term neonate:
    <14 days old: 3 mg/kg/dose PO once daily × 5 days
    ≥14–28 days old: 3 mg/kg/dose PO BID × 5 days

Continued

OSELTAMIVIR PHOSPHATE continued

Child <1 yr: see following table

Age (Months)	Dosage for 5 Days	Volume of Oral Suspension (6 mg/mL)
<3	12 mg PO BID	2 mL
3–5	20 mg PO BID	3.33 mL
6–11	25 mg PO BID	4.2 mL

Child ≥1–12 yr: see following table

Weight (kg)	Dosage for 5 Days	Volume of Oral Suspension (6 mg/mL)
≤5	30 mg PO BID	5 mL
>15–23	45 mg PO BID	7.5 mL
>23–40	60 mg PO BID	10 mL
>40	75 mg PO BID	12.5 mL

≥13 yr and adult: 75 mg PO BID × 5 days

Prophylaxis of influenza (initiate therapy within 2 days of exposure; see remarks):
Child 3 mo–<1 yr: 3 mg/kg/dose PO once daily; alternative dosage based on age:
  3–5 mo: 20 mg PO once daily
  6–11 mo: 25 mg PO once daily
Child 1–12 yr:
  ≤15 kg: 30 mg PO once daily
  16–23 kg: 45 mg PO once daily
  24–40 kg: 60 mg PO once daily
  >40 kg: 75 mg PO once daily
≥13 yr and adult: 75 mg PO once daily for a minimum of 7 days and up to 6 wk; initiate therapy within 2 days of exposure

Currently indicated for the treatment of influenza A and B strains. Use in children <1 yr has not been recommended due to concerns of excessive CNS penetration and fatalities in 7-day-old rats.

Nausea and vomiting generally occur within the first 2 days and are the most common adverse effects. Insomnia, vertigo, seizures, hypothermia, neuropsychiatric events (may result in fatal outcomes), arrhythmias, rash, and toxic epidermal necrolysis have also been reported. Reduce dosage treatment dose if GFR is 10–30 mL/min to 75 mg PO once daily × 5 days for adults. (See Chapter 30).

PROPHYLACTIC USE: Oseltamivir is not a substitute for annual flu vaccination. Safety and efficacy have been demonstrated for ≤6 wk of therapy; duration of protection lasts for as long as dosing is continued. Adjust prophylaxis dose if GFR is 10–30 mL/min by extending the dosage interval to once every other day.

Probenecid increases oseltamivir levels. Oseltamivir decreases the efficacy of the nasal influenza vaccine (live attenuated influenza vaccine, FluMist); avoid administration of vaccine within 2 wk before or 48 hrs after oseltamivir administration, unless medically indicated.

Dosage adjustments in hepatic impairment, severe renal disease and dialysis have not been established for either treatment or prophylactic use. The safety and efficacy of repeated treatment or prophylaxis courses have not been evaluated. Doses may be administered with or without food.

OXACILLIN
Various generics
Antibiotic, penicillin (penicillinase resistant)

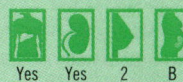
Yes   Yes   2   B

Injection: 1, 2, 10 g
Injection, premixed in iso-osmotic dextrose: 1 g/50 mL, 2 g/50 mL
Injectable products contain 2.8–3.1 mEq Na per 1 g drug

Neonate (IM/IV):
  ≤7 days old:
    <2 kg: 50 mg/kg/24 hr ÷ Q12 hr
    ≥2 kg: 75 mg/kg/24 hr ÷ Q8 hr
  8–28 days old:
    <1 kg:
      8–14 days old: 50 mg/kg/24 hr ÷ Q12 hr
      15–28 days old: 75 mg/kg/24 hr ÷ Q8 hr
    1–2 kg: 75 mg/kg/24 hr ÷ Q8 hr
    ≥2 kg: 100 mg/kg/24 hr ÷ Q6 hr
  Meningitis (IV):
    ≤7 days old: 75 mg/kg/24 hr ÷ Q8–12 hr
    8–28 days old: 150–200 mg/kg/24 hr ÷ Q6–8 hr
Infant and child (IM/IV): 100–200 mg/kg/24 hr ÷ Q4–6 hr (**max. dose:** 12 g/24 hr); use 200 mg/kg/24 hr for endocarditis and severe infections
Adult (IM/IV): 250–2000 mg/dose Q4–6 hr; use higher dosage range for endocarditis or severe infections
  Max. dose (all ages): 12 g/24 hr

Rash and GI disturbances are common. Leukopenia, reversible hepatotoxicity, and acute interstitial nephritis has been reported. Hematuria and azotemia have occurred in neonates and infants with high doses. May cause false-positive urinary and serum proteins.

Probenecid increases serum oxacillin levels. Tetracyclines may antagonize bactericidal effects of oxacillin.

CSF penetration is poor unless meninges are inflamed. Use the lower end of the usual dosage range for patients with creatinine clearances <10 mL/min. **Adjust dose in renal failure (see Chapter 30).**

OXCARBAZEPINE
Trileptal, Oxtellar XR, and generics
Anticonvulsant

Yes   Yes   2   C

Tabs: 150, 300, 600 mg
Extended-release tabs (Oxtellar XR): 150, 300, 600 mg
Oral suspension: 300 mg/5 mL (250 mL); contains saccharin, ethanol, and propylene glycol

IMMEDIATE-RELEASE PRODUCT:
  Child (2–<4 yr):
    Adjunctive therapy: Start with 8–10 mg/kg/24 hr PO ÷ BID up to a **max. dose** of 600 mg/24 hr. For children <20 kg, may consider using a starting dose of 16–20 mg/kg/24 hr PO ÷ BID; gradually increase the dose over a 2–4-wk period and do not exceed 60 mg/kg/24 hr ÷ BID

Continued

OXCARBAZEPINE continued
IMMEDIATE-RELEASE PRODUCT:
Child (4–16 yr, see remarks):
  Adjunctive therapy: Start with 8–10 mg/kg/24 hr PO ÷ BID up to a **max. dose** of 600 mg/24 hr. Then gradually increase the dose over a 2-wk period to the following maintenance doses:
    20–29 kg: 900 mg/24 hr PO ÷ BID
    29.1–39 kg: 1200 mg/24 hr PO ÷ BID
    >39 kg: 1800 mg/24 hr PO ÷ BID
  Conversion to monotherapy: Start with 8–10 mg/kg/24 hr PO ÷ BID and simultaneously initiate dosage reduction of concomitant AEDs and withdrawal completely over 3–6 wk. Dose may be increased at weekly intervals, as clinically indicated, by a **maximum** of 10 mg/kg/24 hr to achieve the recommended monotherapy maintenance dose as described in the following table.
  Initiation of monotherapy: Start with 8–10 mg/kg/24 hr PO ÷ BID. Then increase by 5 mg/kg/24 hr every 3 days up to the recommended monotherapy maintenance dose as described in the following table:

RECOMMENDED MONOTHERAPY MAINTENANCE DOSES FOR CHILDREN BY WEIGHT

Weight (kg)	Daily Oral Maintenance Dose (mg/24 hr) Divided BID
20–<25	600–900
25–<35	900–1200
35–<45	900–1500
45–<50	1200–1500
50–<60	1200–1800
60–<70	1200–2100
≥70	1500–2100

Adult:
  Adjunctive therapy: Start with 600 mg/24 hr PO ÷ BID. Dose may be increased at weekly intervals, as clinically indicated, by a **maximum** of 600 mg/24 hr. Usual maintenance dose is 1200 mg/24 hr PO ÷ BID. Doses ≥2400 mg/24 hr are generally not well tolerated due to CNS side effects.
  Conversion to monotherapy: Start with 600 mg/24 hr PO ÷ BID and simultaneously initiate dosage reduction of concomitant AEDs. Dose may be increased at weekly intervals, as clinically indicated, by a **maximum** of 600 mg/24 hr to achieve a dose of 2400 mg/24 hr PO ÷ BID. Concomitant AEDs should be terminated gradually over approximately 3–6 wk.
  Initiation of monotherapy: Start with 600 mg/24 hr PO ÷ BID. Then increase by 300 mg/24 hr every 3 days up to 1200 mg/24 hr PO ÷ BID.

EXTENDED-RELEASE TABS (Oxtellar XR; see remarks):
Child 6–17 yr:
  Adjunctive therapy: Start with 8–10 mg/kg/24 hr PO once daily up to a **max. dose** of 600 mg/24 hr. Then gradually increase at weekly intervals in 8–10-mg/kg/24 hr increments (**max. dosage increment:** 600 mg) to the following maintenance doses:
    20–29 kg: 900 mg PO once daily
    29.1–39 kg: 1200 mg PO once daily
    ≥39.1 kg: 1800 mg PO once daily
Adult:
  Adjunctive therapy: Start with 600 mg PO once daily (consider using 900 mg if receiving concomitant enzyme-inducing antiepileptic drugs). Then gradually increase at weekly intervals in 600-mg/24 hr increments to a maintenance dose of 1200–2400 mg once daily.

Clinically significant hyponatremia may occur; generally seen within the first 3 mo of therapy. May also cause headache, dizziness, drowsiness, ataxia, fatigue, nystagmus,

OXCARBAZEPINE continued

urticaria, diplopia, abnormal gait, and GI discomfort. About 25%–30% of patients with carbamazepine hypersensitivity will experience a cross reaction with oxcarbazepine. Serious dermatological reactions (Stevens–Johnson and TEN), multiorgan hypersensitivity reactions, bone marrow depression, osteoporosis, pancreatitis, folic acid deficiency, hypothyroidism, rare cases of anaphylaxis and angioedema, and suicidal behavior or ideation have been reported.

Inhibits CYP450 2C19 and induces CYP450 3A4/5 drug-metabolizing enzymes. Carbamazepine, cyclosporine, phenobarbital, phenytoin, valproic acid, and verapamil may decrease oxcarbazepine levels. Oxcarbazepine may increase phenobarbital and phenytoin levels. Oxcarbazepine can decrease the effects of oral contraceptives, cyclosporine, felodipine, and lamotrigine.

If GFR < 30 mL/min, adjust dosage by administering 50% of the normal starting dose (**max. dose**: 300 mg/24 hr) followed by a slower than normal increase in dose if necessary **(see Chapter 30).** No dosage adjustment is required in mild/moderate hepatic impairment. Use is **not recommended** in severe hepatic impairment due to lack of information.

Extended- and immediate-release products are not bioequivalent as higher doses of the extended-release product may be necessary. Doses may be administered with or without food.

OXYBUTYNIN CHLORIDE
Ditropan XL, Oxytrol, and generics; previously available as Ditropan
Anticholinergic agent, antispasmodic

Yes   Yes   ?   B

Tabs: 5 mg
Tabs, extended release (Ditropan XL and generics): 5, 10, 15 mg
Syrup: 1 mg/mL (473 mL); contains parabens
Transdermal system (Oxytrol): delivers 3.9 mg/24 hr (1, 2s, 4s, 8s); contains 36 mg per system

Child ≤ 5 yr:
  Immediate release: 0.2 mg/kg/dose BID–TID PO; **max. dose**: 15 mg/24 hr
Child > 5 yr:
  Immediate release: 5 mg/dose BID–TID PO; **max. dose**: 15 mg/24 hr
  Extended release (≥6 yr): Start with 5 mg/dose once daily PO; if needed, increase as tolerated by 5 mg increments up to a **maximum** of 20 mg/24 hr
Adult:
  Immediate release: 5 mg/dose BID–TID PO; **max. dose**: 5 mg QID
  Extended release (Ditropan XL): 5–10 mg/dose once daily PO, adjust in 5 mg weekly increments, if needed, up to a **max. dose** of 30 mg/dose once daily PO
  Transdermal system: 1 patch (3.9 mg/24 hr) every 3–4 days (twice weekly)

Use with caution in hepatic or renal disease, hyperthyroidism, IBD, or cardiovascular disease. Anticholinergic side effects may occur, including drowsiness, confusion, and hallucinations. **Contraindicated** in glaucoma, GI obstruction, megacolon, myasthenia gravis, severe colitis, hypovolemia, and GU obstruction. Memory impairment, angioedema, and QT-interval prolongation have been reported. Oxybutynin is a CYP450 3A4 substrate; inhibitors and inducers of CYP450 3A4 may increase and decrease the effects of oxybutynin, respectively. May antagonize the effects of metoclopramide.

Dosage adjustments for the extended-release dosage form are at weekly intervals. **Do not** crush, chew, or divide the extended-release tablets. Apply transdermal system on dry intact skin on the abdomen, hip, or buttock by rotating the site and avoiding same-site application within 7 days.

OXYCODONE
OxyContin, Roxicodone, Xtampza ER, and many others including generics
Narcotic, analgesic

Yes   Yes   2   B/D

Expressed as hydrochloride salt unless indicated otherwise
Oral solution: 1 mg/mL (5, 15, 473 mL); contains alcohol
Concentrated oral solution: 20 mg/mL (15, 30 mL); may contain saccharin
Tabs: 5, 10, 15, 20, 30 mg
Controlled-release tabs (OxyContin and generics): 10, 15, 20, 30, 40, 60, 80 mg (80 mg strength for opioid-tolerant patients only)
Caps: 5 mg
Extended-release caps (Xtampza ER): 9, 13.5, 18, 27, 36 mg oxycodone base; equivalent to 10, 15, 20, 30, and 40 mg oxycodone hydrochloride salt, respectively

Opioid-naïve doses based on oxycodone hydrochloride salt:
  Child: 0.05–0.15 mg/kg/dose Q4–6 hr PRN up to 5 mg/dose PO
  Adolescent (≥50 kg) and adult: 5–10 mg Q4–6 hr PRN PO; see remarks for use of controlled-release tablets

Abuse potential, CNS and respiratory depression, increased ICP, histamine release, constipation, and GI distress may occur. **Use with caution** in severe renal impairment (increases $T_{1/2}$) and mild/moderate hepatic dysfunction (using 1/3 to 1/2 of usual dose has been recommended). **Naloxone is the antidote.** See Chapter 6 for equianalgesic dosing. Check dosages of acetaminophen or aspirin when using combination products (e.g., Percocet, Percodan). Oxycodone is metabolized by the CYP450 3A4 (major) and 2D6 (minor) isoenzyme.

When using controlled-release tablets (e.g., Oxycontin), determine patient's total 24-hr requirements and divide by 2 to administer on a Q12-hr dosing interval. Oxycontin 80-mg tablet is **USED ONLY** for opioid tolerant patients; this strength can cause fatal respiratory depression in opioid-naïve patients. Controlled-release dosage form **should not be used** as a PRN analgesic and must be swallowed whole.

Pregnancy category changes to "D" if used for prolonged periods or in high doses at term.

OXYCODONE AND ACETAMINOPHEN
Endocet, Roxilox, Percocet, Roxicet, and many others including generics
Combination analgesic with a narcotic

Yes   Yes   2   C

Tabs (Percocet, Endocet, and others including generics):
  Most common strength: oxycodone HCl 5 mg + acetaminophen 325 mg
  Other strengths:
    Oxycodone HCl 2.5 mg + acetaminophen 325 mg
    Oxycodone HCl 7.5 mg + acetaminophen 325 mg
    Oxycodone HCl 10 mg + acetaminophen 325 mg
Oral solution (Roxicet and generics): Oxycondone HCl 5 mg + acetaminophen 325 mg/5 mL (500 mL); may contain 0.4% alcohol and saccharin

Dose based on amount of oxycodone and acetaminophen. Do not exceed 4 g/24 hr of acetaminophen.

See *Oxycodone* and *Acetaminophen*. Check dosages of acetaminophen when using these combination products.

OXYCODONE AND ASPIRIN
Various generics; previously available as Percodan and Endodan
Combination analgesic (narcotic and salicylate)

Yes   Yes   2   D

Tabs: Oxycodone 4.8355 mg and aspirin 325 mg

Dose based on amount of oxycodone and aspirin. Do not exceed 4 g/24 hr of aspirin.

See *Oxycodone* and *Aspirin*. **Do not use** in children <16 yr because of risk for Reye's Syndrome. Check dosages of aspirin when using these combination products.

OXYMETAZOLINE
Afrin 12 Hour, Neo-Synephrine 12-Hour Nasal, Nostrilla, and many others including generics
Nasal decongestant, vasoconstrictor

No   No   2   C

Nasal spray [OTC]: 0.05% (15, 30 mL); may contain benzalkonium chloride and propylene glycol

Nasal decongestant (not to exceed 3 days in duration):
≥6 yr–adult: 2–3 sprays or 2–3 drops in each nostril BID. **Do not exceed** 2 doses/24-hr period.

Contraindicated in patients on MAO inhibitor therapy. Rebound nasal congestion may occur with excessive use (>3 days) via the nasal route. Systemic absorption may occur. Headache, insomnia, hypertension, transient burning, stinging, dryness, nasal mucosa ulceration, and sneezing have occurred.

Accidental ingestion in children <5 yr has been reported and required hospitalization for adverse events (nausea, vomiting, lethargy, tachycardia, respiratory depression, bradycardia, hypotension, hypertension, sedation, mydriasis, stupor, hypothermia, drooling and coma).

PALIVIZUMAB
Synagis
Monoclonal antibody

No   No   ?   C

Injection, solution: 100 mg/mL (0.5, 1 mL; single use); contains glycine and histidine

RSV prophylaxis during RSV season for the following age and clinical criteria (see latest edition of Red Book for most recent indications).
Following recommendations are from *Pediatrics.* 2014;134(2):415-420.
    Candidates for recommended use:
        <12 mo of age (one of the following):
            Born at ≤28 wk gestation; OR
            With chronic lung disease (CLD) of prematurity (<32 wk gestation requiring >21% oxygen for at least 28 days after birth); OR
            With hemodynamically significant congenital heart disease
        <24 mo of age with CLD requiring medical therapy (e.g., supplemental oxygen, bronchodilator, diuretics, or chronic steroids) within 6 mo prior to start of RSV season

Continued

PALIVIZUMAB continued

Candidates for consideration:
  <12 mo of age (one of the following):
    With congenital airway abnormalities or neuromuscular disorders that decrease ability to manage airway secretions; OR
    With cystic fibrosis with clinical evidence of CLD and/or nutritional compromise
  ≤24 mo of age (one of the following):
    With cystic fibrosis with severe lung disease (previous pulmonary exacerbation in first year of life or abnormal chest x-ray) or weight for length < the 10th percentile; OR
    Profoundly immunocompromised; OR
    Undergoing cardiac transplantation during RSV season

DOSE:
  ≤24 months old: 15 mg/kg/dose IM Q monthly just prior to and during the RSV season. Max. of five doses per RSV season is recommended by the AAP. Therapy should be discontinued if child experiences breakthrough RSV hospitalization.

RSV season is typically November through April in the northern hemisphere but may begin earlier or persist later in certain communities. IM is currently the only route of administration, so **use with caution** in patients with thrombocytopenia or any coagulation disorder. The following adverse effects have been reported at slightly higher incidences when compared with placebo: rhinitis, rash, pain, increased liver enzymes, pharyngitis, cough, wheeze, diarrhea, vomiting, conjunctivitis, and anemia. Rare acute hypersensitivity reactions have been reported (first or subsequent doses).

Does not interfere with the response to routine childhood vaccines. May interfere with immunologic-based RSV diagnostic tests (some antigen detection–based assays and viral culture assays) but not with reverse transcriptase–polymerase chain reaction (PCR)-based assays.

Palivizumab is currently indicated for RSV prophylaxis in high-risk infants only. Efficacy and safety have not been demonstrated for treatment of RSV.

Each dose should be administered IM in the anterolateral aspect of the thigh. It is recommended to divide doses with total injection volumes > 1 mL. **Avoid** injection in the gluteal muscle because of risk of damage to the sciatic nerve.

PANCRELIPASE/PANCREATIC ENZYMES
Creon, Pancreaze, Pertzye, Ultresa, Viokace, and Zenpep
Pancreatic enzyme

No   No   2   C

Delayed-release, enterically coated beads, microspheres, or minitabs in capsules (porcine derived):

Product	Lipase (USP) Units	Amylase (USP) Units	Protease (USP) Units
CREON[2]			
3	3000	15,000	9500
6	6000	30,000	19,000
12	12,000	60,000	38,000
24	24,000	120,000	76,000
36	36,000	180,000	114,000
PANCREAZE[3]			
MT 2	2600	10,850	6200
MT 4	4200	24,600	14,200
MT 10	10,500	61,500	35,500
MT 16	16,800	98,400	56,800
MT 20	21,000	83,900	54,700

PANCRELIPASE/PANCREATIC ENZYMES continued

Product	Lipase (USP) Units	Amylase (USP) Units	Protease (USP) Units
PERTZYE[2,4]			
4	4000	15,125	14,375
8	8000	30,250	28,750
16	16,000	60,500	57,500
ULTRESA[3]			
4	4000	8000	8000
13	13,800	27,600	27,600
20	20,700	41,400	41,400
23	23,000	46,000	46,000
ZENPEP[1]			
3	3000	16,000	10,000
5	5000	27,000	17,000
10	10,000	55,000	34,000
15	15,000	82,000	51,000
20	20,000	109,000	68,000
25	25,000	136,000	85,000
40	40,000	218,000	136,000

1. Enteric-coated beads
2. Enteric-coated microspheres
3. Enteric-coated mini-tabs
4. Contains bicarbonate

Tabs (porcine derived):

Product	Lipase (USP) Units	Amylase (USP) Units	Protease (USP) Units
VIOKACE			
10	10,440	39,150	39,150
20	20,880	78,300	78,300

Initial doses (actual requirements are patient specific):
Enteric-coated microspheres and microtabs:
  Infant: 2000–4000 U lipase per 120 mL (formula or breast milk)
  Child < 4 yr: 1000 U lipase/kg/meal
  Child ≥ 4 yr and adult: 500 U lipase/kg/meal
  Max. dose (Child–adult): 2500 U lipase/kg/meal, or 10,000 U lipase/kg/24 hr, or 4000 U lipase/g fat/24 hr

Total daily dose should include approximately three meals and two to three snacks per day. Snack doses are approximately half of meal doses, depending on the amount of fat and food consumed.

May cause occult GI bleeding, allergic reactions to porcine proteins, hyperuricemia, and hyperuricosuria with high doses. Dose should be titrated to eliminate diarrhea and to minimize steatorrhea. **Do not** chew microspheres or microtabs. Concurrent administration with H₂ antagonists or gastric acid pump inhibitors may enhance enzyme efficacy. Doses higher than 6000 U lipase/kg/meal have been associated with colonic strictures in children <12 yr. Powder dosage form is not preferred owing to potential GI mucosal ulceration.

Avoid use of generic pancreatic enzyme products because they have been associated with treatment failures. Products not approved by the FDA are no longer allowed to be distributed in the United States.

Continued

PANCRELIPASE/PANCREATIC ENZYMES continued

Patients requiring enzyme supplementation, who receive enteral feeding via a feeding tube, may alternatively use a digestive enzyme cartridge (RELiZORB).

PANCURONIUM BROMIDE
Various generic brands
Nondepolarizing neuromuscular blocking agent

Yes   Yes   ?   C

Injection: 1 mg/mL (10 mL), 2 mg/mL (2, 5 mL); contains benzyl alcohol

Intermittent dosing (see remarks):
  Neonate:
    Initial: 0.02 mg/kg/dose IV
    Maintenance: 0.05–0.1 mg/kg/dose IV Q0.5–4 hr PRN
  1 mo–adult:
    Initial: 0.04–0.1 mg/kg/dose IV
    Maintenance: 0.015–0.1 mg/kg/dose IV Q30–60 min
Continuous IV infusion (see remarks):
  Neonate: 0.02–0.04 mg/kg/hr
  Child: 0.03–1 mg/kg/hr
  Adolescent and adult: 0.02–0.04 mg/kg/hr

Onset of action is 1–2 min. May cause tachycardia, salivation, and wheezing. Severe anaphylactic reactions have been reported; crossreactivity between neuromuscular blocking agents has been reported.

Drug effects may be accentuated by hypothermia, acidosis, neonatal age, decreased renal function, halothane, succinylcholine, hypokalemia, hyponatremia, hypocalcemia, clindamycin, tetracycline, and aminoglycoside antibiotics. Drug effects may be antagonized by alkalosis, hypercalcemia, peripheral neuropathies, diabetes mellitus, demyelinating lesions, carbamazepine, phenytoin, theophylline, anticholinesterases (e.g., neostigmine and pyridostigmine), and azathioprine. For obese patients, use of lean body weight for dose calculation has been recommended to prevent intense block of long duration and possible overdose.

Antidote is neostigmine (with atropine or glycopyrrolate). **Avoid** use in severe renal impairment (<10 mL/min). Patients with cirrhosis may require a high initial dose to achieve adequate relaxation, but muscle paralysis will be prolonged.

PANTOPRAZOLE
Protonix and generics
Gastric acid pump inhibitor

Yes   Yes   2   B

Tab, delayed release: 20, 40 mg
Injection: 40 mg; contains edetate sodium
Oral suspension: 2 mg/mL ; contains 0.25 mEq sodium bicarbonate per 1 mg drug
Enterically coated granules for delayed-release oral suspension (Protonix): 40 mg packets (30s); contains polysorbate 80

Child (see remarks):
  GERD (limited data):
    Infant and <5 yr: 1.2 mg/kg/24 hr PO once daily. **Note:** Pantoprazole did not significantly improve GERD symptom scores in an open-label trial in 128 infants (1–11 mo) receiving

PANTOPRAZOLE continued

1.2 mg/kg/24 hr PO once daily × 4 wk, followed by a 4-wk, double-blinded, placebo-controlled withdrawal phase.

≥5 yr and adolescent: 20 or 40 mg PO once daily.

GERD with erosive esophagitis:

1–5 yr (limited data): 0.3, 0.6, or 1.2 mg/kg/24 hr PO once daily all improved GERD symptoms in an 8-wk, multicenter, randomized, placebo-controlled trial for 60 subjects with GERD and histologic/erosive esophagitis

≥5 yr (up to 8-wk therapy):
  15–<40 kg: 20 mg PO once daily
  ≥40 kg: 40 mg PO once daily

IV (data limited to pharmacokinetic trials): Some doses ranging from 0.32 to 1.88 mg/kg/dose have been reported from three separate trials (N = 31; 0.01–16.4 yr). Patients with Systemic Inflammatory Response Syndrome (SIRS) cleared the drug more slowly, resulting in higher $T_{1/2}$ and AUC, than those without SIRS. Despite limited data, 1–2 mg/kg/24 hr ÷ Q12–24 hr have been used. Additional studies are needed.

Adult:

GERD with erosive esophagitis:
  PO: 40 mg once daily × 8–16 wk
  IV: 40 mg once daily × 7–10 days

Peptic ulcer: 40–80 mg PO once daily × 4–8 wk

Hypersecretory conditions:
  PO: 40 mg BID; dose may be increased as needed up to a **max. dose** of 240 mg/24 hr.
  IV: 80 mg Q12 hr; dose may be increased as needed to Q8 hr (**max. dose**: 240 mg/24 hr).
  Therapy > 7 days at 240 mg/24 hr has not been evaluated.

Convert from IV to PO therapy as soon as patient is able to tolerate PO. Common side effects include diarrhea and headache. May cause transient elevation in LFTs. Like other PPIs, may increase risk for *C. difficile*-associated diarrhea. Hypomagnesemia has been reported with long-term use. Hypersensitivity reactions (e.g., anaphylaxis, shock, angioedema, bronchospasm, acute interstitial nephritis, and urticaria), agranulocytosis, pancytopenia, and taste disorders have been reported.

Drug is a substrate for CYP450 2C19 (major), 2D6 (minor), and 3A3/4 (minor) isoenzymes. May decrease the absorption of itraconazole, ketoconazole, iron salts, and ampicillin esters. May increase the effect/toxicity of methotrexate.

Children aged 1–2 yr have demonstrated more rapid clearance of pantoprazole in pharmacokinetic studies; this age group may require higher doses. All oral doses may be taken with or without food. **Do not** crush or chew tablets. The extemporaneously compounded oral suspension may be less bioavailable owing to the loss of the enteric coating. Granules for delayed-release oral suspension product may be mixed with 5 mL apple juice (administer immediately followed by rinsing container with more apple juice) or sprinkled on 1 teaspoonful of apple sauce (administer within 10 min); see package insert for NG administration.

For IV infusion, doses may be administered over 15 min at a concentration of 0.4–0.8 mg/mL or over 2 min at a concentration of 4 mg/mL. Midazolam and zinc are **not compatible** with the IV dosage form. Parenteral routes other than IV are **not recommended**.

PAROMOMYCIN SULFATE
Generics; previously available as Humatin
Amebicide, antibiotic (aminoglycoside)

No   No   1   ?

Caps: 250 mg

Intestinal amebiasis (Entamoeba histolytica), Dientamoeba fragilis, and Giardia lamblia infection:
  Child and adult: 25–35 mg/kg/24 hr PO ÷ Q8 hr × 7 days
Tapeworm (Taenia saginata, Taenia solium, Diphyllobothrium latum, and Dipylidium caninum):
  Child: 11 mg/kg/dose PO Q15 min × 4 doses
  Adult: 1 g PO Q15 min × 4 doses
Tapeworm (Hymenolepis nana):
  Child and adult: 45 mg/kg/dose PO once daily × 5–7 days
Cryptosporidial diarrhea:
  Adult: 1.5–2.25 g/24 hr PO ÷ 3–6 × daily. Duration varies from 10–14 days to 4–8 wk. Maintenance therapy has also been used. Alternatively, 1 g PO BID × 12 wk in conjunction with azithromycin 600 mg PO once daily × 4 wk has been used in patients with AIDS.

Contraindicated in intestinal obstruction. **Use with caution** in ulcerative bowel lesions to avoid renal toxicity via systemic absorption. Drug is generally poorly absorbed and therefore **not** indicated for sole treatment of extraintestinal amebiasis. Side effects include GI disturbance, hematuria, rash, ototoxicity, and hypocholesterolemia. Bacterial overgrowth of nonsusceptible organisms, including fungi, may occur. May decrease the effects of digoxin. Pregnancy category has not been formally assigned by the FDA.

PAROXETINE
Paxil, Pexeva, Paxil CR, Brisdelle, and generics
Antidepressant, selective serotonin reuptake inhibitor

Yes   Yes   2   X

Tabs: 10, 20, 30, 40 mg
Caps (Brisdelle): 7.5 mg
Controlled-release tabs (Paxil CR and generics): 12.5, 25, 37.5 mg
Oral suspension: 10 mg/5 mL (250 mL); contains saccharin and parabens

Child:
  Depression: Well-controlled clinical trials have failed to demonstrate efficacy in children. The FDA recommends paroxetine not to be used for this indication.
  Obsessive compulsive disorder (limited data, based on a 10-wk randomized controlled trial in 207 children 7–17 yr; mean age 11.1 + 3.03 yr): Start with 10 mg PO once daily. If needed, adjust upwards by increasing dose no more than 10 mg/24 hr no more frequently than Q7 days up to a **max. dose** of 50 mg/24 hr. Mean doses of 20.3 mg/24 hr (children) and 26.8 mg/24 hr (adolescents) were used.
  Social anxiety disorder (8–17 yr): Start with 10 mg PO once daily. If needed, increase dose by 10 mg/24 hr no more frequently than Q7 days up to a **max. dose** of 50 mg/24 hr.
Adult:
  Depression: Start with 20 mg PO QAM × 4 wk. If no clinical improvement, increase dose by 10 mg/24 hr Q7 days PRN up to a **max. dose** of 50 mg/24 hr
    Paxil CR: Start with 25 mg PO QAM × 4 wk. If no improvement, increase dose by 12.5 mg/24 hr Q7 days PRN up to a **max. dose** of 62.5 mg/24 hr

PAROXETINE continued

Obsessive compulsive disorder: Start with 20 mg PO once daily; increase dose by 10 mg/24 hr Q7 days PRN up to a **max. dose** of 60 mg/24 hr. Usual dose is 40 mg PO once daily

Panic disorder: Start with 10 mg PO QAM; increase dose by 10 mg/24 hr Q7 days PRN up to a **max. dose** of 60 mg/24 hr

Paxil CR: Start with 12.5 mg PO QAM; increase dose by 12.5 mg/24 hr Q7 days PRN up to a **max. dose** of 75 mg/24 hr.

Contraindicated in patients taking MAO inhibitors (within 14 days of discontinuing MAO inhibitors), linezolid, methylene blue, pimozide, or thioridazine. **Use with caution** in patients with history of seizures, renal or hepatic impairment, cardiac disease, suicidal concerns, mania/hypomania, and diuretic use. Patients with severe renal or hepatic impairment should initiate therapy at 10 mg/24 hr and increase dose as needed up to a **max. dose** of 40 mg/24 hr.

Common side effects include anxiety, nausea, anorexia, and decreased appetite. Monitor for clinical worsening of depression and suicidal ideation/behavior following the initiation of therapy or after dose changes. Stevens–Johnson syndrome has been reported.

Paroxetine is an inhibitor and substrate for CYP450 2D6. May increase the effects/toxicity of tricyclic antidepressants, theophylline, and warfarin. May decrease the effects of tamoxifen. Cimetidine, ritonavir, MAO inhibitors (fatal serotonin syndrome), dextromethorphan, phenothiazines and type 1C antiarrhythmics may increase the effect/toxicity of paroxetine. Weakness, hyperreflexia, and poor coordination have been reported when taken with sumatriptan.

Do not discontinue therapy abruptly, may cause sweating, dizziness, confusion and tremor. May be taken with or without food.

PENICILLIN G PREPARATIONS—AQUEOUS POTASSIUM AND SODIUM
Pfizerpen-G and generics
Antibiotic, aqueous penicillin

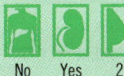

No | Yes | 2 | B

Injection (K⁺): 5, 20 million units (contains 1.7 mEq K and 0.3 mEq Na/1 million units penicillin G)
Premixed frozen injection (K⁺): 1 million units in 50 mL dextrose 4%; 2 million units in 50 mL dextrose 2.3%; 3 million units in 50 mL dextrose 0.7% (contains 1.7 mEq K and 0.3 mEq Na/1 million units penicillin G)
Injection (Na⁺): 5 million units (contains 2 mEq Na/1 million units penicillin G)
Conversion: 250 mg = 400,000 units

Neonate (IM/IV; use higher end of dosage range for meningitis and severe infections):
≤*7 days old:* 50,000–100,000 units/kg/24 hr ÷ Q12 hr
8–28 days old:
 <*1 kg:*
  8–≤14 days old: 50,000–100,000 units/kg/24 hr ÷ Q12 hr
  15–28 days old: 75,000–150,000 units/kg/24 hr ÷ Q8 hr
 ≥*1 kg:* 75,000–150,000 units/kg/24 hr ÷ Q8 hr
Group B streptococcal meningitis:
 ≤*7 days:* 250,000–450,000 units/kg/24 hr ÷ Q8 hr
 8–28 days: 450,000–500,000 units/kg/24 hr ÷ Q4–6 hr
Congenital syphilis (total of 10 days of therapy; if > 1 day of therapy is missed, restart the entire course):
 ≤*7 days:* 100,000 units/kg/24 hr ÷ Q12 hr IV; increase to dosage below at day 8 of life.
 8–28 days: 150,000 units/kg/24 hr ÷ Q8 hr IV

Continued

PENICILLIN G PREPARATIONS—AQUEOUS POTASSIUM AND SODIUM
continued

Infant and child:
  IM/IV (use higher end of dosage range and Q4 hr interval for meningitis and severe infections):
  100,000–400,000 units/kg/24 hr ÷ Q4–6 hr; max. dose: 24 million units/24 hr
  Neurosyphilis: 200,000–300,000 units/kg/24 hr ÷ Q4–6 hr IV × 10–14 days; max. dose: 24 million units/24 hr
Adult:
  IM/IV: 8–24 million units/24 hr ÷ Q4–6 hr
  Neurosyphilis: 18–24 million units/24 hr ÷ Q4–6 hr IV × 10–14 days.

Use penicillin V potassium for oral use. Side effects: anaphylaxis, urticaria, hemolytic anemia, interstitial nephritis, Jarisch–Herxheimer reaction (syphilis). Preparations containing potassium and/or sodium salts may alter serum electrolytes. $T_{1/2}$ = 30 min; may be prolonged by concurrent use of probenecid. For meningitis, use higher daily dose at shorter dosing intervals. For the treatment of anthrax (Bacillus anthracis), see www.bt.cdc.gov for additional information. **Adjust dose in renal impairment (see Chapter 30).**
Tetracyclines, chloramphenicol, and erythromycin may antagonize penicillin's activity. Probenecid increases penicillin levels. May cause false-positive or -negative urinary glucose (Clinitest method), false-positive direct Coombs test, and false-positive urinary and/or serum proteins.

PENICILLIN G PREPARATIONS—BENZATHINE
Bicillin L-A
Antibiotic, penicillin (very long-acting IM)

No　　Yes　　2　　B

Injection: 600,000 units/mL (1, 2, 4 mL); contains parabens and povidone
Injection should be IM only.

Group A streptococci:
  Infant and child: 25,000–50,000 units/kg/dose IM × 1. **Max. dose:** 1.2 million units/dose *OR:*
    >1 mo and <27 kg: 600,000 units/dose IM × 1
    ≥27 kg and adult: 1.2 million units/dose IM × 1
Rheumatic fever prophylaxis (Q3 week administration is recommended for high-risk situations):
  Infant and child (>1 mo and <27 kg): 600,000 units/dose IM Q3–4 wk
  Child ≥ 27 kg and adult: 1.2 million units/dose IM Q3–4 wk
Syphilis (if > 1 day of therapy is missed, restart the entire course; divided total dose into two injection sites):
  Infant and child:
    Primary, secondary, and early latent syphilis (<1 yr duration): 50,000 units/kg/dose × 1
    Late latent syphilis or latent syphilis of unknown duration: 50,000 units/kg/dose Q7 days × 3 doses.
    Max. dose: 2.4 million units/dose
  Adult:
    Primary, secondary, and early latent syphilis: 2.4 million units/dose IM × 1
    Late latent syphilis or latent syphilis of unknown duration: 2.4 million units/dose IM Q7 days × 3 doses.

Provides sustained levels for 2–4 wk. **Use with caution** in renal failure, asthma, and cephalosporin hypersensitivity. Side effects and drug interactions same as for Penicillin G Preparations–Aqueous Potassium and Sodium. Injection site reactions are common.
Deep IM administration only. Do not administer intravenously (cardiac arrest and death may occur) and **do not inject** into or near an artery or nerve (may result in permanent neurological damage).

PENICILLIN G PREPARATIONS—PENICILLIN G BENZATHINE AND PENICILLIN G PROCAINE
Bicillin C-R, Bicillin C-R 900/300
Antibiotic, penicillin (very long-acting IM)

   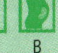
No   Yes   2   B

Bicillin CR: 300,000 units penicillin G procaine + 300,000 units penicillin G benzathine/mL to provide 600,000 units penicillin per 1 mL (2 mL tubex syringe)
Bicillin CR (900/300): 150,000 units penicillin G procaine + 450,000 units penicillin G benzathine/mL (2 mL tubex syringe)
All preparations contain parabens and povidone
Injection should be for IM use only

Dosage based on total amount of penicillin
Group A streptococci:
 Child <14 kg: 600,000 units/dose IM × 1
 Child 14–27 kg: 900,000–1,200,000 units/dose IM × 1
 Child >27 kg and adult: 2,400,000 units/dose IM × 1
Pneumococcal infection (non-CNS): dosed Q2–3 days until afebrile for 48 hr
 Child:
  Bicillin C-R: 600,000 units/dose IM
  Bicillin C-R 900/300: 1,200,000 units/dose IM

This preparation provides early peak levels in addition to prolonged levels of penicillin in the blood. **Do not use this product to treat syphilis; treatment failure can occur.** Use with caution in renal failure, asthma, significant allergies, and cephalosporin hypersensitivity. The addition of procaine penicillin has not been shown to be more efficacious than benzathine alone. However, it may reduce injection discomfort.
Deep IM administration only. Do not administer intravenously (cardiac arrest and death may occur) and **do not** inject into or near an artery or nerve (may result in permanent neurological damage).
Side effects and drug interactions same as for Penicillin G Preparations—Aqueous Potassium and Sodium. Immune hypersensitivity reaction has been reported.

PENICILLIN G PREPARATIONS—PROCAINE
Generics; previously available as Wycillin
Antibiotic, penicillin (long-acting IM)

No   Yes   2   B

Injection: 600,000 units/mL (1, 2 mL); may contain parabens, phenol, povidone, and formaldehyde)
Contains 120 mg procaine per 300,000 units penicillin
Injection should be for IM use only

Newborn (see remarks): 50,000 units/kg/24 hr IM once daily
Infant and child: 25,000–50,000 units/kg/24 hr ÷ Q12–24 hr IM. **Max. dose:** 4.8 million units/24 hr
Adult: 0.6–4.8 million units/24 hr ÷ Q12–24 hr IM
Congenital syphilis, syphilis (if >1 day of therapy is missed, restart the entire course):
 Neonate, infant, and child: 50,000 units/kg/dose once daily IM × 10 days.
Neurosyphilis:
 Adult: 2.4 million units IM once daily and Probenecid 500 mg Q6 hr PO × 10–14 days (both medications)

Continued

PENICILLIN G PREPARATIONS—PROCAINE continued

Inhaled anthrax: Postexposure prophylaxis (total duration of therapy with all forms of therapy is 60 days; switch to an alternative form of therapy after 2 wk of procaine penicillin because of the risk for adverse effects):
Child: 25,000 units/kg/dose (**max. dose**: 1.2 million units/dose) IM Q12 hr
Adult: 1.2 million units IM Q12 hr

Provides sustained levels for 2–4 days. **Use with caution** in renal failure, asthma, significant allergies, cephalosporin hypersensitivity, and neonates (higher incidence of sterile abscess at injection site and risk of procaine toxicity). Side effects and drug interactions similar to Penicillin G Preparations–Aqueous Potassium and Sodium. In addition, may cause CNS stimulation and seizures. Immune hypersensitivity reaction has been reported.
Deep IM administration only. Do not administer intravenously (cardiac arrest and death may occur) and **do not inject** into or near an artery or nerve (may result in permanent neurological damage). Large doses may be administered in two injection sites. No longer recommended for empiric treatment of gonorrhea due to resistant strains.

PENICILLIN V POTASSIUM
Generics; previously available as Veetids
Antibiotic, penicillin

No   Yes   2   B

Tabs: 250, 500 mg
Oral solution: 125 mg/5 mL, 250 mg/5 mL (100, 200 mL); may contain saccharin
Contains 0.7 mEq potassium/ 250 mg drug
250 mg = 400,000 units

Child: 25–75 mg/kg/24 hr ÷ Q6–8 hr PO; **max. dose**: 2 g/24 hr
Adolescent and adult: 125–500 mg/dose PO Q6–8 hr
Acute group A streptococcal pharyngitis (use BID dosing regimen ONLY if good compliance is expected):
  Child <27 kg: 250 mg PO BID–TID × 10 days
  ≥27 kg, adolescent and adult: 500 mg PO BID–TID × 10 days
Rheumatic fever prophylaxis and pneumococcal prophylaxis for sickle cell disease and functional or anatomical asplenia (regardless of immunization status):
  2 mo–<3 yr: 125 mg PO BID
  3–5 yr: 250 mg PO BID; for sickle cell and asplenia, use may be discontinued after 5 yr of age if child received recommended pneumococcal immunizations and did not experience invasive pneumococcal infection
Recurrent rheumatic fever prophylaxis:
  Child and adult: 250 mg PO BID

See *Penicillin G Preparations*–Aqueous Potassium and Sodium for side effects and drug interactions. GI absorption is better than penicillin G. **Note**: Must be taken 1 hr before or 2 hr after meals. Penicillin will prevent rheumatic fever if started within 9 days of the acute illness. **Adjust dose in renal failure (see Chapter 30).**

PENTAMIDINE ISETHIONATE
Pentam 300, NebuPent
Antibiotic, antiprotozoal

No   Yes   3   C

Injection (Pentam 300): 300 mg
Inhalation (NebuPent): 300 mg

Treatment (child and adult):
  Pneumocystis jiroveci (carinii): 4 mg/kg/24 hr IM/IV once daily × 14–21 days (IV is the preferred route)
  Trypanosomiasis (Trypanosoma gambiense, Trypanosoma rhodesiense without CNS involvement): 4 mg/kg/24 hr IM/IV once daily × 10 days
  Visceral leishmaniasis (Leishmania donovani, L. infantum, L. chagasi): 4 mg/kg/dose IM/IV once daily, or once every other day × 15–30 doses
  Cutaneous leishmaniasis (Leishmania [Viannia] panamensis): 2–4 mg/kg/dose IM/IV once or twice a week until lesions healed
Prophylaxis (child and adult):
  Pneumocystis jiroveci (carinii):
    IM/IV: 4 mg/kg/dose Q2–4 wk; max. single dose: 300 mg
    Inhalation (use with Respigard II nebulizer):
    <5 yr: 9 mg/kg (**max. dose**: 300 mg/dose) Q month
    ≥5 yr: 300 mg Q month

Use with caution in ventricular tachycardia, Stevens–Johnson syndrome, and daily doses > 21 days. May cause hypoglycemia, hyperglycemia, hypotension (both IV and IM administration), nausea, vomiting, fever, mild hepatotoxicity, pancreatitis, megaloblastic anemia, nephrotoxicity, hypocalcemia, and granulocytopenia. Additive nephrotoxicity with aminoglycosides, amphotericin B, cisplatin, and vancomycin may occur. Aerosol administration may also cause bronchospasm, cough, oxygen desaturation, dyspnea, and loss of appetite. Infuse IV over 1–2 hr to reduce the risk of hypotension. Sterile abscess may occur at IM injection site.
Adjust dose in renal impairment (see Chapter 30) with systemic use.

PENTOBARBITAL
Nembutal
Barbiturate

Yes   No   3   D

Injection: 50 mg/mL (20, 50 mL); contains propylene glycol and 10% alcohol

Hypnotic
  Child:
    IM: 2–6 mg/kg/dose. **Max. dose:** 100 mg
  Adult:
    IM: 150–200 mg
Preprocedure sedation
  Child:
    IV/IM: 3–6 mg/kg/dose. **Max. dose:** 150 mg

Continued

PENTOBARBITAL continued

Barbiturate coma
Child and adult:
IV: loading dose: 10–15 mg/kg given slowly over 1–2 hr
Maintenance: Begin at 1 mg/kg/hr. Dose range: 1–3 mg/kg/hr as needed

Contraindicated in liver failure and history of porphyria. **Use with caution** in hypovolemic shock, CHF, hypotension, and hepatic impairment. No advantage over phenobarbital for control of seizures. Adjunct in treatment of ICP. May cause drug-related isoelectric EEG. **Do not administer** for >2 wk in treatment of insomnia. May cause hypotension, arrhythmias, hypothermia, respiratory depression, and dependence.
Onset of action: IM: 10–15 min; IV: 1 min. Duration of action: IV: 15 min.
Administer IV at a rate of <50 mg/min.
Therapeutic serum levels: Sedation: 1–5 mg/L; Hypnosis: 5–15 mg/L; Coma: 20–40 mg/L (steady state is achieved after 4–5 days of continuous IV dosing).

PERMETHRIN
Elimite, Nix, and generics
Scabicidal agent

No   No   2   B

Cream (Elimite and generics): 5% (60 g); contains 0.1% formaldehyde
Liquid cream rinse (Nix Lice Killing Crème Rinse-OTC and generics): 1% (59 mL with comb); contains 20% isopropyl alcohol
Lotion (OTC): 1% (59 mL with comb)
Additional OTC permethrin products for use on bedding, furniture, and garments include the following:
Liquid spray (Nix Lice Control Spray): 0.25% (150 mL)
Spray (Rid Home Lice Bedbug and Dust Mite Spray): 0.5% (141.8 g)

Pediculus humanus capitis, Phthirus pubis (>2 mo):
Head lice: Saturate hair and scalp with 1% cream rinse after shampooing, rinsing, and towel drying hair. Leave on for 10 min, then rinse. May repeat in 7 days. May be used for lice in other areas of the body (e.g., pubic lice) in same fashion. If the 1% cream rinse is resistant, the 5% cream may be used after shampooing, rinsing, and towel drying hair. Leave on for 8–14 hr overnight under a shower cap; then rinse off. May repeat in 7 days.
Scabies: Apply 5% cream from neck to toe (head to toe for infants and toddlers) wash off with water in 8–14 hr. May repeat in 7 days. Use in infants <1 mo is safe and effective when applied for a 6 hr period.

Ovicidal activity generally makes single-dose regimen adequate. However, resistance to permethrin has been reported. **Avoid** contact with eyes during application. Shake well before using. May cause pruritus, hypersensitivity, burning, stinging, erythema, and rash. For either lice or scabies, instruct patient to launder bedding and clothing. For lice, treat symptomatic contacts only. For scabies, treat all contacts even if asymptomatic. Topical cream dosage form contains formaldehyde. Dispense 60 g per adult or two small children.

PHENAZOPYRIDINE HCL
Pyridium, Azo-Urinary Pain Relief [OTC], Azo-Urinary Pain Relief Maximum Strength [OTC], and generics
Urinary analgesic

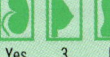
Yes   Yes   3   B

Tabs: 95 mg [OTC] (12s, 30s), 97.5 mg [OTC] (12s, 24s), 100 mg, 200 mg
Oral suspension: 10 mg/mL

UTI (use with an appropriate antibacterial agent):
  Child 6–<12 yr: 12 mg/kg/24 hr ÷ TID PO until symptoms of lower urinary tract irritation are controlled or for 2 days. **Max. dose:** 200 mg/dose.
  ≥12 yr and adult: 190–200 mg TID PO until symptoms are controlled or for 2 days.

May cause pruritus, rash, GI distress, vertigo, and headache. Anaphylactoid-like reaction, methemoglobinemia, hemolytic anemia, and renal and hepatic toxicity have been reported usually at overdosage levels. Colors urine orange; stains clothing. May also stain contact lenses and interfere with urinalysis tests based on spectrometry or color reactions. Give doses with or after meals.
Avoid use in moderate/severe renal impairment; adjust dose in mild renal impairment (see Chapter 30).

PHENOBARBITAL
Generics; previously available as Luminal
Barbiturate

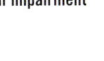
Yes   Yes   2   D

Tabs: 15, 16.2, 30, 32.4, 60, 64.8, 97.2, 100 mg
Elixir or oral solution: 20 mg/5 mL; may contain alcohol
Injection: 65, 130 mg/mL (1 mL); may contain 10% alcohol and propylene glycol

Status epilepticus:
  Loading dose, IV:
    Neonate, infant, and child: 15–20 mg/kg/dose (**max. loading dose:** 1000 mg) in a single or divided dose. May give additional 5 mg/kg doses Q15–30 min to a **max. total** of 40 mg/kg
  Maintenance dose, PO/IV: Monitor levels
    Neonate: 3–5 mg/kg/24 hr ÷ once daily–BID
    Infant: 5–6 mg/kg/24 hr ÷ once daily–BID
    Child 1–5 yr: 6–8 mg/kg/24 hr ÷ once daily–BID
    Child 6–12 yr: 4–6 mg/kg/24 hr ÷ once daily–BID
    >12 yr: 1–3 mg/kg/24 hr ÷ once daily–BID
Hyperbilirubinemia (limited data; <12 yr): 3–8 mg/kg/24 hr PO ÷ BID–TID. Doses up to 12 mg/kg/24 hr have been used. Not recommended for biliary cirrhosis.
Preoperative sedation (child): 1–3 mg/kg/dose IM/IV/PO × 1. Give 60–90 min before procedure.

Contraindicated in porphyria, severe respiratory disease with dyspnea or obstruction. **Use with caution** in hepatic or renal disease (reduce dose). IV administration may cause respiratory arrest or hypotension. Side effects include drowsiness, cognitive impairment, ataxia, hypotension, hepatitis, rash, respiratory depression, apnea, megaloblastic anemia, and anticonvulsant hypersensitivity syndrome. Paradoxical reaction in children (not dose related) may cause hyperactivity, irritability, insomnia. Induces several liver enzymes (CYP450 1A2, 2A6, 2B6, 2C8/9, 3A4), P-glycoprotein, and glucuronidation (UGT1A1), thus decreases blood levels of many drugs (e.g., anticonvulsants). **IV push not to exceed 1 mg/kg/min.**

Continued

PHENOBARBITAL continued

$T_{1/2}$ is variable with age: neonates, 45–100 hr; infants, 20–133 hr; children, 37–73 hr. Owing to long half-life, consider other agents for sedation during procedures.

Therapeutic levels: 15–40 mg/L. Recommended serum sampling time at steady-state: trough level obtained within 30 min prior to the next scheduled dose after 10–14 days of continuous dosing.

Adjust dose in renal failure (see Chapter 30).

PHENTOLAMINE MESYLATE
OraVerse and generics; previously available as Regitine
Adrenergic blocking agent (α); antidote, extravasation

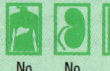
No   No   ?   C

Injection: 5 mg vial; may contain mannitol
Injection in solution for submucosal use:
  OraVerse: 0.4 mg/1.7 mL (1.7 mL in dental cartridges) (10s, 50s); contains edetate disodium

Treatment of α-adrenergic drug extravasation (most effective within 12 hr of extravasation):
All doses are 5 doses administered SC around the site of extravasation within 12 hr of extravasation. See below for weight-based dosing and recommended drug concentration.

Patient Weight	Drug Concentration (Diluted With Preservative-Free NS)	Dose for Each Syringe × 5 Syringes	Total Dose From all 5 Syringes
<1 kg	0.2 mg/mL	0.05 mL	0.05 mg
1–<2.5 kg	0.2 mg/mL	0.1 mL	0.1 mg
2.5–<5 kg	0.2 mg/mL	0.25 mL	0.25 mg
5–<10 kg	1 mg/mL	0.1 mL	0.5 mg
10–20 kg	1 mg/mL	0.2 mL	1 mg
20–<30 kg	1 mg/mL	0.4 mL	2 mg
30–<40 kg	1 mg/mL	0.6 mL	3 mg
40–<50 kg	1 mg/mL	0.8 mL	4 mg
≥50 kg	1 mg/mL	1 mL	5 mg

Max. total dose:
  Neonate: 2.5 mg; monitor BP when total dose exceeds 0.1 mg/kg
  Infant, child, adolescent, and adult: 0.1–0.2 mg/kg/dose or 5 mg
Diagnosis of pheochromocytoma, IM/IV:
  Child: 0.05–0.1 mg/kg/dose up to a **max. dose** of 5 mg
  Adult: 5 mg/dose
Hypertension, prior to surgery for pheochromocytoma, IM/IV:
  Child: 0.05–0.1 mg/kg/dose up to a **max. dose** of 5 mg 1–2 hr *before* surgery; repeat Q2–4 hr PRN
  Adult: 5 mg/dose 1–2 hr *before* surgery; repeat Q2–4 hr PRN

Contraindicated in MI, coronary insufficiency and angina. **Use with caution** in hypotension, arrhythmias, and cerebral vascular spasm/occlusion

For diagnosis of pheochromocytoma, patient should be resting in a supine position. A blood pressure reduction of more than 35 mm Hg systolic and 24 mm Hg diastolic is considered a positive test for pheochromocytoma. For treatment of extravasation, use 27- to 30-gauge needle with multiple small injections and monitor site closely as repeat doses may be necessary.

PHENYLEPHRINE HCL
Neo-Synephrine, many others, and generics
Adrenergic agonist

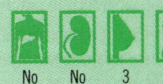
No No 3 C

Injection: 10 mg/mL (1%) (1, 5, 10 mL); may contain bisulfites
Nasal spray [OTC]:
  0.25% (Afrin Childrens, Neo-Synephrine Cold and Sinus Mild Strength, Rhinall): 0.25% (15, 30, 40 mL)
  0.5% (Neo-Synephrine Cold and Sinus Regular Strength): 0.5% (15 mL)
  1% (4-Way, Nasal Four, Neo-Synephrine Cold and Sinus Extra Strength): 1% (15, 30 mL)
NOTE: For Neo-Synephrine 12-hr Nasal, see Oxymetazoline
Ophthalmic drops (Altafrin and generics): 2.5% (2, 3, 5, 15 mL), 10% (5 mL); contains benzalkonium chloride
Tabs (Medi-Pheny, Sudafed PE, and others) [OTC]: 5, 10 mg
Oral solution (Sudafed PE Childrens; OTC): 2.5 mg/5 mL (118 mL)
Oral drops (Little Colds Decongestant; OTC): 2.5 mg/1 mL (30 mL); contains sodium benzoate

Hypotension:
NOTE: the IV drip dosage units for children are in mcg/kg/min, compared to mcg/min for adults. To prepare infusion: See inside front cover.
  Child:
    IV bolus: 5–20 mcg/kg/dose (initial **max. dose**: 500 mcg/dose, subsequent **max. dose**: 1000 mcg/dose) Q10–15 min PRN
    IV drip: 0.1–0.5 mcg/kg/min; titrate to effect
    IM/SC: 0.1 mg/kg/dose Q1–2 hr PRN; **max. dose**: 5 mg
  Adult:
    IV bolus: 0.1–0.5 mg/dose Q10–15 min PRN
    IV drip: Initial rate at 100–180 mcg/min; titrate to effect. Usual maintenance dose: 40–60 mcg/min
Pupillary dilation:
  <1 yr: 2.5% solution; 1 drop in each eye 15–30 min before exam.
  Child (≥1 yr) and adult: 2.5% or 10% solution; 1 drop in each eye 10–60 min before exam.
Nasal decongestant (in each nostril; give up to 3 days):
  Child 6–12 yr: 2–3 sprays to each nostril of 0.25% solution Q4 hr PRN
  >12 yr–adult: 2–3 sprays to each nostril of 0.5% or 1% solution Q4 hr PRN
Oral decongestant (see remarks):
  4–<6 yr:
    Oral drops (2.5 mg/mL): 1 mL (2.5 mg) PO Q4 hr PRN; not to exceed six doses (15 mg) in 24 hr
    Oral solution (2.5 mg/5 mL): 5 mL (2.5 mg) PO Q4 hr PRN, up to 30 mL (15 mg) per 24 hr
  ≥6–<12 yr:
    Oral solution (2.5 mg/5 mL): 10 mL (5 mg) PO Q4 hr PRN up to 60 mL (30 mg) per 24 hr
  ≥12 yr and adult: 10 mg PO Q4 hr PRN up to 60 mg/24 hr

Use with caution in presence of arrhythmias, hyperthyroidism, or hyperglycemia. May cause tremor, insomnia, palpitations. Metabolized by MAO. **Contraindicated** in pheochromocytoma and severe hypertension. Injectable product may contain sulfites.
Nasal decongestants may cause rebound congestion with excessive use (>3 days). The 1% nasal spray can be used in adults with extreme congestion.
Oral phenylephrine is found in a variety of combination cough and cold products and has replaced pseudoephedrine and phenylpropanolamine. OTC or nonprescription use of this

Continued

PHENYLEPHRINE HCL continued

product is **not recommended** for children aged <6 yr; reports of serious adverse effects (cardiac and respiratory distress, convulsions, and hallucinations) and fatalities (from unintentional overdosages, including combined use of other OTC products containing the same active ingredients) have been made.

PHENYTOIN
Dilantin, Dilantin Infatab, Phenytek, and generics
Anticonvulsant, class Ib antiarrhythmic

Yes Yes 2 D

Chewable tabs (Dilantin Infatab and generics): 50 mg
Extended-release caps:
  Dilantin and generics: 30, 100 mg
  Phenytek: 200, 300 mg
Oral suspension: 125 mg/5 mL (240 mL); contains ≤0.6% alcohol
Injection: 50 mg/mL (2, 5 mL); contains alcohol and propylene glycol

Status epilepticus: See Chapter 1.
 Loading dose (all ages): 15–20 mg/kg IV
 Max. dose: 1500 mg/24 hr
 Maintenance for seizure disorders (initiate 12 hr after administration of loading dose):
  Neonate: start with 5 mg/kg/24 hr PO/IV ÷ Q12 hr; usual range 4–8 mg/kg/24 hr PO/IV ÷ Q8–12 hr
  Infant/child: start with 5 mg/kg/24 hr ÷ BID–TID PO/IV; usual dose range (doses divided BID–TID):
   6 mo–3 yr: 8–10 mg/kg/24 hr
   4–6 yr: 7.5–9 mg/kg/24 hr
   7–9 yr: 7–8 mg/kg/24 hr
   10–16 yr: 6–7 mg/kg/24 hr
   Note: Use once daily–BID dosing with extended-release caps
  Adult: Start with 100 mg/dose Q8 hr IV/PO and carefully titrate (if needed) by 100 mg increments Q2–4 wk to 300–600 mg/24 hr (or 6–7 mg/kg/24 hr) ÷ Q8–24 hr IV/PO
Antiarrhythmic (secondary to digitalis intoxication):
 Load (all ages): 1.25 mg/kg IV Q5 min up to a **total** of 15 mg/kg
 Maintenance:
  Child (IV/PO): 5–10 mg/kg/24 hr ÷ Q8–12 hr
  Adult: 250 mg PO QID × 1 day, then 250 mg PO Q12 hr × 2 days, then 300–400 mg/24 hr ÷ Q6–24 hr

Contraindicated in patients with heart block or sinus bradycardia and those who are receiving delavirdine (decrease virologic response). IM administration is **not recommended** because of erratic absorption and pain at injection site; consider fosphenytoin. Side effects include gingival hyperplasia, hirsutism, dermatitis, blood dyscrasia, ataxia, lupus-like and Stevens–Johnson syndromes, lymphadenopathy, liver damage, and nystagmus. Suicidal behavior or ideation and multiorgan hypersensitivity (DRESS) have been reported. An increased risk for serious skin reactions (e.g., TEN and Stevens–Johnson syndrome) may occur in patients with the HLA-B*1502 allele.

Many drug interactions; levels may be increased by cimetidine, chloramphenicol, INH, sulfonamides, trimethoprim, etc. Levels may be decreased by some antineoplastic agents. Phenytoin induces hepatic microsomal enzymes (CYP450 1A2, 2C8/9/19, and 3A3/4), leading to decreased effectiveness of oral contraceptives, fosamprenavir (used without ritonavir), quinidine, valproic

PHENYTOIN continued

acid, theophylline, and other substrates to the previously listed CYP450 hepatic enzymes. May increase levels of amprenavir when administered with fosamprenavir and ritonavir. May cause resistance to neuromuscular blocking action of nondepolarizing neuromuscular blocking agents (e.g., pancuronium, vecuronium, rocuronium, and cisatracurium).

Suggested dosing intervals for specific oral dosage forms: extended-release caps (once daily–BID); chewable tablets, and oral suspension (TID). Oral absorption reduced in neonates. $T_{1/2}$ is variable (7–42 hr) and dose-dependent. Drug is highly protein-bound; free fraction of drug will be increased in patients with hypoalbuminemia.

For seizure disorders, therapeutic levels: 10–20 mg/L (free and bound phenytoin) **OR** 1–2 mg/L (free only). Monitor free phenytoin levels in hypoalbuminemia or renal insufficiency. Recommended serum sampling times: trough level (PO/IV) within 30 min prior to the next scheduled dose; peak or postload level (IV) 1 hr after the end of IV infusion. Steady state is usually achieved after 5–10 days of continuous dosing. For routine monitoring, measure trough.

IV push/infusion rate: **Not to exceed** 0.5 mg/kg/min in neonates, or 1 mg/kg/min infants, children, and adults with **max. dose** of 50 mg/min; may cause cardiovascular collapse. Consider fosphenytoin in situations of tenuous IV access and risk for extravasation.

PHOSPHORUS SUPPLEMENTS
K-PHOS Neutral, Av-Phos 250 Neutral, Phospha 250 Neutral, PHOS-NaK, Sodium Phosphate, Potassium Phosphate, and many generics for injections
Electrolyte supplement

No   Yes   2   C

Oral: (reconstitute in 75 mL H₂O per tablet or packet of powder)
Na and K phosphate:
  PHOS-NaK; powder (OTC): 250 mg (8 mM) P, 6.96 mEq (160 mg) Na, 7.16 mEq (280 mg) K per packet of powder (100s)
  K-PHOS Neutral, Av-Phos 250 Neutral, or Phospha 250 Neutral; tabs: 250 mg P (8 mM), 13 mEq Na, 1.1 mEq K
  K-PHOS No. 2; tabs: 250 mg P (8 mM), 5.8 mEq Na, 2.3 mEq K
Injection:
  Na phosphate: 3 mM (93 mg) P, 4 mEq Na/mL
  K phosphate: 3 mM (93 mg) P, 4.4 mEq K/mL
Conversion: 31 mg P = 1 mM P

Acute hypophosphatemia: 0.16–0.32 mM/kg/dose (or 5–10 mg/kg/dose) IV over 6 hr
Maintenance/replacement:
  Child:
    IV: 0.5–1.5 mM/kg (or 15–45 mg/kg) over 24 hr
    PO: 30–90 mg/kg/24 hr (or 1–3 mM/kg/24 hr) ÷ TID–QID
  Adult:
    IV: 50–65 mM (or 1.5–2 g) over 24 hr
    PO: 3–4.5 g/24 hr (or 100–150 mM/24 hr) ÷ TID–QID
Recommended IV infusion rate: ≤0.1 mM/kg/hr (or 3.1 mg/kg/hr) of phosphate. When potassium salt is used, the rate will be limited by the **max.** potassium infusion rate. **Do not** coinfuse with calcium containing products.

May cause tetany, hyperphosphatemia, hyperkalemia, hypocalcemia. **Use with caution** in patients with renal impairment. Be aware of sodium and/or potassium load when

Continued

PHOSPHORUS SUPPLEMENTS continued

supplementing phosphate. IV administration may cause hypotension and renal failure or arrhythmias, heart block, and cardiac arrest with potassium salt. PO dosing may cause nausea, vomiting, abdominal pain, or diarrhea. See Chapter 21 for daily requirements and Chapter 11 for additional information on hypophosphatemia and hyperphosphatemia.

PHYSOSTIGMINE SALICYLATE
Generics; previously available as Antilirium
Cholinergic agent

No   No   ?   C

Injection: 1 mg/mL (2 mL); contains 2% benzyl alcohol and 0.1% sodium bisulfite

Reversal of toxic anticholinergic effects from antihistamine or anticholinergic agents:
  Child: 0.02 mg/kg/dose IM or IV (administered no >0.5 mg/min), dose may be repeated every 5–10 min if no response or return of anticholinergic symptoms up to a **max. total** of 2 mg
  Adult: 0.5–2 mg IM or IV (administered no >1 mg/min), if needed repeat dose every 10–30 min until response is seen or when adverse effects occurs

Physostigmine antidote: Atropine always should be available. **Contraindicated** in asthma, gangrene, diabetes, cardiovascular disease, GI or GU tract obstruction, any vagotonic state, and patients receiving choline esters or depolarizing neuromuscular blocking agents (e.g., decamethonium, succinylcholine). May cause seizures, arrhythmias, bradycardia, GI symptoms, and other cholingeric effects. Rapid IV administration can cause bradycardia and hypersalivation leading to respiratory distress and seizures.

PHYTONADIONE/VITAMIN K₁
Mephyton and generics
Vitamin, fat soluble

No   No   2   C

Tabs (Mephyton): 5 mg
Oral suspension: 1 mg/mL
Injection, emulsion:
  2 mg/mL (0.5 mL); preservative free
  10 mg/mL (1 mL); contains 0.9% benzyl alcohol

Neonatal hemorrhagic disease (Vitamin K deficiency bleeding):
  Prophylaxis: 0.5–1 mg IM × 1 within 1 hr after birth. For preterm neonates <1 kg birth weight, use 0.3–0.5 mg/kg IM × 1
  Treatment: 1–2 mg/24 hr IM/SC/IV
Oral anticoagulant (warfarin) overdose (see remarks):
  No significant bleeding:
    INR 4–4.5: Consider PO vitamin K at dosage indicated for INR >4.5–<10 below and monitor INR Q24 hr.
    NR > 4.5–<10: Monitor INR Q24 hr until INR <4.
      <40 kg: 0.03 mg/kg PO × 1
      ≥40 kg: 1–2.5 mg PO × 1
    INR ≥ 10: Monitor INR Q12 hr and repeat vitamin K dose Q12–24 hr PRN
      <40 kg: 0.06 mg/kg PO × 1
      ≥40 kg: 5–10 mg PO × 1

PHYTONADIONE/VITAMIN K₁ continued

Minor bleeding (any elevated INR): Monitor INR Q12–24 hr, repeat vitamin K dose in 24 hr if full correction not achieved and bleeding persists.

PO:
  <40 kg: 0.03 mg/kg × 1
  ≥40 kg: 1–2.5 mg × 1
IV: 0.5–2.5 mg × 1

Significant or Life-threatening bleeding (any elevated INR): 5–10 mg IV × 1; use in combination with FFP (10–15 mL/kg) or prothrombin complex concentrate. Monitor INR Q4–6 hr, repeat vitamin K dose if full correction not achieved at 12–24 hr and bleeding persists

Vitamin K deficiency:
  Infant and child:
    PO: 2.5–5 mg/24 hr
    IM/SC/IV: 1–2 mg/dose × 1
  Adolescent and adult:
    PO: 2.5–25 mg/24 hr
    IM/SC/IV: 2.5–10 mg/dose × 1

Monitor PT/PTT. Large doses (10–20 mg) in newborns may cause hyperbilirubinemia and severe hemolytic anemia. Blood coagulation factors increase within 6–12 hr after oral doses and within 1–2 hr following parenteral administration. Use of higher doses for warfarin overdose may cause warfarin resistance for ≥1 wk.

IV injection rate **not to exceed** 3 mg/m^2/min or 1 mg/min. IV or IM doses may cause flushing, dizziness, cardiac/respiratory arrest, hypotension, and anaphylaxis. IV or IM administration is indicated only when other routes of administration are not feasible (or in emergency situations).

Concurrent administration of oral mineral oil may decrease GI absorption of vitamin K. Protect product from light. **See Chapter 21 for multivitamin preparations.**

PILOCARPINE HCL
Isopto Carpine, Salagen, Pilopine HS, and generics
Cholinergic agent

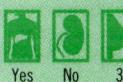
Yes   No   3   C

Ophthalmic solution (Isopto Carpine and generics): 1% (15 mL), 2% (15 mL), 4% (15 mL); may contain benzalkonium chloride
Ophthalmic gel (Pilopine HS): 4% (4 g); contains benzalkonium chloride
Tab:
  Salagen: 5 mg
  Generics: 5, 7.5 mg

For elevated intraocular pressure:
  Child and adult:
    Drops: 1–2 drops in each eye 4–6 times a day; adjust concentration and frequency as needed.
    Gel: 0.5-inch ribbon applied to lower conjunctival sac QHS. Adjust dose as needed.

Xerostomia:
  Adult: 5 mg/dose PO TID, dose may be titrated to 10 mg/dose PO TID in patients who do not respond to lower dose and who are able to tolerate the drug. 5 mg/dose PO QID has been used in Sjogren's syndrome.

OPHTHALMIC USE: Contraindicated in acute iritis or anterior chamber inflammation and uncontrolled asthma. May cause stinging, burning, lacrimation, headache, and retinal

Continued

PILOCARPINE HCL continued

detachment. **Use with caution** in patients with corneal abrasion or significant cardiovascular disease. Use with topical NSAIDs (e.g., ketorolac) may decrease topical pilocarpine effects.

ORAL USE: Sweating, nausea, rhinitis, chills, flushing, urinary frequency, dizziness, asthenia, and headaches have also been reported. Reduce oral dosing in the presence of mild hepatic insufficiency (Child-Pugh score of 5–6); **avoid use** in severe hepatic insufficiency.

PIMECROLIMUS
Elidel
Topical immunosuppressant, calcineurin inhibitor

No   No   3   C

Cream: 1% (30, 60, 100 g); contains benzyl alcohol and propylene glycol

Atopic dermatitis (second-line therapy):
≥*2 yr and adult (see remarks):* Apply a thin layer to affected area BID and rub in gently and completely. Reevaluate patient in 6 wk if lesions are not healed.

Do not use in children < 2 yr (higher rate of upper respiratory infections), immunocompromised patients, or with occlusive dressings (promotes systemic absorption). **Avoid use** on malignant or premalignant skin conditions as rare cases of lymphoma and skin malignancy have been reported with topical calcineurin inhibitors. Approved as a second-line therapy for atopic dermatitis for patients who fail to respond, or do not tolerate, other approved therapies. Use medication for short periods of time by using the minimum amounts to control symptoms; long-term safety is unknown. **Avoid** contact with eyes; nose; mouth; and cut, infected, or scraped skin. Minimize and **avoid** exposure to natural and artificial sunlight, respectively.

Most common side effects include burning at the application site, headache, viral infections, and pyrexia. Skin discoloration, skin flushing associated with alcohol use, anaphylactic reactions, ocular irritation after application to the eye lids or near the eyes, angioneurotic edema, and facial edema have been reported. Drug is a CYP450 3A3/4 substrate.

PIPERACILLIN WITH TAZOBACTAM
Zosyn and generics
Antibiotic, penicillin (extended spectrum with β-lactamase inhibitor)

No   Yes   2   B

8:1 ratio of piperacillin to tazobactam:
Injection, powder: 2 g piperacillin and 0.25 g tazobactam; 3 g piperacillin and 0.375 g tazobactam; 4 g piperacillin and 0.5 g tazobactam; 36 g piperacillin and 4.5 g tazobactam
Injection, premixed in iso-osmotic dextrose: 2 g piperacillin and 0.25 g tazobactam in 50 mL; 3 g piperacillin and 0.375 g tazobactam in 50 mL; 4 g piperacillin and 0.5 g tazobactam in 100 mL
Contains 2.84 mEq Na/g piperacillin

All doses based on piperacillin component.
Neonate: 100 mg/kg/dose IV at the following intervals:
  <1 kg:
    ≤*14 days old:* Q12 hr
    15–28 days old: Q8 hr
  ≥*1 kg:*
    ≤*7 days old:* Q12 hr
    8–28 days old: Q8 hr

PIPERACILLIN WITH TAZOBACTAM *continued*

Severe infections (IV; shortening the dosing interval to Q6 hr and lengthening the dose administration time (see remarks) may enhance the pharmacodynamic properties):
  <2 mo (currently undefined by manufacturer; extrapolated from piperacillin dosing): 80 mg/kg/dose Q6 hr; some recommend using 80 mg/kg/dose Q4 hr
  2–9 mo: 80 mg/kg/dose Q6–8 hr
  >9 mo: 100 mg/kg/dose Q6–8 hr
  Max. dose (all ages): 16 g/24 hr

Appendicitis or peritonitis (IV route for 7–10 days; dosing interval may be shorten to Q6 hr to enhance pharmacodynamic properties):
  2–9 mo: 80 mg/kg/dose Q6–8 hr
  >9 mo–adolescent:
    ≤40 kg: 100 mg/kg/dose (max. 3000 mg/dose) Q6–8 hr
    >40 kg: 3 g/dose Q6 hr
  Max. dose (all ages): 16 g/24 hr

Adult:
  Intra-abdominal or soft tissue infections: 3 g IV Q6 hr
  Nosocomial pneumonia: 4 g IV Q6 hr
Cystic fibrosis (antipseudomonal): 350–600 mg/kg/24 hr IV ÷ Q4–6 hr; **max. dose:** 24 g/24 hr

Tazobactam is a β-lactamase inhibitor, thus extending the spectrum of piperacillin. Like other penicillins, CSF penetration occurs only with inflamed meninges. GI disturbances, pruritus, rash, and headaches are common. Abnormal platelet aggregation and prolonged bleeding, serious skin reactions (e.g., Stevens–Johnson, DRESS, acute generalized exanthematous pustulosis, and TEN) have been reported. Cystic Fibrosis patients have an increased risk for fever and rash. Increase incidence of acute kidney injury has been reported when used in combination with IV vancomycin.

Coagulation parameters should be tested more frequently and monitored regularly with high doses of heparin, warfarin, or other drugs affecting blood coagulation or thrombocyte function. May falsely decrease aminoglycoside serum levels if the drugs are infused close to one another; allow a minimum of 2 hr between infusions to prevent this interaction. May prolong the neuromuscular blockade effects of vecuronium.

Prolonging the dose administration time to 4 hr will maximize the pharmacokinetic/pharmacodynamic properties by prolonging the time of drug concentration above the MIC. **Adjust dose in renal impairment (see Chapter 30).**

POLYCITRA

See Citrate Mixtures

POLYETHYLENE GLYCOL—ELECTROLYTE SOLUTION
Bowel cleansing products: GoLYTELY, CoLyte, NuLYTELY, TriLyte, and generics
Laxative products: MiraLax, GaviLAX, GlycoLax, HealthyLax, PegyLax, and many others including generics
Bowel evacuant, osmotic laxative

No   No   ?   C

Powder for oral solution:
  Bowel cleansing products:
   GoLYTELY and others: Polyethylene glycol 3350 236 g, Na sulfate 22.74 g, Na bicarbonate 6.74 g, NaCl 5.86 g, KCl 2.97 g (mixed with water to 4 L). Contents may vary. See package insert for specific contents of other products

Continued

POLYETHYLENE GLYCOL—ELECTROLYTE SOLUTION continued

Laxative products:
MiraLax [OTC], GaviLAX [OTC], Glycolax [OTC], HealtyLax [OTC], PegyLax [Rx], and generics [OTC and Rx]: Polyethylene glycol 3350 (17, 119, 238, 250, 255, 500, 510, 527, 765, 850 g)

Bowel cleansing (use products containing supplemental electrolytes for bowel cleansing such as GoLYTELY, CoLyte, NuLYTELY, TriLyte and others; and patients should be NPO 3–4 hr prior to dosing):
Child:
  Oral/nasogastric: 25–40 mL/kg/hr until rectal effluent is clear (usually in 4–10 hr)
Adult:
  Oral: 240 ml PO Q10 min up to 4 L or until rectal effluent is clear
  Nasogastric: 20–30 mL/min (1.2–1.8 L/hr) up to 4 L
Constipation (MiraLax and others):
  Child (limited data in 20 children with chronic constipation, 18 mo–11 yr; see remarks): a mean effective dose of 0.84 g/kg/24 hr PO ÷ BID for 8 wk (range: 0.25–1.42 g/kg/24 hr) was used to yield two soft stools per day. Do not exceed 17 g/24 hr. If patient weighs > 20 kg, use adult dose.
  Adult: 17 g (one heaping tablespoonful) mixed in 240 mL of water, juice, soda, coffee, or tea PO once daily
Fecal impaction (Miralax and others):
  >3 yr: 1–1.5 g/kg/24 hr (**max. dose**: 100 g/24 hr) PO × 3 days. Following disimpaction, give a maintenance dose of 0.4 g/24 hr ≥2 months.

Contraindicated in polyethylene glycol hypersensitivity. Monitor electrolytes, BUN, serum glucose, and urine osmolality with prolonged administration. Seizures resulting from electrolyte abnormalities have been reported.
BOWEL CLEANSING: Contraindicated in toxic megacolon, gastric retention, colitis, and bowel perforation. **Use with caution** in patients prone to aspiration or with impaired gag reflex. Effect should occur within 1–2 hr. Solution generally more palatable if chilled.
CONSTIPATION (MiraLax and others): Contraindicated in bowel obstruction.
Child: Dilute powder using the ratio of 17 g powder to 240 mL of water, juice, or milk. An onset of action within 1 wk in 12 of 20 patients, with the remaining 8 patients reporting improvement during the second wk of therapy. Side effects reported in this trial included diarrhea, flatulence, and mild abdominal pain. [See *J Pediatr* 2001;139(3):428-432 for additional information.]
Adult: 2–4 days may be required to produce a bowel movement. Most common side effects include nausea, abdominal bloating, cramping, and flatulence. Use beyond 2 wk has not been studied.

POLYMYXIN B SULFATE AND BACITRACIN

See Bacitracin ± Polymyxin B

POLYMYXIN B SULFATE AND TRIMETHOPRIM SULFATE
Polytrim Ophthalmic Solution and generics
Topical antibiotic (ophthalmic preparations listed)

No   No   2   C

Ophthalmic solution: Polymyxin B sulfate 10,000 U/mL, and trimethoprim sulfate 1 mg/mL (10 mL); some preparations may contain 0.04 mg/mL benzalkonium chloride

≥2 mo and adult: Instill 1 drop in the affected eye(s) Q3 hr (**max.** of 6 doses/24 hr) × 7–10 days.

POLYMYXIN B SULFATE AND TRIMETHOPRIM SULFATE continued

Active against susceptible strains of *S. aureus, S. epidermidis, S. pneumoniae, S. viridans, H. influenzae,* and *P. aeruginosa.* **Not indicated** for the prophylaxis or treatment of ophthalmia neonatorum. Local irritation consisting of redness, burning, stinging, and/or itching is common. Hypersensitivity reactions consisting of lid edema, itching, increased redness, tearing, and/or circumocular rash have been reported.

Apply finger pressure to lacrimal sac during and for 1–2 min after dose application.

POLYMYXIN B SULFATE, NEOMYCIN SULFATE, HYDROCORTISONE OTIC
Generics; previously available as Cortisporin Otic
Topical otic antibiotic

No   No   2   C

Otic solution or suspension: Polymyxin B sulfate 10,000 U/mL, neomycin sulfate 5 mg/mL (3.5 mg/mL neomycin base), hydrocortisone 10 mg/mL (10 mL); some preparations may contain thimerosol and metabisulfite.
For ophthalmic suspension, see NEOMYCIN/POLYMYXIN B OPHTHALMIC PRODUCTS

Otitis externa:
≥2 yr–adult: 3–4 drops TID–QID × 7–10 days. If preferred, a cotton wick may be saturated and inserted into ear canal. Moisten wick with antibiotic every 4 hr. Change wick Q24 hr.

Contraindicated in patients with active varicella and herpes simplex and in cases with perforated eardrum (possible ototoxicity). Use with caution in chronic otitis media and when the integrity of the tympanic membrane is in question. Metabisulfite containing products may cause allergic reactions to susceptible individuals. Hypersensitivity (itching, skin rash, redness, swelling, or other sign of irritation in or around the ear) may occur. Neomycin may cause sensitization. Prolonged treatment may result in overgrowth of nonsusceptible organisms and fungi. May cause cutaneous sensitization.
Shake suspension well before use. Warm the medication to body temperature prior to use.

POLYTRIM OPHTHALMIC SOLUTION

See Polymixin B Sulfate and Trimethoprim Sulfate

POLYSPORIN

See Bacitracin ± Polymyxin B

PORACTANT ALFA

See Surfactant, pulmonary

POTASSIUM IODIDE
Iosat, SSKI, ThyroShield, ThyroSafe, and others
Antithyroid agent

No   Yes   X   D

Tabs:
 Iosat [OTC]: 65 mg (50 mg iodine), 130 mg
 ThyroSafe [OTC]: 65 mg

Continued

POTASSIUM IODIDE continued

Oral solution:
 ThyroShield [OTC]: 65 mg/mL (30 mL); contains parabens and saccharin
 Saturated solution (SSKI): 1000 mg/mL (30, 240 mL); 10 drops = 500 mg potassium iodide
Potassium content is 6 mEq (234 mg) K⁺/gram potassium iodide

Neonatal Grave's disease: 50–100 mg (about 1–2 drops of SSKI) PO once daily
Thyrotoxicosis:
 Child: 50–250 mg (about 1–5 drops of SSKI) PO TID
 Adult: 50–500 mg (1–10 drops of SSKI) PO TID
Cutaneous or lymphocutaneous sporotrichosis (treat for 4–6 wk after lesions have completely healed; increase dose until either max. dose is achieved or signs of intolerance appear):
 Child and adolescent (limited data): 50 mg PO TID. Dose may be gradually increased as tolerated to the **max. dose** of the lesser of 50 mg/kg/dose or 2000–2500 mg PO TID.
 Adult: Start with 250 mg PO TID. Doses may be gradually increased as tolerated to the **max. dose** of 2000–2500 mg PO TID.

Contraindicated in pregnancy, hyperkalemia, iodine-induced goiter, and hypothyroidism. **Use with caution** in cardiac disease and renal failure. GI disturbance, metallic taste, rash, salivary gland inflammation, headache, lacrimation, and rhinitis are symptoms of iodism. Give with milk or water after meals. Monitor thyroid function tests. Onset of antithyroid effects: 1–2 days.
Lithium carbonate and iodide-containing medications may have synergistic hypothyroid activity. Potassium-containing medications, potassium-sparing diuretics, and ACE inhibitors may increase serum potassium levels.
For use as a thyroid blocking agent in nuclear or radiation emergencies, see http://www.fda.gov/drugs/emergencypreparedness/bioterrorismanddrugpreparedness/ucm319791.htm.

POTASSIUM SUPPLEMENTS
Many brand names and generics
Electrolyte

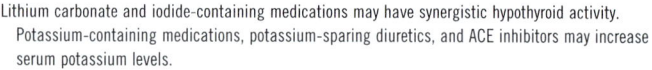

No Yes 1 C

Potassium chloride (40 mEq K = 3 g KCl):
 Sustained-release caps: 8, 10 mEq
 Sustained-release tabs: 8, 10, 15, 20 mEq
 Powder: 20, 25 mEq/packet
 Oral solution/liquid: 10% (6.7 mEq/5 mL), 20% (13.3 mEq/5 mL) (473 mL)
 Concentrated injection: 2 mEq/mL
Potassium gluconate (40 mEq K = 9.4 g K gluconate):
 Tabs: 465 mg (2 mEq), 581 mg (2.5 mEq)
 Caps [OTC as K-99]: 595 mg (2.56 mEq)
Potassium acetate (40 mEq K = 3.9 g K acetate):
 Concentrated injection: 2, 4 mEq/mL
Potassium bicarbonate/citric acid (10 mEq K = 1 g K bicarbonate):
 Effervescent tab for oral solution (Effer-K): 10, 20, 25 mEq; each 10 mEq K contains 0.84 g citric acid
Potassium phosphate:
 See *Phosphorus Supplements*

Normal daily requirements: See Chapter 21
Replacement: Determine based on maintenance requirements, deficit, and ongoing losses. See Chapter 11.

POTASSIUM SUPPLEMENTS continued

Hypokalemia:
  Oral:
   Child: 1–4 mEq/kg/24 hr ÷ BID–QID. Monitor serum potassium
   Adult: 40–100 mEq/24 hr ÷ BID–QID
  IV: MONITOR SERUM K CLOSELY
   Child: 0.5–1 mEq/kg/dose given as an infusion of 0.5 mEq/kg/hr × 1–2 hr
   Max. IV infusion rate: 1 mEq/kg/hr. This may be used in critical situations (i.e., hypokalemia with arrhythmia)
   Adult:
     Serum K ≥2.5 mEq/L: Replete at rates up to 10 mEq/hr. **Total dosage not to exceed** 200 mEq/24 hr
     Serum K <2 mEq/L: Replete at rates up to 40 mEq/hr. **Total dosage not to exceed** 400 mEq/24 hr
  Max. peripheral IV solution concentration: 40 mEq/L
  Max. concentration for central line administration: 150–200 mEq/L

PO administration may cause GI disturbance and ulceration. Oral liquid supplements should be diluted in water or fruit juice prior to administration. Sustained-release tablets must be swallowed whole and **NOT** dissolved in the mouth or chewed.

Do not administer IV potassium undiluted. IV administration may cause irritation, pain, and phlebitis at the infusion site. **Rapid or central IV infusion may cause cardiac arrhythmias.** Patients receiving infusion >0.5 mEq/kg/hr (>20 mEq/hr for adults) should be placed on an ECG monitor.

PRALIDOXIME CHLORIDE
Protopam, 2-PAM, and generics
In combination with atropine: Duodote, ATNAA
Antidote, organophosphate poisoning

No   Yes   ?   C

Injection (Protopam): 1000 mg
Injection for intramuscular injection, in auto-injector device: 600 mg/2 mL (2 mL); dispenses 600 mg; contains benzyl alcohol
In combination with atropine (Duodote, ATNNA): 600 mg/2 mL of pralidoxime and 2.1 mg/0.7 mL of atropine; contains benzyl alcohol. Duodote or ATNNA must be administered by emergency medical services personnel who have had adequate training in the recognition and treatment of nerve agent or insecticide intoxication

Organophosphate poisoning (use with atropine):
  Child:
   IV intermittent: 20–50 mg/kg/dose (**max. dose:** 2000 mg) × 1 IV. May repeat in 1–2 hr if muscle weakness is not relieved, then at Q10–12 hr PRN if cholinergic signs reappear
   IV continuous infusion: loading dose of 20–50 mg/kg/dose (**max. dose:** 2000 mg) IV over 15–30 min followed by 10–20 mg/kg/hr
   IM:
     <40 kg: 15 mg/kg/dose × 1 IM. May repeat Q15 min PRN up to a **max. total dose** of 45 mg/kg for mild symptoms; may repeat twice in rapid succession for severe symptoms (**max. total dose** of 45 mg/kg). For persistent symptoms, may repeat another max. 45 mg/kg series (in three divided doses) approximately 1 hr after the last injection
     ≥40 kg: 600 mg × 1 IM. May repeat Q15 min PRN up to a **max. total dose** of 1800 mg for mild symptoms; may repeat twice in rapid succession for severe symptoms (**max. total dose** of

Continued

PRALIDOXIME CHLORIDE continued

1800 mg). For persistent symptoms, may repeat another **max.** 1800 mg series (in three divided doses) approximately 1 hr after the last injection.
Adult:
   IV intermittent: 1–2 g/dose × 1 IV. May repeat in 1–2 hr if muscle weakness is not relieved, then at Q10–12 hr PRN if cholinergic signs reappear
   IM: Use ≥ 40 kg child IM dosage from above

Contraindicated in poisoning due to phosphorus, inorganic phosphates, or organic phosphates without anticholinesterase activity. **Do not use** as an antidote for carbamate classes of pesticides. Removal of secretions and maintaining a patent airway is critical. May cause muscle rigidity, laryngospasm, and tachycardia after rapid IV infusion. Drug is generally ineffective if administered 36–48 hr after exposure. Additional doses may be necessary.
For IV administration, dilute to 50 mg/mL or less and infuse over 15–30 min (**not to exceed** 200 mg/min). Reduce dosage in renal impairment because 80%–90% of the drug is excreted unchanged in the urine 12 hr after administration.

PREDNISOLONE
Oral products:
  Orapred ODT, Prelone, Pediapred, Millipred, Veripred 20, and generics
Ophthalmic products:
  Pred Forte, Pred Mild, Omnipred and generics
Corticosteroid

No   No   2   C/D

Tabs: 5 mg
Syrup (Prelone and generics): 15 mg/5 mL (240 mL); may contain alcohol and saccharin
Tablets, orally disintegrating (as Na phosphate) (Orapred ODT and generics): 10, 15, 30 mg
Oral solution (as Na phosphate):
  Pediapred and generics: 5 mg/5 mL (120 mL); alcohol and dye free
  Generics: 15 mg/5 mL (237 mL); may contain 2% alcohol and is dye free
  Millipred: 10 mg/5 mL (237 mL); contains parabens and is dye free
  Veripred 20: 20 mg/5 mL (237 mL); alcohol and dye free; and contains parabens
Ophthalmic suspension (as acetate; both strengths contain benzalkonium chloride and may contain bisulfites):
  Pred Mild: 0.12% (5, 10 mL)
  Omnipred, PredForte, and generics: 1% (5, 10, 15 mL)
Ophthalmic solution (as Na phosphate): 1% (10 mL); may contain benzalkonium chloride

See *Prednisone* for oral dosing (equivalent dosing).
Ophthalmic (consult ophthalmologist before use):
  Child and adult: Start with 1–2 drops Q1 hr during the day and Q2 hr during the night until favorable response, then reduce dose to 1 drop Q4 hr. Dose may be further reduced to 1 drop TID–QID.

See *Prednisone* for remarks. See Chapter 10 for relative steroid potencies. Pregnancy category changes to "D" if used in the first trimester.
OPHTHALMIC USE: Contraindicated in viral (e.g., herpes simplex, vaccinia, and varicella), fungal, and mycobacterial infections of the cornea and conjunctiva. Increase in intraocular pressure, cataract formation, and delayed wound healing may occur.

PREDNISONE
Deltasone, Rayos, and generics
Corticosteroid

Yes   No   2   C/D

Tabs (Deltasone and generics): 1, 2.5, 5, 10, 20, 50 mg
Delayed-release tabs (Rayos): 1, 2, 5 mg
Oral solution: 1 mg/mL (120, 500 mL); may contain 5% alcohol and saccharin
Concentrated solution: 5 mg/mL (30 mL); contains 30% alcohol

Antiinflammatory/immunosuppressive:
  Child: 0.5–2 mg/kg/24 hr PO ÷ once daily–BID
Acute asthma:
  Child: 2 mg/kg/24 hr PO ÷ once daily–BID × 5–7 days; **max. dose**: 80 mg/24 hr. Patients may benefit from tapering if therapy exceeds 5–7 days.
Asthma exacerbations (2007 National Heart, Lung, and Blood Institute Guideline Recommendations; dose until peak expiratory flow reaches 70% of predicted or personal best):
  Child ≤12 yr: 1–2 mg/kg/24 hr PO ÷ Q12 hr (**max. dose:** 60 mg/24 hr)
  >12 yr and adult: 40–80 mg/24 hr PO ÷ Q12–24 hr
Outpatient asthma exacerbation burst therapy (longer durations may be necessary):
  Child ≤12 yr: 1–2 mg/kg/24 hr PO ÷ Q12–24 hr (**max. dose:** 60 mg/24 hr) × 3–10 days
  Child >12 yr and adult: 40–60 mg/24 hr PO ÷ Q12–24 hr × 5–10 days
Nephrotic syndrome:
  Child: Starting dose of 2 mg/kg/24 hr PO (**max. dose:** 60 mg/24 hr) ÷ once daily–TID is recommended. Further treatment plans are individualized. Consult a nephrologist

See Chapter 10 for physiologic replacement, relative steroid potencies, and doses based on body surface area. Methylprednisolone is preferable in hepatic disease because prednisone must be converted to methylprednisolone in the liver.

Side effects may include: mood changes, seizures, hyperglycemia, diarrhea, nausea, abdominal distension, GI bleeding, HPA axis suppression, osteopenia, cushingoid effects, and cataracts with prolonged use. Prednisone is a CYP450 3A3/4 substrate and inducer. Barbiturates, carbamazepine, phenytoin, rifampin, isoniazid, may reduce the effects of prednisone, whereas estrogens may enhance the effects. Pregnancy category changes to "D" if used in the first trimester.

PRIMAQUINE PHOSPHATE
Various generics
Antimalarial

No   No   ?   C

Tabs: 26.3 mg (15 mg base)
Oral suspension: 10.52 mg (6 mg base)/5 mL

Doses expressed in mg of primaquine base:
Malaria:
  Prevention of relapses for P. vivax or P. ovale only (initiate therapy during the last 2 wk of, or following a course of, suppression with chloroquine or comparable drug):
    Child: 0.5 mg/kg/dose (**max. dose:** 30 mg/dose) PO once daily × 14 days
    Adult: 30 mg PO once daily × 14 days

Continued

PRIMAQUINE PHOSPHATE continued

Malaria:
  Prevention of chloroquine-resistant strains (initiate 1 day prior to departure and continue until 3–7 days after leaving endemic area):
    Child: 0.5 mg/kg/dose PO once daily; **max. dose:** 30 mg/24 hr
    Adult: 30 mg PO once daily
Pneumocystis jiroveci (carinii) pneumonia (in combination with clindamycin):
    Child: 0.3 mg/kg/dose (**max. dose:** 30 mg/dose) PO once daily × 21 days
    Adult: 30 mg PO once daily × 21 days

Contraindicated in granulocytopenia (e.g., rheumatoid arthritis and lupus erythematosus) and bone marrow suppression. **Avoid use** with quinacrine and with other drugs that have a potential for causing hemolysis or bone marrow suppression. **Use with caution** in G6PD and NADH methemoglobin-reductase deficient patients due to increased risk for hemolytic anemia and leukopenia, respectively. Monitor ECG for QTc prolongation in patients with cardiac disease, history of arrhythmias, uncorrected hypokalemia and/or hypomagnesemia, bradycardia, and receiving concomitant QTc prolonging medications. Use in pregnancy is **not recommended** by the AAP *Red Book*. Cross sensitivity with iodoquinol.

May cause headache, visual disturbances, nausea, vomiting, and abdominal cramps. Hemolytic anemia, leukopenia, cardiac arrhythmia, QTc interval prolongation, and methemoglobinemia have been reported. Administer all doses with food to mask bitter taste.

PRIMIDONE
Mysoline and generics
Anticonvulsant, barbiturate

Yes Yes 2 D

Tabs: 50, 250 mg

Neonate: 12–20 mg/kg/24 hr PO ÷ BID–QID; initiate therapy at the lower dosage range and titrate upwards

Child, adolescent, and adult:

Day of Therapy	<8 yr	≥8 yr and Adult
Days 1–3	50 mg PO QHS	100–125 mg PO QHS
Days 4–6	50 mg PO BID	100–125 mg PO BID
Days 7–9	100 mg PO BID	100–125 mg PO TID
Day 10 and thereafter	125–250 mg PO TID or 10–25 mg/kg/ 24 hr ÷ TID–QID	250 mg PO TID–QID; **max. dose:** 2 g/24 hr

Use with caution in renal or hepatic disease and pulmonary insufficiency. Primidone is metabolized to phenobarbital and has the same drug interactions and toxicities (see *Phenobarbital*). Additionally, primidone may cause vertigo, nausea, leukopenia, malignant lymphoma-like syndrome, diplopia, nystagmus, systemic lupus-like syndrome. Monitor for suicidal behavior or ideation. Acetazolamide may decrease primidone absorption. **Adjust dose in renal failure (see Chapter 30).**

Follow both primidone and phenobarbital levels. Therapeutic levels: 5–12 mg/L of primidone and 15–40 mg/L of phenobarbital. Recommended serum sampling time at steady-state: trough level obtained within 30 min prior to the next scheduled dose after 1–4 days of continuous dosing.

PROBENECID
Various generics
Penicillin therapy adjuvant, uric acid lowering agent

No   Yes   ?   B

Tabs: 500 mg

To prolong penicillin levels.
  Child (2–14 yr): 25 mg/kg PO × 1, then 40 mg/kg/24 hr ÷ QID; **max. single dose:** 500 mg/dose. Use adult dose if >50 kg
  Adult: 500 mg PO QID
Hyperuricemia:
  Adult: 250 mg PO BID × 1 wk, then 500 mg PO BID; may increase by 500 mg increments Q4 wk PRN up to a **max. dose** of 2–3 g/24 hr ÷ BID
Gonorrhea, antibiotic adjunct (administer just prior to antibiotic):
  ≤45 kg: 23 mg/kg/dose PO × 1
  >45 kg: 1 g PO × 1
Prevention of nephrotoxicity from cidofovir: see Cidofovir.

Use with caution in patients with peptic ulcer disease. **Contraindicated** in children <2 yr and patients with renal insufficiency. **Do not use** if GFR < 30 mL/min.
Increases uric acid excretion. Inhibits renal tubular secretion of acyclovir, ganciclovir, ciprofloxacin, levofloxacin, nalidixic acid, moxifloxacin, organic acids, penicillins, cephalosporins, AZT, dapsone, methotrexate, nonsteroidal antiinflammatory agents, and benzodiazepines. Salicylates may decrease probenecid's activity. Alkalinize urine in patients with gout. May cause headache, GI symptoms, rash, anemia, and hypersensitivity. False-positive glucosuria with Clinitest may occur.

PROCAINAMIDE
Various generics
Antiarrhythmic, class Ia

Yes   Yes   X   C

Injection: 100 mg/mL (10 mL), 500 mg/mL (2 mL); may contain methylparabens and bisulfites

Child (limited data):
  IV: Load with 15 mg/kg/dose IV or IO × 1 over 30–60 min. Then followed by maintenance continuous IV infusion of 20–80 mcg/kg/min; **max. dose:** 2 g/24 hr
  IM: 20–30 mg/kg/24 hr ÷ Q4–6 hr; **max. dose:** 4 g/24 hr (peak effect in 1 hr)
Adult:
  IV: Load: 50–100 mg/dose; repeat dose Q5 min PRN to a max. total dose of 1000–1500 mg
    Maintenance: 1–6 mg/min by continuous infusion
  IM: 50 mg/kg/24 hr ÷ Q3–6 hr
NOTE: The IV infusion dosage units for adults are in mg/min compared with mcg/kg/min for children.

Contraindicated in myasthenia gravis, complete heart block, SLE, and torsade de pointes. **Use with caution** in asymptomatic premature ventricular contractions, digitalis intoxication, CHF, and renal or hepatic dysfunction. **Adjust dose in renal failure (see Chapter 30).**
May cause lupus-like syndrome, positive Coombs test, thrombocytopenia, arrhythmias, GI complaints, and confusion. Increased LFTs and liver failure have been reported. Monitor BP and ECG when using IV. QRS widening by >0.02 sec suggests toxicity.
Do not use with desipramine and other TCAs. Cimetidine, ranitidine, amiodarone, β-blockers, and trimethoprim may increase procainamide levels. Procainamide may enhance the effects of skeletal

Continued

PROCAINAMIDE *continued*

muscle relaxants and anticholinergic agents. Therapeutic levels: 4–10 mg/L of procainamide or 10–30 mg/L of procainamide and NAPA levels combined.

Recommended serum sampling times:
IM intermittent dosing: Trough level within 30 min prior to the next scheduled dose after 2 days of continuous dosing (steady state).
IV continuous infusion: 2 and 12 hr after start of infusion and at 24-hr intervals thereafter.

PROCHLORPERAZINE
Compro and generics; previously available as Compazine
Antiemetic, phenothiazine derivative

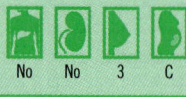

No   No   3   C

Tabs (as maleate): 5, 10 mg
Suppository (Compro and generics): 25 mg (12s)
Injection (as edisylate): 5 mg/mL (2 mL); may contain benzyl alcohol

Antiemetic doses:
  Child (>10 kg or >2 yr):
    PO or PR: 0.4 mg/kg/24 hr ÷ TID–QID or alternative dosing by weight:
      10–14 kg: 2.5 mg once daily–BID; **max. dose:** 7.5 mg/24 hr
      15–18 kg: 2.5 mg BID–TID; **max. dose:** 10 mg/24 hr
      19–39 kg: 2.5 mg TID or 5 mg BID; **max. dose:** 15 mg/24 hr
      >39 kg: Use adult dose
    IM: 0.1–0.15 mg/kg/dose BID–TID; **max. dose:** 10 mg/single dose or 40 mg/24 hr
  Adult:
    PO: 5–10 mg/dose TID–QID; **max. dose:** 40 mg/24 hr
    PR: 25 mg/dose BID
    IM: 5–10 mg/dose Q3–4 hr
    IV: 2.5–10 mg/dose; may repeat Q3–4 hr
    Max. IM/IV dose: 40 mg/24 hr
Psychoses:
  Child 2–12 yr and >9 kg:
    PO: Start with 2.5 mg BID–TID with a **max. first day dose** of 10 mg/24 hr. Dose may be increased as needed to 20 mg/24 hr for children 2–5 yr and 25 mg/24 hr for 6–12 yr.
    IM: 0.13 mg/kg/dose × 1 and convert to PO immediately.
  Adult:
    PO: 5–10 mg TID–QID; may be increased as needed to a **max. dose** of 150 mg/24 hr
    IM: 10–20 mg Q2–4 hr PRN convert to PO immediately.
Intractable migraines:
  Child (5–18 yr, limited data): 0.15 mg/kg/dose IV over 10 min was effective in migraine headaches presenting in the emergency departments (see *Ann Emerg Med.* 2004;43:256-262).

Toxicity as for other phenothiazines (see *Chlorpromazine*). Extrapyramidal reactions (reversed by diphenhydramine) or orthostatic hypotension may occur. May mask signs and symptoms of overdosage of other drugs and may obscure the diagnosis and treatment of conditions such as intestinal obstruction, brain tumor, and Reye's syndrome. May cause false-positive test for phenylketonuria, urinary amylase, uroporphyrins, and urobilinogen. **Do not use** IV route in children. Use only in management of prolonged vomiting of known etiology.

PROMETHAZINE
Phenergan and generics
Antihistamine, antiemetic, phenothiazine derivative

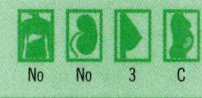
No   No   3   C

Tabs: 12.5, 25, 50 mg
Oral solution/syrup: 6.25 mg/5 mL (118, 473 mL); contains alcohol
Suppository: 12.5, 25, 50 mg (12s)
Injection: 25, 50 mg/mL (1 mL); may contain sulfites and phenol

Antihistaminic:
  Child ≥ 2 yr: 0.1 mg/kg/dose (**max. dose**: 12.5 mg/dose) Q6 hr PO during the day hours and 0.5 mg/kg/dose (**max. dose**: 25 mg/dose) QHS PO PRN
  Adult: 6.25–12.5 mg PO/PR TID and 25 mg QHS
Nausea and vomiting PO/IM/IV/PR (see remarks):
  Child ≥ 2 yr: 0.25–1 mg/kg/dose Q4–6 hr PRN; **max. dose**: 25 mg/dose
  Adult: 12.5–25 mg Q4–6 hr PRN
Motion sickness: (1st dose 0.5–1 hr before departure):
  Child ≥ 2 yr: 0.5 mg/kg/dose Q12 hr PO/PR PRN; **max. dose**: 25 mg/dose
  Adult: 25 mg PO Q8–12 hr PRN

Avoid use in children <2 yr because of risk for fatal respiratory depression. Toxicity similar to other phenothiazines (see *Chlorpromazine*). **Do not** administer SC or intra-arterially because of severe local reactions. IV route of administration is **not recommended** (IM preferred) due to severe tissue injury (tissue necrosis and gangrene). If using IV route, dilute 25 mg/mL strength product with 10–20 mL NS and administer over 10–15 min, consider lower initial doses, administer through a large-bore vein and check patency of line before administering, administer through an IV line at the port farthest from the patient's vein, and monitor for burning or pain during or after injection. Administer oral doses with meals to decrease GI irritation.

May cause profound sedation, blurred vision, respiratory depression (use lowest effective dose in children and **avoid** concomitant use of respiratory depressants), and dystonic reactions (reversed by diphenhydramine). Cholestatic jaundice and neuroleptic malignant syndrome has been reported. May interfere with pregnancy tests (immunological reactions between hCG and anti-hCG). **For nausea and vomiting, use only in management of prolonged vomiting of known etiology.**

PROPRANOLOL
Inderal, Inderal LA, Hemangeol, and generics
Adrenergic blocking agent (β), class II antiarrhythmic

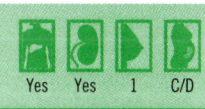
Yes   Yes   1   C/D

Tabs: 10, 20, 40, 60, 80 mg
Extended-release caps (Inderal LA and others including generics): 60, 80, 120, 160 mg
Oral solution: 20 mg/5 mL, 40 mg/5 mL; contains parabens and saccharin
  Hemangeol: 4.28 mg/mL (120 mL); alcohol, sugar and parben free; contains saccharin
Injection: 1 mg/mL (1 mL)

Arrhythmias:
  Child:
    IV: 0.01–0.1 mg/kg/dose IV push over 10 min, repeat Q6–8 hr PRN; **max. dose**: 1 mg/dose for infant; 3 mg/dose for child
    PO: Start at 0.5–1 mg/kg/24 hr ÷ Q6–8 hr; increase dosage Q3–5 days PRN. Usual dosage range: 2–4 mg/kg/24 hr ÷ Q6–8 hr; **max. dose**: 60 mg/24 hr or 16 mg/kg/24 hr

Continued

PROPRANOLOL continued

Arrhythmias:
Adult:
  IV: 1 mg/dose Q5 min up to total 5 mg
  PO: 10–30 mg/dose TID–QID; increase PRN. Usual dosage range: 30–160 mg/24 hr ÷ TID–QID

Hypertension:
Child:
  PO: Initial: 0.5–1 mg/kg/24 hr ÷ Q6–12 hr. May increase dose Q5–7 days PRN; **max. dose**: 8 mg/kg/24 hr
Adult:
  PO: 40 mg/dose PO BID or 60–80 mg/dose (sustained-release capsule) PO once daily. May increase 10–20 mg/dose Q3–7 days; **max. dose**: 640 mg/24 hr

Migraine prophylaxis:
Child:
  <35 kg: 10–20 mg PO TID
  ≥35 kg: 20–40 mg PO TID
Adult: 80 mg/24 hr ÷ Q6–8 hr PO; increase dose by 20–40 mg/dose Q3–4 wk PRN. Usual effective dose range: 160–240 mg/24 hr

Tetralogy spells:
IV: 0.15–0.25 mg/kg/dose slow IV push. May repeat in 15 min × 1. See also Chapter 7.
PO: Start at 2–4 mg/kg/24 hr ÷ Q6 hr PRN. Usual dose range: 4–8 mg/kg/24 hr ÷ Q6 hr PRN. Doses as high as 15 mg/kg/24 hr have been used with careful monitoring.

Thyrotoxicosis:
Neonate: 2 mg/kg/24 hr PO ÷ Q6–12 hr
Adolescent and adult:
  IV: 1–3 mg/dose over 10 min. May repeat in 4–6 hr
  PO: 10–40 mg/dose PO Q6 hr

Infantile hemangioma (see remarks):
Infant (5 wk–5 mo and ≥2 kg; labelled dosing information for Hemangeol product): 0.6 mg/kg/dose BID PO (at least 9 hr apart) × 7 days, then increase to 1.1 mg/kg/dose BID PO × 14 days, followed by 1.7 mg/kg/dose BID PO × 6 mo
Alternative dosing: Start at 1 mg/kg/24 hr ÷ Q8 hr PO. If tolerated after one day, increase dose to 2 mg/kg/24 hr ÷ Q8 hr PO

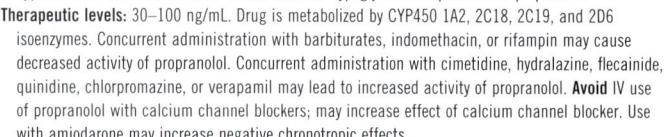

Contraindicated in asthma, Raynaud's syndrome, heart failure, and heart block. **Not indicated** for the treatment of hypertensive emergencies. **Use with caution** in presence of obstructive lung disease, diabetes mellitus, and renal or hepatic disease. May cause hypoglycemia, hypotension, nausea, vomiting, depression, weakness, impotence, bronchospasm, and heart block. Cutaneous reactions, including Stevens–Johnson, TEN, exfoliative dermatitis, erythema multiforme, and utricaria have been reported. Acute hypertension has occurred after insulin-induced hypoglycemia in patients on propranolol.

Therapeutic levels: 30–100 ng/mL. Drug is metabolized by CYP450 1A2, 2C18, 2C19, and 2D6 isoenzymes. Concurrent administration with barbiturates, indomethacin, or rifampin may cause decreased activity of propranolol. Concurrent administration with cimetidine, hydralazine, flecainide, quinidine, chlorpromazine, or verapamil may lead to increased activity of propranolol. **Avoid** IV use of propranolol with calcium channel blockers; may increase effect of calcium channel blocker. Use with amiodarone may increase negative chronotropic effects.

For infantile hemangioma, monitor BP and HR 2 hr after initiating therapy and after dose increases. To reduce risk of hypoglycemia, administer doses during or right after a feeding; hold doses if child is not eating or is vomiting. Infants <6 mo must be fed every 4 hr. Readjust dose periodically with changes (increases) in child's body weight. Successful use in infantile hepatic hemangiomas has also been reported.

Pregnancy category changes to "D" if used in second or third trimesters.

PROPYLTHIOURACIL
PTU and generics
Antithyroid agent

Yes   Yes   2   D

Tabs: 50 mg
Oral suspension: 5 mg/mL
100 mg PTU = 10 mg methimazole

Dosages should be adjusted as required to achieve and maintain T₄, TSH levels in normal ranges.
Neonate: 5–10 mg/kg/24 hr ÷ Q8 hr PO
Child:
  Initial: 5–7 mg/kg/24 hr ÷ Q8 hr PO, OR by age
    6–10 yr: 50–150 mg/24 hr ÷ Q8 hr PO
    >10 yr: 150–300 mg/24 hr ÷ Q8 hr PO
  Maintenance: Generally begins after 2 mo. Usually 1/3–2/3 the initial dose in divided doses (Q8–12 hr) when the patient is euthyroid
Adult:
  Initial: 300–400 mg/24 hr ÷ Q6–8 hr PO; some may require larger doses of 600–900 mg/24 hr
  Maintenance: 100–150 mg/24 hr ÷ Q8 hr PO

Generally reserved for patients who are unable to tolerate methimazole and for whom radioactive iodine or surgery are not appropriate. May be the antithyroid treatment of choice during or just prior to the first trimester of pregnancy because of risk for fetal abnormalities associated with methimazole.

May cause blood dyscrasias, fever, liver disease, dermatitis, urticaria, malaise, CNS stimulation or depression, and arthralgias. Glomerulonephritis, severe liver injury/failure, agranulocytosis, interstitial pneumonitis, exfoliative dermatitis, and erythema nodosum have also been reported. May decrease the effectiveness of warfarin. Monitor thyroid function. A dose reduction of β-blocker may be necessary when the hyperthyroid patient becomes euthyroid.

For neonates, crush tablets, weigh appropriate dose, and mix in formula/breast milk. **Adjust dose in renal failure (see Chapter 30).**

PROSTAGLANDIN E₁

See Alprostadil

PROTAMINE SULFATE
Various generics
Antidote, heparin

No   No   ?   C

Injection: 10 mg/mL (5, 25 mL); preservative free

Heparin antidote, IV:
1 mg protamine will neutralize 115 U porcine intestinal heparin, or 100 U (1 mg) low-molecular-weight heparin.
  Consider time since last heparin dose:
    If <0.5 hr: give 100% of specified dose
    If within 0.5–1 hr: give 50%–75% of aforementioned dose
    If within 1–2 hr: give 37.5%–50% of aforementioned dose

Continued

PROTAMINE SULFATE continued

Heparin antidote IV (continued; time since last heparin dose):
  If ≥2 hr: give 25%–37.5% of aforementioned dose
  Max. dose: 50 mg/dose IV
  Max. infusion rate: 5 mg/min
  Max. IV concentration: 10 mg/mL
If heparin was administered by deep SC injection, give 1–1.5 mg protamine per 100 U heparin as follows:
  Load with 25–50 mg via slow IV infusion followed by the rest of the calculated dose via continuous infusion over 8–16 hr or the expected duration of heparin absorption.
Enoxaparin overdosage, IV (see remarks): Approximately 1 mg protamine will neutralize 1 mg enoxaparin.
  Consider time since last enoxaparin dose:
    If <8 hr: give 100% of aforementioned dose.
    If within 8–12 hr: Give 50% of aforementioned dose.
    If >12 hr: Protamine not required but if serious bleeding is present, give 50% of aforementioned dose.
    If aPTT remains prolonged 2–4 hr after the first protamine dose, a second infusion of 0.5 mg protamine per 1 mg enoxaparin may be given.
  Max. dose: 50 mg/dose. See *Heparin* antidote IV dosage for **max.** administration concentration and rate.

Risk factors for protamine hypersensitivity include known hypersensitivity to fish and exposure to protamine-containing insulin or prior protamine therapy.
May cause hypotension, bradycardia, dyspnea, and anaphylaxis. Monitor aPTT or ACT. Heparin rebound with bleeding has been reported to occur 8–18 hr later.
Use in enoxaparin overdose may not be complete despite using multiple doses of protamine.

PSEUDOEPHEDRINE
Sudafed, Sudafed 12 Hour, Sudafed 24 Hour, and generics
Sympathomimetic, nasal decongestant

No Yes 2 C

Tabs (OTC): 30, 60 mg
Extended-release tab (OTC):
  Sudafed 12 Hour and generics: 120 mg
  Sudafed 24 Hour: 240 mg
Oral liquid (OTC): 15 mg/5 mL, 30 mg/5 mL (120 mL); may contain sodium benzoate
Oral syrup (OTC): 30 mg/5 mL (473 mL); contains parabens and sodium benzoate
Purchases of OTC products are limited to behind the pharmacy counter sales with monthly sale limits due to the methamphetamine epidemic.

Child <12 yr: 4 mg/kg/24 hr ÷ Q6 hr PO or by age
  <4 yr: 4 mg/kg/24 hr ÷ Q6 hr PO; **max. dose**: 60 mg/24 hr
  4–5 yr: 15 mg/dose Q4–6 hr PO; **max. dose**: 60 mg/24 hr
  6–12 yr: 30 mg/dose Q4–6 hr PO; **max. dose**: 120 mg/24 hr
Child ≥12 yr and adult:
  Immediate release: 30–60 mg/dose Q4–6 hr PO; **max. dose**: 240 mg/24 hr
  Sustained release:
    Sudafed 12 Hour and generics: 120 mg PO Q12 hr
    Sudafed 24 Hour: 240 mg PO Q24 hr

Contraindicated with MAO inhibitor drugs and in severe hypertension and severe coronary artery disease. **Use with caution** in mild/moderate hypertension, hyperglycemia,

PSEUDOEPHEDRINE continued

hyperthyroidism, and cardiac disease. May cause dizziness, nervousness, restlessness, insomnia, and arrhythmias. Pseudoephedrine is a common component of OTC cough and cold preparations and is combined with several antihistamines; these products are not recommended for children <6 yr. Because drug and active metabolite are primarily excreted renally, **doses should be adjusted in renal impairment.** May cause false-positive test for amphetamines (EMIT assay).

PSYLLIUM
Metamucil, Geri-Mucil, Konsyl, Reguloid, and many others including some generics
Bulk-forming laxative

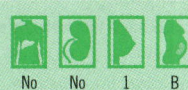

No   No   1   B

Granules [OTC]: 100% psyllium (Konsyl: 4.3 g psyllium/rounded teaspoon) (300 g); contains maltodextrin; sugar and gluten free
Powder [OTC]: 100% psyllium, some versions containing sucrose (sugar-free version available) (Metamucil and Geri-Mucil: 3.4 g psyllium/rounded teaspoon); for other products check label for the amount of psyllium per unit of measurement
Caps:
  Generics: 0.4 g
  Konsyl and Reguloid: 0.52 g
3.4 g psyllium hydrophilic mucilloid is equivalent 2 g soluble fiber

Constipation (granules or powder must be mixed with a full glass (240 mL) of water or juice):
<6 yr: 1.25–2.5 g/dose PO once daily–TID; **max. dose:** 7.5 g/24 hr
6–11 yr: 2.5–3.75 g/dose PO once daily–TID; **max. dose:** 15 g/24 hr
≥12 yr and adult: 2.5–7.5 g/dose PO once daily–TID; **max. dose:** 30 g/24 hr

Contraindicated in cases of fecal impaction or GI obstruction. **Use with caution** in patients with esophageal strictures and rectal bleeding. Phenylketonurics should be aware that certain preparations may contain aspartame. Should be taken or mixed with a full glass (240 mL) of liquid. Onset of action: 12–72 hr.

PYRANTEL PAMOATE
Reese's Pinworm, Pin-Rid, Pin-X, and other generics
Anthelmintic

Yes   No   2   C

Oral suspension (OTC): 50 mg/mL pyrantel base (144 mg/mL pyrantel pamoate) (30, 60 mL); may contain sodium benzoate, parabens, and saccharin
Tabs (OTC): 62.5 mg pyrantel base (180 mg pyrantel pamoate)
Chewable tabs (OTC): 250 mg pyrantel base (720.5 mg pyrantel pamoate); contains aspartame

All doses expressed in terms of pyrantel base.
Child (≥2 yr) and adult:
  Ascaris (roundworm) and Trichostrongylus: 11 mg/kg/dose PO × 1
  Enterobius (pinworm): 11 mg/kg/dose PO × 1. Repeat same dose 2 wk later
  Hookworm or eosinophilic enterocolitis: 11 mg/kg/dose PO once daily × 3 days
  Moniliformis: 11 mg/kg/dose PO × 1. Repeat twice 2 weeks apart
  Max. dose (all indications): 1 g/dose

Use with caution in liver dysfunction. **Do not use** in combination with piperazine because of antagonism. May cause nausea, vomiting, anorexia, transient AST elevations, headaches, rash, and muscle weakness. Limited experience in children <2 yr. May increase theophylline levels. Drug may be mixed with milk or fruit juice and may be taken with food.

PYRAZINAMIDE
Pyrazinoic acid amide and generics
Antituberculous agent

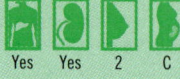
Yes Yes 2 C

Tab: 500 mg
Oral suspension: 10, 100 mg/mL
In combination with isoniazid and rifampin (Rifater):
  Tab: 300 mg with 50 mg isoniazid and 120 mg rifampin; contains povidone and propylene glycol

Tuberculosis: Use as part of a multidrug regimen for tuberculosis. See latest edition of the AAP Red Book for recommended treatment for tuberculosis.
  Child:
    Daily dose: 15–30 mg/kg/24 hr PO once daily; **max. dose:** 2 g/24 hr
    Twice-weekly dose: 50 mg/kg/dose PO 2 × per week; **max. dose:** 2 g/dose
  Adult:
    Daily dose: 15–30 mg/kg/24 hr PO once daily; **max. dose:** 2 g/24 hr
    Twice-weekly dose: 50–70 mg/kg/dose PO 2 × per week; **max. dose:** 4 g/dose

See latest edition of the AAP Red Book for recommended treatment for tuberculosis. **Contraindicated** in severe hepatic damage and acute gout. The CDC and ATS **do not recommend** the combination of pyrazinamide and rifampin for latent TB infections. **Use with caution** in patients with renal failure (dosage reduction has been recommended), gout or diabetes mellitus. Monitor liver function tests (baseline and periodic) and serum uric acid.
Hepatotoxicity is most common dose-related side effect; doses ≤30 mg/kg/24 hr minimize effect. Hyperuricemia, maculopapular rash, arthralgia, fever, acne, porphyria, dysuria, and photosensitivity may occur. Severe hepatic toxicity may occur with rifampin use. May decrease isoniazid levels.

PYRETHRINS WITH PIPERONYL BUTOXIDE
A-200, Pronto, RID, LiceMD, Licide, and others
Pediculicide

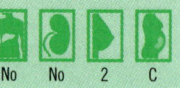
No No 2 C

All products are available without a prescription.
Gel (LiceMD): 0.3% pyrethrins and 3% piperonyl butoxide (30, 118 mL)
Shampoo (RID, Pronto, Licide, A-200): 0.33% pyrethrins and 4% piperonyl butoxide (60, 120, 240 mL); may contain alcohol

Pediculosis (≥2 yr and adult): Apply to hair or affected body area for 10 min, then wash thoroughly and comb with fine-tooth comb or nit-removing comb; repeat in 7–10 days.

Contraindicated in ragweed hypersensitivity; drug is derived from chrysanthemum flowers. For topical use only. **Avoid** use in and around the eyes, mouth, nose, or vagina. **Avoid** repeat applications in <24 hr. Low ovicidal activity requires repeat treatment. Dead nits require mechanical removal. Wash bedding and clothing to eradicate infestation.
Local irritation including erythema, pruritis, urticaria, edema, and eczema may occur.

PYRIDOSTIGMINE BROMIDE
Mestinon, Regonol, and other generics
Cholinergic agent

No Yes 1 B

Oral syrup (Mestinon): 60 mg/5 mL (480 mL); contains 5% alcohol and sodium benzoate
Tabs (Mestinon and generics): 60 mg

PYRIDOSTIGMINE BROMIDE continued

Sustained-release tab (Mestinon and generics): 180 mg
Injection (Regonol): 5 mg/mL (2 mL); may contain 0.2% parabens and benzyl alcohol

Myasthenia gravis:
  Neonate:
    PO: 5 mg/dose Q4–6 hr
    IM/IV: 0.05–0.15 mg/kg/dose Q4–6 hr; **max.** single IM/IV dose: 10 mg
  Child:
    PO: 7 mg/kg/24 hr in 5–6 divided doses
    IM/IV: 0.05–0.15 mg/kg/dose Q4–6 hr; **max.** single IM/IV dose: 10 mg
  Adult:
    PO (immediate release): 60 mg TID; increase Q48 hr PRN. Usual effective dose: 60–1500 mg/24 hr
    PO (sustained release): 180–540 mg once daily–BID
    IM/IV (use when PO therapy is not practical): Give 1/30 of the usual PO

Contraindicated in mechanical intestinal or urinary obstruction. **Use with caution** in patients with epilepsy, asthma, bradycardia, hyperthyroidism, arrhythmias, or peptic ulcer. May cause nausea, vomiting, diarrhea, rash, headache, and muscle cramps. Pyridostigmine is mainly excreted unchanged by the kidney. Therefore, lower doses titrated to effect in renal disease may be necessary.
Changes in oral dosages may take several days to show results. **Atropine is the antidote.**

PYRIDOXINE
Vitamin B$_6$ and various names including generics
Vitamin, water soluble

No   No   1   A/C

Tabs (HCl) [OTC]: 25, 50, 100, 250, 500 mg
Oral solution (HCl): 1 mg/mL
Injection (HCl): 100 mg/mL (1 mL); some products may contain aluminum

Deficiency, IM/IV/PO (PO preferred):
  Child: 5–25 mg/24 hr × 3 wk, followed by 2.5–5 mg/24 hr as maintenance therapy (via multivitamin preparation)
  Adolescent and adult: 10–20 mg/24 hr × 3 wk, followed by 2–5 mg/24 hr as maintenance therapy (via multivitamin preparation)
Drug-induced neuritis (PO):
  Prophylaxis:
    Child: 1 mg/kg/24 hr or 10–50 mg/24 hr
    Adolescent and adult: 25–50 mg/24 hr
  Treatment (optimal dose not established):
    Child: 50–200 mg/24 hr
    Adolescent and adult: 50–300 mg/24 hr
Pyridoxine-dependent seizures:
  Neonate and infant:
    Initial: 50–100 mg/dose IM or rapid IV × 1
    Maintenance: 50–100 mg/24 hr PO
Recommended daily allowance: See Chapter 21

Use caution with concurrent levodopa therapy. Chronic administration has been associated with sensory neuropathy. Nausea, headache, increased AST, decreased serum folic acid

Continued

PYRIDOXINE continued

level, and allergic reaction may occur. May lower phenobarbital and phenytoin levels. See Chapter 20 for management of neonatal seizures.

Pregnancy category changes to "C" if dosage exceeds U.S. RDA recommendation.

PYRIMETHAMINE
Daraprim
Antiparasitic agent

Yes Yes 2 C

Tabs: 25 mg
Oral suspension: 2 mg/mL
Combination product with sulfadoxine (Fansidar) is no longer available in the United States.

Congenital toxoplasmosis (administer with sulfadiazine and leucovorin; see remarks):
  Load: 2 mg/kg/24 hr PO ÷ Q12 hr × 2 days
  Maintenance: 1 mg/kg/24 hr PO once daily × 2–6 mo, then 1 mg/kg/24 hr 3 × per wk to complete total 12 mo of therapy

Toxoplasmosis (administer with sulfadiazine or trisulfapyrimidines and leucovorin):
  Child:
    Load: 2 mg/kg/24 hr PO ÷ BID (**max. dose:** 100 mg/24 hr) × 2 days for non-HIV exposed/positive or × 3 days for HIV exposed/positive
    Maintenance: 1 mg/kg/24 hr PO once daily (**max. dose:** 25 mg/24 hr) × 3–6 wk for non-HIV exposed/positive or ≥6 wk for HIV exposed/positive
  Adult: 200 mg PO × 1 followed by 50–75 mg/24 hr once daily × 3–6 wk for non-HIV exposed/positive or ≥6 wk for HIV exposed/positive

Pyrimethamine is a folate antagonist. Supplementation with folinic acid leucovorin at 5–15 mg/24 hr is recommended. **Contraindicated** in megaloblastic anemia secondary to folate deficiency. **Use with caution** in G6PD deficiency, malabsorption syndromes, alcoholism, pregnancy, and renal or hepatic impairment. Pyrimethamine can cause glossitis, bone marrow suppression, seizures, rash, and photosensitivity. For congenital toxoplasmosis, see *Clin Infect Dis* 1994;18:38-72. Zidovudine and methotrexate may increase risk for bone marrow suppression. Aurothioglucose, trimethoprim, and sulfamethoxazole may increase risk for blood dyscrasias. Administer doses with meals. Most cases of acquired toxoplasmosis **do not** require specific antimicrobial therapy.

QUETIAPINE
Seroquel, Seroquel XR, and generics
Antipsychotic, second generation

Yes No 2 C

Tabs: 25, 50, 100, 200, 300, 400 mg
Extended-release tabs: 50, 150, 200, 300, 400 mg
Oral suspension: 40 mg/mL

Bipolar Mania (continue therapy at lowest dose to maintain efficacy and periodically assess maintenance treatment needs; PO):

QUETIAPINE continued

Immediate-release dosage forms:

Age	Dose Titration	Recommended Dose	Maximum Dose
Child ≥10 yr and adolescent	Day 1: 25 mg BID Day 2: 50 mg BID Day 3: 100 mg BID Day 4: 150 mg BID Day 5: 200 mg BID ≥Day 6: If needed, additional increases should be ≤100 mg/24 hr up to 600 mg/24 hr. Total daily doses may be divided TID based on response and tolerability.	400–600 mg/24 hr	600 mg/24 hr
Adult	Day 1: 50 mg BID Day 2: 100 mg BID Day 3: 150 mg BID Day 4: 200 mg BID ≥Day 5: If needed, additional increases ≤200 mg/24 hr up to 800 mg/24 hr by Day 6.	400–800 mg/24 hr	800 mg/24 hr

Extended-release tabs (see remarks):

Age	Dose Titration	Recommended Dose	Maximum Dose
Child ≥10 yr and adolescent	Day 1: 50 mg once daily Day 2: 100 mg once daily Day 3–5: increase by 100 mg/24 hr increments each day until 400 mg once daily is achieved on day 5.	400–600 mg once daily	600 mg/24 hr
Adult	Day 1: 300 mg once daily Day 2: 600 mg once daily Day 3: Adjust dose to 400–800 mg once daily based on efficacy and tolerance	400–800 mg once daily	800 mg/24 hr

Continued

QUETIAPINE continued

Schizophrenia (continue therapy at lowest dose to maintain efficacy and periodically assess maintenance treatment needs; PO):

Immediate-release dosage forms:

Age	Dose Titration	Recommended Dose	Maximum Dose
Adolescent (13–17 yr)	Day 1: 25 mg BID Day 2: 50 mg BID Day 3: 100 mg BID Day 4: 150 mg BID Day 5: 200 mg BID ≥Day 6: If needed, additional increases should be ≤100 mg/24 hr up to 800 mg/24 hr. Total daily doses may be divided TID based on response and tolerability.	400–800 mg/24 hr	800 mg/24 hr
Adult	Day 1: 25 mg BID Day 2 and 3: increase in increments of 25–50 mg divided 2–3 doses daily to 300–400 mg/24 hr divided BID–TID by day 4. If needed, increase dose by 50–100 mg/24 hr at intervals of at least 2 days.	150–750 mg/24 hr	750 mg/24 hr

Extended-release tabs (see remarks):

Age	Dose Titration	Recommended Dose	Maximum Dose
Adolescent (13–17 yr)	Day 1: 50 mg once daily Day 2: 100 mg once daily Day 3: 200 mg once daily Day 4: 300 mg once daily Day 5: 400 mg once daily	400–800 mg once daily	800 mg/24 hr
Adult	Day 1: 300 mg once daily If needed, increase dose in increments of up to 300 mg/24 hr.	400–800 mg once daily	800 mg/24 hr

Avoid use in patients with history of cardiac arrhythmias or prolonged QTc syndrome, concurrent medications that can prolong the QTc interval, and alcohol use. **Use with caution** in hypovolemia and diabetes mellitus.

Suicidal ideation/behavior or worsening depression may occur especially in children and young adults during the first few months of therapy or during dosage changes.

Common side effects in children include hypertension, hyperglycemia, hyperprolactenemia, and significant weight gain. Other common side effects include orthostatic hypotension, tachycardia, hypercholesterolemia, hypertriglyceridemia, abdominal pain, GI disturbances, increase appetite, xerostomia, increase serum transaminases, EPS, headache, dizziness, agitation, and fatigue. Anaphylactic reactions, DRESS, TEN, SIADH, cardiomyopathy, priapism, DKA, pancreatitis, eosinophilia, agranulocytosis, leukopenia, neutropenia, cataracts, hypothyroidism, neuroleptic malignant syndrome, and seizures have been reported.

Do not abruptly discontinue medication as acute withdrawal symptoms may occur. Dosage adjustment in hepatic impairment may be necessary as it is primarily heptically metabolized. Quetiapine is a major substrate for CYP450 3A4 and minor substrate for 2D6. Opiods and other CNS depressants

QUETIAPINE continued

may enhance CNS depressant effects. Carbamazepine may decrease the effects of quetiapine. Quetiapine may decrease dopamine agonist effects (e.g., antiparkinson agents) but may enhance the anticholinergic and QTc prolongation effects to those medications pocessing these risks. Always check for drug interactions as effects can be mild to severe.

Nonextended-release dosage forms may be administered with or without food. Extended-release tabs must be swallowed whole and administered preferably in the evening without food (a light meal of ≤300 calories is allowed). May convert patients from immediate-release to extended-release tabs at the equivalent total daily dose and administer once daily; individual dosage adjustments may be necessary.

QUINIDINE
Various generics
Class Ia antiarrhythmic

   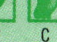

Yes   Yes   2   C

As gluconate (62% quinidine):
  Slow-release tabs: 324 mg
  Injection: 80 mg/mL (50 mg/mL quinidine) (10 mL); contains phenol
As sulfate (83% quinidine):
  Tabs: 200, 300 mg
  Oral suspension: 10 mg/mL
Equivalents: 200 mg sulfate = 267 mg gluconate
All doses expressed as salt forms.

Antiarrhythmic:
  Child (Give PO as sulfate; give IM/IV as gluconate):
    Test dose: 2 mg/kg × 1 IM/PO; **max. dose:** 200 mg
    Therapeutic dose:
      IV (as gluconate): 2–10 mg/kg/dose Q3–6 hr PRN
      PO (as sulfate): 15–60 mg/kg/24 hr ÷ Q6 hr
  Adult (Give PO as sulfate; give IM as gluconate):
    Test dose: 200 mg × 1 IM/PO.
    Therapeutic dose:
    As sulfate:
      PO, immediate release: 100–600 mg/dose Q4–6 hr. Begin at 200 mg/dose and titrate to desired effect.
    As gluconate:
      IM: 400 mg/dose Q4–6 hr
      IV: 200–400 mg/dose, infused at a rate of ≤10 mg/min
      PO: 324–972 mg Q8–12 hr
Malaria:
  Child and adult (give IV as gluconate; see remarks):
    Loading dose: 10 mg/kg/dose (**max. dose:** 600 mg) IV over 1–2 hr followed by maintenance dose. Omit or decrease load if patient has received quinine or mefloquine.
    Maintenance dose: 0.02 mg/kg/min IV as continuous infusion until oral therapy can be initiated. If more than 48 hr of IV therapy is required, reduce dose by 30%–50%.

Test dose is given to assess for idiosyncratic reaction to quinidine. Toxicity indicated by increase of QRS interval by ≥0.02 s (skip dose or stop drug). May cause GI symptoms, hypotension, tinnitus, TTP, rash, heart block, and blood dyscrasias. When used alone, may

Continued

QUINIDINE continued

cause 1:1 conduction in atrial flutter, leading to ventricular fibrillation. Patients may get idiosyncratic ventricular tachycardia with low levels, especially when initiating therapy.

Quinidine is a substrate of CYP450 3A3/4 and 3A5–7 enzymes and an inhibitor of CYP450 2D6 and 3A3/4 enzymes. Can cause increase in digoxin levels. Quinidine potentiates the effect of neuromuscular blocking agents, β-blockers, anticholinergics, and warfarin. Amiodarone, antacids, delavirdine, diltiazem, grapefruit juice, saquinavir, ritonavir, verapamil, or cimetidine may enhance the drug's effect. Barbiturates, phenytoin, cholinergic drugs, nifedipine, sucralfate, or rifampin may reduce quinidine's effect. **Use with caution** in renal insufficiency (15%–25% of drug is eliminated unchanged in the urine), myocardial depression, sick sinus syndrome, G6PD deficiency, and hepatic dysfunction.

Therapeutic levels: 3–7 mg/L. Recommended serum sampling times at steady state: trough level obtained within 30 min prior to the next scheduled dose after 1–2 days of continuous dosing (steady-state).

MALARIA USE: Continuous monitoring of ECG, blood pressure, and serum glucose are recommended, especially in pregnant women and young children.

QUINUPRISTIN AND DALFOPRISTIN
Synercid
Antibiotic, streptogramin

Yes   No   ?   B

Injection: 500 mg (150 mg quinupristin and 350 mg dalfopristin)

Doses expressed in mg of combined quinupristin and dalfopristin.
Vancomycin-resistant Enterococcus faecium (VREF):
  Child <16 yr (limited data), ≥16 yr and adult: 7.5 mg/kg/dose IV Q8 hr
Complicated skin infections:
  Child <16 yr (limited data), ≥16 yr and adult: 7.5 mg/kg/dose IV Q12 hr for at least 7 days
VREF endocarditis:
  Child and adult: 7.5 mg/kg/dose IV Q8 hr for at least 8 weeks

Not active against *Enterococcus faecalis*. **Use with caution** in hepatic impairment; dosage reduction may be necessary. Most common side effects include pain, burning, inflammation, and edema at the IV infusion site; thrombophlebitis and thrombosis; GI disturbances; rash; arthralgia; myalgia; increased liver enzymes; hyperbilirubinemia; and headache. Dose frequency reductions (Q8 hr to Q12 hr) or discontinuation can improve severe cases of arthralgia and myalgia. Use total body weight for obese patients when calculating dosages.

Drug is an inhibitor to the CYP450 3A4 isoenzyme. **Avoid use** with CYP450 3A4 substrates, which can prolong QTc interval. May increase the effects/toxicity of cyclosporine, tacrolimus, sirolimus, delavirdine, nevirapine, indinavir, ritonavir, diazepam, midazolam, carbamazepine, methylprednisolone, vinca alkaloids, docetaxel, paclitaxel, quinidine, and some calcium channel blockers.

Pediatric (<16 yr) pharmacokinetic studies have not been completed. Reduce dose for patients with hepatic cirrhosis (Child–Pugh A or B).

Drug is compatible with $D5_W$ and incompatible with saline and heparin. Infuse each dose over 1 hr using the following **max. IV concentrations:** peripheral line: 2 mg/mL; central line: 5 mg/mL. If injection site reaction occurs, dilute infusion to <1 mg/mL.

RANITIDINE HCL
Zantac, Zantac 75 [OTC], Zantac 150 Maximum Strength [OTC], Deprizine, and generics
Histamine-2-antagonist

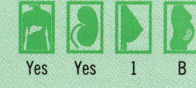
Yes   Yes   1   B

Tabs: 75 [OTC], 150 [OTC and Rx], 300 mg
Caps: 150, 300 mg
Oral syrup: 15 mg/mL (480 mL); may contain 7.5% alcohol and parabens
Oral suspension (Deprizine): 25 mg/mL (250 mL); sugar, dye, and paraben free; contains sodium benzoate
Injection: 25 mg/mL (2, 6, 40 mL); may contain 0.5% phenol

Neonate:
  PO: 2–4 mg/kg/24 hr ÷ Q8–12 hr
  IV: 2 mg/kg/24 hr ÷ Q6–8 hr
≥1 mo–16 yr:
  Duodenal/gastric ulcer (see remarks):
    PO:
      Treatment: 4–8 mg/kg/24 hr ÷ Q12 hr; **max. dose**: 300 mg/24 hr
      Maintenance: 2–4 mg/kg/24 hr ÷ Q12 hr; **max. dose**: 150 mg/24 hr
    IV/IM: 2–4 mg/kg/24 hr ÷ Q6–8 hr; **max. dose**: 200 mg/24 hr
  GERD/erosive esophagitis:
    PO: 5–10 mg/kg/24 hr ÷ Q8–12 hr; GERD **max. dose**: 300 mg/24 hr, erosive esophagits **max. dose**: 600 mg/24 hr
    IV/IM: 2–4 mg/kg/24 hr ÷ Q6–8 hr; **max. dose**: 200 mg/24 hr
Adolescent and adult:
  PO: 150 mg/dose BID or 300 mg/dose QHS
  IM/IV: 50 mg/dose Q6–8 hr; **max. dose**: 400 mg/24 hr
Continuous infusion, all ages: Administer daily IV dosage over 24 hr (may be added to parenteral nutrition solutions).

May cause headache and GI disturbance, malaise, insomnia, sedation, arthralgia, and hepatotoxicity. Acute interstitial nephritis has been reported. May increase levels of nifedipine and midazolam. May decrease levels of ketoconazole, itraconazole, and delavirdine. May cause false-positive urine protein test (Multistix).

Duodenal/gastric ulcer doses for ≥1 mo–16 yr are extrapolated from clinical adult trials and pharmacokinetic data in children. Extemporaneously compounded carbohydrate-free oral solution dosage form is useful for patients receiving the ketogenic diet. The syrup dosage form has a peppermint flavor and may not be tolerated. **Adjust dose in renal failure (see Chapter 30).**

RASBURICASE
Elitek
Antihyperuricemic agent

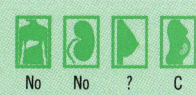
No   No   ?   C

Injection: 1.5, 7.5 mg; contains mannitol

Hyperuricemia: 0.1–0.2 mg/kg/dose (rounded down to the nearest whole 1.5 mg multiple) IV over 30 min × 1. Patients generally respond to 1 dose, but if needed, dose may be repeated Q24 hr for up to four additional doses.

Continued

RASBURICASE continued

Contraindicated in G6PD deficiency or history of hypersensitivity, hemolytic reactions, or methemoglobinemia with rasburicase. **Use with caution** in asthma, allergies, hypersensitivity with other medications, and children <2 yr (decreased efficacy and increased risk for rash, vomiting, diarrhea, and fever).

Common side effects include nausea, vomiting, abdominal pain, discomfort, diarrhea, constipation, mucositis, fever, and rash. Serious and fatal hypersensitivity reactions, including anaphylaxis, have been reported in <1% of patients and can occur at anytime; discontinue use immediately and permanently.

During therapy, uric acid blood samples must be sent to the laboratory immediately. Blood should be collected in prechilled tubes containing heparin and placed in an ice-water bath to avoid potential falsely low uric acid levels (degradation of plasma uric acid occurs in the presence of rasburicase at room temperature). Centrifugation in a precooled centrifuge (4°C) is indicated. Plasma samples must be assayed within 4 hr of sample collection.

RH$_0$ (D) IMMUNE GLOBULIN INTRAVENOUS (HUMAN)
WinRho-SDF, Rhophylac
Immune Globulin

No Yes 1 C

Injection (WinRho-SDF): 1500 IU (1.3 mL), 2500 IU (2.2 mL), 5000 IU (4.4 mL), 15,000 IU (13 mL); may contain polysorbate 80
Prefilled injection (Rhophylac): 1500 IU (2 mL)
Conversion: 1 mcg = 5 IU

All doses based on international units (IU).
Immune thrombocytopenic purpura [nonsplenectomized Rh$_0$(D)-positive patients]:
  Initial dose (may be given in two divided doses on separate days or as a single dose):
    Hemoglobin ≥ 10 mg/dL: 250 IU/kg/dose IV × 1
    Hemoglobin < 10 mg/dL: 125–200 IU/kg/dose IV × 1. See remarks for hemoglobin < 8 mg/dL
  Additional doses:
    Responders to initial dose: 125–300 IU/kg/dose IV; actual dose and frequency of administration is determined by the patient's response and subsequent hemoglobin level.
    Nonresponders to initial dose:
      Hemoglobin < 8 g/dL: alternative therapy should be used
      Hemoglobin 8–10 g/dL: 125–200 IU/kg/dose IV × 1
      Hemoglobin > 10 g/dL: 250–300 IU/kg/dose × 1

WinRho SDF is currently the only Rh$_0$ (D) immune globulin product indicated for ITP. **Contraindicated** in IgA deficiency. **Use with extreme caution** in patients with hemoglobin < 8 mg/dL and thrombocytopenia or bleeding disorders. Adverse events associated with ITP include headache, chills, fever, and reduction in hemoglobin [due to the destruction of Rh$_0$ (D) antigen-positive red cells]. Intravascular hemolysis resulting in anemia and renal insufficiency has been reported. May interfere with immune response to live virus vaccines (e.g., MMR, varicella). Rh$_0$(D)-positive patients should be monitored for signs and symptoms of intravascular hemolysis, anemia, and renal insufficiency. Administer IV doses over 3–5 min.

RIBAVIRIN
Oral: Rebetol, Copegus, Ribasphere, Ribasphere Ribapak,
Moderiba, and generics
Inhalation: Virazole
Antiviral agent

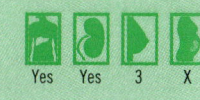
Yes Yes 3 X

Oral solution (Rebetol): 200 mg/5 mL (100 mL); contains sodium benzoate and propylene glycol
Oral caps (Rebetol, Ribasphere and generics): 200 mg
Tabs:
  Copegus and generics: 200 mg
  Ribasphere and Moderiba: 200, 400, 600 mg
  BID dose packs:
    Moderiba: 200 mg/400 mg (7 tabs each, 28 tabs each), 400 mg/400 mg (14, 56 tabs),
    600 mg/400 mg (7 tabs each, 28 tabs each), 600 mg/600 mg (14, 56 tabs)
    Ribasphere Ribapak: 200 mg/400 mg (7 tabs each, 28 tabs each), 400 mg/400 mg (14 tabs), 600 mg/400 mg
    (7 tabs each, 28 tabs each), 600 mg/600 mg (14 tabs)
Aerosol (Virazole): 6 g

Hepatitis C (PO, see remarks):
Child ≥3 yr (in combination with interferon alfa-2b at 3 million units 3 × per wk SC; use ribavirin oral solution or capsule):
  <25 kg: 15 mg/kg/24 hr ÷ BID; use oral solution
  25–36 kg: 200 mg BID
  37–49 kg: 200 mg QAM and 400 mg QPM
  50–61 kg: 400 mg BID
  >61–75 kg: 400 mg QAM and 600 mg QPM
  >75 kg: 600 mg BID
  Duration of therapy:
    Genotype 1: 48 weeks; consider discontinuing combination therapy at 12 weeks if a 2 log decrease in viral load is not achieved or if virus is still detectable at 24 weeks
    Genotypes 2 and 3: 24 weeks
  Dosage modification for toxicity: See remarks.
  Copegus tabs [PO; in combination with PEGASYS at 180 mcg/1.73 m² × BSA (max. dose 180 mcg/dose) once weekly SC]:
    23–33 kg: 200 mg BID
    34–46 kg: 200 mg QAM and 400 mg QPM
    47–59 kg: 400 mg BID
    60–74 kg: 400 mg QAM and 600 mg QPM
    ≥75 kg: 600 mg BID
    Duration of therapy: 24 wk for genotype 2 or 3 and 48 wk for other genotypes
Adult:
  Oral capsules in combination with interferon alfa-2b at 3 million units 3 × per week SC:
    ≤75 kg: 400 mg QAM and 600 mg QPM
    >75 kg: 600 mg BID
  Oral capsules or solution in combination with Peginterferon alfa-2b:
    <66 kg: 400 mg BID
    66–80 kg: 400 mg QAM and 600 mg QPM
    81–105 kg: 600 mg BID
    >105 kg: 600 mg QAM and 800 mg QPM

Continued

RIBAVIRIN continued

Adult:
Oral tablets in combination with Peginterferon alfa-2a for hepatitis C genotype 1, 4:
≤*75 kg:* 500 mg BID × 48 wk
>*75 kg:* 600 mg BID × 48 wk
Oral tablets in combination with Peginterferon alfa-2a for genotype 2, 3: 400 mg BID × 24 wk
Oral tablets in combination with Peginterferon alfa-2a for HIV coinfected patient (regardless of hepatitis C genotype): 400 mg BID × 48 wk
Dosage modification for toxicity: See remarks

Inhalation:
Continuous: Administer 6 g by aerosol over 12–18 hr once daily for 3–7 days. The 6 g ribavirin vial is diluted in 300 mL preservative-free sterile water to a final concentration of 20 mg/mL. Must be administered with Viratek Small Particle Aerosol Generator (SPAG-2)
Intermittent (for nonventilated patients): Administer 2 g by aerosol over 2 hr TID for 3–7 days. The 6 g ribavirin vial is diluted in 100 mL preservative-free sterile water to a final concentration of 60 mg/mL. The intermittent use is not recommended in patients with endotracheal tubes

ORAL RIBAVIRIN: Contraindicated in pregnancy, significant or unstable cardiac disease, autoimmune hepatitis, hepatic decompensation (Child-Pugh score > 6; class B or C), hemoglobinopathies, and creatinine clearance < 50 mL/min. **Use with caution** in preexisiting cardiac disease, pulmonary disease, and sarcoidosis. Anemia (most common), insomnia, depression, irritability, and suicidal behavior (higher in adolescent and pediatric patients) have been reported with the oral route

Tinnitus, hearing loss, vertigo, severe hypertriglyceridemia, and homicidal ideation have been reported in combination with interferon. Pancytopenia has been reported in combination with interferon and azathoprine. Increased risk for hepatic decompensation with cirrhotic chronic hepatitis C patients treated with α-interferons or with HIV co-infection receiving HAART and interferon alfa-2a. Growth inhibition (delays in weight and height gain) was observed in children (5–17 yr old) receiving combination therapy for up to 48 weeks.

May decrease the effects of zidovudine and stavudine and increase risk for lactic acidosis with nucleoside analogues. **Reduce or discontinue dosage for toxicity as follows (for Copegus, see package insert):**

Patient with no cardiac disease:
Hgb < 10 g/dL and ≥8.5 g/dL:
Child: 12 mg/kg/dose PO once daily; may further reduce to 8 mg/kg/dose PO once daily
Adult: 600 mg PO once daily (capsules or solution) or 200 mg PO QAM and 400 mg PO QPM (tablets)
Hgb < 8.5 g/dL: Discontinue therapy permanently

Patient with cardiac disease:
≥*2 mg/dL decrease in Hgb during any 4-wk period during therapy:*
Child: 12 mg/kg/dose PO once daily; may further reduce to 8 mg/kg/dose PO once daily (monitor weekly)
Adult: 600 mg PO once daily (capsules or solution) or 200 mg PO QAM and 400 mg PO QPM (tablets)
Hgb < 12 g/dL after 4 wk of reduced dose: Discontinue therapy permanently

INHALED RIBAVIRIN: Use of ribavirin for RSV is controversial and **not** routinely indicated. Aerosol therapy may be considered for selected infants and young children at high risk for serious RSV disease (see most recent edition of the *AAP Redbook*). Most effective if begun early in course of RSV infection; generally in the first 3 days. May cause worsening respiratory distress, rash, conjunctivitis, mild bronchospasm, hypotension, anemia, and cardiac arrest. **Avoid** unnecessary occupational exposure to ribavirin due to its teratogenic effects. Drug can precipitate in the respiratory equipment.

RIBOFLAVIN
Vitamin B₂ and various brands and generics
Water-soluble vitamin

No | No | 2 | A/C

Tabs [OTC]: 25, 50, 100 mg
Caps [OTC]: 50, 400 mg

Riboflavin deficiency:
  Child: 2.5–10 mg/24 hr ÷ once daily–BID PO
  Adult: 5–30 mg/24 hr ÷ once daily–BID PO
U.S. RDA requirements: see Chapter 21.

Hypersensitivity may occur. Administer with food. Causes yellow to orange discoloration of urine. For multivitamin information, see Chapter 21.
Pregnancy category changes to "C" if used in doses above the RDA.

RIFABUTIN
Mycobutin and generics
Antituberculous agent

Yes | Yes | 3 | B

Caps: 150 mg
Oral suspension: 20 mg/mL

MAC primary prophylaxis for first episode of opportunistic disease in HIV (see remarks for interactions and www.aidsinfo.nih.gov/guidelines):
  >5 yr and adult: 300 mg PO once daily; doses may be administered as 150 mg PO BID if GI upset occurs
MAC secondary prophylaxis for recurrence of opportunistic disease in HIV [in combination with ethambutol and a macrolide antibiotic (clarithromycin or azithromycin)]:
  Infant and child: 5 mg/kg/24 hr PO once daily; **max. dose:** 300 mg/24 hr
  Adolescent and adult: 300 mg PO once daily; doses may be administered 150 mg PO BID if GI upset occurs
MAC treatment:
  Child: 10–20 mg/kg/24 hr PO once daily; **max. dose:** 300 mg/24 hr as part of a multi-drug regimen for severe disease
  Adult: 300 mg PO once daily; may be used in combination with azithromycin and ethambutol
    In combination with non-nucleoside reverse transcriptase inhibitors:
      With efavirenz and no concomitant protease inhibitor: 450 mg PO once daily or 600 mg PO 3 × per wk
      With nevirapine: 300 mg PO 3 × per wk
    In combination with protease inhibitors:
      With amprenavir, indinavir, or nelfinavir: 150 mg PO once daily or 300 mg PO 3 × per wk
      With ritonavir boosted regimens (e.g., saquinavir/ritonavir, or lopinavir/ritonavir): 150 mg PO once every other day or 150 mg PO 3 × per week

Should not be used for MAC prophylaxis with active TB. May cause GI distress, discoloration of skin and body fluids (brown-orange color) and marrow suppression. Rash, eosinophilia, and bronchospasm have been reported. Use with caution in renal and liver impairment.
Adjust dose in renal impairment (see Chapter 30). May permanently stain contact lenses.

Continued

RIFABUTIN continued

Uveitis can occur when using high doses (>300 mg/24 hr in adults) in combination with macrolide antibiotics.

Rifabutin is an inducer of CYP450 3A enzyme and is structurally similar to rifampin (similar drug interactions, see *Rifampin*). Clarithromycin, fluconazole, itraconazole, nevirapine, and protease inhibitors increase rifabutin levels. Efavirenz may decrease rifabutin levels. May decrease effectiveness of dapsone, delavirdine, nevirapine, amprenavir, indinavir, nelfinavir, saquinavir, itraconazole, warfarin, oral contraceptives, digoxin, cyclosporine, ketoconazole, and narcotics.

Doses may be administered with food if patient experiences GI intolerance.

RIFAMPIN
Rifadin and generics
Antibiotic, antituberculous agent, rifamycin

Yes   Yes   2   C

Caps: 150, 300 mg
Oral suspension: 10, 15, 25 mg/mL
Injection: 600 mg

Staphylococcus aureus *infections (as part of synergistic therapy with other antistaphylococcal agents):*
0–1 mo: 10–20 mg/kg/24 hr ÷ Q12 hr IV/PO
>1 mo: 10–20 mg/kg/24 hr ÷ Q12 hr IV/PO; **max. dose:** 600 mg/24 hr
  Prosthetic valve endocarditis:
    Early infection (≤1 yr surgery): 20 mg/kg/24 hr ÷ Q8 hr IV/PO; **max. dose:** 900 mg/24 hr
    Late infection (>1 yr surgery): 15–20 mg/kg/24 hr ÷ Q12 hr IV/PO; **max. dose:** 600 mg/24 hr
  Adult: 600 mg once daily, or 300–450 mg Q12 hr IV/PO
    Prosthetic valve endocarditis: 300 mg Q8 hr IV/PO for a minimum of 6 wk in combination with antistaphylococcal penicillin with or without gentamicin for first 2 wk
Tuberculosis (see latest edition of the AAP Red Book, for duration of therapy and combination therapy): Twice weekly therapy may be used after 1–2 months of daily therapy.
Infant, child, and adolescent:
  Daily therapy: 10–20 mg/kg/24 hr ÷ Q12–24 hr IV/PO
  Twice weekly therapy: 10–20 mg/kg/24 hr PO twice weekly
  Max. daily dose: 600 mg/24 hr
Adult:
  Daily therapy: 10 mg/kg/24 hr once daily PO
  Twice weekly therapy: 10 mg/kg/24 hr once daily twice weekly
  Max. daily dose: 600 mg/24 hr
Prophylaxis for N. meningitidis (see latest edition of the AAP Red Book for additional information):
0–<1 mo: 10 mg/kg/24 hr ÷ Q12 hr PO × 2 days
≥1 mo: 20 mg/kg/24 hr ÷ Q12 hr PO × 2 days
Adult: 600 mg PO Q12 hr × 2 days
Max. dose (all ages): 1200 mg/24 hr

Never use as monotherapy except when used for prophylaxis. Patients with latent tuberculosis infection should NOT be treated with rifampin and pyrazinamide because of the risk of severe liver injury. Use is **NOT recommended** in porphyria. **Use with caution** in diabetes.

RIFAMPIN continued

May cause GI irritation, allergy, headache, fatigue, ataxia, muscle weakness, confusion, fever, hepatitis, transient LFT abnormalities, blood dyscrasias, interstitial nephritis, and elevated BUN and uric acid. Causes red discoloration of body secretions such as urine, saliva, and tears (which can permanently stain contact lenses). Induces hepatic enzymes (CYP450 2C9, 2C19, and 3A4), which may decrease plasma concentration of digoxin, corticosteroids, buspirone, benzodiazepines, fentanyl, calcium channel blockers, β-blockers, cyclosporine, tacrolimus, itraconazole, ketoconazole, oral anticoagulants, barbiturates, and theophylline. May reduce the effectiveness of oral contraceptives and antiretroviral agents (protease inhibitors and non-nucleoside reverse transcriptase inhibitors). Hepatotoxicity is a concern when used in combination with pyrazinamide and ritonavir-boosted saquinavir (**use is contraindicated**).

Adjust dose in renal failure (see Chapter 30). Reduce dose in hepatic impairment. Give oral doses 1 hr before or 2 hr after meals.

For *H. influenza* prophylaxis, see latest edition of the *Red Book*.

RIMANTADINE
Flumadine and generics
Antiviral agent

Yes   Yes   3   C

Tabs: 100 mg
Oral suspension: 10 mg/1 mL

Influenza A prophylaxis (for at least 10 days after known exposure; usually for 6–8 wk during influenza A season or local outbreak):
Child:
  1–9 yr: 5 mg/kg/24 hr PO once daily–BID; **max. dose:** 150 mg/24 hr
  ≥10 yr:
    <40 kg: 5 mg/kg/24 hr PO ÷ BID; **max. dose:** 150 mg/24 hr
    ≥40 kg: 100 mg/dose PO BID
Adult: 100 mg PO BID
Influenza A treatment (within 48 hr of illness onset):
  Use the aforementioned prophylaxis dosage × 5–7 days

Resistance to influenza A and recommendations against the use for treatment and prophylaxis have been reported by the CDC. Check with local microbiology laboratories and the CDC for seasonal susceptibility/resistance.

Preferred over amantadine for influenza due to lower incidence of adverse events. Individuals immunized with live attenuated influenza vaccine (e.g., FluMist) should not receive rimantadine prophylaxis for 14 days after the vaccine. Chemoprophylaxis does not interfere with immune response to inactivated influenza vaccine.

May cause GI disturbance, xerostoma, dizziness, headache, and urinary retention. CNS disturbances are less than those with amantadine. **Contraindicated** in amantadine hypersensitivity. **Use with caution** in renal or hepatic insufficiency; dosage reduction may be necessary. A dosage reduction of 50% has been recommended in severe hepatic or renal impairment. Subjects with severe renal impairment have been reported to have an 81%

RISPERIDONE
Risperdal, Risperdal M-Tab, Risperidone M-Tab, Risperdal Consta, and generics
Atypical antipsychotic, serotonin (5-HT₂), and dopamine (D₂) antagonist

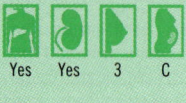

Yes   Yes   3   C

Tabs: 0.25, 0.5, 1, 2, 3, 4 mg
Oral solution: 1 mg/mL (30 mL); may contain benzioc acid
Orally disintegrating tabs (Risperdal M-Tab, Risperidone M-Tab, and generics): 0.25, 0.5, 1, 2, 3, 4 mg; contains phenylalanine
IM Injection (Risperdal Consta): 12.5, 25, 37.5, 50 mg (prefilled syringe with 20 G, 2 inch needle and 2 mL diluent); for IM administration only

Irritability associated with autistic disorder:
5–16 yr (PO daily doses may be administered once daily–BID; patients experiencing somnolence may benefit from QHS or BID dosing or dose reduction):
  Initial dose:
    <20 kg: 0.25 mg/24 hr PO for a minimum of 4 days; use with caution if <15 kg as dosing recommendation is not established
    ≥20 kg: 0.5 mg/24 hr PO for a minimum of 4 days
  Dose increment (if needed) after 4 days of initial dose:
    <20 kg: 0.5 mg/24 hr PO for a minimum of 14 days, if additional increments needed, increase dose by 0.25 mg/24 hr at intervals of at least 14 days
    ≥20 kg: 1 mg/24 hr PO for a minimum of 14 days, if additional increments needed, increase dose by 0.5 mg/24 hr at intervals of at least 14 days
  Max. daily dose for plateau of therapeutic effect (from one pivotal clinical trial):
    <20 kg: 1 mg/24 hr
    ≥20–45 kg: 2.5 mg/24 hr
    >45 kg: 3 mg/24 hr

Bipolar mania: Oral doses may be administered once daily–BID, and patients experiencing somnolence may benefit from QHS or BID dosing or dose reduction. Long-term use beyond 3 wk and doses (all ages) >6 mg/24 hr have not been evaluated.
  Child (10–17 yr): Start with 0.5 mg/24 hr PO once daily (QAM or QHS). If needed, increase dose at intervals ≥24 hr in increments of 0.5 or 1 mg/24 hr, as tolerated, up to a recommended dose of 2.5 mg/24 hr. Although efficacy has been demonstrated between 0.5–6 mg/24 hr, no additional benefit was seen above 2.5 mg/24 hr. Higher doses were associated with more adverse effects.
  Adult: Start with 2–3 mg PO once. Dosage increases or decreases of 1 mg/24 hr can be made at 24-hr intervals. Dosage range: 1–6 mg/24 hr.

Schizophrenia: Oral doses may be administered once daily–BID, and patients experiencing somnolence may benefit from BID dosing (see remarks).
  Adolescent (13–17 yr): No data are available to support long-term use of >8 wk.
    PO: Start with 0.5 mg once daily (QAM or QHS). If needed, increase dose at intervals ≥24 hr in increments of 0.5 to 1 mg/24 hr, as tolterated, to a recommended dose of 3 mg/24 hr. Although efficacy has been demonstrated between 1–6 mg/24 hr, no additional benefit and greater side effects were seen above 3 mg/24 hr. Doses >6 mg/24 hr have not been studied.
  Adult:
    PO: Start with 1 mg BID on day 1; if tolerated, increase to 2 mg BID on day 2 and to 3 mg BID thereafter. Dosage increases or decreases of 1–2 mg can be made on a weekly basis if needed. Usual effective dose: 2–8 mg/24 hr. Doses above 16 mg/24 hr have not been evaluated.
    IM: Start with 25 mg Q2 wk; if no response, dose may be increased to 37.5 mg or 50 mg at 4-wk intervals. Max. IM dose: 50 mg Q2 wk. PO risperidone should also be administered with the

RISPERIDONE continued

initial IM dose and continued × 3 wk and discontinued to provide adequate plasma concentrations during the initial IM dosing.

Use with caution in cardiovascular disorders, diabetes, renal or hepatic impairment (dose reduction necessary), hypothermia or hyperthermia, seizures, breast cancer or other prolactin dependent tumors, and dysphagia. Common side effects include abdominal pain and other GI disturbances, arthralgia, anxiety, dizziness, headache, insomnia, somnolence (use QHS dosing), EPS, cough, fever, pharyngitis, rash, rhinitis, sexual dysfunction, tachycardia, and weight gain. Weight gain, somnolence, and fatigue were common side effects reported in the autism studies. Priapism, hypothermia, sleep apnea syndrome, ileus, urinary retention, diabetes mellitus, and hypoglycemia have been reported in post marketing reports. Very rare cases of anaphylaxis have been reported with use of the IM dosage form in patients who have previously tolerated the oral dosage form.

In the presence of severe renal or hepatic impairment or risk for hypotension, the following adult dosing has been recommended: Start with 0.5 mg PO BID. Increase dose, if needed and tolerated, in increments no more than 0.5 mg BID. Increases to doses > 1.5 mg BID should occur at intervals of at least 1 wk; slower titration may be required in some patients.

Limited studies in pediatric related Tourette's syndrome, schizophrenia, and aggressive behavior in psychiatric disorders are reported. Autistic disorder safety and efficacy in children <5 yr have not been established. If therapy has been discontinued for a period of time, therapy should be reinitiated with the same initial titration regimen.

Drug is a CYP450 2D6 and 3A4 isoenzyme substrate. Concurrent use of isoenzyme inhibitors (e.g., fluoxetine, paroxetine, sertraline, and cimetidine) and inducers (e.g., carbamazepine, rifampin, phenobarbital, and phenytoin) may increase and decrease the effects of risperidone, respectively. Alcohol, CNS depressants, and St. John's wort may potentiate the drug's side effect. Risperidone may enhance the hypotensive effects of levodopa and dopamine agonists.

Oral dosage forms may be administered with or without food. Oral solution can be mixed in water, coffee, orange juice, or low-fat milk but is incompatible with cola or tea. **Do not** split or chew the orally disintegrating tablet. Use IM suspension preparation within 6 hr after reconstitution.

RIZATRIPTAN BENZOATE
Maxalt, Maxalt-MLT, and generics
Antimigraine agent, selective serotonin agonist

Yes Yes 3 C

Tabs:
  Maxalt and generics: 5 mg, (6s, 18s), 10 mg (6s, 18s)
Orally disintegrating tabs (ODT):
  Maxalt-MLT and generics: 5, 10 mg (18s); contains aspartame

Treatment of acute migraines with or without aura (tabs and ODT):
  Child 6–17 yr (efficacy and safety with > 1 dose within 24 hr has not been established):
    <40 kg: 5 mg PO \x 1
    ≥40 kg: 10 mg PO \x 1
  Adult (safety of an average of > 4 headaches in a 30 day period has not been established; see remarks): 5–10 mg PO \x 1. If needed in 2 hrs, a second dose may be administered. Max. daily dose: 30 mg/24 hr.

Continued

RIZATRIPTAN BENZOATE continued

Dosage adjustment if receiving propranolol:
Child 6–17 yr:
<40 kg: DO NOT USE
≥40 kg: 5 mg PO\x 1; max. dose: 5 mg/24 hr period.
Adult: 5 mg PO up to a maximum of 3 doses in 2 hr intervals; max. dose: 15 mg/24 hr period.

Contraindicated in hemiplegic or basilar migraine, coronary artery vasospasm, uncontrolled hypertension, ischemic bowel or coronary artery disease, peripheral vascular disease, and history of stroke or TIA.

Do not administer with any ergotamine-containing medication ergot-type medication, any other 5-HT1 agonist (e.g., triptans), methylene blue, or with/within 2 weeks of discontinuing a MAO inhibitor or linezolid.

Use with **caution** in renal and hepatic impairment as a 44% increase in AUC for patients receiving hemodialysis and a 30% increase plasma concentration for patients with moderate hepatic dysfunction were reported.

Common adverse effects include nausea, asthenia, dizziness, somnolence and fatigue. Serious adverse effects include chest pain, coronary artery spasm, hypertension, MI, peripheral ischemia, ventricular arrhythmia, ischemic colitis, anaphylaxis, angioedema, cerebrovascular accident, and serotonin syndrome. Transient and permanent vision loss have been reported.

When using the oral disintegrating tablet (ODT), place the whole tablet on the tongue, allow the tablet to dissolve and swallow with saliva. Administration with liquids is optional. Do not break the ODT tablet.

ROCURONIUM
Generics; previously available as Zemuron
Nondepolarizing neuromuscular blocking agent

Yes   No   ?   C

Injection: 10 mg/mL (5, 10 mL)

Use of a peripheral nerve stimulator to monitor drug effect is recommended
Infant:
IV: 0.5 mg/kg/dose; may repeat Q20–30 min PRN
Child (3 mo– 14 yr):
IV: 0.6 mg/kg/dose × 1; if needed, give maintenance doses of 0.075–0.125 mg/kg/dose Q20–30 min PRN when neuromuscular blockade returns to 25% of control. Alternatively, a maintenance continuous IV infusion may be used starting at 7–12 mcg/kg/min (use lower end for children 2–11 yr) when neuromuscular blockade returns to 10% of control.
Adolescent and adult:
IV: Start with 0.6–1.2 mg/kg/dose × 1; if needed, maintenance doses at 0.1–0.2 mg/kg/dose Q20–30 min PRN. Alternatively, a maintenance continuous IV infusion may be used starting at 10–12 mcg/kg/min (range: 4–16 mcg/kg/min).

Use with **caution** in hepatic impairment and history of anaphylaxis with other neuromuscular blocking agents. Hypertension, hypotension, arrhythmia, tachycardia, nausea, vomiting, bronchospasm, wheezing, hiccups, rash, and edema at the injection site may occur. Myopathy after long term use in an ICU, and QT interval prolongation in pediatric patients receiving general anestetic agents have been reported. Increased neuromuscular blockade may occur with concomitant use of aminoglycosides, clindamycin, tetracycline, magnesium sulfate, quinine, quinidine, succinylcholine, and inhalation anesthetics (for continuous infusion, reduce infusion by 30%–50% at 45–60 min after intubating dose).

Caffeine, calcium, carbamazepine, phenytoin, phenylephrine, azathioprine, and theophylline may reduce neuromuscular blocking effects.

ROCURONIUM continued

Use must be accompanied by adequate anesthesia or sedation. Peak effects occur in 0.5–1 min for children and in 1–3.7 min for adults. Duration of action: 30–40 min in children and 20–94 min in adults (longer in geriatrics). Recovery time in children 3 mo to 1 yr is similar to adults. To prevent residual paralysis, extubate patient **only** after the patient has sufficiently recovered from neuromuscular blockade. In obese patients, use actual body weight for dosage calculation.

RUFINAMIDE
Banzel
Anticonvulsant, triazole derivative

Yes Yes ? C

Tabs: 200, 400 mg
Oral suspension: 40 mg/mL (460 mL); contains parabens and propylene glycol

Lennox-Gastaut Syndrome (it is not known if doses lower than the targeted dosages are effective):
    Child 1–< 17 yr (see remarks): Start at 10 mg/kg/24 hr PO ÷ BID, then increase dose by ~10 mg/kg/24 hr every other day up to the **maximum** targeted dose of 45 mg/kg/24 hr ÷ BID **not to exceed** 3200 mg/24 hr.
    Child ≥ 17 yr and adult: Start at 400–800 mg/24 hr PO ÷ BID, then increase dose by 400–800 mg/24 hr every other day up to the **maximum** targeted dose of 3200 mg/24 hr ÷ BID.

Contraindicated in Familial Short QT syndrome. Use is **not recommended** in severe hepatic impairment (Child-Pugh 10 to 15). Use with **caution** when taking other medications that can shorten the QT interval, performing tasks requiring mental alertness, and in mild/moderate hepatic impairment (Child-Pugh 5 to 9), .

Common side effects include fatigue, blurred vision, diplopia, ataxia, dizziness, headache, somnolence, nausea, vomiting and shortening of cardiac QT interval. Serious side effects of leukopenia, severe dermatological reactions (e.g., Stevens Johnson syndrome), multiorgan hypersensitivity reactions (e.g., DRESS), and suicidal ideation have been reported.

Rufinamide is a weak inhibitor of CYP 450 2E1 and weak inducer of 3A4. May decrease levels/effects of nifedipine, nimodipine, piperaquine, calcifediol, clozapine, carbamazepine, lamotrigine, triazolam, orlistat, and hormonal contraceptives. May increase the levels/effects of phenytoin and phenobarbital. Primidone, phenobarbital, phenytoin, and carbamazepine may decrease the levels/effects of rufinamide. Whereas, valproic acid may increase the levels/effects of rufinamide.

The effectiveness data for 1–4 year old children is based on bridging pharmacokinetic (PK) and safety data as their PK and safety data are similar to children \ge 4 yr and adults.

Consider dose adjustment for drug loss in patients receiving hemodialysis (rufinamide is dialyzable). Tablets may be crushed and all doses may be administered with or without food.

SALMETEROL
Serevent Diskus
β₂-adrenergic agonist (long acting)

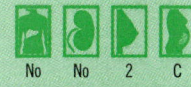
No No 2 C

Dry powder inhalation (DPI; Diskus): 50 mcg/inhalation (28, 60 inhalations); contains lactose
In combination with fluticasone: see *Fluticasone Propionate and Salmeterol*

Persistent asthma (see remarks):
    ≥4 yr and adult: 1 inhalation (50 mcg) Q12 hr

Continued

SALMETEROL continued

Prevention of exercise-induced bronchospasm:
  ≥*4 yr and adult:* 1 inhalation 30–60 min before exercise. Additional dose should not be used for another 12 hr. Patients who are already using Q12 hr dosing for persistent asthma should not use additional salmeterol doses for this indication and use alternative therapy (e.g., albuterol) prior to exercise.

For long-term asthma control, should be used in combination with inhaled corticosteroids. **Should not be used to relieve symptoms of acute asthma.** It is long acting and has its onset of action in 10–20 min, with a peak effect at 3 hr. May be used QHS (1 inhalation of the DPI) for nocturnal symptoms. Salmeterol is a chronic medication and is not used in similar fashion to short-acting β-agonists (e.g., albuterol). Patients already receiving salmeterol Q12 hr should not use additional doses for prevention of exercise-induced bronchospasm; consider alternative therapy. Asthma exacerbations or hospitalizations were reported to be lower when used with an inhaled corticosteroid.

WARNING: Long-acting β₂-agonists may increase the risk for asthma-related death. A subgroup analysis suggested higher risk in African-American patients compared with Caucasians. Use salmeterol only as additional therapy for patients not adequately controlled on other asthma-controller medications (e.g., low- to medium-dose inhaled corticosteroids) or whose disease severity clearly requires initiation of treatment with two maintenance therapies.

Should not be used in conjunction with an inhaled, long-acting β₂-agonist and is **not** a substitute for inhaled or systemic corticosteroid. Use with strong CYP 450 3A inhibitors (e.g., ketoconazole, HIV protease inhibitors, clarithromycin, itraconazole, nefazodone, and telithromycin) is not recommended due to risk for cardiovascular adverse events (e.g., QTc prolongation, tachycardia). Salmeterol is a CYP 450 3A substrate.

Proper patient education is essential. Side effects are similar to those of albuterol. Hypertension and arrhythmias have been reported. See Chapter 24 for recommendations for asthma controller therapy.

SCOPOLAMINE HYDROBROMIDE
Transderm Scop and generics
Anticholinergic agent

Yes   Yes   2   C

Injection: 0.4 mg/mL (1 mL); may contain alcohol
Transdermal (Transderum Scop): 1.5 mg/patch (4s, 10s, and 24s); delivers ~1 mg over 3 days

Antiemetic (SC/IM/IV):
  Child: 6 mcg/kg/dose Q6–8 hr PRN; **max. dose**: 300 mcg/dose
Transdermal (≥12 yr) (see remarks):
  Motion sickness: Apply patch behind the ear at least 4 hr prior to exposure to motion; remove after 72 hr.
  Antiemetic prior to surgery: Apply patch behind the ear the evening before surgery. Remove patch 24 hr after surgery.
  Antiemetic prior to cesarean section: Apply patch behind the ear 1 hr prior to surgery to minimize infant exposure. Remove patch 24 hr after surgery.

Toxicities similar to those of atropine. **Contraindicated** in urinary or GI obstruction and glaucoma. **Use with caution** in hepatic or renal dysfunction, cardiac disease, seizures, or psychoses. May cause dry mouth, drowsiness, and blurred vision.

Transdermal route should **NOT** be used in children < 12 yr. Drug withdrawal symptoms (nausea, vomiting, headache, and vertigo) have been reported following removal of transdermal patch in patients using the patch for >3 days. For perioperative use, the patch should be kept in place for 24 hr following surgery.

SELENIUM SULFIDE
Selsun Blue, Tersi, and generics
Topical antiseborrheic agent

No   No   2   C

Shampoo: 1% [OTC] (207, 325, 400, 420 mL), 2.25% (180 mL); some OTC shampoo products are available with conditioner
Topical lotion: 2.5% (120 mL)
Topical aerosol foam (Tersi): 2.25% (70 g)

≥2 yr and adult:
  Seborrhea/Dandruff: Massage 5–10 mL of shampoo into wet scalp and leave on scalp for 2–3 min. Rinse thoroughly and repeat. Shampoo twice weekly × 2 weeks. Maintenance applications once every 1–4 wk.
  Tinea versicolor: Apply 2.5% lotion to affected areas of skin. Allow to remain on skin × 10 min. Rinse thoroughly. Repeat once daily × 7 days. Follow with monthly applications for 3 mo to prevent recurrences.

Rinse hands and body well after treatment. May cause local irritation, hair loss, and hair discoloration. **Avoid** eyes, genital areas, and skin folds. Shampoo may be used for tinea capitis to reduce risk of transmission to others (does not eradicate tinea infection).
For tinea versicolor, 15%–25% sodium hyposulfite or thiosulfate (Tinver lotion) applied to affected areas BID × 2–4 wk is an alternative. Topical antifungals (e.g., clotrimazole, miconazole) may be used for small, focal infections. **Do not use** for tinea versicolor during pregnancy.

SENNA/SENNOSIDES
Senokot, Senna-Gen, Lax-Pills, and many others
Laxative, stimulant

No   No   1   C

Based on mg of senna (all products are OTC):
  Oral powder: 284 g
  Oral syrup: 176 mg/5 mL, 218 mg/5 mL (60 mL, 240 mL)
  Tabs: 187, 217, 374 mg
  187 mg senna extract is approximately 8.6 mg sennosides.
Based on mg of sennosides (all products are OTC):
  Oral syrup: 8.8 mg/5 mL (40 mL)
  Tabs: 8.6, 15, 17.2, 25 mg
  Chewable tabs: 15 mg
  8.6 mg sennosides is approximately 187 mg senna extract.

Constipation:
Dosing based on mg senna:
  Child:
    Oral: 10–20 mg/kg/dose PO QHS (**max. dose**: as shown below) or dosage by age:
      1 mo–1 yr: 55–109 mg PO QHS to **max. dose**: 218 mg/24 hr
      1–5 yr: 109–218 mg PO QHS to **max. dose**: 436 mg/24 hr
      5–15 yr: 218–436 mg PO QHS to **max. dose**: 872 mg/24 hr
  Adult:
    Oral powder: 1/2 to 1 tsp PO once daily–BID
    Syrup: 436–654 mg PO at bedtime; **max. dose**: 654 mg (15 mL) BID
    Tabs: 374 mg PO at bedtime; **max. dose**: 748 mg BID

Continued

SENNA/SENNOSIDES continued

Dosing based on mg sennosides:
Child:
  Syrup:
    1 mo–2 yr: 2.2–4.4 mg (1.25–2.5 mL) PO QHS to **max. dose**: 8.8 mg/24 hr
    2–5 yr: 4.4–6.6 mg (2.5–3.75 mL) PO QHS to **max. dose**: 6.6 mg BID
    6–12 yr: 8.8–13.2 mg (5–7.5 mL) PO QHS to **max. dose**: 13.2 mg BID
  Tabs:
    2–5 yr: 4.3 mg PO QHS to **max. dose**: 8.6 mg BID
    6–12 yr: 8.6 mg PO QHS to **max. dose**: 17.2 mg BID
>12 yr and adult:
  Granules: 15 mg PO QHS to **max. dose**: 30 mg BID
  Syrup: 17.6–26.4 mg (10–15 mL) PO QHS to **max. dose**: 26.4 mg BID
  Tabs: 17.2 mg PO QHS to **max. dose**: 34.4 mg BID

Effects occur within 6–24 hr after oral administration. Prolonged use (>1 wk) should be **avoided** as it may lead to dependency. May cause nausea, vomiting, diarrhea, and abdominal cramps. Active metabolite stimulates Auerbach's plexus. Syrup may be administered with juice or milk or mixed with ice cream.

SERTRALINE HCL
Zoloft and generics
Antidepressant (selective serotonin reuptake inhibitor)

Yes   Yes   2   C

Tabs: 25, 50, 100 mg
Oral concentrate solution: 20 mg/mL (60 mL); may contain alcohol and menthol

Depression (see remarks):
  Child ≥ 6–12 yr (data limited in this age group): Start at 12.5–25 mg PO once daily. May increase dosage by 25 mg at 1-wk intervals up to a **max. dose** of 200 mg/24 hr.
  Child ≥ 13 yr and adult: Start at 25–50 mg PO once daily. May increase dosage by 50 mg at 1-wk intervals up to a **max. dose** of 200 mg/24 hr.
Obsessive compulsive disorder (see remarks):
  Child ≥ 6–12 yr: Start at 25 mg PO once daily. May increase dosage by 25 mg at 3–4-day intervals or by 50 mg at 7-day intervals up to a **max. dose** of 200 mg/24 hr.
  Child ≥ 13 yr and adult: Start at 50 mg PO once daily. May increase dosage by 50 mg at 1-wk intervals up to a **max. dose** of 200 mg/24 hr.

Drug is **contraindicated** in combination (or within 14 days of discontinuing use) with an MAO inhibitor (e.g., linezolid or IV methylene blue) or pimozide (increases adverse/toxic effects of pimozide). **Use with caution** in patients with abnormal bleeding, SIADH, and hepatic or renal impairment. Adverse effects include nausea, diarrhea, tremor, and increased sweating. Hyponatremia, diabetes mellitus, and platelet dysfunction have been reported. Monitor for clinical worsening of depression and suicidal ideation/behavior following the initiation of therapy or after dose changes. Use during the late third trimester of pregnancy may increase risk for newborn withdrawal symptoms and persistent pulmonary hypertension in the newborn.

Use with drugs that interfere with hemostasis (e.g., NSAIDs, aspirin, and warfarin) may increase risk for GI bleeds. Use with warfarin may increase PT. Inhibits the CYP450 2D6 drug metabolizing enzyme. Serotonin syndrome may occur when taken with selective serotonin reuptake inhibitors (e.g., amitriptyline, amphetamines, buspirone, dihydroergotamine, sumatriptan, and sympathomimetics).

Do not abruptly discontinue use; gradually taper dose (4–6 wk has been recommended) to reduce risk for withdrawal symptoms.

SERTRALINE HCL continued

Mix oral concentrate solution with 4 oz. of water, ginger ale, lemon/lime soda, lemonade, or orange juice. After mixing, a slight haze may appear; this is normal. This dosage form should be **used cautiously** in patients with latex allergy because the dropper contains dry natural rubber.

SILDENAFIL
Revatio, Viagra, and generics
Phosphodiesterase type-5 (PDE5) inhibitor

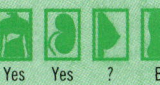
Yes   Yes   ?   B

Tabs:
  Revatio and generics: 20 mg
  Viagra: 25, 50, 100 mg
Oral suspension: 2.5 mg/mL
  Revatio: 10 mg/mL (112 mL)
Injection:
  Revatio and generics: 0.8 mg/mL (12.5 mL)

Pulmonary hypertension:
  Neonate (limited data from case reports and small clinical trials):
    PO: Several dosages have been reported and have ranged from 0.5–3 mg/kg/dose Q6–12 hr PO. A single ~0.3 mg/kg/dose PO has been used in selected patients to facilitate weaning from inhaled nitric oxide.
    IV (case report from four neonates >34-wk gestation and <72-hr old): Start with 0.4 mg/kg/dose IV over 3 hr followed by a continuous infusion of 1.6 mg/kg/24 hr (0.067 mg/kg/hr) for up to 7 days.
  Infant and child (limited data):
    PO: Start at 0.25 mg/kg/dose Q6 hr or 0.5 mg/kg/dose Q8 hr; if needed, titrate dose up to 1–2 mg/kg/dose Q6–8 hr. A single ~0.4 mg/kg/dose PO has been used in selected patients to facilitate weaning from inhaled nitric oxide.
  Child 1–17 yr (higher doses and long-term use are associated with increased risk for mortality; see remarks):
    PO:
      ≥8–20 kg: 10 mg TID
      >20–45 kg: 20 mg TID
      >45 kg: 40 mg TID
Pulmonary arterial hypertension:
  Adult:
    PO: 20 mg TID (take at least 4–6 hr apart)
    IV: 10 mg TID

Contraindicated with concurrent use of nitrates (e.g., nitroglycerin) and other nitric oxide donors; potentiates hypotensive effects. **Use with caution** in sepsis (high levels of cGMP may potentiate hypotension), hypotension, and sickle cell anemia (use not established) and with concurrent CYP450 3A4 inhibiting medications (see discussion that follows) and antihypertensive medications. Hepatic insufficiency or severe renal impairment (GFR < 30 mL/min) significantly reduces sildenafil clearance.

Findings from a dose-ranging study in 1–17-year olds with pulmonary arterial hypertension showed an association of increased mortality risk with long-term use (>2 yr). Headache, pyrexia, URTIs,

Continued

SILDENAFIL continued

vomiting, and diarrhea were the most frequently reported side effects in this study. Optimal dosing based on age and body weight still needs to be determined. Hazard ratios for mortality were 3.95 (95% CI: 1.46–10.65) for high versus low doses and 1.92 (95% CI: 0.65–5.65) for medium versus low doses in follow up study for those receiving therapy for ≥3 yr. A subsequent extension open-label study on the same population for an additional 16 weeks reported a greater hazard ratio for mortality with high dose vs. low dose therapy (p = 0.007).

In adults, a transient impairment of color discrimination may occur; this effect could increase risk of severe retinopathy of prematurity in neonates. Common side effects reported in adults include flushing, rash, diarrhea, indigestion, headache, abnormal vision, and nasal congestion. Hearing loss has been reported.

Sildenafil is substrate for CYP450 3A4 (major) and 2C8/9 (minor). Azole antifungals, cimetidine, ciprofloxacin, clarithromycin, erythromycin, nicardipine, propofol, protease inhibitors, quinidine, verapamil, and grapefruit juice may increase the effects/toxicity of sildenafil. Bosentin, efavirenz, carbamazepine, phenobarbital, phenytoin, rifampin, St. John's wort, and high-fat meals may decrease sildenafil effects.

SILVER SULFADIAZINE
Silvadene, Thermazene, SSD Cream, and generics
Topical antibiotic

Yes Yes 3 B

Cream: 1% (20, 25, 50, 85, 400, 1000 g); contains methylparabens and propylene glycol

Child (≥2 mo) and adult: Cover affected areas completely once daily–BID. Apply cream to a thickness of 1/16 inch using sterile technique.

Contraindicated in premature infants and infants ≤2 mo of age due to concerns of kernicterus and in pregnancy (approaching term). **Use with caution** in G6PD and renal and hepatic impairment. Discard product if cream has darkened. Significant systemic absorption may occur in severe burns. Adverse effects include pruritus, rash, bone marrow suppression, hemolytic anemia, hepatitis, interstitial nephritis, and life-threatening cutaneous reactions (e.g., Stevens–Johnson syndrome, TEN, and exfoliative dermatitis). **NOT** for ophthalmic use. Dressing may be used but is **not** necessary. See Chapter 4 for more information.

SIMETHICONE
Mylicon, Phazyme, Mylanta Gas, Gas-X, and generics
Antiflatulent

No No 1 C

All dosage forms available OTC
Oral drops: 40 mg/0.6 mL (30 mL)
Caps: 125, 180, 250 mg
Tabs: 60, 95 mg
Chewable tabs: 80, 125 mg
Strip, orally disintegrating: 40 mg (16s), 62.5 mg (18s, 30s); may contain alcohol

Infant and child < 2 yr: 20 mg PO QID PRN; **max. dose:** 240 mg/24 hr
2–12 yr: 40 mg PO QID PRN
>12 yr and adult: 40–250 mg PO QPC and QHS PRN; **max. dose:** 500 mg/24 hr

Efficacy has not been demonstrated for treating infant colic. **Avoid** carbonated beverages and gas-forming foods. Oral liquid may be mixed with water, infant formula, or other suitable liquids for ease of oral administration.

SIROLIMUS
Rapamune and generics
Immunosuppressant agent

Yes   Yes   3   C

Tabs: 0.5, 1, 2 mg
Oral solution (Rapamune): 1 mg/mL (60 mL); contains 1.5%–2.5% ethanol

Child ≥ 13 yr:
  <40 kg: 3 mg/m²/dose PO × 1 immediately after transplantation, followed by 1 mg/m²/24 hr PO ÷ Q12–24 hr on the next day. Adjust dose to achieve desired trough blood levels.
  ≥40 kg: use adult (low/moderate immunologic risk) ≥40 kg dosage below.

Adult:
  Patients at low/moderate immunologic risk:
    In combination with cyclosporine (adjust dose to achieve desired trough blood levels):
      <40 kg: 3 mg/m²/dose PO × 1 immediately after transplantation, followed by 1 mg/m²/dose PO once daily on the next day
      ≥40 kg: 6 mg PO × 1 immediately after transplantation, followed by 2 mg PO once daily on the next day.
  Patients at high immunologic risk:
    In combination with cyclosporine (withdrawal of cyclosporine is not recommended): 15 mg PO × 1 immediately after transplantation, followed by 5 mg PO once daily on the next day. Adjust dose to achieve desired trough blood levels.

Increased susceptibility to infection and development of lymphoma may result from immunosuppression. **Fatal** bronchial anastomotic dehiscence has been reported in lung transplantation. Excess mortality, graft loss, and hepatic artery thrombosis have been reported in liver transplantation when used with tacrolimus. Patients with the greatest amount of urinary protein excretion prior to sirolimus conversion were those whose protein excretion increased the most after conversion. Increase risk of BK virus-associated nephropathies has been reported. Increased mortality in stable liver transplant patients has been reported after conversion from a calcineurin inhibitor-based regimen to sirolimus.

Monitor whole blood trough levels (just prior to a dose at steady state), especially with pediatric patients, hepatic impairment, concurrent use of CYP450 3A4 and/or P-gp inducers and inhibitors, and/or if cyclosporine dosage is markedly changed or discontinued. Steady state is generally achieved after 5–7 days of continuous dosing. **Interpretation will vary based on specific treatment protocol and assay methodology (HPLC vs. immunoassay vs. LC/MS/MS).** Younger children may exhibit faster sirolimus clearance compared with adolescents.

Sirolimus is a substrate for CYP450 3A4 and P-gp. Cyclosporine, diltiazem, protease inhibitors, erythromycin, grapefruit juice, and other inhibitors of CYP450 3A4 may increase the toxicity of sirolimus. Phenobarbital, carbamazepine, phenytoin, and St John's wort may decrease the effects of sirolimus. Strong inhibitors (e.g., azole antifungals and clarithromycin) and strong inducers (e.g., rifamycins) are **not recommended**.

Hypertension, peripheral edema, increase serum creatinine, dyspnea, epistaxis, headache, anemia, thrombocytopenia, hyperlipidemia, hypercholesterolemia, and arthralgia may occur. Progressive multifocal leukoencephalopathy (PML), diabetes mellitus, posterior reversible encephalopathy syndrome, ovarian cysts, and menstrual disorders have been reported. Urinary tract infections have been reported in pediatric renal transplant patients with high immunologic risk.

Two mg of the oral solution has been demonstrated to be clinically equivalent to 2 mg tablets. However, it is not known whether they are still therapeutically equivalent at higher doses. Reduce maintenance dosage by 1/3 in the presence of hepatic function impairment. Administer doses

Continued

SIROLIMUS continued

consistently with or without food. When administered with cyclosporine, give dose 4 hr after cyclosporine. **Do not** crush or split tablets. Measure the oral liquid dosage form with an amber oral syringe and dilute in a cup with 60 mL of water or orange juice only. Take dose immediately after mixing, add/mix additional 120 mL diluent into the cup, and drink immediately after mixing.

SODIUM BICARBONATE
Neut and generics
Alkalinizing agent, electrolyte

No   Yes   1   C

Injection: 4% (Neut) (0.48 mEq/mL) (5 mL), 4.2% (0.5 mEq/mL) (5, 10 mL), 7.5% (0.89 mEq/mL) (50 mL), 8.4% (1 mEq/mL) (10, 50 mL)
Tabs: 325 mg (3.8 mEq), 650 mg (7.6 mEq)
Powder: 1, 120, 500 g; contains 30 mEq Na$^+$ per 1/2 teaspoon
Each 1 mEq bicarbonate provides 1 mEq Na$^+$.

Cardiac arrest: See inside front cover
Correction of metabolic acidosis: Calculate patient's dose with the following formulas
  Neonate, infant, and child:
    HCO_3^- (mEq) = 0.3 × weight (kg) × base deficit (mEq/L), **OR**
    HCO_3^- (mEq) = 0.5 × weight (kg) × [24 − serum HCO_3^- (mEq/L)]
  Adult:
    HCO_3^- (mEq) = 0.2 × weight (kg) × base deficit (mEq/L), **OR**
    HCO_3^- (mEq) = 0.5 × weight (kg) × [24 − serum HCO_3^- (mEq/L)]
Urinary alkalinization (titrate dose accordingly to urine pH):
  Child: 84–840 mg (1–10 mEq)/kg/24 hr PO ÷ QID
  Adult: 4 g (48 mEq) × 1 followed by 1–2 g (12–24 mEq) PO Q4 hr. Doses up to 16 g (192 mEq)/24 hr have been used.

Contraindicated in respiratory alkalosis, hypochloremia, and inadequate ventilation during cardiac arrest. **Use with caution** in CHF, renal impairment, cirrhosis, hypocalcemia, hypertension, and concurrent corticosteroids. Maintain high urine output. Monitor acid–base balance and serum electrolytes. May cause hypernatremia (contains sodium), hypokalemia, hypomagnesemia, hypocalcemia, hyperreflexia, edema, and tissue necrosis (extravasation). Oral route of administration may cause GI discomfort and gastric rupture from gas production.
For direct IV administration (cardiac arrest) in neonates and infants, use the 0.5 mEq/mL (4.2%) concentration or dilute the 1 mEq/mL (8.4%) concentration 1:1 with sterile water for injection and infuse at a rate **no greater than** 10 mEq/min. The 1 mEq/mL (8.4%) concentration may be used in children and adults for direct IV administration.
For IV infusions (for all ages), dilute to a **max. concentration** of 0.5 mEq/mL in dextrose or sterile water for injection and infuse over 2 hr using a **max. rate** of 1 mEq/kg/hr.
Sodium bicarbonate should **not** be mixed with or be in contact with calcium, norepinephrine, or dobutamine.

SODIUM CHLORIDE—INHALED PREPARATIONS
Hypersal, Simply Saline, Ocean, Ayr Saline, Rhinaris, and many other brands and generics
Electrolyte, inhalation

No   No   1   C

Nebulized solution: 0.9% (3, 5, 15 mL), 3% (4, 15 mL), 6% (4 mL), 7% (4 mL), 10% (4, 15 mL)
  Hypersal (preservative free): 3.5% (4 mL), 7% (4 mL)
Nasal solution spray/drops/mist (OTC): 0.125% (15 mL), 0.2% (30 mL), 0.65% (15, 30, 45 mL), 0.9% (45, 90 mL), 3% (44 mL)

SODIUM CHLORIDE—INHALED PREPARATIONS continued

Intranasal as moisturizer:
Child and adult:
  Spray/Mist: 2–6 sprays into each nostril Q2 hr PRN
  Drops: 2–6 drops into each nostril Q2 hr PRN
Cystic Fibrosis (Pretreatment with albuterol is recommended to prevent bronchospasms; see remarks):
  ≥6 yr and adult: Nebulize 4 mL of 7% solution once daily–BID. If unable to tolerate the 7% strength, lower strengths of 3%, 3.5%, or 5% may be used
Acute viral bronchiolitis (for hospitalized patients only; pretreatment with albuterol is recommended to prevent bronchospasms; see remarks):
  Infant (>34 week gestation up to 18 mo old): Nebulize 4 mL of 3% solution Q2 hr × 3 doses followed by Q4 hr × 5 doses, followed by Q6 hr until discharge

INTRANASAL USE: May be used as a nasal wash for sinuses, restore moisture, thin nasal secretions, or relieve dry, crusted, and inflamed nasal membranes from colds, low humidity, allergies, nasal decongestant overuse, minor nose bleeds, and other irritations. Nasal administration instructions:
  Nasal drops: tilt head back and hold bottle upside down
  Nasal spray: hold head in upright position and give short, firm squeezes into each nostril. Sniff deeply
NEBULIZATION: Hypertonic solutions lowers sputum viscosity and enhances mucociliary clearance
  Cystic Fibrosis: Improves FEV_1 and reduces pulmonary exacerbation frequency. May cause bronchospasm, cough, pharyngitis, hemoptysis, and acute decline in pulmonary function (administer first dose in a medical facility). It is recommended to withhold therapy in the presence of massive hemoptysis
  Acute viral bronchiolitis: Reduces length of hospitalization when compared with normal saline. May cause acute bronchospasm and local irritation

---

SODIUM PHENYLACETATE AND SODIUM BENZOATE
Ammonul and generics
Ammonium detoxicant, Urea Cycle Disorder Treatment Agent

Yes   Yes   ?   C

Injection: 100 mg sodium phenylacetate and 100 mg sodium benzoate per 1 mL (50 mL)

IV via central line (administered with IV arginine, continue infusion until ammonia levels are in the normal range): See Chapter 13 for dosing information

Use with caution in renal and hepatic impairment. Significant amounts of sodium may be administered with prolonged durations of therapy. Ammonia clearance is most efficient with hemodialysis.

Side effects include hypotension, hypokalemia, hyperglycemia, injection site reaction, nausea/vomiting, altered mental status, fever, metabolic acidosis, cerebral edema, seizures, anemia, and disseminated intravascular coagulation. CNS side effects are more frequent with ornithine transcarbamylase (OTC) and carbamyl phosphate synthetase (CPS). Blood and lymphatic system disorders and hypotension are common in patients ≤ 30 days old, whereas nausea, vomiting, and diarrhea are common in patients > 30 days old.

Although no formal drug interaction studies have been completed, penicillin antibiotics and probenecid may increase serum concentrations of sodium phenylacetate and sodium benzoate by competing for renal tubular secretion. Use of valproic acid or corticosteroids may increase plasma ammonia levels.

Must be diluted and administered IV via central line; peripheral line administration may result in burning.

SODIUM PHOSPHATE
Fleet Enema, Fleet Pedia-Lax, Fleet Enema Extra, Fleet Phospho-Soda, OsmoPrep, and generics
Laxative, enema/oral

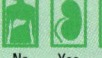   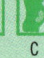
No   Yes   2   C

Enema [OTC]:
 7 g dibasic sodium phosphate and 19 g monobasic sodium phosphate/118 mL; contains 4.4 g sodium per 118 mL
   Pediatric size (Fleet Pedia-Lax): 66 mL
   Adult size (Fleet Enema): 133 mL
 7 g dibasic sodium phosphate and 19 g monobasic sodium phosphate/197 mL; contains 4.4 g sodium per 197 mL
   Fleet Enema Extra: 230 mL
Oral solution (Fleet Phospho-Soda and generics) [OTC]: 2.4 g monobasic sodium phosphate and 0.9 g dibasic sodium phosphate/5 mL (45 mL); contains 96.4 mEq Na per 20 mL and 62.25 mEq phosphate/5 mL
Oral tablets (OsmoPrep): 1.5 g

Not to be used for phosphorus supplementation (see Phosphorus Supplements).
Enema (see remarks):
 2–4 yr: 33 mL enema (half of Fleet Pedia-Lax) × 1
 5–11 yr: 66 mL enema (Fleet Pedia-Lax) × 1
 ≥12 yr and adult: 133 mL enema (Fleet Enema) OR 230 mL enema (Fleet enema Extra) × 1
Oral laxative (Fleet Phospho-Soda or generic); mix with a full glass of water:
 5–9 yr: 7.5 mL PO × 1
 10–11 yr: 15 mL PO × 1
 ≥12 yr and adult: 15–45 mL PO × 1

Contraindicated in patients with severe renal failure, megacolon, bowel obstruction, and congestive heart failure. May cause hyperphosphatemia, hypernatremia, hypocalcemia, hypotension, dehydration, and acidosis. **Avoid** retention of enema solution and **do not exceed** recommended doses, as this may lead to severe electrolyte disturbances due to enhanced systemic absorption. Colonic mucosal aphthous ulceration should be considered when interpreting colonoscopy findings with use in patients with known or suspected IBD. Rare but serious form of kidney failure (acute phosphate nephropathy) has been reported with the use of bowel cleansing preparations such as Fleet Phospho-Soda.
Onset of action: PO, 3–6 hr; PR, 2–5 min.

SODIUM POLYSTYRENE SULFONATE
Kayexalate, SPS, Kalexate, Kionex, and generics
Potassium-removing resin

No   Yes   1   C

Powder: 454 g
Oral suspension: 15 g/60 mL (60, 120, 500 mL); contains 21.5 mL sorbitol per 60 mL and 0.1%–0.3% alcohol
Rectal suspension: 30 g/120 mL (120 mL), 50 g/200 mL (200 mL)
Contains 4.1 mEq Na$^+$/g drug.

Note: Suspension may be given PO or PR. Practical exchange ratio is 1 mEq K per 1 g resin. May calculate dose according to desired exchange (see remarks).

SODIUM POLYSTYRENE SULFONATE continued

Infant and child:
PO: 1 g/kg/dose Q6 hr
PR: 1 g/kg/dose Q2–6 hr. Dosing by practical exchange (1 mEqK per 1 g resin) has been recommended for infants and smaller children

Adult:
PO: 15 g once daily–QID
PR: 30–50 g Q6 hr

Contraindicated in obstructive bowel disease, neonates with reduced gut motility, and oral administration in neonates. **Use cautiously** in presence of renal failure, CHF, hypertension, or severe edema. May cause hypokalemia, hypernatremia, hypomagnesemia, and hypocalcemia. Cases of colonic necrosis, GI bleeding, ischemic colitis, and perforation have been reported with the concomitant use of sorbitol in patients with GI risk factors (prematurity, history of intestinal disease or surgery hypovolemia, and renal insufficiency/failure). Use in neonates generally **not recommended** due to complication concerning hypernatremia and NEC.

1 mEq Na delivered for each mEq K removed. **Do not administer** with antacids or laxatives containing Mg^{2+} or Al^{3+}. Systemic alkalosis may result. Retain enema in colon for at least 30–60 min.

SPIRONOLACTONE
Aldactone and generics
Diuretic, potassium sparing

Yes   Yes   2   C/D

Tabs: 25, 50, 100 mg
Oral suspension: 1, 2.5, 5, 25 mg/mL

Diuretic:
Neonate: 1–3 mg/kg/24 hr ÷ once daily–BID PO
Child: 1–3.3 mg/kg/24 hr ÷ BID–QID PO; **max. dose:** 100 mg/24 hr
Adult: 25–200 mg/24 hr ÷ once daily–BID PO (see remarks); **max. dose:** 200 mg/24 hr

Diagnosis of primary aldosteronism:
Child: 125–375 mg/m²/24 hr ÷ once daily–BID PO
Adult: 400 mg once daily PO × 4 days (short test) or 3–4 wk (long test), then 100–400 mg once daily–BID maintenance.

Hirsutism in women:
Adult: 50–200 mg/24 hr ÷ once daily–BID PO

Contraindicated in Addison's disease, hyperkalemia, use with eplerenone, or severe renal failure (see Chapter 30). **Use with caution** in dehydration, hyponatremia, and renal or hepatic dysfunction. May cause hyperkalemia (especially with severe heart failure), GI distress, rash, lethargy, dizziness, and gynecomastia. May potentiate ganglionic blocking agents and other antihypertensives. Monitor potassium levels and be aware of other K^+ sources, K^+-sparing diuretics, and angiotensin-converting enzyme inhibitors (all can increase K^+).

Do not use with other medications known to cause hyperkalemia (e.g., ACE inhibitors, angiotensin II antagonists, aldosterone blockers, and other potassium sparing diuretics). Hyperkalemic metabolic acidosis has been reported with concurrent cholestyramine use. May cause false elevation in serum digoxin levels measured by radioimmunoassay.

Although TID–QID regimens have been recommended, data suggests once daily–BID dosing to be adequate. Pregnancy category changes to "D" if used in pregnancy induced hypertension.

STREPTOMYCIN SULFATE
Generics
Antibiotic, aminoglycoside; antituberculous agent

No Yes 2 D

Powder for injection: 1 g

MDR Tuberculosis: Use as part of a multidrug regimen; see latest edition of AAP Red Book). IM route is preferred. Monitor levels.
Infant, child, and adolescent (<15 yr or ≤40 kg):
  Daily therapy: 20–40 mg/kg/24 hr IM/IV once daily
    Max. daily dose: 1 g/24 hr
  Twice weekly therapy (under direct observation): 20 mg/kg/dose IM/IV twice weekly
    Max. daily dose: 1 g/24 hr
Child, adolescent, and adult (≥15 yr or >40 kg):
  Daily therapy: 15 mg/kg/24 hr IM/IV once daily; max. daily dose: 1 g/24 hr
  Twice weekly therapy (under direct observation): 15 mg/kg/dose IM/IV twice weekly; **max. daily dose:** 1 g/24 hr
Brucellosis, tularemia, plague, and rat bite fever: See latest edition of the Red Book.

Contraindicated with aminoglycoside and sulfite hypersensitivity. **Use with caution** in preexisting vertigo, tinnitus, hearing loss, and neuromuscular disorders. Drug is administered via deep IM injection **only**. Follow auditory status. May cause CNS depression, other neurologic problems, myocarditis, serum sickness, nephrotoxicity, and ototoxicity. Concomitant neurotoxic, ototoxic, or nephrotoxic drugs and dehydration may increase risk for toxicity.
Therapeutic levels: peak 15–40 mg/L; trough: <5 mg/L. Recommended serum sampling time at steady-state: trough within 30 min prior to the third consecutive dose and peak 30–60 min after the administration of the third consecutive dose. Therapeutic levels are **not** achieved in CSF.
Adjust dose in renal failure (see Chapter 30).

SUCCIMER
Chemet, DMSA [dimercaptosuccinic acid]
Chelating agent

Yes Yes ? C

Cap: 100 mg

Lead chelation, child:
10 mg/kg/dose (or 350 mg/m^2/dose) PO Q8 hr × 5 days, then 10 mg/kg/dose (or 350 mg/m^2/dose) PO Q12 hr × 14 days.
Manufacturer recommendation (see following table):

Weight (kg)	Dose (mg) Q8 hr × 5 Days Followed by Same Dose Q12 hr × 14 Days
8–15	100
16–23	200
24–34	300
35–44	400
≥45	500

Use caution in patients with compromised renal or hepatic function. Repeated courses may be necessary. Follow serum lead levels. Allow minimum of 2 wk between courses, unless blood levels require more aggressive management. Side effects: GI symptoms, increased LFTs (10%), rash, headaches, and dizziness. **Coadministration with other chelating agents**

SUCCIMER continued

is not recommended. Treatment of iron deficiency is recommended as well as environmental remediation. Contents of capsule may be sprinkled on food for those who are unable to swallow capsule.

SUCCINYLCHOLINE
Anectine, Quelicin
Neuromuscular blocking agent

Yes   No   ?   C

Injection:
Anectine, Quelicin: 20 mg/mL (10 mL); contains parabens

Paralysis for intubation (see remarks):
Infant, child, and adolescent:
  Initial:
    IV:
      Infant and younger child: 2 mg/kg/dose × 1
      Older child and adolescent: 1 mg/kg/dose × 1
    IM: 3–4 mg/kg/dose × 1
    Max. dose: 150 mg/dose
Adult:
  Initial:
    IV: 0.3–1.1 mg/kg/dose × 1
    IM: 2.5–4 mg/kg/dose × 1
    Max. dose: 150 mg/dose
Maintenance for long surgical procedures: 0.04–0.07 mg/kg/dose IV Q5–10 min PRN. Continuous infusion **not recommended**.

Pretreatment with atropine is recommended to reduce incidence of bradycardia. For rapid sequence intubation, see Chapter 1.

Contraindicated after the acute phase of an injury following major burns, multiple trauma, extensive denervation of skeletal muscle, or upper motor neuron injury because severe hyperkalemia and subsequent **cardiac arrest** may occur.

Cardiac arrest has been reported in children and adolescents primarily with skeletal muscle myopathies (e.g., Duchenne's muscular dystrophy). Identify developmental delays suggestive of a myopathy prior to use. Predose creatine kinase may be useful for identifying patients at risk. Monitoring of ECG for peaked T-waves may be useful in detecting early signs of this adverse effect.

May cause malignant hyperthermia (use dantrolene to treat), bradycardia, hypotension, arrhythmia, and hyperkalemia. Severe anaphylactic reactions have been reported; **use caution** if previous anaphylactic reaction to other neuromuscular blocking agents. **Use with caution** in patients with severe burns, paraplegia, or crush injuries and in patients with preexisting hyperkalemia. Beware of prolonged depression in patients with liver disease, malnutrition, pseudocholinesterase deficiency, hypothermia, and those receiving aminoglycosides, phenothiazines, quinidine, β-blockers, amphotericin B, cyclophosphamide, diuretics, lithium, acetylcholine, and anticholinesterases. Diazepam may decrease neuromuscular blocking effects. Prior use of succinylcholine may enhance the neuromuscular blocking effect of vecuronium and its duration of action.

Duration of action 4–6 min IV, 10–30 min IM. Must be prepared to intubate within 1 min.

SUCRALFATE
Carafate and generics
Oral antiulcer agent

No   Yes   1   B

Tabs: 1 g
Oral suspension: 100 mg/mL (420 mL); contains sorbitol and parabens

Child:
  Duodenal or gastric ulcer: 40–80 mg/kg/24 hr ÷ Q6 hr PO; **max. dose:** 1000 mg/dose
  Stomatitis: 5–10 mL (500–1000 mg of suspension), swish and spit or swish and swallow QID
Adult:
  Duodenal ulcer:
    Treatment: 1 g PO QID (1 hr before meals and QHS) or 2 g PO BID × 4–8 wk.
    Maintenance/prophylaxis: 1 g PO BID
  Stress ulcer:
    Prophylaxis: 1 g PO QID
  Stomatitis: 10 mL (1000 mg of suspension), swish and spit or swish and swallow QID
  Proctitis (use oral suspension as rectal enema): 20 mL (2 g) PR once daily–BID

May cause vertigo, constipation, and dry mouth. Hypersensitivity, including anaphylactic reactions, and hyperglycemia in diabetic patients have been reported. Aluminum may accumulate in patients with renal failure. This may be augmented by the use of aluminum-containing antacids. **Use with caution** in patients with dysphagia or other conditions that may alter gag or cough reflexes or diminish oropharyngeal coordination/motility receiving the oral tablet dosage form; cases of tablet aspiration with respiratory complications have been reported.

Decreases absorption of phenytoin, digoxin, theophylline, cimetidine, fat-soluble vitamins, ketoconazole, omeprazole, quinolones, and oral anticoagulants. Administer these drugs at least 2 hr before or after sucralfate doses.

Drug requires an acidic environment to form a protective polymer coating for damaged GI tract mucosa. Administer oral doses on an empty stomach (1 hr before meals and QHS).

SULFACETAMIDE SODIUM OPHTHALMIC
Bleph-10 and generics
Ophthalmic antibiotic, sulfonamide derivative

No   No   ?   C

Ophthalmic solution: 10% (5, 15 mL); may contain thimerosol or benzalkonium chloride
Ophthalmic ointment: 10% (3.5 g)

Conjunctivitis (usual duration of therapy for ophthalmic use is 7–10 days):
  >2 mo and adult:
    Ointment: Apply 0.5 inch ribbon into conjunctival sac Q3–4 hr and QHS initially, and reduce the dosing frequency with adequate response
    Drops: 1–2 drops to affected eye(s) Q2–3 hr initially and reduce the dosing frequency with adequate response

Hypersensitivity reactions between different sulfonamides can occur regardless of route of administration. May cause local irritation, stinging, burning, conjunctival hyperemia, excessive tear production, and eye pain. Rare toxic epidermal necrolysis and Stevens–Johnson syndrome have been reported. Sulfacetamide preparations are incompatible with silver preparations.

To reduce risk of systemic absorption with ophthalmic solution, apply finger pressure to lacrimal sac during and 1–2 min after instillation.

SULFADIAZINE
Various generics
Antibiotic, sulfonamide derivative

Yes   Yes   3   C/D

Tabs: 500 mg
Oral suspension: 100, 200 mg/mL

Infant ≥ 2 mo, child, and adolescent: 75 mg/kg/dose or 2000 mg/m^2/dose PO × 1, followed by 150 mg/kg/24 hr or 4000 mg/m^2/24 hr ÷ Q4–6 hr (**max. dose:** 6000 mg/24 hr)
Adult: 2–4 g/dose × 1, followed by 2–4 g/24 hr PO ÷ Q4–8 hr
Congenital toxoplasmosis (administer with pyrimethamine and folinic acid; see pyrimethamine for dosage information):
  Infant: 100 mg/kg/24 hr PO ÷ BID × 12 mo
Toxoplasmosis (administer with pyrimethamine and folinic acid; see pyrimethamine for dosage information):
  Infant ≥ 2 mo and child: 100–200 mg/kg/24 hr ÷ Q6 hr PO × 3–4 wk; **max. dose:** 6000 mg/24 hr
  Adult: 4–6 g/24 hr PO ÷ Q6 hr × 3–4 wk
Rheumatic fever prophylaxis:
  ≤27 kg: 500 mg PO once daily
  >27 kg: 1000 mg PO once daily

Most cases of acquired toxoplasmosis do not require specific antimicrobial therapy.
  Contraindicated in porphyria and hypersensitivity to sulfonamides. **Use with caution** in premature infants and infants <2 mo because of risk of hyperbilirubinemia and in hepatic or renal dysfunction (30%–44% eliminated in urine). Maintain hydration. May cause fever, rash, hepatitis, SLE-like syndrome, vasculitis, bone marrow suppression and hemolysis in patients with G6PD deficiency, and Stevens–Johnson syndrome.
May cause increased effects of warfarin, methotrexate, thiazide diuretics, uricosuric agents, and sulfonylureas due to drug displacement from protein binding sites. Large quantities of vitamin C or acidifying agents (e.g., cranberry juice) may cause crystalluria. Pregnancy category changes from "C" to "D" if administered near term. Administer on an empty stomach with plenty of water.

SULFAMETHOXAZOLE AND TRIMETHOPRIM
Trimethoprim-sulfamethoxazole, Co-Trimoxazole, TMP-SMX;
Bactrim, Septra, Sulfatrim, and others
Antibiotic, sulfonamide derivative

Yes   Yes   2   D

Tabs (reg strength): 80 mg TMP/400 mg SMX
Tabs (double strength): 160 mg TMP/800 mg SMX
Oral suspension: 40 mg TMP/200 mg SMX per 5 mL (100, 480 mL)
Injection: 16 mg TMP/mL and 80 mg SMX/mL (5, 10, 30 mL); some preparations may contain propylene glycol and benzyl alcohol

Doses based on TMP component.
Minor/moderate infections (PO or IV):
  Child: 8–12 mg/kg/24 hr ÷ BID; **max. dose** 160 mg/dose
  Adult (>40 kg): 160 mg/dose BID
Severe infections (PO or IV):
  Child and adult: 20 mg/kg/24 hr ÷ Q6–8 hr

Continued

SULFAMETHOXAZOLE AND TRIMETHOPRIM continued

UTI prophylaxis:
  Child: 2–4 mg/kg/24 hr PO once daily
Pneumocystic jiroveci (carinii) pneumonia (PCP):
  Treatment (≥2 mo and adult, PO or IV): 15–20 mg/kg/24 hr ÷ Q6–8 hr × 21 days
  Prophylaxis (PO or IV):
    ≥1 mo and child: 150 mg/m^2/24 hr ÷ BID for 3 consecutive days/wk; **max. dose**: 320 mg/24 hr
    Adolescent and adult: 80 or 160 mg once daily or 160 mg 3 days/wk

Not recommended for use in infants <2 mo (excluding PCP prophylaxis). **Contraindicated** in patients with sulfonamide or trimethoprim hypersensitivity and megaloblastic anemia due to folate deficiency. May cause kernicterus in newborns; may cause blood dyscrasias, crystalluria, glossitis, renal or hepatic injury, GI irritation, rash, Stevens–Johnson syndrome, hemolysis in patients with G6PD deficiency. Severe hyponatremia may occur during treatment of pneumocystic jiroveci pneumonia. Hyperkalemia may appear in HIV/AIDS patients. **Use with caution** in renal and hepatic impairment and G6PD deficiency. QT prolongation resulting in ventricular tachycardia has been reported.

Epidemiological studies suggest use during pregnancy may be associated with increased risk of congenital malformations (particularly neural tube defects), cardiovascular malformations, urinary tract defects, oral clefts, and club foot.

Sulfamethoxazole is a CYP450 2C9 substrate and inhibitor. Trimethoprim is a CYP450 2C9, 3A4 substrate and 2C8/9 inhibitor. **Reduce dose in renal impairment (see Chapter 30). See Chapter 17 for PCP prophylaxis guidelines.**

SULFASALAZINE
Azulfidine, Azulfidine EN-tabs, Salicylazosulfapyridine, and generics
Antiinflammatory agent

Yes Yes 2 B/D

Tabs: 500 mg
Delayed release tabs (Azulfidine EN-tabs, Sulfazine EC, and generics): 500 mg
Oral suspension: 100 mg/mL

Inflammatory bowel disease:
  Child ≥ 6 yr:
    Initial dosing:
      Mild: 40–50 mg/kg/24 hr ÷ Q6 hr PO
      Moderate/severe: 50–75 mg/kg/24 hr ÷ Q4–6 hr PO
      Max. initial dose: 4 g/24 hr
    Maintenance: 30–70 mg/kg/24 hr ÷ Q4–8 hr PO; **max. dose**: 4 g/24 hr
  Adult:
    Initial: 3–4 g/24 hr ÷ Q4–8 hr PO
    Maintenance: 2 g/24 hr ÷ Q6 hr PO
    Max. dose: 6 g/24 hr
Juvenile idiopathic arthritis:
  Child 6–16 yr: Start with 10 mg/kg/24 hr ÷ BID PO and increase by 10 mg/kg/24 hr Q7 days until planned maintenance dose is achieved. Usual maintenance dose is 30–50 mg/kg/24 hr ÷ BID PO up to a **max.** of 2 g/24 hr.

Contraindicated in sulfa or salicylate hypersensitivity, porphyria, and GI or GU obstruction. Discontinue use if a serious infection develops. **Use with caution** in renal impairment, blood dyscrasias, or asthma. Maintain hydration. May cause orange-yellow discoloration of urine and skin. May permanently stain contact lenses. May cause photosensitivity, hypersensitivity

SULFASALAZINE continued

(which may result in hepatitis and nephritis), blood dyscrasias, CNS changes, nausea, vomiting, anorexia, diarrhea, and renal damage. Hepatotoxicity/hepatic failure, anaphylaxis, angioedema, severe drug rash with eosinophilia and systemic symptoms (DRESS), and interstitial lung disease have been reported. May cause hemolysis in patients with G6PD deficiency. Pseudomononucleosis, myocarditis, folate deficiency (decreases folic acid absorption), nephrolithiasis, and oropharyngeal pain have been reported.

Reduces serum digoxin and cyclosporine levels. Slow acetylators may require lower dosage due to accumulation of active sulfapyridine metabolite. May cause false-positive test for urinary normetanephrine if using liquid chromatography methods.

Pregnancy category changes to "D" if administered near term. Bloody stools or diarrhea have been reported in breast fed infants of mothers receiving sulfasalazine.

SUMATRIPTAN SUCCINATE
Imitrex, Imitrex STAT dose, Sumavel Dose Pro, Zembrace SymTouch, and generics
Antimigraine agent, selective serotonin agonist

Yes　Yes　2　C

Injection, for subcutaneous use:
　Zembrace SymTouch: 3 mg/0.5 mL (0.5 mL)
　Imitrex STAT dose, Sumavel DosePro, and generics: 4 mg/0.5 mL (0.5 mL)
　Imitrex, Imitrex STAT dose, and generics: 6 mg/0.5 mL (0.5 mL)
Tabs: 25, 50, 100 mg
Oral suspension: 5 mg/mL
Nasal spray (as a unit-dose spray device): 5 mg dose in 100 microliters (6 units per pack); 20 mg dose in 100 microliters (6 units per pack)

Adolescent and adult (see remarks):
　PO: 25 mg as soon as possible after onset of headache. If no relief in 2 hr, give 25–100 mg Q2 hr up to a daily **max.** of 200 mg.
　　Max. single dose: 100 mg/dose.
　　Max. daily dose: 200 mg/24 hr (with exclusive PO dosing or with an initial SC dose and subsequent PO dosing).
　SC: 4–6 mg × 1 as soon as possible after onset of headache. If no response, may give an additional dose 1 hr later; **max. daily dose:** 12 mg/24 hr.
　Nasal: 5–20 mg/dose into one nostril or divided into each nostril after onset of headache Dose may be repeated in 2 hr up to a **max.** of 40 mg/24 hr.

Contraindicated with concomitant administration of ergotamine derivatives, MAO inhibitors (and use within the past 2 wk) or other vasoconstrictive drugs. **Not** for migraine prophylaxis. **Use with caution** in renal or hepatic impairment. **A max. single dose** of 50 mg has been recommended in adults with hepatic dysfunction. Acts as selective agonist for serotonin receptor. Induration and swelling at the injection site; flushing; dizziness; and chest, jaw, and neck tightness may occur with SC administration. Weakness, hyperreflexia, incoordination, and serotonin syndrome (may be life-threatening) have been reported with use in combination with selective serotonin reuptake inhibitors (e.g., fluoxetine, fluvoxamine, paroxetine, and sertraline).

May cause coronary vasospasm if administered IV. **Use injectable form SC only!** Onset of action is 10–120 min SC and 60–90 min PO. For nasal use, the safety of treating more than 4 headaches in a 30-day period has not been established.

Continued

SUMATRIPTAN SUCCINATE continued

Efficacy studies were not conclusive in clinical trials for children. Some **do not recommend** use in patients < 18 yr owing to poor efficacy and reports of serious adverse events (e.g., stroke, visual loss, and death) in both children and adults with all dosage forms.

To minimize infant exposure to sumatriptan, avoid breast feeding for 12 hr after treatment.

SURFACTANT, PULMONARY/BERACTANT
Survanta
Bovine lung surfactant

No   No   ?   ?

Suspension for inhalation: 25 mg/mL phospholipids (4, 8 mL); contains 0.5–1.75 mg triglycerides, 1.4–3.5 mg free fatty acids and <1 mg protein per 1 mL drug

Prophylactic therapy: 4 mL/kg/dose intratracheally as soon as possible; up to 4 doses may be given at intervals no shorter than Q6 hr during the first 48 hr of life.

Rescue therapy (treatment): 4 mL/kg/dose intratracheally, immediately following the diagnosis of respiratory distress syndrome (RDS). May repeat dose as needed Q6 hr to **max.** of 4 doses total.

Method of administration for previously listed therapies (see remarks): Suction infant prior to administration. Each dose is divided into four 1 mL/kg aliquots; administer 1 mL/kg in each of four different positions (slight downward inclination with head turned to the right and head turned to the left; slight upward inclination with the head turned to the right and head turned to the left).

Transient bradycardia, O_2 desaturation, pallor, vasoconstriction, hypotension, endotracheal tube blockage, hypercarbia, hypercapnia, apnea, and hypertension may occur during the administration process. Other side effects may include pulmonary interstitial emphysema, pulmonary air leak, and posttreatment nosocomial sepsis. Monitor heart rate and transcutaneous O_2 saturation during dose administration and arterial blood gases for postdose hyperoxia and hypocarbia after administration.

All doses are administered intratracheally via a 5 french feeding catheter. If the suspension settles during storage, gently swirl the contents—**do not shake.** Drug is stored in the refrigerator, protected from light, and needs to be warmed by standing at room temperature for at least 20 min or warmed in the hand for at least 8 min. Artificial warming methods should **NOT** be used.

SURFACTANT, PULMONARY/CALFACTANT
Infasurf
Bovine lung surfactant

No   No   ?   ?

Intratracheal suspension: 35 mg/mL phospholipids (3, 6 mL); contains 26 mg phosphatidylcholine, 0.7 mg protein, and 0.26 mg surfactant protein B per 1 mL

Prophylactic therapy: 3 mL/kg/dose intratracheally as soon as possible; up to a total of 3 doses may be given Q12 hr.

Rescue therapy (treatment; see remarks): 3 mL/kg/dose intratracheally immediately after the diagnosis of respiratory distress syndrome (RDS). May repeat dose as needed Q12 hr to **max.** of 3 doses total.

Method of administration for previously listed therapies (see remarks): Suction infant prior to administration. Manufacturer recommends administration through a side-port adapter into the endotracheal tube with two attendants (one to instill drug and another to monitor and position patient). Each dose is divided into two 1.5-mL/kg aliquots; administer 1.5 mL/kg in each of the two different positions (infant positioned to the right or left-side dependent). Drug is administered while ventilation is continued over 20–30 breaths for each aliquot, with small bursts timed only during

SURFACTANT, PULMONARY/CALFACTANT continued

the inspiratory cycles. A pause followed by evaluation of respiratory status and repositioning should separate the two aliquots. The drug has also been administered by dividing dose into four equal aliquots and administered with repositioning in the prone, supine, right, and left lateral positions.

Common adverse effects include cyanosis, airway obstruction, bradycardia, reflux of surfactant into the ET tube, requirement for manual ventilation, and reintubation. Monitor O_2 saturation and lung compliance after each dose such that oxygen therapy and ventilator pressure are adjusted as necessary.

All doses administered intratracheally via a 5 french feeding catheter. If suspension settles during storage, gently swirl the contents—**do not shake.** Drug is stored in the refrigerator, protected from light, and does not need to be warmed before administration. Unopened vials that have been warmed to room temperature (once only) may be refrigerated within 24 hours and stored for future use.

For rescue therapy, repeat doses may be administered as early as 6 hr after the previous dose for a total of up to 4 doses if the infant is still intubated and requires at least 30% inspired oxygen to maintain a $PaO_2 \geq 80$ torr.

SURFACTANT, PULMONARY/PORACTANT ALFA
Curosurf
Porcine lung surfactant

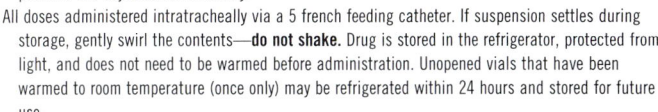
No No ? ?

Intratracheal suspension: 80 mg/mL (1.5, 3 mL): contains 76 mg phospholipids, 1 mg and 0.45 mg surfactant protein B per 1 mL drug

Rescue therapy (treatment): 2.5 mL/kg/dose × 1 intratracheally, immediately following the diagnosis of respiratory distress syndrome (RDS). May administer 1.25 mL/kg/dose Q12 hr × 2 doses as needed up to a **max. total dose** of 5 mL/kg.

Method of administration (see remarks): Suction infant prior to administration. Each dose is divided into two aliquots, with each aliquot administered into one of the two main bronchi by positioning the infant with either the right or left side dependent. After the first aliquot is administered, remove the catheter from the ET tube and manually ventilate the infant with 100% oxygen at a rate of 40–60 breaths/min for 1 min. When the infant is stable, reposition the infant and administer the second dose with the same procedures. Then remove the catheter without flushing.

Currently FDA approved for the treatment (rescue therapy) of RDS. Transient episodes of bradycardia, decreased oxygen saturation, reflux of surfactant into the ET tube, and airway obstruction have occurred during dose administration. Monitor O_2 saturation and lung compliance after each dose, and adjust oxygen therapy and ventilator pressure as necessary. Pulmonary hemorrhage has been reported.

All doses administered intratracheally via a 5 french feeding catheter. Suction infant prior to administration and 1 hr after surfactant instillation (unless signs of significant airway obstruction).

Drug is stored in the refrigerator and protected from light. Each vial of drug should be slowly warmed to room temperature and gently turned upside down for uniform suspension **(do not shake)** before administration. Unopened vials that have been warmed to room temperature (once only) may be refrigerated within 24 hr and stored for future use.

TACROLIMUS
Prograf, Astragraf XL, Envarsus XR, Protopic, FK506, and generics
Immunosuppressant

Yes   Yes   2   C

Caps (Prograf and generics): 0.5, 1, 5 mg
Extended-release caps (Astragraf XL): 0.5, 1, 5 mg (see remarks)
Extended-release tabs (Envarsus XR): 0.75, 1, 4 mg (see remarks)
Oral suspension: 0.5, 1 mg/mL
Injection (Prograf): 5 mg/mL (1 mL); contains alcohol and polyoxyl 60 hydrogenaed castor oil (cremophor)
Topical ointment (Protopic and generics): 0.03%, 0.1% (30, 60, 100 g)

SYSTEMIC USE:
Child:
  Liver transplantation without preexisting renal or hepatic dysfunction (initial doses; titrate to therapeutic levels):
  IV: 0.03–0.05 mg/kg/24 hr by continuous infusion
  PO: 0.15–0.2 mg/kg/24 hr ÷ Q12 hr
Adult (initial doses; titrate to therapeutic levels):
  IV: 0.01–0.05 mg/kg/24 hr by continuous infusion
  PO: 0.075–0.2 mg/kg/24 hr ÷ Q12 hr
  Liver transplantation: 0.1–0.15 mg/kg/24 hr ÷ Q12 hr
  Kidney transplantation: 0.1–0.2 mg/kg/24 hr ÷ Q12 hr
  Cardiac transplantation: 0.075 mg/kg/24 hr ÷ Q12 hr

TOPICAL USE:
Atopic dermatitis (continue treatment for 1 wk after clearing of signs and symptoms; see remarks):
  Child ≥ 2–15 yr old: Apply a thin layer of the 0.03% ointment to the affected skin areas BID and rub in gently and completely.
  Adolescent ≥ 16 yr and adult: Apply a thin layer of the 0.03% or 0.1% ointment to the affected skin areas BID and rub in gently and completely.

Avoid use in patients with prolonged cardiac QT intervals. IV dosage form **contraindicated** in patients allergic to polyoxyl 60 hydrogenated castor oil (cremophor). Experience in pediatric kidney transplantation is limited. Pediatric patients may require higher mg/kg doses than adults. For BMT use (beginning 1 day before BMT), dose and therapeutic levels similar to those in liver transplantation have been used.

Major adverse events include tremor, headache, insomnia, diarrhea, constipation, hypertension, nausea, and renal dysfunction. Hypokalemia, hypomagnesemia, hyperglycemia, confusion, depression, infections, lymphoma, liver enzyme elevation, and coagulation disorders may also occur. GI perforation, agranulocytosis, and hemolytic anemia have been reported.

Tacrolimus is a substrate of the CYP450 3A4 drug metabolizing enzyme. Calcium channel blockers, imidazole antifungals (ketoconazole, itraconazole, fluconazole, clotrimazole, and posaconazole), macrolide antibiotics (erythromycin, clarithromycin, and troleandomycin), cisapride, cimetidine, cyclosporine, danazol, herbal products containing schisandra sphenanthera extracts, methylprednisolone, and grapefruit juice can increase tacrolimus serum levels. In contrast, carbamazepine, caspofungin, phenobarbital, phenytoin, rifampin, rifabutin, and sirolimus may decrease levels. Use with sirolimus may increase risk for hepatic artery thrombosis. Use with other CYP450 3A inhibitors and substrates has the potential to prolong the cardiac QT interval. Reduce dose in renal or hepatic insufficiency.

TACROLIMUS continued

Monitor trough levels (just prior to a dose at steady state). Steady state is generally achieved after 2–5 days of continuous dosing. Interpretation will vary based on treatment protocol and assay methodology (whole-blood ELISA vs. MEIA vs. HPLC). Whole-blood trough concentrations of 5–20 ng/mL have been recommended in liver transplantation at 1–12 mo. Trough levels of 7–20 ng/mL (whole blood) for the first 3 mo and 5–15 ng/mL after 3 mo have been recommended in renal transplantation.

Tacrolimus therapy generally should be initiated 6 hr or more after transplantation. PO is the preferred route of administration, and administration should be done on an empty stomach. Safety and efficacy of the extended-release capsules (Astragraf XL) have not been established for kidney transplant patients < 16 yr old. Extended-release tablets (Envarsus XR) are currently labelled for use in adult kidney transplant patients being converted from an immediate-release tacrolimus formulation. An 80% conversion factor has been recommended for African-Americans converted from immediate-release dosage form to Envarsus XR. All extended-release formulations are NOT interchangeable. IV infusions should be administered at concentrations between 0.004 and 0.02 mg/mL diluted with NS or D_5W.

TOPICAL USE: Not recommended for use in patients with skin conditions with a skin barrier defect with the potential for systemic absorption. **Do not use** in children < 2 yr, immunocompromised patients, or patients with occlusive dressings (promotes systemic absorption). Approved as a second-line therapy for short-term and intermittent treatment of atopic dermatitis for patients who fail to respond or do not tolerate other approved therapies. Long-term safety is unknown. Skin burn sensation, pruritus, flu-like symptoms, allergic reaction, skin erythema, headache, and skin infection are the most common side effects. Application site edema has been reported. Although the risk is uncertain, the FDA has issued an alert about the potential cancer risk with the use of this product. See www.fda.gov/medwatch for the latest information.

TAZAROTENE
Avage, Fabior, Tazorac
Topical retinoid acid prodrug, keratolytic agent for acne or psoriasis

No No 3 X

Topical Cream:
  Tazorac: 0.05%, 0.1% (30, 60 g); contains benzyl alcohol
  Avage: 0.1% (30 g); contains benzyl alcohol
Topical Foam:
  Fabior: 0.1% (50, 100 g)
Topical Gel:
  Tazorac: 0.05%, 0.1% (30, 100 g); contains benzyl alcohol

Acne:
  ≥12 yr and adult: Apply a small amount of 0.1%-strength dosage forms to affected areas QHS. Use thin film (2 mg/cm^2) for cream or gel dosage form and small amount for foam dosage form.
Psoriasis:
  ≥12 yr and adult: Apply a small amount of 0.05% gel (2 mg/cm^2) to affected areas QHS initially. If needed and tolerated, increase to 0.1% gel QHS. The cream dosage form may also be used the same way as the gel, but it is currently labelled for use in adults (≥18 yr).

Contraindicated in pregnancy. Pregnancy testing 2 wk prior to use and initiation of use during menstrual period have been recommended. **Avoid** use in abraded or eczematous

Continued

TAZAROTENE continued

skin, with other medications or cosmetics with drying effects, or medications that can cause photosensitivity.

Tazarotene is a retinoid prodrug, which is converted to its active form, the cognate carboxylic acid of tazarotene (AGN 190299), by rapid deesterification in animals and man.

Common side effects include erythema, dry skin, skin irritation/pain, pruritus, and worsening of psoriasis.

Avoid contact with mucous membranes. The foam dosage form is flammable; avoid fire, flame, or smoking during or immediately after use.

TERBUTALINE
Various generics; previously available as Brethine
β_2-adrenergic agonist

No　Yes　2　C

Tabs: 2.5, 5 mg
Oral suspension: 1 mg/mL
Injection: 1 mg/mL (1 mL)

Oral:
　≤12 yr: Initial: 0.05 mg/kg/dose Q8 hr, increase as required. **Max. dose**: 0.15 mg/kg/dose Q8 hr or total of 5 mg/24 hr
　>12 yr and adult: 2.5–5 mg/dose PO Q6–8 hr
　　Max. dose:
　　　12–15 yr: 7.5 mg/24 hr
　　　>15 yr: 15 mg/24 hr
Nebulization (use IV dosage form):
　<2 yr: 0.5 mg in 2.5 ml NS Q4–6 hr PRN
　2–9 yr: 1 mg in 2.5 ml NS Q4–6 hr PRN
　>9 yr: 1.5–2.5 mg in 2.5 ml NS Q4–6 hr PRN
SC injection:
　≤12 yr: 0.005–0.01 mg/kg/dose (**max. dose**: 0.4 mg/dose) Q15–20 min × 3; if needed, Q2–6 hr PRN.
　>12 yr and adult: 0.25 mg/dose Q20 min PRN × 3; **max. total dose:** 0.75 mg.
Continuous infusion, IV: 2–10 mcg/kg loading dose followed by infusion of 0.1–0.4 mcg/kg/min. May titrate in increments of 0.1–0.2 mcg/kg/min Q30 min depending on clinical response. Doses as high as 10 mcg/kg/min have been used.
To prepare infusion: See *IV infusions* on page i.

The IV and PO route should **not** be used for the prevention or prolonged treatment of preterm labor because of the potential for serious maternal **cardiac events and even death.** Nervousness, tremor, headache, nausea, tachycardia, arrhythmias, and palpitations may occur. Paradoxical bronchoconstriction may occur with excessive use; if it occurs, discontinue drug immediately. Injectable product may be used for nebulization. For acute asthma, nebulization may be given more frequently than Q4–6 hr.

Monitor heart rate, blood pressure, respiratory rate, and serum potassium when using the continuous IV infusion route of administration. **Adjust dose in renal failure (see Chapter 30).**

TETRACYCLINE HCL
Various generics; previously available as Sumycin
Antibiotic

Yes   Yes   2   D

Caps: 250, 500 mg
Oral suspension: 25 mg/mL

Do not use in children < 8 yr
Child ≥ 8 yr: 25–50 mg/kg/24 hr PO ÷ Q6 hr; **max. dose:** 3 g/24 hr
  Acne: 500 mg PO BID
Adult: 250–500 mg PO Q6–12 hr

Not recommended in patients < 8 yr owing to tooth staining and decreased bone growth. Also **not recommended** for use in pregnancy because these side effects may occur in the fetus. The risk for these adverse effects are highest with long-term use. May cause nausea, GI upset, hepatotoxicity, stomatitis, rash, fever, and superinfection. Photosensitivity reaction may occur. **Avoid** prolonged exposure to sunlight.

Never use outdated tetracyclines because they may cause Fanconi-like syndrome. **Do not** give with dairy products or with any divalent cations (i.e., Fe^{2+}, Ca^{2+}, and Mg^{2+}). Give 1 hr before or 2 hr after meals. May decrease the effectiveness of oral contraceptives, increase serum digoxin levels, and increase effects of warfarin. Use with methoxyflurane increases risk for nephrotoxicity and use with isotretinoin is associated with pseudotumor cerebri. **Adjust dose in renal failure (see Chapter 30).**

Short-term maternal use is not likely to cause harm to breastfeeding infants.

THEOPHYLLINE
Theo-24, Theochron, Elixophyllin, and generics
Bronchodilator, methylxanthine

Yes   No   2   C

Other dosage forms may exist.
Immediate release:
  Elixir (Elixophyllin): 80 mg/15 mL (473 mL); may contain up to 20% alcohol.
Sustained/extended release (see remarks):
  Tabs:
    Q12 hr dosing (Theochron and generics): 100, 200, 300, 450 mg
    Q24 hr dosing (generics): 400, 600 mg
  Caps (Q24 hr dosing: Theo-24): 100, 200, 300, 400 mg
  Sustained-release forms should **not** be chewed or crushed. Capsules may be opened and contents may be sprinkled on food.

Dosing intervals are for immediate-release preparations.
For sustained-release preparations, divide daily dose > Q8–24 hr based on product.
Neonatal apnea:
  Loading dose: 5 mg/kg/dose PO × 1
  Maintenance: 3–6 mg/kg/24 hr PO ÷ Q6–8 hr
Bronchospasm; PO:
  Loading dose: 1 mg/kg/dose for each 2 mg/L desired increase in serum theophylline level
  Maintenance, infant (<1 yr):
    Preterm:
      <24 days old (postnatal): 1 mg/kg/dose PO Q12 hr
      ≥24 days old (postnatal): 1.5 mg/kg/dose PO Q12 hr

Continued

THEOPHYLLINE continued

Bronchospasm; PO:
  Full-term up to 1 yr old: Total daily dose (mg) = [(0.2 × age in weeks) + 5] × (kg body weight)
    ≤6 mo: Divide daily dose Q8 hr
    >6 mo: Divide daily dose Q6 hr
  Maintenance, child > 1 yr and adult without risk factors for altered clearance (see remarks):
    <45 kg: Begin therapy at 12–14 mg/kg/24 hr ÷ Q4–6 hr up to **max. dose** of 300 mg/24 hr. If needed based on serum levels, gradually increase to 16–20 mg/kg/24 hr ÷ Q4–6 hr. **Max. dose:** 600 mg/24 hr.
    ≥45 kg: Begin therapy with 300 mg/24 hr ÷ Q6–8 hr. If needed based on serum levels, gradually increase to 400–600 mg/24 hr ÷ Q6–8 hr.

Drug metabolism varies widely with age, drug formulation, and route of administration. Most common side effects and toxicities are nausea, vomiting, anorexia, abdominal pain, gastroesophageal reflux, nervousness, tachycardia, seizures, and arrhythmias.

Serum levels should be monitored. Therapeutic levels: bronchospasm: 10–20 mg/L; apnea: 7–13 mg/L. Half-life is age dependent: 30 hr (newborns); 6.9 hr (infants); 3.4 hr (children); 8.1 hr (adults). See *Aminophylline* for guidelines for serum level determinations. Liver impairment, cardiac failure, and sustained high fever may increase theophylline levels. Theophylline is a substrate for CYP450 1A2. Levels are increased with allopurinol, alcohol, ciprofloxacin, cimetidine, clarithromycin, disulfiram, erythromycin, estrogen, isoniazid, propranolol, thiabendazole, and verapamil. Levels are decreased with carbamazepine, isoproterenol, phenobarbital, phenytoin, and rifampin. May cause increased skeletal muscle activity, agitation, and hyperactivity when used with doxapram and increases quinine levels/toxicity.

Use ideal body weight in obese patients when calculating dosage because of poor distribution into body fat. Risk factors for increased clearance include: smoking, cystic fibrosis, hyperthyroidism, and high-protein diet. Factors for decreased clearance include CHF, correction of hyperthyroidism, fever, viral illness, sepsis, and high carbohydrate diet.

Suggested dosage intervals for sustained-released products (see following table):

THEOPHYLLINE SUSTAINED-RELEASE PRODUCTS

Trade Name	Available Strengths	Dosage Interval
CAPSULES:		
Theo-24	100, 200, 300, 400 mg	Q24 hr
TABLETS:		
Theochron and generics	100, 200, 300, 450 mg	Q12 hr
Generics	400, 600 mg	Q24 hr

THIAMINE
VITAMIN B₁, many generic products
Water-soluble vitamin

| No | No | 1 | A/C |

Tabs (OTC): 50, 100, 250 mg
Caps (OTC): 50 mg
Injection: 100 mg/mL (2 mL); may contain benzyl alcohol

For US RDA, see Chapter 21.
Beriberi (thiamine deficiency):
  Child: 10–25 mg/dose IM/IV once daily (if critically ill) or 10–50 mg/dose PO once daily × 2 wk, followed by 5–10 mg/dose once daily × 1 mo.
  Adult: 5–30 mg/dose IM/IV TID (if critically ill) × 2 wk, followed by 5–30 mg/24 hr PO ÷ once daily or TID × 1 mo.

THIAMINE continued

Wernicke's encephalopathy syndrome:
   Adult: 100 mg IV × 1, then 50–100 mg IM/IV once daily until patient resumes a normal diet. (Administer thiamine before starting glucose infusion.)

Multivitamin preparations contain amounts meeting RDA requirements. Allergic reactions and anaphylaxis may occur, primarily with IV administration. Therapeutic range: 1.6–4 mg/dL. High carbohydrate diets or IV dextrose solutions may increase thiamine requirements. Large doses may interfere with serum theophylline assay. Pregnancy category changes to "C" if used in doses above the RDA.

THIORIDAZINE
Various generics, previously available as Mellaril
Antipsychotic, phenothiazine derivative

Yes   No   ?   C

Tabs: 10, 25, 50, 100 mg

Child 2–12 yr: Start with 0.5 mg/kg/24 hr PO ÷ BID–TID; dosage range: 0.5–3 mg/kg/24 hr PO ÷ BID–TID. **Max. dose**: 3 mg/kg/24 hr.
>12 yr and adult: Start with 75–300 mg/24 hr PO ÷ TID. Then gradually increase PRN to **max. dose** 800 mg/24 hr ÷ BID–QID.

Indicated for schizophrenia unresponsive to standard therapy. **Contraindicated** in severe CNS depression, brain damage, narrow-angle glaucoma, blood dyscrasias, and severe liver or cardiovascular disease. **DO NOT** co-administer with drugs that may inhibit the CYP450 2D6 isoenzymes (e.g., SSRIs such as fluoxetine, fluvoxamine, paroxetine; and β-blockers such as propranolol and pindolol); drugs that may widen the QTc interval (e.g., disopyramide, procainamide, and quinidine); and in patients with known reduced activity of CYP450 2D6.
May cause drowsiness, extrapyramidal reactions, autonomic symptoms, ECG changes (QTc prolongation in a dose-dependent manner), arrhythmias, paradoxical reactions, and endocrine disturbances. Long-term use may cause tardive dyskinesia. Pigmentary retinopathy may occur with higher doses; a periodic eye exam is recommended. More autonomic symptoms and less extrapyramidal effects than chlorpromazine. Concurrent use with epinephrine can cause hypotension. Increased cardiac arrhythmias may occur with tricyclic antidepressants.
In an overdose situation, monitor ECG and avoid drugs that can widen QTc interval.

TIAGABINE
Gabitril and generics
Anticonvulsant

Yes   No   3   C

Tabs: 2, 4, 12, 16 mg
Oral suspension: 1 mg/mL

Adjunctive therapy for refractory seizures (see remarks):
   Child ≥ 2 yr (limited data from a safety and tolerability study in 52 children 2–17 yr, mean 9.3 ± 4.1): Initial dose of 0.25 mg/kg/24 hr PO ÷ TID × 4 wk. Dosage was increased at 4-wk intervals to 0.5, 1, and 1.5 mg/kg/24 hr until an effective and well-tolerated dose was established. Criteria for dose increase required tolerance of the current dosage level and <50% reduction in seizures. Patients receiving enzyme-inducing antiepileptic drugs (AEDs) received a **max. daily dose** of 0.73 ± 0.44 mg/kg/24 hr and patients receiving non–enzyme-inducing AEDs received a **max.** of 0.61 ± 0.32 mg/kg/24 hr.

Continued

TIAGABINE continued

Adjunctive therapy for partial seizures (dosage based on use with enzyme-inducing AEDs; see remarks). NOTE: patients receiving non–enzyme-inducing AEDs results in tiagabine blood levels about two times higher than patients receiving enzyme-inducing AEDs.
- **≥12 yr and adult:** Start at 4 mg PO once daily × 7 days. If needed, increase dose to 8 mg/24 hr PO ÷ BID. Dosage may be increased further by 4–8 mg/24 hr at weekly intervals (daily doses may be divided BID–QID) until a clinical response is achieved or up to specified **max. dose**.
  Max. dose:
    12–18 yr: 32 mg/24 hr
    Adult: 56 mg/24 hr

Use with caution in hepatic insufficiency (may need to reduce dose and/or increase dosing interval). Most common side effects include dizziness, somnolence, depression, confusion, and asthenia. Nervousness, tremor, nausea, abdominal pain, confusion, and difficulty in concentrating may also occur. Cognitive/neuropsychiatric symptoms resulting in nonconvulsive status epilepticus requiring subsequent dose reduction or drug discontinuation have been reported. Suicidal behavior or ideation, bullous dermatitis, and blurred vision have been reported. **Off-label use in patients WITHOUT epilepsy is discouraged** due to reports of seizures in these patients.

Tiagabine's clearance is increased by concurrent hepatic enzyme-inducing antiepileptic drugs (e.g., phenytoin, carbamazepine, and barbiturates). Lower doses or a slower titration for clinical response may be necessary for patients receiving non–enzyme-inducing drugs (e.g., valproate, gabapentin, and lamotrigine). **Avoid** abrupt discontinuation of drug.

TID dosing schedule may be preferred since BID schedule may not be well tolerated. Doses should be administered with food.

TIOTROPIUM
Spiriva HandiHaler, Spiriva Respimat
Anticholinergic agent, long acting

No | Yes | ? | C

Aerosol inhaler:
  Spiriva Respimat: 1.25 mcg/actuation (60 actuations/inhaler) (4 g), 2.5 mcg/puff (60 actuations/inhaler) (4 g)
Inhalational capsules:
  Spiriva HandiHaler: 18 mcg (boxes of 5s, 30s, or 90s with one HandiHaler device); contains milk protein

Asthma (maintenance therapy):
  Child (1–12 yr): See remarks.
  Child ≥ 12 and adult (Spiriva Respimat): Inhale 2.5 mcg once daily.

Contraindicated in patients with ipratropium hypersensitivity reactions (e.g., angioedema, itching, or rash). Common side effects include headache, constipation, xerostomia, UTI, bronchitis, cough, pharyngitis, sinusitis, and URI. Bowel obstruction, angle-closure glaucoma, urinary retention, and bronchospasm have been reported.

Use as an add on maintenance therapy for asthma along with inhaled corticosteroid. Maximum benefits may take up to 4–8 wk of continuous use. Doses > 2.5 mcg/24 hr were not associated with greater efficacy in FEV_1 for asthmatic adults. Studies in children 1–17 yr with inhaled Spriva Respimat dosed at 2.5 or 5 mcg once daily have demonstrated efficacy and safety for patients whose asthma were not well controlled despite treatment with inhaled corticosteroids.

Monitor for anticholinergic side effects in patients with moderate/severe renal impairment (eGFR < 60 mL/min).

TOBRAMYCIN
Tobrex, TOBI, TOBI Podhaler, Bethkis, Kitabis Pak, and generics; previously available as Nebcin
Antibiotic, aminoglycoside

Injection: 10 mg/mL (2 mL), 40 mg/mL (2, 30, 50 mL); may contain phenol and bisulfites
Premixed injection: 80 mg in 100 mL NS
Powder for injection: 1.2 g; preservative free
Ophthalmic ointment (Tobrex): 0.3% (3.5 g)
  In combination with dexamethasone (TobraDex): 0.3% tobramycin with 0.1% dexamethasone (3.5 g); contains 0.5% chlorbutanol
Ophthalmic solution (Tobrex): 0.3% (5 mL)
  In combination with dexamethasone (both products contains 0.01% benzalkonium chloride and EDTA):
    TobraDex and generics: 0.3% tobramycin with 0.1% dexamethasone (2.5, 5, 10 mL)
    TobraDex ST: 0.3% tobramycin with 0.05% dexamethasone (5 mL)
Nebulizer solution:
  Bethkis: 300 mg/4 mL (56s); preservative free
  TOBI, Kitabis Pak, and generic: 300 mg/5 mL (56s); preservative free
  170 mg/3.4 mL (mixed in 0.45% NS, preservative free, use with eFlow/Trio nebulizer)
Powder for inhalation:
  TOBI Podhaler: 28 mg capsules (224 capsules in 4 weekly packs with inhalation device)

Initial empiric dosage; patient specific dosage defined by therapeutic drug monitoring (see remarks).
Neonate/Infant, IM/IV (see following table):

Postconceptional age (wk)	Postnatal Age (Days)	Dose (mg/kg/dose)	Interval (hr)
≤29*	0–7	5	48
	8–28	4	36
	>28	4	24
30–34	0–7	4.5	36
	>7	4	24
≥35	ALL	4	24†

*Or significant asphyxia, PDA, indomethacin use, poor cardiac output, reduced renal function
†Use Q36 hr interval for HIE patients receiving whole-body therapeutic cooling.

Child: 7.5 mg/kg/24 hr ÷ Q8 hr IV/IM
Cystic fibrosis (if available, use patient's previous therapeutic mg/kg dosage):
  Conventional Q8 hr dosing: 7.5–10.5 mg/kg/24 hr ÷ Q8 hr IV
  High-dose extended-interval (once daily) dosing: 10–12 mg/kg/dose Q24 hr IV
Adult: 3–6 mg/kg/24 hr ÷ Q8 hr IV/IM
Ophthalmic:
  Tobramycin:
    Child and adult:
      Ophthalmic ointment: Apply 0.5-inch ribbon into conjunctival sac(s) BID–TID; for severe infections, apply Q3–4 hr
      Ophthalmic drop: Instill 1–2 drops of solution to affected eye(s) Q4 hr; for severe infections, instill 2 drops Q30–60 min initially and then reduce dosing frequency

Continued

TOBRAMYCIN continued

Ophthalmic:
   Tobramycin with dexamethasone:
      ≥2 yr and adult:
         Ophthalmic ointment: Apply 0.5-inch ribbon of ointment into conjunctival sac(s) TID–QID.
         Ophthalmic drop: Instill 1–2 drops of solution to affected eye(s) Q2 hr × 24–48 hr, then 1–2 drops Q4–6 hr.

Inhalation:
   Cystic fibrosis prophylaxis therapy:
      ≥6 yr and adult:
         TOBI, Bethkis, and generic product: 300 mg Q12 hr administered in repeated cycles of 28 days on drug followed by 28 days off drug.
         Use with eFlow/Trio nebulizer: 170 mg Q12 hr administered in repeated cycles of 28 days on drug followed by 28 days off drug.
         TOBI Podhaler: Four 28-mg capsules (112 mg) Q12 hr administered in repeated cycles of 28 days on drug followed by 28 days off drug.

Use with caution in combination with neurotoxic, ototoxic, or nephrotoxic drugs; anesthetics or neuromuscular blocking agents; preexisting renal, vestibular or auditory impairment; and in patients with neuromuscular disorders. May cause ototoxicity, nephrotoxicity, and neuromuscular blockade. Serious allergic reactions including anaphylaxis and dermatologic reactions including exfoliative dermatitis, toxic epidermal necrolysis, erythema multiforme, and Stevens–Johnson syndrome have been reported rarely. **Ototoxic effects synergistic with furosemide.**

Higher doses are recommended in patients with cystic fibrosis, neutropenia, or burns. **Adjust dose in renal failure (see Chapter 30).** Monitor peak and trough levels.

Therapeutic peak levels with conventional Q8 hr dosing:
   6–10 mg/L in general
   8–10 mg/L in pulmonary infections, neutropenia, osteomyelitis, and severe sepsis

Therapeutic trough levels with conventional Q8 hr dosing: <2 mg/L. Recommended serum sampling time at steady-state; trough within 30 min prior to the third consecutive dose and peak 30–60 min after the administration of the third consecutive dose.

Therapeutic peak and trough goals for high-dose extended-interval dosing for cystic fibrosis:
   Peak: 20–40 mg/L; recommended serum sampling time at 30–60 min after the administration of the first dose.
   Trough: <1 mg/L; recommended serum sampling time within 30 min before the second dose.

Serum levels should be rechecked with changing renal function, poor clinical response, and at a minimum of once weekly for prolonged therapies.

To maximize bactericidal effects, an individualized peak concentration to target a peak/MIC ratio of 8–10:1 may be applied.

For initial dosing in obese patients, use an adjusted body weight (ABW). ABW = Ideal Body Weight + 0.4 (Total Body Weight − Ideal Body Weight).

INHALATIONAL USE: Transient voice alteration, bronchospasm, dyspnea, pharyngitis, and increased cough may occur. Transient tinnitus, decreased appetite, and hearing loss have been reported nebulized dosage form. Aphonia, discolored sputum, and malaise have been reported with the powder for inhalation. Use is not recommended with nephrotoxic, neurotoxic, or ototoxic medications. Use with other inhaled medications in cystic fibrosis, use the following order of administration: bronchodilator first, chest physiotherapy, other inhaled medications (if indicated), and tobramycin last. For TOBI Podhaler, inhale the entire contents of each capsule.

Pregnancy category is "D" for injection and inhalation routes of administration and "B" for the ophthalmic route.

TOLNAFTATE
Tinactin, many other brands, and generics
Antifungal agent

No No ? ?

Topical aerosol liquid [OTC]: 1% (128, 150 g); may contain 29% vol/vol or 41% wt/wt alcohol
Aerosol powder [OTC]: 1% (133 g); contains 11% vol/vol alcohol and talc
Cream [OTC]: 1% (15, 30, 114 g)
Topical powder [OTC]: 1% (45, 108 g)
Topical solution [OTC]: 1% (10, 15, 30 mL)

Child (≥2 yr) and adult:
Topical: apply 1–3 drops of solution or small amount of liquid, cream, or powder to affected areas BID–TID for 2–4 wk.

May cause mild irritation and sensitivity. Contact dermatitis has been reported. **Avoid** eye contact. **Do not use** for nail or scalp infections. Discontinue use if sensitization develops. Pregnancy category not formally assigned by FDA.

TOPIRAMATE
Topamax, Topomax Sprinkle, Trokendi XR, Qudexy XR, and generics
Anticonvulsant

Yes Yes 2 D

Caps, sprinkle:
  Topamax Sprinkle and generics: 15, 25 mg
Tabs: 25, 50, 100, 200 mg
Extended-release caps, sprinkle (Q24 hr dosing; see remarks):
  Qudexy XR and generics: 25, 50, 100, 150, 200 mg
Extended-release caps (Q24 hr dosing; see remarks):
  Trokendi XR: 25, 50, 100, 200 mg
Oral suspension: 6 mg/mL

Adjunctive therapy for partial onset seizures or Lennox-Gastaut syndrome:
  Child 2–16 yr: Start with 1–3 mg/kg/dose (**max. dose:** 25 mg/dose) PO QHS × 7 days, then increase by 1–3 mg/kg/24-hr increments at 1- to 2- wk intervals (divided daily dose BID) to response. Usual maintenance dose is 5–9 mg/kg/24 hr PO ÷ BID.
  ≥17 yr and adult: Start with 25–50 mg PO QHS × 7 days, then increase by 25–50 mg/24 hr increments at 1-wk intervals until adequate response. Doses >50 mg should be divided BID. Usual maintenance dose: 100–200 mg/24 hr. Doses above 1600 mg/24 hr have not been studied.
Adjunctive therapy for primary generalized tonic–clonic seizures:
  Child 2–16 yr: Use above initial dose and slower titration rate by reaching 6 mg/kg/24 hr by the end of 8 wk.
  ≥17 yr and adult: Use above initial dose and slower titration rate by reaching 200 mg BID by the end of 8 wk; **max. dose:** 1600 mg/24 hr.
Monotherapy for partial onset seizures or primary generalized tonic–clonic seizures:
  Child 2–<10 yr: Start with 25 mg PO QHS × 7 days, if needed and tolerated, may increase dose to 25 mg PO BID. May further increase by 25–50 mg/24 hr at weekly intervals over 5–7 wk up to the lower end of the following daily target maintenance dosing range (if needed and tolerated, increase to higher end of dosing range by increasing by 25–50 mg/24 hr at weekly intervals):
    ≤11 kg: 150–250 mg/24 hr ÷ BID
    12–22 kg: 200–300 mg/24 hr ÷ BID

Continued

TOPIRAMATE continued

Monotherapy for partial onset seizures or primary generalized tonic clonic seizures: (cont.)
- **23–31 kg:** 200–350 mg/24 hr ÷ BID
- **32–38 kg:** 250–350 mg/24 hr ÷ BID
- **>38 kg:** 250–400 mg/24 hr ÷ BID

Child ≥ 10 yr and adult: Start with 25 mg PO BID × 7 days, then increase by 50 mg/24 hr increments at 1-wk intervals up to a **max. dose** of 100 mg PO BID at wk 4. If needed, dose may be further increased at weekly intervals by 100 mg/24 hr up to a recommended **max. dose** of 200 mg PO BID.

Migraine prophylaxis:
≥12 yr and adult: titrate dosage to 50 mg PO BID with the following schedule:

	Morning PO Dose	Evening PO Dose
Week 1	None	25 mg
Week 2	25 mg	25 mg
Week 3	25 mg	50 mg
Week 4 and beyond	50 mg	50 mg

Use clinical outcome to guide dose and titration. Longer intervals between dose adjustments can be used.

Use with caution in renal and hepatic dysfunction (decreased clearance) and sulfa hypersensitivity. **Reduce dose by 50% when creatinine clearance is < 70 mL/min.** Common side effects (incidence lower in children) include ataxia, cognitive dysfunction, dizziness, nystagmus, paresthesia, sedation, visual disturbances, nausea, dyspepsia, and kidney stones (incidence higher in children). Secondary angle closure glaucoma characterized by ocular pain, acute myopia, and increased intraocular pressure has been reported and may lead to blindness if left untreated. Patients should be instructed to seek immediate medical attention if they experience blurred vision or periorbital pain. Oligohidrosis and hyperthermia have been reported primarily in children and should be monitored especially during hot weather and with use of drugs that predispose patients to heat-related disorders (e.g., carbonic anyhdrase inhibitors and anticholinergics). Low serum bicarbonate levels have been reported in pediatric clinical trials. Hyperchloremic, non–anion gap metabolic acidosis has also been reported. Suicidal behavior or ideation has been reported.

Drug is metabolized by and inhibits the CYP450 2C19 isoenzyme. Phenytoin, valproic acid, and carbamazepine may decrease topiramate levels. Topiramate may decrease valproic acid, digoxin, and ethinyl estradiol (to decrease oral contraceptive efficacy), but may increase phenytoin levels. Alcohol and CNS depressants may increase CNS side effects. Carbonic anhydrase inhibitors (e.g., acetazolamide) may increase risk of metabolic acidosis, nephrolithiasis, or paresthesia. Use with valproic acid may result in the development of hyperammonemia.

Safety and efficacy in migraine prophylaxis in pediatrics have not been established; an increase in serum creatinine has been reported in a clinical trial.

Qudexy XR and Trokendi XR are not bioequivalent and should not be interchanged. Doses may be administered with or without food. Capsule may be opened and sprinkled on small amount of food (e.g., 1 teaspoonful of applesauce) and swallowed whole **(do not chew)**. Maintain adequate hydration to prevent kidney stone formation.

TRAZODONE
Generics, previously available as Desyrel
Antidepressant, triazolopyridine derivative

Yes Yes 2 C

Tabs: 50, 100, 150, 300 mg
Oral suspension: 10 mg/mL

TRAZODONE continued

Depression (titrate to lowest effective dose; see remarks):
  Child (6–18 yr): Start at 1.5–2 mg/kg/24 hr PO ÷ BID–TID; if needed, gradually increase dose Q3–4 days up to a **maximum** of 6 mg/kg/24 hr ÷ TID.
    Alternative dosing for adolescent: Start at 25–50 mg/24 hr; if needed, increase to 100–150 mg/24 hr in divided doses.
  Adult: Start at 150 mg/24 hr PO ÷ TID; if needed, increase by 50 mg/24 hr Q3–4 days up to a **max.** of 600 mg/24 hr for hospitalized patients (400 mg/24 hr for ambulatory patients).
Insomnia with comorbid psychiatric disorders (limited data):
  18 mo–<3 yr: Start at 25 mg PO QHS. If needed, increase by 25 mg Q2 wk up to a max. of 100 mg/24 hr.
  3–5 yr: Start at 50 mg PO QHS, if needed, increase by 25 mg Q2 wk up to a max. of 150 mg/24 hr.
  5 yr–adolescent: 25–50 mg PO QHS, if needed, increase by 25–50 mg Q2 wk up to a max. of 200 mg/24 hr. Daily dose may be divided BID–TID when used for palliative care.

Use with caution in preexisting cardiac disease, initial recovery phase of MI, in patients receiving antihypertensive medications, renal and hepatic impairment (has not been evaluated), and electroconvulsive therapy. Common side effects include dizziness, drowsiness, dry mouth, and diarrhea. May cause angle-closure glaucoma in patients with anatomically narrow angles who do not have an iridectomy. Seizures, tardive dyskinesia, EPS, arrhythmias, priapism, blurred vision, neuromuscular weakness, anemia, orthostatic hypotension, and rash have been reported. Monitor for clinical worsening of depression and suicidal ideation/behavior following the initiation of therapy or after dose changes.

Trazodone is a CYP450 3A4 isoenzyme substrate (may interact with inhibitors and inducers) and may increase digoxin levels and increase CNS effects of alcohol, barbiturates, and other CNS depressants. Max. antidepressant effect is seen at 2–6 wk.

TRETINOIN—TOPICAL PREPARATIONS
Retin-A, Retin-A Micro, Avita, Renova, Tretin-X, and many others
In combination with clindamycin: Veltin, Ziagen, and generics
Retinoic acid derivative, topical acne product

No   No   2   C

Cream: 0.02% (40, 60 g), 0.025% (20, 45 g), 0.05% (20, 40, 60 g), 0.075% (35 g), and 0.1% (20, 45 g); may contain parabens
Topical gel: 0.01% (15, 45 g), 0.025% (15, 20, 45 g), 0.04% (20, 45, 50 g), 0.05% (45 g), 0.8% (50 g), and 0.1% (20, 45, 50 g); may contain 90% alcohol, benzyl alcohol, and propylene glycol
In combination with clindamycin:
Topical gel: 0.025% tretinoin and 1.2% clindamycin (30, 60 g)

Topical:
  Child > 12 yr and adult: Gently wash face with a mild soap, pat the skin dry, and wait for 20 30 min before use. Initiate therapy with either 0.02% or 0.025% cream, or 0.01% gel and apply a small pea-sized amount to the affected areas of the face QHS or on alternate days. See remarks.
In combination with clindamycin:
  ≥12 yr and adult: Gently wash face with a mild soap, pat the skin dry, and wait 20 to 30 min before use. Apply a pea-size amount to entire face QHS.

Contraindicated in sunburns. **Avoid** excessive sun exposure. If stinging or irritation occurs, decrease frequency of administration to every other day. **Avoid** contact with eyes, ears, nostrils, mouth, or open wounds. Local adverse effects include irritation, erythema, excessive dryness, blistering, crusting, hyperpigmentation or hypopigmentation, and acne

Continued

TRETINOIN—TOPICAL PREPARATIONS continued

flare-ups. Concomitant use of other topical acne products may lead to significant skin irritation. Onset of therapeutic benefits may be experienced within 2–3 wk with optimal effects in 6 wk. The gel dosage form is flammable and should not be exposed to heat or temperatures > 120°F.

TRIAMCINOLONE
Nasal preparations: Nasacort Allergy 24HR Children, Nasacort Allergy 24HR, Nasal Allergy 24 Hour, and generics
Topical preparations: Triderm, Kenalog, Oralone, and generics
Injection preparations: Kenalog-10, Kenalog-40 and others in kits
Corticosteroid

Yes   Yes   2   C/D

Nasal spray:
　Nasacort Allergy 24 HR, Nasal Allergy 24 Hour, and generics [OTC]: 55 mcg/actuation (60 actuations per 10.8 mL, 120 actuations per 16.9 mL); contains benzalkonium chloride and EDTA.
　Nasacort Allergy 24 HR Children [OTC]: 55 mcg/actuation (60 actuations per 10.8 mL); contains benzalkonium chloride and EDTA.

Cream:
　Triderm and generics: 0.1% (15, 28.4, 30, 85.2, 454 g)
　Generics: 0.025% (15, 80, 454 g), 0.5% (15 g)

Ointment: 0.025%, 0.1% (15, 80, 454 g), 0.5% (15 g)
Lotion: 0.025%, 0.1% (60 mL)
Topical aerosol (Kenalog and generics): 0.2 mg/2 second spray, each g of spray contains 0.147 mg triamcinolone acetate (63, 100 g); contains 10.3% alcohol
Dental paste (Oralone and generics): 0.1% (5 g)
See Chapter 10 for potency rankings and sizes of topical preparations.
Injection as acetonide: 10 mg/mL (Kenalog-10) (5 mL), 40 mg/mL (Kenalog-40) (1, 5, 10 mL); contains benzyl alcohol and polysorbate 80
　Kits (all contain benzyl alcohol and polysorbate 80):
　　ReadySharp Triamcinolone: 40 mg/mL (1 × 1 mL)
　　Pro-C-Dure 5: 40 mg/mL (2 × 1 mL)
　　Arze-Ject-A, Pro-C-Dure 6: 40 mg/mL (3 × 1 mL)

Intranasal (titrate to lowest effective dose after symptoms are controlled; discontinue use if no relief of symptoms occur after 3 wk of use):
　Child 2–5 yr: 1 spray in each nostril once daily (110 mcg/24 hr; starting and **max. dose**).
　Child 6–11 yr: Start with 1 spray in each nostril once daily (110 mcg/24 hr). If no benefit in 1 wk, dose may be increased to the **max. dose** of 2 sprays in each nostril once daily (220 mcg/24 hr). Decrease dose to 1 spray each nostril when symptoms are controlled.
　≥12 yr and adult: 2 sprays in each nostril once daily (220 mcg/24 hr; starting and **max. dose**). Decrease dose to 1 spray each nostril when symptoms are controlled.
Topical cream/ointment/lotion:
　Child and adult: Apply a thin film to affected areas BID–TID for topical concentrations of 0.1% or 0.5% and BID–QID for 0.025% or 0.05%.
Topical spray:
　Child and adult: Spray to affected area TID–QID
SYSTEMIC USE:
　Antiinflammatory and allergic condition:
　　Child and adolescent (IM): 0.11–1.6 mg/kg/24 hr ÷ TID–QID

TRIAMCINOLONE continued

Intralesional for dermatosis:
≥12 yr and adult (Kenalog-10, 10 mg/mL): Inject up to 1 mg/site at intervals of 1 wk or more. May give separate doses in sites >1 cm apart, **not to exceed** 30 mg.

Rare reports of bone mineral density loss and osteoporosis has been reported with prolonged use of inhaled dosage form. Nasal preparations may cause epistaxis, cough, fever, nausea, throat irritation, dyspepsia, and fungal infections (rarely). Topical preparations may cause dermal atrophy, telangiectasias, and hypopigmentation. Anaphylaxis has been reported with use of the injectable dosage form. Topical steroids should be **used with caution** on the face and in intertriginous areas. See Chapter 8.

Dosage adjustment for hepatic failure with systemic use may be necessary. **Use with caution** in thyroid dysfunction, respiratory TB, ocular herpes simplex, peptic ulcer disease, osteoporosis, hypertension, CHF, myasthenia gravis, ulcerative colitis, and renal dysfunction. With systemic use, pregnancy category changes to "D" if used in the first trimester. Pregnancy category is "D" with the ophthalmic route.

Shake intranasal dosage forms before each use. **Avoid** SC and IV administration with injectable dosage forms. Injectable forms contain benzyl alcohol. **Avoid** spraying the eye or inhaling the topical aerosol dosage form.

TRIAMTERENE
Dyrenium
Diuretic, potassium sparing

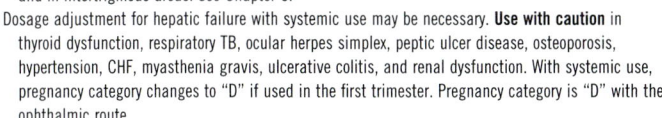
Yes Yes ? C/D

Caps: 50, 100 mg

Hypertension:
Child: 1–2 mg/kg/24 hr ÷ BID PO. May increase up to a **max.** of 3–4 mg/kg/24 hr up to 300 mg/24 hr.
Adult: 50–100 mg/24 hr ÷ once daily–BID PO; **max. dose**: 300 mg/24 hr.

Do not use if GFR < 10 mL/hr or in severe hepatic disease. **Adjust dose in renal impairment (see Chapter 30)** and cirrhosis. Monitor serum electrolytes. May cause hyperkalemia, hyponatremia, hypomagnesemia, and metabolic acidosis. Interstitial nephritis, thrombocytopenia, and anaphylaxis have been reported.

Concurrent use of ACE inhibitors may increase serum potassium. **Use with caution** when administering medications with high potassium load (e.g., some penicillins) and in patients with hepatic impairment or on high potassium diets. Cimetidine may increase effects. This drug is also available as a combination product with hydrochlorothiazide; erythema multiforme and toxic epidermal necrolysis have been reported with this combination product. Administer doses with food to minimize GI upset. Pregnancy category changes to "D" if used in pregnancy induced hypertension.

TRIFLURIDINE
Viroptic and generics
Antiviral, ophthalmic

No No ? C

Ophthalmic solution: 1% (7.5 mL); contains thimerosal

Herpes keratoconjunctivitis:
≥6 yr, adolescent, and adult: Instill 1 drop into affected eye(s) Q2 hr while awake up to a **maximum** of 9 drops/24 hr. Reduce dose when there is reepithelialization of the corneal ulcer

Continued

TRIFLURIDINE continued

to 1 drop Q4 hr (minimum 5 drops/24 hr) × 7 days. If improvement does not occur in 7–14 days, consider alternative therapy. **DO NOT EXCEED** 21 days of treatment.

Burning sensation in eyes and palpebral edema are common side effects. Rare cross sensitivity with idoxuridine, increased intraocular pressure, keratoconjunctivitis, and ocular hyperemia have been reported.

Avoid touching the applicator tip to eyes, fingers, or other surfaces and do not wear contact lenses during treatment of ocular infections. Apply pressure to the lacrimal sac during and for 1–2 min after dose administration to reduce risk of systemic absorption.

Store medication in the refrigerator (2–8°C). Storage at room temperature will result in a decrease in pH to cause stinging and ocular discomfort when in use.

TRILISATE

See Choline Magnesium Trisalicylate

TRIMETHOBENZAMIDE HCL
Tigan and generics
Antiemetic

Yes   Yes   ?   ?

Caps: 300 mg
Injection (Tigan): 100 mg/mL (2, 20 mL); may contain phenol or parabens

Child (PO): 15–20 mg/kg/24 hr ÷ TID–QID
  Alternative dosing:
    <13.6 kg: 100 mg TID–QID
    13.6–40 kg: 100–200 mg/dose TID–QID
    >40 kg: 300 mg/dose TID–QID
Adult:
  PO: 300 mg/dose TID–QID
  IM: 200 mg/dose TID–QID

Do not use in premature or newborn infants. **Avoid** use in patients with hepatotoxicity, acute vomiting, or allergic reaction. CNS disturbances are common in children (extrapyramidal symptoms, drowsiness, confusion, and dizziness). Hypotension, especially with IM use, may occur. **IM not recommended in children.** Consider reducing dosage in the presence of renal impairment since a significant amount of drug is excreted and eliminated by the kidney.
FDA pregnancy category has not been formally assigned.

TRIMETHOPRIM AND SULFAMETHOXAZOLE

See Sulfamethoxazole and Trimethoprim

URSODIOL
Actigall, Urso 250, Urso Forte, and generics
Gallstone solubilizing agent, cholelitholytic agent

Yes   No   1   B

Oral suspension: 20, 25, 50, 60 mg/mL
Caps (Actigall and generics): 300 mg

URSODIOL continued

Tabs:
  Urso 250 and generics: 250 mg
  Urso Forte and generics: 500 mg

Biliary atresia:
  Infant and child (limited data): 10–20 mg/kg/24 hr ÷ BID–TID PO
Pruritis from cholestasis:
  Infant, child, and adolescent (limited data): 15–30 mg/kg/24 hr ÷ once daily–BID PO
TPN-induced cholestasis:
  Infant and child [limited data, Gastroenterology. 1996;111(3):716–719]: 30 mg/kg/24 hr ÷ TID PO
Cystic fibrosis (to improve fatty acid metabolism in liver disease):
  Child: 15–30 mg/kg/24 hr ÷ BID–TID PO
Gallstone dissolution:
  Adult: 8–10 mg/kg/24 hr ÷ BID–TID PO

Contraindicated in calcified cholesterol stones, radiopaque stones, bile pigment stones, or stones > 20 mm in diameter. **Use with caution** in patients with nonvisualizing gallbladder and chronic liver disease. May cause GI disturbance, rash, arthralgias, anxiety, headache, and elevated liver enzymes (elevated ALT, AST, alkaline phosphatase, bilirubin, and GGT). Monitor LFTs every month for the first 3 months after initiating therapy and every 6 months thereafter. Thrombocytopenia has been reported in clinical trials.

Aluminum-containing antacids, cholestyramine, and oral contraceptives decrease ursodiol effectiveness. Dissolution of stones may take several months. Stone recurrence occurs in 30%–50% of patients within 5 yr.

VALACYCLOVIR
Valtrex and generics
Antiviral agent

Yes Yes 1 B

Tabs/Caplets: 500, 1000 mg
Oral suspension: 50 mg/mL

Child: Recommended dosages based on steady-state pharmacokinetic data in immunocompromised children. Efficacy data is incomplete.
  To mimic an IV acyclovir regimen of 250 mg/m²/dose or 10 mg/kg/dose TID:
    30 mg/kg/dose PO TID OR alternatively by weight:
      4–12 kg: 250 mg PO TID
      13–21 kg: 500 mg PO TID
      22–29 kg: 750 mg PO TID
      ≥30 kg: 1000 mg PO TID
  To mimic a PO acyclovir regimen of 20 mg/kg/dose 4 or 5 times a day:
    20 mg/kg/dose PO TID OR alternatively by weight:
      6–19 kg: 250 mg PO TID
      20–31 kg: 500 mg PO TID
      ≥32 kg: 750 mg PO TID
Chickenpox (immunocompetent patient; initiate therapy at earliest signs or symptoms, within 24 hr of rash onset):
  2–<18 yr: 20 mg/kg/dose PO TID × 5 days; **max. dose:** 1 g/dose TID.
HSV treatment (immunocompetent):
  3 mo–11 yr: 20 mg/kg/dose PO BID; **max. dose:** 1000 mg/dose.

Continued

VALACYCLOVIR continued

Herpes zoster (see remarks):
  Adult (immunocompetent): 1 g/dose PO TID × 7 days within 48–72 hr of onset of rash.
Genital herpes:
  Adolescent and adult:
   Initial episodes: 1 g/dose PO BID × 10 days.
   Recurrent episodes: 500 mg/dose PO BID × 3 days.
   Suppressive therapy:
    Immunocompetent patient: 500–1000 mg/dose PO once daily × 1 year, then reassess for recurrences. Patients with <9 recurrences per yr may be dosed at 500 mg/dose PO once daily × 1 yr.
Herpes labialis (cold sores; initiated at earliest symptoms):
  ≥12 yr and adult: 2 g/dose PO Q12 hr × 1 day.

This prodrug is metabolized to acyclovir and L-valine with better oral absorption than acyclovir. **Use with caution in hepatic or renal insufficiency (adjust dose; see Chapter 30).** Thrombotic thrombocytopenic purpura/hemolytic uremic syndrome (TTP/HUS) has been reported in patients with advanced HIV infection and in bone marrow and renal transplant recipients. Probenecid or cimetidine can reduce the rate of conversion to acyclovir.
Headache, nausea, and abdominal pain are common adverse events in adults. Headache is common in children. See Acyclovir for additional drug interactions and adverse effects.
For initial episodes of genital herpes, therapy is most effective when initiated within 48 hr of symptom onset. Therapy should be initiated immediately after the onset of symptoms in recurrent episodes (no efficacy data when initiating therapy > 24 hr after onset of symptoms). Data are not available for use as suppressive therapy for periods > 1 yr.
Valacyclovir **CANNOT** be substituted for acyclovir on a one-to-one basis. Doses may be administered with or without food.

VALGANCICLOVIR
Valcyte and generics
Antiviral agent

Yes   Yes   3   C

Tabs: 450 mg
Oral solution: 50 mg/mL (88 mL); contains saccharin and sodium benzoate
Oral suspension: 60 mg/mL

Neonate and infant:
  Symptomatic congenital CMV [from pharmacokinetic (PK) data in 8 infants 4–90 days old (mean: 20 days) and 24 neonates 8–34 days old]: 15–16 mg/kg/dose PO BID produced similar levels to IV ganciclovir 6 mg/kg/dose BID. A comparison of 6 weeks vs. 6 months of therapy in 96 neonates (>32-wk gestation and ≥1.8 kg) showed modest improvement in long-term hearing and developmental outcomes at 1–2 yr of age with the longer duration of therapy of 6 months.
Child (1 mo–16 yr):
  CMV prophylaxis in kidney (4 mo–16 yr), heart (1 mo–16 yr), or liver (4 mo–16 yr) transplantation (see remarks): Once daily PO dosage is calculated with the following equation. Daily mg dose (**max. dose:** 900 mg) = 7 × BSA × CrCl. BSA is determined by the Mosteller equation and CrCl is determined by a modified Schwartz equation (**max. value:** 150 mL/min/1.73 m^2).

VALGANCICLOVIR *continued*

Mosteller BSA (m^2) equation: square root of [(height (cm) × weight (kg)) ÷ 3600]
Modified Schwartz (mL/min/1.73 m^2) equation (max. value: 150 mL/min/1.73 m^2): k × height (cm) ÷ serum creatinine (mg/dL); where k = 0.33 if patient is < 1 yr old with low birth weight for gestational age; k = 0.45 if patient is < 1 yr old with birth weight appropriate for gestational age or if patient is 1–<2 yr old; k = 0.55 for boys 2–<13 yr old and girls 2–<16 yr old; or k = 0.7 for boys 13–16 yr old.
Duration of therapy:
    Kidney transplantation (≥4 mo–16 yr): 200 days
    Heart transplantation (≥1 mo–16 yr): 100 days
    Liver transplantation: see remarks.
Adolescent (>16 yr) and adult:
CMV retinitis:
    Induction therapy: 900 mg PO BID × 21 days with food
    Maintenance therapy: 900 mg PO once daily with food
CMV prophylaxis in heart, kidney, and kidney-pancreas transplantation: 900 mg PO once daily starting within 10 days of transplantation until 100 days post heart or kidney–pancreas transplantation, or until 200 days post kidney transplantation.

This prodrug is metabolized to ganciclovir, with better oral absorption than ganciclovir. **Contraindicated** with hypersensitivity to valganciclovir/ganciclovir; ANC < 500 mm^3; platelets < 25,000 mm^3; hemoglobin < 8 g/dL; and patients on hemodialysis. **Use with caution in renal insufficiency (adjust dose; see Chapter 30)**, preexisting bone marrow suppression, or in those receiving myelosupressive drugs or irradiation. Has not been evaluated in hepatic impairment. May cause headache, insomnia, peripheral neuropathy, diarrhea, vomiting, neutropenia, anemia, and thrombocytopenia. Neutropenia incidence is greater at day 200 vs day 100 in pediatric kidney transplant patients.

Use effective contraception during and for at least 90 days after therapy; may impair fertility in men and women. See *Ganciclovir* for drug interactions and additional adverse effects.

CMV prophylaxis data in liver transplantation is limited. A retrospective review in 10 pediatric patients, mean age 4.9 ± 5.6 yr, showed that 15–18 mg/kg/dose PO once daily × 100 days following liver transplantation resulted in 1 case of asymptomatic CMV infection detected by CMV antigenemia at day 7 of therapy. This patient then received a higher dose of 15 mg/kg/dose BID until three consecutive negative CMV antigenemia were achieved. The dose was switched back to a prophylactic regimen at day 46 posttransplant.

Monitor serum creatinine levels regularly and consider body changes to height and body weight for prophylaxis dosing.

Valganciclovir **CANNOT** be substituted for ganciclovir on a one-to-one basis. All doses are administered with food. **Avoid** direct skin or mucous membrane contact with broken or crushed tablets.

VALPROIC ACID
Depakene, Depacon, and generics
[Depakote: See Divalproex Sodium]
Anticonvulsant

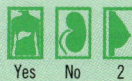
Yes   No   2   D/X

Caps (Depakene and generics): 250 mg
Oral solution or syrup (Depakene and generics): 250 mg/5 mL (473 mL); may contain parabens
Injection (Depacon and generics): 100 mg/mL (5 mL)

Continued

VALPROIC ACID continued

Oral:
Initial: 10–15 mg/kg/24 hr ÷ once daily–TID.
Increment: 5–10 mg/kg/24 hr at weekly intervals to **max. dose** of 60 mg/kg/24 hr.
Maintenance: 30–60 mg/kg/24 hr ÷ BID–TID. Due to drug interactions, higher doses may be required in children on other anticonvulsants. If using divalproex sodium, administer BID.

Intravenous (use only when PO is not possible):
Use same PO daily dose ÷ Q6 hr. Convert back to PO as soon as possible.

Rectal (use syrup diluted 1:1 with water, given PR as a retention enema):
Load: 20 mg/kg/dose
Maintenance: 10–15 mg/kg/dose Q8 hr

Migraine prophylaxis:
Child (limited data): 15–30 mg/kg/24 hr PO ÷ BID; alternative dosing for children ≥ 12 yr is 250 mg PO BID (**max. dose**: 1000 mg/24 hr).
Adult: Start with 500 mg/24 hr ÷ PO BID. Dose may be increased to a **max.** of 1000 mg/24 hr ÷ PO BID. If using divalproex sodium extended-release tablets, administer daily dose once daily.

Contraindicated in hepatic disease, pregnancy (for migraine indication), mitochondrial disorders with mutations in DNA polymerase gamma (e.g., Alpers-Huttenlocher Syndrome), and children < 2 yr suspected of the aforementioned mitochondrial disorder. May cause GI, liver, blood, and CNS toxicity; weight gain; transient alopecia; pancreatitis (potentially life-threatening); nausea; sedation; vomiting; headache; thrombocytopenia (dose-related); platelet dysfunction; rash (especially with lamotrigine); and hyperammonemia. Hepatic failure has occurred especially in children < 2 yr (especially those receiving multiple anticonvulsants, with congenital metabolic diseases, with severe seizure disorders with mental retardation, and with organic brain disease). Idiosyncratic life-threatening pancreatitis has been reported in children and adults. Hyperammonemic encephalopathy has been reported in patients with urea cycle disorders. Suicidal behavior or ideation, male infertility, elevated testosterone, decreased bone mineral density, DRESS, hair texture/color changes, and nail/nail bed disorders have been reported.

Valproic acid is a substrate for CYP450 2C19 isoenzyme and an inhibitor of CYP450 2C9, 2D6, and 3A3/4 (weak). It increases amitriptyline/nortriptyline, rufinamide, phenytoin, diazepam, and phenobarbital levels. Concomitant phenytoin, phenobarbital, topiramate, meropenem, cholestyramine, and carbamazepine may decrease valproic acid levels. Amitriptyline or nortriptyline may increase valproic acid levels. May interfere with urine ketone and thyroid tests.

Do not give syrup with carbonated beverages. Use of IV route has not been evaluated for >14 days of continuous use. Infuse IV over 1 hr up to a **max. rate** of 20 mg/min. Depakote and Depakote ER are **NOT** bioequivalent; see package insert for dose conversion.

Therapeutic levels: 50–100 mg/L. Recommendations for serum sampling at steady-state: Obtain trough level within 30 min prior to the next scheduled dose after 2–3 days of continuous dosing. Levels of 50–60 mg/L and as high as 85 mg/L have been recommended for bipolar disorders. Monitor CBC and LFTs prior to and during therapy.

Valproic acid and divalproex should not be used in pregnant women. Increased risk of neural tube defects, decreased child IQ scores, craniofacial defects, and cardiovascular malformations have been reported in babies exposed to valproic acid and divalproex sodium.

Pregnancy category is "X" when used for migraine prophylaxis and is a "D" for all other indications.

VALSARTAN
Diovan
Angiotensin II Receptor Blocker, antihypertensive agent

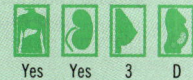
Yes Yes 3 D

Tabs: 40, 80, 160, 320 mg
Oral suspension: 4 mg/mL

Hypertension (see remarks):
  Child 1–5 yr (≥8 kg; limited data): A reported range of 0.4–3.4 mg/kg/dose PO once daily with the following maximum doses:
   <18 kg: 40 mg/24 hr
   ≥18 kg: 80 mg/24 hr
  Child 6–16 yr: Start at 1.3 mg/kg/dose (**max. dose**: 40 mg) PO once daily. Dose may be increased up to the 2.7 mg/kg/dose up to 160 mg (whichever is lower); doses greater than this have not been studied.
  Adolescent ≥ 17 yr and adult (non–volume-depleted status): Start 80 or 160 mg PO once daily; usual dose range is 80–320 mg once daily. **Max. dose**: 320 mg/24 hr.

Contraindicated with aliskiren use in diabetic patients. Discontinue use immediately after when pregnancy is detected. **Use with caution** in renal and liver insufficiency (no data are available), heart failure, postmyocardial infarction, renal artery stenosis, renal function changes, and volume depletion.

Hypotension, dizziness, headache, cough, and increases in BUN and sCr are common side effects. Hyperkalemia (consider salt substitutes, foods, and medications that may increase potassium levels), bullous dermatitis, angioedema, acute renal failure, and dysgeusia have been reported. May increase lithium levels, resulting in toxicity for those receiving concurrent lithium therapy; monitor lithium levels closely.

Onset of initial antihypertensive effects is 2 hr with maximum effects after 2–4 wk of chronic use. Patients may require higher doses of oral tablet dosage form than with the oral suspension due to increased bioavailability with the oral suspension.

VANCOMYCIN
Vancocin, First-Vancomycin 25, First-Vancomycin-50, Vancomycin+SyrSpend SF PH4, and generics
Antibiotic, glycopeptide

No Yes 1 C/B

Injection: 5, 10 g
Premixed injection: 500 mg/100 mL in dextrose; 750 mg/150 mL in dextrose; 1000 mg/200 mL in dextrose (iso-osmotic solutions)
Caps: 125, 250 mg
Oral solution: 25 mg/mL
  First Vancomycin-25: 25 mg/mL (150, 300 mL)
  First Vancomycin-50: 50 mg/mL (150, 210, 300 mL)
Oral suspension (Vancomycin+SyrSpend SF PH4): 50 mg/mL (120, 240 mL)

Initial empiric dosage; patient specific dosage defined by therapeutic drug monitoring (see remarks).

Continued

VANCOMYCIN continued

Neonate, IV (see following table for dosage interval):
Bacteremia: 10 mg/kg/dose
Meningitis, pneumonia: 15 mg/kg/dose

Postmenstrual Age (Weeks)*	Postnatal Age (Days)	Dosage Interval (hr)
≤29	0–14	18
	>14	12
30–36	0–14	12
	>14	8
37–44	0–7	12
	>7	8
≥45	All	6

*Postmenstrual age = gestational age + postnatal age

Infant, child, adolescent, and adult, IV:

Age	General Dosage	CNS Infections, Endocarditis, Osteomyelitis, Pneumonia, and MRSA Bacteremia
1 mo–12 yr	15 mg/kg Q6 hr	20 mg/kg Q6 hr
Adolescent (>12–<18 yr)	15 mg/kg Q6–8 hr	20 mg/kg Q6–8 hr
Adult (≥18 yr)	15 mg/kg Q8–12 hr	20 mg/kg Q8–12 hr

Clostridium difficile colitis (PR route of administration may be preferable for complete ileus):
Child: 40–50 mg/kg/24 hr ÷ Q6 hr PO × 7–10 days.
  Max. dose: 500 mg/24 hr; higher maximum of 2 g/24 hr have also been used.
Adult: 125 mg/dose PO Q6 hr × 7–10 days; dosages as high as 2 g/24 hr ÷ Q6–8 hr have also been used.

Endocarditis prophylaxis for GU or GI (excluding esophageal) procedures (complete all antibiotic dose infusion(s) within 30 min of starting procedure):
Moderate-risk patients allergic to ampicillin or amoxicillin:
  Child: 20 mg/kg/dose IV over 1–2 hr × 1
  Adult: 1 g/dose IV over 1–2 hr × 1
High-risk patients allergic to ampicillin or amoxicillin:
  Child and adult: Same dose as moderate-risk patients plus gentamicin 1.5 mg/kg/dose (**max. dose**: 120 mg/dose) IV/IM ×1

Ototoxicity and nephrotoxicity may occur and may be exacerbated with concurrent aminoglycoside use. Greater nephrotoxicity risk has been associated with higher therapeutic serum trough concentrations (≥15 mg/mL), concurrent piperacillin/tazobactam therapy, and receiving furosemide in the intensive care unit. **Adjust dose in renal failure (see Chapter 30).** Use total body weight for obese patients when calculating dosages. Low concentrations of the drug may appear in CSF with inflamed meninges. Nausea, vomiting, and drug-induced erythroderma are common with IV use. "Red man syndrome" associated with rapid IV infusion may occur. Infuse over 60 min (may infuse over 120 min if 60 min infusion is not tolerated). **NOTE:** Diphenhydramine is used to reverse red man syndrome. Allergic reactions [including drug rash with eosinophilia and systemic symptoms (DRESS)], neutropenia, and immune-mediated thrombocytopenia have been reported.

Although current extrapolated adult guidelines suggest measuring only trough levels, an additional postdistributional level may be useful in characterizing enhanced/altered drug clearance for quicker dosage modification to attain target levels; this may be useful for infants with known faster clearance and patients in renal compromise. Consult a pharmacist.

VANCOMYCIN continued

The following therapeutic trough level recommendations are based on the assumption that the pathogen's Vancomycin MIC is ≤ 1 mg/L.

Indication	Goal Trough Level
Uncomplicated skin and soft tissue infection, non-MRSA bacteremia, febrile neutropenia	10–15 mg/L
CNS infections, endocarditis, pneumonia, osteomyelitis, MRSA bacteremia	15–20 mg/L

Peak level measurement (20–50 mg/L) has also been recommended for patients with burns, clinically nonresponsive in 72 hr of therapy, with persistent positive cultures, and with CNS infections (≥30 mg/L).

Recommended serum sampling time at steady-state: Trough within 30 min prior to the fourth consecutive dose and peak 60 min after the administration of the fourth consecutive dose. Infants with faster elimination (shorter $T_{1/2}$) may be sampled around the third consecutive dose.

ORAL USE: Metronidazole (PO) is the drug of choice for *C. difficile colitis*; vancomycin should be avoided due to the emergence of vancomycin resistant enterococcus. Common adverse effects with oral vancomycin capsules in adults include nausea, abdominal pain, and hypokalemia.

Pregnancy category "C" for the intravenous route and "B" for the oral route of administration.

VARICELLA-ZOSTER IMMUNE GLOBULIN (HUMAN)
VariZig, VZIG
Hyperimmune globulin, varicella-zoster

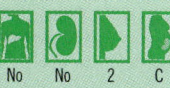

No   No   2   C

Injection: 125 U (1.2 mL); contains 10% maltose, 0.03% polysorbate 80, and <40 mcg/mL IgA; preservative free. May contain low levels of anti-Protein S antibodies.

Dose should be given within 48 hr of varicella exposure and no later than 96 hr post exposure. IM administration:
- *<2 kg:* 62.5 U
- *2.1–10 kg:* 125 U
- *10.1–20 kg:* 250 U
- *20.1–30 kg:* 375 U
- *30.1–40 kg:* 500 U
- *>40 kg:* 625 U
- Max. dose: 625 U/dose

If patient is at high risk and reexposed to varicella for more than 3 weeks after a prior dose, another full dose may be given.

Contraindicated in severe thrombocytopenia due to IM injection, immunoglobulin A deficiency (anaphylactic reactions may occur), and known immunity to varicella-zoster virus. See Chapter 16 for indications. Local discomfort, redness and swelling at the injection site, and headache may occur.

Hyperviscosity of the blood may increase risk for thrombotic events. Interferes with immune response to live virus vaccines such as measles, mumps, and rubella; defer administration of live vaccines 6 mo or longer after VZIG dose. See latest AAP *Red Book* for additional information.

Avoid IM injection into the gluteal region due to risk for sciatic nerve damage and **do not exceed** age-specific **single max. IM injection** volume.

VASOPRESSIN
Pitressin, Vasostrict and generics, 8-Arginine Vasopressin
Antidiuretic hormone analog

Yes   No   2   C

Injection: 20 U/mL (aqueous) (1 mL); may contain 0.5% chlorobutanol

Diabetes insipidus: Titrate dose to effect (see remarks).
 SC/IM:
  Child: 2.5–10 U BID–QID
  Adult: 5–10 U BID–QID
 Continuous infusion (adult and child): Start at 0.5 milliunit/kg/hr (0.0005 U/kg/hr). Increase dosage by 0.5 milliunit/kg/hr every 10 min PRN up to **max. dose** of 10 milliunit/kg/hr (0.01 U/kg/hr).
Growth hormone and corticotropin provocative tests:
  Child: 0.3 U/kg IM; **max. dose:** 10 U
  Adult: 10 U IM
GI hemorrhage (IV; NOTE: dosage metric is U/kg/min for children and U/min for adults):
  Child: Start at 0.002–0.005 U/kg/min. Increase dose as needed to **max. dose** of 0.01 U/kg/min.
  Adult: Start at 0.2–0.4 U/min. Increase dose as needed to **max. dose** of 0.8 U/min.
Cardiac arrest, ventricular fibrillation, and pulseless ventricular tachycardia:
  Child (use following 2 doses of epinephrine; limited data): 0.4 U/kg IV × 1
  Adult: 40 U IV or IO × 1
Vasodilatory shock with hypotension (unresponsive to fluids and pressors; NOTE: dosage metric is U/kg/min for children and U/min for adults):
  Infant, child, adolescent (various reports): 0.00017–0.008 U/kg/min via continuous IV infusion in combination with pressors.
  Adult: 0.01–0.04 U/min via continuous IV infusion in combination with pressors.

Use with caution in seizures; migrane; asthma; and renal, cardiac, or vascular diseases. Side effects include tremor, sweating, vertigo, abdominal discomfort, nausea, vomiting, urticaria, anaphylaxis, hypertension, and bradycardia. May cause vasoconstriction, water intoxication, and bronchoconstriction. Drug interactions: lithium, demeclocycline, heparin, and alcohol reduce activity; carbamazepine, tricyclic antidepressants, fludrocortisone, and chlorpropamide increase activity.

Do not abruptly discontinue IV infusion (taper dose). Patients with variceal hemorrhage and hepatic insufficiency may respond to lower dosages. Monitor fluid intake and output, urine specific gravity, urine and serum osmolality, plasma osmolality, and sodium.

VECURONIUM BROMIDE
Various generics; previously available as Norcuron
Nondepolarizing neuromuscular blocking agent

Yes   Yes   ?   C

Injection: 10, 20 mg

Neonate:
  Initial: 0.1 mg/kg/dose IV
  Maintenance: 0.03–0.15 mg/kg/dose IV Q1–2 hr PRN
Infants (>7 wk–1 yr) (see remarks):
  Initial: 0.08–0.1 mg/kg/dose IV
  Maintenance: 0.05–0.1 mg/kg/dose IV Q1 hr PRN; may administer via continuous infusion at 0.06–0.09 mg/kg/hr IV

VECURONIUM BROMIDE continued

>1 yr–adult (see remarks):
  Initial: 0.08–0.1 mg/kg/dose IV
  Maintenance: 0.05–0.1 mg/kg/dose IV Q1 hr PRN; may administer via continuous infusion at 0.09–0.15 mg/kg/hr IV

Use with caution in patients with renal or hepatic impairment, and neuromuscular disease. Dose reduction may be necessary in hepatic insufficiency. Infants (7 wk to 1 yr) are more sensitive to the drug and may have a longer recovery time. Children (1–10 yr) may require higher doses and more frequent supplementation than adults. Enflurane, isoflurane, aminoglycosides, β-blockers, calcium channel blockers, clindamycin, furosemide, magnesium salts, quinidine, procainamide, and cyclosporine may increase the potency and duration of neuromuscular blockade. Calcium, caffeine, carbamazepine, phenytoin, steroids (chronic use), acetylcholinesterases, and azthioprine may decrease effects. May cause arrhythmias, rash, and bronchospasm. Severe anaphylactic reactions have been reported.

Neostigmine, pyridostigmine, or edrophonium are antidotes. Onset of action within 1–3 min. Duration is 30–40 min. **See Chapter 1 for rapid sequence intubation.**

VERAPAMIL
Calan, Calan SR, Verelan, Verelan PM, and generics
Calcium channel blocker

Yes Yes 2 C

Tabs: 40, 80, 120 mg
Extended/sustained-release tabs (Calan SR and generics): 120, 180, 240 mg
Extended/sustained-release caps (Verelan, Verelan PM, and generics; for q24 hr dosing): 100, 120, 180, 200, 240, 300, 360 mg
Injection: 2.5 mg/mL (2, 4 mL)
Oral suspension: 50 mg/mL

IV for dysrhythmias: Give over 2–3 min. May repeat once after 30 min.
  1–16 yr, for PSVT: 0.1–0.3 mg/kg/dose × 1 may repeat dose in 30 min; **max. dose:** 5 mg first dose, 10 mg second dose.
  Adult, for SVT: 5–10 mg (0.075–0.15 mg/kg) × 1 may administer second dose of 10 mg (0.15 mg/kg) 15–30 min later.

PO for hypertension:
  Child: 4–8 mg/kg/24 hr ÷ TID or by age:
    1–5 yr: 40–80 mg Q8 hr
    >5 yr: 80 mg Q6–8 hr
    Max. dose: 480 mg/24 hr
  Adult: 240–480 mg/24 hr ÷ TID–QID or divide once daily–BID for sustained-release preparations.

Contraindications include hypersensitivity, cardiogenic shock, severe CHF, sick sinus syndrome, or AV block. **Use with caution** in hepatic and renal (**reduce dose in renal insufficiency; see Chapter 30**) impairment. Owing to negative inotropic effects, **verapamil should not be used to treat SVT in an emergency setting in infants. Avoid IV use** in neonates and young infants due to apnea, bradycardia, and hypotension. May cause constipation, headache, dizziness, edema, and hypotension. EPS has been reported.

Monitor ECG. **Have calcium and isoproterenol available to reverse myocardial depression.** May decrease neuromuscular transmission in patients with Duchenne's muscular dystrophy and worsen myasthenia gravis.

Continued

VERAPAMIL continued

Drug is a substrate of CYP450 1A2, and 3A3/4; and an inhibitor of CYP3A4 and P-gp transporter. Barbiturates, sulfinpyrazone, phenytoin, vitamin D, and rifampin may decrease serum levels/effects of verapamil; quinidine and grapefruit juice may increase serum levels/effects. Verpamil may increase effects/toxicity of β-blockers (severe myocardial depression), carbamazepine, cyclosporine, digoxin, ethanol, fentanyl, lithium, nondepolarizing muscle relaxants, prazosin, and tizanidine. Use with telithromycin has resulted in hypotension, bradyarrythmias, and lactic acidosis. Bradycardia has been reported with concurrent use of clonidine; and increased bleeding times has been reported with use with aspirin.

VIGABATRIN
Sabril
Anticonvulsant

Yes   Yes   ?   C

Tabs: 500 mg
Powder for oral solution: 500 mg per packet to be dissolved in 10 mL water (50s)

Infantile spams (1 mo–2 yr; see remarks for discontinuation of therapy): Start at 50 mg/kg/24 hr ÷ BID PO; if needed and tolerated, may titrate dosage upwards by 25–50-mg/kg/24 hr increments Q3 days up to a **maximum** of 150 mg/kg/24 hr ÷ BID. Withdrawal therapy if no clinical benefit is seen in 2–4 weeks.

Adjunctive therapy for refractory complex partial seizures (withdraw therapy if no clinical benefit is seen in 3 months; see remarks for discontinuation of therapy):
  Child (≥10 kg): Start at 40 mg/kg/24 hr ÷ BID PO, if needed and tolerated, adjust dose to the following maintenance dose:
   10–15 kg: 500–1000 mg/24 hr ÷ BID
   16–30 kg: 1000–1500 mg/24 hr ÷ BID
   31–50 kg: 1500–3000 mg/24 hr ÷ BID
   >50 kg: 2000–3000 mg/24 hr ÷ BID
  Adolescent (≥16 yr) and adult (see remarks for discontinuation of therapy): Start at 500 mg BID PO, if needed and tolerated, increase daily dose by 500 mg increments at 7 day intervals. Usual dose: 1500 mg BID; **max. dose:** 6000 mg/24 hr. Doses > 3 g/24 hr have not been shown to provide additional benefit and are associated with more side effects.

Use with caution in renal impairment **(reduce dose; see Chapter 30)** and other CNS depressants (enhanced effects). Can cause progressive and permanent vision loss (risk increases with dose and duration); periodic vision testing is required. Common side effects in children and adults include rash, weight gain, GI disturbances, arthralgia, visual disturbances, vertigo, sedation, headache, confusion, and URIs. Liver failure, anemia, psychotic disorder, angioedema, Stevens–Johnson syndrome, TEN, and suicidal ideation have been reported. Dose-dependent abnormal MRIs have been reported in infants treated for infantile spasms.
Ketorolac, naproxen, and mefloquine may decrease the effect of vigabitrin. Vigabitrin may decrease the effects/levels of phenytoin but increase the levels/toxicity of carbamazepine.
Use in adjunctive therapy for refractory complex partial seizure has labeled indication for ≥10-yr-old patients when potential benefits outweigh the risk of vision loss.
DO NOT rapidly withdraw therapy. Dosage needs to be tapered when discontinuing therapy to minimize increased seizure frequency. The following tapering guidelines have been recommended:
  Infant: decrease by 25–50 mg/kg every 3–4 days
  Child: decrease dose by 1/3 every 7 days for 3 weeks
  Adult: decrease by 1 g/24 hr every 7 days

VIGABATRIN continued

Doses may be administered with or without food. Access to this medication is restricted to prescribers and pharmacies registered under a special restricted distribution program (SABRIL REMS Program) in the United States. Call 888–457–4273 or see www.SabrilREMS.com for more information.

VITAMIN A
Aquasol A and generics
Vitamin, fat soluble

No | No | 2 | A/X

Caps [OTC]: 8,000, 10,000, 25,000 IU
Tabs [OTC]: 5,000, 10,000 IU
Injection (Aquasol A): 50,000 IU/mL (2 mL); contains polysorbate 80 and chlorobutanol

US RDA: See Chapter 21.
Supplementation in measles (a third dose may be administered 2–4 wk after the second dose if patient has ocular signs of vitamin A deficiency or is severely malnourished; see remarks):
  <6 mo: 50,000 IU/dose once daily PO × 2 days
  6 mo–<1 yr: 100,000 IU/dose once daily PO × 2 days
  1–5 yr: 200,000 IU/dose once daily PO × 2 days
Malabsorption syndrome prophylaxis:
  Child > 8 yr and adult: 10,000–50,000 IU/dose once daily PO of water miscible product.

High doses above the U.S. RDA are teratogenic (category X). The use of vitamin A in measles is recommended in children aged 6 mo–2 yr who are either hospitalized or who have any of the following risk factors: immunodeficiency, ophthalmologic evidence of vitamin A deficiency, impaired GI absorption, moderate to severe malnutrition, and recent immigration from areas with high measles mortality. May cause GI disturbance, rash, headache, increased ICP (pseudotumor cerebri), papilledema, and irritability. Large doses may increase the effects of warfarin. Mineral oil, cholestyramine, and neomycin will reduce vitamin A absorption. Do not access vitamin A levels during an acute inflammatory condition as falsely low levels have been reported. **See Chapter 21 for multivitamin preparations.**

VITAMIN B₁

See Thiamine

VITAMIN B₂

See Riboflavin

VITAMIN B₃

See Niacin

VITAMIN B₆

See Pyridoxine

VITAMIN B$_{12}$

See Cyanocobalamin

VITAMIN C

See Ascorbic Acid

VITAMIN D$_2$

See Ergocalciferol

VITAMIN D$_3$

See Cholecalciferol

VITAMIN E/α-TOCOPHEROL
Aqueous Vitamin E, Nutr-E-Sol, and many others including generics
Vitamin, fat soluble

No   No   2   A/C

Tabs [OTC]: 100, 200, 400 IU
Caps [OTC]: 100, 200, 400, 1000 IU
Oral solution (Aqueous Vitamin E and generics [OTC]): 50 IU/mL (12, 30 mL); may contain propylene glycol, polysorbate 80, and saccharin
Oral liquid (Nutr-E-sol) [OTC]: 400 IU/15 mL (473 mL)

US RDA: See Chapter 21.
Vitamin E deficiency, PO: Follow levels.
Use water miscible form with malabsorption.
   Neonate: 25–50 IU/24 hr × 1 week followed by recommended dietary intake.
   Child: 1 IU/kg/24 hr.
   Adult: 60–75 IU/24 hr.
Cystic fibrosis (use water miscible form): 5–10 IU/kg/24 hr PO once daily; max. dose: 400 IU/24 hr.

Adverse reactions include GI distress, rash, headache, gonadal dysfunction, decreased serum thyroxine, and triiodothyronine, and blurred vision. Necrotizing enterocolitis has been associated with large doses (>200 units/24 hr) of a hyperosmolar product administered to low birth weight infants. May increase hypoprothrombinemic response of oral anticoagulants (e.g., warfarin), especially in doses > 400 IU/24 hr.
One unit of vitamin E = 1 mg of DL-α-tocopherol acetate. In malabsorption, water miscible preparations are better absorbed. Therapeutic levels: 6–14 mg/L.
Pregnancy category changes to "C" if used in doses above the RDA. **See Chapter 21 for multivitamin preparations.**

VITAMIN K

See Phytonadione

VORICONAZOLE
Vfend and generics
Antifungal, triazole

Yes   Yes   ?   D

Tabs: 50, 200 mg; contains povidone
Oral suspension: 40 mg/mL (75 mL); may contain sodium benzoate
Injection: 200 mg; contains 3200 mg sulfobutyl ether β-cyclodextrin (SBECD) (see remarks)

Empiric doses. Between patient and interoccasion pharmacokinetic variability is high.
Monitor trough level and adjust dose accordingly. See www.clinicaltrials.gov for updated dosing information.

<2 yr (limited data): 9 mg/kg/dose IV/PO Q12 hr.

2–11 yr (limited data; see remarks): 7–9 mg/kg/dose IV/PO Q12 hr; **max. initial dose:** 350 mg/dose.
   Invasive aspergillosis, invasive candidiasis, or other rare molds (e.g., Scedosporium and Fusarium) (including 12–14 yr olds weighing <50 kg; dosing based on a previous clinical trial that was terminated due to slow enrollment): 9 mg/kg/dose IV Q12 hr × 2 doses followed by 8 mg/kg/dose IV Q12 hr. Convert to oral therapy when significant clinical improvement after 1 wk of IV therapy at a dose of 9 mg/kg/dose PO Q12 hr (max. dose: 350 mg Q12 hr).
   Esophageal candidiasis (including 12–14 yr olds weighing <50 kg); dosing based on a previous clinical trial that was terminated due to slow enrollment:
      IV: 4 mg/kg/dose Q12 hr.
      PO: 9 mg/kg/dose Q12 hr; **max. dose:** 350 mg Q12 hr.
   Prophylaxis pediatric acute leukemia (regimen currently being evaluated): 6 mg/kg/dose PO Q12 hr × 2 doses followed by 4 mg/kg/dose PO Q12 hr.

≥12 yr and adolescent:
   Invasive aspergillosis, invasive candidiasis, or other rare molds (e.g., Scedosporium and Fusarium); excluding 12–14-yr olds weighing <50 kg (dosing based on a previous clinical trial that was terminated due to slow enrollment): 6 mg/kg/dose IV Q12 hr × 2 doses followed by 4 mg/kg/dose IV Q12 hr. Convert to oral therapy when significant clinical improvement after 1 wk of IV therapy at a dose of 200 mg PO Q12 hr. For patients weighing <50 kg, use 2–11-yr dosing regimen. Alternatively, use adult PO dosage.
   Esophageal candidiasis (excluding 12–14 yr olds weighing <50 kg, use 2–11-yr dosing regimen for patients < 50 kg); dosing based on a previous clinical trial that was terminated due to slow enrollment:
      IV: 3 mg/kg/dose Q12 hr
      PO: 200 mg Q12 hr; alternatively use adult PO dosage
   Prophylaxis pediatric acute leukemia (up to 15 yr old); regimen currently being evaluated:
   6 mg/kg/dose PO Q12 hr × 2 doses followed by 4 mg/kg/dose PO Q12 hr.

Adult:
   Invasive aspergillosis, candidemia, Fusarium/Scedosporiosis, or other serious fungal infections:
      Loading dose: 6 mg/kg/dose Q12 hr × 2 doses
      Maintenance dose:
         Candidemia: 3–4 mg/kg/dose IV Q12 hr.
         Invasive aspergillosis, Fusarium/Scedosporiosis, or other serious fungal infections: 4 mg/kg/dose IV Q12 hr; if patient is unable to tolerate, reduce dose to 3 mg/kg/dose IV Q12 hr.
      PO maintenance dose: Initial dose may be increased to the maximum dose when response is inadequate; if dose is not tolerated, reduce dose by 50 mg increments, until tolerated, with minimum of the initial recommended dose.
         <40 kg: 100 mg Q12 hr; **max. dose**: 300 mg/24 hr
         ≥40 kg: 200 mg Q12 hr; **max. dose**: 600 mg/24 hr

Continued

VORICONAZOLE continued
Adult:
Esophageal candidiasis (treat for a minimum of 14 days and until 7 days after resolution of symptoms): Initial dose may be increased to the maximum dose when response is inadequate; if dose is not tolerated, reduce dose by 50 mg increments, until tolerated, with minimum of the initial recommended dose.
  <40 kg: 100 mg Q12 hr; **max. dose**: 300 mg/24 hr
  ≥40 kg: 200 mg Q12 hr; **max. dose**: 600 mg/24 hr

Contraindicated with concomitant administration with rifampin, carbamazepine, long acting barbiturates, ritonavir, efavirenz, rifabutin, ergot alkaloids, or St. John's Wort (decreases voriconazole levels); and with terfenadine, astemizole, cisapride, pimozide, quinidine, or sirolimus (voriconazole increases levels of these drugs to increase side effects). **Use with caution** in proarrhythmic conditions (e.g., congenital/acquired QTc prolongation, cardiomyopathy, and sinus bradycardia), severe hepatic disease, galactose intolerance, and concurrent use with CYP450 3A4 substrates that can lead to prolonged QTc interval (e.g., cisapride, pimozide, and quinidine).
Drug is a substrate and inhibitor for CYP450 2C9, 2C19 (major substrate), and 3A4 isoenzymes.
Currently approved for use in invasive aspergillosis, candidal esophagitis, and *Fusarium* and *Scedosporium apiospermum* infections. Common side effects include GI disturbances, fever, headache, hepatic abnormalities, photosensitivity (avoid direct sunlight and use protective measures), rash (6%), and visual disturbances (30%). Serious but rare side effects include anaphylaxis, liver or renal failure, and Stevens–Johnsons syndrome. Pancreatitis has been reported in children. Monitor serum transaminase and bilirubin levels weekly for the first month of therapy followed by reduced frequency has been recommended.
Correct potassium, magnesium, and calcium levels before and during voriconzole therapy. **Adjust dose in hepatic impairment** by decreasing only the maintenance dose by 50% for patients with a Child-Pugh Class A or B. **Do not use** IV dosage form for patients with GFR <50 mL/min because of accumulation of the cyclodextrin excipient; switch to oral therapy if possible. Patients receiving concurrent phenytoin should increase their voriconazole maintenance doses (IV: 5 mg/kg/dose Q 12 hr; PO: double the usual dose).
See www.clinicaltrials.gov for updated Pediatrics clinical trial information. Interoccasion pharmacokinetic variability is high, thus requiring serum level monitoring. Therapeutic levels: trough: 1–5.5 mg/L. Levels <1 mg/L have resulted in treatment failures and levels >5.5 mg/L have resulted in neurotoxicity such as encephalopathy. Recommended serum sampling time: obtain trough within 30 min prior to a dose. Steady state is typically achieved after 5–7 days of initiating therapy.
Administer IV over 1–2 hr with a **max. rate** of 3 mg/kg/hr at a concentration ≤ 5 mg/mL. Administer oral doses 1 hr before and after meals.

WARFARIN
Coumadin, Jantoven, and generics
Anticoagulant

Yes   Yes   1   D/X

Tabs: 1, 2, 2.5, 3, 4, 5, 6, 7.5, 10 mg

Infant and child (see remarks): To achieve an INR between 2 and 3
  Loading dose on day 1:
    Baseline INR ≤ 1.3: 0.2 mg/kg/dose PO; **max. dose**: 7.5 mg/dose
    Liver dysfunction, baseline INR > 1.3, cardiopulmonary bypass within previous 10 days, NPO status/poor nutrition, receiving broad spectrum antibiotics, receiving medications that significantly inhibit CYP450 2C9, or slow metabolizers of warfarin (see remarks): 0.05–0.1 mg/kg/dose PO; **max. dose**: 5 mg/dose

WARFARIN continued

Immediate postoperative period after a Fontan procedure: 0.05 mg/kg/dose PO; **max. dose**: 2.5 mg/dose

Loading dose on days 2–4:

Day 2		Days 3 & 4	
INR level	**Dose Adjustment**	**INF Level**	**Dose Adjustment**
1.1–1.3	Repeat day 1 loading dose	1.1–1.4	Increase previous dose by 20%–50%
1.4–1.9	Decrease day 1 loading dose by 50%	1.5–1.9	Continue current dose
≥2	Hold dose for 24 hr, then give 50% of day 1 loading dose on day 3	2–3	Use 25%–50% of day 1 loading dose
		3.1–3.5	Use 25% of day 1 loading dose
		>3.5	Hold dose until INR < 3.5, then restart at ≤25% of day 1 loading dose

Maintenance dose (therapy day ≥ 5):

Goal INR 2–3		Goal INR 2.5–3.5	
INR	**Dose Adjustment**	**INR**	**Dose Adjustment**
1.1–1.4	Increase previous dose by 20%	1.1–1.9	Increase previous dose by 20%
1.5–1.9	Increase previous dose by 10%	2–2.4	Increase previous dose by 10%
2–3	No Change	2.5–3.5	No change
3.1–3.5	Decrease previous dose by 10%	3.6–4	Decrease previous dose by 50% for one dose, then restart at a dose (prior to 50% dose decrease) decreased by 20% the next day
>3.5	Hold dose until INR < 3.5, then restart at 20% less than the last dose	>4	Hold dose for one day, then restart at a dose decreased by 20% of the last dose

Usual maintenance dose: ~0.1 mg/kg/24 hr PO once daily; range: 0.05–0.34 mg/kg/24 hr. See remarks.

Adult (see remarks): 5–10 mg PO once daily × 2–5 days. Adjust dose to achieve the desired INR or PT. Maintenance dose range: 2–10 mg/24 hr PO once daily.

Contraindicated in severe liver or kidney disease, uncontrolled bleeding, GI ulcers, and malignant hypertension. Acts on vitamin K–dependent coagulation factors II, VII, IX, and X. Side effects include fever, skin lesions, skin necrosis (especially in protein C deficiency), anorexia, nausea, vomiting, diarrhea, hemorrhage, and hemoptysis.

Warfarin is a substrate for CYP450 1A2, 2C8, 2C9, 2C18, 2C19, and 3A3/4. Chloramphenicol, chloral hydrate, cimetidine, delavirdine, fluconazole, fluoxetine, metronidazole, indomethacin, large doses of vitamins A or E, nonsteroidal antiinflammatory agents, omeprazole, oxandrolone, quinidine, salicylates, SSRIs (e.g., fluoxetine, paroxetine, and sertraline), sulfonamides, and zafirlukast may increase warfarin's effect. Ascorbic acid, barbiturates, carbamazepine, cholestyramine, dicloxacillin, griseofulvin, oral contraceptives, rifampin, spironolactone, sucralfate, and vitamin K (including foods with high content) may decrease warfarin's effect.

Younger children generally require higher doses to achieve desired effect. A cohort study of 319 children found that infants < 1 yr required an average daily dose of 0.33 mg/kg and teenagers 11–18 yr required 0.09 mg/kg to maintain a target INR of 2–3. Children receiving Fontan cardiac surgery may require smaller doses than children with either congenital heart disease (without

Continued

WARFARIN continued

Fontan) or no congenital heart disease. [See Chest. 2004;126:645–687S and Blood. 1999;94(9):3007–3014 for additional information.]

Lower initial doses should be considered for patients with pharmacogenetic variations in CYP2C9 (e.g., *2 and *3 alleles) and VKORC1 (e.g., 1639G>A allele) enzymes, elderly and/or debilitated patients, and patients with a potential to exhibit greater than expected PT/INR response to warfarin.

The international normalized ratio (INR) is the recommended test to monitor warfarin anticoagulant effect. It takes 5–7 days for an INR to reach steady state on a consistent dosing schedule. The particular INR desired is based upon the indication and has been extrapolated from adults. An INR of 2–3 has been recommended for prophylaxis and treatment of DVT, pulmonary emboli, and bioprosthetic heart valves. An INR of 2.5–3.5 has been recommended for mechanical prosthetic heart valves and the prevention of recurrent systemic emboli. If PT is monitored, it should be 1.5–2 times the control. Patients at high risk for bleeding may benefit from more frequent INR monitoring.

Onset of action occurs within 36–72 hr and peak effects occur within 5–7 days. IV dosing is equivalent to PO doses and is used in situations where oral dosing is not possible. **The antidote is vitamin K and fresh frozen plasma.**

Pregnancy category is "D" for women with mechanical heart valves and "X" for all others indications.

ZIDOVUDINE
Retrovir, AZT, and generics
Antiviral agent, nucleoside analogue reverse transcriptase inhibitor

Yes   Yes   2   C

Caps: 100 mg
Tabs: 300 mg
Oral syrup: 50 mg/5 mL (240 mL); contains 0.2% sodium benzoate
Injection: 10 mg/mL (20 mL); preservative free
In combination with lamivudine (3TC) as Combivir and generics:
  Tabs: 300 mg zidovudine + 150 mg lamivudine
In combination with abacavir and lamivudine (3TC) as Trizivir and generics:
  Tabs: 300 mg zidovudine + 300 mg abacavir + 150 mg lamivudine

HIV: See www.aidsinfo.nih.gov/guidelines.
Prevention of HIV vertical transmission:
  14–34 weeks of pregnancy (maternal dosing):
    Until labor: 600 mg/24 hr PO ÷ BID–TID
  During labor: 2 mg/kg/dose IV over 1 hr followed by 1 mg/kg/hr IV infusion until umbilical cord clamped
  Premature infant:

Gestational Age (wk)	Oral (PO) Dosage	Intravenous (IV) Dosage*
<30	2 mg/kg/dose Q12 hr, increase to 3 mg/kg/dose Q12 hr at 4 wk of age	1.5 mg/kg/dose Q12 hr, increase to 2.3 mg/kg/dose Q12 hr at 4 wk of age
30–34	2 mg/kg/dose Q12 hr, increase to 3 mg/kg/dose Q12 hr at postnatal age of 15 days	1.5 mg/kg/dose Q12 hr, increase to 2.3 mg/kg/dose Q12 hr at postnatal age of 15 days
≥35	4 mg/kg/dose Q12 hr	3 mg/kg/dose Q12 hr

*Convert to PO route when possible

ZIDOVUDINE continued

Term neonate and infant < 6 wk (initiate therapy within 12 hr of birth and continue untill 6 wk of age):
  PO: 2 mg/kg/dose Q6 hr, or 4 mg/kg/dose Q12 hr
  IV: 1.5 mg/kg/dose Q6 hr or 3 mg/kg/dose Q12 hr, administered over 60 min

HIV postexposure prophylaxis (all therapies to begin within 2 hr of exposure if possible):
  ≥12 yr and adult: 200 mg/dose PO TID or 300 mg/dose PO BID × 28 days. Use in combination with lamivudine or emtricitabine and with either one of the following: lopinavir/ritonavir, atazanavir/ritonavir, darunavir/ritonavir, raltegravir, etravirine, or etravirine × 28 days. Many other regimens exist; see www.aidsinfo.nih.gov/guidelines for the most recent information.

HIV treatment (see www.aidsinfo.nih.gov/guidelines for additional antiretroviral therapies and dosing information):
  Neonate:

Gestational age (wk)	Oral (PO) Dosage	Intravenous (IV) Dosage*
<30	**Birth to 4 wk of age:** 2 mg/kg/dose Q12 hr **4 wk to 8–10 wk of age:** 3 mg/kg/dose Q12 hr **>8–10 wk of age:** 12 mg/kg/dose Q12 hr	**Birth to 4 wk of age:** 1.5 mg/kg/dose Q12 hr **4 wk to 8–10 wk of age:** 2.3 mg/kg/dose Q12 hr **>8–10 wk of age:** 9 mg/kg/dose Q12 hr
30–34	**Birth to 2 wk of age:** 2 mg/kg/dose Q12 hr **>2 wk to 6–8 wk of age:** 3 mg/kg/dose Q12 hr **>6–8 wk of age:** 12 mg/kg/dose Q12 hr	**Birth to 2 wk of age:** 1.5 mg/kg/dose Q12 hr **>2 wk to 6–8 wk of age:** 2.3 mg/kg/dose Q12 hr **>6–8 wk of age:** 9 mg/kg/dose Q12 hr
≥35	**Birth to 4 wk of age:** 4 mg/kg/dose Q12 hr **>4 wk of age:** 12 mg/kg/dose Q12 hr	**Birth to 4 wk of age:** 3 mg/kg/dose Q12 hr **>4 wk of age:** 9 mg/kg/dose Q12 hr

*Convert to PO route when possible

  Infant (≥35 wk PCA, >4 wk of age, and ≥4 kg), child, and adolescent:
  PO: 180–240 mg/m^2/dose BID or the following by weight category:
    4–<9 kg: 12 mg/kg/dose BID or 8 mg/kg/dose TID
    9–<30 kg: 9 mg/kg/dose BID or 6 mg/kg/dose TID
    ≥30 kg: 300 mg BID or 200 mg TID
  IV:
    Infant (≥3 mo), child, and adolescent (<30 kg): 120 mg/m^2/dose Q6 hr; **max. dose:** 160 mg/dose
    Adolescent ≥ 30 kg: 1–2 mg/kg/dose Q4 hr

See www.aidsinfo.nih.gov/guidelines for additional remarks.
Use with caution in patients with impaired renal or hepatic function. Dosage reduction is recommended in severe renal impairment and may be necessary in hepatic dysfunction. Drug penetrates well into the CNS. Most common side effects include anemia, granulocytopenia, nausea, and headache (dosage reduction, erythropoietin, filgrastim/GCSF, or discontinuance may be required depending on event). Seizures, confusion, rash, myositis, myopathy (use > 1 yr), hepatitis, and elevated liver enzymes have been reported. Macrocytosis is noted after 4 wk of therapy and can be used as an indicator of compliance.

Continued

ZIDOVUDINE continued

Lactic acidosis and severe hepatomegaly with steatosis, including fatal cases have been reported. Neutropenia and severe anemia has been reported in advanced HIV disease.

Do not use in combination with stavudine because of poor antiretroviral effect. Effects of interacting drugs include increased toxicity (acyclovir and trimethoprim-sulfamethoxazole); increased hematological toxicity (ganciclovir, interferon-α, and marrow suppressive drugs); and granulocytopenia (drugs which affect glucuronidation). Methadone, atovaquone, cimetidine, valproic acid, probenecid, and fluconazole may increase levels of zidovudine. Whereas, rifampin, rifabutin, and clarithromycin may decrease levels.

Do not administer IM. IV form is incompatible with blood product infusions and should be infused over 1 hr (intermittent IV dosing). Despite manufacturer recommendations of administering oral doses 30 min prior to or 1 hr after meals, doses may be administered with food.

ZINC SALTS, SYSTEMIC
Galzin, Orazinc, and generics
Trace mineral

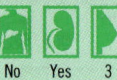
No   Yes   3   A/C

Tabs as sulfate (Orazinc and generics) [OTC], 23% elemental: 66, 110, 220 mg
Caps as sulfate (Orazinc, and generics) [OTC], 23% elemental: 220 mg
Caps as acetate (Galzin): 25, 50 mg elemental per capsule
Liquid as acetate: 5 mg elemental Zn/mL
Liquid as sulfate: 10 mg elemental Zn/mL
Injection as sulfate: 5 mg elemental Zn/mL (5 mL); may contain benzyl alcohol
Injection as chloride: 1 mg elemental Zn/mL (10 mL)

Zinc deficiency (see remarks):
 Infant and child: 0.5–1 mg elemental Zn/kg/24 hr PO ÷ once daily–TID
 Adult: 25–50 mg elemental Zn/dose (100–220 mg Zn sulfate/dose) PO TID
Wilson's disease:
 Child (≥10 yr): 75 mg/24 hr elemental Zn PO ÷ TID; if needed, may increase to 150 mg/24 hr elemental Zn PO ÷ TID
U.S. RDA: See Chapter 21.
For supplementation in parenteral nutrition, see Chapter 21.

Nausea, vomiting, GI disturbances, leukopenia, and diaphoresis may occur. Gastric ulcers, hypotension, and tachycardia may occur at high doses. Patients with excessive losses (burns) or impaired absorption require higher doses. Therapeutic levels: 70–130 mcg/dL.

Parenteral products may contain aluminum; **use with caution** in renal impairment. May decrease the absorption of penicillamine, tetracycline, and fluoroquinolones (e.g., ciprofloxacin). Drugs that increase gastric pH (e.g., H₂ antagonists and proton pump inhibitors) can reduce the absorption of zinc. Excessive zinc administration can cause copper deficiency.

Approximately 20%–30% of oral dose is absorbed. Oral doses may be administered with food if GI upset occurs. Pregnancy category is "A" for zinc acetate and "C" for all other salt forms.

ZOLMITRIPTAN
Zomig
Antimigraine agent, selective serotonin agonist

Yes   Yes   3   C

Tabs: 2.5 mg (scored), 5 mg
Oral disintegrating tabs (ODT): 2.5, 5 mg; contains aspartame
Nasal spray: 2.5 mg single unit nasal spray (6s), 5 mg single unit nasal spray (6s)

ZOLMITRIPTAN continued

Treatment of acute migraines with or without aura:
Oral (Safety of an average of >3 headaches in a 30-day period has not been established; see remarks):
 Adult:
  PO tabs: Start with 1.25–2.5 mg PO × 1. If needed in 2 hr, a second dose may be administered. Dose may be increased to a **maximum** single dose of 5 mg if needed. **Max. daily dose:** 10 mg/24 hr.
  ODT tabs: Use the same dosage recommendation for PO tabs but with a 2.5 mg initial dose.
Nasal (safety of an average of >4 headaches in a 30 day period has not been established; see remarks):
 ≥12 yr and adult: Start with 2.5 mg inhaled into a single nostril × 1. If needed in 2 hr, a second dose may be administered. Dose may be increased to a **maximum** single dose of 5 mg if needed. **Max. daily dose:** 10 mg/24 hr.
  Patients receiving concurrent cimetidine: Limit **maximum** doses to 2.5 mg as the **max. single dose** and **do not exceed** 5 mg in any 24 hr period.

Contraindicated in ischemic bowel disease; ischemic coronary artery disease; uncontrolled hypertension; peripheral vascular disease; history of stroke or TIA, arrhythmias, and hemiplegic or basilar migraine; significant cardiovascular disease; and coronary artery vasospasm.

Do not administer with any ergotamine-containing medication ergot-type medication, any other 5-HT1 agonist (e.g., triptans), methylene blue, or with/within 2 wk of discontinuing a MAO inhibitor or linezolid. Patients with multiple cardiovascular risk factors and negative cardiovascular evaluation should have their first dose administered in a medically supervised facility.

Use **not** recommended in moderate/severe hepatic impairment. Severe renal impairment (CrCl 5–25 mL/min) reduces zolmitriptan clearance by 25%.

Common adverse reactions for all dosage forms unless otherwise indicated include nausea, taste alteration (nasal route), xerostomia, dizziness, hyperesthesia (nasal route), paresthesia, somnolence, sensation of hot and cold, throat pain, and asthenia (oral route). Hypertension, coronary artery spasm, MI, cerebral hemorrhage, and headaches have been reported.

For intranasal use, blow nose gently prior to dosing. Block opposite nostril while administering dose by breathing in gently.

When using the oral disintegrating tablet (ODT), place the whole tablet on the tongue, allow the tablet to dissolve, and swallow with saliva. Administration with liquids is optional. Do not break the ODT tablet.

ZONISAMIDE
Zonegran and generics
Anticonvulsant

Yes   Yes   3   C

Caps: 25, 50, 100 mg
Oral syrup: 10 mg/mL

Infant and child (data is incomplete):
 Suggested dosing from a review of Japanese open-label studies for partial and generalized seizures: Start with 1–2 mg/kg/24 hr ÷ BID PO. Increase dosage by 0.5–1 mg/kg/24 hr Q2 wk to the usual dosage range of 5–8 mg/kg/24 hr ÷ BID PO.
 Recommended higher alternative dosing: Start with 2–4 mg/kg/24 hr PO ÷ BID-TID. Gradually increase dosage at 1- to 2-wk intervals to 4–8 mg/kg/24 hr; **max. dose**: 12 mg/kg/24 hr.

Continued

ZONISAMIDE continued

Infantile spasms (regimen that was effective in a small study from Japan; additional studies needed): Start with 2–4 mg/kg/24 hr PO ÷ BID. Then increase by 2–5 mg/kg/24 hr every 2–4 day until seizures disappear, up to a **maximum** of 20 mg/kg/24 hr.

>16 yr–adult:

Adjunctive therapy for partial seizures: 100 mg PO once daily × 2 wk. Dose may be increased to 200 mg PO once daily × 2 wk. Additional dosage increments of 100 mg/24 hr can be made at 2 wk intervals to allow attainment of steady-state levels. Effective doses have ranged from 100 to 600 mg/24 hr ÷ once daily–BID (BID dosing may provide better efficacy). No additional benefit has been shown for doses >400 mg/24 hr.

Because zonisamide is a sulfonamide, it is **contraindicated** in patients allergic to sulfonamides (may result in Stevens–Johnson syndrome or TEN). Common side effects of drowsiness, ataxia, anorexia, gastrointestinal discomfort, headache, rash, and pruritis usually occur early in therapy and can be minimized with slow dose titration. Children are at increased risk for hyperthermia and oligohydrosis, especially in warm or hot weather. Suicidal behavior or ideation, acute pancreatitis, urolithiasis, metabolic acidosis (more frequent and severe in younger patients), DRESS/multiorgan hypersensitivity, rhabdomyolysis and elevated creatinine phosphokinase have been reported.

Although not fully delineated, therapeutic serum levels of 20–30 mg/L have been suggested as higher rates of adverse reactions have been seen at levels > 30 mg/L.

Zonisamide is a CYP450 3A4 substrate. Phenytoin, carbamazepine, and phenobarbital can decrease levels of zonisamide.

Use with caution in renal or hepatic impairment; slower dose titration and more frequent monitoring is recommended. **Do not use** if GFR is < 50 mL/min. **Avoid** abrupt discontinuation or radical dose reductions. Shallow capsules whole and **do not** crush or chew.

Bibliography

1. Daily Med: Current Medication Information. National Library of Medicine. National Institutes of Health. Bethesda, MD. <http://dailymed.nlm.nih.gov/dailymed>.
2. Drugs and Lactation Database (LactMed). United States National Library of Medicine, Toxicology Data Network. <http://toxnet.nlm.nih.gov/cgi-bin/sis/htmlgen?LACT>.
3. Pickering LK, ed. *Red Book: 2015 Report of the Committee on Infectious Diseases.* 30th ed. Elk Grove Village, IL: American Academy of Pediatrics; 2015 <http://aapredbook.aappublications.org>.
4. AIDSinfo: Information on HIV/AIDS Treatment, Prevention, and Research. U.S. Department of Health and Human Services. <www.aidsinfo.nih.gov>.
5. Young TE, Mangum OB. Pediatrics and Neofax electronic version. New York, NY: Thomson Healthcare, USA. <http://neofax.micromedexsolutions.com/neofax/neofax.php?strTitle=NeoFax&area=1&subarea=0>.

6. McEvoy GK, Snow EK, eds. AHFS Drug Information. Stat!Ref electronic version. Bethesda, MD: American Society of Health-System Pharmacists. <www.ahfsdruginformation.com>.
7. Micromedex® Healthcare Series 2.0. electronic database. New York, NY: Thomson Healthcare USA. Updated periodically. <http://www.micromedexsolutions.com/micromedex2/librarian>.
8. Takemoto CK, Hodding JH, Kraus DM Pediatric Dosage Handbook, electronic intranet database. Hudson, OH: Lexi-Comp, Inc. Updated periodically. <www.crlonline.com/crlsql/servlet/crlonline>.
9. National Institutes of Health: National Heart, Lung and Blood Institute –Expert Panel. Clinical practice guidelines: Guidelines for the Diagnosis and Management of Asthma. <http://www.nhlbi.nih.gov/guidelines/asthma/asthsumm.htm>.
10. Bradley JS, Byington CL, Shah SS, et al. The Management of Community-Acquired Pneumonia in Infants and Children Older Than 3 Months of Age: Clinical Practice Guidelines by the Pediatric Infectious Disease Society and the Infectious Diseases Society of America. *Clin Infect Dis.* 2011;53(7):617-630.
11. Committee on Infectious Diseases and Bronchiolitis Guidelines Committee. Updated Guidance for Palivizumab Prophylaxis Among Infants and Young Children at Increased Risk of Hospitalization for Respiratory Syncytial Virus Infection. *Pediatrics.* 2014;134(2):415-420.
12. National High Blood Pressure Education Program Working Group on High Blood Pressure in Children and Adolescents. The Fourth Report on the Diagnosis, Evaluation, and Treatment of High Blood Pressure in Children and Adolescents. *Pediatrics.* 2004;114:555-576.
13. Flynn JT, Daniels SR. Pharmacologic Treatment of Hypertension in Children and Adolescents. *Journal of Pediatrics.* 2006;149:746-754.
14. Lande MB, Flynn JT. Treatment of hypertension in children and adolescents. *Pediatric Nephrology.* 2009;24:1939-1949.
15. Monagle P, Chan AKC, Goldenberg NA, et al. Antithrombotic Therapy in Neonates and Children: American College of Chest Physicians Evidence-Based Clinical Practice Guidelines (9th Edition). *Chest.* 2012;141(2 suppl):e737S-e801S.
16. Yin T, Miyata T. Warfarin dose and the pharmacogenomics of CYP2C9 and VKORC1 – Rationale and perspectives. *Thromb Res.* 2007;120:1-10.
17. American Thoracic Society. Targeted Tuberculin Testing and Treatment of Latent Tuberculosis Infection. *American Journal of Respiratory Critical Care Medicine.* 2000;161:1376-1395.
18. Food and Drug Administration Drug Safety Labeling Changes. <www.fda.gov/Safety/MedWatch/SafetyInformation/Safety-RelatedDrugLabelingChanges/default.htm>.
19. Abrams SA, the Committee on Nutrition. Clinical Report: Calcium and Vitamin D Requirements of Enterally Fed Preterm Infants. *Pediatrics.* 2013;131:e1676-e1683.
20. Registry and results database of publicly and privately supported clinical studies of human participants conducted around the world. U.S. National Institute of Health. <www.clinicaltrials.gov>.
21. New Pediatric Drug Labeling Database. U.S. Food and Drug Administration. Silver Spring, MD. <www.fda.gov/NewPedLabeling>.

Chapter 30

Drugs in Renal Failure

Elizabeth A.S. Goswami, PharmD, BCPS, BCPPS, and Helen K. Hughes, MD, MPH

I. DOSE ADJUSTMENT METHODS

A. Maintenance Dose

In patients with renal insufficiency, the dose may be adjusted using the following methods:

1. **Interval extension (I):** Lengthen intervals between individual doses, keeping dose size normal. For this method, a suggested interval is shown.
2. **Dose reduction (D):** Reduce amount of individual doses, keeping interval between doses normal; recommended when relatively constant blood level of drug is desired. For this method, percentage of usual dose is shown. For some medications and indications, specific dosing is provided.
3. **Interval extension and dose reduction (DI):** Both lengthen interval and reduce dose.
4. **Interval extension or dose reduction (D, I):** In some instances, either dose or interval can be changed.

   NOTE: These dose adjustment methods do not apply to patients in the neonatal period. For neonatal renal dosing, please consult a neonatal dosage reference. Dose modifications given are only approximations and may not be appropriate for all patients or indications. **Each patient must be monitored closely for signs of drug toxicity, and serum levels must be measured when available; drug doses and intervals should be adjusted accordingly.** When in doubt, always consult a nephrologist or pharmacist who has expertise in renal dosing.

B. Dialysis

General recommendations are provided when available. However, factors such as patient age, indication for use, residual native kidney function, specific peritoneal dialysis (PD) or intermittent hemodialysis (IHD) settings, etc., will affect the medication dosing needs of each individual patient. **Consult with a nephrologist or pharmacist who is very familiar with medication dosing in dialysis prior to prescribing medications for a dialysis patient.**

II. ANTIMICROBIALS REQUIRING ADJUSTMENT IN RENAL FAILURE (Table 30.1)

TABLE 30.1
ANTIMICROBIALS REQUIRING ADJUSTMENT IN RENAL FAILURE[1-5]

Drug	Pharmacokinetics		Normal Dose Interval	Method	Adjustments in Renal Failure		
	Route of Excretion*	Normal $t_{1/2}$ (h)			CrCl (mL/min/1.73 m²)	Percentage of Usual Dose	Interval
Acyclovir (IV)	Renal (60%–90%)	2–3	Q8 hr	D, I	25–50	100%	Q12 hr
					10–25	100%	Q24 hr
					<10/IHD α/PD	50%	Q24 hr
Amantadine† **Note:** On day 1, normal dose should be given, then decreased for subsequent doses based on renal insufficiency.	Renal (80%–90%)	10–30	Q12–24 hr	D, I	30–50	50%	Q24 hr
					15–29	50%	Q48 hr
					<15/IHD/PD	100%	Q7 days
Amikacin	Renal (>95%)	1.5–3	Q8–12 hr	I	<60/IHD/PD	Administer a standard initial dose. Determine the appropriate interval for redosing based on serum concentrations. For IHD, redose when predialysis concentration is <10 mg/L or postdialysis level is <6–8 mg/L[1]	
Amoxicillin **Note:** Do not administer 875 mg immediate release or 77 mg extended release tablets.	Renal (60%)	1–2	Q8–12 hr	I	10–30	20 mg/kg	Q12 hr
					<10/IHD Σ/PD	20 mg/kg	Q24 hr

Continued

TABLE 30.1
ANTIMICROBIALS REQUIRING ADJUSTMENT IN RENAL FAILURE—cont'd

Drug	Pharmacokinetics		Normal Dose Interval	Method	Adjustments in Renal Failure		
	Route of Excretion*	Normal $t_{1/2}$ (h)			CrCl (mL/min/1.73 m^2)	Percentage of Usual Dose	Interval
Amoxicillin/clavulanate **Note:** Do not administer 875 mg tablet	Renal (60%/25%–40%)	1	Q8–12 hr	I	10–30 <10/IHD Σ/PD	20 mg/kg 20 mg/kg	Q12 hr Q24 hr
Amphotericin B	Renal (40%)	Initial: 12–40.3 hr Terminal: 15 days	Q24 hr	D, I	Dosage adjustments are unnecessary with preexisting renal impairment. If decreased renal function is due to amphotericin B, daily dose can be decreased by 50%, or dose can be given every other day.[1]		
Amphotericin B lipid complex (Abelcet®)	Renal (1%)	Terminal: 173	Q24 hr		No guidelines established.		
Amphotericin B, liposomal (AmBisome®)	Renal (10%)	Initial: 7–10 Terminal: 100–153	Q24 hr		No guidelines established.		
Ampicillin (IV)	Renal (90%)	1–2	Q4–6 hr	I	10–30 <10/IHD Σ/PD	100% 100%	Q8 hr Q12 hr
Ampicillin/sulbactam	Renal (75%–85%)	1–2/1	Q4–6 hr	I	15–29 <15/IHD Σ/PD	100% 100%	Q12 hr Q24 hr
Aztreonam **Note:** Administer full dose for initial dose, then adjust subsequent doses for kidney function.	Renal (60%–70%) [hepatic]	1.3–2.2	Q6–8 hr	D, I	10–30 <10/IHD/PD IHD: Administer 12% of the full dose as an additional supplemental dose after dialysis in severe infections.[5]	50%–75% 25%–33%	Q8 hr Q12 hr
Cefaclor	Renal (80%)	0.5–1	Q8–12 hr	D	<10/IHD Σ/PD	50%	Q8–12 hr

Cefadroxil	Renal (>90%)	1–2	Q12 hr	I	10–25/IHD α	100%	Q24 hr
					<10/PD	100%	Q36 hr
Cefazolin	Renal (80%–100%)	1.5–2.5	Q6–8 hr	D, I	35–54	100%	Q8 hr
Note: Administer full dose for initial dose, then adjust subsequent doses for kidney function.					11–34	50%	Q12 hr
					≤10	50%	Q18–24 hr
					IHD α/PD	25 mg/kg	Q24 hr
Cefdinir	Renal (10%–20%)	1–2	Q12–24 hr	D, I	<30	7 mg/kg (max 300 mg)	Q24 hr
					IHD Σ/PD	7 mg/kg (max 300 mg)	Q48 hr
Cefepime	Renal (85%)	1.8–2	Q8 hr	D, I	10–50/IHD α/PD	100%	Q24 hr
Note: Administer full dose for initial dose, then adjust subsequent doses for kidney function.					<10	50%	Q24 hr
Cefixime[†]	Renal (50%)/[biliary]	3–4	Q12–24 hr	D	21–60/IHD	65%	Q12–24 hr
					<20/PD	45%	Q12–24 hr
Cefotaxime	Renal (60%)	1–1.5	Q6–8 hr	D	30–50	100%	Q8–12 hr
					10–29	100%	Q12 hr
					<10/IHD α/PD	100%	Q24 hr
Cefotetan	Renal (50%–80%)/[biliary]	3–4.5	Q12 hr	D	10–30	50%	Q12 hr
					<10	25%	Q12 hr
					IHD Σ	25%	Q24 hr
					PD	50%	Q24 hr

Continued

TABLE 30.1
ANTIMICROBIALS REQUIRING ADJUSTMENT IN RENAL FAILURE—cont'd

Drug	Pharmacokinetics			Adjustments in Renal Failure			
	Route of Excretion*	Normal $t_{1/2}$ (h)	Normal Dose Interval	Method	CrCl (mL/min/1.73 m^2)	Percentage of Usual Dose	Interval
Cefoxitin	Renal (85%)	0.75–1.5	Q4–8 hr	I	30–50	100%	Q8 hr
					10–30	100%	Q12 hr
					<10/IHD α/PD	100 %	Q24 hr
Cefpodoxime	Renal (30%)	2.2	Q12 hr	I	<30	100%	Q24 hr
					IHD	Administer thrice weekly after dialysis sessions	
Cefprozil	Renal (61%)	1.5	Q12–24 hr	D	<30/IHD/PD	50%	Q12–24 hr
					Administer 5 mg/kg supplement after IHD.[2]		
Ceftaroline†	Renal (88%)	1.5–2.5	Q8–12 hr	D, I	31–50	66%	Q8–12 hr
					15–30	50%	Q8–12 hr
					<15	33%	Q8–12 hr
					IHD α	33%	Q12 hr
Ceftazidime **Note:** Administer full dose for initial dose, then adjust subsequent doses for kidney function.[3]	Renal (80%–90%)	1.5–2	Q8 hr	D, I	30–50	100%	Q12 hr
					10–30	100%	Q24 hr
					<10/IHD α/PD	50%	Q24 hr
Ceftibuten	Renal (60%–70%)	2–2.5	Q24 hr	D	30–49	50%	Q24 hr
					5–29	25%	Q24 hr
					IHD	9 mg/kg (maximum 400 mg)	After each dialysis session.

Drug	Elimination	Half-life (hr)	Normal dose	Method	GFR (mL/min)	Dose adjustment	Interval
Cefuroxime (IV)	Renal (>90%)	1.5–2	Q8 hr	I	10–20	100%	Q12 hr
					<10/IHD Σ/PD	100%	Q24 hr
Cephalexin	Renal (>90%)	0.5–1.2	Q6–8 hr	I	30–50	100%	Q8 hr
					10–29	100%	Q12 hr
					<10/IHD α/PD	100%	Q24 hr
Ciprofloxacin	Renal (30%–50%) [hepatic]	1.3–5	Q8–12 hr	D, I	10–29	100%	Q18 hr
					<10/IHD α/PD	100%	Q24 h
Clarithromycin	Renal (20%–40%) [hepatic]	3–7	Q12 hr	D, I	<30	50%	Q12 hr
					<10/IHD α/PD	25%	Q24 hr
Ertapenem†	Renal (80%) [hepatic]	2.5–4	Q12–24 hr	D	≤30/IHD/PD	50%	Q24 hr
					IHD: If administered within 6 hr before dialysis, administer 30% of the daily dose after dialysis		
Erythromycin	Hepatic [renal (<15%)]	1.5–2	Q6–12 hr	D	<10/IHD/PD	50%–75%	Q8–12 hr
Ethambutol	Renal (50%) [hepatic]	2.5–3.5	Q24 hr	I	10–50	100%	Q24–36 hr
					<10	100%	Q48 hr
					IHD	100%	3 times weekly after dialysis
					PD	Data are not available. Begin with IHD dosing. Monitor closely and consider therapeutic drug monitoring.[6]	

Continued

TABLE 30.1
ANTIMICROBIALS REQUIRING ADJUSTMENT IN RENAL FAILURE—cont'd

Drug	Route of Excretion*	Pharmacokinetics Normal t½ (h)	Normal Dose Interval	Method	Adjustments in Renal Failure CrCl (mL/min/1.73 m²)	Percentage of Usual Dose	Interval
Famciclovir[†]	Renal (73%) [hepatic]	2–3	Q8 hr	D, I	**Herpes Zoster Treatment**[†]		
					40–59	500 mg	Q12 hr
					20–39	500 mg	Q24 hr
					<20	250 mg	Q24 hr
					IHD	250 mg	After each dialysis session
					Recurrent Genital Herpes Treatment—Single Day Regimen[†]		
					40–59	500 mg	Q12 hr × 1 day
					20–39	500 mg	Once
					<20	250 mg	Once
					IHD	250 mg	Once after dialysis
					Recurrent Genital Herpes Suppression[†]		
					20–39	125 mg	Q12 hr
					<20	125 mg	Q24 hr
					IHD	125 mg	After each dialysis session
					Recurrent Herpes Labialis—Single Dose Regimen[†]		
					40–59	750 mg	Once
					20–39	500 mg	Once
					<20	250 mg	Once
					IHD	250 mg	Once after dialysis

Drug				Recurrent Orolabial or Genital Herpes in HIV–Infected Patients†		
Fluconazole **Note:** Alternative IHD recommendation: Provide standard loading then administer 50% dose Q48 hr, administering after dialysis on dialysis days[1]	Renal (80%)	15–25	Q24 hr	D, I	20–39 <20 IHD	500 mg 250 mg 250 mg	Q24 hr Q24 hr After each dialysis session
					10–50 <10/PD IHD	50% 50% 100%	Q24 hr Q48 hr After each dialysis session
Flucytosine[7] **Note:** If available, therapeutic drug monitoring should be used to guide optimal dosing. Avoid flucytosine in children with severe kidney impairment.[8]	Renal (90%)	3–8	Q6 hr	I	20–40 10–50 <10/PD IHD	100% 100% 100% 100%	Q12 hr Q24 hr Q48 hr After each dialysis session
Foscarnet	Renal (80%–90%)	2–4.5	Induction: Q8 h Maintenance: Q24 hr	D, I	See package insert for adjustments for induction and maintenance.		

Continued

TABLE 30.1
ANTIMICROBIALS REQUIRING ADJUSTMENT IN RENAL FAILURE—cont'd

Drug	Pharmacokinetics			Adjustments in Renal Failure		
	Route of Excretion*	Normal t₁/₂ (h)	Normal Dose Interval	Method	CrCl (mL/min/1.73 m²)	Percentage of Usual Dose	Interval

Drug	Route of Excretion*	Normal t₁/₂ (h)	Normal Dose Interval	Method	CrCl (mL/min/1.73 m²)	Percentage of Usual Dose	Interval
Ganciclovir	Renal (>80%)	2.5–3.6	Induction: Q12 hr IV Maintenance: Q24 hr IV	D, I	**Induction IV**		
					50–69	2.5 mg/kg	Q12 hr
					25–49	2.5 mg/kg	Q24 hr
					10–24	1.25 mg/kg	Q24 hr
					<10/PD	1.25 mg/kg	Q48–72 hr
					IHD	1.25 mg/kg	Thrice weekly after IHD
					Maintenance IV		
					50–69	2.5 mg/kg	Q24 hr
					25–49	1.25 mg/kg	Q24 hr
					10–24	0.625 mg/kg	Q24 hr
					<10/PD	0.625 mg/kg	Q48–72 hr
					IHD	0.625 mg/kg	Thrice weekly after IHD
Gentamicin	Renal	1.5–3	Q8–12 hr	I	<50/IHD/PD	Administer standard initial dose. Determine appropriate interval for redosing based on serum concentrations.	
Imipenem/cilastatin **Note:** Manufacturer recommends patients with CrCl ≤5 not receive imipenem/cilastatin unless dialysis will be initiated within 48 hr	Renal (70%)	1–1.2	Q6–8 hr	D, I	30–50	50%	Q8 hr
					10–29	50%	Q12 hr
					<10/IHD α/PD	50%	Q24 hr

Isoniazid	Renal (75%–95%) [hepatic]	2–5 slow acetylator 0.5–1.5 fast acetylator	Q24 hr		100%	Q24 hr
Lamivudine[9†] **Note:** Administer full dose for initial dose, then adjust subsequent doses for kidney function. If CrCl <5, administer 50% of full dose as initial dose.	Renal	2	Q12 hr	D, I	30–49 15–29 5–14 <5/IHD/PD	100% 66% 33% 17%	Q24 hr Q24 hr Q24 hr Q24 hr
Levofloxacin	Renal (87%)	5–8	Q12–24 hr	I	10–29 <10/IHD/PD	100% 100%	Q24 hr Q48 hr
Meropenem	Renal (70%)	1–1.5	Q8 hr	D, I	26–50 10–25 <10/IHD α/PD	100% 50% 50%	Q12 hr Q12 hr Q24 hr
Metronidazole	Hepatic [renal 15%)]	6–12	Q6–12 hr	D	<10	No dose adjustments are available from the manufacturer. Metabolites may accumulate; monitor for adverse events. Some use a dose of 4 mg/kg at standard intervals.[1,2]	
					IHD Σ PD	4 mg/kg 4 mg/kg	Q6 hr Q6 hr
Norfloxacin[†]	Hepatic [renal (30%)]	3–4	Q12 hr	I	<30	100%	Q24 hr

Continued

TABLE 30.1
ANTIMICROBIALS REQUIRING ADJUSTMENT IN RENAL FAILURE—cont'd

Drug	Pharmacokinetics			Adjustments in Renal Failure			
	Route of Excretion*	Normal $t_{1/2}$ (h)	Normal Dose Interval	Method	CrCl (mL/min/1.73 m²)	Percentage of Usual Dose	Interval
Oseltamivir[†]	Renal (>99%)	6–10	Q12–24 hr	D, I	**Influenza Treatment**		
					31–60	50%	Q12 hr
					11–30	50%	Q24 hr
					<10/IHD	Administer weight based dosing as follows after each dialysis session:		
					≤15 kg	7.5 mg	
					16–23 kg	10 mg	
					24–40 kg	15 mg	
					>40 kg	30 mg	
					PD	50%	Once
					Influenza Prophylaxis		
					31–60	50%	Q24 hr
					10–30	50%	Q48 hr
					<10	No recommended dosage regimen.	
					IHD	50%	After every other dialysis session
					PD	50%	Weekly for duration of prophylaxis

Drug	Route of Elimination (Normal) [Alternative]	Half-Life (Normal)	Dose Adjustment Method	GFR (mL/min)	Dose Adjustment	Interval
Penicillin G—and aqueous K+Na+ (IV) **Note:** Administer full dose for initial dose, then adjust subsequent doses for kidney function.	Renal (60%–85%) [hepatic]	0.5–1.2 hr	D	10–50 <10/IHD α/PD	75% 20%–50%	Q4–6 hr Q4–6 hr
Penicillin V K+ (PO)	Renal (hepatic)	0.5 hr	I	<10/IHD α/PD	100%	Q8 hr
Pentamidine	Renal	5–9	I	10–30 <10/IHD α/PD	100% 100%	Q36 hr Q48 hr
Piperacillin/tazobactam[1,2]	Renal (75%–90%/>80%)	0.7–1.2/0.7–1.6	D, I	30–50 <30 IHD/PD IHD: Administer 25% of standard dose as supplemental dose after dialysis	50%–75% 50%–75% 50%–75%	Q6 hr Q8 hr Q12 hr
Rifabutin	Renal (53%) [hepatic]	36–45	D	<30	50%	Q12–24 hr
Streptomycin sulfate[†] **Note:** Interval extension is preferred to dose decrease to preserve concentration–dependent bactericidal activity. Use serum concentrations to determine optimal patient-specific dosing for efficacy and safety.[4]	Renal (30%–90%)	2.5	I	10–50 <10 IHD/PD	100% 100% 100%	Q24–72 hr Q72–96 Administer 2–3 times weekly after dialysis

Continued

TABLE 30.1
ANTIMICROBIALS REQUIRING ADJUSTMENT IN RENAL FAILURE—cont'd

Drug	Pharmacokinetics			Adjustments in Renal Failure		
	Route of Excretion*	Normal $t_{1/2}$ (h)	Normal Dose Interval	Method	CrCl (mL/min/1.73 m^2)	Percentage of Usual Dose	Interval
Sulfamethoxazole/trimethoprim	Renal (85%)/Renal (65%)	Sulfamethoxazole: 9–12 Trimethoprim: 3–6	Q12 hr	D	15–30 <15 IHD α/PD	50% Not recommended. If needed administer 5–10 mg/kg Q24 hr. Not recommended. If needed administer 5–10 mg/kg Q24 hr.	Q12 h
Tetracycline	Renal (60%) [hepatic]	6–12	Q6 hr	I	50–80 10–50 <10	100% 100% 100%	Q8–12 hr Q12–24 hr Q24 hr
Tobramycin	Renal (>90%)	1.5–3	Q8–24 hr	I	<60	Administer standard initial dose. Determine appropriate interval for redosing based on serum concentrations.	
Valacyclovir[†] **Note:** For IHD for all indications, dose for CrCl <10 and administer dose after dialysis. For PD for all indications, administer 500 mg Q48 hr.[4]	Hepatic to acyclovir.	Valacyclovir: ~30 min Acyclovir: 2–3	Q8–24 hr	D, I	**Herpes Zoster (Adults)** 30–49 10–29 <10 **Genital Herpes (Adolescents/Adults): Initial Episode** 10–29 <10 **Genital Herpes (Adolescents/Adults): Recurrent Episode** <30	 100% 100% 50% 100% 50% 100%	 Q12 hr Q24 hr Q24 hr Q24 hr Q24 hr Q24 hr

Drug	Route	Dose	Category
Valganciclovir **Note:** For dosing in children, a maximum CrCl value of 150 mL/min/1.73 m² should be used to calculate the dose. Calculate CrCl using a modified Schwartz formula where k = 0.33 in infants aged <1 year, with low birth weight appropriate for gestational age, 0.45 in infants aged <1 year, with birth weight appropriate for gestational age, 0.45 in children aged 1 to <2 years, 0.55 in boys aged 2 to <13 years and girls aged 2 to <16 years, and 0.7 in boys aged 13 to 16 years.	Renal (>80%)	Valganciclovir: 0.4–0.6 Ganciclovir: 2.5–3.6	Q12–24 hr	D

Genital Herpes (Adolescents/Adults): Suppressive

<30	500 mg	Q24 hr (for usual dose of 1 g Q24 hr)
	OR	
	500 mg	Q48 hr (for usual dose of 500 mg Q24 hr)

Herpes Labialis (Adolescents/Adults)

30–49	50%	Q12 hr × 2 doses
10–29	25%	Q12 hr × 2 doses
<10	25%	Single dose

Children

Normal dosing accounts for kidney function:
Once daily dose (mg) = 7 × body surface area × creatinine clearance.

Adults—Induction

40–59	450 mg Q12 hr
25–39	450 mg Q24 hr
10–24	450 mg Q48 hr
<10/IHD α	Use of renally adjusted ganciclovir preferred. May consider dose of 200 mg thrice weekly.

Adults—Maintenance

40–59	450 mg Q24 hr
25–39	450 mg Q48 hr
10–24	450 mg Twice weekly
<10/IHD α	Use of renally adjusted ganciclovir preferred. May consider dose of 200 mg thrice weekly.

Continued

TABLE 30.1
ANTIMICROBIALS REQUIRING ADJUSTMENT IN RENAL FAILURE—cont'd

Drug	Pharmacokinetics			Adjustments in Renal Failure		
	Route of Excretion*	Normal t$_{1/2}$ (h)	Normal Dose Interval	Method	CrCl (mL/min/1.73 m^2)	Percentage of Usual Dose Interval
Vancomycin	Renal (80%–90%)	2.2–8	Q6–12 hr	I	<50	Administer standard initial dose. Determine appropriate interval for redosing based on serum concentrations.
					IHD/PD	Administer standard initial dose. Obtain serum concentration after dialysis to determine need to redose. Obtain levels 4–6 hr after dialysis to allow for redistribution from peripheral compartment. If patient is unstable may obtain sooner with knowledge that concentration may be lower than steady state.

CrCl, Creatinine clearance; D, dose reduction; GFR, glomerular filtration rate; HIV, human immunodeficiency virus; I, interval extension; IHD, intermittent hemodialysis; IM, intramuscular; IV, intravenous; K⁺, potassium; Na⁺, sodium; PD, peritoneal dialysis; PO, oral; t$_{1/2}$, half–life with normal renal function.
*Percentage in parenthesis represents the amount of drug and/or metabolites excreted in the urine. Route in brackets indicates secondary route of excretion.
†In adults: guidelines not established in children.
α For IHD administer after dialysis on dialysis days
Σ Administer a supplemental dose after dialysis

III. NONANTIMICROBIALS REQUIRING ADJUSTMENT IN RENAL FAILURE (Table 30.2)

TABLE 30.2
NONANTIMICROBIALS REQUIRING ADJUSTMENT IN RENAL FAILURE[1-5]

Drug	Route of Excretion*	Pharmacokinetics Normal $t_{1/2}$ (h)	Normal Dose Interval	Method	Adjustments in Renal Failure CrCl (mL/min/1.73 m^2)	Percentage of Usual Dose	Interval
Acetaminophen	Hepatic	2–4	Q4–6 hr	I	10–50	100%	Q6 hr
					<10	100%	Q8 hr
Acetazolamide	Renal (>70%)	2.4–5.8	Q6–24 hr	I	10–50	100%	Q12 hr
					IHD α	12.5%–titrate to effect	Q12–24 hr
					<10/PD	Avoid use	
Allopurinol	Renal	1–3	Q6–12 hr	D	10–50	50%	Q6–12 hr
					<10/IHD/PD	30%	Q6–12 hr
Aminocaproic acid	Renal (76%)	1–2	Q4–6 hr, continuous	D	Oliguria/ESRD	12%–25%	Q4–6 hr, continuous
Aspirin	Hepatic (renal)	Dose dependent: 3–10	Q4–24 hr	I	10–50	100%	Q4–24 hr
					IHD α	100%	Q24 hr
					<10/PD	Avoid use for analgesia and anti-inflammatory indications	
Atenolol	Renal (50%)	3.5–7	Q24 hr	D, I	15–35	1 mg/kg up to 50 mg	Q24 hr

Continued

TABLE 30.2
NONANTIMICROBIALS REQUIRING ADJUSTMENT IN RENAL FAILURE —cont'd

Drug	Pharmacokinetics			Adjustments in Renal Failure		
	Route of Excretion*	Normal $t_{1/2}$ (h)	Normal Dose Interval	Method	CrCl (mL/min/1.73 m²)	Percentage of Usual Dose	Interval
Azathioprine	Hepatic to 6-mercaptopurine [renal]	2	Q24 hr	D	<15/IHD α/PD 10–50 <10/IHD α/PD	1 mg/kg up to 50 mg 75% 50%	Q48 hr Q24 hr Q24 hr
Bismuth subsalicylate	Hepatic [renal]	Salicylate: 2–5 Bismuth: 21–72 days	Q3–4 hr		Avoid use in patients with renal failure.		
Calcium supplements	GI [renal (20%)]	Variable	Variable		<25	May require dosage adjustment depending on calcium level.	
Captopril	Renal (95%) [hepatic]	1.5–2	Q6–24 hr	D	10–50 <10/IHD α/PD	75% 50%	Q6–24 hr Q6–24 hr
Carbamazepine **NOTE:** Avoid use of IV product in moderate to severe kidney dysfunction. Solubilizing agent may accumulate and lead to toxicity.	Hepatic (renal)	Initial: 25–65 Subsequent: 8–17	Q6–12 hr	D	<10/IHD α/PD	75%	Q6–12 hr

Drug	Elimination	Half-life (hr)	Normal interval	Method	GFR (mL/min/1.73 m²)	Dose	Interval
Cetirizine	Renal (70%) [hepatic]	6.2–8	Q12–24 hr	D	<6 yrs of age with Renal Impairment Use not recommended. 6–11 yrs of age		
					11–50	2.5–5 mg	Q24 hr
					<11	Use not recommended.	
					≥12 yrs of age		
					11–30/IHD/PD	5 mg	Q24 hr
					<11	Use not recommended.	
Chloroquine	Renal (70%) [hepatic]	3–5 days	Weekly	D	<10	50%	Weekly
Chlorothiazide	Renal (>90%)	0.75–2	Q12–24 hr	NA	<40	May be ineffective.	
					<10	Use not recommended.	
Cimetidine	Renal (48%) [(hepatic)]	1.4–2	Q6–12 hr	D, I	>40	100%	Q6 hr
					20–40	100% OR 75%	Q8 hr Q6 hr
					<20	100% OR 50%	Q12 hr Q6 hr
					IHD a/PD	100%	Q12 hr
Clobazam	Renal (82%) [Hepatic, GI]	Children: 16 Adults: 36–42	Q12–24 hr	D	<30	Use with caution; has not been studied.	
Desloratadine†	Renal (87%) [GI]	27	Q24 hr	I	<50	100%	Q48 hr

Continued

TABLE 30.2
NONANTIMICROBIALS REQUIRING ADJUSTMENT IN RENAL FAILURE—cont'd

	Pharmacokinetics			Adjustments in Renal Failure		
Drug	Route of Excretion*	Normal $t_{1/2}$ (h)	Normal Dose Interval	Method	CrCl (mL/min/1.73 m²)	Percentage of Usual Dose	Interval

Drug	Route of Excretion*	Normal $t_{1/2}$ (h)	Normal Dose Interval	Method	CrCl (mL/min/1.73 m²)	Percentage of Usual Dose	Interval
Digoxin	Renal (50%–70%)	18–48		D, I	**Digitalizing Dose**		
					ESRD	50%	NA
					Maintenance Dose		
					30–50	75%	Q12–24 hr
					10–30	50%	Q12–24 hr
						OR 100%	Q36 hr
					<10/HD/PD	25%	Q12–24 hr
						OR 100%	Q48 hr
Disopyramide†	Renal (40%–60%) [GI]	3–10	Q6 hr	I	30–40	100%	Q8 hr
					15–30	100%	Q12 hr
					<15	100%	Q24 hr
EDTA calcium disodium†	Renal	1.5 (IM) 0.3–1 (IV)	Q4 hr IM Q12 hr IV	D, I	**Serum Creatinine: IV Dose**		
					≤2 mg/dL	1 g/m²	Q24 hr × 5 days
					2–3 mg/dL	500 mg/m²	Q24 hr × 5 days
					3–4 mg/dL	500 mg/m²	Q48 hr × 3 doses
					>4 mg/dL	500 mg/m²	Once weekly
Enalapril (IV: enalaprilat)	Renal (60%–80%) [hepatic]	1.5–6 (PO) 5–20 (IV)	Q6–24 hr	D	10–50	75%	Q6–24 hr
					<10	50%	Q6–24 hr
					Manufacturer does not recommended in infants and children aged ≤16 yr, with GFR <30 mL/min/1.73 m².		

Enoxaparin[†]	Renal (40%)	4.5–7	Q12–24 hr	I	<30	100%	Q24 hr
					IHD/PD	Serious bleeding complications may occur in this population. Avoid use. If used, reduce dose and monitor anti-Xa activity.[5]	
Famotidine	Renal (70%)	2–3	Q12–24 hr	D, I	30–50	100%	Q24 hr
					10–29	50%	Q24 hr
					<10/IHD/PD	25%	Q24 hr
Felbamate[†]	Renal (50%)	20–30	Q6–8 hr	D	<50	50%	Q6–8 hr
Fentanyl	Hepatic [renal (75%)]	Single dose: 2–4 Prolonged infusion: 21	Q30 min–1 hr, continuous Patch: Q72 hr	D	**Injection** <50	Manufacturer does not recommend dose reduction. Titrate to clinical effect.	
					Patch Mild–moderate impairment	Initial dose: 50%	Q72 hr
					Severe impairment	Not recommended.	
Fexofenadine	GI [renal (12%)]	14	Q12 hr	I	<50	100%	Q24 hr
Flecainide[†]	Hepatic [Renal (>80%)]	8–20	Q8–12 hr	D	<35	50%	Q12 hr
Furosemide	Renal (50%–80%) [hepatic]	0.5	Q6–24 hr PO Q6–12 hr IV		Avoid use in oliguric states.		
Gabapentin	Renal (>75%) [GI]	5	Q8 hr	D, I	30–50	75%	Q12 hr
					15–29	75%	Q24 hr
					<15/IHD/PD	75%	Q48 hr

Continued

TABLE 30.2
NONANTIMICROBIALS REQUIRING ADJUSTMENT IN RENAL FAILURE—cont'd

Drug	Pharmacokinetics			Adjustments in Renal Failure		
	Route of Excretion*	Normal t₁/₂ (h)	Normal Dose Interval	Method	CrCl (mL/min/1.73 m²)	Percentage of Usual Dose	Interval

Drug	Route of Excretion*	Normal t_{1/2} (h)	Normal Dose Interval	Method	CrCl (mL/min/1.73 m²)	Percentage of Usual Dose	Interval
Hydralazine#	Hepatic [renal 14%]	2–8	Q4–6 hr (IV) Q6–12 hr (PO)	I	10–50 <10/IHD/PD	100% 100%	Q8 hr (fast acetylator) Q8–16 hr Q12–24 hr (slow acetylator)
Insulin (regular)**	Hepatic (renal)	IV: 0.5–1 Subcutaneous: 1.5	Variable	D	10–50 <10/IHD/PD	75% 50%	No change No change
Lacosamide†	Renal (95%) [GI]	13	Q12 hr	D	<30 IHD	Maximum dose: 300 mg/24 hr period Administer 50% dose supplementation after 4-hr dialysis session.	
Levetiracetam	Renal (66%)	5–8	Q12 hr	D	**Children** <50 IHD ΣPD **Adults** 50–80 30–50 <30 IHD ΣPD	50% 50% 500–1000 mg 250–750 mg 250–500 mg 500–1000 mg	Q12 hr Q24 hr Q12 hr Q12 hr Q12 hr Q24 hr
Lisinopril	Renal	11–13	Q24 hr	D	10–50 <10/IHD α/PD	50% 25%	Q24 hr Q24 hr
					Per manufacturer, use not recommended for children with CrCl < 30 mL/min/1.73 m².		

Drug	Route of Elimination	Half-life (hr)	Normal Dose	Method	GFR (mL/min)	Dose %	Interval
Lithium **Note:** Monitor serum concentrations. Due to high volume of distribution, lithium concentrations rebound after dialysis.[2]	Renal (>90%)	18–24	Q6-8 hr	D	10–50 <10 IHD	50–75% 25–50% Dose after dialysis. Doses may vary, use serum concentrations to guide.	Q6-8 hr Q6-8 hr
Loratadine	Hepatic [renal (80%)]	Loratadine: 8.4 Metabolite: 28	Q24 hr	I	<30	100%	Q48 hr
Meperidine **Note:** Accumulation of normeperidine can lead to tremors and seizures. Limit duration to ≤48 hr in all patients. Avoid use in patients with kidney dysfunction.[1]	Renal (hepatic) (normeperidine, renal)	Meperidine: 2.3–4 Normeperidine: 6–18	Q3-4 hr	D	10–50 <10 IHD/PD	75% 50% Avoid use.	Avoid use, especially repeat administrations. Avoid use, especially repeat administrations.
Methadone	Hepatic (renal < 10%)	20–35	Q6-12 hr	D	<10/IHD/PD	50%–75%	Q6-12 hr
Methyldopa	Hepatic [renal (70%)]	1–3	Q6-12 hr PO Q6-8 hr IV	I	>50 10–50 <10/IHD ΣPD	100% 100% 100%	Q8 hr Q8-12 hr Q12-24 hr
Metoclopramide	Renal (85%)	2.5–6	Q6 hr PO Q6-8 hr IV	D	30–50 10–30 <10/IHD/PD	75% 50% 25%	No change No change No change

Continued

TABLE 30.2
NONANTIMICROBIALS REQUIRING ADJUSTMENT IN RENAL FAILURE—cont'd

Drug	Pharmacokinetics			Adjustments in Renal Failure			
	Route of Excretion*	Normal $t_{1/2}$ (h)	Normal Dose Interval	Method	CrCl (mL/min/1.73 m²)	Percentage of Usual Dose	Interval
Midazolam **Note:** Metabolite α–hydroxy–midazolam can accumulate in kidney failure, leading to prolonged sedation after midazolam is discontinued.[4]	Hepatic [renal (>60% as α–hydroxy–midazolam)]	2.5–4.5	Variable	D	10–29 <10	25% 50%	No change No change
Milrinone	Renal (>85%)	1.5–2.5	Continuous infusion	D	50 40 30 20 10 5		0.43 mcg/kg/min 0.38 mcg/kg/min 0.33 mcg/kg/min 0.28 mcg/kg/min 0.23 mcg/kg/min 0.2 mcg/kg/min
Morphine	Hepatic [renal (5%–15%)]	1–8	Variable	D	10–50 <10/IHD/PD	75% 50%	No change No change
Neostigmine	Hepatic [renal (50%)]	0.5–2	Variable	D	10–50 <10	50% 25%	No change No change

Oxcarbazepine	Hepatic [Renal]	Oxcarbazepine: 2 MHD metabolite: 9	Q12 hr	D	<30	Initial dose: 50%. Titrate slowly.	Q12 hr
Pancuronium bromide	Renal (40%) [hepatic]	1.5–2.5	Q30–60 min OR continuous infusion	D	10–50 <10/IHD/PD	50% Avoid use.	No change
Phenazopyridine	Renal (65%) [hepatic]	Unavailable	Q8 hr for 2 days	I	50–80 <50	100% Contraindicated	Q8–16 hr
Phenobarbital	Hepatic [renal, 20%–50%]	35–140	Q8–12 hr	I	<10/IHD α/PD α	100%	Q24 hr
Primidone **Note:** Due to complex metabolism, it is preferred to use other options when available for patients with kidney failure.[5]	Hepatic [renal (20%)]	Primidone: 10–12 PEMA metabolite: 16 Phenobarbital: 35–140	Q6–12 hr	I	>50 10–50 <10/IHD α	100% 100% 100%	Q12 hr Q12–24 hr Q24 hr
Procainamide	Hepatic [renal (25% as NAPA)]	Procainamide: 1.7–4.7 NAPA: 6	PO: Q4–6 hr IV: continuous	D	**IV Loading Dose** <10 **IV Maintenance**[†] <10 IHD	 12 mg/kg Initiate at low end of dosing range and titrate to effect. Monitor levels. Supplementation may be needed.	Once
Quinidine	Renal (15%–25%)	2.5–8	Q4–12 hr	D	<10/IHD ΣPD	75%	Q4–12 hr

Continued

TABLE 30.2
NONANTIMICROBIALS REQUIRING ADJUSTMENT IN RENAL FAILURE—cont'd

Drug	Pharmacokinetics			Adjustments in Renal Failure		
	Route of Excretion*	Normal $t_{1/2}$ (h)	Normal Dose Interval	Method	CrCl (mL/min/1.73 m²)	Percentage of Usual Dose	Interval
Ranitidine	Renal (30%–70%) [hepatic]	1.7–2.5	Q12 hr PO Q6–8 hr IV/IM	D	30–50 10–29 <10/IHD α/PD	100% 50% 50%	Q12 hr Q12 hr Q24 hr
Sodium phenylacetate and sodium benzoate	Renal	Unavailable	Continuous	D	<50	Use with caution and close monitoring.	
Spironolactone	Renal (hepatic/biliary)	Spironolactone: 1.3–1.4 Metabolite: 13–24	Q6–24 hr	I	10–50 <10	100% Avoid use	Q12–24 hr
Terbutaline	Renal (60%) [hepatic]	2.9–14	Oral: Q8 hr Subcutaneous: Q2–6 hr IV: Continuous	D	<50	Manufacturer does not recommend dose reduction. Use with caution.	

Triamterene	Hepatic [renal (21%)]	1.6–2.5	Q12–24 hr	I	<10	Do not use due to risk of hyperkalemia.[4]
Verapamil	Renal (70%) [hepatic]	2–8	Variable	D	<10	Dose reduction may be needed; use caution. Monitor blood pressure, ECG for PR prolongation, and other signs of overdose.
Vigabatrin	Renal (80%)	5–10	Q12 hr	D	50–80 30–50 10–30	75% Q12 hr 50% Q12 hr 25% Q12 hr

*Percentage in parentheses represents the amount of drug and/or metabolites excreted in the urine. Route in brackets indicates secondary route of excretion.

[†] In adults; guidelines not established in children

α For IHD administer after dialysis on dialysis days

Σ Administer a supplemental dose after dialysis

‖ Administer supplemental dose after every 4 hours of dialysis, based on daily dose as follows (daily dose/recommended supplemental dose): 100 mg/125 mg; 125 mg/150 mg; 150 mg/200 mg; 200 mg/250 mg; 300 mg/350 mg.

¶ Dose interval varies for rapid and slow acetylators with normal and impaired renal function.

**Renal failure may cause hyposensitivity or hypersensitivity to insulin. Empiric dosing recommendations may not be appropriate for all patients; adjust to clinical response and blood glucose.

CrCl, Creatinine clearance; D, dose reduction; EDTA, ethylenediaminetetraacetic acid; ECG, electrocardiogram; ESRD, end-stage renal disease; GFR, glomerular filtration rate; GI, gastrointestinal; I, interval extension; IHD, hemodialysis; IM, intramuscular; IV, intravenous; MHD, 10-monohydroxy metabolite; PD, peritoneal dialysis; PO, oral; $t_{1/2}$, half-life.

REFERENCES

1. Lexicomp Online, Pediatric and Neonatal Lexi-Drugs Online. *Electronic database*. Hudson, OH: Lexi-Comp, Inc.; 2016 Available at: <http://www.crlonline.com>; Accessed 19 April 2016.
2. Aronoff GR, Bennett WM, Berns JS, et al. *Drug Prescribing in Renal Failure: Dosing Guidelines for Adults*. 5th ed. Philadelphia: American College of Physicians; 2007.
3. Veltri M, Neu AM, Fivush BA, et al. Dosing during intermittent hemodialysis and continuous renal replacement therapy: special considerations in pediatric patients. *Paediatr Drugs*. 2004;6:45-66.
4. Micromedex® Healthcare Series 2.0, (electronic version). Truven Health Analytics, Greenwood Village, Colorado, USA. Available at <http://www.micromedexsolutions.com>. Accessed 19 April 2016.
5. Lexicomp Online, Lexi-Drugs Online. *Electronic database*. Hudson, Ohio: Lexi-Comp, Inc.; 2016 Available at: <http://www.crlonline.com>; Accessed 19 April 2016.
6. Blumberg HM, Burman WJ, Chaisson RE, et al. American Thoracic Society/Centers for Disease Control and Prevention/Infectious Diseases Society of America. Treatment of tuberculosis. *Am J Respir Crit Care Med*. 2003;167:603-662.
7. Panel on Opportunistic Infections in HIV-Infected Adults and Adolescents. Guidelines for the prevention and treatment of opportunistic infection in HIV-infected adults and adolescents: recommendations from the Centers for Disease Control and Prevention, the National Institutes of Health, and the HIV Medicine Association of the Infectious Disease Society of America. Available at <http://aidsinfo.nih.gov/contentfiles/lvguidelines/adult_oi.pdf>. Accessed 31 Mar 2016.
8. Department of Health and Human Services. Panel on Opportunistic Infections in HIV-Exposed and HIV-Infected Children 2013. Available from: <https://aidsinfo.nih.gov/contentfiles/lvguidelines/OI_Guidelines_Pediatrics.pdf>. Accessed: 25 Nov 2016.
9. Panel on Antiretroviral Guidelines for Adults and Adolescents. Guidelines for the use of antiretroviral agents in HIV-1-infected adults and adolescents. Department of Health and Human Services. Available at <http://www.aidsinfo.nih.gov/ContentFiles/AdultandAdolescentGL.pdf>. Accessed 1 Apr 2016.

Index

Note: Page numbers followed by *f*, *t*, or *b* indicate figures, tables, or boxes, respectively.

A

A, B, C, D, and Es, 2
A-200. *See* Pyrethrins with piperonyl butoxie
A-a gradient (alveolar-arterial oxygen gradient), 93
AAP. *See* American Academy of Pediatrics
Abacavir, 1104
Abatacept, 692
Abbreviations, acronyms, and symbols, 733*t*
A-B-C pathway, 2
ABCs (airway, breathing, circulation), 73
ABC DON'T (Airway, Breathing, Circulation, D-stick, Oxygen, Naloxone, Thiamine), 14
ABCDDS (or ABCDs) mnemonic, 667
Abdomen
   adolescent examination, 112
   secondary survey of, 74*t*–75*t*
Abdominal imaging, 676–678
   contrast-enhanced CT, 79, 923
   in intussusception, 678, 679*f*
   in pyloric stenosis, 677–678, 677.e3*f*
   radiography
      intussusception on, 678, 679*f*
      in UTIs, 521
   after trauma, 678
   in trauma, 678
   ultrasound, 677–678, 677.e3*f*
      in UTIs, 521
Abdominal pain
   acute, 317–318, 318*t*
   in HSP, 698
Abdominal paracentesis, 57, 57*f*
Abdominal trauma
   blunt, 78–80
   emergency treatment of, 79–80
   imaging, 678
   intraabdominal injury (IAI), 79
   laboratory studies in, 79
Abelcet. *See* Amphotericin B lipid complex
ABI (absolute benefit increase), 727
Abilify. *See* Aripiprazole
ABLC. *See* Amphotericin B lipid complex

Abscesses
   dental, 461*t*–468*t*
   peritonsillar, 461*t*–468*t*, 470
   retropharyngeal, 461*t*–468*t*, 470, 669*t*
   soft tissue, 62, 62*f*–63*f*
   tubo-ovarian (TOA), 680
Absence seizures, 558*b*, 559*t*–560*t*
Absolute benefit increase (ABI), 727
Absolute risk reduction (ARR), 727
Absorica. *See* Isotretinoid
Abuse. *See* Child abuse; Drug abuse
AC ventilation. *See* Assist control ventilation
Academy of Nutrition and Dietetics, 570
Acanthosis nigracans, 225, 225.e7*f*–225.e8*f*
Acanya. *See* Benzoyl peroxide with clindamycin
AccuNeb. *See* Albuterol
Accutane. *See* Isotretinoid
Acetadote. *See* Acetylcysteine
Acetaminophen (Tylenol, Tempra, Panadol, Feverall, Anacin Aspirin Free, Paracetamol, Ofirmev)
   analgesic properties, 138–139, 139.e1*t*
   dose adjustment in renal failure, 1125*t*–1134*t*
   formulary entry, 757–758
   overdose, 22–26, 23*t*–24*t*, 25*f*
   oxycodone and acetaminophen (Endocet, Roxilox, Percocet, Roxicet), 1002
Acetazolamide (Diamox)
   dose adjustment in renal failure, 1125*t*–1134*t*
   formulary entry, 758–759
   for hydrocephalus, 564
Acetone odor, 21.e1*t*–21.e3*t*
Acetylcysteine (Acetadote)
   for acetaminophen overdose, 25–26
   formulary entry, 759–760
ACHES mnemonic, 125
Achondroplasia, 352–353
Acid-base disorders, 312–314
   analysis of, 639
   etiology of, 313*f*–314*f*
   rules for determining, 312–314

1138 Index

Acidemia
  glutaric type 1 (GAI), 341
  isovaleric, 341
  lactic, 343
  methylmalonic (MMA), 341–342
  organic, 341–342
  propionic (PA), 341
Acidosis, 312
  dialysis for, 529
  ketoacidosis, 256, 517
    diabetic (DKA), 256–259
  lactic, 960
  metabolic. *See* Metabolic acidosis
  renal tubular, 537, 538*t*
  respiratory. *See* Respiratory acidosis
Acid-suppressant therapy
  with metronidazole, 968
  for reflux, 324
ACIP. *See* Advisory Committee on Immunization Practices
Acne
  cystic, 929
  neonatal, 219
  nodular, 929
  treatment of, 973, 1075
Acne vulgaris, 213–216, 215*t*, 847
Acquired immunodeficiency syndrome (AIDS), 470–484, 882
Acral melanoma, 225.*e*2*f*
Acrodermatitis enteropathica, 218*f*
Acronyms, 733*t*
ACT. *See* Airway clearance therapy
ACTH (adrenocorticotropic hormone). *See* Corticotropin
ACTH stimulation test, 268–269, 1096
ActHIB. *See* PRP-T
AC-THIB, 415*f*–418*f*
Actigall. *See* Ursodiol
Actinomycin D. *See* Dactinomycin
Actiq. *See* Fentanyl
Activase. *See* Alteplase
Activated charcoal
  contraindications to, 21
  for ingestions, 21
Activated partial thromboplastin time (aPTT), 376
  age-specific values, 377*t*–378*t*
Activated protein C resistance, 379*b*
Activities of daily living (ADLs), 229
Acular. *See* Ketorolac
Acute abdominal pain, 317–318, 318*t*
Acute adrenal crisis, 272
Acute agitation, 911, 993
Acute asthma, 1029
Acute ataxia, 565*b*
Acute bacterial sinusitis, 942

Acute bacterial skin and skin structure infection (ABSSSI), 820
Acute blood loss, 926
Acute chest syndrome, 370*t*–371*t*
Acute dialysis, 529
Acute diarrhea, 950
Acute dystonic reaction, 795
Acute gastroenteritis, 997
Acute graft-versus-host disease (aGVHD), 621, 621.*e*1*t*
Acute group A streptococcal pharyngitis, 1012
Acute headache, 551*b*
Acute hemolytic reaction, 385
Acute hypophosphatemia, 1019
Acute interstitial nephritis, 532*f*
Acute iron poisoning, 850
Acute kidney injury (AKI), 526–530
  clinical presentation of, 526–528
  etiology of, 526, 527*t*
  postrenal, 526, 527*t*
  prerenal, 526, 527*t*
  radiographic imaging considerations, 529–530
  renal, 526, 527*t*
Acute leukemia, 1101
Acute liver failure (ALF), 325–327
Acute lymphocytic leukemia (ALL), 609*t*–610*t*
Acute mastoiditis, 461*t*–468*t*
Acute maxillary sinusitis, 819, 835–836
Acute migraine, 1053–1054, 1107
Acute myeloid leukemia (AML), 609*t*–610*t*
Acute myocardial infarction, 182
Acute nephritic syndrome, 530
Acute otitis externa, 834
Acute otitis media
  initial management of, 461*t*–468*t*
  recurrent or persistent, 942
  treatment of, 834–835, 942, 992
Acute pain, 136
Acute pancreatitis, 328–329, 330*t*
Acute pelvic inflammatory disease, 790
Acute pulmonary hypertensive crisis, 88–89
Acute renal failure, 601*t*–602*t*
Acute respiratory alkalosis, 641*t*
Acute severe encephalopathy, 861
Acute sinusitis, 461*t*–468*t*, 789
Acute spinal cord injury, 965
Acute stabilization, 96–100
Acute stroke, 566*b*
Acute transfusion reactions, 385–390
Acute tubular necrosis (ATN), 526, 527*t*, 528

Acute viral bronchiolitis, 1063
Acute-onset focal neurologic deficit, 566b
Acute-phase reactants, 701–702
Acuvail. See Ketorolac
Acyclovir (Zovirax)
  dose adjustment in renal failure, 1111t–1124t
  for eczema herpeticum superinfection, 222
  formulary entry, 760–761
  for herpes, 115t–116t, 457t–458t, 471t–476t
  for HSV, 457t–458t, 760–761
  neonatal dosing, 513t–514t
  for oncology patients, 626t
  for varicella, 440, 457t–458t, 471t–476t, 761
Acyclovir-resistant herpes simplex, 900
Acylcarnitine profile, 336t
Aczone. See Dapsone
Adacel. See Tdap (tetanus, diphtheria, & acellular pertussis) vaccine
Adalat CC. See Nifedipine
Adalimumab, 692
Adapalene (Differin)
  formulary entry, 762
  formulations and concentrations, 216t
Adapalene + benzoyl peroxide (Epiduo), 762
Adaptive skills, 229, 231t–232t
Adcetris. See Brentuximab
Adderall. See Dextroamphetamine + amphetamine
Addison disease, 271
Adenocard. See Adenosine
Adenoid hypertrophy, 396
Adenoidectomy, 138
Adenosine (Adenocard), 762–763
Adenotonsillectomy, 658
Adenovirus infection, 832, 624.e1t
Adequate intake (AI), 583
ADHD. See Attention-deficit/hyperactivity disorder
ADHD Medication Guide, 229, 248
Adhesives, tissue, 68
Adolescent medicine, 108–135
  access to services for STIs, 114
  arterial catheters, 34
  asthma care, 649f
  contraception, 125
  emergency management, 3t
  guidelines for, 110, 113, 123
  health maintenance, 110–123
  immunizations, 123, 124t
  medication for depression, 250
Adolescent medicine (Continued)
  pain assessment, 136
  physical examination, 112–113
  screening laboratory tests and procedures, 113–123
  transitioning into adult care, 134
  web resources, 108
Adolescents, 108–110
  advance directives for, 631
  hypertension in, 540t–541t
  mental health of, 132–134
  participation in memory making, 632
  psychosocial development of, 109–110, 109.e1t
  pubertal development of, 108–109
  reference values for, 709t–716t
  septic arthritis in, 461t–468t
  sexual health of, 123–131
  suicide among, 132
  transgender, 285–286
Adoxa. See Doxycycline
Adrenal crisis, 269–270, 272
Adrenal function, 267–273
Adrenal hyperplasia, congenital, 269–271, 269f, 270t
Adrenal insufficiency, 267–273
  acute, 914
  management of, 271–272
  primary, 271
Adrenal medulla, 273
Adrenalin. See Epinephrine HCl
Adrenocorticotropic hormone (ACTH). See Corticotropin
Adrenocorticotropin hormone (ACTH) stimulation test, 268–269, 1096
Adrenoleukodystrophy (ALD), 347.e1
Adrenomyeloneuropathy (AMN), 347.e1
Adriamycin. See Doxorubicin
Advair. See Fluticasone propionate and salmeterol
Advance directives, 631
Advanced Life Support (ALS), 490
Advanced Trauma Life Support (ATLS), 73
Advil. See Ibuprofen
Advisory Committee on Immunization Practices (ACIP), 419–420
Adzenys XR-ODT. See Amphetamine
AEDs (automated external defibrillators), 3
Aerobic bacteria, 444f–445f
Aerosolized medications, 656
Aerospan. See Flunisolide
AFI (amniotic fluid index), 490.e1, 490.e2b
Afrin 12 Hour. See Oxymetazoline

Agammaglobulinemia, X-linked, 403t–404t
Age
  bone age, 683
  gestational, 490.e1–490.e3
  postmenstrual, 490.e3
Agency for Healthcare Quality and Research, 721.e1
Ages and Stages Questionnaire (ASQ), 236, 237t–238t
Aggression, 233t–235t
Agitation
  acute, 911
  associated with bipolar disorder or schizophrenia, 993
  medications for palliative care, 634t
  in serotonin syndrome, 23t–24t
  treatment of, 910, 993
AGMA. See Anion gap metabolic acidosis
AHI (apnea–hypopnea index), 658
AIDS (acquired immunodeficiency syndrome), 470–484, 882
Airway
  assessment of, 4
  emergency management of, 4–8
  foreign bodies in, 670
  Mallampati classification system, 147, 146.e2f
  monitoring, 148
  radiographic imaging of, 667, 669f–670f
  radiologic examination of, 667–670, 669t
Airway (with cervical spine immobilization), Breathing, Circulation, D-stick, Oxygen, Naloxone, Thiamine (ABC DON'T), 14
Airway clearance therapy (ACT), 656
Airway disease, reactive, 770, 954
Airway edema, 852
Airway pressure, mean (PAW), 90
AKI. See Acute kidney injury
AK-Poly-Bac Ophthalmic. See Bacitracin + polymyxin B
Alamast. See Pemirolast
Alanine aminotransferase (ALT), 326t, 709t–716t
Alavert. See Loratadine
Albinism, 218f
Albumin (Albuminar, Albutein, Buminate, Plasbumin, Normal Serum Albumin)
  formulary entry, 763
  reference values, 709t–716t
Albumin solution, 302t
Albutein. See Albumin
Albuterol (VoSpire ER, ProAir HFA, Proventil HFA, Ventolin HFA, ProAir RespiClick, AccuNeb)
  for allergic emergencies, 10
  formulary entry, 763–764
  for hyperkalemia, 308f
  ipratropium bromide + albuterol (Combivent Respimat), 924–925
  for prevention of bronchospasms, 1063
Alcaftadine (Lastacaft), 397
Alclometasone dipropionate, 223t
Alcohol abuse, 235
  fetal alcohol syndrome (FAS), 185t, 496, 225.e6f
Alcohol dependence, 235
Alcohol odor, 21.e1t–21.e3t
ALD (adrenoleukodystrophy), 347.e1
Aldactone. See Spironolactone
Aldolase, 704, 709t–716t
Aldosterone, 271t
Aldosteronism, 1065
Alemtuzumab (Campath), 613t–615t
Alert, Vocal stimulation response, Painful stimulation response, Unresponsive (AVPU) pathway, 74t–75t
Alevazol. See Clotrimazole
Aleve. See Naproxen sodium
ALF. See Acute liver failure
Alfamino formulas, 594t–602t
Alimentum formulas, 570, 601t–602t
Alkaline phosphatase, 326t, 709t–716t
Alkalinization, 616
Alkalosis, 312
  metabolic, 312, 313f–314f, 641t
  respiratory, 312, 313f–314f, 641t
Alkeran. See Melphalan
Alkylating agents
  characteristics of, 613t–615t
  late effects of, 625.e1t–625.e2t
Alkylators, 613t–615t
ALL (acute lymphocytic leukemia), 609t–610t
Allegra. See Fexofenadine and pseudoephedrine
Allergens, 400
Allergen-specific IgE, 400
Allergic conjunctivitis, 994
Allergic dermatitis, 221
Allergic emergencies, 9–10
Allergic eosinophilic gastroenteritis, 398

Allergic reactions
  to drugs, 401
  to foods, 397–401, 842
  severe, 862
  skin lesions, 220–224
  treatment of, 862, 1086
Allergic rhinitis (AR), 395–397
  perennial, 395, 788
  seasonal, 395, 788, 925, 976
  treatment of, 831, 976, 994
Allergic salute, 395
Allergies, Medications, Past illnesses, Last meal, Events (AMPLE) history, 73
Alloimmune thrombocytopenia, neonatal (NAIT), 374–375
Allopurinol (Zyloprim, Aloprim)
  dose adjustment in renal failure, 1125t–1134t
  formulary entry, 764–765
  for hyperleukocytosis/leukocytosis, 616
  for hyperuricemia, 616
Almacone. *See* Aluminum hydroxide with magnesium hydroxide
Almond, bitter, 21.e1t–21.e3t
Almotriptan (Axert)
  formulary entry, 765
  for migraine, 554–555, 554t
Alocril (nedocromil), 397
Alomide. *See* Lodoxamide
Alopecia
  traction, 212
  treatment of, 974
Alopecia areata, 212
Aloprim. *See* Allopurinol
α (alpha), 723
α-adrenergic drug extravasation, 1016
α-agonists
  for hypertension, 544t–545t
  with PCA, 145
α-blockers
  for hypertension, 544t–545t
  for nephrolithiasis, 542–543
α-fetoprotein, maternal, 490.e1b
Alphanate, 387t–388t
α-tocopherol. *See* Vitamin E
AlphaTrex. *See* Betamethasone
Alport syndrome, 532f
Alprostadil (Prostin VR Pediatric), 765–766
Alteplase (Activase, Cathflo Activase), 766
Altered states of consciousness
  differential diagnosis of, 14b
  emergency management of, 13–15

ALTEs (apparent life-threatening events), 644–646
Aluminum hydroxide (Amphojel), 767
Aluminum hydroxide with magnesium hydroxide (Maalox, Mylanta, Almacone, RuLox), 141t, 767–768
Alveolar gas equation, 92–93
Alveolar-arterial oxygen gradient (A-a gradient), 93
Alvesco. *See* Ciclesonide
Amantadine hydrochloride (Symmetrel)
  dose adjustment in renal failure, 1111t–1124t
  formulary entry, 768
Ambiguous genitalia, 284–285
AmBisome. *See* Amphotericin B, liposomal
Amcinonide, 223t
Amebiasis, 968, 1008
Amenorrhea, 277, 956
Amerge. *See* Naratriptan
American Academy of Allergy, Asthma and Immunology, 637
American Academy of Child and Adolescent Psychiatry (AACAP) Physicians Med Guide, 250
American Academy of Clinical Toxicology, 20
American Academy of Family Physicians (AAFP), 349–350
American Academy of Hospice and Palliative Medicine, 628
American Academy of Neurology Practice Guidelines, 548
American Academy of Pediatrics (AAP)
  Children's Health Topics, 570
  Committee on Infectious Diseases, 419–420
  guidelines for health supervision in fragile X syndrome, 357
  guidelines for health supervision in Marfan syndrome, 351
  guidelines for health supervision in Noonan syndrome, 356
  guidelines for health supervision in trisomy 21, 348–349
  Provider Resources for Vaccine Conversations with Parents, 420
  recommendations for TB screening, 484
  Red Book: 2015 Report of the Committee on Infectious Diseases, 412
  Urinary Tract Infection (UTI) Practice Guidelines for Children 2-24 months, 516, 519

American Academy of Pediatrics (AAP) (Continued)
  web resources, 229, 412, 516, 570
  websites for clinicians, 108
American Association of Poison Control Centers, 20
American Burn Association, 73
American College of Gastroenterology, 316
American College of Medical Genetics, 333
American College of Obstetricians and Gynecologists (ACOG), 114
American College of Radiology Appropriateness Criteria, 663
American College of Rheumatology, 688, 693, 694t
American College of Surgeons Advanced Trauma Life Support (ATLS), 73
American Diabetes Association, 255
American Heart Association (AHA)
  Pediatric Advanced Life Support (PALS), 73
  recommendations for cardiovascular screening of competitive athletes, 201.e1b
  Statement on Management of Stroke in Infants and Children, 548
American Lung Association, 637
American Pain Society, 136
American Psychological Association (APA) Physicians Med Guide, 250
American Society for Parenteral and Enteral Nutrition, 570
American Society of Anesthesiologists (ASA), 136, 147, 146.e3t
American Society of Human Genetics, 357.e1
American Thoracic Society, 637
Americans with Disabilities Act (ADA), 246
America's Store Brand formulas, 570, 594t–602t
Amethopterin. See Methotrexate
Amicar. See Aminocaproic acid
Amifostine, 613t–615t
Amikacin sulfate (Amikin)
  dose adjustment in renal failure, 1111t–1124t
  formulary entry, 769
  spectrum of activity, 451t
Amiloride, 544t–545t
Amino acid 8.5% (Travasol), 302t
Amino acid–based formulas components, 302t, 594t–600t
Amino acids, 336t

Aminoacidopathies, 342
Aminocaproic acid (Amicar)
  dose adjustment in renal failure, 1125t–1134t
  formulary entry, 770
  for vWD, 387t–388t
Aminoglycosides
  for catheter-related bloodstream infections, 461t–468t
  for gastroenteritis, 461t–468t
  for osteomyelitis, 461t–468t
  for parotitis, 461t–468t
  spectrum of activity, 451t
Aminopenicillins, 447t–449t
Aminophylline, 770–771
5-Aminosalicylic acid (5-ASA). See Mesalamine
Amiodarone HCl (Cordarone, Pacerone, Nexterone)
  formulary entry, 771–772
  warfarin interactions, 385b
Amitriptyline (Elavil)
  formulary entry, 772–773
  for migraine prevention, 556t
AML (acute myeloid leukemia), 609t–610t
Amlodipine (Norvasc)
  formulary entry, 773
  for hypertension, 544t–545t
Ammonia
  reference values, 709t–716t
  sample collection for, 336t
Ammonium chloride, 774
Ammonul. See Sodium phenylacetate and sodium benzoate
AMN (adrenomyeloneuropathy), 347.e1
Amniocentesis, 490.e1
Amniotic fluid index (AFI), 490.e1, 490.e2b
Amniotic fluid volume estimation, 490.e1, 490.e2b
Amobarbital, 385b
Amoxicillin (Moxatag)
  for chlamydia, 115t–116t
  combined with metronidazole, 968
  dose adjustment in renal failure, 1111t–1124t
  endocarditis prophylaxis regimen, 192t
  formulary entry, 774–775
  for gastroenteritis, 461t–468t
  for Lyme disease, 479t–480t
  for otitis media, 461t–468t
  for pharyngitis, 461t–468t
  for pneumonia, 461t–468t

Amoxicillin (Moxatag) *(Continued)*
for septic arthritis, 461t–468t
for sinusitis, 461t–468t
spectrum of activity, 447t–449t
Amoxicillin-clavulanic acid (Augmentin)
for bites, 461t–468t
for cellulitis, 461t–468t
for dental abscess infection, 461t–468t
dose adjustment in renal failure, 1111t–1124t
formulary entry, 775–776
for lymphadenitis, 461t–468t
for otitis media, 461t–468t
for sinusitis, 461t–468t
spectrum of activity, 447t–449t
Amphadase. *See* Hyaluronidase
Amphetamine (Evekeo, Adzenys XR-ODT, Dyanavel XR)
formulary entry, 776–777
overdose, 23t–24t
urine toxicology screen, 21t
Amphetamine + dextroamphetamine (Adderall)
ages of FDA approval, 245t
formulary entry, 854–855
Amphojel. *See* Aluminum hydroxide
Amphotericin B
dose adjustment in renal failure, 1111t–1124t
formulary entry, 777–778
for sinusitis, 461t–468t
Amphotericin B, liposomal (AmBisome)
dose adjustment in renal failure, 1111t–1124t
formulary entry, 778–779
Amphotericin B lipid complex (Abelcet, ABLC)
dose adjustment in renal failure, 1111t–1124t
formulary entry, 778
Ampicillin
dose adjustment in renal failure, 1111t–1124t
endocarditis prophylaxis regimen, 192t
formulary entry, 779–780
for gastroenteritis, 461t–468t
for meningitis, 461t–468t
neonatal dosing, 513t–514t
for pneumonia, 461t–468t
spectrum of activity, 447t–449t
Ampicillin/sulbactam (Unasyn)
for abscess infection, 461t–468t
for bites, 461t–468t
for cellulitis, 461t–468t

Ampicillin/sulbactam (Unasyn) *(Continued)*
dose adjustment in renal failure, 1111t–1124t
formulary entry, 780
spectrum of activity, 447t–449t
AMPLE (Allergies, Medications, Past illnesses, Last meal, Events) history, 73
Amylase, 709t–716t
Amyloid A, serum, 701
Anabolic steroids, 385b
Anacin Aspirin Free. *See* Acetaminophen
Anakinra, 692
Analgesia, 138–142
adjuncts, 919
aspirin, 784
augmented, 772
for burns, 100
carbamide peroxide, 811
for chemotherapy patients, 625
hydromorphone HCl, 915
ibuprofen, 917–918
for joint pain, 698
local anesthetics, 30, 139–142, 141t–142t
for low-birth-weight infants, 143
methadone HCl, 961
morphine sulfate, 977
naproxen/naproxen sodium, 981
nonopioid analgesics, 138–139
nonpharmacologic measures for, 142–143
opioids, 139
oral, 811
otic, 781
for palliative care, 634t
patient-controlled, 143–144, 143t
procedural sedation, 30, 145–148, 931
example protocols, 148, 153t
limits for targeted depth and length, 146.e1f
quick reference, 139.e1t
safety of, 138
suggested protocols, 153t
web resources, 136
Analysis of variance (ANOVA)
Kruskall-Wallis, 724t
one-way (F test), 724t
two-way, 724t
Anaphylactic shock, 86.e1t
Anaphylaxis
emergency management of, 9–10
treatment of, 400, 862

Anaplasmosis, 479t–480t
Anaprox. *See* Naproxen sodium
Anatomic considerations, 78–80
Ancef. *See* Cefazolin
Ancobon. *See* Flucytosine
Ancylostoma caninum, 955
Androstenedione, 287, 287.e3t
Anectine. *See* Succinylcholine
Anemia, 364–368
 aplastic, 367
 associated with chemotherapy, 848–849
 in cancer, 874–875
 in chemotherapy patients, 624
 of chronic inflammation, 367
 in chronic renal failure, 848–849, 873–875
 classification of, 366t
 Cooley's, 372
 Diamond–Blackfan, 367
 Fanconi, 367
 hemolytic, 367–368
 of infancy, 366
 iron-deficiency
  screening for, 584
  treatment of, 926–928
 macrocytic, 366t
 microcytic, 366t
 normocytic, 366t
 pernicious, 843
 of prematurity, 874
 screening for, 123
 sickle cell, 368
Anesthesia
 fasting recommendations for, 146–147, 147t
 lidocaine, 944
 local, 139–142
  injectable, 142, 142t
  topical, 139, 141t
 for oral ulcers, 700
Aneuploidy syndromes, 347–350
Angelman syndrome, 354
Angina, 987
Angioedema
 food allergy, 397
 treatment of, 400
Angiofibroma, facial, 352
Angioma, 532f
Angiomyolipoma, renal, 352
Angiotensin-converting enzyme (ACE), 701.e2
Angiotensin-converting enzyme (ACE) inhibitors
 for hypertension, 544t–545t
 for renal disease, 701.e3

Angiotensin-receptor blockers, 544t–545t
Animal bites, 93–95, 94t
 closure, 94–95
 deep, 93
 high infection risk, 93–95
 infections in, 461t–468t
 inpatient care for, 95
 outpatient care for, 95
 periorbital, 93
 wound considerations, 93–95
 wound hygiene, 94
Anion gap (AG), 312
 calculation of, 312–314
 nonelevated anion gap metabolic acidosis (NAGMA), 312–314, 313f–314f
 urine (UAG), 537
Anion gap metabolic acidosis (AGMA), 312–314, 339f
 etiology of, 313f–314f
 in poisoning, 21.e1t–21.e3t
Ankle splints, 71f, 70.e2
Ankylosing spondylitis, 881, 981
Anogenital ratio, 284
Anorchia, 285
Anorexia nervosa, 250, 278f
ANOVA (analysis of variance)
 Kruskall-Wallis, 724t
 one-way (F test), 724t
 two-way, 724t
Antacids
 aluminum hydroxide, 767
 aluminum hydroxide with magnesium hydroxide (Maalox, Mylanta, Almacone, RuLox), 767
 calcium carbonate (Tums, Children's Pepto), 805
 magnesium hydroxide, 953
Anterior propping, 236.e6t
Anthracyclines
 chemotherapeutic agents, 613t–615t
 late effects of, 625.e1t–625.e2t
Anthrax
 inhalational, 942, 1012
 post exposure prophylaxis against, 833–834
 treatment of, 833–834, 866
Anthropometric measurements, 570–571
Antiarrhythmics
 lidocaine, 944
 phenytoin, 1018
 quinidine, 1043

Antibiotics. *See also specific agents*
  for acne vulgaris, 214, 215*t*, 217*t*
  aminoglycosides, 451*t*
  bacterial endocarditis prophylaxis, 191, 192*b*, 192*t*
  β-Lactams, 447*t*–449*t*
  chemotherapeutic agents, 613*t*–615*t*
  choosing, 443
  for cystic fibrosis, 656
  dose adjustment in renal failure, 1111*t*–1124*t*
  fluoroquinolones, 450*t*
  for idiopathic pneumonia syndrome, 623
  for lymphadenitis, 454
  macrolides, 450*t*
  for morphea, 701.e3
  neonatal dosing, 513*t*–514*t*
  for neutropenia, 624
  for PPHN, 502
  prophylaxis for oncology patients, 625, 626*t*
  sensitivities, 443
  single drug class, 452*t*
  spectrum of activity, 443, 447*t*–452*t*
  tetracyclines, 451*t*
  topical, 100.e1*b*
  for UTIs, 521–523
Antibodies, 477*f*
Antibody deficiency
  evaluation for, 403*t*–404*t*
  HIV infection with, 405
  replacement therapy for, 401, 406, 920
Anticholinergics
  for allergic rhinitis, 397
  poisoning with, 22*t*–24*t*
  reversal of, 1020
Anticholinesterase overdose, 23*t*–24*t*
Anticoagulation therapy
  and coagulation tests, 382
  for stroke, 567
  for thrombosis, 382
Anticonvulsants
  for migraine prevention, 556*t*
  for seizures, 562*t*
Anticyclic citrullinated peptide (anti-CCP) antibodies, 703
Antidepressants
  ages of FDA approval, 245*t*
  amitriptyline, 772
  for depressive disorders, 249
  imipramine, 919
  for migraine prevention, 556*t*
Antidiarrheal agents, 320

Antidiuretic hormone (ADH), 537–538
  increased release of, 292–293, 293*b*
  syndrome of inappropriate antidiuretic hormone (SIADH), 274–276
Anti-DNA antibody, 694*t*
Antidopaminergics, 555
Antidotes, 21–22
Anti-ds (double-stranded DNA) antibody, 694
Antiemetic therapy, 626*t*
  adjunct therapy, 951
  chlorpromazine, 828–829
  dexamethasone, 852
  dronabinol, 867
  droperidol, 867
  hydroxyzine, 916
  metoclopramide, 966
  prochlorperazine, 1032
  scopolamine hydrobromide, 1056
Antifungals, 481*t*
Antihistamines
  for allergic emergencies, 10
  for allergic rhinitis, 396–397
  for antiemetic therapy, 626*t*
  for atopic dermatitis (eczema), 222
  cyproheptadine, 845
  intranasal, 396
  for migraine, 555, 556*t*
  oral, 396
  poisoning with, 23*t*–24*t*
  promethazine, 1033
  for reflux, 324
  reversal of, 1020
  sedating, 149*b*–150*b*
Antihypertensive drugs, 544*t*–545*t*
Antiinflammatory agents. *See also* Nonsteroidal anti-inflammatory drugs (NSAIDs)
  aspirin, 784
  betamethasone, 796
  corticotropin, 841
  cortisone acetate, 841
  for cystic fibrosis, 789–790
  dexamethasone, 852
  hydrocortisone, 914
  indomethacin, 922
  methylprednisolone, 965
  prednisone, 1029
  triamcinolone, 1086
Antilirium. *See* Physostigmine salicylate
Antimicrobials. *See* Antibiotics
Antimotility agents, 320
Antinuclear antibody (ANA), 702
  reference values, 709*t*–716*t*
  in SLE, 693, 694*t*
Antiphospholipid antibodies, 379*b*

α_2-Antiplasmin, 377t–378t
α_2-Antiplasmin deficiency, 386f
Antiplatelet therapy, 567
Antipsychotics
  ages of FDA approval, 245t
  antiemetic agents, 626t
Antipyretics
  aspirin, 784
  ibuprofen, 917–918
Antiretroviral therapy, 481t, 483
Anti-Smith (Sm) antibody, 694, 694t
Antistreptolysin O titer, 709t–716t
Antithrombin III, 377t–378t
Antithrombin III deficiency, 379b
Antithymocyte globulin, 621
Anti-TNF agents. See Tumor necrosis factor inhibitors
α_2-Antitrypsin, 377t–378t
Antipyrine and benzocaine (Antipyrine and Benzocaine Otic), 781
Antizol. See Fomepizole
Anuria, 955
Anxiety, 132
  screening for, 237t–238t
  separation anxiety, 233t–235t
  stranger anxiety, 233t–235t
  treatment of, 916
Anxiety disorders, 248–249, 1008
Anxiolysis, 145–146
Anxiolytics
  ages of FDA approval, 245t
  lorazepam, 951
Anzemet. See Dolasetron
Aortic arch, 675, 677f
Aortic stenosis, 186t–187t
  heart sounds in, 166b
  sports restrictions, 199.e1t
Apgar scores, 493, 493t
Apidra (insulin glulisine), 260t
Aplasia cutis congenita, 218f
Aplastic crisis, 370t–371t
Apnea
  definition of, 502–503
  in newborns, 502–503, 503f
    management of, 770, 802, 865, 1077
  methylxanthine-refractory, 865
  obstructive sleep apnea syndrome (OSAS), 656–658, 657b
  of prematurity, 502
Apnea–hypopnea index (AHI), 658
Apparent life-threatening events (ALTEs), 644–646
Appendicitis, 1023
Appetite stimulation, 845, 867

Aprepitant
  for antiemetic therapy, 626t
  warfarin interactions, 385b
Apresoline. See Hydralazine hydrochloride
Apriso. See Mesalamine
Aptensio XR. See Methylphenidate HCl
aPTT. See Activated partial thromboplastin time
AquADEKs, 588t–590t
Aquasol A. See Vitamin A
Aqueous Vitamin E. See Vitamin E
AR. See Allergic rhinitis
Ara-C. See Cytarabine
Aralen. See Chloroquine phosphate
Aranesp. See Darbepoietin alfa
Arbinoxa. See Carbinoxamine
The Arc, 242
Arestin. See Minocycline
Arginine, 340
Arginine chloride, injectable (R-Gene 10), 781
8-Arginine vasopressin. See Vasopressin
Arginosuccinase deficiency
  differential diagnosis of, 337f
  treatment of, 340
Arginosuccinic acid synthetase deficiency, 337f
Aripiprazole (Abilify)
  ages of FDA approval, 245t
  formulary entry, 782–783
Arm recoil, 494f, 495
Arm splints, 71f, 70.e1–70.e2
Arnuity Ellipta. See Fluticasone furoate
ARR (absolute risk reduction), 727
Array CGH, 358t
Arrhythmias
  nonventricular, 174t–175t
  secondary to digitalis intoxication, 1018
  supraventricular, 174t–175t, 176f
  tachyarrhythmia, 771
  treatment of, 1018, 1033–1034. See also Antiarrhythmics
  ventricular, 177f, 177t, 771–772
Arsenic poisoning, 861
Arterial blood gas (ABG), 639, 640f
  reference values, 709t–716t
Arterial catheters, 34
Arterial O_2 saturation (SaO_2), 637–638
Arterial switch procedure, 191
Arteriovenous malformation, 532f
Arteriovenous O_2 difference ($AVDO_2$), 93.e1

Arthritis, 688–693
  in Behçet disease, 700
  definition of, 688
  health maintenance in, 693
  juvenile idiopathic (JIA), 688–693, 689*t*
    associated autoantibodies, 695*t*
    treatment of, 881, 1070
  juvenile rheumatoid (JRA), 688–693
    synovial fluid characteristics, 718*t*
    treatment of, 981
  management of, 691–693
  migratory polyarthritis, 698
  nonerosive, 694*t*
  psoriatic (PsA), 688–691, 881
  reactive, 691
  rheumatoid, 881
  septic, 704
    initial management of, 461*t*–468*t*
    synovial fluid characteristics, 718*t*
  synovial fluid characteristics, 718*t*
  traumatic, 718*t*
  tuberculous, 718*t*
Arthrocentesis, knee, 59–61
ASA. *See* Aspirin
5-ASA (5-aminosalicylic acid). *See* Mesalamine
Asacol. *See* Mesalamine
Ascaris, 955, 1037
Ascorbic acid (vitamin C)
  formulary entry, 783
  in infant multivitamin drops, 588*t*
  in multivitamin tablets, 589*t*–590*t*
  recommended intakes, 586*t*
  reference values, 709*t*–716*t*
ASD. *See* Atrial septal defect; Autism spectrum disorder
Ash leaf macules, 218*f*, 352
Ask-Tell-Ask method, 630
Asmanex. *See* Mometasone furoate
Asparaginase (L-Asp, PEG-Asp, Elspar, Erwinia), 613*t*–615*t*
Aspartate aminotransferase (AST), 326*t*, 704, 709*t*–716*t*
Asperger's disorder, 244
Aspergillosis, 930
  invasive, 969, 1101
Aspiration
  bladder. *See* Bladder aspiration
  foreign-body (FBA), 13
  soft tissue, 61
Aspirin (ASA)
  analgesic properties, 139
  dose adjustment in renal failure, 1125*t*–1134*t*

Aspirin (ASA) *(Continued)*
  formulary entry, 783–784
  for Kawasaki disease, 198, 198.e1*t*
  oxycodone and aspirin, 1003
  for stroke, 567
Asplenia
  immunoprophylaxis guidelines for, 367, 422
  pneumococcal prophylaxis for, 1012
ASQ (Ages and Stages Questionnaire), 237*t*–238*t*
Assessment
  of ABCs (airway, breathing, circulation), 73
  burn assessment chart, 98*f*
  Focused Assessment with Sonography for Trauma (FAST), 79
  newborn, 493–496
  nutritional, 570–577
  pain, 136
  tools for, 236
Assist control (AC) ventilation, 91
Astelin. *See* Azelastine
Astepro. *See* Azelastine
Asthma, 646
  acute, 1029
  allergic, 651*f*–652*f*
  assessment of, 10
  classification of, 647*f*–649*f*
  clinical presentation of, 646
  definition of, 646
  emergency management of, 10–12
  exercise-induced, 900
  initial treatment for, 647*f*–649*f*
  maintenance therapy for, 1080
  NIH guideline recommendations for, 801
  persistent, 1055
  spirometry and lung volume readings in, 643*f*
  stepwish approach to, 646, 647*f*–652*f*
  treatment of, 646, 831, 895–897, 899, 976, 1029, 1055
  web resources ffor, 637
Asthma action plans, 646
Asthma exacerbations
  prevention of, 646
  therapy for, 770, 852, 965, 1029
    guidelines for, 965, 1029
    outpatient burst therapy, 965, 1029
Asthma Guideline 2007 (NIH), 801
Asthmanefrin. *See* Epinephrine, racemic
Astragraf XL. *See* Tacrolimus

Asymmetrical tonic neck reflex (ATNR), 236.e4t–236.e5t
Asystole, 872
Ataxia, 564
  acute, 565b
  differential diagnosis of, 565b
  evaluation of, 565b
  in poisoning, 21.e1t–21.e3t
Atazanavir, 385b
Atelectasis, 672
Atenolol (Tenormin)
  dose adjustment in renal failure, 1125t–1134t
  formulary entry, 784
  for hypertension, 544t–545t
Athletes. See Sports
Ativan. See Lorazepam
ATLS (Advanced Trauma Life Support), 73
ATNAA. See Pralidoxime chloride with atropine
ATNR (asymmetrical tonic neck reflex), 236.e4t–236.e5t
Atomoxetine (Strattera), 785
Atonic seizures, 558b
Atopic dermatitis (eczema), 221–222
  with allergic rhinitis, 395
  food allergy, 398
  treatment of, 400, 1022, 1074
Atopic nails, 225.e3f
Atopy patch testing (APT), 399
Atovaquone (Mepron)
  formulary entry, 785–786
  for oncology patients, 626t
Atrial enlargement, 172f
Atrial fibrillation, 174t–175t, 176f, 888
Atrial flutter, 174t–175t, 176f
Atrial septal defect (ASD), 186t–187t
  heart sounds in, 166b
  sports restrictions, 199.e1t
Atrial septostomy, 190–191
Atrial tachycardia, ectopic, 174t–175t
Atrioventricular (AV) block, 178f, 179t
Atrioventricular reentrant tachycardia, 174t–175t
Atrioventricular septal defects, 186t–187t
Atropine sulfate (AtroPen)
  formulary entry, 786–787
  ketazolam (ketamine + midazolam + atropine), 153t
  for physostigmine antidote, 1020
  pralidoxime chloride with atropine (Duodote, ATNAA), 1027–1028
  for procedural sedation, 153t
  for RSI, 7t–8t

Atrovent. See Ipratropium bromide
ATRT (atypical teratoid rhabdoid tumor), 611t
Attention-deficit/hyperactivity disorder (ADHD), 201, 247–248
  screening for, 237t–238t
  subtypes, 247
  treatment of, 247–248, 776, 840, 854–855, 909–910, 947, 963–964
  web resources, 229
Attributable risk, 727
Atypical teratoid rhabdoid tumor (ATRT), 611t
Augmentin. See Amoxicillin-clavulanic acid
Aura, 553
  acute migraine with, 1053–1054, 1107
Auralgan. See Antiyprine and benzocaine
Auro Ear Wax Remover. See Carbamide peroxide
Auscultation, respiratory, 637, 638t
Autism, 244, 879
Autism screening tests, 237t–238t
Autism spectrum disorders (ASDs), 244
  diagnostic criteria for, 244
  screening for, 237t–238t, 244
Autistic disorder, 244
  irritability associated with, 782, 1052
Autoantibodies, 702–703
  associated rheumatologic diseases, 695t
  diabetes, 256
  in SLE, 693–694, 694t
Autoimmune bullous diseases, 220–221
Autoimmune skin lesions, 220–224
Automated external defibrillators (AEDs), 3
Automatisms, 559t–560t
Autopsy consent, 635
Autosomal dominant disease, 334.e1
Autosomal recessive disease, 334.e1
Avage. See Tazarotene
Avascular necrosis of femoral head, 681, 681.e2f
AVDo$_2$ (arteriovenous O$_2$ difference), 93.e1
Avinza. See Morphine sulfate
Avita. See Tretinoin
Av-Phos 250 Neutral. See Phosphorus supplements

AVPU (Alert, Vocal stimulation response, Painful stimulation response, Unresponsive) pathway, 73, 74t–75t
Axert. *See* Almotriptan
Ayr Saline. *See* Sodium chloride
Azactam. *See* Aztreonam
Azasite. *See* Azithromycin
Azathioprine (Imuran, Azasan)
   for Behçet disease, 700
   dose adjustment in renal failure, 1125t–1134t
   formulary entry, 787–788
   for granulomatous disease, 701.e2
   toxicity, 691.e1t
Azelastine (Astelin, Astepro, Optivar)
   for allergic rhinitis, 396–397
   formulary entry, 788
Azithromycin (Zithromax, Zmax, Azasite)
   for chancroid, 120t
   for chlamydia, 115t–116t
   for conjunctivitis, 461t–468t
   endocarditis prophylaxis regimen, 192t
   formulary entry, 789–790
   for gastroenteritis, 461t–468t
   for gonorrhea, 115t–116t
   for pertussis, 461t–468t
   for pneumonia, 461t–468t
   spectrum of activity, 450t
   for traveler's diarrhea, 461t–468t
Azo-Urinary Pain Relief. *See* Phenazopyridine HCl
AZT. *See* Zidovudine
Aztreonam (Azactam, Cayston)
   formulary entry, 790–791
   spectrum of activity, 447t–449t
Azulfidine. *See* Sulfasalazine

B

B lymphocytes, 408t
B-12 Compliance. *See* Cyanocobalamin
BabyBIG. *See* Botulinum IVIG
Bacille Calmette-Guérin (BCG) vaccine, 439.e1
   administration, 439.e1
   for children with HIV diease, 423
   routine vaccination, 439.e1
   side effects of, 439.e1
Bacitracin
   for burns, 100.e1b
   formulary entry, 791–792
Bacitracin + neomycin/polymyxin B (Neosporin, Neo To Go, Neo-Polycin, Triple Antibiotic), 983–984
Bacitracin + neomycin/polymyxin B + hydrocortisone (Neo-Polycin HC), 983
Bacitracin + polymyxin B (AK-Poly-Bac Ophthalmic, Double Antibiotic Topical, Polysporin Topical), 791–792
Back: secondary survey of, 74t–75t
Baclofen (Lioresal, Gablofen, Kemstro), 792–793
Bacteremia
   chronic, 532f
   treatment of, 947, 952, 1094
Bacteria
   aerobic, 444f–445f
   anaerobic, 446f
Bacterial endocarditis prophylaxis, 191, 774, 781, 815, 822, 824, 835–837
   for cardiac conditions, 192b
   for dental procedures, 192b, 192t, 198, 815, 822, 824
   for respiratory tract procedures, 192b, 192t
Bacterial infections
   COPD exacerbation, 789
   gastroenteritis, 461t–468t
   initial management of, 455–470
   of skin, 211
Bacterial pneumonia, community-acquired (CABP), 820
Bacterial sinusitis, acute, 942
Bacterial skin and skin structure infection, acute (ABSSSI), 820
Bacterial superinfection, 222
Bacterial vaginosis
   diagnostic features of, 118t
   management of, 118t
   treatment of, 837, 968
Bacteriuria, asymptomatic, 523
Bactrim. *See* Sulfamethoxazole and trimethoprim
Bactroban. *See* Mupirocin
Bag-mask ventilation, 4, 9
BAL (British Anti-Lewisite). *See* Dimercaprol
Ballard score, 493–495
Baltimore criteria, 623
Banzel. *See* Rufinamide
Barbiturate coma, 1014
Barbiturates, 149b–150b, 151t
Barrier methods of contraception, 130
Basal calorie method, 291
Basal energy expenditure (BEE), 578, 581.e1
Basal metabolic rate (BMR), 578–581
Battle's sign, 74t–75t, 77

Bayes nomogram, 728, 728.e1f
BCG vaccine. *See* Bacille Calmette-Guérin vaccine
Beau lines, 225, 225.e4f
Beclomethasone dipropionate (QVar, Beconase AQ, Qnasl)
  converting from fluticasone to, 794
  dosages, 646.e1t–646.e2t
  formulary entry, 793–794
BECTS (benign epilepsy of childhood with centrotemporal spikes), 559t–560t
Bedside Chronic Kidney Disease in Children (CKiD) cohort, 524
Bedtime limits, 658
Bedtime resistance, 658
BEE (basal energy expenditure), 578
Behavior
  age-appropriate issues, 233t–235t
  guidelines for, 230
  response to pain, 136
  screening for problems, 237t–238t
  web resources for, 229
Behavioral history, 236
Behavioral modifications, 322
Behçet disease, 699–700
Bell's staging system, modified, 507.e1t
Benadryl. *See* Diphenhydramine
Benazepril, 544t–545t
Benign epilepsy, 559t–560t
Benign heart murmurs, 165–166
Benign vascular tumors, 203–207
BenzaClin. *See* Benzoyl peroxide with clindamycin
Benzamycin. *See* Benzoyl peroxide with erythromycin
Benzathine penicillin G (Bicillin L-A)
  formulary entry, 1010
  for pharyngitis, 461t–468t
  for syphilis, 115t–116t
Benzathine penicillin G and procaine penicillin G (Bicillin C-R), 1011
Benzodiazepines, 151t
  antiemetic agents, 626t
  poisoning or overdose, 23t–24t, 891
  properties of, 149b–150b
  reversal of, 891
  urine toxicology screen, 21t
Benzoyl peroxide (BPO, Desquam-DX, NeoBenz Micro, Oxy-5, Oxy-10, PanOxyl)
  for acne vulgaris, 214, 215t
  formulary entry, 794–795
Benzoyl peroxide with adapalene (Epiduo, Epiduo Forte), 762

Benzoyl peroxide with clindamycin (BenzaClin, Duac, Acanya), 794
Benzoyl peroxide with erythromycin (Benzamycin), 794
Benztropine mesylate (Cogentin), 795
Bepotastine (Bepreve), 397
Beractant (Survanta), 1072
Bereavement, 636
Bereavement coordinators, 628
Bereavement services, 636
Beriberi (vitamin B_1 deficiency), 1078
β (beta), 723
Beta$_2$-agonists, 647f–649f
  long-acting (LABAs), 650f–652f, 900
  short-acting (SABAs), 647f–652f
β-blockers
  for hypertension, 544t–545t
  for Kawasaki disease, 198.e1t
  for migraine prevention, 556t
  poisoning or overdose, 23t–24t, 906
β-lactamases, extended-spectrum, 447t–449t
β-lactams, 447t–449t
Betamethasone (AlphaTrex, Celestone Soluspan, Diprolene, Luxiq, Sernivo)
  formulary entry, 796–797
  potency, 223t, 271t
Bethkis. *See* Tobramycin
Bexsero (MenB-4C). *See* Meningococcal B vaccine
Bias, 722
Bicarbonate. *See also* Sodium bicarbonate
  fractional excretion of (FeHCO$_3$), 537
  for metabolic crisis, 340
  reference values, 709t–716t
Bicarbonate reabsorption, 526
Bicillin C-R. *See* Penicillin G
Bicillin L-A. *See* Penicillin G
Bigeminy, 177t
Bile, 304t
Biliary atresia, 678, 1089
Biliary obstruction, 518t
Bilious emesis, 508.e1t
Bilious emesis differential, 508
Bilirubin, 327
  reference values, 709t–716t
  unconjugated hyperbilirubinemia in the newborn, 504–506
  urinalysis for, 518, 518t
Bilitool, 490
Biological agents
  for arthritis, 692, 691.e1t
  for SLE, 695
  toxicity, 691.e1t

Biological agents *(Continued)*
  vaccines for patients on, 423–424
  web resources, 412
Biophysical profile test, 490.e2*t*
Bio-Statin. *See* Nystatin
Biostatistics, 723–728
Biotin
  in multivitamin tablets, 589*t*–590*t*
  recommended intakes, 586*t*
Bioxiverz. *See* Neostigmine
Bipolar disorder, 132
  acute agitation associated with, 993
  therapy, 782
  treatment of, 938, 993
Bipolar mania, 1040–1041, 1052
Birth trauma, 495
Birth weight, normal, 493
Birth-related extradural fluid collection, 495*t*, 496*f*
Bisacodyl (Dulcolax, Fleet Laxative, Fleet Bisacodyl), 797
Bismuth subsalicylate (Pepto-Bismol, Kaopectate, Kao-Tin, Stomach Relief)
  dose adjustment in renal failure, 1125*t*–1134*t*
  formulary entry, 797–798
Bites
  animal bites, 93–95, 94*t*
  in child abuse, 101
  human, 94*t*
  infections in, 461*t*–468*t*
Bitter almond odor, 21.e1*t*–21.e3*t*
BK virus hemorrhagic cystitis, 832
BK virus infection, 624.e1*t*
Black dot tinea capitis, 211
Blackheads, 213
Bladder aspiration, suprapubic, 59, 520
  landmarks for, 60*f*
  ultrasound-guided, 59.e1, 59.e1*f*
Bladder dysfunction, 527*t*
Bladder irrigation, 777
Bladder ultrasound, 521
Blalock-Taussig (BT) shunt, 190
  modified, 190*f*, 191
Blaschkoid dyspigmentation, 227, 227.e1*f*
Blaschko's lines, 227
Blastomycosis, 930
Bleeding
  abnormal uterine, 956
  gastrointestinal, 316–317, 317*t*
  vitamin K deficiency, 1020
Bleeding diathesis, 48, 532*f*
Bleeding disorders, 382, 386*f*

Bleeding time (BT), 376–379
  age-specific values, 377*t*–378*t*
Bleomycin (Blenoxane)
  characteristics of, 613*t*–615*t*
  late effects of, 625.e1*t*–625.e2*t*
Bleph-10. *See* Sulfacetamide sodium ophthalmic
Block skills, 236, 236.e3*f*
Blood
  CMV-negative, 391
  HBV prophylaxis after percutaneous exposure, 430*t*
  occult bood test, 330
Blood cell indices, 365*t*
Blood chemistry, 708–720
Blood component replacement, 385–393
Blood culture
  specimen collection for, 443
  specimen preparation for, 443
Blood donors
  reasons not to consider directed donors, 390
  reasons to consider directed donors, 390
Blood gases, 639
  arterial (ABG), 639, 640*f*
  capillary (CBG), 639
  reference values, 709*t*–716*t*
  venous (VBG), 639
Blood loss, acute, 926
Blood pressure (BP), 156–163
  abnormalities, 156–163
  assessment of, 2
  in headaches, 551.e1*t*
  high-normal, 539
  measurement of, 539–541
  normal values, 156, 157*t*–162*t*, 163*f*–165*f*, 539–541, 156.e1*t*
  systolic (SBP), 165*f*
Blood products
  components, 390–392
  immunoprophylaxis guidelines for patients treated with, 426
  irradiated, 391
  platelet products, 391–392
  for TTP, 623
Blood sampling, 31–48
  repeat blood lead testing, 27*t*
Blood smears, 393
Blood transfusions
  complications of, 385–390
  exchange transfusion, 392–393, 505–506
  for hyperleukocytosis/leukocytosis, 616

Blood transfusions *(Continued)*
   PRBC transfusion, 390–393, 624, 426.e1t
   with RBCs, 390–392
Blood urea nitrogen/creatinine (BUN/Cr) ratio, 528
Blood volume, estimated (EBV), 389t
Bloodborne pathogens, 486–487
Bloodstream infections, catheter-related, 461t–468t
Blunt trauma, 78–80
BMJ Statistics at Square One, 721
BMR (basal metabolic rate), 578–581
Body fluids, 708
   electrolyte composition of, 304t
   evaluation of, 717t
   sampling, 48–64
Body image, 109.e1t
Body mass index (BMI), 571
   formula for, 571
   growth charts for boys, 579f
   growth charts for girls, 577f
Body mass index (BMI) percentile, 571
Body surface area (BSA), 291, 291.e1t
   nomogram and equation, 736, 736f
Bone age, 683
Bone cysts, 681, 684f
Bone infections, 947, 952
Bone lesions, 681–683
Bone marrow transplantation (BMT)
   complications of, 621–624
   IVIG for, 405, 920
   prophylaxis for, 889
   treatment regimens, 625
   viral infections in, 426.e1t
Bone sarcoma, 609t–610t
Boost formulas, 570, 594t–602t
Boosters, 421–422
Boostrix. *See* Tdap (tetanus, diphtheria, & acellular pertussis) vaccine
Bordeaux bottle, 669f
Borrelia burgdorferi, 198
Botulinum IVIG (BabyBIG), 426.e1t
Bowel cleansing products (GoLYTELY, CoLyte, NuLYTELY, TriLyte), 1023–1024
Bowel conditions, 318–325
Bowel movements, 321–322
Bowel obstruction, 678
Bowel prep, 982
Boys
   BEE calculation, 581.e1
   body mass index, 579f
   delayed puberty in, 277
   EER equations, 581.e1

Boys *(Continued)*
   growth charts, 574f–575f, 578f–579f, 571.e2f
   head circumference, 575f, 571.e3f
   height velocity, 571.e2f
   length-to-weight ratio, 575f
   normal blood pressure values, 160t–162t, 163f
   physical activity coefficient (PA), 580.e1t
   recommended element intakes, 591t
   recommended vitamin intakes, 586t
   sample EERs, 582t
   stature and weight, 578f
   target height range for, 276
BP. *See* Blood pressure
BPD (bronchopulmonary dysplasia), 653–654
BPO. *See* Benzoyl peroxide
Brachial plexus injury, 495
Bradycardia, 174t–175t
   in newborns, 503
   in poisoning, 21.e1t–21.e3t
   treatment of, 786, 872
   without central apnea, 503
Bradypnea, 21.e1t–21.e3t
Brain MRI, 558
Brain tumors
   management of, 612, 852
   signs and symptoms of, 609t–611t
Breakthrough seizures, 561
Breast(s)
   adolescent examination, 112
   in newborn, 494f
   Tanner stages of development, 109f
Breastfed infants, 267
Breastfeeding, 585–588. *See also* Lactation
   contraindications to, 592t
   drug formulary categories, 735
   newborn care, 492
   video instruction, 588
   web resources, 570
Breath-holding spells, 557t
Breathing
   assessment of, 9
   emergency management of, 9
   mouth-to-mouth, 9
   mouth-to-nose, 9
Breech delivery, 511
Brentuximab (Adcetris), 613t–615t
Breo Ellipta. *See* Fluticasone furoate and vilanterol
Brethine. *See* Terbutaline
Brevibloc. *See* Esmolol HCl

Brief interventions, 133
Brief unresolved unexplained events (BRUEs), 644–646
 differential diagnosis of, 644, 644b–645b
 management of, 644–646
Bright Beginnings formulas, 570, 594t–602t
Bright Futures Guidelines, 110, 113, 229
Brisdelle. *See* Paroxetine
British Anti-Lewisite (BAL). *See* Dimercaprol
Brompheniramine with phenylephrine (Dimetapp Children's Cold and Allergy), 798–799
Bronchiolitis, 653, 1063
Bronchitis, 816, 819, 821, 836
Bronchodilators
 adjunctive therapy, 954
 epinephrine HCl, 872
 formoterol, 899
Bronchopulmonary dysplasia (BPD), 653–654
Bronchoscopy, 667
Bronchospasms
 exercise-induced, 976, 1056
 prevention of, 976, 1056, 1063
 treatment of, 787, 1077–1078
Brucellosis, 1066
BRUEs (brief unresolved unexplained events), 644–646
Bruises, 101
BSA (body surface area), 291, 291.e1t
BT. *See* Bleeding time
Bucket-handle fractures, 683
Budesonide (Pulmicort, Rhinocort Aqua Nasal Spray, Entocort EC, Uceris)
 dosages, 646.e1t–646.e2t
 for eosinophilic esophagitis, 325
 formulary entry, 798–799
Budesonide and formoterol (Symbicort)
 dosages, 646.e1t–646.e2t
 formulary entry, 801
Bulimia, 893
Bulimia nervosa, 250
Bulla(e), 203, 204f–205f
Bullous diseases, autoimmune, 220–221
Bullous impetigo, 211, 218f
Bullous pemphigoid, 220
Bumetanide
 formulary entry, 801
 for hypertension, 544t–545t

Buminate. *See* Albumin
Bupivacaine
 injectable, 142, 142t
 toxicity, 142
Buprenorphine, 21t
Burns, 95–100, 96t
 assessment chart, 98f
 in child abuse, 101
 classification of, 97t, 95.e1f
 closed-space, 96
 dressings for, 100
 electrolyte composition of, 304t
 emergency management of, 96–100
 inpatient management of, 100
 mapping, 95
 outpatient management of, 96
 pain management in, 100
 prevention of, 100
 secondary survey, 98–100
 types of, 96t
 web resources, 73
Busulfan (Myleran)
 characteristics of, 613t–615t
 late effects of, 625.e1t–625.e2t
Butabarbital, 385b
Butorphanol, 802
BVL. *See* Vinblastine

C

C1-inh, 377t–378t
C-A-B (Circulation Airway, and Breathing) pathway, 2, 73
CABP (community-acquired bacterial pneumonia), 820. *See also* Pneumonia
Cafcit. *See* Caffeine citrate
Café-au-lait spots, 218f, 225, 225.e7f
Cafergot. *See* Ergotamine tartrate with caffeine
Caffeine citrate (Cafcit)
 formulary entry, 802–803
 for migraine, 554
Calan. *See* Verapamil
Calcidio. *See* Ergocalciferol
Calciferol. *See* Ergocalciferol
Calcijex. *See* Calcitriol
Calcineurin inhibitors
 for atopic dermatitis (eczema), 222
 for nephrotic syndrome, 536–537
Calcitonin—salmon (Miacalcin, Fortical Nasal Spray), 803
Calcitrate. *See* Calcium citrate

Calcitriol (1,25-dihydroxycholecalciferol, Rocaltrol, Calcijex), 803–804
Calcium
  in multivitamin tablets, 589t–590t
  for osteopenia, 693
  recommended intakes, 591t
  reference values, 709t–716t
  urinary, 526
Calcium acetate (PhosLo, Calphron, Eliphos, Phoslyra), 804
Calcium carbonate (Tums, Children's Pepto), 805
Calcium channel blockers
  for hypertension, 544t–545t
  poisoning or overdose, 23t–24t, 805, 906
  for Raynaud phenomenon, 701
Calcium chloride, 805–806
Calcium citrate (Calcitrate, Citracal), 806
Calcium disodium versenate, 868
Calcium disturbances, 307–309, 529
Calcium glubionate, 806–807
Calcium gluconate (Cal-Glu)
  formulary entry, 807
  for hyperkalemia, 308f
Calcium lactate (Cal-Lac), 807–808
Calcium phosphate, tribasic (Posture-D), 808
Calcium supplements, 1125t–1134t
Calcium/creatinine (Ca/Cr) ratio, 526
  age-adjusted values, 527t
Caldolor. *See* Ibuprofen
Calfactant (Infasurf), 1072–1073
Cal-Glu. *See* Calcium gluconate
Cal-Lac. *See* Calcium lactate
Caloric calculations, 291
Caloric modulars, 592, 593t
Calories
  formulas high in, 601t–602t
  newborn requirements for, 499t
Calphron. *See* Calcium acetate
Campath (alemtuzumab), 613t–615t
Campylobacter, 691
Canakinumab, 692
Canasa. *See* Mesalamine
Cancer. *See also* Oncology
  anemia in, 874–875
  duodenal, 1068
  gastric, 1068
  liver, 609t–610t
Cancer pain, 886
Cancer survivors
  follow-up guidelines for, 607
  treatment for, 625
Cancidas. *See* Caspofungin

Candida, 224–225
Candida albicans, 118t
  antimicrobial prophylaxis against, 626t
  germ tube screen for, 470
Candidemia, 1101
Candidiasis
  diagnosis of, 218f
  diaper, 219–220
  esophageal, 889, 969, 1101–1102
  invasive, 969, 1101
  local, 218f
  oral, 481t, 841
  oropharyngeal, 889, 991
  prophylaxis against, 626t, 969
  skin infections, 481t
  treatment of, 889, 930
  vaginal, 889
  vulvovaginal, 118t
Cannabinoids
  antiemetic agents, 626t
  synthetic overdose, 23t–24t
  urine toxicology screen, 21t
CaO_2. *See* Oxygen content
Capillariasis, 955
Capillary blood gas (CBG), 639
Capillary refill, 2
Capnography, 638–639
Capoten. *See* Captopril
Captopril
  dose adjustment in renal failure, 1125t–1134t
  formulary entry, 808–809
  for hypertension, 544t–545t
Caputo Scales, 236, 237t–238t
Carafate. *See* Sucralfate
Carbamate poisoning, 787
Carbamazepine (Epitol, Tegretol, Carbatrol, Equetro, Carnexiv)
  dose adjustment in renal failure, 1125t–1134t
  formulary entry, 809–810
  for seizures, 562t
  warfarin interactions, 385b
Carbamide peroxide (Debrox, Auro Ear Wax Remover, Thera-Ear, Gly-Oxide), 811
Carbamylphosphate synthetase (CPS) deficiency, 342
  differential diagnosis of, 337f
  management of, 340, 342
Carbapenems, 447t–449t
Carbatrol. *See* Carbamazepine
Carbinoxamine (Arbinoxa, Karbinal ER), 811–812
Carbohydrate intolerance, 601t–602t

Carbohydrate metabolism disorders, 343–344
Carbon dioxide (CO_2 content), 709t–716t
Carbon dioxide, end-tidal ($ETCO_2$), 638
Carbon monoxide, 709t–716t
Carbon monoxide poisoning, 96
Carboplatin (CBDCA, Paraplatin), 613t–615t
Carboxyhemoglobin, 709t–716t
Carcinoma. See Cancer
Cardene. See Nicardipine
Cardiac anatomy, 671f–674f
Cardiac arrest
 pulseless, 872
 sudden, 2
 treatment of, 805, 807, 872, 1096
Cardiac catheterization, 184, 184.e2f
Cardiac defects, 185t
Cardiac diseases, 503–504
Cardiac examination, 112
Cardiac imaging, 183–184
Cardiac rhabdomyoma, 352
Cardiac shunts, 190, 190f
Cardiac surgery, 190–191
Cardiac system
 changes as death approaches, 633
 late effects of cancer treatment on, 625.e1t–625.e2t
 review of, 111
Cardiac tamponade, 195–196
Cardiac valves, prosthetic, 192b
Cardiogenic shock, 86, 86.e1t
Cardiogenic syncope, 557t
Cardiology, 156–202
Cardiomyopathy
 dilated, 193–194
 hypertrophic, 193–194, 987, 199.e1t
 restrictive, 194
 sports restrictions, 199.e1t
Cardiopulmonary bypass, 1102
Cardiopulmonary failure, 86.e2t
Cardiopulmonary resuscitation (CPR), 632, 786
Cardiovascular screening, 200–201, 201.e1b
Cardizem. See Diltiazem
Carnation formulas, 570, 594t–602t
Carnexiv. See Carbamazepine
Carnitine (Levocarnitine, Carnitor, Carnitor SF, L-Carnitine)
 formulary entry, 812
 for metabolic crisis, 340
 for organic acidemia, 341
 quantitative, 336t

Carnitine deficiency, 341, 812
Carnitine metabolism disorders, 341–347
Carnitor. See Carnitine
Carnitor SF. See Carnitine
Carotid bruit, 167t
Cartia XT. See Diltiazem
Carvedilol (Coreg)
 formulary entry, 812–813
 for hypertension, 544t–545t
Case managers, 628
Case-control studies, 726t
Casein-based formulas, 594t–600t
Caspofungin (Cancidas), 813–814
CAST (Childhood Autism Screening Test), 237t–238t
CAT (Clinical Adaptive Test), 237t–238t
Cat bites, 94t, 461t–468t
Catapres. See Clonidine
Catch-up growth, 582–583
 requirements for, 582–583, 583b
Catch-up immunization schedule, 412, 414f
Catecholamines
 normal values, 287, 287.e1t–287.e2t
 tumors that produce, 82.e1
Cathartics, 953
Catheter-associated urinary tract infections, 520
Catheterization
 cardiac, 184, 184.e2f
 radial artery, 34–36
 transurethral, 520
 umbilical artery (UA), 45–48, 47f
 umbilical vein (UV), 45–48
 urinary bladder, 58–59
Catheter-related bloodstream infections, 461t–468t
Catheters, arterial, 34
Cathflo Activase. See Alteplase
Catog bites, 94t
CAVH/D (continuous arteriovenous hemofiltration/hemodialysis), 529
Cayston. See Aztreonam
CBT. See Cognitive-behavioral therapy
CCNU. See Lomustine
CDC. See Centers for Disease Control and Prevention
CDDP. See Cisplatin
Ceclor. See Cefaclor
Cedax. See Ceftibuten
Cefaclor
 dose adjustment in renal failure, 1111t–1124t
 formulary entry, 814

Cefadroxil (Duricef)
dose adjustment in renal failure, 1111t–1124t
formulary entry, 815
Cefazolin
dose adjustment in renal failure, 1111t–1124t
endocarditis prophylaxis regimen, 192t
formulary entry, 815
for lymphadenitis, 461t–468t
spectrum of activity, 447t–449t
Cefdinir
dose adjustment in renal failure, 1111t–1124t
formulary entry, 816
for otitis media, 461t–468t
spectrum of activity, 447t–449t
Cefepime (Maxipime)
for catheter-related bloodstream infections, 461t–468t
dose adjustment in renal failure, 1111t–1124t
formulary entry, 816–817
for sinusitis, 461t–468t
spectrum of activity, 447t–449t
for tracheitis, 461t–468t
for UTI, 461t–468t
for ventriculoperitoneal shunt infection, 461t–468t
Cefixime (Suprax)
dose adjustment in renal failure, 1111t–1124t
formulary entry, 817
for gonorrhea, 115t–116t
for sinusitis, 461t–468t
spectrum of activity, 447t–449t
Cefotaxime (Claforan)
for abscess infection, 461t–468t
for conjunctivitis, 461t–468t
dose adjustment in renal failure, 1111t–1124t
formulary entry, 817–818
for gonorrhea, 115t–116t
for meningitis, 461t–468t
neonatal dosing, 513t–514t
for pneumonia, 461t–468t
for septic arthritis, 461t–468t
for sinusitis, 461t–468t
spectrum of activity, 447t–449t
Cefotetan (Cefotan)
dose adjustment in renal failure, 1111t–1124t
formulary entry, 818

Cefotetan (Cefotan) *(Continued)*
for pelvic inflammatory disease, 115t–116t
spectrum of activity, 447t–449t
Cefoxitin
formulary entry, 819
for pelvic inflammatory disease, 115t–116t
spectrum of activity, 447t–449t
Cefpodoxime
dose adjustment in renal failure, 1111t–1124t
formulary entry, 819
for otitis media, 461t–468t
for sinusitis, 461t–468t
spectrum of activity, 447t–449t
Cefprozil
dose adjustment in renal failure, 1111t–1124t
formulary entry, 820
Ceftaroline fosamil (Teflaro)
formulary entry, 820–821
spectrum of activity, 447t–449t
Ceftazidime (Fortaz, Tazicef)
for catheter-related bloodstream infections, 461t–468t
dose adjustment in renal failure, 1111t–1124t
formulary entry, 821
for osteomyelitis, 461t–468t
spectrum of activity, 447t–449t
Ceftibuten (Cedax)
dose adjustment in renal failure, 1111t–1124t
formulary entry, 821
Ceftin. *See* Cefuroxime
Ceftriaxone (Rocephin)
for abscess infection, 461t–468t
for cellulitis, 461t–468t
for chancroid, 120t
for conjunctivitis, 461t–468t
endocarditis prophylaxis regimen, 192t
for fever without localizing signs, 453f
formulary entry, 822
for gastroenteritis, 461t–468t
for gonorrhea, 115t–116t
for intra-abdominal infections, 461t–468t
for meningitis, 461t–468t
for otitis media, 461t–468t
for parotitis, 461t–468t
for PID, 115t–116t
for pneumonia, 461t–468t
for pyelonephritis, 461t–468t

Ceftriaxone (Rocephin) *(Continued)*
  for septic arthritis, 461*t*–468*t*
  for sickle cell disease, 461*t*–468*t*
  for sinusitis, 461*t*–468*t*
  spectrum of activity, 447*t*–449*t*
  for tracheitis, 461*t*–468*t*
Cefuroxime (Zinacef, Ceftin)
  dose adjustment in renal failure, 1111*t*–1124*t*
  formulary entry, 823
  for Lyme disease, 479*t*–480*t*
  spectrum of activity, 447*t*–449*t*
Cefzil. *See* Cefprozil
Celecoxib (Celebrex)
  analgesic properties, 139
  formulary entry, 824
Celestone Soluspan. *See* Betamethasone
Celiac disease, 325
CellCept. *See* Mycophenolate mofetil
Cellulitis
  initial management of, 461*t*–468*t*
  orbital, 461*t*–468*t*, 666, 666*f*
  periorbital (preseptal), 461*t*–468*t*, 666
  soft tissue, 62, 62*f*–63*f*
Celsius, 708
Center for Epidemiological Studies Depression Scale for Children (CES-DC), 237*t*–238*t*, 249
Center of Excellence for Transgender Health (UCSF), 255
Centers for Disease Control and Prevention (CDC)
  Catch-up immunization schedule, 414*f*, 426
  growth charts and nutrition information, 570
  Guidelines: HEADS UP to Youth Sports, 73, 78
  guidelines for adolescent and school health, 113
  immunization schedules, 412, 413*f*–418*f*, 426
  Morbidity and Mortality Weekly Reports, 412
  Prevention of Child Maltreatment, 73
  Provider Resources for Vaccine Conversations with Parents, 420
  Section on Environmental Health, 20
  Travelers' Health website, 412, 426
  vaccine information statement (VIS) forms, 412
  web resources, 412
  websites for clinicians, 108

Central hypotonia, 356
Central line placement, 674, 675*f*–676*f*. *See also* Central venous catheter placement
Central nervous system (CNS) injury
  ECG effects of, 180*t*
  late effects of cancer treatment, 625.*e*1*t*–625.*e*2*t*
Central venous catheter placement, 36–42
  access sites for, 37
  femoral venous, 41–42, 43*f*–44*f*
  image-guided, 674
  internal jugular vein, 37–41, 38*f*–41*f*
  landmark approach, 39–41
  Seldinger technique, 37
  subclavian venous, 37, 41, 42*f*
  ultrasound-guided, 37, 39, 40*f*–41*f*, 41–42, 44*f*
Centre for Evidence Based Medicine, 721
Centrum Kids, 589*t*–590*t*
Centrum Tablet, 589*t*–590*t*
Cephalexin (Keflex)
  for cellulitis, 461*t*–468*t*
  for cystitis, 461*t*–468*t*
  for dacrocystitis, 461*t*–468*t*
  dose adjustment in renal failure, 1111*t*–1124*t*
  endocarditis prophylaxis regimen, 192*t*
  formulary entry, 824–825
  for lymphadenitis, 461*t*–468*t*
  for pyelonephritis, 461*t*–468*t*
  spectrum of activity, 447*t*–449*t*
Cephalosporins
  for bites, 461*t*–468*t*
  for catheter-related bloodstream infections, 461*t*–468*t*
  for cellulitis, 461*t*–468*t*
  for otitis media, 461*t*–468*t*
  for pharyngitis, 461*t*–468*t*
  spectrum of activity, 447*t*–449*t*
Cephamycins, 447*t*–449*t*
Cephulac. *See* Lactulose
CER (crossed extension reflex), 236.*e*4*t*–236.*e*5*t*
CeraLyte solutions, 603*t*
Cerebellar function tests, 551
Cerebral edema
  brain tumor–associated, 852
  in diabetic ketoacidosis, 257
Cerebral palsy (CP), 242–244
  classification of, 243, 243*t*
  web resources, 229

Cerebral Palsy Foundation, 229
Cerebral perfusion pressure (CPP), 82, 567
Cerebrospinal fluid (CSF) evaluation, 717t
Cerebrospinal fluid (CSF) leak, 421
Cerebrospinal fluid (CSF) shunting, 564
Cerebrovascular accident, 617–618
Cerebyx. See Fosphenytoin
Cerumenolytics
 antiyprine and benzocaine, 781
 carbamide peroxide, 811
Cervarix. See Human papillomavirus (HPV) vaccine
Cervical cancer, 122–123
Cervical infections, 817
Cervical lymph nodes, 455.e1f
Cervical lymphadenopathy, 454–455, 454f
Cervical spine (C-spine) imaging, 78, 666–667, 668f
Cervical spine (C-spine) injuries, 78
Cervicitis
 chlamydial, 790
 gonococcal, 790
Cesarean section, 1056
CES-DC (Center for Epidemiological Studies Depression Scale for Children), 237t–238t, 249
Cetirizine (Zyrtec)
 for allergic rhinitis, 396
 dose adjustment in renal failure, 1125t–1134t
 formulary entry, 825–826
Cetirizine + pseudoephedrine (Zyrtec-D 12 Hour), 825–826
Cetraxal. See Ciprofloxacin
CF. See Cystic fibrosis
CGH (comparative genomic hybridization) array, 358t
Chancroid, 120t, 822
CHARGE syndrome, 185t, 496
Chédiak-Higashi syndrome, 403t–404t
Chemet. See Succimer
Chemical burns, 96t, 99
Chemoprophylaxis
 for influenza A and B, 432
 for meningococcus, 435
Chemotherapy
 adjuncts, 613t–615t
 agent characteristics of, 613t–615t
 anemia associated with, 848–849
 complications of, 624–625
 immunizations during, 625.e3
 late effects of, 625.e1t–625.e2t
 maintenance, 423

Chemotherapy (Continued)
 molecularly targeted agents, 613t–615t
 myeloablative, 619
 treatment regimens, 625
 vaccinations during, 423
Chemotherapy-induced nausea and vomiting, 625
 prevention of, 996
 treatment of, 864, 908
Chest compressions, 3–4, 3t
Chest examination, 74t–75t
Chest radiography, 183–184, 670–674
 anteroposterior (AP) images, 671f–672f
  central line placement on, 675f–676f
  of heart and vessels, 677f
 central line placement on, 674
 in congenital heart disease, 675
 ETT placement on, 674
 lateral images, 670, 673f–674f, 675
 posteroanterior (PA) images, 670, 675
Chest tube placement, 51–55, 52f
Chest wall abnormalities, 637
Chest wall compression, 656
$\chi 2$ (chi square) test, 724t
Chickenpox. See Varicella
Chief complaint, 110
Child abuse, 101–103, 683
 classic findings, 683, 685f–686f
 documentation of, 103
 fractures suspicious for, 102, 103t
 Prevention of Child Maltreatment (CDC), 73
 reporting, 102
 sexual abuse, 102
 skeletal findings, 103t
 skeletal survey for, 102, 683
 skin findings, 101
Child and Adolescent Psychiatry Practice Parameters, 229
Child life specialists, 143, 628
Child Neurology Society, 548
Childhood Autism Screening Test (CAST), 237t–238t, 244
Childhood disintegrative disorder, 244
Childhood-onset fluency disorder, 242
Children with Diabetes (website), 255
The Children's Hospital of Philadelphia (CHOP), 412
Children's Nephrotic Syndrome Consensus, 535–536
Children's Oncology Camping Association, 607

Children's Pepto. *See* Calcium carbonate
Chlamydia, 691
　management of, 115*t*–116*t*, 461*t*–468*t*, 790, 973
　screening guidelines for sexually active adolescents, 114–117
Chlamydia trachomatis, 973
Chlamydial cervicitis, 790
Chloral hydrate, 1125*t*–1134*t*
Chlorambucil, 700
Chloramphenicol
　formulary entry, 826
　for meningitis, 461*t*–468*t*
　warfarin interactions, 385*b*
Chlorhexidine, 700
Chloride
　in multivitamin tablets, 589*t*–590*t*
　reference values, 709*t*–716*t*
Chloroquine phosphate (Aralen)
　dose adjustment in renal failure, 1125*t*–1134*t*
　formulary entry, 826–827
Chloroquine-resistant malaria, 1030
Chlorothiazide (Diuril)
　dose adjustment in renal failure, 1125*t*–1134*t*
　formulary entry, 827–828
Chlorpheniramine maleate (Chlor-Trimeton), 828
Chlorpromazine (Thorazine), 828–829
Chlorthalidone, 544*t*–545*t*
Chlor-Trimeton. *See* Chlorpheniramine maleate
Cholecalciferol (vitamin D_3, D-3, Decara, D Drops, Emfamil D-Vi-Sol), 829–830
Cholestasis, 325
　pruritus from, 1089
　TPN-induced, 1089
Cholesterol
　goals for, 200
　high-density lipoprotein (HDL), 200
　low-density lipoprotein (LDL), 200
　reference values, 709*t*–716*t*
Cholesterol screening
　for adolescents, 123
　recommendations for, 199–200
Cholesterol supplementation, 347
Cholesterol synthesis disorders, 346–347
Cholestyramine (Questran, Cholestyramine Light, Prevalite), 830
Choline, 586*t*

Choline magnesium trisalicylate
　analgesic properties, 139
　formulary entry, 830–831
Cholinergic poisoning with, 22*t*
CHOP. *See* The Children's Hospital of Philadelphia
Chorionic villus sampling (CVS), 490.*e*1
Choroid plexus papilloma/carcinoma, 611*t*
Christmas disease, 387*t*–388*t*
Chromium
　in multivitamin tablets, 589*t*–590*t*
　recommended intakes, 591*t*
Chromosome microarray, 336*t*
Chronic bacteremia, 532*f*
Chronic bronchitis exacerbation, 819, 821
Chronic diarrhea, 950
Chronic graft-versus-host disease (cGVHD), 622, 625.*e*3
Chronic granulomatous disease, 403*t*–404*t*
Chronic headaches, 552*b*
Chronic hepatitis B, 935–936
Chronic hypertension, 539–542, 913
Chronic inflammation: anemia of, 367
Chronic iron overload, 850
Chronic kidney disease (CKD), 538–539
　Bedside Chronic Kidney Disease in Children (CKiD) cohort, 524
　classification of, 538–539
　clinical manifestations of, 539, 540*t*
　etiology of, 539
　iron deficiency anemia in, 926
　radiographic imaging considerations, 529–530
　urine specific gravity, 516
Chronic Kidney Disease Epidemiology Collaboration (CKD-EPI), 524
Chronic lung disease of infancy, 653–654
Chronic lung disease of prematurity, 653–654
Chronic myositis, 704
Chronic obstructive pulmonary disease (COPD) exacerbation, 789
Chronic pain
　augmented analgesia for, 772
　in infants, 136
　management of, 919
Chronic pancreatitis, 329–330, 329.*e*1*t*
Chronic pulmonary hypertension, 89
Chronic renal failure
　anemia in, 848, 873–875
　treatment of, 849
Chronic respiratory alkalosis, 641*t*

Chronic sinusitis, 461t–468t
Chronic spasticity, 846
Chronic suppurative otitis media, 992
Chronic uveitis, 689t
Chronulac. See Lactulose
Churg-Strauss syndrome, 697t
Chvostek's sign, 307, 21.e1t–21.e3t
Chylothorax, 601t–602t
Ciclesonide (Alvesco, Omnaris, Zetonna)
   dosages, 646.e1t–646.e2t
   formulary entry, 831
Cidofovir (Vistide)
   for adenovirus, 624.e1t
   for BK virus, 624.e1t
   formulary entry, 832
Cilastatin and imipenem (Primaxin), 918
Ciloxan. See Ciprofloxacin
Cimetidine (Tagamet)
   dose adjustment in renal failure, 1125t–1134t
   formulary entry, 832–833
   warfarin interactions, 385b
Ciprofloxacin (Cipro, Ciloxan, Cetraxal, Ciprodex, Otovel Otic)
   for cystitis, 461t–468t
   dose adjustment in renal failure, 1111t–1124t
   formulary entry, 833–834
   for intra-abdominal infections, 461t–468t
   for otitis externa, 461t–468t
   spectrum of activity, 450t
   for traveler's diarrhea, 461t–468t
   for UTI, 461t–468t
   warfarin interactions, 385b
Circulation
   allergic emergencies, 9
   assessment of, 2
   changes as death approaches, 633
   emergency management of, 2–4, 3t
Circulation Airway, and Breathing (C-A-B) pathway, 2, 73
Cisplatin (cis-platinum, CDDP, Platinol), 613–615t
Citracal. See Calcium citrate
Citrate mixtures, 835
Citrullinemia, 337f, 340
CKD. See Chronic kidney disease
Claforan. See Cefotaxime
CLAMS (Clinical Linguistic and Auditory Milestone Scale), 237t–238t
Claravis. See Isotretinoid
Clarithromycin (Biaxin)
   dose adjustment in renal failure, 1111t–1124t

Clarithromycin (Biaxin) *(Continued)*
   endocarditis prophylaxis regimen, 192t
   formulary entry, 835–836
   with metronidazole, 968
   spectrum of activity, 450t
   warfarin interactions, 385b
Claritin. See Loratadine
Claritin-D. See Loratadine with pseudoephedrine
Clavicle, fractured, 495
Clavulanate
   amoxicillin-clavulanate. See Amoxicillin-clavulanic acid (Augmentin)
   for sinusitis, 461t–468t
Clean catch urine culture, 520
Clear liquid diet, 601t–602t
Cleft lip and palate (CLP), 355, 355.e1f
Clindamycin (Cleocin, ClindaMax, Evoclin)
   for abscess infection, 461t–468t
   for acne vulgaris, 214
   for bacterial vaginosis, 118t
   for bites, 461t–468t
   for cellulitis, 461t–468t
   for dacrocystitis, 461t–468t
   for endocarditis prophylaxis, 192t
   formulary entry, 836–837
   for lymphadenitis, 461t–468t
   for mastoiditis, 461t–468t
   for osteomyelitis, 461t–468t
   for otitis media, 461t–468t
   for parotitis, 461t–468t
   for pharyngitis, 461t–468t
   for PID, 115t–116t
   for pneumonia, 461t–468t, 1030
   for septic arthritis, 461t–468t
   for sinusitis, 461t–468t
   spectrum of activity, 452t
Clindamycin with benzoyl peroxide (BenzaClin, Duac, Acanya), 794
Clindamycin with tretinoin (Veltin, Ziagen), 1085–1086
Clinical Adaptive Test (CAT), 237t–238t
Clinical Linguistic and Auditory Milestone Scale (CLAMS), 237t–238t
Clinical questions, 721
Clinical Trial Database (NCI), 607
Clinical trials, 726t
   grid for calculations in, 727t
   grid for evaluating tests, 728t
   Pediatric Study Characteristics Database, 732
   study designs, 726t

Clinicians' Postexposure Prophylaxis (PEP) Line, 486
Clinistix, 517
Clinitest, 517
Clitoromegaly, 284
Clobazam (Onfi)
  dose adjustment in renal failure, 1125t–1134t
  formulary entry, 837–838
  for seizures, 562t
Clobetasol propionate, 223t
Clocortolone pivalate, 223t
Clofarabine (Clolar), 613t–615t
Clonazepam (Klonopin)
  formulary entry, 838–839
  for seizures, 562t
Clonic seizures, 558b
Clonidine (Catapres, Kapvay, Duraclon, Nexiclon XR)
  formulary entry, 839–840
  for hypertension, 544t–545t
  for hypertensive urgency, 84t
  overdose, 23t–24t
  with PCA, 145
Closed head trauma (CHT), 75–78
Clostridium difficile infection, 316
  treatment of, 968, 1094
Clotrimazole (Alevazol, Lotrimin AF, Gyne-Lotrimin)
  for candidiasis, 481t
  formulary entry, 840–841
  for ringworm, 481t
Clubbing, nail, 225, 225.e4f
CMV. *See* Cytomegalovirus
Coagulation, 376–382
  age-specific values, 377t–378t
Coagulation cascade, 376f
Coagulation disorders, 387b, 387t–388t
Coagulation inhibitors, 377t–378t
Coagulation tests, 376–379, 382
Coarctation of the aorta, 186t–187t
Cobalamin (vitamin B$_{12}$). *See also* Cyanocobalamin
  in infant multivitamin drops, 588t
  in multivitamin tablets, 589t–590t
  recommended intakes, 586t
  reference values, 709t–716t
Cocaine ingestion
  management considerations, 82.e1
  overdose, 23t–24t
  urine toxicology screen, 21t
Coccidioides, 930
Cochlear implants, 421
Cochrane Reviews, 721
Codeine, 21t, 138
Codman triangles, 684f

Coefficient of absorption (CA), 330.e1
Cogentin. *See* Benztropine mesylate
Cognitive development
  milestones of early literacy, 233t
  screening tests for, 237t–238t
Cognitive-behavioral therapy (CBT)
  for depressive disorders, 249
  for mental health issues, 251
Cohort studies, 726t
Colace. *See* Docusate
Colchicine
  for Behçet disease, 700
  for scleroderma, 701.e3
Cold, common, 924
Cold injury, 96t
Cold (septic) shock, 87f, 86.e1t
Cold sores, 1090
Colic, 233t–235t
Colitis
  C difficile, 1094
  enterocolitis. *See* Enterocolitis
  infantile proctocolitis, 398
  ulcerative. *See* Ulcerative colitis
Collagen vascular disease, 180t
Collodion baby, 218f
Colloids
  for hypovolemic/distributive shock, 87f
  for inhalation injury, 97
Colocort. *See* Hydrocortisone
Color, 493t
Color Doppler flow imaging, 675
CoLyte. *See* Polyethylene glycol (PEG) electrolyte solutions
Coma
  barbiturate, 1014
  emergency management of, 14–15
  Glasgow Coma Scale, 15t
  Modified Coma Scale for infants, 15t
  myxedema, 943
  in poisoning, 21.e1t–21.e3t
  treatment of, 943, 1014
Combivax, 425f
Combivent Respimat. *See* Ipratropium bromide + albuterol
Combivir. *See* Zidovudine with lamivudine
Comedones
  closed, 213
  open, 213
Common variable immunodeficiency, 403t–404t
Communication, 628–631
  Ask-Tell-Ask method, 630
  family meetings, 629–630
  NURSE method for, 630–631

Communication *(Continued)*
tools for difficult conversations, 630–631
Communication and Symbolic Behavior Scales and Developmental Profile (CSBS DP), 237t–238t
Communication disorders, 242
Community resources, 628
Community-acquired bacterial pneumonia (CABP), 820. *See also* Pneumonia
Community-acquired pneumonia. *See also* Pneumonia
  exacerbation of, 819
  treatment of, 779, 789–790, 816, 942
Comparative genomic hybridization (CGH), 358t
Compartment syndrome, 74t–75t, 80–81
Compazine. *See* Prochlorperazine
Compensated shock, 84
Compensatory responses, 639, 641t
Competitive athletes, 201.e1b
Compleat formulas, 594t–600t
Complement, 701, 703–704
  decreased levels of, 703
  increased levels of, 704
  serum levels, 408t
  total hemolytic level (CH_{50}), 703
Complement C3, 703
Complement C4, 703
Complement deficiency
  congenital, 703
  immunoprophylaxis guidelines for, 367
Complement pathway, 409f
Complement-mediated thrombotic microangiopathy, 375
Complex febrile seizures, 556
Complex partial seizures, 1098
Computed tomography (CT)
  abdominal, 79, 678, 923
  advantages and disadvantages of, 664t
  of airway, 667
  in bowel obstruction, 678
  contrast-enhanced, 79, 666–667, 674, 678, 923
  of eyes, 665–666
  of head, 664
  head imaging, 76, 76b, 665
  judicious use of, 663
  noncontrast, 665
  parenchymal findings, 674

Computed tomography (CT) *(Continued)*
  PECARN clinical decision rule for, 76, 76b
  in vessel abnormalities, 675–676
COMVAX. *See* PRP-OMP
Concerta. *See* Methylphenidate HCl
Concussions
  postconcussive symptoms, 77
  in sports-related injuries, 77–78
Conduction blocks, 178f
  nonventricular, 178t
  ventricular, 179t
Confidence intervals, 725
Confidentiality, 110
Confounding, 725
Confounding bias, 722
Congenital adrenal hyperplasia, 269–271, 269f
  diagnosis of, 270t
  newborn screening for, 270–271
  treatment of, 890
Congenital complement deficiency, 703
Congenital dermal melanocytosis, 219
Congenital heart disease, 185–191
  acyanotic, 186t–187t
  bacterial endocarditis prophylaxis for, 192b
  cyanotic, 185–187, 188t–189t
  exercise recommendations for, 199.e1t
  imaging of, 675
  newborn screening for, 493
  pulse oximetry screening for, 185
  sports restrictions, 199.e1t
  syndromes associated with, 185t
Congenital hip dislocation, 681, 681.e1f
Congenital hypopigmented macules, 226.e3f
Congenital infections, 455, 457t–458t
  CMV infection, 1090
  imaging of, 665
  syphilis, 1009
  toxoplasmosis, 1069
  treatment of, 1009, 1069, 1090
Congenital ingrown toenails, 225, 225.e5f
Congenital malformations, 665
Congenital nail disorders, 225, 225.e6f
Congestive heart failure, 166b
Conjugated hyperbilirubinemia, 506–507
Conjunctivitis
  allergic, 994
  exudative, 461t–468t
  initial management of, 461t–468t

Conjunctivitis *(Continued)*
  neonatal, 461*t*–468*t*
  suppurative, 461*t*–468*t*
  treatment of, 878, 905, 942, 992, 994, 1068
Connective tissue diseases, 350–351, 695*t*
Conners' Rating Scales-Revised, 237*t*–238*t*
Conscious sedation, 145
Consciousness: altered states
  differential diagnosis of, 14*b*
  emergency management of, 13–15
Consent, 30, 110
  for autopsy, 635
  to medical care for STIs, 114
  for minors, 114
Constipation, 321–322
  definition of, 321
  differential diagnosis of, 321*t*
  functional, 321–322, 321.e1*t*
  in infants, 322
  maintenance therapy for, 322
  medications for, 322
  nonfunctional, 321, 321*t*
  treatment of, 322, 907, 935, 972, 1024, 1037, 1057
Constitutional growth delay, 277, 278*f*
Contact dermatitis, 218*f*, 221
Contact injury, thermal, 96*t*
Continuous arteriovenous hemofiltration/hemodialysis (CAVH/D), 529
Continuous positive airway pressure (CPAP), 658
Continuous venovenous hemofiltration/hemodialysis (CVVH/D), 529
Contraception, 125–131
  barrier methods, 130
  emergency, 130–131
  fertility awareness-based methods, 130
  follow-up recommendations, 131
  hormonal, 125
  initiation of, 125–127
  long-acting reversible (LARC), 125
  medroxyprogesterone, 956
  methods of, 125, 126*f*, 127–130
  quick start, 127, 128*f*
  selection of, 125–127
  for sickle cell disease, 372*t*
  special considerations for adolescents, 125
  websites for clinicians, 108
Contraception counseling, 125
Contrast enemas, 678

Contrast media, radiographic iodinated (RICM), 529
Conversion formulas, 708
Cooley's anemia, 372
Coombs test
  direct, 368
  indirect, 368
Coordination, 551
Copegus. *See* Ribavirin
Copper
  in multivitamin tablets, 589*t*–590*t*
  recommended intakes, 591*t*
Copper IUD, 130
Cordarone. *See* Amiodarone
Coreg. *See* Carvedilol
Cori disease, 344
Corneal ulcers, 942, 992
Corner fractures, 683
Corrected reticulocyte count (CRC), 367
Correlation, 723
Cortef. *See* Hydrocortisone
Cortenema. *See* Hydrocortisone
Cortical tuber, 352
Corticosporin Otic. *See* Polymyxin B sulfate, neomycin sulfate, hydrocortisone otic
Corticosteroids
  for allergic emergencies, 10
  for allergic rhinitis, 396
  for arthritis, 692
  for asthma, 647*f*–652*f*
    dosages, 646.e1*t*–646.e2*t*
  for Behçet disease, 700
  for GVHD, 621–622
  for idiopathic pneumonia syndrome, 623
  inhaled (ICS), 648*f*, 650*f*–652*f*
    dosages, 646.e1*t*–646.e2*t*
  for ITP, 374
  late effects of, 625.e1*t*–625.e2*t*
  for nephrotic syndrome, 535–537
  for OSAS, 658
  for seizures, 559*t*–560*t*
  for SLE, 695
  topical, 223*t*
  vaccines for patients on, 423, 424*t*
Corticotropin (HP Acthar), 841
Corticotropin provocative tests, 268–269, 1096
Cortifoam. *See* Hydrocortisone
Cortisol
  AM levels, 268*t*
  potency of, 271*t*
  salivary levels, 273

Cortisone acetate
 formulary entry, 841
 potency of, 271*e*2*f*
Cosa magna, 681.*e*2*f*
Co-Trimoxazole. *See* Sulfamethoxazole and trimethoprim
Cough syncope, 557*t*
Coumadin. *See* Warfarin
Counseling
 contraception, 125
 about EC, 131
 pretest, 360
Cow's milk–based formulas, 594*t*–600*t*
Coxsackie A virus, 471*t*–476*t*
Coxsackie B virus, 471*t*–476*t*
Cozaar. *See* Losartan
CP. *See* Cerebral palsy
CPAP (continuous positive airway pressure), 658
C-peptide, 256
CPP (cerebral perfusion pressure), 82, 567
CPS (carbamylphosphate synthetase) deficiency, 342
Crackles (rales), 638*t*
Cradle cap, 219
CRAFFT Questionnaire, 133, 133*b*, 251
Cranial bruits, 551.*e*1*t*
Cranial nerves, 549*t*
Craniopharyngioma, 611*t*
Craniosynostosis, 353, 665
C-reactive protein (CRP), 701–702, 709*t*–716*t*
Creatine kinase (CK), 704, 709*t*–716*t*
Creatine phosphokinase, 709*t*–716*t*
Creatinine
 blood urea nitrogen/creatinine (BUN/Cr) ratio, 528
 calcium/creatinine (Ca/Cr) ratio, 526, 527*t*
 eGFR from, 523–524
 reference values, 709*t*–716*t*
Creatinine clearance (CCr), 523
Creon. *See* Pancrelipase
Cricoid pressure (Sellick maneuver), 4
Critical care
 emergencies, 81–93
 reference data, 92–93
 web resources, 73
Crohn's disease, 323, 800
Cromolyn (Nasalcrom, Gastrocrom, Opticrom)
 for allergic rhinitis, 396–397
 for asthma, 650*f*–652*f*
 formulary entry, 842

Crossed extension reflex (CER), 236.*e*4*t*–236.*e*5*t*
Cross-sectional studies, 726*t*
Croup (laryngotracheobronchitis)
 emergency management of, 12–13
 radiographic findings, 669*t*
 treatment of, 852, 873
Crust, 203, 209*f*
Cryoprecipitate, 392
Cryptococcal meningitis, 778, 889
Cryptococcus neoformans, 930
Cryptorchidism, 285
Cryptosporidial diarrhea, 1008
CSBS DP (Communication and Symbolic Behavior Scales and Developmental Profile), 237*t*–238*t*
C-spine (cervical spine) imaging, 78, 666–667, 668*f*
CT. *See* Computed tomography
CTX. *See* Cyclophosphamide
Culture
 blood, 443
 urine, 520
Curosurf (poractant alfa). *See* Surfactant
Cushing disease, 278*f*
Cushing evaluation, 273
Cushing syndrome, 272–273
Cushing triad, 75, 82
Cutaneous emergencies, allergic, 9
Cutaneous leishmaniasis, 1013
Cutaneous pathergy, 700
Cutaneous sporotrichosis, 1026
Cutis marmorata, 218*f*
Cutivate. *See* Fluticasone propionate
Cuvposa. *See* Glycopyrrolate
CVS (chorionic villus sampling), 490.*e*1
CVVH/D (continuous venovenous hemofiltration/hemodialysis), 529
Cyanocobalamin (B-12 Compliance, Physicians EZ Use B-12, Nascobal), 842–843. *See also* Cobalamin
Cyanosis
 in newborns, 497–500
 in poisoning, 21.*e*1*t*–21.*e*3*t*
Cyanotic congenital heart disease, 188*t*–189*t*
Cyanotic lesions, 185–187
Cyanotic spells, 977
Cyclic citrullinated peptide antibodies, 703
Cyclogyl. *See* Cyclopentolate
Cyclomydril. *See* Cyclopentolate wth phenylephrine
Cyclopentolate (Cyclogyl), 843

Cyclopentolate wth phenylephrine (Cyclomydril), 844
Cyclophosphamide (CTX, Cytoxan)
  characteristics of, 613t–615t
  late effects of, 625.e1t–625.e2t
  for nephrotic syndrome, 536–537
  for SLE, 695
  toxicity, 691.e1t
Cyclosporine (Sandimmune, Gengraf, Neoral, Restasis)
  for arthritis, 692
  for Behçet disease, 700
  formulary entry, 844–845
  for GVHD, 621
  for SLE, 695
  toxicity, 691.e1t
Cyproheptadine
  formulary entry, 845–846
  for migraine prevention, 556t
Cystic acne, 929
Cystic fibrosis (CF), 654–656
  antiinflammatory agents for, 789–790
  clinical manifestations of, 655t
  complications of, 759
  formulas for, 601t–602t
  prophylaxis therapy for, 791, 1082
  pulmonary exacerbations, 958
  screening for, 655
  spirometry and lung volume readings in, 643t
  therapy for, 769, 791, 816, 820–821, 833, 865, 918, 1023, 1063, 1081, 1089, 1100
Cystic Fibrosis Foundation, 637
Cystitis, 532f
  hemorrhagic, 623, 832
  management of, 461t–468t, 833
Cysts
  bone, 681, 684f
  polycystic kidney, 532f
  polycystic ovary, 282
Cytarabine (Ara-C), 613t–615t
Cytochrome P450: example inducers and inhibitors of, 756t
Cytokine interactions, 423–424
Cytomegalovirus (CMV) immunoglobulin, 624.e1t
Cytomegalovirus (CMV) infection, 457t–458t, 471t–476t
  antimicrobial prophylaxis against, 626t
  in BMT recipients, 624.e1t
  congenital, 1090
  imaging of, 665
  pneumonia, 624.e1t
  prevention of, 904, 1090–1091

Cytomegalovirus (CMV) infection (Continued)
  retinitis, 832, 900, 1091
  treatment of, 832, 900, 904, 1090–1091
Cytotoxic therapy
  for arthritis, 692, 691.e1t
  for SLE, 695
  toxicity, 691.e1t
Cytovene. See Ganciclovir
Cytoxan. See Cyclophosphamide

D

D Drops. See Cholecalciferol
D Vi-Sol, 588t
D-3. See Cholecalciferol
Dacryocystitis, 461t–468t
Dactinomycin (actinomycin D)
  characteristics of, 613t–615t
  late effects of, 625.e1t–625.e2t
Dalfopristin and quinupristin (Synercid), 1044
Dandruff, 932, 1057
Dantrolene (Dantrium, Revonto, Ryanodex), 846
Dapsone (Aczone, diaminodiphenylsulfone, DDS)
  for acne vulgaris, 214
  formulary entry, 847
  for oncology patients, 626t
Daptacel. See DTaP (diphtheria, tetanus, & acellular pertussis) vaccine
Daraprim. See Pyrimethamine
Darbepoietin alfa (Aranesp), 848–849
Daunorubicin, 613t–615t
Day treatment, 251
Daytrana. See Methylphenidate HCl
DCC (deoxycorticosterone) acetate, 271t
DCSS (diffuse cutaneous systemic scleroderma), 701.e3
DDAVP. See Desmopressin acetate
D-dimer, 377t–378t
DDS (diaminodiphenylsulfone). See Dapsone
Death
  acceptable causes of, 635
  changes as death approaches, 633–634
  concepts of, 631, 631t
  documentation of, 635
Death certificates, 635
Death pronouncement, 634–635
  preparation for, 635
  procedure for, 635
Debrox. See Carbamide peroxide

Decadron. *See* Dexamethasone
Decara. *See* Cholecalciferol
Decision making, 628–631
  child participation in, 631
  guides or principles for, 630
  to limit interventions, 632–633
Decision-making tools (DMTs), 628–629
Decongestants, 1017
Decontamination, 21
Deep animal bites, 93
Deep neck infections, 455–470
Deep-vein thrombosis (DVT)
  imaging of, 675
  prophylaxis of, 567, 870–871, 911
  treatment of, 870
Deferoxamine mesylate (Desferal), 850
Defibrotide, 623
Deficit replacement strategy, 297–301
Deficit repletion, 293–301
Dehydration
  in cardiogenic shock, 86
  clinical observations in, 294*t*
  deficit replacement strategies for, 298*b*–300*b*, 299–301
  hypernatremic, 297, 298*b*, 300–301, 300*b*
  hyponatremic, 294, 296*b*, 297, 299–300, 299*b*
  isonatremic, 293–294, 295*b*, 299
  management of, 86
  mild, 301
  moderate, 301
Dehydroepiandrosterone (DHEA), 283*t*
Dehydroepiandrosterone sulfate (DHEA-S), 284*t*
Delavirdine, 385*b*
Delayed puberty, 109, 277–281, 280*f*
Delayed sleep phase syndrome, 659
Delayed transfusion reaction, 389–390
Delirium, 21.e1*t*–21.e3*t*
Delivery room, 491*f*
Delta gap, 314
Deltasone. *See* Prednisone
Delzicol. *See* Mesalamine
Dennie-Morgan lines, 395
Dental abscesses, 461*t*–468*t*
Dental procedures: bacterial endocarditis prophylaxis for, 192*b*, 192*t*, 198, 815, 822, 824
Dentition examination, 112
Deoxycorticosterone (DCC) acetate, 271*t*
Depacon. *See* Valproic acid
Depakene. *See* Valproic acid
Depakote. *See* Divalproex sodium
Depigmentation, 226–227
Depo-Medrol. *See* Methylprednisolone

Depo-Provera. *See* Medroxyprogesterone
Depot medroxyprogesterone acetate (DMPA). *See* Medroxyprogesterone
Depression, 132
  HEADSSS assessment, 111*b*
  medication for, 250, 879, 893, 990, 1008, 1058, 1085
  in poisoning, 21.e1*t*–21.e3*t*
  screening for, 237*t*–238*t*
Depressive disorders, 249–250
Deprizine. *See* Ranitidine HCl
Dermal melanocytosis, 219
Dermal melanosis, 226
Dermatitis
  allergic, 221
  atopic (eczema), 221–222, 398, 400, 1022, 1074
  contact, 218*f*, 221
  irritant, 221
  seborrheic, 218*f*, 219
Dermatitis herpetiformis, 220–221
Dermatology, 203–228
  neonatal conditions, 216–220
  system review, 111
  web resources, 490
Dermatomes, 550*f*
Dermatomyositis
  associated autoantibodies, 695*t*
  diagnosis of, 699
  juvenile, 699
Dermatosis, 1087
Derotational righting, 236.e6*t*
Desensitization, 401, 402*f*
Desferal. *See* Deferoxamine mesylate
Desloratadine, 1125*t*–1134*t*
Desmoplastic infantile glioma (DIG), 611*t*
Desmopressin acetate (DDAVP, Stimate)
  for coagulation disorders, 387*t*–388*t*
  for diabetes insipidus, 276
  formulary entry, 850–851
Desonide, 223*t*
Desoximetasone, 223*t*
Desquamation, 218*f*
Desquam-DX. *See* Benzoyl peroxide
Desyrel. *See* Trazodone
Detergent pods, 23*t*–24*t*
Detoxification, 133–134
Development
  abnormal, 230
  guidelines for, 230
  milestones, 231*t*–232*t*
  pubertal, 108–109
  red flags, 240*t*
  streams, 229
  web resources, 229

Developmental delay, 230
Developmental disorders, 241–244
  diagnosis of, 241
  interventions for, 246
  medical evaluation of, 236–241
  red flags, 240t
  state support for, 246
Developmental evaluation, 230–236
Developmental hip dysplasia, 681, 681.e1f
Developmental history, 235–236
Developmental night waking, 233t–235t
Developmental quotient (DQ), 230
Developmental referral, 246
Developmental screening, 230–236
  guidelines for, 230–235
  standardized, 235
  tests and tools, 236, 237t–238t
Developmental surveillance, 230–235
Deviancy, 230
Dexamethasone (Dexpak Taperpak, Maxidex)
  for antiemetic therapy, 626t
  for asthma, 10
  for brain tumors, 612
  for croup, 13
  formulary entry, 851–852
  for increased ICP, 84, 617
  for meningitis, 461t–468t
  potency, 223t, 271t
  for spinal cord compression, 617
Dexamethasone suppression test, 273
Dexamethasone with ciprofloxacin (Ciprodex), 833
Dexamethasone with tobramycin (TobraDex), 1081–1082
Dexedrine. See Dextroamphetamine
DexFerrum. See Iron, injectable preparations
Dexmedetomidine (Precedex)
  formulary entry, 852–853
  with PCA, 145
  properties of, 149b–150b, 139.e1t
Dexmethylphenidate (Focalin)
  ages of FDA approval, 245t
  formulary entry, 853–854
Dexpak Taperpak. See Dexamethasone
Dexrazoxane, 613t–615t
Dextroamphetamine (Dexedrine, ProCentra, Zenzedi), 854–855
Dextroamphetamine + amphetamine (Adderall)
  ages of FDA approval, 245t
  formulary entry, 854–855

Dextrose solution
  for coma, 14
  composition of, 302t
  for hyperkalemia, 308f
  for metabolic crisis, 339, 341
  for newborn hypoglycemia, 498t
  for sulfonylureas poisoning, 23t–24t
  for tumor lysis syndrome, 616
DHT. See Dihydrotestosterone
Diabetes, 255–260
  autoantibodies to, 256
  classification of, 256–257
  increased risk, 255
  infant of diabetic mother, 496
  matury-onset diabetes of youth (MODY), 257
  monitoring, 260
  monogenic, 256
  neonatal, 257
  polygenic, 256–257
  screening for, 123
  symptoms, 255
Diabetes insipidus (DI), 274–276
  central, 275–276, 275t, 538
  diagnosis of, 274–275, 275t
  nephrogenic, 275t, 276, 537–538
  normal (psychogenic), 275t
  treatment of, 851, 1096
Diabetes mellitus. See also Infant of diabetic mother (IDM)
  type 1, 256–257, 256t
  type 2, 256–257, 256t, 259–260, 261f
Diabetic ketoacidosis (DKA), 256–259, 258f
Dialysis, 1110
  acute, 529
  continuous arteriovenous hemofiltration/hemodialysis (CAVH/D), 529
  continuous venovenous hemofiltration/hemodialysis (CVVH/D), 529
  formulas for, 601t–602t
  hemodialysis
    for ingestions, 22
    intermittent, 529
    for metabolic crisis, 340
  peritoneal, 529
  for TTP, 623
Diaminodiphenylsulfone (DDS). See Dapsone
Diamond–Blackfan anemia, 367
Diamox. See Acetazolamide
Diaper candidiasis, 219–220

Diarrhea, 319–321
  acute, 319–321, 950
  chronic, 319–321, 950
  cryptosporidial, 1008
  differential diagnosis of, 320t
  electrolyte composition of, 304t
  intractable, 991–992
  osmotic, 319
  secretory, 319
  treatment of, 798, 950, 982, 991–992
Diastat. *See* Diazepam
Diastolic heart murmurs, 168b
Diazepam (Valium, Diastat), 151t, 139.e1t
  formulary entry, 855–856
  for palliative care, 634t
  for seizures, 16t
Diazoxide (Proglycem), 857
Diclofenac, 139
Dicloxacillin
  formulary entry, 857
  for lymphadenitis, 461t–468t
  spectrum of activity, 447t–449t
  warfarin interactions, 385b
Dientamoeba fragilis, 1008
Dietary evaluation, 571
Dietary modifications
  for constipation, 322
  for diarrhea, 320
  elimination diets, 400
  formulas for clinical conditions that require, 602
  for kidney stones, 545
  for reflux, 324
  for seizures, 559t–560t, 561
Dietary reference intakes (DRIs), 583, 586t, 591t
Diethylenetriamine pentaacetic acid (DTPA)/mercaptoacetyl triglycine (MAG-3) scan, 522
Differin. *See* Adapalene
Diffuse cutaneous systemic scleroderma (DCSS), 701.e3
Diffuse infrapontine glioma (DIPG), 611t
Diflorasone diacetate, 223t
Diflucan. *See* Fluconazole
DIG (desmoplastic infantile glioma), 611t
DiGeorge syndrome, 356–357
  dominant cardiac defects, 185t
  evaluation for, 403t–404t
DigiFab. *See* Digoxin immune FAB

Digitalis intoxication
  ECG effects, 180t
  treatment of arrhythmia secondary to, 1018
Digoxin (Lanoxin)
  dose adjustment in renal failure, 1125t–1134t
  formulary entry, 857–858
Digoxin immune FAB (DigiFab), 859
Dihydroergotamine, 555
Dihydrotestosterone (DHT), 287, 287.e1t
Dihydroxyanthracenedione dihydrochloride (mitoxantrone), 613t–615t
1,25-Dihydroxycholecalciferol. *See* Calcitriol
1,25-Dihydroxy-vitamin D, 709t–716t
Dilantin. *See* Phenytoin
Dilated cardiomyopathy, 193–194
Dilated fundoscopic examination, 512
Dilaudid. *See* Hydromorphone HCl
Diltiazem (Cardizem, Cartia XT, Matzim LA, Taztia XT, Tiazac)
  formulary entry, 859–860
  for Raynaud phenomenon, 701
Dimenhydrinate (Dramamine, Friminate), 860–861
Dimercaprol (BAL)
  formulary entry, 861
  for lead poisoning, 27
Dimercaptosuccinic acid (DMSA). *See* Succimer
Dimercaptosuccinic acid (DMSA) scans, 520–521, 680
Dimetapp Children's Cold and Allergy. *See* Brompheniramine with phenylephrine
Dinutuximab, 613t–615t
Diovan. *See* Valsartan
DIPG (diffuse infrapontine glioma), 611t
Diphenhydramine (Benadryl)
  for allergic emergencies, 10
  for allergic rhinitis, 396
  for antiemetic therapy, 626t
  formulary entry, 861–862
  for migraine, 555
  for palliative care, 634t
  properties of, 141t, 149b–150b, 139.e1t
Diphtheria/tetanus/pertussis vaccines, 426–427
  diphtheria, tetanus, & acellular pertussis (DTaP) vaccine. *See* DTaP

Diphtheria/tetanus/pertussis vaccines (*Continued*)
- diphtheria and tetanus toxoid (DT), 426–427
- tetanus, diphtheria, & acellular pertussis (Tdap) vaccine. *See* Tdap

Diphyllobothrium latum, 1008
Diprolene. *See* Betamethasone
Dipylidium caninum, 1008
Dipyridamole, 198
Directed donors
- reasons not to consider, 390
- reasons to consider, 390

Disability Programs and Services (website), 229
Discharge criteria, 148
Disclosure
- of familial genetic information, 360, 357.e1
- of incidental findings, 360

Discoid rash, 694*t*
Discontinuing interventions, 632
Disease-modifying antirheumatic drugs (DMARDs), 692
- for SLE, 695
- toxicity, 691.e1*t*

Disimpaction, 322
Dislocation
- congenital hip dislocation, 681, 681.e1*f*
- finger/toe, 70

Disomy, uniparental, 334.e1
Disopyramide, 1125*t*–1134*t*
Disordered eating, 132
Displacement of the ETT, Obstruction, Pneumothorax, or Equipment failure (DOPE), 9
Disseminated intravascular coagulation (DIC), 387*b*
Dissociation, 230
Dissociative sedation, 146
Distal intestinal obstruction syndrome, 759
Distal tubule functional tests, 526
Distraction, 143
Distributive shock, 86, 87*f*
Disulfiram, 385*b*
Ditropan XL. *See* Oxybutynin chloride
Diuretics
- for hypertension, 544*t*–545*t*
- spironolactone, 1065

Diuril. *See* Chlorothiazide

Divalproex sodium (Depakote)
- formulary entry, 862
- for migraine prevention, 556*t*
- for seizures, 559*t*–560*t*, 562*t*

Diverticulum, Meckel's, 678
DKA. *See* Diabetic ketoacidosis
DMPA (depot medroxyprogesterone acetate). *See* Medroxyprogesterone
DMSA (dimercaptosuccinic acid). *See* Succimer
DMSA (dimercaptosuccinic acid) scans, 520–521, 680
DMTs (decision-making tools), 628–629
DNA cross-linkers, 613*t*–615*t*
DNA intercalators, 613*t*–615*t*
DNA methylation disorders, 353–355
DNA strand breakers, 613*t*–615*t*
DNA-based testing. *See also* Genetic testing
- for cystic fibrosis, 655
- sample collection for, 336*t*

DNAR (Do Not Attempt Resuscitation) orders, 632
DNase. *See* Dornase alfa
DNET (dysembryoplastic neuroepithelial tumor), 611*t*
Do Not Attempt Resuscitation (DNAR) orders, 632
Do Not Escalate Treatment requests, 632
"Do Not Use" List (TJC), 733*t*
Dobutamine, 862–863
Dobutrex. *See* Dobutamine
Documentation
- of child abuse, 103
- of death, 635
- state forms, 633

Docusate (Colace, DocuSol, Kao-Tin, Sur-Q-Lax, Enemeez Mini), 863
Dog bites, 94*t*, 461*t*–468*t*
Dolasetron (Anzemet), 864
Dolophine. *See* Methadone HCl
Doose syndrome, 561
Dopamine
- formulary entry, 864–865
- normal plasma levels, 287.e2*t*
- normal urine levels, 287.e1*t*
- for shock, 87*f*

Dopamine antagonists, 626*t*
DOPE (Displacement of the ETT, Obstruction, Pneumothorax, or Equipment failure), 9
Doppler ultrasound, 184.e1
- intussusception findings, 678
- power imaging, 675

Doppler ultrasound *(Continued)*
  in sickle cell disease, 372*t*
  in testicular pathology, 680
  transcranial (TCD), 372*t*, 675
Dopram. *See* Doxapram HCl
Doripenem, 447*t*–449*t*
Dornase alfa (DNase, Pulmozyme)
  for CF, 656
  formulary entry, 864–865
Dorsalis pedis artery puncture, 36
Doryx. *See* Doxycycline
Dose adjustment methods, 1110
Dose reduction (D) dose adjustment method, 1110
Double Antibiotic Topical. *See* Bacitracin + polymyxin B
Double-bubble sign, 677.*e2f*
Double-volume exchange transfusion, 505–506
Doughnut sign, 677.*e3f*
Downward thrust (DT) reflex, 236.*e4t*–236.*e5t*
Doxapram HCl (Dopram), 865–866
Doxazosin, 544*t*–545*t*
Doxorubicin (Adriamycin), 613*t*–615*t*
Doxycycline (Adoxa, Vibramycin, Doryx, Monodox, Oracea)
  for acne vulgaris, 217*t*
  for chlamydia, 115*t*–116*t*
  for conjunctivitis, 461*t*–468*t*
  for ehrlichiosis, 479*t*–480*t*
  formulary entry, 866–867
  for gonorrhea, 115*t*–116*t*
  for Lyme disease, 479*t*–480*t*
  for PID, 115*t*–116*t*, 818–819
  for Rocky Mountain spotted fever, 479*t*–480*t*
  for septic arthritis, 461*t*–468*t*
  spectrum of activity, 451*t*
  for syphilis, 115*t*–116*t*
DQ (developmental quotient), 230
Dramamine. *See* Dimenhydrinate
Dravet syndrome, 561
Dressings, 100
DRIs (dietary reference intakes), 583
Dronabinol (Marinol, tetrahydrocannabinol, THC)
  for antiemetic therapy, 626*t*
  formulary entry, 867
Droperidol (Inapsine), 867–868
Drug abuse or dependence, 235. *See also* Substance use
  websites for patients, 108
Drug allergy, 401
  evaluation and management of, 402*f*
  management of, 401

Drug index, 737–755
Drug interactions. *See specific drugs*
Drug intolerance, 401
Drug resistance
  extensive (XDR), 486
  multidrug (MDR), 486
Drug Safety Reporting Updates, 732
Drug-induced lupus, 695*t*, 696
Drug-induced neuritis, 1039
Drugs. *See also specific drugs*
  abbreviations, acronyms, and symbols, 733*t*
  administration of, 64–65
  aerosolized, 656
  breastfeeding categories, 735
  dosages, 732–1109
  dose adjustment methods for, 1110
  HEADSSS assessment, 111*b*
  information data sources, 732
  in NICU, 513
  nonantimicrobials that require dose adjustment in renal failure, 1125*t*–1134*t*
  Official "Do Not Use" List (TJC), 733*t*
  for palliative care, 634*t*
  pregnancy categories, 735
  in renal failure, 1110–1136
  sample formulary entry, 734
DT (downward thrust) reflex, 236.*e4t*–236.*e5t*
DTaP (diphtheria, tetanus, & acellular pertussis) vaccine (Infanrix, Daptacel), 426
  administration, 427
  catch-up schedule for, 414*f*
  after chemotherapy, 625.*e3*
  contraindications to, 426–427
  after HSCT, 625.*e3*
  precautions, 426–427
  recommended schedule for, 413*f*, 415*f*–418*f*
  routine vaccination, 426
  side effects of, 427
DTaP/HepB/IPV combination (Pediarix), 441
DTaP/IPV combination (Kinrix), 441
DTaP/IPV combination (Quadracel), 442
DTaP/IPV/PRP-T combination (Pentacel), 415*f*–418*f*, 428, 441
Duac. *See* Benzoyl peroxide with clindamycin
Duchenne muscular dystrophy, 180*t*
Ductus arteriosus closure, 917–918, 922
Dulcolax. *See* Bisacodyl

Dulera. *See* Mometasone furoate + formoterol
Duodenal atresia, 677.*e2f*
Duodenal cancer, 1068
Duodenal ulcers
 prophylaxis of, 1068
 treatment of, 884, 939, 995, 1045, 1068
Duodote. *See* Pralidoxime chloride with atropine
Duraclon. *See* Clonidine
Duragesic. *See* Fentanyl
Duricef. *See* Cefadroxil
DVT. *See* Deep-vein thrombosis
Dyanavel XR. *See* Amphetamine
Dycill. *See* Dicloxacillin
Dyrenium. *See* Triamterene
Dysembryoplastic neuroepithelial tumor (DNET), 611*t*
Dysentery, 461*t*–468*t*
Dysmenorrhea, 917, 981
Dysmorphology, 347–357, 358*t*
Dyspigmentation, 227, 227.*e1f*
Dyspnea, 634*t*
Dysrhythmia, 1097
Dystonic reactions
 acute, 795
 treatment of, 862

E

Ear(s), newborn, 494*f*
Early childhood, 233*t*–235*t*
Early Head Start, 246
Early intervention services, 246
Early literacy milestones, 233*t*
Eating assessment, 111*b*
Eating disorders, 132, 250
Ebstein anomaly, 166*b*
EC (emergency contraception), 130–131
ECG. *See* Electrocardiography
Echocardiography, 184, 184.*e1*
 in congenital heart disease, 675
 M mode, 184.*e1*
 transesophageal, 184
 transthoracic, 184
 two-dimensional, 184.*e1*
 in vessel abnormalities, 675–676
Echovirus, 471*t*–476*t*
Ecstasy overdose, 23*t*–24*t*
Eculizumab (Soliriis), 415*f*–418*f*
Eczema. *See* Atopic dermatitis
Eczema herpeticum superinfection, 222
Edema
 airway, 852
 angioedema, 397, 400

Edema *(Continued)*
 cerebral, 257, 852
 in CKD, 539
 myxedema coma, 943
 treatment of, 913, 966
Edetate (EDTA) calcium disodium
 dose adjustment in renal failure, 1125*t*–1134*t*
 formulary entry, 868
 for lead poisoning, 27
Edrophonium chloride (Enlon)
 formulary entry, 868–869
 for vecuronium bromide overdose, 1097
EDTA. *See* Edetate
Educational assessment, 111*b*
Educational history, 236
EER (estimated energy requirements), 580–581
EES (erythromycin ethyl succinate). *See* Erythromycin
Efavirenz, 385*b*
Effect modification (interaction), 725
Effusions
 parapneumonic, 672–674
 pericardial, 195
 pleural. *See* Pleural effusion
EGD (esophagogastroduodenoscopy), 316
Ehlers-Danlos syndrome, 184, 351
Ehrlichiosis, 479*t*–480*t*
Elavil. *See* Amitriptyline
Elbow injury, 70
EleCare formulas, 570, 594*t*–602*t*
Electrical burns, 96*t*, 98
Electrocardiography (ECG), 166–182
 abnormalities, 172–173
 lead placement, 169*f*
 normal parameters, 170*t*
 systematic approach for evaluating, 167–172, 171*f*
 systemic effects on, 180*t*
Electroencephalography (EEG)
 polysomnography, 657–658
 for seizures, 557, 559*t*–560*t*
Electrolyte disturbances. *See also specific disturbances*
 dialysis for, 529
 in poisoning, 21.*e1t*–21.*e3t*
 serum, 304–311
Electrolyte management. *See* Fluid and electrolyte management
Electromyography (EMG), 657–658
Electrooculography (EOG), 657–658
Elements, 591*t*
Elestat. *See* Epinastine

Eletriptan (Relpax), 554*t*
Elidel. *See* Pimecrolimus
Elimination diets, 400
Elimite. *See* Permethrin
Eliphos. *See* Calcium acetate
Elitek. *See* Rasburicase
Elixophyllin. *See* Theophylline
Ella. *See* Ulipristal
Elocon. *See* Mometasone furoate
Elspar. *See* Asparaginase
Emedastine (Emadine), 397
Emergency and crisis services, 251
Emergency contraception (EC), 130–131
Emergency management, 2–19
  of airway, 4–8
  in anaphylaxis, 9–10
  in blunt thoracic and abdominal trauma, 79–80
  of breathing, 9
  in burns, 96–100
  of circulation, 2–4, 3*t*
  critical care, 81–93
  in hypovolemic/distributive shock, 87*f*
  in mental health issues, 251
  in neurologic conditions, 13–17
  oncologic emergencies, 612–619
  in respiratory conditions, 10–13
  in trauma, 73
Emergency plans, 147
Emesis. *See also* Nausea and vomiting
  antiemetic therapies, 626*t*
  in chemotherapy patients, 625
  medications for palliative care, 634*t*
Emfamil D-Vi-Sol. *See* Cholecalciferol
EMLA (eutectic mixture of local anesthetics). *See* Lidocaine and prilocaine
Emollients, 701.*e*3
Emotional changes as death approaches, 633
Employment assessment, 111*b*
Empyema, 672–674
Emverm. *See* Mebendazole
E-Mycin. *See* Erythromycin
Enalapril maleate (Vasotec, Epaned)
  dose adjustment in renal failure, 1125*t*–1134*t*
  formulary entry, 869
  for hypertension, 544*t*–545*t*
  for hypertensive emergency, 83*t*
Enalaprilat
  dose adjustment in renal failure, 1125*t*–1134*t*
  formulary entry, 869
Enbrel. *See* Etanercept

Encephalitis, 760
Encephalopathy
  hepatic, 982
  treatment of, 861, 982, 1079
  Wernicke's, 1079
Encopresis, 321–322
End of life care
  home care, 632
  memory making, 631–632
Endocarditis, 191
  bacterial. *See* Bacterial endocarditis prophylaxis
  prophylaxis of, 191, 192*b*, 192*t*, 789–790, 1050, 1094
  prosthetic valve, 192*b*, 1050
  treatment of, 952, 1050
Endocet. *See* Oxycodone and acetaminophen
Endocrinology, 255–289
  late effects of cancer treatment, 625.*e*1*t*–625.*e*2*t*
  web resources, 255
Endodan. *See* Oxycodone and aspirin
Endometriosis, 532*f*
Endometriosis-associated pain, 956
Endoscopic third ventriculostomy (ETV), 564
Endothelial damage, 379*b*
Endotracheal tube (ETT), 5
  Displacement of the ETT, Obstruction, Pneumothorax, or Equipment failure (DOPE), 9
  image-guided placement of, 674
  indications for, 12
  size and depth, 492*t*
End-tidal CO_2 (ET_{CO_2}), 638
Enemas
  bisacodyl, 797
  contrast, 678
  for disimpaction, 322
  fluoroscopy-guided therapeutic, 678
  mesalamine, 959
  sodium phosphate, 1064
Enemeez Mini. *See* Docusate
Energy deposition, 579
Energy expenditure
  basal (BEE), 578, 581.*e*1
  total (TEE), 579
Energy needs
  definition of, 578–581
  estimation of, 578–583
Enfacare, 570
Enfagrow formulas, 594*t*–602*t*
Enfalyte solutions, 603*t*
Enfamil formulas, 570, 594*t*–602*t*
Enfaport formula, 594*t*–602*t*

Engerix-B. *See* Hepatitis B vaccine
Enion. *See* Edrophonium chloride
Enoxaparin (Lovenox)
   dose adjustment in renal failure, 1125*t*–1134*t*
   formulary entry, 870–871
   overdose, 1036
Ensure formulas, 570, 594*t*–602*t*
Entamoeba histolytica, 1008
Enteral nutrition, 592–602
   caloric modulars, 592, 593*t*
   formulas for, 592, 594*t*–602*t*
Enterobius, 955, 1037
Enterococcus, 191, 520
Enterococcus faecium infections, vancomycin-resistant (VRE or VREF), 947, 952, 1044
Enterocolitis
   eosinophilic, 955, 1037
   food-induced, 398
   neonatal, 676
   neutropenic, 618
Enterovirus infection, 457*t*–458*t*, 471*t*–476*t*, 691
Entocort EC. *See* Budesonide
Enulaose. *See* Lactulose
Enuresis, nocturnal, 851, 990
Envarsus XR. *See* Tacrolimus
Enzyme replacement therapy, pancreatic (PERT), 656
Enzymes
   chemotherapeutic agents, 613*t*–615*t*
   serum muscle enzymes, 704
Eosinophilia, 396
Eosinophilic enterocolitis, 955, 1037
Eosinophilic esophagitis (EE), 324–325, 895
Eosinophilic gastroenteritis, allergic, 398
Eosinophils, 373*t*
Epaned. *See* Enalapril maleate
Ependymoma, 611*t*
Ephelides (freckles), 225
Epidermal melanosis, 225–226
Epidermal nevus, 218*f*
Epidermolysis bullosa, 218*f*
Epidermolytic hyperkeratosis, 218*f*
Epididymitis, 532*f*
Epiduo. *See* Adapalene + benzoyl peroxide
Epigenetic disorders, 353–355
Epiglottitis
   emergency management of, 12
   radiographic findings, 669*t*
EpiInfo, 721.e1

Epilepsy, 558
   benign, 559*t*–560*t*
   classification of, 558*b*
   evaluation of, 557
   formulas for, 601*t*–602*t*
   juvenile myoclonic, 559*t*–560*t*
   recurrent events that mimic, 557*t*
Epinastine (Elestat), 397
Epinephrine, racemic (Asthmanefrin), 13
   for allergic emergencies, 10
   formulary entry, 871
Epinephrine HCl (Adrenalin, EpiPen)
   for allergic emergencies, 9–10
   for asthma, 11
   auto-injectors, 400
   formulary entry, 872–873
   injectable, 142, 142*t*
   LET (lidocaine, epinephrine, tetracaine), 141*t*, 153*t*
   normal levels, 287.e1*t*–287.e2*t*
   topical, 141*t*
Epi-Pen, 10
EpiPen. *See* Epinephrine HCl
Epi-Pen Junior, 10
Epithelial cell nevus, 226
Epithelial cells, urinary, 518
Epitol. *See* Carbamazepine
Epivir. *See* Lamivudine
Epivir-HBV. *See* Lamivudine
Epoetin alfa (Epogen, Procrit)
   conversion to darbepoetin alfa, 849
   formulary entry, 873–875
Epstein-Barr virus infection, 471*t*–476*t*, 477*f*, 691
Equetro. *See* Carbamazepine
Equipment, 4–5
Erb-Duchenne palsy, 511*t*
Ergocalciferol (Calciferol, Calcidio, vitamin D_2), 875–876
Ergotamine tartrate (Ergomar), 876
Ergotamine tartrate with caffeine (Cafergot, Migergot), 876
Erosive esophagitis, 880, 939, 1007, 1045
Errors
   type I, 723
   type II, 723
Ertapenem (Invanz)
   dose adjustment in renal failure, 1111*t*–1124*t*
   formulary entry, 876–877
   spectrum of activity, 447*t*–449*t*
Erwinia. *See* Asparaginase
Erygel. *See* Erythromycin
EryPed. *See* Erythromycin

Ery-Tab. *See* Erythromycin
Erythema, reactive, 208, 209*f*
Erythema infectiosum, 471*t*–476*t*
Erythema toxicum neonatorum (ETN), 216, 218*f*
Erythroblastopenia, transient, of childhood (TEC), 367
Erythrocin. *See* Erythromycin
Erythrocyte sedimentation rate (ESR), 701–702, 709*t*–716*t*
Erythromycin (Erythrocin, Pediamycin, EES, E-Mycin, EryPed, Ery-Tab, PCE, Erygel)
 for acne vulgaris, 214, 217*t*
 for chlamydia, 115*t*–116*t*
 for conjunctivitis, 461*t*–468*t*
 dose adjustment in renal failure, 1111*t*–1124*t*
 formulary entry, 877–878
 for gastroenteritis, 461*t*–468*t*
 for pertussis, 461*t*–468*t*
 for pneumonia, 461*t*–468*t*
 spectrum of activity, 450*t*
Erythromycin ethyl succinate (EES). *See* Erythromycin
Erythromycin with benzoyl peroxide (Benzamycin), 794
Erythropoietin. *See* Epoetin Alfa
Escherichia coli, 520
Escitalopram (Lexapro)
 ages of FDA approval, 245*t*
 formulary entry, 878–879
Eskalith. *See* Lithium
Esmolol HCl (Brevibloc), 879–880
Esomeprazole (Nexium), 880–881
Esophageal atresia, 677, 677.e1*f*
Esophageal candidiasis, 889, 969, 1101–1102
Esophageal conditions, 318–325
Esophageal foreign bodies, 670
Esophageal impedance monitoring, 324
Esophageal pH monitoring, 324
Esophagitis
 eosinophilic, 324–325, 895
 erosive, 880, 939, 1007, 1045
 food allergy, 398
 treatment of, 884, 995
Esophagogastroduodenoscopy (EGD), 316
Estimated blood volume (EBV), 389*t*
Estimated energy requirements (EER), 580–581
 calculations, 581
 equations, 581.e1
 samples, 582*t*
 under stressed conditions, 581.e1

Estimated glomerular filtration rate (eGFR), 523–524
Estradiol, 282*t*
Estrostep. *See* Oral contraceptives
Etanercept (Enbrel)
 for arthritis, 692
 formulary entry, 881–882
 for idiopathic pneumonia syndrome, 623
Ethambutol HCl (Myambutol)
 dose adjustment in renal failure, 1111*t*–1124*t*
 formulary entry, 882
Ethanol
 overdose, 23*t*–24*t*
 urine toxicology screen, 21*t*
Ethics, 357
Ethosuximide (Zarontin)
 formulary entry, 882–883
 for seizures, 559*t*–560*t*, 562*t*
Ethylene glycol/methanol poisoning, 23*t*–24*t*
Etiquette, 636
ETN (erythema toxicum neonatorum), 216
Etomidate
 for deep sedation, 145
 for intubation, 6*f*
 for RSI, 7*t*–8*t*
Etoposide (VP-16, VePesid), 613*t*–615*t*
ETT. *See* Endotracheal tube
ETV (endoscopic third ventriculostomy), 564
Eutectic mixture of lidocaine and prilocaine. *See* Lidocaine and prilocaine
Eutectic mixture of local anesthetics (EMLA). *See* Lidocaine and prilocaine
Evekeo. *See* Amphetamine
Evidence-based medicine, 721–722
Evoclin. *See* Clindamycin
Evzio. *See* Naloxone
Ewing sarcoma, 609*t*–610*t*, 683, 684*f*
Exalgo. *See* Hydromorphone HCl
Exchange transfusion
 double-volume, 505–506
 for hyperleukocytosis/leukocytosis, 616
 in infants, 505–506, 506*f*
Excitation, 21.e1*t*–21.e3*t*
Excoriation, 203, 209*f*
Exercise recommendations, 199.e1*t*
Exercise-induced asthma, 900
Exercise-induced bronchospasm, 976, 1056

Expiratory pressure, maximal, 640–641
Exposure history, 20
Extensive drug resistance (XDR), 486
External jugular puncture, 32–34, 33f
Extina. *See* Ketoconazole
Extracellular fluid, 294.e1, 294.e1t
Extracellular fluid compartment, 294.e1
Extracorporeal membrane oxygenation, 502
Extracorporeal shock wave lithotripsy, 543
Extradural fluid collection, birth-related, 495t, 496f
Extraglomerular hematuria, 530–531
Extrapyramidal symptoms, 795
Extremely low-birth-weight (ELBW) infants, 493
Extremities
  imaging, 680–683
  secondary survey of, 74t–75t
Extremity pain, 690t
Extubation, 92
Eye(s), newborn, 494f
Eye examination
  in diabetes, 260
  imaging, 665–666
  secondary survey, 100

F

F test, 724t
Fabior. *See* Tazarotene
FACES pain scale, 136, 138f
Facial angiofibroma, 352
Factor II, 377t–378t
Factor II deficiency, 386f
Factor IX
  age-specific values, 377t–378t
  for factor IX deficiency, 387t–388t
  for hemophilia, 389t
  recombinant, 392
Factor IX deficiency, 386f, 387t–388t
Factor V, 377t–378t
Factor V deficiency, 386f
Factor V Leiden, 379b
Factor VII, 377t–378t
Factor VII deficiency, 386f
Factor VIIa, 384t
Factor VIII
  age-specific values, 377t–378t
  for factor VIII deficiency, 387t–388t
  for hemophilia, 389t
  monoclonal, 392
  recombinant, 392
Factor VIII deficiency, 386f, 387t–388t
Factor X, 377t–378t
Factor X deficiency, 386f
Factor XI, 377t–378t
Factor XI deficiency, 386f
Factor XII, 377t–378t
Factor XII deficiency, 386f
Factor XIII deficiency, 386f
Factor XIIIa, 377t–378t
Fahrenheit, 708
Failure to thrive, 582–583
Famciclovir (Famvir)
  dose adjustment in renal failure, 1111t–1124t
  formulary entry, 883–884
  for herpes zoster, 471t–476t
  for varicella, 440
Familial genetic information, 360, 357.e1
Familial short stature, 276, 278f
Family consent, 635
Family history, 112, 236
Family meetings, 629–630
Family participation, 631–632
Family planning. *See* Contraception
Famotidine (Pepcid)
  dose adjustment in renal failure, 1125t–1134t
  formulary entry, 884
Famvir. *See* Famciclovir
Fanatrex FusePaq. *See* Gabapentin
Fanconi anemia, 367
Fanconi syndrome, 537
FAS (fetal alcohol syndrome), 185t, 496, 225.e6f
FAST (Focused Assessment with Sonography for Trauma), 79
Fasting, 146–147, 147t
Fat, fecal, 330
Fat malabsorption, 601t–602t
Fat requirements, 585t
Fatty acid oxidation (FAO) disorders, 341–347
FBA (foreign-body aspiration), 13
5-FC (5-fluorocytosine). *See* Flucytosine
FDA. *See* U.S. Food and Drug Administration
FDPs (fibrin degradation products), 377t–378t
Fears, nighttime, 659
Febrile illness–associated seizures, 555–556
Febrile neutropenia, 778
Febrile nonhemolytic reaction, 385–389
Febrile seizures
  complex, 556
  simple, 555
Fecal fat, quantitative, 330
Fecal impaction, 1024

Feeding
  newborn care, 492
  trained night feeding, 233t–235t
Feeding disorders, 250
Feet
  puncture of, 461t–468t
  ringworm of, 481t
FEF$_{25-75}$ (forced expiratory flow), 643, 643f, 643t
FeHCO$_3$ (fractional excretion of bicarbonate), 537
Felbamate (Felbatol)
  dose adjustment in renal failure, 1125t–1134t
  formulary entry, 885
  for seizures, 562t
Felodipine, 544t–545t
Femoral head: avascular necrosis of, 681, 681.e2f
Femoral vein
  cannulation, 41–42, 43f
  central venous catheter placement via, 41–42, 44f
FENa (fractional excretion of sodium), 525
Fentanyl (Sublimaze, Duragesic, Fentora, Actiq, Lanzanda), 140t, 139.e1t
  for analgesia and sedation, 153t
  dose adjustment in renal failure, 1125t–1134t
  formulary entry, 885–887
  for intubation, 6f
  opioid tapering, 146b
  for PCA, 143t
  for procedural sedation, 153t
  for RSI, 7t–8t
Fentora. See Fentanyl
Ferate. See Iron, oral preparations
Fer-In-Sol. See Iron, oral preparations
FeroSul. See Iron, oral preparations
Ferretts. See Iron, oral preparations
Ferric gluconate. See Iron, injectable preparations
Ferritin, 701, 709t–716t
Ferrlecit. See Iron, injectable preparations
Ferrous fumarate. See Iron, oral preparations
Ferrous gluconate. See Iron, oral preparations
Ferrous sulfate. See Iron, oral preparations
Fertility awareness, 130
Fetal alcohol syndrome (FAS), 185t, 496, 225.e6f

Fetal anomaly screening, 490.e1
Fetal heart rate (FHR)
  accelerations, 490.e3
  decelerations, 490.e3
  intrapartum monitoring, 490.e3
  normal, 490.e3
Fetal karyotyping, 490.e1
Fetal ultrasound, 490.e1
FEurea (fractional excretion of urea), 525
FEV$_1$ (forced expiratory volume in 1 second), 643, 643f, 643t
Fever
  empiric therapy for, 958
  management of, 816
  oncologic emergency, 618–619, 620f
  in sickle cell disease, 370t–371t
  of unknown origin (FUO), 445–446
  without localizing signs, 444–446, 453f
Feverall. See Acetaminophen
Fexofenadine, 1125t–1134t
Fexofenadine and pseudoephedrine (Allegra), 887–888
FFP. See Fresh frozen plasma
FHR. See Fetal heart rate
Fiber requirements, 592t
Fibersource formulas, 594t–600t
Fibrillation
  atrial, 174t–175t, 176f
  ventricular, 177f, 177t
Fibrin degradation products (FDPs), 377t–378t
Fibrinogen, 701
  age-specific values, 377t–378t
  reference values, 709t–716t
Fibrinogen deficiency, 386f
Fibrinolytic system, 377t–378t
Fibroma
  nonossifying, 681, 681.e5f
  periungal, 225, 225.e6f
FICA acronym, 630
Fifth disease, 471t–476t
Filgrastim (Neupogen, Granix, Zarxio)
  formulary entry, 888
  for neutropenia, 624
Fine-motor skills, 229
Fingerstick, 31
Finger/toe dislocation reduction, 70
FiO$_2$ (inspired oxygen concentration), 90, 91.e1
First-Lansoprazole. See Lansoprazole
First-Metronidazole. See Metronidazole
First-Omeprazole. See Omeprazole
First-Vancomycin. See Vancomycin

FISH (fluorescence *in situ* hybridization), 358*t*, 347.*e*1
Fisher's exact test, 724*t*
Fissures, 203, 209*f*
Fistula, tracheoesophageal, 677, 677.*e*1*f*
Five Ps, 111.*e*1*b*
FK506. *See* Tacrolimus
FLACC scale, 136, 137*t*
Flagyl. *See* Metronidazole
Flame injury, 96*t*
Flecainide acetate
  dose adjustment in renal failure, 1125*t*–1134*t*
  formulary entry, 888–889
Fleet Bisacodyl. *See* Bisacodyl
Fleet Enema. *See* Sodium phosphate
Fleet Laxative. *See* Bisacodyl
Fleet Liquid Glycerin Supp. *See* Glycerin
Fleet Mineral Oil. *See* Mineral oil
Fleet Pedia-Lax. *See* Sodium phosphate
Fleet Phospho-Soda. *See* Sodium phosphate
Flintstones Complete, 589*t*–590*t*
Flintstones Sour Gummies, 589*t*–590*t*
Flonase. *See* Fluticasone propionate
Flonase Sensimist. *See* Fluticasone furoate
Florinef. *See* Fludrocortisone acetate
Flovent. *See* Fluticasone; Fluticasone propionate
Flow-volume curves, 641–643, 642*f*
Floxin. *See* Ofloxacin
Floxin Otic. *See* Ofloxacin
Fluconazole (Diflucan)
  dose adjustment in renal failure, 1111*t*–1124*t*
  formulary entry, 889–890
  neonatal dosing, 513*t*–514*t*
  for oncology patients, 626*t*
  for ringworm, 481*t*
  for tinea capitis, 481*t*
  for vulvovaginal candidiasis, 118*t*
  warfarin interactions, 385*b*
Flucytosine (Ancobon, 5-fluorocytosine, 5-FC)
  dose adjustment in renal failure, 1111*t*–1124*t*
  formulary entry, 890
Fludarabine (Fludara), 613*t*–615*t*
Fludrocortisone, 271*t*
Fludrocortisone acetate
  for adrenal insufficiency, 272
  formulary entry, 890–891
  potency of, 271*t*

Fluid and electrolyte management, 290–315
  deficit replacement strategy, 297–301
  deficit repletion, 293–301
  fluid deficit assessment, 293
  guidance for, 290
  maintenance fluid volume, 291
  maintenance requirements, 290–293, 291*f*
  maintenance solute, 292–293
  newborn care, 496–497
  newborn requirements, 498*t*
  normal electrolyte composition, 304*t*
  ongoing losses, 301
  serum electrolyte disturbances, 304–311
  for TTP, 623
  volume overload, 529
Fluid restriction, 274, 623
Fluid resuscitation
  in acute pulmonary hypertensive crisis, 89
  in burns, 97, 99*f*
  calculation of fluids for, 292–293, 301
  in cardiogenic shock, 86, 86.*e*1*t*
  in diabetic ketoacidosis, 258*f*
  in poor perfusion and shock, 3–4
  rapid, 297
  sample calculations, 295*b*–296*b*
Flumadine. *See* Rimantadine
Flumazenil
  formulary entry, 891
  for procedural sedation reversal, 148
Flunisolide (Aerospan)
  dosages, 646.*e*1*t*–646.*e*2*t*
  formulary entry, 892
Fluocinolone acetonide, 223*t*
Fluocinolone with ciprofloxacin (Otovel Otic), 833
Fluocinonide, 223*t*
Fluocinonide acetonide, 223*t*
Fluorabon. *See* Fluoride
Fluor-A-Day. *See* Fluoride
Fluorescence *in situ* hybridization (FISH), 358*t*, 347.*e*1
Fluorescent treponemal antibody absorption (FTA-ABS), 455.*e*2*t*
Fluoride (Fluorabon, Fluor-A-Day, Fluoritab, Lozi-Flur)
  formulary entry, 892–893
  in infant multivitamin drops, 588*t*
  recommended intakes, 591*t*
Fluoride supplementation, 585
Fluoritab. *See* Fluoride
9α–Fluorocortisone. *See* Fludrocortisone

5-Fluorocytosine (5-FC). *See* Flucytosine
9-Fluorohydrocortisone. *See* Fludrocortisone acetate
Fluoroquinolones
  for chlamydia, 115t–116t
  for conjunctivitis, 461t–468t
  for gastroenteritis, 461t–468t
  spectrum of activity, 450t
Fluoroscopy, 664t
Fluoroscopy-guided therapeutic enema, 678
Fluoxetine hydrochloride (Prozac, Sarafem)
  ages of FDA approval, 245t
  formulary entry, 893–894
Flurandrenolide, 223t
Flushing, 21.e1t–21.e3t
Fluticasone furoate (Veramyst, Flonase Sensimist, Arnuity Ellipta), 894–896
Fluticasone furoate and vilanterol (Breo Ellipta), 894
Fluticasone propionate (Flonase, Cutivate, Flovent)
  for allergic rhinitis, 397
  converting to beclomethasone, 794
  dosages, 646.e1t–646.e2t
  for eosinophilic esophagitis, 325
  formulary entry, 894–896
  potency, 223t
  recommended dosages for asthma, 895
Fluticasone propionate and salmeterol (Advair)
  dosages, 646.e1t–646.e2t
  formulary entry, 896–897
Fluvoxamine, 897–898
Focal neurologic deficit, acute-onset, 566b
Focal segmental glomerulosclerosis (FSGS), 535–536
Focal seizures, 558, 558b
Focalin. *See* Dexmethylphenidate
Focused Assessment with Sonography for Trauma (FAST), 79
Folate
  in multivitamin tablets, 589t–590t
  recommended intakes, 586t
  reference values, 709t–716t
Folate antagonists, 613t–615t
Folex (methotrexate), 613t–615t
Folic acid (Folvite), 898–899
Folic acid deficiency, 898
Folic acid supplementation, 372t
Folinic acid, 457t–458t
Follicle-stimulating hormone, 279t
Follow-up plans, 630

Folvite. *See* Folic acid
Fomepizole (Antizol), 899
Fontan procedure, 1103
Fontan shunt, 190–191, 190f
  modified, 191
Fontanels, 353.e1f
Food: thermic effect of (TEF), 579
Food allergy, 397–401
  diagnosis of, 398–400, 399f
  evaluation of, 399f
  management of, 399f
  treatment of, 842
Food challenges, 400
Food intolerance, 400
Food-induced enterocolitis, 398
Food-specific immunotherapy, 400
Foot puncture, 461t–468t
Foradil Aerolizer. *See* Formoterol
Forced expiratory flow (FEF$_{25-75}$), 643, 643f, 643t
Forced expiratory volume in 1 second (FEV$_1$), 643, 643f, 643t
Forced vital capacity (FVC), 642, 643f, 643t
Forearm splint, 71f, 70.e1
Foreign bodies
  esophageal, 670
  lower airway, 670
Foreign travel: immunoprophylaxis guidelines for, 426
Foreign-body aspiration (FBA), 13
Formoterol (Foradil Aerolizer, Perforomist), 899–900
Formoterol and budesonide (Symbicort), 801, 646.e1t–646.e2t
Formoterol and mometasone (Dulera)
  dosages, 646.e1t–646.e2t
  formulary entry, 974–975
Formulas
  for clinical conditions that require special diets, 602
  company websites, 570
  enteral, 592
  for newborns, 492
  for special clinical circumstances, 601t–602t
Fortamet. *See* Metformin
Fortaz. *See* Ceftazidime
Fortical Nasal Spray. *See* Calcitonin—salmon
Fortifiers, 594t–600t
Foscarnet (Foscavir)
  for CMV, 471t–476t
  dose adjustment in renal failure, 1111t–1124t
  formulary entry, 900–901

Fosinopril, 544t–545t
Fosphenytoin (Cerebyx)
  formulary entry, 901–902
  for seizures, 16t
Fractional excretion of bicarbonate (FeHCO₃), 537
Fractional excretion of sodium (FENa), 525
Fractional excretion of urea (FEurea), 525
Fractures, 80–81
  bucket-handle, 683
  in child abuse, 102, 103t, 683, 685f–686f
  clavicle, 495
  corner, 683
  imaging, 683
  patterns unique to children, 80–81, 80f
  Salter-Harris classification of, 680t
  stress, 681
Fragile X syndrome, 357
FRC (functional residual capacity), 643f, 643t
Freckles (ephelides), 225
Free and appropriate public education (FAPE), 246
Free water deficit (FWD), 297
Fresh frozen plasma (FFP), 392
  for cerebrovascular accident, 617
  for excessive warfarin anticoagulation, 384t
  for hyperleukocytosis/leukocytosis, 616
Friedreich ataxia, 180t
Friminate (dimenhydrinate). See Dimenhydrinate
Frog-leg lateral hip radiographs, 681
Frostbite, 96t
Frovatriptan (Frova), 554t
FSGS (focal segmental glomerulosclerosis), 535–536
Functional residual capacity (FRC), 643f, 643t
Funding bias, 722
Funduscopic examination
  dilated, 512
  in headaches, 551.e1t
Fungal infections, 470
  community-acquired, 481t
  of skin, 210
  treatment of, 778, 1101
Fungizone. See Amphotericin B
FUO (fever of unknown origin), 445–446

Furadantin. See Nitrofurantoin
Furosemide (Lasix)
  dose adjustment in renal failure, 1125t–1134t
  formulary entry, 902
  for hydrocephalus, 564
  for hypertension, 544t–545t
Fusarium, 1101
FVC (forced vital capacity), 642, 643f, 643t
FWD (free water deficit), 297
Fycompa (parampanel), 562t

G

G6PD (glucose-6-phosphate dehydrogenase) assay, 368
Gabapentin (Neurontin, Fanatrex FusePaq, Gralise, Horizant)
  dose adjustment in renal failure, 1125t–1134t
  formulary entry, 903–904
  for seizures, 562t
Gabitril. See Tiagabine
Gablofen. See Baclofen
Gadolinium, 530
Galactose, 709t–716t
Galactosemia, 343
Galant reflex, 236.e4t–236.e5t
Gallstones, 1089
Galzin. See Zinc salts
Gamma globulin, 194
Gamma-genzene hexachloride. See Lindane
Gamma-glutamyl transferase (GGT), 326t, 709t–716t
Ganciclovir (Cytovene, Zirgan)
  for CMV, 457t–458t, 471t–476t, 624.e1t
  dose adjustment in renal failure, 1111t–1124t
  formulary entry, 904
Gangliocytoma, 611t
Ganglioglioma, 611t
Garamycin. See Gentamicin
Gardasil. See Human papillomavirus (HPV) vaccine
Gardnerella vaginalis, 118t
Garlic odor, 21.e1t–21.e3t
Gas exchange evaluation, 637–639
Gastric cancer, 1068
Gastric fluid, 304t
Gastric infection, 798
Gastric lavage, 316
Gastric ulcers, 880, 939, 995, 1045
Gastrocrom. See Cromolyn

Gastroenteritis
  allergic eosinophilic, 398
  bacterial, 461*t*–468*t*
  initial management of, 461*t*–468*t*
  vomiting in, 997
Gastroenterology, 316–332
  tests, 330
  web resources, 316
Gastroesophageal reflux (GER), 323–324
  differential diagnosis of, 557*t*
  treatment of, 965
Gastroesophageal reflux disease (GERD), 323–324
  with erosive esophagitis, 1007
  short-term treatment of, 939
  treatment of, 880, 884, 939, 995, 1006–1007, 1045
Gastrointestinal (GI) bleeding, 316–317, 317*t*, 1096
Gastrointestinal (GI) conditions, 318–325
  as death approaches, 633
  food allergy, 398
  in newborns, 507–508
Gastrointestinal (GI) dysmotility, 965
Gastrointestinal (GI) emergencies, 316–318
  allergic, 9
  secondary survey, 99
Gastrointestinal (GI) procedures, 1094
Gastroschisis, 508.*e*1*t*
Gas-X. *See* Simethicone
Gatifloxacin (Zymaxid, Zymar), 905
Gaucher disease, 345–346
GaviLAX. *See* Polyethylene glycol (PEG) electrolyte solutions
GCS (Glasgow Coma Scale), 73
GCSF (granulocyte colony-stimulating factor). *See* Filgrastim
Gender dysphoria, 285–286
Gender expression, 123–125
Gender identity, 123–125
Gender nonconforming, 125
GeneReviews, 333, 343, 347–357
GeneTests, 333
Genetic testing
  considerations for, 357.*e*1
  for cystic fibrosis, 655
  diagnostic, 347, 357–360, 358*t*
  disclosure of familial genetic information, 360, 357.*e*1
  disclosure of incidental findings, 360
  ethics of, 357
  pretest counseling, 360

Genetics, 333–363
Genetics Home Reference, 333
Gengraf. *See* Cyclosporine
Genital examination
  adolescent, 113
  in child abuse, 102
Genital herpes, 120*t*
  recurrent, 883
  treatment of, 883, 1090
Genital HSV, 761
Genital ulcers and warts
  in Behçet disease, 700
  diagnostic features of, 120*t*
  management of, 120*t*
Genitalia
  ambiguous, 284–285
  development of, 110*t*
  newborn, 494*f*
  ringworm of, 481*t*
Genitourinary infections (STIs), 115*t*–116*t*
Genitourinary procedures, 1094
Genitourinary system
  imaging of, 679–680
  review of, 111
  secondary survey of, 74*t*–75*t*, 100
Genodermatosis, 225
Genomic imprinting, 334.*e*1
Gentamicin (Garamycin)
  dose adjustment in renal failure, 1111*t*–1124*t*
  formulary entry, 905–906
  neonatal dosing, 513*t*–514*t*
  for PID, 115*t*–116*t*
  for pneumonia, 461*t*–468*t*
  for septic arthritis, 461*t*–468*t*
  spectrum of activity, 451*t*
GER. *See* Gastroesophageal reflux
Gerber formulas, 594*t*–602*t*
GERD. *See* Gastroesophageal reflux disease
Geri-Mucil. *See* Psyllium
Germ tube screen, 470
Germinal matrix hemorrhage, 665
Germinoma, 611*t*
Gesell block skills, 236, 236.*e*3*f*
Gesell figures, 236, 239*f*
Gestational age
  Ballard score, 493–495
  estimation of, 493–495, 490.*e*1–490.*e*3
GGT (gamma-glutamyl transferase), 326*t*, 709*t*–716*t*
Giant cell astrocytoma, 611*t*
Giant cell vasculitis, 697*t*
Giardia lamblia (giardiasis), 968, 1008

Girls
  BEE calculation, 581.e1
  blood pressure values, 157t–159t, 164f
  body mass index, 577f
  delayed puberty in, 277
  EER equations, 581.e1
  growth charts, 572f–573f, 576f–577f, 571.e1f
  head circumference, 573f, 571.e3f
  height velocity, 571.e1f
  length-to-weight ratio, 573f
  physical activity coefficient (PA), 580.e1t
  recommended element intakes, 591t
  recommended vitamin intakes, 586t
  sample EERs, 582t
  stature and weight, 576f
  target height range for, 276
Glasgow Coma Scale (GCS), 15t, 73
Glaucoma, 758
Gleevec. See Imatinib
Glenn shunt, 190–191, 190f
Glioma, 611t
Glomerular disease
  causes of, 531t
  with proteinuria, 535b
Glomerular filtration rate (GFR)
  estimated (eGFR), 523–524
  measurement of, 525, 525t
  normal values, 524t
Glomerular function tests, 523–525
Glomerular hematuria, 530–531
Glomerulogenesis, 523–525
Glomerulonephritis, 527t, 532f, 698
Glomerulosclerosis, focal segmental (FSGS), 535–536
Glucagon HCl (GlucaGen, Glucagon Emergency Kit), 906
Glucagon stimulation test, 286–287
Glucerna formulas, 594t–602t
Glucocorticoids
  effects of, 271t
  for granulomatous disease, 701.e2
  maintenance, 271
  for scleroderma, 701.e3
  for Sjögren syndrome, 701.e4
  stress-dose, 272
Glucophage. See Metformin
Glucose
  CSF levels, 717t
  for hypoglycemia, 286, 498t, 499f
  newborn requirements, 496–497
  reference values, 709t–716t
Glucose control, 260
Glucose infusion rate (GIR), 496–497

Glucose reabsorption, 525–526
Glucose tolerance
  impaired, 601t–602t
  oral glucose tolerance test (OGTT), 255–256
Glucose-6-phosphate dehydrogenase (G6PD) assay, 368
Glucosuria, 517, 525–526
Glumetza. See Metformin
GLUT1 deficiency, 561
Glutaric acidemia type 1 (GA1), 341
Glycerin (Pedia-Lax, Sani-Supp, Fleet Liquid Glycerin Supp)
  for disimpaction, 322
  formulary entry, 907
Glycine, 341
Glycogen storage disease (GSD), 343–344
  type I (Von Gierke disease), 343–344
  type II (Pompe disease), 344
  type III (Cori disease), 344
GlycoLax. See Polyethylene glycol (PEG) electrolyte solutions
Glycopyrrolate (Robinul, Cuvposa), 907
Gly-Oxide. See Carbamide peroxide
Glytrol formula, 601t–602t
GnRH (gonadotropin-releasing hormone) stimulation test, 281
Gold poisoning, 861
GoLYTELY. See Polyethylene glycol (PEG) electrolyte solutions
Gonadal system, 625.e1t–625.e2t
Gonadal tumors, 609t–610t
Gonadotropin-releasing hormone (GnRH) stimulation test, 281
Gonococcal cervicitis or urethritis, 790
Gonococcal ophthalmia, 822, 878
Gonorrhea infections
  antibiotic adjunctive therapy, 1031
  management of, 115t–116t, 461t–468t, 818–819, 822
  screening for, 117
Good Start, 570
Goodenough–Harris Draw-a-Person Test, 236, 236.e1b–236.e2b
Goodpasture's syndrome, 532f
Graded challenge, 401
Graft-versus-host disease (GVHD)
  acute, 621, 621.e1t
  chronic, 622, 625.e3
Gralise. See Gabapentin
Gram stain, urine, 518
Gramicidin + neomycin/polymyxin B (Neosporin Ophthalmic Solution), 983

Granisetron (Sancuso, Sustol)
for antiemetic therapy, 626t
formulary entry, 908
Granix. *See* Filgrastim
Granulocyte colony-stimulating factor (GCSF). *See* Filgrastim
Granulocyte transfusion, 624
Granulomatosis with polyangiitis, 532f, 697t
Grasp reflex, 236.e4t–236.e5t
Grave's disease, 265, 1026
Gray patch tinea capitis, 211
Grifulvin V. *See* Griseofulvin
Griseofulvin (Gris-PEG)
formulary entry, 909
for ringworm, 481t
for tinea capitis, 212, 481t
warfarin interactions, 385b
Gross motor skills, 229, 231t–232t
Group A streptococcal (GAS) infection, 1010–1012
Group B streptococcal (GBS) infection, 455
meningitis, 1009
secondary prevention of, 460f
treatment of, 461t–468t, 1009
UTIs, 520
Growth, 276–277, 570–606
catch-up, 582–583, 583b
estimate velocity, 277t
evaluation of, 571–574
incomplete, 943
premature, 490
web resources, 570
Growth charts, 570–574, 573f, 571.e1f–571.e2f
for boys, 574f–575f, 578f–579f
for girls, 572f–573f, 576f–577f
interpretation of, 571
for preterm infants, 580f–581f
Growth delay, constitutional, 277, 278f
Growth failure, 582–583
Growth hormone deficiency, 278f
Growth hormone provocative tests, 1096
Growth parameters, 551.e1t
Growth plate injury, 680t
Guanfacine (Intuniv, Tenex), 909–910
Guidelines: HEADS UP to Youth Sports (CDC), 73, 78
Gums, 112
Guttmacher Institute, 110, 114
GVHD. *See* Graft-versus-host disease
Gynecological system, 111
Gynecomastia, 108
Gyne-Lotrimin. *See* Clotrimazole

H
Habit spasms, 557t
Haemophilus ducreyi, 120t
Haemophilus influenzae, 191
Haemophilus influenzae type b (Hib) infection, 428
children at high risk for, 422
immunoprophylaxis against, 427–428
Haemophilus influenzae type b (Hib) vaccine
catch-up schedule for, 414f
after chemotherapy, 625.e3
DTaP/IPV/PRP-T combination (Pentacel), 415f–418f, 428, 441
after HSCT, 625.e3
recommended schedule for, 413f, 415f–418f
routine vaccination, 428
Hair, pubic, 110t
Hair loss, 211–213
Hair Regrowth for Treatment Men. *See* Minoxidil
Halcinonide, 223t
Haldol. *See* Haloperidol
Halobetasol propionate, 223t
Haloperidol (Haldol)
ages of FDA approval, 245t
formulary entry, 910–911
for palliative care, 634t
Hand(s): animal bites to, 93, 95
Hand-eye coordination, 229
Hand-foot-mouth disease, 471t–476t
Haptoglobin, 367–368, 701, 709t–716t
Harlequin baby, 218f
Hashimoto thyroiditis, 265
HAV. *See* Hepatitis A virus
HBV. *See* Hepatitis B virus
HCTZ. *See* Hydrochlorothiazide
HDCV (Imovax), 436
HDL. *See* High-density lipoprotein
Head and neck bites, 94–95
Head circumference, 551.e1t
for girls and boys (growth charts), 573f, 575f, 571.e3f
for preterm infants, 580f–581f
Head imaging, 664–665
CT, 76, 76b, 558
PECARN clinical decision rule for, 76, 76b
in seizures, 558
in trauma, 665
ultrasound, 558
Head lice, 1014
Head righting, 236.e6t
Head Start, 246

Head trauma, 75–78
  acute, 14
  imaging of, 665
  minor closed head trauma, 75–78
  secondary survey of, 74t–75t
Headaches, 551–555
  acute, 551b
  differential diagnosis of, 551b–552b
  evaluation of, 551–553, 551.e1t
  important historical information, 552b
  migraine, 553–555. See also Migraine headache
  recurrent or chronic, 552b
  warning signs on history, 552b
HEADS UP to Youth Sports (CDC Guidelines), 73, 78
HEADSSS assessment, 110, 111b
Health care decisions, 631. See also Decision making
Health insurance, 125–131
Healthy Eating Guidelines (USDA), 570
HealthyLax. See Polyethylene glycol (PEG) electrolyte solutions
Hearing, 625.e1t–625.e2t
Hearing screening
  for adolescents, 112, 123
  dysmorphology evaluation, 347
Heart
  evaluation of, 183
  imaging of, 675–676, 677f
  radiological contours, 183, 183f
  situs, 675
Heart block, 178f, 178t
Heart disease
  acquired, 191–198
  congenital, se congenital heart disease
  rheumatic, 198
Heart failure, 813
  congestive, 166b
Heart murmurs, 165–166
  benign, 165–166
  diastolic, 168b
  grading of, 165
  innocent, 167t
  pathologic, 166
  systolic, 168b
Heart rate (HR)
  Apgar scores, 493t
  assessment of, 2
  fetal heart rate (FHR), 490.e3
  normal newborn, 493
  normal values, 170t
  systematic approach for evaluating ECGs, 167
Heart rhythm, 2

Heart size, 675
Heart sounds, 164, 166b
Heart transplantation, 192b, 1074, 1091
Heat rash (miliaria), 219
Heated humidified high-flow nasal cannula (HHFNC), 90
Heelstick, 31
Heel-to-ear maneuver, 494f, 495
Height, 276–277
  growth charts for boys, 571.e2f
  growth charts for girls, 571.e1f
  target range, 276–277
  waist/height ratio, 572–574
Heinz body preparation, 368
Helicobacter pylori infection, 798, 835–836, 968
Helium
  for asthma, 11
  for croup, 13
Hemangeol. See Propranolol
Hemangioblastoma, 611t
Hemangioma, 203–207, 532f
  diagnosis of, 218f
  infantile, 1034
Hematocrit (Hct), 365t
Hematologic diseases
  in newborns, 504–507
  in SLE, 694t
Hematology, 364–394
Hematoma, subungal, 225
Hematopoietic stem cell transplantation (HSCT), 619–621
  Candida prophylaxis in, 969
  immunoprophylaxis after, 423
  preparative regimens, 619
  types of, 619–621
Hematuria, 530–531
  causes of, 531t
  diagnostic strategy for, 532f
  extraglomerular, 530–531
  glomerular, 530–531
  gross, 530
  management of, 533f
  microscopic, 530
  persistent, 530
Hemi-Fontan shunt, 190–191
Hemodialysis
  continuous arteriovenous hemofiltration/hemodialysis (CAVH/D), 529
  continuous venovenous hemofiltration/hemodialysis (CVVH/D), 529
  for ingestions, 22
  intermittent, 529
  for metabolic crisis, 340

Hemoglobin (Hb)
  age-specific values, 365*t*
  carboxyhemoglobin, 709*t*–716*t*
  urine, 517
Hemoglobin A_{1c} (HbA_{1c})
  interpreting, 255
  reference values, 709*t*–716*t*
  in type 2 DM, 260
Hemoglobin Bart/hydrops fetalis, 369
Hemoglobin electrophoresis, 368, 369*t*
Hemoglobin F, 709*t*–716*t*
Hemoglobin H (HbH) disease, 369
Hemoglobinopathies, 368–372
Hemoglobinuria, 517
Hemolytic anemia, 367–368
Hemolytic reactions, acute, 385
Hemolytic-uremic syndrome (HUS), 375, 532*f*, 623
Hemophilia, 389*t*
Hemophilia A, 387*t*–388*t*, 851
Hemophilia B, 387*t*–388*t*
Hemorrhage
  categorization of, 86.e2*t*
  gastrointestinal, 1096
  germinal matrix, 665
  intraventricular (IVH), 510, 922
  traumatic subungal, 225.e1*f*
Hemorrhagic cystitis, 623, 832
Hemorrhagic disease, 1020
Hemorrhoids, 914
Hemothorax, 79
Henoch-Schönlein purpura (HSP), 532*f*, 696–699, 697*t*
Heparin sodium
  antidote for, 912, 1035–1036
  for cerebrovascular accident, 618
  and coagulation tests, 382
  formulary entry, 911–912
  low-molecular-weight heparin (LMWH). *See* Low-molecular-weight heparin
  unfractionated (UFH). *See* Unfractionated heparin
Hepatic encephalopathy, 982
Hepatic impairment, 880
Hepatitis A (HepA) vaccine
  administration, 429
  catch-up schedule for, 414*f*
  HepA/Hep B combination (Twinrix), 442
  for pre-teens and adolescents, 124*t*
  recommended schedule for, 413*f*, 415*f*–418*f*
  routine vaccination, 428
  for travelers, 429

Hepatitis A virus (HAV)
  immunoprophylaxis against, 405, 428–429
    after Ig or blood product administration, 426.e1*t*
    intramuscular immunoglobulin (IMIG), 429
  postexposure prophylaxis against, 429
Hepatitis B, 457*t*–458*t*, 487, 532*f*
  chronic, 935–936
  serologic markers, 328*t*
Hepatitis B immune globulin (HBIG), 429
  after Ig or blood product administration, 426.e1*t*
  after percutaneous exposure to blood, 430*t*
Hepatitis B surface antigen (HbsAg), 425*f*
Hepatitis B (HepB) vaccine, 429
  catch-up schedule for, 414*f*
  DTaP/HepB/IPV combination (Pediarix), 441
  Engerix-B, 430
  HepA/Hep B combination (Twinrix), 442
  after HSCT, 625.e3
  for neonates of mothers with HbsAg status unknown or positive, 425*f*
  after percutaneous exposure to blood, 430*t*
  for pre-teens and adolescents, 124*t*
  for preterm and low-birth-weight infants, 424
  Recombivax, 429
  recommended schedule for, 413*f*–418*f*
  routine vaccination, 429
Hepatitis B virus (HBV):
  immunoprophylaxis against, 429–430
  postexposure, 430*t*, 487
Hepatitis C, 457*t*–458*t*, 487, 1047–1048
Hepatobiliary scintigraphy with 99mTc-iminodiacetate (HIDA), 678
Hepatoblastoma, 609*t*–610*t*
Hepatocellular carcinoma, 609*t*–610*t*
Hepatolenticular degeneration, 347.e1
Hereditary nail disorders, 225
Hereditary tyrosinemia (HT1), 342
Heroin, 21*t*

Herpangina, 471t–476t
Herpes
  genital, 120t, 761, 883, 1090
  management of, 115t–116t
  mucocutaneous, 883
Herpes keratoconjunctivitis, 1087
Herpes labialis, 761, 883, 1090
Herpes simplex virus (HSV) infection, 457t–458t
  acyclovir-resistant, 900
  antimicrobial prophylaxis against, 626t
  diagnosis of, 218f
  eczema herpeticum superinfection, 222
  encephalitis, 760
  imaging of, 665
  mucocutaneous, 760–761
  prophylaxis of, 761
  treatment of, 760–761, 1089
Herpes zoster, 471t–476t
  in BMT recipients, 624.e1t
  treatment of, 761, 883, 1090
Herpetic keratitis, 904
Heteroplasmy, 334.e1
Hexadrol. *See* Dexamethasone
HFOV (high-frequency oscillatory ventilation), 90.e1
HHFNC (heated humidified high-flow nasal cannula), 90
HHS. *See* U.S. Department of Health and Human Services
Hiberix, 428
Hib-MenCY (MenHibrix). *See* Meningococcal vaccine
HIDA (hepatobiliary scintigraphy with 99mTc-iminodiacetate), 678
High-density lipoprotein (HDL) cholesterol
  reduced, 200
  reference values, 709t–716t
High-frequency chest wall compression devices (vest therapy), 656
High-frequency jet ventilation, 91, 90.e1
High-frequency oscillatory ventilation (HFOV), 90.e1
High-frequency ventilation, 91–92
High-molecular-weight kininogen (HMWK), 377t–378t
Hip disorders
  congenital hip dislocation, 681, 681.e1f
  imaging, 681
Hirsutism, 1065

Histamine-1 (H_1) receptor antagonists. *See also* Antihistamines
  for allergic emergencies, 10
  for allergic rhinitis, 397
  for antiemetic therapy, 626t
Histamine-2 (H_2) receptor antagonists (H_2RAs), 324. *See also* Antihistamines
Histiocytic disease, 609t–610t
Histoplasma capsulatum, 930
Histoplasmosis, nonmeningeal, 930
History
  AMPLE (Allergies, Medications, Past illnesses, Last meal, Events) history, 73
  behavioral, 236
  for chronic HTN, 541
  developmental, 235–236
  educational, 236
  exposure, 20
  family, 112, 236
  focused, 146–147
  for headache, 552b
  medical, 112
  medicosocial, 109–110
  psychosocial, 109–110
  sexual, 111.e1b
  for UTIs, 519
HIV. *See* Human immunodeficiency virus
HLA-B27, 691
Holliday-Segar method, 291, 292b, 292t
  sample calculations, 295b–296b, 298b
Holt-Oram syndrome
  ECG changes in, 180t
  sternal abnormalities in, 184
Home assessment, 111b
Home care, 632
Homocystinemia, 379b
Homovanillic acid, 287.e1t
Hookworms, 955, 1037
Horizant. *See* Gabapentin
Hormonal contraception, 125
Hormonal therapy, 214, 215t
Hospice palliative care specialists, 628
HP Acthar. *See* Corticotropin
HSCT. *See* Hematopoietic stem cell transplantation
HSP (Henoch-Schönlein purpura), 532f, 696–699, 697t
HT1 (hereditary tyrosinemia), 342
HTS. *See* Hypertonic saline
Humalog. *See* Insulin lispro

Humalog Mix. See Insulin lispro
Human albumin. See Albumin
Human bites, 94t, 461t–468t
Human immunodeficiency virus (HIV)
　exposure to, 486–487
　immunoprophylaxis guidelines for, 422–423
　postexposure prophylaxis (PEP), 486–487, 1105
　pre-exposure prophylaxis (PrEP), 486
　prevention of vertical transmission of, 1104–1105
Human immunodeficiency virus (HIV) infection, 457t–458t, 470–484, 532f
　with antibody deficiency, 405
　cryptococcal meningitis in, 778
　MAC in, 789–790, 1049
　management of, 470–484, 482t, 889, 1105
　mucocutaneous herpes in, 883
　opportunistic disease in, 930
　perinatal management of, 482t
　prophylaxis for recurrence of opportunistic disease in, 930
　in utero exposure, 482t
Human milk, 585–588, 594t–600t
Human papillomavirus (HPV) infection, 120t
　immunoprophylaxis against, 430–431
Human papillomavirus (HPV) vaccine (Cervarix, Gardasil), 430
　catch-up schedule for, 414f
　for pre-teens and adolescents, 124t
　recommended schedule for, 413f, 415f–418f
　routine vaccination, 430–431
Humate-P, 387t–388t
Humatin. See Paromomycin sulfate
Humulin 70/30. See Insulin
Humulin N. See Isophane insulin
Hunter syndrome, 334, 344–345
Hurler syndrome, 344–345
Hurler-Scheie type mucopolysaccharidosis, 345
HUS (hemolytic-uremic syndrome), 375, 532f, 623
Hyaluronidase (Amphadase, Hydase, Hylenex, Vitrase), 912
Hydralazine hydrochloride
　dose adjustment in renal failure, 1125t–1134t
　formulary entry, 913
　for hypertension, 544t–545t
　for hypertensive emergency, 83t

Hydration
　for HSP, 698
　for hyperleukocytosis/leukocytosis, 616
　for tumor lysis syndrome, 616
Hydrocarbon odors, 21.e1t–21.e3t
Hydrocephalus, 564, 758
Hydrochlorothiazide (HCTZ, Microzide)
　formulary entry, 913–914
　for hypertension, 544t–545t
Hydrocodone, 139.e1t
Hydrocortisone (Solu-Cortef, Cortef, Cortifoam, Colocort, Cortenema, NuCort)
　for adrenal crisis, 272
　for adrenal insufficiency, 271–272
　formulary entry, 914
　for hypercalcemia associated with hyperparathyroidism, 267
　potency, 223t, 271t
　for shock, 87f
　stress-dose, 272
Hydrocortisone with ciprofloxacin (Cipro HC Otic), 833
Hydrocortisone with neomycin/polymyxin B, 983, 1025
Hydrocortisone with neomycin/polymyxin B + bacitracin (Neo-Polycin HC), 983
Hydrodiuril. See Hydrochlorothiazide
Hydrometroculpos, 680
Hydromorphone HCl (Dilaudid, Exalgo), 140t, 139.e1t
　formulary entry, 915
　for PCA, 143t
　urine toxicology screen, 21t
25-Hydroxy vitamin D, 268t
Hydroxychloroquine (Plaquenil)
　for arthritis, 692
　formulary entry, 915–916
　for SLE, 695
　toxicity, 691.e1t
21-Hydroxylase deficiency, 269
17-Hydroxyprogesterone, 270, 270t
Hydroxyurea, 372t
Hydroxyzine (Vistaril), 139.e1t
　formulary entry, 916–917
　properties of, 149b–150b
Hylenex. See Hyaluronidase
Hymenolepis nana, 1008
Hyoscyamine, 634t
Hyperactivity. See Attention-deficit/hyperactivity disorder
Hyperammonemia, 334, 337f, 340
Hyperandrogenism, 282

Hyperbilirubinemia, 327
 conjugated, 506–507
 differential diagnosis of, 329t
 treatment of, 1015
 unconjugated, 504–506
Hypercalcemia, 307–309, 532f, 701.e2
 associated with hyperparathyroidism, 267
 ECG changes in, 180t
 etiology of, 309b
 treatment of, 803
Hypercalciuria, 526
Hypercoagulable states, 379–382, 379b–380b
Hyperglycemia, 497, 498t
Hyperglycinemia, nonketotic (NKH), 340
Hypergonadotropic hypogonadism, 280
Hyperimmune globulins, 406
Hyperinsulinemia, 286
Hyperinsulinemic hypoglycemia, 857
Hyperkalemia, 306–307, 308f
 causes of, 306t
 dialysis for, 529
 ECG changes in, 179, 180t
Hyperleukocytosis, 612–616, 618
Hyperlipidemia
 management of, 200
 screening for, 260
Hypermagnesemia, 310
 ECG changes in, 180t
 etiology of, 310b
Hypernatremia, 304, 305t
Hypernatremic dehydration, 297
 deficit replacement for, 297, 300–301
 sample calculations, 298b, 300b
 severe, 297, 300b
Hyperoxia test, 187.e1t
Hyperparathyroidism, 266–267
Hyperphosphatemia, 311, 311b, 767, 804
Hyperpigmentation, 225–226, 226.e1f
Hyperpyrexia
 in poisoning, 21.e1t–21.e3t
 supportive care for, 21
Hypersal. *See* Sodium chloride
Hypersecretory conditions, 880, 939, 995, 1007
Hypersensitivity reactions
 insect bite-induced, 224
 treatment of, 872–873
Hypertension, 273
 causes of, 541–542, 541t
 chronic, 539–542, 913
 classification of, 540t
 clinical evaluation of, 541–542

Hypertension *(Continued)*
 definition of, 539
 delayed, 21.e1t–21.e3t
 monitoring for, 260
 persistent pulmonary hypertension of the newborn (PPHN), 501–502
 in poisoning, 21.e1t–21.e3t
 postoperative, 879
 prior to surgery for pheochromocytoma, 1016
 pulmonary, 88–89, 1059
 treatment of, 542, 544t–545t, 773, 784, 813, 839, 869, 913, 948, 952, 962, 966–967, 986–987, 1016, 1034, 1087, 1093, 1097
Hypertensive crisis, 81–82, 962
 management of, 913, 82.e1
 pulmonary, 88–89
Hypertensive emergency, 81
 injectable medications for, 83t
 management of, 82, 933
Hypertensive urgency, 81
 enteral medications for, 84t
 management of, 82, 987
Hyperthermia, malignant, 846
Hyperthyroidism, 262–266
 ECG changes in, 180t
 treatment of, 961
Hypertonic saline (HTS)
 for elevated ICP, 85t
 nasal rinsing with, 397
 phase I deficit replacement, 297
 for SIADH, 274
Hypertrophic cardiomyopathy, 193–194
 sports restrictions, 199.e1t
 treatment of, 987
Hypertrophic pyloric stenosis, 677.e3f
Hypertrophic subaortic stenosis, idiopathic, 193–194
Hyperuricemia
 management of, 616, 1031, 1045
 prevention of, 616
Hyperviscosity, 379b, 501
Hypnotics, 139.e1t
 pentobarbital, 1013
 poisoning with, 22t
 for RSI, 7t–8t
Hypoalbuminemia, 763
Hypoaldosteronism, 538t
Hypocalcemia, 307–309
 etiology of, 309b
 treatment of, 805–808, 954
Hypocarbia, 501
Hypochloremia, 781
Hypogammaglobulinemia, severe, 401

Hypoglycemia, 334
  definition of, 286
  evaluation of, 338f
  hyperinsulinemic, 857
  management of, 497, 498t, 499f, 906
  neonatal evaluation of, 286–287
  newborn screening for, 499f
  in poisoning, 21.e1t–21.e3t
Hypogonadotropic hypogonadism, 280–281
Hypokalemia, 304–307, 306t
  ECG changes in, 180t
  treatment of, 1027
Hypomagnesemia, 309–310, 310b
  ECG changes in, 180t
  treatment of, 954
Hyponatremia, 274, 304, 305t
Hyponatremic dehydration, 294
  deficit replacement for, 297, 299–300
  sample calculations, 296b, 299b
  severe symptomatic, 299b
Hyponatremic hypovolemia, 294
Hypoparathyroidism, 266
  management of, 875
  treatment of, 804
Hypoperfusion, 21.e1t–21.e3t
Hypophosphatemia, 310–311, 311b, 1019
Hypopigmentation, 226–227
  diffuse, 227
  localized, 226–227
  postinflammatory, 227, 227.e1f
Hypopigmented macules, 226–227, 226.e3f
Hypopituitarism, 287
Hypotension, 2
  in poisoning, 21.e1t–21.e3t
  supportive care for, 21–22
  treatment of, 1017, 1096
  vasodilatory shock with, 1096
Hypothermia
  criteria for, 508
  in poisoning, 21.e1t–21.e3t
  protocol for neonates, 508
Hypothyroidism, 262, 264t
  differential diagnosis of, 278f
  ECG changes in, 180t
  newborn screening for, 262
Hypotonia, 355–356
Hypotonic fluids, 292–293
Hypoventilation, obstructive, 656
Hypovolemia, 763
  hyponatremic, 294
Hypovolemic shock, 86, 87f, 86.e1t
Hypoxia, 21.e1t–21.e3t

Hypoxic-ischemic encephalopathy (HIE), 508, 509t

I

IAI (intraabdominal injury), 79
IBD (inflammatory bowel disease), 323, 842, 1070
IBIH (insect bite-induced hypersensitivity), 224
Ibuprofen (Advil, Motrin, NeoProfen, Caldolor)
  analgesic properties, 139
  for arthritis, 691
  formulary entry, 917–918
Ice pick view, 184.e1
ICS. See Inhaled corticosteroids
ICU sedation, 853
ID. See Intellectual disability
Identity development, 109.e1t
Idiopathic hypertrophic subaortic stenosis, 193–194
Idiopathic pneumonia syndrome, 623
Idiopathic thrombocytopenic purpura (ITP), 373–375
IDM. See Infant of diabetic mother
IEP (Individualized Education Program), 246
Ifex. See Ifosfamide
Ifosfamide (isophosphamide, Ifex)
  characteristics of, 613t–615t
  late effects of, 625.e1t–625.e2t
IGF-BP3 (insulin-like growth factor–binding protein), 287, 287.e2t
IGRA (interferon gamma release assay), 484
IIV (inactivated influenza vaccine), 415f–418f
Ileocolic intussusception, 678, 679f
Ileoileal intussusception, 698
Ileostomy fluid, 304t
Image Gently Alliance, 663
Imaging. See also specific modalities
  abdominal, 676–678
  of airway, 667–670
  cardiac, 183–184
  of chest, 670–674
  dysmorphology evaluation, 347
  of extremities, 680–683
  of eyes, 665–666
  genitourinary, 679–680
  of head, 664–665
  of heart and vessels, 675–676
  spinal, 666–667
  in UTIs, 521–522
Imatinib (Gleevec), 613t–615t
Iminodiacetate, 678

Imipenem, 447t–449t
Imipenem and cilastatin (Primaxin)
  dose adjustment in renal failure, 1111t–1124t
  formulary entry, 918
Imipramine (Tofranil), 919
Imitrex. *See* Sumatriptan
Immune globulin
  formulary entry, 920–921
  immunoprophylaxis guidelines for patients on, 426
  indications for, 422
  intramuscular (IMIG), 405–406, 920
  intravenous (IVIG), 401–405, 920
    for ITP, 374
    for Kawasaki disease, 198
  subcutaneous, 406, 920–921
  therapeutic, 401–406
Immune globulin A (IgA), 407t–408t
Immune globulin A (IgA) deficiency, 325, 403t–404t
Immune globulin A (IgA) nephropathy, 532f
Immune globulin E (IgE)
  allergen-specific, 400
  serum levels, 407t
Immune globulin G (IgG), 407t–408t
Immune globulin M (IgM), 407t–408t
Immune thrombocytopenic purpura (ITP), 405, 920, 1046
Immunizations. *See also specific vaccines*
  administration of, 64–65, 419
  for adolescents, 123, 124t
  in arthritis, 693
  catch-up schedule, 414f
  during chemotherapy, 423
  for chemotherapy patients, 625.e3
  for children at high risk for Hib disease, 422
  for children at high risk for meningococcal disease, 421–422
  for children at high risk for pneumcoccal disease, 420–421
  for children with asplenia or HIV, 422
  for children with asplenia or persistent complement deficiency, 422
  for children with congenital immunodeficiency disorders, 422
  for children with functional or anatomic asplenia, 422
  for children with HIV disease, 422–423
  combination vaccines, 441–442

Immunizations *(Continued)*
  contraindications to, 419, 422–424
  during corticosteroid therapy, 423
  guidelines for, 412–420, 426–442
  for HSCT recipients, 423, 625.e3
  after Ig or blood product administration, 426, 426.e1t
  and immunosuppressive therapy, 423
  informed consent for, 412
  live vaccines, 419, 422, 424
    during corticosteroid therapy, 424t
    for patients on biological response modifiers, 423–424
  for low-birth-weight infants, 424
  misconceptions about, 420
  for neonates, 493
  for neonates of mothers with HbsAg status unknown or positive, 425f
  nonlive, 419
  not considered contraindications to, 420
  for oncology patients, 625
  for patients on biological response modifiers, 423–424
  precautions, 419
  preferred sites for, 419
  during pregnancy, 424
  for pre-teens, 124t
  for preterm infants, 424
  schedules, 412, 413f, 415f–418f
  for solid organ transplant recipients, 423
  supplied in vials or syringes that contain natural rubber, 419
  for travelers to foreign countries, 426
  types of, 419
  web resources, 412
Immunocompromise, 420–421
Immunodeficiency
  congenital, 422
  evaluation for, 403t–404t
  radiographic findings, 669t
  when to suspect, 403t
Immunofluorescence assay, 709t–716t
Immunoprophylaxis, 412–442. *See also* Immunizations
  against GVHD, 621
Immunosuppressants
  for arthritis, 692
  azathioprine, 787
  cortisone acetate, 841
  hydrocortisone, 914
  methylprednisolone, 965
  prednisone, 1029
  for scleroderma, 701.e3
  vaccines and, 423

Immunotherapy
 for allergic rhinitis, 397
 food-specific, 400
Imodium. See Loperamide
Imovax. See HDCV
Impetigo, 211
 bullous, 218f
 treatment of, 823
Implants, subdermal, 127
Imprinting, genomic, 334.e1
Imuran. See Azathioprine
IMV (intermittent mandatory ventilation), 90–91
Inactivated influenza vaccine (IIV), 415f–418f
Inactivated poliovirus (IPV) vaccine, 435
 catch-up schedule for, 414f
 after chemotherapy, 625.e3
 DTaP/HepB/IPV combination (Pediarix), 441
 DTaP/IPV combination (Kinrix), 441
 DTaP/IPV combination (Quadracel), 442
 DTaP/IPV/PRP-T combination (Pentacel), 415f–418f, 441
 after HSCT, 625.e3
 PRP-T (Hiberix), 415f–418f, 428, 441
 recommended schedule for, 413f, 415f–418f
Inapsine. See Droperidol
Incidence, 725
Incontinentia pigmenti, 218f
Independence, 109.e1t
Inderal. See Propranolol
Individualized Education Program (IEP), 246
Individuals with Disabilities Education Improvement Act (IDEA), 229, 246
Indomethacin (Indocin, Tivorbex), 922
Infancy: chronic lung disease of, 653–654
Infanrix (DTaP), 426
Infant formulas, 601t–602t
 company websites, 570
 enteral nutrition components, 594t–600t
 preparation of, 593t
Infant multivitamin drops, 588t
Infant of diabetic mother (IDM), 496
 dominant cardiac defects, 185t
 hypoglycemia in, 499f
Infant skull, 353.e1f
Infant Toddler Checklist (CSBS DP), 237t–238t
Infantile hemangioma, 1034

Infantile proctocolitis, 398
Infantile spasms, 559t–560t
 dietary therapy for, 561
 treatment of, 841, 1098, 1108
Infants
 age-appropriate behavioral issues, 233t–235t
 arterial catheters for, 34
 asthma in, 647f, 650f
 caloric requirements, 499t
 coagulation values, 377t–378t
 constipation in, 322
 disimpaction for, 322
 EER equations, 581.e1
 emergency management for, 3t
 hypertension in, 541t
 large-for-gestational-age (LGA), 493, 499f
 low-birth-weight. See Low-birth-weight (LBW) infants
 mean TSH and T$_4$ values, 263t
 Modified Coma Scale for, 15t
 newborn. See Newborn care; Newborns
 normal blood pressure values, 156.e1t
 normal bowel movements, 321–322
 organic acidemia in, 341
 pain assessment in, 136
 peripheral blood T and B cells, 408t
 physiologic anemia of infancy, 366
 premature. See Preterm infants
 preterm. See Preterm infants
 recommended element intakes, 591t
 recommended vitamin intakes, 586t
 reference values, 709t–716t
 routine newborn care for, 492–493
 serum complement levels, 408t
 serum immunoglobulin levels, 407t–408t
 small-for-gestational-age (SGA), 493, 499f
 sodium requirements, 498t
 trisomy 21 in, 348
 with in utero HIV exposure, 482t
 very low-birth-weight (VLBW), 493
Infasurf. See Surfactant
Infections. See also specific infections
 anaerobic, 968
 in animal bite wounds, 93–95
 bacterial, 211, 455–470
 in bites, 461t–468t
 catheter-related bloodstream, 461t–468t
 congenital, 457t–458t, 665

Infections *(Continued)*
  deep neck, 455–470
  fungal, 210, 470, 481*t*
  initial management of, 461*t*–468*t*
  intra-abdominal, 461*t*–468*t*, 818, 958, 1023
  intrauterine (congenital), 455
  joint, 947, 952
  mild/moderate, 779–780, 818–819, 822–824, 833, 958, 980
  minor/moderate, 1069
  moderate, 791
  neonatal, 455–470, 461*t*–468*t*
  parasitic infestations, 208–210, 968
  perinatal, 455, 457*t*–458*t*
  serious, 816
  severe, 779–780, 791, 816, 818–819, 823–824, 833, 930, 958, 980, 1010, 1023, 1069
  skin, 207–211, 816
  skin and soft tissue, 789, 1023
  spinal fusion, 461*t*–468*t*
  tickborne, 470, 479*t*–480*t*
  treatment of, 816, 957, 973
  viral, 207–208, 455, 470, 471*t*–476*t*
  yeast, 470
Infectious disease, 390, 444–487
Infectious mononucleosis, 471*t*–476*t*
Infectious rhinitis, 396
INFeD. *See* Iron, injectable preparations
Infertility, 656
Infestations, parasitic, 208–210, 968
Infiltrates, 672
Inflammation, chronic, 367
Inflammatory bowel disease (IBD), 323, 842, 1070
Inflammatory disease, 917
Infliximab, 692
Influenza, 471*t*–476*t*
  chemoprophylaxis for, 432
  immunoprophylaxis of, 431–432
  prophylaxis of, 432, 654, 768, 998, 1051
  treatment of, 768, 997–998, 1051
Influenza vaccine
  administration of, 432
  inactivated (IIV), 415*f*–418*f*
  live attenuated (LAIV), 415*f*–418*f*, 420, 422–423, 431–432
  in pregnancy, 424
  for pre-teens and adolescents, 124*t*
  recommended schedule for, 413*f*, 415*f*–418*f*
  routine vaccination, 431

Influenza vaccine *(Continued)*
  in sickle cell disease, 372*t*
  web resources, 412
Informed consent
  for genetic testing, 360
  vaccine, 412
Ingestions, 21–22
Ingrown toenails, congenital, 225, 225.*e*5*f*
INH. *See* Isoniazid
Inhalation injury
  acute stabilization in, 96
  thermal, 96*t*
Inhalational anthrax, 942, 1012
Inhaled corticosteroids (ICS)
  for asthma, 648*f*, 650*f*–652*f*
  dosages, 646.*e*1*t*–646.*e*2*t*
Inheritance patterns, 334
Injectable local anesthetics, 142, 142*t*
Injections
  intramuscular, 64
  subcutaneous, 64
Injury
  cervical spine, 78
  cold, 96*t*
  head, 14, 75–78
  skeletal, 103*t*
  spinal cord, without radiographic abnormality (SCIWORA), 667
  thermal, 95–100, 96*t*
  traumatic, 75–81
Inpatient care
  for animal bites, 95
  for burns, 100
  for mental health issues, 251
INR, 377*t*–378*t*
Insect bite-induced hypersensitivity (IBIH), 224
Insecticide poisoning, 787
Insomnia, 658, 1085
Inspiratory pressure, maximal, 640–641
Inspiratory time (Ti), 90–91, 91.*e*1
Inspired oxygen concentration (FiO_2), 90–91, 91.*e*1
Insulin, 256
  for CCB overdose, 23*t*–24*t*
  for DKA, 258*f*
  dosages, 259, 259*t*
  dose adjustment in renal failure, 1125*t*–1134*t*
  formulary entry, 922–923
  for hyperkalemia, 308*f*
  isophane (NPH, Humulin N/Novolin N), 260*t*
  preparations, 922–923

Insulin *(Continued)*
  products, 260*t*
  regular (Humulin 70/30), 260*t*, 1125*t*–1134*t*
  requirements for, 259
  subcutaneous, 259, 259*t*
Insulin aspart (NovoLog, NovoLog Mix), 260*t*
Insulin detemir (Levemir), 260*t*
Insulin glargine (Lantus), 260*t*
Insulin glulisine (Apidra), 260*t*
Insulin lispro (Humalog, Humalog Mix), 260*t*
Insulin-like growth factor 1 (IGF-1), 279*t*
Insulin-like growth factor–binding protein (IGF-BP3), 287, 287.*e*2*t*
Intellectual developmental disorder, 242.*e*1*t*–242.*e*2*t*
Intellectual disability (ID), 241–242
  diagnostic criteria for, 242
  severity levels, 242.*e*1*t*–242.*e*2*t*
  web resources, 229
Interferon alfa-2a, 700
Interferon gamma release assay (IGRA), 484
Interleukin (IL)-1 receptor antagonists, 692
Intermittent hemodialysis, 529
Intermittent mandatory ventilation (IMV), 90–91
Internal jugular vein: central venous catheter placement via, 37–41, 38*f*–39*f*
  ultrasound-guided, 39, 40*f*–41*f*
International Association for the Study of Pain, 136
International Pediatric Hypertension Association, 516
International Society for Pediatric and Adolescent Diabetes, 255
Interstitial fibrosis, 643*t*
Interstitial nephritis, 527*t*, 532*f*
Interval extension (I) dose adjustment method, 1110
Interval extension and dose reduction (DI) dose adjustment method, 1110
Interval extension or dose reduction (D, I) dose adjustment method, 1110
Interventions
  discontinuing, 632
  limiting, 632–633
Intestinal amebiasis, 1008
Intestinal obstruction
  distal intestinal obstruction syndrome, 759

Intestinal obstruction *(Continued)*
  formulas for, 601*t*–602*t*
  high, 677
Intoxication. *See also* Poisoning
  acetaminophen, 22
  opiate, 980
Intraabdominal infections, 461*t*–468*t*, 958, 1023
Intraabdominal injury (IAI), 79
Intracellular fluid, 294.*e*1, 294.*e*1*t*
Intracranial pressure (ICP)
  decreased, 551*b*
  increased, 48, 82–84, 85*f*, 551*b*, 617
Intramuscular immune globulin (IMIG), 405–406, 920
Intramuscular injections, 64
Intramuscular vaccines
  administration of, 419
  preferred sites for, 419
Intranasal antihistamines, 396
Intranasal combination agents, 397
Intranasal corticosteroids
  for allergic rhinitis, 396
  for OSAS, 658
Intraocular pressure, elevated, 1021
Intraosseous (IO) access, 43–45, 44*f*
Intrapartum fetal heart rate (FHR) monitoring, 490.*e*3
Intrapulmonary shunt fraction (Qs/Qt), 93.*e*1
Intraspinal lesions, 548
Intrauterine device (IUD), 127, 130
Intrauterine (congenital) infections, 455
Intravenous immune globulin (IVIG), 401–405, 920
  for enterovirus, 457*t*–458*t*, 471*t*–476*t*
  after Ig or blood product administration, 426.*e*1*t*
  for ITP, 374
  for Kawasaki disease, 198
  for parvovirus, 471*t*–476*t*
  for unconjugated hyperbilirubinemia in the newborn, 505
  for varicella, 457*t*–458*t*
Intravenous placement
  central line placement, 674, 675*f*–676*f*. *See also* Central venous catheter placement
  peripheral, 32
Intraventricular hemorrhage (IVH)
  in neonates, 510
  prophylaxis for, 922
Intubation, 4–8
  for asthma, 11–12
  paralysis for, 1067

Intubation *(Continued)*
  rapid sequence (RSI), 5, 7*t*–8*t*
  treatment algorithm for, 6*f*
Intuniv. *See* Guanfacine
Intussusception, 678, 679*f*, 698
Invanz. *See* Ertapenem
Invasive aspergillosis, 969, 1101
Invasive candidiasis, 969, 1101
IO (intraosseous) access, 43–45, 44*f*
Iodide. *See* Potassium iodide
Iodine
  in multivitamin tablets, 589*t*–590*t*
  recommended intakes, 591*t*
Iohexol (Omnipaque), 923–924
Iosat. *See* Potassium iodide
Ipratropium bromide (Atrovent)
  for allergic rhinitis, 397
  formulary entry, 924–925
Ipratropium bromide + albuterol (Combivent Respimat), 924–925
IPV. *See* Inactivated poliovirus vaccine
Iquix. *See* Levofloxacin
Irbesartan, 544*t*–545*t*
Iron
  in infant multivitamin drops, 588*t*
  injectable preparations (Ferrlecit, INFeD, DexFerrum, Venofer), 925–927
  in multivitamin tablets, 589*t*–590*t*
  oral preparations (Fer-In-Sol, FeroSul, Slow FE, Slow Iron, Ferate, Ferretts), 588*t*, 927–928
  overdose, 23*t*–24*t*, 850
  polysaccharide-iron complex (Myferon 150, PIC 200, Poly-Iron 150, NovaFerrum), 927–928
  recommended intakes, 591*t*
  reference values, 709*t*–716*t*
  total iron-binding capacity (TIBC), 709*t*–716*t*
Iron deficiency anemia
  in CKD, 926
  prophylaxis for, 928
  treatment of, 926–927
Iron dextran. *See* Iron, injectable preparations
Iron sucrose. *See* Iron, injectable preparations
Iron supplements, 497, 584–585
Iron-deficiency anemia, 364–368, 584
Irradiated blood products, 391
Irritability, 782, 1052
Irritant dermatitis, 221
Isonatremic dehydration
  deficit replacement strategy for, 299
  sample calculations, 295*b*

Isoniazid (INH, Nydrazid, Laniazid)
  dose adjustment in renal failure, 1111*t*–1124*t*
  formulary entry, 928–929
  for hyperkalemia, 308*f*
  for TB, 485
  warfarin interactions, 385*b*
Isoniazid + rifampin (Rifamate, IsonRif), 928–929
Isoniazid + rifampin + pyrazinamide (Rifater), 928–929, 1038
IsonRif. *See* Isoniazid + rifampin
Isophane insulin (NPH, Humulin N/Novolin N), 260*t*
Isoproterenol (Isuprel), 929
Isopto Carpine. *See* Pilocarpine HCl
Isosource formulas, 594*t*–600*t*
Isosthenuria, 517
Isotonic saline
  for hypovolemic/distributive shock, 87*f*
  phase I deficit replacement, 297
Isotretinoid (Absorica, Claravis, Myorisan, Zenatane)
  for acne vulgaris, 214–216, 215*t*
  formulary entry, 929–930
Isovaleric acidemia, 341
Isradipine, 544*t*–545*t*
Isuprel. *See* Isoproterenol
ITP. *See* Idiopathic thrombocytopenic purpura; Immune thrombocytopenic purpura
Itraconazole (Sporanox, Onmel)
  formulary entry, 930–931
  for ringworm, 481*t*
  warfarin interactions, 385*b*
IUD (intrauterine device), 127, 130
Ivermectin, 210
IVIG. *See* Intravenous immune globulin

J
J depression, 169, 171*f*
JAMA evidence, 721.e1
Jantoven. *See* Warfarin
Japanese encephalitis (JE) immunoprophylaxis, 432
Japanese encephalitis (JE) vaccine (JE-VC), 432.e1
Jaundice, 21.e1*t*–21.e3*t*
JE. *See* Japanese encephalitis
Jet ventilation, high-frequency, 91, 90.e1
Jevity formulas, 594*t*–600*t*
JIA. *See* Juvenile idiopathic arthritis
The Joint Commission Official "Do Not Use" List, 733*t*

Joint fluid analysis, 691, 692f, 704
Joint infections, 947, 952
Joint pain
  analgesia for, 698
  differential diagnosis of, 690t
Jones criteria, 199b
JPA (juvenile pilocytic astrocytoma), 611t
JRA. See Juvenile rheumatoid arthritis
Junctional rhythm, 174t–175t
Junctional supraventricular tachycardia, 174t–175t
Juvenile dermatomyositis, 699
Juvenile idiopathic arthritis (JIA), 688–693, 689t
  associated autoantibodies, 695t
  treatment of, 881, 1070
Juvenile myoclonic epilepsy, 559t–560t
Juvenile pilocytic astrocytoma (JPA), 611t
Juvenile rheumatoid arthritis (JRA), 688–693
  synovial fluid characteristics, 718t
  treatment of, 916–917, 981
Juvenile xanthogranuloma, 218f

K

Kadian. See Morphine sulfate
Kalexate. See Sodium polystyrene sulfonate
Kaopectate. See Bismuth subsalicylate
Kao-Tin. See Bismuth subsalicylate; Docusate
Kapvay. See Clonidine
Karbinal ER. See Carbinoxamine
Karyotyping, 358t, 347.e1
  fetal, 490.e1
  sample collection for, 336t
Kawasaki disease, 196–198, 697t
  guidelines for treatment and follow-up, 198.e1t
  incomplete, 196, 197f
  IVIG for, 405
  treatment of, 784, 920
Kayexalate. See Sodium polystyrene sulfonate
Keflex. See Cephalexin
Kemstro. See Baclofen
Kenalog. See Triamcinolone
Keppra. See Levetiracetam
Keratitis, herpetic, 904
Keratoconjunctivitis, herpes, 1087
Keratoconjunctivitis sicca, 701.e3
Keratolytics, 208
Kerion, 211

Ketamine (Ketalar)
  for analgesia and sedation, 153t, 139.e1t
  formulary entry, 931
  for intubation, 6f
  for procedural sedation, 153t
  properties of, 149b–150b
  for RSI, 7t–8t
  for TET spells, 189t
Ketamine + midazolam + atropine (ketazolam), 153t
Ketoacidosis, 256, 517
KetoCal formulas, 570, 594t–602t
Ketoconazole (Nizoral, Xolegel, Extina, Ketodan)
  formulary entry, 931–932
  for ringworm, 481t
Ketodan. See Ketoconazole
Ketogenic diet, 559t–560t, 561
Ketones, urinary, 517
Ketonuria, 517
Ketorolac (Acular, Acuvail)
  analgesic properties, 139, 139.e1t
  formulary entry, 932–933
  morphine equivalence, 139
Ketotifen fumarate (Zaditor), 397
Kidney and bladder ultrasonography, 521
Kidney disease
  chronic. See Chronic kidney disease (CKD)
  late effects of cancer treatment, 625.e1t–625.e2t
  management of, 701.e3
  in SLE, 694t
Kidney function tests, 523–526
Kidney injury, acute. See Acute kidney injury (AKI)
Kidney stones, 542–545
Kidney transplantation
  allograft rejection in, 532f
  management of, 978, 1074, 1090–1091
Kidney-pancreas transplantation, 1091
Kidney-related disease, 531t
Kinrix. See DTaP/IPV combination
Kionex. See Sodium polystyrene sulfonate
Kitabis Pak. See Tobramycin
Klebsiella, 520
Klinefelter syndrome, 350
Klonopin. See Clonazepam
Klumpke's paralysis, 511t
Knee arthrocentesis, 59–61
Koilonychia, 225, 225.e5f
Kondremul. See Mineral oil

Konsyl. *See* Psyllium
K-PHOS Neutral. *See* Phosphorus supplements
Krabbe disease, 345–346
Kristalose. *See* Lactulose
Kruskall-Wallis analysis of variance by ranks, 724t
Kytril. *See* Granisetron

L

LABAs (long-acting beta$_2$-agonists), 650f–652f, 900
Labetalol
 formulary entry, 933–934
 for hypertension, 544t–545t
 for hypertensive emergency, 83t
 for hypertensive urgency, 84t
Laboratory studies
 normal ranges, 708
 nutritional assessment, 571
 reference values, 708, 709t–716t
 for rheumatic disease, 701–704
Lacerations, 65–68
Lacosamide (Vimpat)
 dose adjustment in renal failure, 1125t–1134t
 formulary entry, 934
 for seizures, 562t
Lactate
 reference values, 709t–716t
 sample collection for, 336t
Lactate dehydrogenase (LDH), 704
 reference values, 709t–716t
 serum levels, 367
Lactated Ringer's (LR) solution, 297, 302t
Lactation. *See also* Breastfeeding
 EER equations, 581.e1
 recommended element intakes, 591t
 recommended vitamin intakes, 586t
Lactic acidemias, 343
Lactic acidosis
 fatal, 960
 mitochondrial encephalomyopathy, lactic acidosis (MELAS) stroke-like episodes, 340
LactMed, 333, 588
Lactose intolerance, 601t–602t
Lactulose (Cephulac, Chronulac, Enuloase, Kristalose)
 for constipation, 322
 formulary entry, 935
LAIV (live, attenuated influenza vaccine), 415f–418f, 420, 422–423, 431

Lamictal. *See* Lamotrigine
Lamivudine (Epivir, Epivir-HBV, 3TC)
 dose adjustment in renal failure, 1111t–1124t
 formulary entry, 935–936
 zidovudine with abacavir and lamivudine (Trizivir), 1104
 zidovudine with lamivudine (Combivir), 1104
Lamotrigine (Lamictal)
 formulary entry, 936–938
 for seizures, 559t–560t, 562t
Landau response, 236.e6t
Langerhans cell histiocytosis (LCH)
 diagnosis of, 218f
 signs and symptoms of, 611t
Language, 229
Language development
 milestones, 231t–232t
 screening tests for, 237t–238t
Laniazid. *See* Isoniazid
Lanoxin. *See* Digoxin
Lansoprazole (Prevacid, First-Lansoprazole), 939
Lantus (insulin glargine), 260t
Lanugo, 494f
Lanzanda. *See* Fentanyl
LARC (long-acting reversible contraception), 125
Large bowel obstruction, 678
Large-for-gestational-age (LGA) infants, 493, 499f
Lariam. *See* Mefloquine HCl
Laryngeal mask airway (LMA), 4
Laryngotracheobronchitis (croup), 12–13
Lasix. *See* Furosemide
Last menstrual period (LMP), 490.e1–490.e3
Lateral propping, 236.e6t
Laxatives
 for constipation, 322
 magnesium hydroxide, 953
 PEG-electrolyte solutions (MiraLax, GaviLAX, GlycoLax, HealthyLax, PegyLax), 1023–1024
 sodium phosphate, 1064
Lax-Pills. *See* Senna
LCH. *See* Langerhans cell histiocytosis
LDL. *See* Low-density lipoprotein
LDs. *See* Learning disabilities
Lead: reference values for, 709t–716t
Lead chelation, 1066
Lead poisoning, 23t–24t, 26–27
 emergency management of, 26t
 management of, 861, 868

Lead poisoning *(Continued)*
  repeat blood lead testing guidelines for, 27t
Lead time bias, 722
Learning disabilities (LDs), 242
Least restrictive environment (LRE), 246
Leflunomide, 691.e1t
Left bundle-branch block (LBBB), 166b, 179t
Left ventricular dysfunction, 199.e1t
Left ventricular hypertrophy (LVH), 173b
Legacy making, 631–632
Legg-Calvé-Perthes disease, 681, 681.e2f
Leishmania chagasi infection, 1013
Leishmania donovani infection, 1013
Leishmania infantum infection, 1013
Leishmania [Viannia] panamensis infection, 1013
Leishmaniasis, 779, 1013
Length and weight
  conversion formulas, 708
  growth chart for boys, 574f
  growth chart for girls, 572f
  for preterm infants, 580f–581f
Length-to-weight ratio
  for boys, 575f
  for girls, 573f
Lennox-Gastaut syndrome, 559t–560t
  adjunctive therapy for, 1083
  therapy for, 837–838, 885, 1055
Lentigines, 218f
LEP (lower extremity placing) reflex, 236.e4t–236.e5t
Leprosy, 847
LET (lidocaine, epinephrine, tetracaine), 141t, 153t
Leucovorin, 613t–615t
Leukapheresis, 618
Leukemia, 532f
  acute, 1101
  acute lymphocytic leukemia (ALL), 609t–610t
  acute myeloid leukemia (AML), 609t–610t
  prophylaxis of, 1101
Leukocyte adhesion deficiency, 403t–404t
Leukocyte esterase test, 520
Leukocyte-poor platelet products, 392
Leukocyte-poor PRBCs, 391
Leukocytes, 373t
Leukomalacia, periventricular, 510
Leukopenia, 694t
Leukostasis, 612–616

Leukotriene inhibitors, 396
Leukotriene receptor antagonists (LTRAs), 651f–652f
Levalbuterol (Xopenex), 940
Levamisol, 536–537
Levaquin. *See* Levofloxacin
Levemir (insulin detemir), 260t
Levetiracetam (Keppra, Roweepra, Spritam)
  dose adjustment in renal failure, 1125t–1134t
  formulary entry, 940–941
  for seizures, 559t–560t, 562t
Levocarnitine. *See* Carnitine
Levofloxacin (Levaquin, Quixin, Iquix)
  dose adjustment in renal failure, 1111t–1124t
  formulary entry, 942–943
  for sinusitis, 461t–468t
  spectrum of activity, 450t
Levonorgestrel (Plan B One Step, Next Choice), 130–131
Levophed. *See* Norepinephrine bitartrate
Levothyroxine (T_4, Synthroid, Levoxyl, Tirosint, Unithroid), 943
Levoxyl. *See* Levothyroxine
Lexapro. *See* Escitalopram
LGA (large-for-gestational-age) infants, 493, 499f
Lialda. *See* Mesalamine
Lice, 1014
LiceMD. *See* Pyrethrins with piperonyl butoxie
Licide. *See* Pyrethrins with piperonyl butoxie
Lidocaine (Xylocaine, L-M-X, Lidoderm)
  for analgesia and sedation, 141t, 153t
  formulary entry, 944–945
  injectable, 142, 142t
  for intubation, 6f
  for local analgesia, 30
  for mucositis pain control, 625
  for RSI, 7t–8t
  topical, 141t
  viscous, 141t
Lidocaine, epinephrine, tetracaine (LET), 141t, 153t
Lidocaine and prilocaine (Oraqix, Eutectic mixture of lidocaine and prilocaine)
  for analgesia and sedation, 141t, 153t
  formulary entry, 945
Lidoderm. *See* Lidocaine

Life expectancy, 656
Lifestyle changes
　for GERD, 324
　for migraine headache, 553–555
Likelihood ratio (LR), 728
Limit setting, 233t–235t
Limiting interventions, 632–633
Lindane (gamma-genzene hexachloride), 946
Linear morphea, 701.e2
Linezolid (Zyvox)
　formulary entry, 946–947
　spectrum of activity, 452t
Lioresal. See Baclofen
Lip, cleft, 355, 355.e1f
Lipase: reference values, 709t–716t
Lipids
　goals for, 200
　recommendations for monitoring, 199–200
　reference values, 709t–716t
　screening, 199–200
Lisdexamfetamine (Vyvanse)
　ages of FDA approval, 245t
　formulary entry, 947–948
Lisinopril (Prinivil, Qbrelis, Zestril)
　dose adjustment in renal failure, 1125t–1134t
　formulary entry, 948
　for hypertension, 544t–545t
Literacy milestones, 233t
Lithium (Lithobid)
　dose adjustment in renal failure, 1125t–1134t
　formulary entry, 948–949
Live, attenuated influenza vaccine (LAIV), 415f–418f, 420, 422–423, 431
Liver cancer, 609t–610t
Liver cell injury, 325
Liver disease, 325–327, 387b
　bilirubin/urobilinogen in, 518t
　differential diagnosis of, 386f
　late effects of cancer treatment, 625.e1t–625.e2t
　warfarin therapy for, 1102
Liver failure
　in acetaminophen overdose, 26
　acute (ALF), 325–327
　severe, 703
Liver function tests, 325, 326t
Liver transplantation, 1074
LMA (laryngeal mask airway), 4
LMP (last menstrual period), 490.e1–490.e3

LMWH (low-molecular-weight heparin). See Low-molecular-weight heparin
LMX. See Lidocaine
LNs. See Lymph nodes
Local anesthetics, 30, 139–142
　injectable, 142, 142t
　topical, 139, 141t
Local candidiasis, 218f
Locomotion, 229
Lodoxamide (Alomide), 949
Lodoxamide-tromethamine, 397
Loeys-Dietz syndrome, 185t
Lomustine (CCNU), 613t–615t
Long arm posterior splint, 71f, 70.e1–70.e2
Long bone trauma, 80–81, 103t
Long QT syndrome, 173–179, 199.e1t
Long-acting beta$_2$-agonists (LABAs), 650f–652f, 900
Long-acting reversible contraception (LARC), 125
Loperamide (Imodium), 950
Lopressor. See Metoprolol
Loratadine (Alavert, Claritin)
　dose adjustment in renal failure, 1125t–1134t
　formulary entry, 950–951
Loratadine with pseudoephedrine (Claritin-D), 950–951
Lorazepam (Ativan), 151t, 139.e1t
　for antiemetic therapy, 626t
　formulary entry, 951–952
　for palliative care, 634t
　for seizures, 16t
Losartan (Cozaar)
　formulary entry, 952
　for hypertension, 544t–545t
Lotrimin AF. See Clotrimazole
Lotrimin AT. See Miconazole
Lovastatin, 385b
Lovenox. See Enoxaparin
Low-birth-weight (LBW) infants, 493
　immunoprophylaxis guidelines for, 424
　pain relief for, 143
　serum immunoglobulin levels, 408t
Low-density lipoprotein (LDL) cholesterol
　elevated levels, 200
　goals for, 200
　reference values, 709t–716t
Lower airway foreign bodies, 670
Lower extremity placing (LEP) reflex, 236.e4t–236.e5t
Lower motor neuron findings, 549t

Low-molecular-weight heparin (LMWH).
  See also Enoxaparin
  for Kawasaki disease, 198.e1t
  for stroke, 567
  for thrombosis, 380–382
Lozi-Flur. See Fluoride
LR (likelihood ratio), 728
LTRAs (leukotriene receptor
    antagonists), 651f–652f
Lucinactant. See Surfactant
Lumbar puncture, 48–50, 553, 553b,
    556
  indications for, 556
  in lateral (recumbent) position, 49,
    50f
  in sitting position, 49, 49f
  ultrasound marking, 49,
    49.e1f–49.e2f
Lumbar (sacral, pelvis) syndrome, 206
Luminal. See Phenobarbital
Lung(s), normal, 671f–674f
Lung fields, 183
Lung volumes, 643f, 643t
Lupus
  drug-induced, 695t
  maternal, 180t
Luteinizing hormone, 279t
Luxiq. See Betamethasone
Lyme disease, 198, 479t–480t
  early, 774
  ECG changes in, 180t
  treatment of, 823
Lymph nodes (LNs)
  cervical, 455.e1f
  direct infection of, 446
  pathologic, 607–611
  reactive, 446
Lymphadenitis, 454
  indolent, 446
  initial management of, 461t–468t
  suppurative, 446
Lymphadenopathy
  cervical, 454–455, 454f
  evaluation of, 446–455
  reactive, 454
Lymphangioma, 218f
Lymphocutaneous sporotrichosis, 1026
Lymphocytes, 373t
Lymphoma, 532f, 609t–610t
Lymphopenia, 694t
Lyrica (pregabalin), 562t
Lysosomal storage diseases, 344–346

M
Maalox. See Aluminum hydroxide with
    magnesium hydroxide
Macrobid. See Nitrofurantoin
Macrodantin. See Nitrofurantoin
α_2-Macroglobulin, 377t–378t
Macrolides
  for pharyngitis, 461t–468t
  spectrum of activity, 450t
Macules, 203, 204f–205f
  ash leaf, 352
  hypopigmented, 226–227, 226.e3f
Mag-200. See Magnesium oxide
Magnacal Renal formula, 601t–602t
Magnesium
  for migraine, 555
  in multivitamin tablets, 589t–590t
  recommended intakes, 591t
  reference values, 709t–716t
Magnesium citrate, 953
Magnesium disturbances, 309–310
Magnesium hydroxide (Milk of
    Magnesia)
  for constipation, 322
  formulary entry, 953
Magnesium hydroxide with aluminum
    hydroxide (Maalox, Mylanta,
    Almacone, RuLox), 767–768
Magnesium oxide (Mag-200, Mag-Ox
    400, Uro-Mag), 954
Magnesium sulfate ($MgSO_4$), 11,
    23t–24t
Magnetic resonance enterography
    (MRE), 316–317
Magnetic resonance imaging (MRI),
    663
  advantages and disadvantages of,
    664t
  of airway, 667
  brain, 558
  C-spine imaging, 667
  in dermatomyositis, 699
  of eyes, 665
  of head, 664–665
  in Legg-Calvé-Perthes disease, 681
  in osteomyelitis, 681
  in osteosarcoma, 682f–683f
  for seizures, 558
  ultrafast, 665
  in vessel abnormalities, 675–676
Mag-Ox 400. See Magnesium oxide
Major depressive disorder (MDD),
    249
Malabsorption, 330.e1
  differential diagnosis of, 278f
  prophylaxis of, 1099
  treatment of, 875
Malabsorption syndromes, 400, 1099
Malar rash, 694t

Malaria
 acute, 916
 chloroquine-resistant, 1030
 prevention of relapses, 1029
 prophylaxis of, 827, 866, 915, 956–957
 treatment of, 827, 916, 957, 1043
Malformations
 arteriovenous, 532f
 congenital, 665
Malignancy. *See also* Cancer
 diagnosis of, 218f
 lymphadenopathy in, 446
 secondary, 625.e1t–625.e2t
 signs and symptoms of, 609t–610t
Malignant hyperthermia, 846
Mallampati classification system, 147, 146.e2f
Malnutrition
 catch-up growth requirements in, 582–583
 treatment of, 1099
Manganese
 in multivitamin tablets, 589t–590t
 recommended intakes, 591t
Mania, bipolar, 1040–1041, 1052
Manic episodes, 993
Mannitol (Osmitrol, Resectisol)
 for elevated ICP, 85f
 formulary entry, 955
Mann-Whitney *U* test, 724t
Manometry, 553b
Maple syrup urine disease (MSUD), 339–341
Mapping, burn, 95
Marfan syndrome, 350–351
 AAP guidelines for, 351
 dominant cardiac defects, 185t
 sternal abnormalities in, 184
Marinol. *See* Dronabinol
Maroteaux-Lamy syndrome, 344–345
Mast cell stabilizers, 396–397
Mastocytosis, 218f, 842
Mastoiditis, 461t–468t
Maternal α-fetoprotein, 490.e1b
Maternal lupus, 180t
Matulane (procarbazine), 613t–615t
Maturity-onset diabetes of youth (MODY), 257
Matzim LA. *See* Diltiazem
Maxalt. *See* Rizatriptan
Maxidex. *See* Dexamethasone
Maxillary sinusitis, 819, 823, 835–836
Maximal expiratory pressure (MEP), 640–641

Maximal inspiratory pressure (MIP), 640–641
Maxipime. *See* Cefepime
3-MCC (3-methylcrotonyl-CoA carboxylase deficiency), 341
M-CHAT-R/F (Modified Checklist for Autism in Toddlers, Revised with Follow-Up), 237t–238t
MDR. *See* Multidrug resistance
Mean airway pressure (PAW), 90, 91.e1
Mean arterial pressure (MAP), 156
Mean cell hemoglobin concentration (MCHC), 365t
Mean corpuscular volume (MCV), 365t
Measles
 postexposure prophylaxis, 433–434
 vitamin A supplementation for, 471t–476t, 1099
Measles, mumps, rubella (MMR) vaccine, 432
 administration, 433
 catch-up schedule for, 414f
 after chemotherapy, 625.e3
 for children with HIV disease, 423
 dose, 433
 after HSCT, 625.e3
 after Ig or blood product administration, 426, 426.e1t
 postexposure, 433–434
 recommended schedule for, 413f, 415f–418f
 routine vaccination, 432–433
Measles, mumps, rubella, and varicella (MMRV) combination vaccine, 423
Measles/mumps/rubella immunoprophylaxis, 405, 432–434
 after Ig or blood product administration, 426.e1t
 intramuscular immune globulin (IMIG), 433–434
 postexposure prophylaxis, 433–434
Measurement bias, 722
Meatitis, 532f
Mebendazole (Emverm), 955
Mechanical ventilation, 971
Meckel's diverticulum, 678
Mediastinal masses, 674
Medical history, 112
Medical literature, 723–728
Medical Orders for Life-Sustaining Treatment (MOLST) forms, 633
Medications. *See* Drugs; *specific medications*
Medicosocial history, 109–110
Medium-chain acyl-CoA dehydrogenase (MCAD) disorders, 341

Medium-large vessel vasculitis, 696, 697t
Medrol. *See* Methylprednisolone
Medroxyprogesterone (Depo-Provera, Provera), 127–129, 128f, 131, 956
Medulloblastoma, 611t
Meetings, family, 629–630
Mefloquine HCl, 956–957
Mefoxin. *See* Cefoxitin
Melanoma, 226, 225.e2f, 226.e2f
Melanonychia, 225.e2f
Melanosis, neonatal pustular, 217–219
MELAS (mitochondrial encephalomyopathy, lactic acidosis) stroke-like episodes, 340
MELAS (mitochondrial encephalomyopathy, lactic acidosis) syndrome, 343
Mellaril. *See* Thioridazine
Melphalan (L-PAM, Alkeran), 613t–615t
Membranoproliferative glomerulonephritis, 532f
Memory making, 631–632
Menactra (MenACWY-D). *See* Meningococcal vaccines
MenHibrix (Hib-MenCY). *See* Meningococcal vaccines
Meningeal inflammation, 551b
Meningioma, 611t
Meningitis
 cryptococcal, 778, 889
 group B streptococcal, 1009
 neonatal, 461t–468t
 treatment of, 461t–468t, 780, 816, 818, 821–822, 826, 958, 999, 1009–1010, 1094
Meningococcal B vaccine (MenB)
 dose, 434
 MenB-4C (Bexsero), 415f–418f, 434
  guidelines for children with asplenia or persistent complement deficiency, 422
  recommended schedule for, 415f–418f
 MenB-FHbp (Trumenba), 415f–418f, 434
  guidelines for children with asplenia or persistent complement deficiency, 422
  recommended schedule for, 415f–418f
 recommended schedule for, 413f, 415f–418f
 side effects of, 434
Meningococcal conjugate vaccine (MCV4)
 for children with asplenia or persistent complement deficiency, 422
 for pre-teens and adolescents, 124t
Meningococcal disease, 421–422
Meningococcal immunoprophylaxis, 421–422, 434–435
Meningococcal vaccines (MenACWY, MPSV4), 434
 administration, 434
 catch-up schedule for, 414f
 for children at high risk for meningococcal disease, 421
 for children at increased risk, 421t
 for children with asplenia or persistent complement deficiency, 422
 for children with HIV disease, 423
 for children with sickle cell disease, 372t
 dose, 434
 Hib-MenCY combination (MenHibrix), 434, 442
  for children at high risk for meningococcal disease, 421
  for children at increased risk, 421t
  dose, 434
  PRP-T (Hiberix), 415f–418f, 428, 441
  recommended schedule for, 415f–418f
  side effects of, 434
 after HSCT, 625.e3
 MenACWY-CRM (Menveo), 434
  for children at increased risk, 421t
  recommended schedule for, 415f–418f
 MenACWY-D (Menactra), 434
  for children at increased risk, 421t
  recommended schedule for, 415f–418f
  in sickle cell disease, 372t
 postexposure, 435
 recommended schedule for, 413f, 415f–418f
 routine vaccination, 434
 side effects of, 434
Men's Rogaine Extra Strength. *See* Minoxidil
Mental health
 adolescent, 132–134
 changes as death approaches, 634
 web resources for, 229

Mental health disorders, 246–251
 referral and intervention for, 251
 screening tests for, 237t–238t
 surveillance for, 246
Mental status assessment, 13–15, 548
Mentzer index, 366
Menveo (MenACWY-CRM). *See* Meningococcal vaccines
MEP (maximal expiratory pressure), 640–641
Meperidine, 138, 1125t–1134t
Mephyton. *See* Phytonadione
Mepron. *See* Atovaquone
Mercaptoacetyl triglycine (MAG-3), 522
Mercaptopurine (6-MP)
 characteristics of, 613t–615t
 late effects of, 625.e1t–625.e2t
Mercury poisoning, 861
Meropenem (Merrem)
 dose adjustment in renal failure, 1111t–1124t
 formulary entry, 957–958
 spectrum of activity, 447t–449t
Mesalamine (Apriso, Asacol, Canasa, Delzicol, Lialda, Pentasa, Rowasa), 958–959
Mesna, 613t–615t
Mestinson. *See* Pyridostigmine bromide
Meta-analysis, 726t
Metabolic acidosis, 312, 334
 anion gap (AGMA), 312–314, 339f
  etiology of, 313f–314f
  in poisoning, 21.e1t–21.e3t
 correction of, 1062
 etiology of, 313f–314f
 expected compensatory response, 641t
 nonelevated anion gap (NAGMA), 312–314, 313f–314f
Metabolic alkalosis, 312
 etiology of, 313f–314f
 expected compensatory response, 641t
Metabolic crisis, 339–341
Metabolic disease
 categories of, 341–347
 clinical presentation of, 334, 336b
 evaluation of, 334–339, 336t
 laboratory testing in, 334–339
 sample collection for, 336t
 special considerations, 334–339
 when to suspect, 336b
Metabolic screening
 newborn, 340, 493

Metabolism, 334–347
Metadate. *See* Methylphenidate HCl
Metamucil. *See* Psyllium
Metanephrines
 plasma levels, 273
 urine levels, 287.e1t
Metastasis
 diagnosis of, 218f
 in osteosarcoma, 682f–683f
 skip, 682f–683f
Metformin (Glucophage, Glumetza, Fortamet, Riomet)
 formulary entry, 960
 with sulfonylureas, 960
Methadone HCl (Dolophine, Methadose), 140t, 139.e1t
 dose adjustment in renal failure, 1125t–1134t
 formulary entry, 961
 urine toxicology screen, 21t
Methadose. *See* Methadone HCl
Methamphetamine, 21t
Methemoglobin, 709t–716t
Methemoglobinemia, 962, 187.e1t
Methicillin-resistant *Staphylococcus aureus* infections, 947, 952
Methimazole (Tapazole)
 formulary entry, 961
 warfarin interactions, 385b
Methohexital, 145, 151t
Methotrexate (MTX, amethopterin, Folex, Mexate)
 for arthritis, 692
 characteristics of, 613t–615t
 for granulomatous disease, 701.e2
 late effects of, 625.e1t–625.e2t
 for SLE, 695
 toxicity, 691.e1t
Methylation analysis, 358t
Methylation disorders, 353–355
3-Methylcrotonyl-CoA carboxylase deficiency (3-MCC), 341
Methyldopa
 dose adjustment in renal failure, 1125t–1134t
 formulary entry, 962
Methylene blue (ProvayBlue), 962
Methylin. *See* Methylphenidate HCl
Methylmalonic acidemia (MMA), 341–342
Methylphenidate HCl (Ritalin, Aptensio XR, Methylin, Metadate, Concerta, QuilliChew ER, Quillivant XR, Daytrana)
 ages of FDA approval, 245t
 formulary entry, 963–964

Methylprednisolone (Medrol, Solu-Medrol, Depo-Medrol)
 for allergic emergencies, 10
 for asthma, 10
 formulary entry, 965
 potency of, 271t
Methylxanthine-refractory neonatal apnea, 865
Methylxanthines, 11
Metoclopramide (Reglan, Metozolv), 555
 for antiemetic therapy, 626t
 dose adjustment in renal failure, 1125t–1134t
 formulary entry, 965–966
 for migraine, 555
Metolazone, 966
Metoprolol (Lopressor, Toprol-XL)
 formulary entry, 966–967
 for hypertension, 544t–545t
Metozolv. *See* Metoclopramide
MetroCream. *See* Metronidazole
MetroGel. *See* Metronidazole
MetroLotion. *See* Metronidazole
Metronidazole (Flagyl, First-Metronidazole, MetroGel, MetroLotion, MetroCream, Rosadan, Noritate, Vandazole, Nuvessa)
 for bacterial vaginosis, 118t
 combined with amoxicillin and acid suppressing agent with/without clarithromycin, 968
 dose adjustment in renal failure, 1111t–1124t
 formulary entry, 967–969
 for gastroenteritis, 461t–468t
 for intra-abdominal infections, 461t–468t
 neonatal dosing, 513t–514t
 for PID, 115t–116t
 spectrum of activity, 452t
 for trichomoniasis, 118t
 warfarin interactions, 385b
Mexate. *See* Methotrexate
Miacalcin. *See* Calcitonin—salmon
Micafungin sodium (Mycamine)
 formulary entry, 969–970
 for oncology patients, 626t
Micatin. *See* Miconazole
Miconazole (Micatin, Lotrimin AT, Monistat, Vagistat-3)
 for candidal skin infections, 481t
 formulary entry, 970
 for ringworm, 481t
 warfarin interactions, 385b

Microalbuminuria
 definition of, 534
 screening for, 260
Microangiopathy, 375
 thrombotic (TMA), 375, 623
Microbiology, 443
Micromedex, 333
Micropenis, 287
Microscopic hematuria, 530
Microscopic polyangiitis, 697t
Microscopy, urinary, 516
Microsporum canis, 211–212
Microtubule inhibitors, 613t–615t
Microzide. *See* Hydrochlorothiazide
Midazolam
 for analgesia and sedation, 151t, 153t, 139.e1t
 dose adjustment in renal failure, 1125t–1134t
 formulary entry, 971–972
 for intubation, 6f
 ketamine + midazolam + atropine (ketazolam), 153t
 for procedural sedation, 153t
 for RSI, 7t–8t
Migergot. *See* Ergotamine tartrate with caffeine
Migraine cocktail, 555
Migraine headache, 553–555
 acute, 765, 1053–1054, 1107
 with aura, 553, 765
 close associations, 553
 confusional, 557t
 diagnostic criteria for, 553–555, 554b
 intractable, 1032
 precursors to, 553
 preventive therapy for, 556t
 prophylaxis of, 773, 845, 1034, 1084, 1092
 treatment of, 765, 1032, 1053–1054, 1107
 triptans for, 554–555, 554t
 without aura, 554b, 765
Migratory polyarthritis, 698
Milia, 219
Miliaria (heat rash, prickly heat), 218f, 219
Milk, human, 585–588, 594t–600t
Milk of Magnesia. *See* Magnesium hydroxide
Milk protein intolerance, 601t–602t
Millipred. *See* Prednisolone
Milrinone
 dose adjustment in renal failure, 1125t–1134t
 formulary entry, 972

Mineral metabolism disorders, 347.e1
Mineral oil (Kondremul, Fleet Mineral Oil)
  for disimpaction, 322
  formulary entry, 972
Mineralocorticoid effects, 271*t*
Mineralocorticoid maintenance, 272
Minerals
  newborn requirements for, 497
  requirements for, 584–585
Minimal change disease (MCD), 535–536
Minimum inhibitory concentration (MIC), 443
Mini-pill, 129
Minitran. *See* Nitroglycerin
Minocin. *See* Minocycline
Minocycline (Minocin, Solodyn, Arestin)
  for acne vulgaris, 217*t*
  formulary entry, 973
Minors, 114
Minoxidil (Minoxidil for Men, Hair Regrowth Treatment for Men, Men's Rogaine Extra Strength)
  formulary entry, 974
  for hypertension, 544*t*–545*t*
  for hypertensive urgency, 84*t*
Minute ventilation (V_E), 92–93
Miosis, 21.e1*t*–21.e3*t*
MIP (maximal inspiratory pressure), 640–641
MiraLax. *See* Polyethylene glycol (PEG) electrolyte solutions
Mitochondrial disease, 343, 334.e1
Mitochondrial encephalomyopathy, lactic acidosis (MELAS) stroke-like episodes, 340
Mitochondrial encephalomyopathy, lactic acidosis (MELAS) syndrome, 343
Mitoxantrone (dihydroxyanthracenedione dihydrochloride, Novantrone), 613*t*–615*t*
Mitral regurgitation, 166*b*
Mitral stenosis, 166*b*
Mitral valve prolapse (MVP), 199.e1*t*
Mixed connective tissue disease, 695*t*
MMA (methylmalonic acidemia), 341–342
MMR. *See* Measles, mumps, rubella (MMR) vaccine
MMRV (measles, mumps, rubella, and varicella) combination vaccine (ProQuad), 423, 441
Moderiba. *See* Ribavirin

Modification of Diet in Renal Disease (MDRD), 524
Modified Atkins diet, 561
Modified Checklist for Autism in Toddlers, Revised with Follow-Up (M-CHAT-R/F), 237*t*–238*t*, 244
Modified Schwartz equation, 1091
MODY (matury-onset diabetes of youth), 257
Moisturizers, sodium chloride, 1063
Molecularly targeted chemotherapeutic agents, 613*t*–615*t*
Moles, 226
Molluscum contagiosum, 208
MOLST (Medical Orders for Life-Sustaining Treatment) forms, 633
Molybdenum
  in multivitamin tablets, 589*t*–590*t*
  recommended intakes, 591*t*
Mometasone furoate (Asmanex, Nasonex, Elocon)
  dosages, 646.e1*t*–646.e2*t*
  formulary entry, 974–975
  potency, 223*t*
Mometasone furoate + formoterol fumarate (Dulera)
  dosages, 646.e1*t*–646.e2*t*
  formulary entry, 974–975
Mongolian spots, 219
Moniliformis, 1037
Monistat. *See* Miconazole
Monobactams, 447*t*–449*t*
Monoclonal antibodies, 406
Monoclonal factor VIII, 392
Monocytes, 373*t*
Monodox. *See* Doxycycline
Monogen formula, 594*t*–602*t*
Monogenic diabetes, 256
Mononucleosis, infectious, 471*t*–476*t*
Montelukast (Singulair)
  for allergic rhinitis, 396
  for asthma, 650*f*
  formulary entry, 976
Morbidity and Mortality Weekly Reports (CDC), 412
Moro reflex, 236.e4*t*–236.e5*t*
Morphea, 701.e2
  linear, 701.e2
  treatment of, 701.e3
Morphine, 140*t*, 139.e1*t*
  analgesic properties, 139
  dose adjustment in renal failure, 1125*t*–1134*t*
  opioid tapering, 146*b*
  for palliative care, 634*t*
  for PCA, 143*t*

Morphine *(Continued)*
 for TET spells, 189*t*
 urine toxicology screen, 21*t*
Morphine equivalents, 139
Morphine sulfate (Roxanol, MS Contin, Oramorph SR, Avinza, Kadian)
 formulary entry, 976–978
 for TET spells, 189*t*
Morquio syndrome, 344–345
Mosteller BSA (m^2) equation, 1091
Motion sickness, 1033, 1056
Motor development, 237*t*–238*t*
Motor examination, 548
Motrin. *See* Ibuprofen
Mouth-to-mouth breathing, 9
Mouth-to-nose breathing, 9
Movement examination, 551
Moxatag. *See* Amoxicillin
Moxifloxacin, 450*t*
6-MP. *See* Mercaptopurine
MPSV4. *See* Meningococcal vaccines
MRE (magnetic resonance enterography), 316–317
MRI. *See* Magnetic resonance imaging
MS Contin. *See* Morphine sulfate
MSUD (maple syrup urine disease), 339–341
MTX. *See* Methotrexate
Mucociliary clearance, 656
Mucocutaneous herpes, 760–761, 883
Mucomyst. *See* Acetylcysteine
Mucopolysaccharidoses, 344–345
Mucosal emergencies, allergic, 9
Mucositis, 624–625
Multidisciplinary intervention, 246
Multidrug resistance (MDR), 486
Multidrug-resistant tuberculosis, 1066
Multiple endocrine neoplasia (MEN) syndromes, 267.e1*b*
Multiple gene panels, 358*t*
Multisystem disease, 531*t*
Multivehicle collisions (MVCs), 76
Multivitamin tablets, 589*t*–590*t*
Mumps, 432–434, 471*t*–476*t*
Mupirocin (Bactroban), 978
Murmurs, 165–166
Muscarinic poisoning, 22*t*
Muscarinic symptoms, 787
Muscle biopsy, 699
Muscle bulk, 548
Muscle disease, 551
Muscle enzymes, 704
Muscle relaxants, 856
Muscle stretch reflexes, 550.e1*t*
Muscle tone, 493*t*, 548

Musculoskeletal exam, 112, 113.e1*f*
Musculoskeletal procedures, 68–70
Musculoskeletal system, 625.e1*t*–625.e2*t*
Mutation analysis, 358*t*
My Family Health Portrait Tool (HHS), 334
Myambutol. *See* Ethambutol HCl
Myasthenia gravis
 diagnosis of, 868, 984
 treatment of, 984, 1039
Mycamin. *See* Micafungin sodium
Mycobacterial infection, nontuberculous, 882
Mycobacterium avium complex
 in AIDS, 882
 in HIV, 789–790
 prophylaxis of, 836, 1049
 treatment of, 789–790, 836, 882, 1049
Mycobutin. *See* Rifabutin
Mycophenolate, 978–979
Mycophenolate mofetil (CellCept)
 for arthritis, 692
 formulary entry, 978–979
 for GVHD, 621
 for nephrotic syndrome, 536–537
 for SLE, 695
Mycophenolic acid (Myfortic), 978–979
Mycoplasma, 691
Mycosis, urinary tract, 777
Mycostatin. *See* Nystatin
Mydriasis, 21.e1*t*–21.e3*t*
Myeloablative chemotherapy, 619
Myelocele, 667
Myelomeningocele, 667
Myferon 150. *See* Polysaccharide-iron complex
Myfortic. *See* Mycophenolic acid
Mylanta. *See* Aluminum hydroxide with magnesium hydroxide
Mylanta Gas. *See* Simethicone
Mylicon. *See* Simethicone
Myocardial disease, 193–194
Myocardial infarction, 182, 182*f*
Myocarditis, 194
Myoclonic epilepsy, 559*t*–560*t*
Myoclonic seizures, 558*b*, 941
Myoclonus, 557*t*
Myofibromatosis, 218*f*
Myoglobin, 517
Myoglobinuria, 517
Myorisan. *See* Isotretinoid
Myositis, 704

Myotonic dystrophy, 180*t*
Mysoline. *See* Primidone
Myxedema coma, 943

N

Nafcillin
  formulary entry, 979–980
  for osteomyelitis, 461*t*–468*t*
  for septic arthritis, 461*t*–468*t*
  spectrum of activity, 447*t*–449*t*
  warfarin interactions, 385*b*
Nafcillin/oxacillin, 461*t*–468*t*
Nägele rule, 490.e1–490.e3
NAGMA (nonelevated anion gap metabolic acidosis), 312–314, 313*f*–314*f*
Nail clubbing, 225, 225.e4*f*
Nail disorders, 224–225
  acquired, 224–225
  congenital/hereditary, 225, 225.e6*f*
  ringworm, 481*t*
Nail dystrophy, 225, 225.e1*f*–225.e3*f*
Nail hypoplasia, congenital, 225, 225.e6*f*
Nail psoriasis, 225, 225.e3*f*
Nails, atopic, 225
Naloxone (Narcan, Evzio)
  for coma, 14
  formulary entry, 980–981
  for procedural sedation reversal, 148, 152*b*
NanoVM, 589*t*–590*t*
Naprelan. *See* Naproxen sodium
Naproxen (Naprosyn)
  analgesic properties, 139
  for arthritis, 691
  formulary entry, 981–982
Naproxen sodium (Anaprox, Naprelan, Aleve), 981–982
Naratriptan (Amerge), 554*t*
Narcan. *See* Naloxone
Narcolepsy, 557*t*, 776–777, 855
NARES (nonallergic rhinitis with eosinophilia syndrome), 396
Nasacort Allergy 24HR. *See* Triamcinolone
Nasal airway, 4
Nasal Allergy 24 Hour. *See* Triamcinolone
Nasal decongestants, 1017
Nasal polyps, 396
Nasal rinsing, 397
Nasalcrom. *See* Cromolyn
Nasalide. *See* Flunisolide
Nasarel. *See* Flunisolide

Nascobal. *See* Cyanocobalamin
Nasoduodenal (ND) tube placement, 678
Nasogastric tube (NGT), 5
Nasonex. *See* Mometasone furoate
Nasopharyngeal airway, 4
Natal sex, 123–125
National Asthma Education and Prevention Program, 637
National Cancer Institute (NCI)
  Clinical Trial Database, 607
  SEER (Surveillance, Epidemiology, and End Results) data, 607
  web resources, 607
National Center for Learning Disabilities, 229
National Dissemination Center for Children with Disabilities (NICHCY), 229
National Early Childhood Technical Assistance Center, 229
National Guideline Clearinghouse, 721
National Heart, Lung, and Blood Institute (NHLBI), 637, 965, 1029
National Hospice and Palliative Care Organization, 628
National Institute of Child Health and Human Development, 570
National Institute of Mental Health (NIMH), 229
National Institutes of Health (NIH)
  Asthma Guideline 2007 recommendations, 801
  LactMed, 588
National Kidney Disease Education Program, 516
National Kidney Foundation
  guidelines for renal failure, 804
  web resources, 516
National Library of Medicine (NLM), 721.e1
  LactMed, 588
National Newborn Screening and Genetics Resource Center, 333
National Organization for Rare Disorders, 333
National Suicide Prevention Lifeline, 251
Nausea and vomiting, 318
  in acute gastroenteritis, 997
  chemotherapy-induced, 625
    prevention of, 996
    treatment of, 864, 908
  differential diagnosis of, 319*t*

Nausea and vomiting *(Continued)*
  medications for palliative care, 634*t*
  postoperative
    prevention of, 996–997
    treatment of, 864, 908, 966
  radiation-induced
    prevention of, 997
    treatment of, 908
  treatment of, 1033
Navelbine. *See* Vinorelbine
NCI. *See* National Cancer Institute
ND (nasoduodenal) tube placement, 678
NDM (neonatal diabetes), 257
Nebcin. *See* Tobramycin
Nebulization, 1076
NebuPent. *See* Pentamidine isethionate
Neck: secondary survey of, 74*t*–75*t*
Necrotizing enterocolitis
  minimizing risk for, 508
  modified Bell's staging system for, 507.e1*t*
  in newborns, 507–508
Nedocromil (Alocril)
  for allergic rhinitis, 397
  for asthma, 651*f*–652*f*
Needle decompression, 51–55
Negative inspiratory force (NIF), 92
Negative predictive value (NPV), 728
Neisseria gonorrhoeae infections, 691
  screening guidelines for sexually active adolescents, 117
  treatment of, 817
Neisseria meningitidis, 1050
Nembutal. *See* Pentobarbital
Neo Polycin. *See* Neomycin/polymyxin B + bacitracin
Neo To Go. *See* Neomycin/polymyxin B + bacitracin
NeoBenz Micro. *See* Benzoyl peroxide
Neocate formulas, 570, 594*t*–602*t*
Neofax, 490
Neo-fradin. *See* Neomycin sulfate
Neomycin sulfate (Neo-fradin), 982
Neomycin sulfate, polymyxin B sulfate, hydrocortisone otic, 1025
Neomycin/polymyxin B (Neosporin GU)
  formulary entry, 984
  for otitis externa, 461*t*–468*t*
Neomycin/polymyxin B + bacitracin (Neosporin, Neo To Go, Neo-Polycin, Triple Antibiotic), 983–984
Neomycin/polymyxin B + bacitracin + hydrocortisone (Neo-Polycin HC), 983
Neomycin/polymyxin B + gramicidin (Neosporin Ophthalmic Solution), 983
Neomycin/polymyxin B + hydrocortisone, 983
Neonatal abstinence syndrome, 510, 840
Neonatal acne, 219
Neonatal Advanced Life Support (NALS), 490
Neonatal alloimmune thrombocytopenia (NAIT), 374–375
Neonatal apnea, 770, 802, 865, 1077
Neonatal dermatology
  conditions, 216–220
  web resources, 490
Neonatal diabetes (NDM), 257
Neonatal enterocolitis, 676
Neonatal gonococcal ophthalmia prophylaxis, 878
Neonatal hypoglycemia evaluation, 286–287
Neonatal hypoxic-ischemic encephalopathy (HIE), 508, 509*t*
Neonatal Infant Pain Scale (NIPS), 136
Neonatal infections
  bacterial, 455–470
  conjunctivitis, 461*t*–468*t*
  initial management of, 455–470, 461*t*–468*t*
  meningitis, 461*t*–468*t*
  pneumonia, 461*t*–468*t*
  septic arthritis, 461*t*–468*t*
Neonatal Intensive Care Unit, 513*t*–514*t*
Neonatal ketoacidosis, 517
Neonatal lupus, 696
Neonatal pustular melanosis, 217–219
Neonatal rash, 218*f*
Neonatal Resuscitation Program (NRP), 490
Neonatal seizures, 338, 559*t*–560*t*
Neonatal thrombocytopenia, 374–375
Neonatal thyrotoxicosis, 266
Neonates. *See* Newborn care; Newborns
Neonatology, 490–515
Neo-Polycin. *See* Neomycin/polymyxin B + bacitracin
Neo-Polycin HC. *See* Neomycin/polymyxin B + bacitracin + hydrocortisone
NeoProfen. *See* Ibuprofen
Neoral. *See* Cyclosporine
Neosporin. *See* Neomycin/polymyxin B + bacitracin
Neosporin GU. *See* Neomycin/polymyxin B

Neosporin Ophthalmic Solution. *See* Neomycin/polymyxin B + gramicidin
Neostigmine (Prostigmin, Bioxiverz)
  dose adjustment in renal failure, 1125t–1134t
  formulary entry, 984–985
  for vecuronium bromide overdose, 1097
NeoSure, 570
Neo-Synephrine. *See* Phenylephrine HCl
Neo-Synephrine 12-Hour Nasal. *See* Oxymetazoline
Nephritis
  acute nephritic syndrome, 530
  interstitial, 527t
  SLE, 693, 693.e1t
Nephrogenic diabetes insipidus, 275t, 276, 537–538
Nephrogenic systemic fibrosis, 530
Nephrolithiasis, 542–545
Nephrolithotomy, percutaneous, 543
Nephrology, 516–547
Nephrotic syndrome, 534–537
  etiology of, 536b, 536t
  frequently relapsing, 536
  idiopathic, 535–537
  management of, 535–537, 978–979, 1029
  steroid-dependent, 536–537
  steroid-resistant, 537
Nephrotic-range proteinuria, 534
Nepro formula, 594t–602t
Nerve agent poisoning, 787
Nervous system instability, 21.e1t–21.e3t
Neupogen. *See* Filgrastim
Neuritis, drug-induced, 1039
Neuroblastoma, 609t–610t, 613t–615t
Neurocutaneous syndromes, 351–352
Neurofibroma, 532f
Neurofibromatosis type I (NF1), 351–352
Neurogenic shock, 86.e1t
Neuroimaging, 553
Neurologic deficit, acute-onset focal, 566b
Neurologic disease
  in newborns, 508–511
  oxygen challenge test findings in, 187.e1t
  in SLE, 694t
Neurologic emergencies, 13–17
Neurologic examination, 548–551
  age-directed, 236
  in headaches, 551.e1t

Neurologic examination *(Continued)*
  in increased ICP, 82
  secondary survey, 74t–75t
  system review, 111
Neurology, 548–569
Neurology consultation, urgent, 567
Neuromuscular blockers
  nondepolarizing, 984
  for RSI, 7t–8t
Neuromuscular disease, 643t
Neuromuscular maturity, 493–495, 494f
Neurontin. *See* Gabapentin
Neuropathic pain, 903
Neurosyphilis, 1010–1011
Neurovascular survey, 74t–75t
Neut. *See* Sodium bicarbonate
Neutropenia, 372–373
  in chemotherapy patients, 624
  differential diagnosis of, 374b
  empiric therapy for, 778, 958
  febrile, 778
  oncologic emergency, 618–619, 620f
  severe, 372–373
Neutropenic enterocolitis, 618
Neutrophils, 373t
Nevi
  nevomelanocytic, 226, 226.e1f
  pigmented, 226
Nevirapine (NVP, Viramune)
  formulary entry, 985–986
  for perinatal HIV exposure, 481t
  reduction of resistance to, 935
Nevomelanocytic nevi, 226, 226.e1f
Nevus depigmentosus, 218f
New Pediatric Labeling Information, 732
Newborn assessment, 493–496
  CSF evaluation, 717t
Newborn care, 492
  exchange transfusion, 505–506, 506f
  exogenous surfactant therapy, 500
  fluid and electrolyte management, 496–497
  in hyperglycemia, 498t
  in hypoglycemia, 498t, 499f
  medications used in NICU, 513
  nutrition, 497
  pain relief, 142–143
  phototherapy, 505, 505f, 505t
  respiratory considerations, 500
  routine, 492–493
  supplemental O_2, 500
  UFH dose initiation guidelines, 381t
  vaccinations, 493
Newborn desquamation, 218f
Newborn resuscitation, 490–492

Newborn screening (NBS)
for congenital adrenal hyperplasia, 270–271
for cystic fibrosis, 655
for hypothyroidism, 262
metabolic, 340, 493
Newborns
cardiac diseases in, 503–504
cyanosis in, 497–500
electrolyte requirements, 498t
extradural fluid collection in, 495t, 496f
gastrointestinal diseases in, 507–508
glucose requirements, 496–497
Grave's disease in, 1026
Hb electrophoresis patterns in, 369t
of HbsAg status unknown or positive mothers, 425f
hematologic diseases in, 504–507
hemorrhagic disease in, 1020
hypertension in, 541t
mineral requirements, 497
neurologic diseases in, 508–511
organic acidemia in, 341
peripheral nerve injuries in, 511
persistent pulmonary hypertension of the newborn (PPHN), 501–502
pulmonary flow murmur of, 167t
reference values, 709t–716t
respiratory diseases in, 500–502
respiratory distress syndrome in, 500–501
total blood volume, 389t
trisomy 21 in, 348
with *in utero* HIV exposure, 482t
vitamin requirements, 497
water requirements, 497t
Nexiclon XR. See Clonidine
Nexium. See Esomeprazole
Next Choice (levonorgestrel), 130
Nexterone. See Amiodarone
Next-generation sequencing, 358t
NF1 (neurofibromatosis type I), 351–352
NGT (nasogastric tube), 5
NH$_2$, 326t
NHL (non-Hodgkin lymphoma), 609t–610t
Niacin (vitamin B$_3$, Niacor, Niaspan, Slo-Niacin, Nicotinic acid)
formulary entry, 986
in infant multivitamin drops, 588t
in multivitamin tablets, 589t–590t
recommended intakes, 586t
Niacor. See Niacin
Niaspan. See Niacin

Nicardipine (Cardene)
formulary entry, 986–987
for hypertensive emergency, 83t
Nicotine poisoning, 23t–24t
Nicotinic acid. See Niacin
Nicotinics, 22t
Niemann-Pick disease, 345–346
NIF (negative inspiratory force), 92
Nifediac CC. See Nifedipine
Nifedipine (Adalat CC, Nifediac CC, Procardia)
extended-release, 544t–545t
formulary entry, 987–988
for hypertension, 544t–545t
for Raynaud phenomenon, 701
Niferex. See Iron, oral preparations
Night feeding, trained, 233t–235t
Night terrors, 233t–235t, 557t
Night waking, 233t–235t, 658
Nightmares, 233t–235t, 659
Nighttime fears, 659
Nilstat. See Nystatin
NIPPV (noninvasive positive-pressure ventilation), 11, 90
Nipride. See Nitroprusside
NIPS (Neonatal Infant Pain Scale), 136
Nitisinone (NTBC), 342
Nitric oxide (NO), inhaled, 88–89, 502
Nitrite test, 519–520
Nitro-Bid. See Nitroglycerin
Nitro-Dur. See Nitroglycerin
Nitrofurantoin (Furadantin, Macrodantin, Macrobid)
for cystitis, 461t–468t
formulary entry, 988
spectrum of activity, 452t
Nitroglycerin (Nitro-Bid, Nitrostat, Nitro-Time, Nitro-Dur, Nitrolingual, Minitran), 989
Nitrolingual. See Nitroglycerin
Nitroprusside (Nitropress), 990
Nitrostat. See Nitroglycerin
Nitro-Time. See Nitroglycerin
Nitrous oxide, 149b–150b
Nix. See Permethrin
Nizoral. See Ketoconazole
NNH (number needed to harm), 727
NNT (number needed to treat), 727
Nocturnal enuresis, 851, 990
Nodal escape/junctional rhythm, 174t–175t
Nodular acne, 929
Nodules, 203, 204f–205f
Nonallergic rhinitis with eosinophilia syndrome (NARES), 396

Nonelevated anion gap metabolic acidosis (NAGMA), 312–314, 313f–314f
Non-Hodgkin lymphoma (NHL), 609t–610t
Noninvasive positive-pressure ventilation (NIPPV), 11, 90
Nonketotic hyperglycinemia (NKH), 340
Nonsteroidal anti-inflammatory drugs (NSAIDs)
  analgesic properties, 139
  for arthritis, 691
  for migraine, 554–555
  overdose, 23t–24t
  for scleroderma, 701.e3
  for Sjögren syndrome, 701.e4
  for SLE, 695
  ulcers induced by
    prevention of, 880
    treatment of, 939
Noonan syndrome, 356
  AAP guidelines for, 356
  differential diagnosis of, 278f
  dominant cardiac defects, 185t
  sternal abnormalities in, 184
Norcuron. See Vecuronium bromide
Norepinephrine
  normal plasma levels, 287.e2t
  normal urine levels, 287.e1t
  for shock, 87f
Norepinephrine bitartrate (Levophed), 990
Norfloxacin, 1111t–1124t
Noritate. See Metronidazole
Normal saline (NS)
  composition of, 302t
  for hypernatremic dehydration, 297
  for metabolic crisis, 339
  rapid fluid resuscitation with, 297
Normal serum albumin (human). See Albumin
Normetanephrines, 287.e1t
Normodyne. See Labetalol
North American Society for Pediatric Gastroenterology, Hepatology, and Nutrition, 316
Nortriptyline hydrochloride (Pamelor)
  formulary entry, 990–991
  for migraine prevention, 556t
Norvasc. See Amlodipine
Norwood shunt, 190f, 191
Nose: animal bites to, 93
Nosocomial pneumonia, 1023
Nostrilla. See Oxymetazoline
NovaFerrum. See Polysaccharide-iron complex

Novantrone. See Mitoxantrone
Novasource Renal formula, 594t–600t
Novolin N (isophane insulin), 260t
NovoLog (insulin aspart), 260t
NovoLog Mix (insulin aspart), 260t
NovoSeven (rhFVIIa), 384t
NPV (negative predictive value), 728
NRP (Neonatal Resuscitation Program), 490
NS. See Normal saline
NSAIDs. See Nonsteroidal anti-inflammatory drugs
Nuclear medicine, 664t
Nucleic acid amplification test (NAAT), 117
5′-Nucleotidase (5′-NT), 326t
Nucleotide analogs, 613t–615t
NuCort. See Hydrocortisone
NuLYTELY. See Polyethylene glycol (PEG) electrolyte solutions
Number needed to harm (NNH), 727
Number needed to treat (NNT), 727
NURSE method, 630–631
Nursemaid's elbow (radial head subluxation) reduction, 70
Nurses, 628
NUTRA Shake, 601t–602t
Nutramigen formulas, 570, 601t–602t
Nutren formulas, 570, 594t–600t
Nutren Junior formulas, 594t–602t
Nutr-E-Sol. See Vitamin E
NutriRenal formula, 601t–602t
Nutrition, 570–606
Nutritional assessment, 570–577
  clinical, 571
  laboratory studies, 571
  systems review, 111
Nutritional rickets, 875
Nutritional support
  for cystic fibrosis, 656
  newborn care, 497
Nuvessa. See Metronidazole
NVP. See Nevirapine
Nydrazid. See Isoniazid
Nystagmus, 21.e1t–21.e3t
Nystatin (Bio-Statin)
  for candidiasis, 481t
  formulary entry, 991

O
Obesity, 571
  hypothyroidism and, 262
  management of, 574–577, 574.e1f
  treatment of, 777
Obsessive-compulsive disorder, 893, 898, 1008–1009, 1058

Obstructive hypoventilation, 656
Obstructive shock, 86, 86.e1t
Obstructive sleep apnea syndrome (OSAS), 656–658, 657b
Occult bood test, 330
Occupational therapy, 693
Ocean. See Sodium chloride
OCPs (oral contraceptive pills), 129, 214
Octreotide acetate (Sandostatin)
   formulary entry, 991–992
   for sulfonylureas poisoning, 23t–24t
Ocuflox. See Ofloxacin
Odds ratio (OR), 727
Odontoid views, 667
Odors, 21.e1t–21.e3t
Ofirmev. See Acetaminophen
Ofloxacin (Floxin Otic, Ocuflox)
   formulary entry, 992
   spectrum of activity, 450t
OGTT (oral glucose tolerance test), 255–256
OI (oxygenation index), 93
Oil of wintergreen odor, 21.e1t–21.e3t
Olanzapine (Zyprexa)
   for antiemetic therapy, 626t
   formulary entry, 993–994
Oligo chromosomal microarrays, 358t
Oligodendroglioma, 611t
Oligohydramnios, 490.e2b
Oliguria, 528, 528t, 955
Olopatadine (Patanol, Pataday, Pazeo, Patanase)
   for allergic rhinitis, 396–397
   formulary entry, 994–995
Omeprazole (Prilosec, First-Omeprazole, Omeprazole and Syrspend SF Alka)
   formulary entry, 995–996
   warfarin interactions, 385b
Omeprazole and Syrspend SF Alka. See Omeprazole
Omeprazole with sodium bicarbonate (Zegerid), 995–996
OMIM (Online Mendelian Inheritance in Man), 333, 347–357
Omnaris. See Ciclesonide
Omnicef. See Cefdinir
Omnipaque. See Iohexol
Omnipred. See Prednisolone
Omphalocele, 508.e1t
Oncologic emergencies, 612–619
Oncology, 607–627. See also Cancer
   antimicrobial prophylaxis in, 625, 626t
   web resources, 607

Oncovin. See Vincristine
Ondansetron (Zofran, Zuplenz)
   for antiemetic therapy, 626t
   formulary entry, 996–997
   for palliative care, 634t
One-sample (paired) t test, 724t
One-tailed tests, 723
Onfi. See Clobazam
Online Mendelian Inheritance in Man (OMIM), 333, 347–357
Onmel. See Itraconazole
Onychomycosis, 225, 225.e1f
Open Epi, 721.e1
Open pneumothorax, 79
Ophthalmic agents, 397
Ophthalmologic examination
   in child abuse, 102
   dysmorphology evaluation, 347
   follow-up, 513.e1t
   screening, 688
   in sickle cell retinopathy, 372t
Opiate withdrawal, 511b
Opiate-induced pruritus, 980
Opioids, 139
   commonly used opiates, 140t
   poisoning or overdose (intoxication), 22t–24t, 980
   properties of, 149b–150b
   tapering, 146b
Optic glioma, 611t
Opticrom. See Cromolyn
Optivar. See Azelastine
OPV. See Oral poliovirus
Oracea. See Doxycycline
Oral airway, 4
Oral allergy syndrome, 398
Oral candidiasis (thrush), 481t, 841
Oral contraceptives (OCPs, Ortho Tri Cyclen, Estrostep, Yaz), 129, 214
Oral food challenges, 400
Oral glucose tolerance test (OGTT), 255–256
Oral poliovirus (OPV) vaccine, 422, 435
   for children with HIV disease, 423
   contraindications to, 435
Oral rehydration salts (WHO), 603t
Oral rehydration solution (ORS), 301, 603t
Oral rehydration therapy (ORT), 301
   composition of fluids, 302t
   for diarrhea, 320
   fluids not recommended for, 302t
Oral ulcers, 694t, 699–700
Oralone. See Triamcinolone
Oramorph SR. See Morphine sulfate

Oraprep ODT. *See* Prednisolone
Oraqix. *See* Lidocaine and prilocaine
OraVerse. *See* Phentolamine mesylate
Orazinc. *See* Zinc salts
Orbital cellulitis
  imaging of, 666, 666*f*
  initial management of, 461*t*–468*t*
Organic acids, urine, 336*t*
Organophosphate overdose, 23*t*–24*t*, 787
Ornithine transcarbamylase (OTC) deficiency, 337*f*, 340, 342
Oropharyngeal candidiasis, 889, 991
ORS (oral rehydration solution), 301
ORT. *See* Oral rehydration therapy
Ortho Tri Cyclen. *See* Oral contraceptives
Orthopedic screening examination, 113.*e1f*
Orthopedic surgery, 693
Orthopedic trauma, 80–81
Orthopedic Trauma Association, 73
Orthostatic proteinuria, 534
OSAS (obstructive sleep apnea syndrome), 656–658, 657*b*
Oscillatory ventilation, high-frequency (HFOV), 90.*e1*
Oseltamivir phosphate (Tamiflu)
  dose adjustment in renal failure, 1111*t*–1124*t*
  formulary entry, 997–998
  for influenza, 471*t*–476*t*
Osmitrol. *See* Mannitol
Osmolality
  reference values, 709*t*–716*t*
  serum, 312
  urine, 526
Osmolar gap
  serum, 312, 21.*e1t*–21.*e3t*
  stool (Stool Osm), 319
Osmolar gap disturbances, 312–314
Osmolarity, 21.*e1t*–21.*e3t*
Osmolite formulas, 594*t*–600*t*
OsmoPrep. *See* Sodium phosphate
Osmotic diarrhea, 319
Osmotic fragility test, 368
Osmotic laxatives, 322
Osteoarthritis, 718*t*
Osteochondroma, 681, 682*f*–683*f*
Osteogenesis imperfecta, 803
Osteoid osteoma, 681, 681.*e5f*
Osteomalacia, 267*t*
Osteomyelitis, 681
  imaging, 681
  initial management of, 461*t*–468*t*

Osteonecrosis, 681.*e2f*
Osteopenia, 693
Osteosarcoma, 609*t*–610*t*, 682*f*–683*f*
OTC (ornithine transcarbamylase) deficiency, 342
Otic analgesia, 781
Otitis externa, 206
  acute, 834
  initial management of, 461*t*–468*t*
  treatment of, 834, 992, 1025
Otitis media
  acute, 461*t*–468*t*, 822, 834–835
    recurrent or persistent, 942
    with tympanostomy tubes, 992
  chronic suppurative, 992
  initial management of, 461*t*–468*t*
  treatment of, 816, 819–821, 823
Otovel Otic. *See* Ciprofloxacin
Outcomes calculator, 490
Outpatient care
  for animal bites, 95
  for burns, 96
Ovarian torsion, 680
Ovaries
  imaging, 680
  polycystic, 282
Overdose. *See* Poisoning
Overweight, 571, 574–577
Oxacillin
  for dacrocystitis, 461*t*–468*t*
  formulary entry, 999
  for lymphadenitis, 461*t*–468*t*
  neonatal dosing, 513*t*–514*t*
  for osteomyelitis, 461*t*–468*t*
  for parotitis, 461*t*–468*t*
  for septic arthritis, 461*t*–468*t*
  spectrum of activity, 447*t*–449*t*
Oxcarbazepine (Trileptal, Oxtellar XR)
  dose adjustment in renal failure, 1125*t*–1134*t*
  formulary entry, 999–1001
  for seizures, 559*t*–560*t*, 562*t*
Oxtellar XR. *See* Oxcarbazepine
Oxy-5. *See* Benzoyl peroxide
Oxy-10. *See* Benzoyl peroxide
Oxybutynin chloride (Ditropan XL, Oxytrol), 1001
Oxycodone (OxyContin, Roxicodone, Xtampza ER)
  analgesic properties, 140*t*, 139.*e1t*
  formulary entry, 1002
Oxycodone and acetaminophen (Endocet, Roxilox, Percocet, Roxicet), 1002
Oxycodone and aspirin, 1003

OxyContin. *See* Oxycodone
Oxygen
 arterial O$_2$ saturation (SaO$_2$), 637–638
 arteriovenous O$_2$ difference (AVDO$_2$), 93.*e*1
Oxygen challenge test, 187.*e*1*t*
Oxygen content (CaO$_2$), 93.*e*1
Oxygen (O$_2$) extraction ratio, 93.*e*1
Oxygen therapy
 for acute pulmonary hypertensive crisis, 88–89
 for asthma, 11
 for croup, 13
 for newborns, 500
Oxygenation index (OI), 93
Oxyhemoglobin dissociation curve, 638, 639*f*
Oxymetazoline (Afrin 12 Hour, Neo-Synephrine 12-Hour Nasal, Nostrilla), 1003
Oxytocin, 273
Oxytrol. *See* Oxybutynin chloride

P
p value, 723
P wave, 166, 169
PA (physical activity coefficient), 580, 580.*e*1*t*
PA (propionic acidemia), 341
PAC. *See* Premature atrial contraction
Pacerone. *See* Amiodarone
Packed red blood cells (PRBCs)
 for cancer patients, 624
 exchange transfusion, 392–393
 leukocyte-poor, 391
 transfusion, 390–391, 624
 transfusion after Ig or blood product administration, 426.*e*1*t*
Paget's disease, 803
Pain
 abdominal, 317–318, 318*t*, 698
 acute, 136
 behavioral response to, 136
 cancer, 886
 chronic, 136, 772, 919
 endometriosis-associated, 956
 extremity pain, 690*t*
 joint pain, 690*t*
 neuropathic, 903
Pain assessment, 136
 in adolescents, 136
 FACES scale, 136, 138*f*
 FLACC tool, 136, 137*t*
 in infants, 136
 in preschoolers, 136
 in school-age children, 136

Pain specialists, 628
Paired (one-sample) *t* test, 724*t*
Paired tests, 723
PAL (physical activity level), 579
Palate, cleft, 355, 355.*e*1*f*
Palivizumab (Synagis), 406, 437–438
 formulary entry, 1003–1004
 for high-risk infants, 653
 after Ig or blood product administration, 426.*e*1*t*
 routine vaccination, 437–438
Palliative care, 628
 medications for symptomatic relief in, 634*t*
 model for, 629*f*
 web resources, 628
Palliative care teams, 628
Palmar grasp, 236.*e*4*t*–236.*e*5*t*
PALS (Pediatric Advanced Life Support), 73
2-PAM. *See* Pralidoxime chloride
L-PAM, 613*t*–615*t*
Pamelor. *See* Nortriptyline hydrochloride
Panadol. *See* Acetaminophen
Pancreas transplantation, 1091
Pancreatic disease, 656
Pancreatic enzyme replacement therapy (PERT), 656
Pancreatic fluid, 304*t*
Pancreatic rest, 328–329
Pancreatitis, 328–330
 acute, 328–329, 330*t*
 chronic, 329–330, 329.*e*1*t*
Pancreaze. *See* Pancrelipase
Pancrelipase (Creon, Pancreaze, Pertzye, Ultresa, Viokace, and Zenpep), 1004–1006
Pancuronium bromide
 dose adjustment in renal failure, 1125*t*–1134*t*
 formulary entry, 1006
Panic disorder, 1009
PanOxyl. *See* Benzoyl peroxide
Panoyiotopoulos syndrome, 559*t*–560*t*
Pantanol. *See* Olopatadine
Pantoprazole (Protonix), 1006–1007
Pantothenic acid
 in multivitamin tablets, 589*t*–590*t*
 recommended intakes, 586*t*
Papanicolaou (Pap) smear, 122–123
Papillary necrosis, 532*f*
Papular urticaria, 224
Papules, 203, 204*f*–205*f*
Papulosquamous eruptions, 218*f*
Paracentesis, 55–58, 57*f*
Paracetamol. *See* Acetaminophen

Parachute reaction, 236.e6t
Paralysis
 for intubation, 1067
 in poisoning, 21.e1t–21.e3t
Paralytics, 7t–8t
Parametric tests, 723, 724t
Parampanel (Fycompa), 562t
Parapharyngeal infections, 455
Paraplatin. *See* Carboplatin
Parapneumonic effusions, 672–674
Parasitic infestations, 208–210, 968
Parasomnias, 660
Parathyroid gland, 266–267
Parathyroid hormone (PTH), 266–267, 543–545
Parenchymal findings, 674
Parental notification, 114
Parental presence, 143
Parenteral nutrition, 602–604
 initiation and advancement of, 603t
 recommended formulations for, 604, 604t
 suggested formulations for, 603
 suggested monitoring schedule for, 605t
 suggested situations for, 603
 total (TPN), 625, 1089
Parenteral rehydration fluids
 calculation of, 301
 composition of, 302t
Parent's Choice Premium Infant Formula, 594t–600t
Parents' Evaluation of Developmental Status (PEDS), 237t–238t
Paromomycin sulfate, 1008
Paronychia, 224–225
 acute, 224, 224.e1f
 chronic, 224–225, 224.e1f
Parotitis, 461t–468t
Paroxetine (Paxil, Pexeva, Brisdelle), 1008–1009
Paroxysmal atrial fibrillation, 888
Paroxysmal dyskinesias, 557t
Paroxysmal events, 555–564
Paroxysmal supraventricular tachycardia, 888, 1097
Paroxysmal vertigo, 557t
Partial anomalous pulmonary venous return (PAPVR), 166b
Partial exchange transfusion, 616
Partial seizures, 558b
 adjunctive therapy for, 940–941, 1080, 1098, 1108
 complex, 1098
 treatment of, 838, 1107

Parvovirus B19 infection, 457t–458t, 471t–476t, 691
Pastoral care, 628
Pataday. *See* Olopatadine
Patanase. *See* Olopatadine
Patanol. *See* Olopatadine
Patch (transdermal) contraceptive, 129
Patches, 203, 204f–205f
Patent ductus arteriosus (PDA), 186t–187t, 503–504
Patent foramen ovale, 187.e1t
Pathocil. *See* Dicloxacillin
Patient care coordinators, 628
Patient Health Questionnaire-2 (PHQ-2), 132, 237t–238t, 249
Patient Health Questionnaire-9 (PHQ-9), 132
Patient history. *See* History
Patient preferences
 for care, 631
 Voicing my choices planning guide, 632
Patient-controlled analgesia (PCA), 143–144
 adjunctive therapy, 145
 with hydromorphone HCl, 915
 for mucositis pain control, 625
 oral regimen, 145
 orders for, 143t
PAW (mean airway pressure), 90
Paxil. *See* Paroxetine
Pazeo. *See* Olopatadine
PCA. *See* Patient-controlled analgesia
PCE. *See* Erythromycin
PCECV (RabAvert), 436
PCOS (polycystic ovary syndrome), 282–284
PCV13. *See* Pneumococcal conjugate vaccine
PDD-NOS. *See* Pervasive developmental disorder not otherwise specified
Peak expiratory flow rate (PEFR), 640, 641t, 643t
Peak inspiratory pressure (PIP), 91, 91.e1
Pear odor, 21.e1t–21.e3t
Pearson's *r* (product moment correlation coefficient), 724t
PECARN clinical decision rule, 76, 76b
Pedia-Lax. *See* Glycerin
Pedialyte, 302t, 570, 603t
Pediamycin. *See* Erythromycin
Pediapred. *See* Prednisolone
Pediarix. *See* DTaP/HepB/IPV
PediaSure formulas, 570, 594t–602t

Pediatric Advanced Life Support (PALS), 73
Pediatric Critical Care Medicine Website, 73
Pediatric Endocrine Society, 255
Pediatric formulas. *See* Formulas
Pediatric Study Characteristics Database, 732
Pediatric Symptom Checklist (PSC), 237*t*–238*t*, 247
Pediatric Trauma Society, 73
Pediatrics Core Curriculum (Orthopedic Trauma Association), 73
Pediavax, 425*f*
Pediculosis, 1038
Pediculosis capitis, 946, 1014
Pediculosis pubis, 946
Pedigree, 334, 335*f*
PedvaxHIB. *See* PRP-OMP
PEEP (positive end-expiratory pressure), 90–91
Peers, 109.e1*t*
PEFR (peak expiratory flow rate), 640, 641*t*, 643*t*
Peginterferon, 457*t*–458*t*
PegyLax. *See* Polyethylene glycol (PEG) electrolyte solutions
Pellagra, 986
Pelvic examination
 in adolescents, 113
 secondary survey, 74*t*–75*t*
Pelvic inflammatory disease, 122
 guidelines for management of, 115*t*–116*t*
 treatment of, 790, 818–819
Pemirolast (Alamast), 397
Pemphigus foliaceus, 220
Pemphigus vulgaris, 220
D-penicillamine
 for lead poisoning, 27
 for scleroderma, 701.e3
Penicillin
 adjuvant therapy, 1031
 anti-*Staphylococcus*–resistant, 447*t*–449*t*
 for oncology patients, 626*t*
 for osteomyelitis, 461*t*–468*t*
 for sickle cell disease, 372*t*
 for syphilis, 120*t*
Penicillin allergy, 401, 402*f*
Penicillin G
 aqueous potassium and sodium preparations (Pfizerpen-G)
  dose adjustment in renal failure, 1111*t*–1124*t*
  formulary entry, 1009–1010

Penicillin G *(Continued)*
 benzathine (Bicillin L-A)
  formulary entry, 1010
  for pharyngitis, 461*t*–468*t*
  for syphilis, 115*t*–116*t*
 benzathine and procaine (Bicillin C-R), 1011
 dose adjustment in renal failure, 1111*t*–1124*t*
 natural, 447*t*–449*t*
 procaine preparations, 1011–1012
 for syphilis, 457*t*–458*t*
Penicillin V potassium
 dose adjustment in renal failure, 1111*t*–1124*t*
 formulary entry, 1012
 natural, 447*t*–449*t*
 for pharyngitis, 461*t*–468*t*
Penis length, 287, 287.e3*t*
Pentacel. *See* DTaP/IPV/PRP-T combination
Pentamidine isethionate (Pentam 300, NebuPent)
 dose adjustment in renal failure, 1111*t*–1124*t*
 formulary entry, 1013
 for oncology patients, 626*t*
Pentasa. *See* Mesalamine
Pentobarbital (Nembutal)
 formulary entry, 1013–1014
 properties of, 151*t*
Pentostatin, 621
Pepcid. *See* Famotidine
Pepdite formulas, 570, 594*t*–602*t*
Peptamen formulas, 570, 594*t*–602*t*
Pepto-Bismol. *See* Bismuth subsalicylate
Perative formula, 594*t*–602*t*
Percocet. *See* Oxycodone and acetaminophen
Percodan. *See* Oxycodone and aspirin
Percutaneous nephrolithotomy, 543
Perennial allergic rhinitis, 395, 788
Perforomist. *See* Formoterol
Perfusion
 assessment of, 2
 hypoperfusion, 21.e1*t*–21.e3*t*
 poor, 3–4
Periactin. *See* Cyproheptadine
Pericardial disease, 194–196
Pericardial effusion, 195
Pericardial fluid, 717*t*
Pericardiocentesis, 55, 56*f*
Pericarditis, 194–196, 694*t*
Perinatal infections, 455, 457*t*–458*t*
Perinatal testing, 481

Periodontitis, 866
Periorbital bites, 93
Periorbital (preseptal) cellulitis, 461*t*–468*t*, 666
Peripheral α-antagonists, 544*t*–545*t*
Peripheral blood, 408*t*
Peripheral hypotonia, 356
Peripheral intravenous placement, 32
Peripheral nerve injuries, 511
Peritoneal dialysis, 529
Peritoneal fluid, 717*t*
Peritonitis, 1023
Peritonsillar abscesses, 461*t*–468*t*, 470
Periungal fibroma, 225, 225.e6*f*
Periventricular leukomalacia, 510
Permethrin (Elimite, Nix)
 formulary entry, 1014
 for scabies, 210
Pernicious anemia, 843
Peroxisomal disorders, 347.e1
Persistent acute otitis media, 942
Persistent asthma, 1055
Persistent complement deficiency, 422
Persistent hematuria, 530
Persistent pulmonary hypertension, 187.e1*t*
Persistent pulmonary hypertension of the newborn (PPHN), 501–502
Persistently high triglycerides, 200
Personal protective equipment (PPE), 486
Personal-social skills, 229, 231*t*–232*t*
Personnel, 147
Pertussis
 initial management of, 461*t*–468*t*
 treatment of, 789, 835–836
Pertussis vaccines
 diphtheria, tetanus, & acellular pertussis (DTaP) vaccine. *See* DTaP
 diphtheria/tetanus/pertussis vaccines, 426–427
 tetanus, diphtheria, & acellular pertussis (Tdap) vaccine. *See* Tdap
Pertzye. *See* Pancrelipase
Pervasive developmental disorder, 879
Pervasive developmental disorder not otherwise specified (PDD-NOS), 244
Pexeva. *See* Paroxetine
Pfizerpen-G. *See* Penicillin G
pH
 determination of, 312–314
 esophageal monitoring, 324
 urine, 517

PHACES syndrome, 206
Pharmacotherapy. *See* Drugs; *specific pharmaceuticals*
Pharyngeal masses, 669*t*
Pharyngitis
 group A streptococcal, 1012
 initial management of, 461*t*–468*t*
 Streptococcal, 824, 1012
 treatment of, 774, 789, 816, 819–821, 823, 835–836, 1012
Phazyme. *See* Simethicone
Phencyclidine (PCP), 21*t*
Phenazopyridine HCl (Pyridium, Azo-Urinary Pain Relief)
 dose adjustment in renal failure, 1125*t*–1134*t*
 formulary entry, 1015
Phenergan. *See* Promethazine
Phenobarbital
 dose adjustment in renal failure, 1125*t*–1134*t*
 formulary entry, 1015–1016
 for seizures, 16*t*, 559*t*–560*t*, 562*t*
 warfarin interactions, 385*b*
Phenothiazines
 ECG effects of, 180*t*
 toxicity, 862
Phentolamine mesylate (OraVerse), 1016
Phenylalanine, 709*t*–716*t*
Phenylbutazone, 385*b*
Phenylephrine HCl (Neo-Synephrine)
 formulary entry, 1017–1018
 for TET spells, 189*t*
Phenylephrine with cyclopentolate (Cyclomydril), 844
Phenylketonuria (PKU), 342
PhenyTek. *See* Phenytoin
Phenytoin (Dilantin, Phenytek)
 ECG effects of, 180*t*
 formulary entry, 1018–1019
 for seizures, 16*t*, 562*t*
 warfarin interactions, 385*b*
Pheochromocytoma, 273
 diagnosis of, 1016
 surgery for, 1016
Phlexy-Vits, 589*t*–590*t*
PhosLo. *See* Calcium acetate
Phoslyra. *See* Calcium acetate
PHOS-NaK. *See* Phosphorus supplements
Phospha 250 Neutral. *See* Phosphorus supplements
Phosphate disturbances, 310–311

Phosphorus
  in multivitamin tablets, 589t–590t
  recommended intakes, 591t
  reference values, 709t–716t
Phosphorus imbalance, 529
Phosphorus supplements (K-PHOS Neutral, Av-Phos 250 Neutral, Phospha 250 Neutral, PHOS-NaK, Sodium Phosphate, Potassium Phosphate), 1019–1020
Photosensitivity, 694t
Phototherapy, 505, 505f, 505t
PHQ-2 (Patient Health Questionnaire-2), 132, 237t–238t, 249
PHQ-9 (Patient Health Questionnaire-9), 132
Phthirus pubis, 1014
Physical abuse. See Child abuse
Physical activity coefficient (PA), 580, 580.e1t
Physical activity level (PAL), 579
Physical changes as death approaches, 633
Physical examination
  adolescent, 112–113
  cardiac, 156–166
  in child abuse, 101–102
  in chronic hypertension, 541
  in developmental disorder, 236–239
  dilated fundoscopic examination, 512
  in dysmorphology, 347
  in food allergy, 398–400
  ophthalmologic
    in child abuse, 102
    follow-up, 513.e1t
  primary survey, 73
  respiratory, 637
  screening orthopedic examination, 113.e1f
  secondary survey, 73, 74t–75t
  before sedation, 147
  in UTIs, 519
Physical maturity, 494f, 495
Physical Status Classification (ASA), 147, 146.e3t
Physical therapy, 693
Physician Orders for Life-Sustaining Treatment (POLST) forms, 633
Physicians EZ Use B-12. See Cyanocobalamin
Physicians Med Guide, 250
Physiologic anemia of infancy, 366
Physostigmine salicylate
  antidote for, 1020
  formulary entry, 1020

Phytonadione (vitamin K$_1$, Mephyton)
  for excessive warfarin anticoagulation, 384t
  formulary entry, 1020–1021
  for hyperleukocytosis/leukocytosis, 616
  in infant multivitamin drops, 588t
  in multivitamin tablets, 589t–590t
  recommended intakes, 586t
PIC 200. See Polysaccharide-iron complex
Piebaldism, 218f
Pigmentation disorders, 225–227
Pigmented nevi or moles, 218f, 226, 226.e3f
Pilocarpine HCl (Isopto Carpine, Salagen, Pilopine HS)
  formulary entry, 1021–1022
  quantitative (sweat chloride test), 654–655
  for sicca, 701.e4
Pilomyxoid astrocytoma, 611t
Pilopine HS. See Pilocarpine HCl
Pimecrolimus (Elidel), 1022
Pineoblastoma, 611t
Pineocytoma, 611t
Pin-Rid. See Pyrantel pamoate
Pinworms, 955, 1037
Pin-X. See Pyrantel pamoate
Piperacillin
  for catheter-related bloodstream infections, 461t–468t
  dose adjustment in renal failure, 1111t–1124t
  for intra-abdominal infections, 461t–468t
Piperacillin with tazobactam (Zosyn)
  dose adjustment in renal failure, 1111t–1124t
  formulary entry, 1022–1023
  for sinusitis, 461t–468t
  for spinal fusion infections, 461t–468t
Pitressin. See Vasopressin
Pituitary adenoma, 611t
Pituitary gland
  posterior pituitary disorders, 274–276
  posterior pituitary function, 273–276
Pituitary hormones, 273
Pivot formula, 601t–602t
PK (prekallikrein), 377t–378t
PKU (phenylketonuria), 342
Plague, 942, 1066
Plan B One Step (levonorgestrel), 130
Plantar grasp, 236.e4t–236.e5t
Plantar surface, 494f
Plantar warts, 208

Plaque psoriasis, 881
Plaquenil. *See* Hydroxychloroquine
Plaques, 203, 204*t*–205*f*
Plasbumin. *See* Albumin
Plasma amino acids, 336*t*
Plasma ammonia, 336*t*
Plasma creatinine, 523–524
Plasma exchange, 623
Plasma or platelet products, 426.e1*t*
Plasmanate, 302*t*
Plasminogen, 377*t*–378*t*
Plasminogen activator inhibitor, 377*t*–378*t*
Plasminogen activator inhibitor deficiency, 386*f*
Platelet count, 701
Platelet dysfunction, 386*f*
Platelet Function Analyzer-100 (PFA-100) system, 376–379
Platelet function testing, 376–379
Platelet products, 391–392
  leukocyte-poor, 392
  single-donor, 392
Platelet transfusions
  for cerebrovascular accident, 617
  for CMV-negative patients, 624
  for hyperleukocytosis/leukocytosis, 616
  after Ig or blood product administration, 426.e1*t*
Platelets
  activation of, 379*b*
  age-specific values, 365*t*
  aggregation of, 376–379
  blood smears, 393
Platinol. *See* Cisplatin
Platinum agents, 625.e1*t*–625.e2*t*
Pleural effusion
  chest tube insertion for, 51
  thoracentesis for, 53, 54*f*
Pleural fluid, 717*t*
Pleuritis, 694*t*
Plexus injuries, 511*t*
PNET (primitive neuroectodermal tumor), 611*t*
Pneumococcal conjugate vaccine (PCV13), 435
  after BMT, 622
  for children at high risk for pneumococcal disease, 420–421
  contraindications to, 435
  dose, 435
  after HSCT, 625.e3
  recommended schedule for, 413*f*, 415*f*–418*f*

Pneumococcal conjugate vaccine (PCV13) *(Continued)*
  routine vaccination, 435
  for solid organ transplant recipients, 423
Pneumococcal infection
  children at high risk for, 420–421
  penicillin-resistant, 822
  prophylaxis of, 420–421, 435, 1012
  treatment of, 1011
Pneumococcal polysaccharide vaccine (PPSV23), 435
  for children at high risk for pneumococcal disease, 420–421
  dose, 435
  after HSCT, 625.e3
  recommended schedule for, 413*f*, 415*f*–418*f*
  for solid organ transplant recipients, 423
Pneumococcal vaccines
  catch-up schedule for, 414*f*
  recommended schedule for, 413*f*, 415*f*–418*f*
  routine vaccination, 435
  in sickle cell disease, 372*t*
Pneumocystis jiroveci (carinii) pneumonia (PCP)
  prophylaxis of, 626*t*, 786, 847, 1013, 1070
  treatment of, 785–786, 847, 1013, 1030, 1070
Pneumonia
  CMV, 624.e1*t*
  community-acquired, 779, 789–790
    exacerbation of, 819
    treatment of, 816, 942
  community-acquired bacterial pneumonia (CABP), 820
  idiopathic syndrome, 623
  imaging in, 672
  initial management of, 461*t*–468*t*
  neonatal, 461*t*–468*t*
  nosocomial, 1023
  P jiroveci (carinii) (PCP)
    prophylaxis of, 626*t*, 786, 847, 1013, 1070
    treatment of, 785–786, 847, 1013, 1030, 1070
  treatment of, 835–836, 947, 952, 1094
Pneumothorax
  chest tube insertion for, 51
  in newborns, 502
  open, 79

Pneumothorax (Continued)
  tension
    signs of, 79
    treatment of, 79
Poison control, 20, 22
Poison ivy, 221
Poisoning, 20–29
  acetaminophen intoxication, 22
  antidotes, 21–22
  commonly ingested agents, 23t–24t
  diagnostic aids, 21.e1t–21.e3t
  ingestions, 21–22
  initial evaluation of, 20–21
  opiate intoxication, 980
  web resources, 20
Poliomyelitis immunoprophylaxis, 435–436
  contraindications to, 435
  inactivated poliovirus vaccine. See Inactivated poliovirus (IPV) vaccine
  oral poliovirus vaccine. See Oral poliovirus (OPV) vaccine
  routine vaccination, 435
Polioviruses, 471t–476t
POLST (Physician Orders for Life-Sustaining Treatment) forms, 633
Polyangiitis
  granulomatosis with, 532f
  microscopic, 697t
Polyarteritis nodosa, 532f, 697t
Polyarthralgia, 698
Polyarthritis, migratory, 698
Polycitra. See Citrate mixtures
Polycystic kidney, 532f
Polycystic ovary syndrome (PCOS), 282–284
Polycythemia, 507
Polyethylene glycol (PEG) electrolyte solutions
  bowel cleansing products (GoLYTELY, CoLyte, NuLYTELY, TriLyte), 1023–1024
  for constipation, 322
  for disimpaction, 322
  formulary entry, 1023–1024
  laxative products (MiraLax, GaviLAX, GlycoLax, HealthyLax, PegyLax), 1023–1024
Polyhydramnios, 490.e2b
Poly-Iron 150. See Polysaccharide-iron complex
Polymorphonuclear leukocytes, 718t
Polymyositis, 695t

Polymyxin B sulfate
  for conjunctivitis, 461t–468t
  neomycin/polymyxin B (Neosporin GU), 984
  neomycin/polymyxin B + bacitracin (Neo Polycin), 983
  neomycin/polymyxin B + bacitracin (Neosporin, Neo To Go, Neo-Polycin, Triple Antibiotic), 984
  neomycin/polymyxin B + bacitracin + hydrocortisone (Neo-Polycin HC), 983
  neomycin/polymyxin B + gramicidin (Neosporin Ophthalmic Solution), 983
  for otitis externa, 461t–468t
Polymyxin B sulfate, neomycin sulfate, hydrocortisone, 983
Polymyxin B sulfate, neomycin sulfate, hydrocortisone otic, 1025
Polymyxin B sulfate and bacitracin (AK-Poly-Bac Ophthalmic, Double Antibiotic Topical, Polysporin Topical), 791–792
Polyneuropathy, 548
Polyps, 532f
Polysaccharide antigen (PRP), 427–428
Polysaccharide-iron complex (Myferon 150, PIC 200, Poly-Iron 150, NovaFerrum), 927–928
Polysomnography, 657–658
Polysporin Topical. See Bacitracin + polymyxin B
Polyuria, 537–538
Poly-Vi-Sol Multivitamin, 588t
Pompe disease, 344
Popliteal angle, 494f, 495
Poractant alfa (Curosurf). See Surfactant
Porcelain, 709t–716t
Portagen formula, 594t–602t
Portal systemic encephalopathy, 935
Port-wine stain, 218f
Positioning
  frog-leg lateral hip radiographs, 681
  tripod, 12
Positive end-expiratory pressure (PEEP), 90–91
Positive expiratory pressure (PEP), 656
Positive predictive value (PPV), 728
Positive purified protein derivative (PPD) tuberculin test, 433
Positive support reflex (PSR), 236.e4t–236.e5t

Positive-pressure ventilation, noninvasive (NIPPV), 11, 90
Posterior ankle splint, 71f, 70.e2
Posterior pituitary disorders, 274–276
Posterior pituitary function, 273–276
Posterior pituitary hormones, 273
Posterior propping, 236.e6t
Posterior tibial artery puncture, 36
Postherpetic neuralgia, 903
Postmaturity desquamation, 218f
Postmenstrual age, 490.e3
Poststreptococcal glomerulonephritis, 532f
Postural reactions, 236.e6t
Posture, 229
  newborn, 493–495, 494f
Posture-D. See Calcium phosphate
Potassium (K⁺)
  for diabetic ketoacidosis, 258f
  in multivitamin tablets, 589t–590t
  newborn requirements for, 498t
  reference values, 709t–716t
Potassium (K⁺) deficit, 294.e1
Potassium (K⁺) disturbances, 304–307
Potassium iodide (Iosat, SSKI, ThyroShield, ThyroSafe), 1025–1026
Potassium Phosphate. See Phosphorus supplements
Potassium supplements, 1026–1027
Power Doppler, 675
Power/strength, 548
PPE (Pre-Participation Examination), 112–113
PPHN (persistent pulmonary hypertension of the newborn), 501–502
PPIs. See Proton-pump inhibitors
PPSV23. See Pneumococcal polysaccharide vaccine
PPV (positive predictive value), 728
PR interval, 169, 170t
Prader-Willi syndrome (PWS), 278f, 353–354
Pralidoxime chloride (2-PAM, Protopam), 1027–1028
Pralidoxime chloride with atropine (Duodote, ATNAA), 1027–1028
PRBCs. See Packed red blood cells
Prealbumin, 709t–716t
Precedex. See Dexmedetomidine
Precocious puberty, 109, 281–282
Pred Forte. See Prednisolone
Pred Mild. See Prednisolone
Prednicarbate, 223t

Prednisolone
  for asthma, 10
  formulary entry, 1028
  ophthalmic products (Pred Forte, Pred Mild, Omnipred), 1028
  oral products (Orapred ODT, Prelone, Pediapred, Millipred, Veripred 20), 1028
  potency of, 271t
Prednisone (Deltasone, Rayos)
  for adrenal insufficiency, 271–272
  for allergic emergencies, 10
  for asthma, 10
  formulary entry, 1029
  for nephrotic syndrome, 535–536
  potency of, 271t
  stress-dose, 272
Pre-exposure prophylaxis (PrEP), 486
Pregabalin (Lyrica), 562t
Pregestimil, 570, 601t–602t
Pregnancy
  drug formulary categories, 735
  EER equations, 581.e1
  immunizations in, 424
  prevention of. See Contraception
  recommended element intakes, 591t
  recommended vitamin intakes, 586t
Prehypertension, 539
Prekallikrein (PK), 377t–378t
Prelone. See Prednisolone
Premature atrial contraction (PAC), 174t–175t, 176f
Premature growth, 490
Premature infants. See also Preterm infants
  iron deficiency anemia in, 927
Premature ventricular contraction (PVC), 177f, 177t
Prematurity
  anemia of, 874
  chronic lung disease of, 653–654
Premenstrual dysphoric disorder, 893
Preoperative prophylaxis, 818
Preoperative (preprocedure) sedation
  pentobarbital, 1013
  phenobarbital, 1015
Pre-Participation Examination (PPE), 112–113
Prepuberty
  emergency management of children in, 3t
  treatment of, 943
Preschoolers
  pain assessment in, 136

Preseptal (periorbital) cellulitis, 461t–468t, 666
Pressure support ventilation (PSV), 91
Pre-teens, 124t
Preterm formulas, 594t–602t
Preterm infants
  caloric requirements, 499t
  coagulation values, 377t–378t
  CSF evaluation, 717t
  glucose requirements, 496–497
  growth charts for, 580f–581f
  hypoglycemia in, 499f
  immunoprophylaxis guidelines for, 424
  insensible water loss, 496.e1t
  iron deficiency anemia in, 927
  iron requirements, 497
  iron supplementation for, 584
  length, weight, and head circumference, 580f–581f
  mean TSH and T_4 values, 263t
  newborn metabolic screening, 340
  normal blood pressure values, 156.e1t
  phototherapy for, 505t
  potassium requirements, 498t
  reference values, 709t–716t
  rotavirus immunoprophylaxis for, 439
  RSV immunoprophylaxis for, 437
  serum immunoglobulin levels, 408t
  total blood volume, 389t
Prevacid. See Lansoprazole
Prevalence, 725
Prevalite. See Cholestyramine
Prevention
  burn, 100
  immunoprophylaxis, 412–442
  of kidney stones, 545
  of migraine, 556t
  of obesity, 574.e1f
Prevention of Child Maltreatment (CDC), 73
Prickly heat (miliaria), 219
Prilocaine, 141t
Prilosec. See Omeprazole
Primacor. See Milrinone
Primaquine phosphate, 1029–1030
Primary survey, 73
Primaxin. See Imipenem and cilastatin
Primidone (Mysoline)
  dose adjustment in renal failure, 1125t–1134t
  formulary entry, 1030
  warfarin interactions, 385b
Primitive neuroectodermal tumor (PNET), 611t

Prinivil. See Lisinopril
ProAir HFA. See Albuterol
ProAir RespiClick. See Albuterol
Probenecid
  formulary entry, 1031
  for neurosyphilis, 1011
Probiotics, 320–321
Problem-solving development, 237t–238t
Procainamide
  dose adjustment in renal failure, 1125t–1134t
  formulary entry, 1031–1032
Procarbazine (Matulane), 613t–615t
Procardia. See Nifedipine
Procedural sedation, 30, 145–148
  dexmedetomidine, 853
  discharge criteria for, 148
  example protocols, 148, 153t
  limits for targeted depth and length, 146.e1f
  midazolam, 971
  monitoring, 148
  pentobarbital, 1013
  phenobarbital, 1015
  preparation for, 146–147
  suggested protocols, 153t
  web resources, 136
Procedures, 30–72
  general guidelines for, 30
  musculoskeletal, 68–70
ProCentra. See Dextroamphetamine
Prochlorperazine (Compro)
  for antiemetic therapy, 626t
  formulary entry, 1032
  for migraine, 555
  for palliative care, 634t
Procrit. See Epoetin alfa
Proctitis, 1068
Proctocolitis, infantile, 398
Product moment correlation coefficient (Pearson's r), 724t
Professional disclosure, 360, 357.e1
Progesterone receptor modulators, 130
Progestin-only pills, 129, 131
Proglycem. See Diazoxide
Prograf. See Tacrolimus
Prokinetic therapy
  erythromycin, 878
  for reflux, 324
Prolactinoma, 611t
Promethazine (Phenergan)
  for antiemetic therapy, 626t
  formulary entry, 1033
Promote formulas, 594t–600t

Pronto. *See* Pyrethrins with piperonyl butoxie
Propafenone, 385*b*
Propionibacterium acnes, 213
Propionic acidemia (PA), 341
　acute management of, 341
　chronic management of, 342
Propofol
　for deep sedation, 145
　properties of, 149*b*–150*b*
　for RSI, 7*t*–8*t*
Propping
　anterior, 236.*e*6*t*
　lateral, 236.*e*6*t*
　posterior, 236.*e*6*t*
Propranolol (Inderal, Hemangeol)
　ECG effects of, 180*t*
　formulary entry, 1033–1034
　for hemangioma, 206–207
　for hypertension, 544*t*–545*t*
　for migraine prevention, 556*t*
　for TET spells, 189*t*
Propylthiouracil (PTU)
　formulary entry, 1035
　warfarin interactions, 385*b*
ProQuad. *See* Measles, mumps, rubella, and varicella (MMRV) combination vaccine
Prostacyclin (prostaglandin I$_2$), 502
Prostaglandin E$_1$. *See* Alprostadil
Prostaglandin I$_2$ (prostacyclin), 502
Prosthetic valve endocarditis
　prophylaxis of, 192*b*
　treatment of, 1050
Prostigmin. *See* Neostigmine
Prostin VR Pediatric. *See* Alprostadil
Protamine sulfate
　formulary entry, 1035–1036
　for heparin sodium antidote, 912
Protein
　CSF levels, 717*t*
　reference values, 709*t*–716*t*
　requirements for, 584*t*
　urine, 517, 534
Protein allergy/intolerance, 601*t*–602*t*
Protein C, 377*t*–378*t*
Protein C deficiency, 379*b*
Protein S, 377*t*–378*t*
Protein S deficiency, 379*b*
Proteinuria, 517, 531–537
　causes of, 535*b*
　detection of, 531–534
　fixed, 534
　glomerular disease with, 535*b*
　nephrotic-range, 534
　orthostatic, 534, 535*b*

Proteinuria *(Continued)*
　significant, 534, 535*b*
　transient, 535*b*
Proteus, 520
Prothrombin time (PT), 376
　age-specific values, 377*t*–378*t*
Prothrombinase complex concentrate, 384*t*
Protonix. *See* Pantoprazole
Proton-pump inhibitors (PPIs)
　for eosinophilic esophagitis, 325
　for reflux, 324
Protopam. *See* Pralidoxime chloride
Protopic. *See* Tacrolimus
ProvayBlue. *See* Methylene blue
Proventil HFA. *See* Albuterol
Provera. *See* Medroxyprogesterone
Provider Resources for Vaccine Conversations with Parents (CDC), 420
Proximal tubule functional tests, 525–526
Proximal tubule reabsorption, 525
Prozac. *See* Fluoxetine hydrochloride
PRP. *See* Polysaccharide antigen
PRP-OMP (PedvaxHIB or COMVAX), 415*f*–418*f*, 428, 441–442
PRP-T (Hiberix), 415*f*–418*f*, 428, 441
Pruritus control, 224, 916, 980, 1089
　medications for palliative care, 634*t*
PSC (Pediatric Symptom Checklist), 237*t*–238*t*, 247
Pseudoephedrine (Sudafed), 1036–1037
Pseudoephedrine + cetirizine (Zyrtec-D 12 Hour), 825–826
Pseudoephedrine + loratadine (Claritin-D), 950–951
Pseudomonas infection
　treatment of, 816
　UTIs, 520
Pseudoseizures, 557*t*
Pseudotumor cerebri, 758
Psoralens plus ultraviolet A photopheresis (PUVA), 621
Psoriasis
　diagnosis of, 218*f*
　nail, 225, 225.*e*3*f*
　plaque, 881
　psoriatic arthritis sine, 690
　treatment of, 1075
Psoriatic arthritis (PsA), 688–691
　sine psoriasis, 690
　treatment of, 881
PSR (positive support reflex), 236.*e*4*t*–236.*e*5*t*

PSV (pressure support ventilation), 91
Psychiatric disorders, comorbid, 1085
Psychiatric drugs, 245t
Psychiatric review, 111
Psychogenic headaches, 552b
Psychosis
  in poisoning, 21.e1t–21.e3t
  treatment of, 828, 910–911, 1032
Psychosocial development, 109.e1t
Psychosocial Development of Adolescents, 109–110
Psychosocial history, 109–110
Psychosocial screening tests, 237t–238t
Psyllium (Metamucil, Geri-Mucil, Konsyl, Reguloid), 1037
PT. See Prothrombin time
PTH (parathyroid hormone), 266–267, 543–545
PTU. See Propylthiouracil
Pubertal development, 108–109
Puberty
  delayed, 109, 277–281, 280f
  precocious, 109, 281–282
Pubic hair, 110t
Pulmicort. See Budesonide
Pulmocare formulas, 594t–602t
Pulmonary disease
  COPD exacerbation, 789
  oxygen challenge test findings in, 187.e1t
Pulmonary ejection murmur, 167t
Pulmonary embolism, 911
Pulmonary flow murmur, 167t
Pulmonary function tests, 639–643
Pulmonary gas exchange, 637–639
Pulmonary hypertension, 88–89
  chronic therapy for, 89
  heart sounds in, 166b
  persistent, 187.e1t
  persistent pulmonary hypertension of the newborn (PPHN), 501–502
  treatment of, 1059
Pulmonary hypertensive crisis, 88–89
Pulmonary insult, direct, 21.e1t–21.e3t
Pulmonary stenosis, 166b, 186t–187t
Pulmonary vascularity, 675
Pulmonary vasodilator therapy, 501–502
Pulmonology, 637–662
  late effects of cancer treatment, 625.e1t–625.e2t
  web resources for, 637
Pulmozyme. See Dornase alfa
Pulse oximetry (SpO$_2$), 148, 637–638
  screening for critical congenital heart disease, 185
Pulse pressure, 156

Pulseless arrest, 872
Pulseless ventricular tachycardia, 1096
Pulsus paradoxus, 163
Pupillary dilation, 1017
PurAmino formula, 594t–602t
Purine analogs, 613t–615t
Purpura
  Henoch-Schönlein (HSP), 532f, 696–699, 697t
  nonthrombocytopenic palpable, 698
  thrombocytopenic. See Thrombocytopenic purpura
Pustular melanosis, neonatal, 217–219
Pustules, 203, 209f
PUVA (psoralens plus ultraviolet A photopheresis), 621
PVC. See Premature ventricular contraction
PWS (Prader-Willi syndrome), 278f, 353–354
Pyelonephritis, 520
  acute, 942
  initial management of, 461t–468t
  treatment of, 521, 833, 942
  uncomplicated, 833
Pyloric stenosis, 677–678, 677.e3f
Pyogenic granuloma, 207
Pyrantel pamoate (Reese's Pinworm, Pin-Rid, Pin-X), 1037
Pyrazinamide (pyrazinoic acid amide), 1038
Pyrazinamide + isoniazid + rifampin (Rifater), 928–929, 1038
Pyrethrins with piperonyl butoxie (A-200, Pronto, RID, LiceMD, Licide), 1038
Pyridium. See Phenazopyridine HCl
Pyridostigmine bromide (Mestinson, Regonol)
  formulary entry, 1038–1039
  for vecuronium bromide overdose, 1097
Pyridoxine (vitamin B$_6$)
  formulary entry, 1039–1040
  in infant multivitamin drops, 588t
  in multivitamin tablets, 589t–590t
  for neonatal seizures, 338
  recommended intakes, 586t
  for seizures, 559t–560t
Pyridoxine-dependent seizures, 1039
Pyrimethamine (Daraprim), 1040
Pyrimethamine + sulfadiazine with folinic acid, 457t–458t
Pyruvate, 709t–716t
Pyruvate dehydrogenase deficiency, 561
Pyuria, 520

Q

Q waves, 169
Qbrelis. *See* Lisinopril
Qnasl. *See* Beclomethasone dipropionate
QRS complex, 166, 169
 normal values, 170*t*
 wide, 23*t*–24*t*, 21.*e*1*t*–21.*e*3*t*
Qs/Qt (intrapulmonary shunt fraction), 93.*e*1
QTc interval, 169
 long, 173–179, 199.*e*1*t*
Quadracel (DTaP/IPV combination), 442
Quality of life, 629
Quantitative carnitine test, 336*t*
Quantitative fecal fat test, 330
Quantitative pilocarpine ionoelectrophoresis (sweat chloride test), 654–655
Qudexy XR. *See* Topiramate
Quelicin. *See* Succinylcholine
Questions, clinical, 721
Questran. *See* Cholestyramine
Quetiapine (Seroquel)
 ages of FDA approval, 245*t*
 formulary entry, 1040–1043
Quick start contraception, 127, 128*f*
QuilliChew ER. *See* Methylphenidate HCl
Quillivant XR. *See* Methylphenidate HCl
Quinapril, 544*t*–545*t*
Quinidine
 dose adjustment in renal failure, 1125*t*–1134*t*
 formulary entry, 1043–1044
 warfarin interactions, 385*b*
Quinupristin and dalfopristin (Synercid), 1044
Quixin. *See* Levofloxacin
QVar. *See* Beclomethasone dipropionate

R

R wave, 169, 170*t*
RabAvert (PCECV), 436
Rabies immune globulin (RIG), 436, 426.*e*1*t*
 administration, 436
 postexposure, 437
Rabies immunoprophylaxis, 95, 405, 436–437
 administration, 436
 after Ig or blood product administration, 426.*e*1*t*
 postexposure, 436–437, 437*t*
 side effects of, 436
Rabies vaccine
 HDCV (Imovax), 436
 PCECV (RabAvert), 436
 routine vaccination, 436
Raccoon eyes, 74*t*–75*t*, 77
Radial artery catheterization, 34–36
 Seldinger technique, 34, 35*f*
 ultrasound-guided, 34–36, 36*f*
Radial head subluxation (nursemaid's elbow) reduction, 70
Radiation nephritis, 532*f*
Radiation therapy
 late effects of, 625.*e*1*t*–625.*e*2*t*
 limiting exposure, 663
 prevention of nausea and vomiting associated with, 908, 997
 total body irradiation (TBI), 619
 treatment regimens, 625
Radiographic iodinated contrast media (RICM), 529
Radiography
 abdominal, 521
 in AKI/CKD, 529–530
 anteroposterior (AP), 680
 central line placement on, 674
 chest imaging, 183–184, 671*f*–672*f*, 674
  anteroposterior (AP), 671*f*–672*f*
  lateral, 670, 673*f*–674*f*
  posteroanterior (PA), 670
 C-spine imaging, 78
  anteroposterior (AP), 666–667
  lateral, 666–667
 ETT placement on, 674
 frog-leg lateral hip radiographs, 681
 lateral, 680
 neck imaging
  anteroposterior (AP), 667, 669*f*
  lateral, 667, 670*f*
 odontoid views, 667
 in osteomyelitis, 681
 in osteosarcoma, 682*f*–683*f*
 in poisoning, 21.*e*1*t*–21.*e*3*t*
 in pyloric stenosis, 678
 skull, 665
 spinal imaging, 666
 in stress fractures, 681
 in trauma, 680
 in UTIs, 521
Radiology, 663–687
 Appropriateness Criteria (ACR), 663
 choosing the right study, 663–664
 general principles, 663
 web resources for, 663
Rages, 557*t*
Rales (crackles), 638*t*

Randomized Intervention for the Management of Vesicoureteral Reflux study (RIVUR), 522–523
Ranitidine HCl (Zantac, Deprizine)
  dose adjustment in renal failure, 1125*t*–1134*t*
  formulary entry, 1045
Rapamune. *See* Sirolimus
Rapid plasma antigen (RPR), 455.*e*2*t*
Rapid sequence intubation (RSI), 5, 7*t*–8*t*
Rasburicase (Elitek)
  formulary entry, 1045–1046
  for hyperuricemia, 616
Rash
  discoid, 694*t*
  malar, 694*t*
  neonatal, 218*f*
Rat bite fever, 1066
Raynaud phenomenon (RP), 700–701
Raynaud syndrome, 700–701
Rayos. *See* Prednisone
RBCs. *See* Red blood cells
RCF formula, 594*t*–600*t*
RDA (Recommended Dietary Allowance), 583
Reach Out and Read
  milestones of early literacy, 233*t*
  web resources, 229
Reactive airway disease, 770, 954
Reactive arthritis, 691
Reactive erythema, 208, 209*f*
Reactive lymph nodes, 446
Reactive lymphadenopathy, 454
Rebetol. *See* Ribavirin
Recall bias, 722
Receptive/expressive language disorder, 242
Recombivax. *See* Hepatitis B vaccine
Recommended Childhood Immunization Schedule, 412, 413*f*
Recommended Dietary Allowance (RDA), 583
Rectal enemas. *See also* Enemas
  bisacodyl, 797
  docusate, 863
Rectal infections, 817
Rectal suppositories, 797. *See also* Suppositories
Rectal temperature, 493
Red blood cells (RBCs)
  blood smears, 393
  blood transfusion with, 390–392
  after Ig or blood product administration, 426.*e*1*t*
  urinalysis for, 518

Red Book: 2015 Report of the Committee on Infectious Diseases (AAP), 412
Red cell aplasia, 367
Red urine, 530
Reese's Pinworm. *See* Pyrantel pamoate
Reference values, 708, 709*t*–716*t*
Referral
  developmental, 246
  mental health, 251
  to pediatric urology, 523
Reflex irritability, 493*t*
Reflexes
  absent, 551
  brisk, 551
  isolated abnormality of, 551
  muscle stretch, 550.*e*1*t*
  primitive, 236.*e*4*t*–236.*e*5*t*
  rating scale for, 550*b*
  tendon, 550–551
Reflux
  gastroesophageal. *See* Gastroesophageal reflux
  gastrointestinal, 323–324
  vesicoureteral, 522–523, 522*f*
Regitine. *See* Phentolamine mesylate
Reglan. *See* Metoclopramide
Regonol. *See* Pyridostigmine bromide
Regression, 723
  by least squares, 724*t*
  multiple, 724*t*
  nonparametric, 724*t*
Reguloid. *See* Psyllium
Rehabilitation Act, 246
Rehydralyte, 302*t*
Rehydration fluids, 302*t*
Reiter syndrome, 718*t*
Relative benefit increase, 727
Relative risk (RR), 725
Relative risk reduction (RRR), 727
Relpax. *See* Eletriptan
Renal allograft rejection, 532*f*
Renal angiomyolipoma, 352
Renal failure
  antimicrobials that require dose adjustment in, 1111*t*–1124*t*
  chronic, 849, 873–875
  dose adjustment methods for, 1110
  drugs in, 1110–1136
  guidelines for, 804
  nonantimicrobials that require dose adjustment in, 1125*t*–1134*t*
  treatment of, 829, 875
Renal insufficiency, 1110
Renal obstruction, 527*t*

Renal tubular acidosis, 526, 537, 538*t*
Renal tubular function tests, 525–526
Renal vein/artery thrombosis, 532*f*
Renal/bladder ultrasound (RBUS), 679–680
Renalcal formula, 594*t*–602*t*
Renova. *See* Tretinoin
Repeat expansion testing, 358*t*
Replacement therapy
  for antibody-deficient disorders, 401
  blood component, 385–393
  deficit replacement strategy, 297–301
  pancreatic enzyme replacement therapy (PERT), 656
Replete formulas, 594*t*–600*t*
Reporting child abuse, 102
Reproductive system, 625.e1*t*–625.e2*t*
Reprotox, 333
Research
  clinical questions, 721
  Clinical Trial Database (NCI), 607
  evidence-based medicine, 721–722
  grid for calculations in clinical studies, 727*t*
  study designs, 726*t*
Resectisol. *See* Mannitol
Residual volume (RV), 641–643, 643*t*
Resource formulas, 570, 594*t*–602*t*
Respiration, 4
Respiratory acidosis, 312
  etiology of, 313*f*–314*f*
  expected compensatory response, 641*t*
Respiratory alkalosis, 312
  etiology of, 313*f*–314*f*
  expected compensatory response, 641*t*
Respiratory antisecretory agents, 907
Respiratory auscultation, 637, 638*t*
Respiratory disease. *See also* Pulmonary disease
  in newborns, 500–502
Respiratory distress, 618
Respiratory distress syndrome, 500–501
Respiratory effort, 493*t*
Respiratory emergencies, 9–13
Respiratory failure, 89–92
Respiratory physical examination, 637
Respiratory rate (RR)
  normal newborn, 493
  normal rates, 638*t*
Respiratory syncytial virus (RSV), 653
  prophylaxis against, 437–438, 653–654, 1003, 426.e1*t*

Respiratory system
  changes as death approaches, 633
  review of, 111
Respiratory tract procedures, 192*b*, 192*t*
Restasis. *See* Cyclosporine
Restrictive cardiomyopathy, 194
Resuscitation
  DNAR orders, 632
  neonatal, 490–492, 491*f*
  Neonatal Resuscitation Program (NRP), 490
  in poor perfusion and shock, 3–4
Resuscitation fluids, 3–4
Reticulocytes
  age-specific counts, 365*t*
  corrected reticulocyte count (CRC), 367
Retina, 512*f*
Retin-A. *See* Tretinoin
Retinal necrosis, 900–901
Retinitis, CMV, 832, 900
Retinoblastoma (Rb), 609*t*–610*t*
Retinoids, topical
  for acne vulgaris, 214, 215*t*
  formulations and concentrations, 216*t*
Retinol (vitamin A), 709*t*–716*t*
Retinopathy of prematurity (ROP), 511–513, 513.e2*f*
  stages of, 512–513, 513.e2*f*
  suggested schedule for follow-up ophthalmologic examination, 513.e1*t*
  type 1, 513
  type 2, 513
Retropharyngeal abscesses, 470
  initial management of, 461*t*–468*t*
  radiographic findings, 669*t*
Retrovir. *See* Zidovudine
Rett syndrome, 354–355
Return to play, 77
Revatio. *See* Sildenafil
Reverse neuromuscular blockade, 907
R-Gene 10. *See* Arginine chloride, injectable
Rhabdomyoma, cardiac, 352
Rhabdomyosarcoma, 532*f*, 609*t*–610*t*
Rheumatic diseases
  heart disease, 198
  laboratory studies for, 701–704
  synovial fluid characteristics, 718*t*
Rheumatic fever
  guidelines for diagnosis of initial attack, 199*b*
  prophylaxis of, 1010, 1012, 1069
  synovial fluid characteristics, 718*t*

Rheumatoid arthritis
  juvenile, 688–693
    synovial fluid characteristics, 718*t*
    treatment of, 916–917, 981
  treatment of, 881, 922, 981
Rheumatoid factor (RF), 702–703, 709*t*–716*t*
Rheumatologic diseases, 688–701
Rheumatology, 688–706
Rhinaris. *See* Sodium chloride
Rhinitis
  allergic. *See* Allergic rhinitis (AR)
  associated with common cold, 924
  associated with seasonal allergies, 925
  infectious, 396
  nonallergic, with eosinophilia syndrome (NARES), 396
  treatment of, 924–925
  vasomotor/nonallergic, 396
Rhinitis medicamentosa, 396
Rhinocort Aqua Nasal Spray. *See* Budesonide
Rhinorrhea, 397
RH_0 (D) immune globulin intravenous (human) (WinRho-SDF, Rhophylac), 374, 1046
Rhonchi, 638*t*
Rhophylac. *See* RH_0 (D) immune globulin intravenous (human)
Rhythm. *See* Heart rhythm
Rib fractures, 685*f*–686*f*
  in child abuse, 103*t*, 683
  posterior, 683
Rib notching, 184
Ribasphere. *See* Ribavirin
Ribavirin (Rebetol, Copegus, Ribasphere, Moderiba, Virazole)
  formulary entry, 1047–1048
  for HCV, 457*t*–458*t*
Riboflavin (vitamin B_2)
  formulary entry, 1049
  in infant multivitamin drops, 588*t*
  in multivitamin tablets, 589*t*–590*t*
  recommended intakes, 586*t*
  reference values, 709*t*–716*t*
Riboflavin deficiency, 1049
Rickets, 267*t*, 829
  nutritional, 875
  vitamin D–dependent, 875
  vitamin D–resistant, 875
RICM (radiographic iodinated contrast media), 529

RID. *See* Pyrethrins with piperonyl butoxie
Rifabutin (Mycobutin)
  dose adjustment in renal failure, 1111*t*–1124*t*
  formulary entry, 1049–1050
  warfarin interactions, 385*b*
Rifadin. *See* Rifampin
Rifamate. *See* Isoniazid + rifampin
Rifampin (Rifadin)
  formulary entry, 1050–1051
  for TB, 485
  warfarin interactions, 385*b*
Rifampin + isoniazid (Rifamate, IsonRif), 928–929
Rifampin + isoniazid + pyrazinamide (Rifater), 928–929, 1038
Rifapentine, 485
Rifater. *See* Isoniazid + rifampin + pyrazinamide
RIG. *See* Rabies immune globulin
Right bundle-branch block (RBBB), 166*b*, 179*t*
Right ventricular hypertrophy (RVH), 173*b*
Righting, head, 236.e6*t*
Rimantadine (Flumadine), 1051
Ringer's solution, 302*t*
Ringworm, 481*t*
Riomet. *See* Metformin
Risk
  attributable, 727
  relative (RR), 725
Risk reduction
  absolute (ARR), 727
  relative (RRR), 727
Risperidone (Risperdal)
  ages of FDA approval, 245*t*
  formulary entry, 1052–1053
Ritalin. *See* Methylphenidate HCl
Ritonavir, 385*b*
Rituals, 632
Rituximab (Rituxan), 406
  for arthritis, 692
  characteristics of, 613*t*–615*t*
  for nephrotic syndrome, 536–537
  for SLE, 695
Rizatriptan (Maxalt)
  formulary entry, 1053–1054
  for migraine, 554*t*
Robinul. *See* Glycopyrrolate
Rocaltrol. *See* Calcitriol
Rocephin. *See* Ceftriaxone
Rocky Mountain spotted fever, 479*t*–480*t*

Rocuronium
  formulary entry, 1054–1055
  for RSI, 7t–8t
Rodent bites, 94t
Rolandic epilepsy, benign, 559t–560t
Rome III Criteria, 321.e1t
ROP. See Retinopathy of prematurity
Rosadan. See Metronidazole
Ross procedure, 191
Rotarix (RV1), 438
RotaTeq (RV5), 438
Rotavirus (RV) immunoprophylaxis, 438–439
  administration, 438
  catch-up schedule for, 414f
  for children with HIV disease, 423
  recommended schedule for, 413f, 415f–418f
  routine vaccination, 438
Roundworms, 955, 1037
Rowasa. See Mesalamine
Roweepra. See Levetiracetam
Roxanol. See Morphine sulfate
Roxicet. See Oxycodone and acetaminophen
Roxicodone. See Oxycodone
Roxilox. See Oxycodone and acetaminophen
RRR (relative risk reduction), 727
RSI (rapid sequence intubation), 5, 7t–8t
RTA. See Renal tubular acidosis
Rubella, 457t–458t, 471t–476t
Rubella immune globulin, 432
Rubella prophylaxis, 405
  measles/mumps/rubella immunoprophylaxis, 432–434
  postexposure, 434
Rubella vaccines
  measles, mumps, rubella, and varicella (MMRV) combination vaccine, 423
  measles, mumps, rubella (MMR) vaccine, 415f–418f
    catch-up schedule for, 414f
    for children with HIV disease, 423
    after Ig or blood product administration, 426, 426.e1t
    recommended schedule for, 413f
Rufinamide (Banzel)
  formulary entry, 1055
  for seizures, 562t
RuLox. See Aluminum hydroxide with magnesium hydroxide

Russell-Silver syndrome, 278f
RV (residual volume), 641–643, 643t

S

S wave, 170t
SABAs (short-acting inhaled beta$_2$-agonists), 647f–652f
Sabril. See Vigabatrin
Safety
  analgesic, 138
  Drug Safety Reporting Updates, 732
  HEADSSS assessment, 111b
Sagging rope sign, 681.e2f
Salagen. See Pilocarpine HCl
Salicylates, 23t–24t
Salicylazosulfapyridine. See Sulfasalazine
Saline enemas, 322
Saline solution
  hypertonic. See Hypertonic saline (HTS)
  isotonic. See Isotonic saline
  normal. See Normal saline (NS)
  for tumor lysis syndrome, 616
Salmeterol (Serevent Diskus), 1055–1056
Salmeterol/fluticasone (Advair), 646.e1t–646.e2t
Salmon patch, 218f
Salmonella infection, 691
Salter-Harris classification, 680t
Sample size, 725
Sampling
  blood, 31–48
  chorionic villus (CVS), 490.e1
  urine, 519
SAMSHA, 251
Sancuso. See Granisetron
Sandimmune. See Cyclosporine
Sandostatin. See Octreotide acetate
Sanfilippo syndrome, 344–345
Sanger sequencing, 358t
Sani-Supp. See Glycerin
Sano modification, 190f
SaO$_2$. See Arterial O$_2$ saturation
Sapropterin, 342
Sarafem. See Fluoxetine hydrochloride
Sarcoidosis, 701.e1
Sarcoma
  Ewing, 683
  osteosarcoma, 681, 682f–683f
  signs and symptoms of, 609t–610t
Sausage digits, 690

Scabies, 208–210
  diagnosis of, 218f
  treatment of, 946, 1014
Scald/contact injury, 96t
Scale, 203, 209f
Scalp ringworm, 481t
Scandishakes, 601t–602t
Scar(s), 203, 209f
SCARED, 248
Scarf sign, 494f, 495
Scedosporiosis, 1101
SCFE (slipped capital femoral epiphysis), 681, 681.e3f
Schizophrenia
  acute agitation associated with, 993
  treatment of, 782, 993, 1042, 1052–1053
School health guidelines, 113
School problems, 132
School-age children
  pain assessment in, 136
Schwartz equation, 524
  modified, 1091
Scintigraphy
  hepatobiliary, 678
  skeletal, 681
SCIWORA (spinal cord injury without radiographic abnormality), 78, 667
Scleroderma, 701.e2–701.e4
  associated autoantibodies, 695t
  diffuse cutaneous systemic (DCSS), 701.e3
  localized (limited), 701.e2–701.e3
Scoliosis
  imaging of, 667
  spirometry and lung volume readings in, 643t
Scopolamine hydrobromide (Transderm Scop)
  for antiemetic therapy, 626t
  formulary entry, 1056
SCRATCH principles, 224
Screening
  in adolescence, 113–123
  cardiovascular, 200–201, 201.e1b
  congenital heart disease, 493
  developmental, 230–236
  fetal anomaly, 490.e1
  for iron-deficiency anemia, 584
  lipid, 199–200
  newborn (NBS), 493
    for congenital adrenal hyperplasia, 270–271
    for hypothyroidism, 262
    metabolic, 340, 493
    universal, 655

Screening *(Continued)*
  ophthalmology, 688
  orthopedic examination, 113.e1f
  recommendations for competitive athletes, 201.e1b
  substance use, 133
  for type 2 DM, 259–260
  for UTIs, 518
Screening tests, 236
Scrotal inflammation, acute, 698
Scrotal pathology, 680
Scurvy, 783
Seasonal allergic rhinitis, 395, 788, 925, 976
Seatbelt sign, 74t–75t
Seattle criteria, modified, 622
Sebaceous nevus, 218f
Seborrhea, 1057
Seborrheic dermatitis, 218f, 219
Secobarbital, 385b
Secondary survey, 73, 74t–75t, 98–100
Secretions
  medications for palliative care, 634t
  pathological hypersecretory conditions, 995
Secretory diarrhea, 319
Sedation
  analgesia with, 931
  benzodiazepine, 891
  conscious, 145
  deep, 145
  dexmedetomidine, 853
  dissociative, 146
  goal of, 148
  ICU, 853
  for intubation, 6f
  lorazepam, 951
  with mechanical ventilation, 971
  mild, 145–146
  moderate, 145
  preoperative or preprocedure. *See also* Procedural sedation
    pentobarbital, 1013
    phenobarbital, 1015
  protocols for, 153t
Sedative-hypnotics, 139.e1t
  diazepam, 856
  droperidol, 867
  poisoning with, 22t
  for procedural sedation, 148
  properties of, 149b–150b
  for RSI, 7t–8t
Sediment, urinary, 518
SEER (Surveillance, Epidemiology, and End Results) data (NCI), 607
Seizure disorders, 558, 1018

Seizure syndromes, 559t–560t
Seizures, 555–564
    absence, 558b, 559t–560t
    acute management of, 16, 16t
    adjunctive therapy for, 936–937
    atonic, 558b
    breakthrough, 561
    caused by ingestions, 21
    clonic, 558b
    epileptic, 558b
    febrile, 555–556
    febrile illness–associated, 555–556
    focal, 558
    with focal onset, 558b
    generalized, 558b, 838, 1107
    medications for, 634t, 758
    myoclonic, 558b, 941
    neonatal, 338, 559t–560t
    nonfebrile, 556–558
    partial. See Partial seizures
    partial-onset, 934, 1083
    pharmacotherapy for, 561, 838, 937
    in poisoning, 21.e1t–21.e3t
    pyridoxine-dependent, 1039
    refractory, 941, 1079
    refractory partial, 934
    supportive care for, 21
    tonic, 558b
    tonic-clonic, 934, 941, 1083
Seldinger technique, 35f
    for central venous catheter placement, 37
    for radial artery catheterization, 34
Selective serotonin-reuptake inhibitors (SSRIs)
    black box warnings, 249–250
    for bulimia nervosa, 250
    for depressive disorders, 249
Selenium
    in multivitamin tablets, 589t–590t
    recommended intakes, 591t
Selenium sulfide (Selsun Blue, Tersi)
    formulary entry, 1057
    for tinea capitis, 212, 481t
Self-help skills, 229
Self-Report for Childhood Anxiety Related Emotional Disorders (SCARED), 237t–238t
Sellick maneuver (cricoid pressure), 4
Selsun Blue. See Selenium sulfide
Senna (Senokot, Senna-Gen, Lax-Pills), 1057–1058
Sensation changes as death approaches, 633
Sensitivity, 727
Sensory examination, 548, 549t

Separation anxiety, 233t–235t
Sepsis
    in newborns, 502
    in transfusion, 390
Septic arthritis, 704
    adolescent, 461t–468t
    initial management of, 461t–468t
    neonatal, 461t–468t
    synovial fluid characteristics, 718t
Septic shock, 87f, 86.e1t
Septic thrombosis, 947, 952
Septra. See Sulfamethoxazole and trimethoprim
Serevent Diskus. See Salmeterol
Sernivo. See Betamethasone
Seronegative spondyloarthropathy, 688
Seroquel. See Quetiapine
Serotonergic poisoning, 22t
Serotonin (5-HT$_3$) antagonists, 626t
Serotonin syndrome, 23t–24t
Sertraline (Zoloft)
    ages of FDA approval, 245t
    formulary entry, 1058–1059
Serum amyloid A, 701
Serum electrolyte disturbances, 304–311
Serum muscle enzymes, 704
Serum osmolality, 312
    formula for, 312
    normal range, 312
Serum osmolar gap, 312, 21.e1t–21.e3t
Severe combined immunodeficiency, 403t–404t
Sex, natal, 123–125
Sex phenotype, 123–125
Sexual abuse, 102
Sexual development, 277–286
Sexual health, 108, 123–131
Sexual history, 111.e1b
Sexual orientation, 123
Sexual victimization prophylaxis, 817
Sexuality, 111b
Sexually transmitted infections (STIs)
    adolescent access to services for, 114
    consent to medical care for, 114
    guidelines for management of, 115t–116t
    screening guidelines for sexually active adolescents, 114–122
    treatment recommendations for sexually active adolescents, 114–122
    websites for clinicians, 108
SfRowasa. See Mesalamine
SGA (small-for-gestational-age) infants, 493, 499f

Shagreen patches, 352
Sharps, 486
Shiga toxin–mediated hemolytic-uremic syndrome (ST-HUS), 375
Shigella, 691
Shock, 84–86
  anaphylactic, 86.e1t
  cardiogenic, 86, 86.e1t
  categorization of, 86.e2t
  compensated, 84, 86.e2t
  decompensated, 86, 86.e2t
  hypovolemic/distributive, 86, 87f, 86.e1t
  neurogenic, 86.e1t
  obstructive, 86, 86.e1t
  resuscitation in, 3–4
  septic, 87f, 86.e1t
  types of, 86, 86.e1t
  vasodilatory, with hypotension, 1096
Short stature, 276–277
  differential diagnosis of, 276–277, 278f
  familial, 276, 278f
  pathologic, 277
Short-acting inhaled beta$_2$-agonists (SABAs), 647t–652f
Shortening fraction (FS), 184, 184.e1
Shuddering attacks, 557t
Shunt nephritis, 532f
Shunts
  cardiac, 190, 190f
  CSF, 564
  intrapulmonary shunt fraction (Qs/Qt), 93.e1
  ventriculoperitoneal. *See* Ventriculoperitoneal shunts
SIADH (syndrome of inappropriate antidiuretic hormone), 274–276
Siblings, 233t–235t
Sicca, 701.e4
Sickle cell anemia, 368
Sickle cell disease
  complications of, 370t–371t
  health maintenance, 372t
  immunoprophylaxis guidelines for children with, 422
  initial management of, 461t–468t
  pneumococcal prophylaxis for, 1012
  stroke in, 567
Sickle cell trait, 532f
SIDS. *See* Sudden infant death syndrome
Significance levels, 723

Sildenafil (Revatio, Viagra)
  for acute pulmonary hypertensive crisis, 89
  formulary entry, 1059–1060
Silvadene. *See* Silver sulfadiazine
Silver sulfadiazine (Silvadene, Thermazene, SSD Cream)
  for burns, 100.e1b
  formulary entry, 1060
Silver-impregnated products, 100.e1b
Simethicone (Mylicon, Phazyme, Mylanta Gas, Gas-X), 1060
Similac formulas, 570, 594t–602t
Simply Saline. *See* Sodium chloride
SIMV (synchronized IMV), 91
Simvastatin, 347
Single gene testing, 358t
Single nucleotide polymorphism (SNP) array, 336t, 358t
Singulair. *See* Montelukast
Sinus rhythm, 167–168
Sinus tachycardia, 174t–175t
Sinusitis
  acute, 461t–468t, 789, 819–820, 942
  bacterial, 942
  chronic, 461t–468t
  differential diagnosis of, 396
  exacerbation of, 819
  initial management of, 461t–468t
  maxillary, 819, 823, 835–836
  treatment of, 790, 816, 823
Sinusoidal obstruction syndrome, 622–623
Sirolimus (Rapamune)
  formulary entry, 1061–1062
  for GVHD, 621
6 Ps, 80–81
Sjögren syndrome, 695t, 701.e3–701.e4
Skeletal anomalies, 184
Skeletal conditions, 352–353
Skeletal injury, 103t
Skeletal scintigraphy, 681
Skeletal survey, 683
  in child abuse, 102
Skin
  in headaches, 551.e1t
  newborn, 494f
Skin and skin structure infections. *See also* Skin infections
  acute bacterial (ABSSSI), 820
  treatment of, 819
Skin and soft tissue infections, 789, 1023
Skin care, 701.e3

Skin examination
  adolescent, 112
  secondary survey, 74t–75t
Skin infections, 207–211
  candidal, 481t
  complicated, 952, 958
  treatment of, 816, 819, 824, 942, 947, 958
  uncomplicated, 820, 835–836
Skin lesions
  allergic, 220–224
  autoimmune, 220–224
  primary, 203, 204f–205f
  secondary, 203, 209f
Skin staples, 67–68
Skin syndromes, 397–398
Skin testing
  for drug allergy, 401
  for food allergy, 398–399
Skip metastasis, 682f–683f
Skull, infant, 353.e1f
Skull fractures, 103t
Skull radiography, 665
SLE. *See* Systemic lupus erythematosus
Sleep aids, 862
Sleep duration, 659f
Sleep hygiene, 658
Sleep needs, 633
Sleep problems
  childhood, 658–660
  delayed sleep phase syndrome, 659
  inadequate sleep, 658
  obstructive sleep apnea syndrome (OSAS), 656–658, 657b
Sleep-onset association disorder, 658
Slipped capital femoral epiphysis (SCFE), 681, 681.e3f
Slo-Niacin. *See* Niacin
Slow FE. *See* Iron, oral preparations
Slow Iron. *See* Iron, oral preparations
Sly syndrome, 344
Small bowel fluid, 304t
Small bowel obstruction, 678
Small vessel vasculitis, 696, 697t
Small-for-gestational-age (SGA) infants, 493, 499f
Smith-Lemli-Opitz disorder, 346–347
Snoring, 657–658
SNP (single nucleotide polymorphism) array, 358t
SOAP-ME (Suction, Oxygen, Airway Supplies, Pharmacology, Monitoring Equipment), 4–5
Social anxiety disorder, 879, 1008
Social skills, 231t–232t

Social workers, 628
Society for Adolescent Medicine, 108
Society for Pediatric Radiology, 663
Sodium
  fractional excretion of (FENa), 525
  in multivitamin tablets, 589t–590t
  newborn requirements for, 498t
  reference values, 709t–716t
Sodium bicarbonate (NaHCO$_3$, Neut)
  formulary entry, 1062
  for hyperkalemia, 308f
  for local analgesia, 30
  rehydration fluids, 302t
  for wide QRS complex, 23t–24t
Sodium bicarbonate with omeprazole (Zegerid), 995–996
Sodium chloride preparations (Hypersal, Simply Saline, Ocean, Ayr Saline, Rhinaris), 1062–1063
Sodium (Na$^+$) deficit, 294.e1
  general equation for, 294
  replacement strategy for, 297
Sodium disturbances, 304
Sodium phenylacetate, 340
Sodium phenylacetate and sodium benzoate (Ammonul), 342
  dose adjustment in renal failure, 1125t–1134t
  formulary entry, 1063
  for metabolic crisis, 340
Sodium phosphate (Fleet Enema, Fleet Pedia-Lax, Fleet Phospho-Soda, OsmoPrep), 1064. *See also* Phosphorus supplements
Sodium polystyrene sulfonate (SPS, Kayexalate, Kalexate, Kionex)
  formulary entry, 1064–1065
  for hyperkalemia, 308f
Sodium restriction, 623
Sodium supplementation, 272
Sodium valproate, 555
Soft tissue abscesses, 62, 62f–63f
Soft tissue aspiration, 61
  ultrasound-guided, 62, 62f–63f
Soft tissue cellulitis, 62, 62f–63f
Soft tissue infections. *See* Skin and soft tissue infections
Solid organ transplant recipients, 423
Solodyn. *See* Minocycline
Solu-Cortef. *See* Hydrocortisone
Solu-Medrol. *See* Methylprednisolone
Solute deficits, 293–294, 297, 301
Solutes, maintenance, 292–293
Sonography, 79
Sorbitol, 322

Soy-based formulas, 593t–600t
Spasms. *See also* Infantile spasms
bronchospasms. *See* Bronchospasms
habit, 557t
Spasticity, chronic, 846
Spearman's rank correlation coefficient (rσ), 724t
Specific gravity, 516
Specificity, 727–728
Specimen collection
for blood culture, 443
timed urine specimens, 523
Speech sound disorders, 242
Spence Children's Anxiety Scale, 237t–238t, 248
Sphingolipidoses, 345–346
Spinal cord compression, 616–617
Spinal cord impairment, 548
Spinal cord injury
acute, 965
examination of, 548
treatment of, 965
without radiographic abnormality (SCIWORA), 78, 667
Spinal dysraphism, 667
Spinal fusion infections, 461t–468t
Spindle cell nevus, 226
Spine examination
adolescent, 112
imaging, 666–667
Spiritual changes as death approaches, 634
Spiriva HandiHaler. *See* Tiotropium
Spiriva Respimat. *See* Tiotropium
Spirometry, 641–643, 643t
Spironolactone (Aldactone)
for acne vulgaris, 214
dose adjustment in renal failure, 1125t–1134t
formulary entry, 1065
for hypertension, 544t–545t
Spitz nevus, 226, 226.e3f
Splenic sequestration, 370t–371t
Splinting, 68–69, 71f
ankle stirrup splint, 71f, 70.e2
long arm posterior splint, 71f, 70.e1–70.e2
posterior ankle splint, 71f, 70.e2
postsplint care, 69
sugar tong forearm splint, 70.e1
thumb spica splint, 71f, 70.e1
ulnar gutter splint, 71f, 70.e1
volar splint, 71f, 70.e1
Spondyloarthropathy, seronegative, 688
Spooning, 225
Sporanox. *See* Itraconazole

Sporotrichosis, cutaneous or lymphocutaneous, 1026
Sports
allowances for cardiac lesions, 199.e1t
cardiovascular screening, 200–201
recommendations for cardiovascular screening for, 201.e1b
Sports-related injuries
concussions in, 77–78
Guidelines: HEADS UP to Youth Sports (CDC), 73, 78
Spot urine, 526
Spritam. *See* Levetiracetam
SPS. *See* Sodium polystyrene sulfonate
Square window, 494f, 495
SR (stepping reflex), 236.e4t–236.e5t
SSD Cream. *See* Silver sulfadiazine
SSKI. *See* Potassium iodide
ST segment, 169, 171f
Stadol. *See* Butorphanol
Stanford Newborn Nursery, 588
Staphylococcal scalded skin syndrome, 218f
Staphylococcus
anti-*Staphylococcus*–resistant penicillins, 447t–449t
pustulosis, 218f
Staphylococcus aureus infections, 191, 520
methicillin-resistant, 947, 952
treatment of, 1050
Staphylococcus epidermidis, 191
Staphylococcus saprophyticus, 520
Staples, skin, 67–68
State forms, 633
State support
for developmental disorders, 246
disabilities that qualify for, 246
Statistical tests, 723, 724t
power of, 723–725
significance level, 723
Statistics
biostatistics, 723–728
resources and software for, 721
Stature
growth charts for boys, 578f
growth charts for girls, 571.e1f
short, 276–277
tall, 277
Status asthmaticus, 914
Status epilepticus, 561
assessment of, 15–16
emergency management of, 15–17
refractory, 971

Status epilepticus (Continued)
  treatment of, 856, 901, 951, 1015, 1018
Stepping reflex (SR), 236.e4t–236.e5t
Sternal abnormalities, 184
Steroid-dependent nephrotic syndrome, 536–537
Steroids. *See also* Corticosteroids
  anabolic, 385b
  for antiemetic therapy, 626t
  for asthma, 10
  for atopic dermatitis (eczema), 222
  biosynthetic pathway for, 269f
  for hemangioma, 207
  for HSP, 698
  for migraine, 555
  topical, 222
  warfarin interactions, 385b
ST-HUS (Shiga toxin–mediated hemolytic-uremic syndrome), 375
Still's murmur, 167t
Stimate. *See* Desmopressin acetate
Stimulants, 245t
Stirrup splint, ankle, 71f, 70.e2
STIs. *See* Sexually transmitted infections
STNR (symmetrical tonic neck reflex), 236.e4t–236.e5t
Stomach conditions, 318–325
Stomach Relief. *See* Bismuth subsalicylate
Stomatitis, 1068
Stool
  normal output, 319–321
  normal patterns, 321–322
Stool hemoccult, 316–317
Stool osmolar gap (Stool Osm), 319
Stranger anxiety, 233t–235t
Strattera. *See* Atomoxetine
Strength rating scale, 549b
Streptococcal pharyngitis, 824
Streptococcus
  group A streptococcal (GAS) infection, 1010–1012
  group B. *See* Group B streptococcal (GBS) infection
Streptococcus pneumoniae, 774
Streptococcus pyogenes, 774
Streptococcus viridans, 191
Streptomycin sulfate
  dose adjustment in renal failure, 1111t–1124t
  formulary entry, 1066
  spectrum of activity, 451t
Stress fractures, 681
Stress ulcers, 1068
Stretch reflexes, 550.e1t

Stridor, 638t
Stroke, 565–567
  acute, 566b
  differential diagnosis of, 566
  initial workup, 566b
  management of, 548, 566–567
  risk factors for, 565–566
  supportive care for, 566–567
Study designs, 726t
Stunting, 571
Stupor, 943
Stuttering, 242
Subclavian vein: central venous catheter placement via, 37, 41, 42f
Subcutaneous fat necrosis, 218f
Subcutaneous injections, 64
Subcutaneous tissue infections, 958
Subcutaneous vaccines
  administration of, 419
  preferred sites for, 419
Subdermal implants, contraceptive, 127
Sublimaze. *See* Fentanyl
Subluxation, radial head (nursemaid's elbow), 70
Submandibular infections, 455
Substance P receptor antagonists, 626t
Substance use, 133–134
  brief intervention for, 133
  screening for, 133
  treatment of, 133–134
  websites for patients, 108
Substance use disorders, 250–251
Substrate reduction therapy (SRT), 346
Subungal hematoma, 225
Subungal hemorrhage, traumatic, 225.e1f
Succimer (Chemet, DMSA [dimercaptosuccinic acid])
  formulary entry, 1066–1067
  for lead poisoning, 26
Succinylcholine (Anectine, Quelicin)
  formulary entry, 1067
  for RSI, 7t–8t
Sucralfate (Carafate), 1068
Sucrose (Sweet Ease), 142–143
Suction, Oxygen, Airway Supplies, Pharmacology, Monitoring Equipment (SOAP-ME), 4–5
Sudafed. *See* Pseudoephedrine
Sudden cardiac arrest, 2
Sudden infant death syndrome (SIDS), 324, 660
  protective factors for, 660b
  risk factors for, 660b
Sugar(s), urinary, 517
Sugar tong forearm splint, 71f, 70.e1

Suicidal ideation, 132
Suicide
  among adolescents, 132
  HEADSSS assessment, 111*b*
Sulbactam/ampicillin (Unasyn)
  for abscess infection, 461*t*–468*t*
  for bites, 461*t*–468*t*
  for cellulitis, 461*t*–468*t*
  dose adjustment in renal failure, 1111*t*–1124*t*
  formulary entry, 780
  spectrum of activity, 447*t*–449*t*
Sulfacetamide sodium ophthalmic (Bleph-10), 1068
Sulfadiazine
  formulary entry, 1069
  for toxoplasmosis, 457*t*–458*t*
Sulfamethoxazole and trimethoprim (Trimethoprim-sulfamethoxazole, TMP-SMX, Co-Trimoxazole, Bactrim, Septra, Sulfatrim)
  for acne vulgaris, 217*t*
  for bites, 461*t*–468*t*
  for cellulitis, 461*t*–468*t*
  for conjunctivitis, 461*t*–468*t*
  for cystitis, 461*t*–468*t*
  dose adjustment in renal failure, 1111*t*–1124*t*
  formulary entry, 1069–1070
  for gastroenteritis, 461*t*–468*t*
  for oncology patients, 626*t*
  for perinatal HIV exposure, 481*t*
  for pertussis, 461*t*–468*t*
  spectrum of activity, 452*t*
  for UTI prophylaxis, 522–523
  warfarin interactions, 385*b*
Sulfasalazine (Azulfidine, salicylazosulfapyridine)
  for arthritis, 692
  formulary entry, 1070–1071
  toxicity, 691.e1*t*
Sulfatrim. *See* Sulfamethoxazole and trimethoprim
Sulfinpyrazone, 385*b*
Sulfisoxazole, 385*b*
Sulfonylureas
  with metformin, 960
  overdose, 23*t*–24*t*
Sumatriptan (Imitrex, Sumavel Dose Pro, Zembrace SymTouch)
  formulary entry, 1071–1072
  for migraine, 554–555, 554*t*
Sumavel Dose Pro. *See* Sumatriptan
Sumycin. *See* Tetracycline HCl

Superinfection
  bacterial, 222
  eczema herpeticum, 222
Superior vena cava syndrome, 618
Superior vena cava–to–pulmonary artery shunts, 190, 190*f*
Suplena formulas, 594*t*–602*t*
Supportive care, 566–567
Suppositories
  bisacodyl, 797
  mesalamine, 958–959
Suppurative conjunctivitis, 461*t*–468*t*
Suppurative lymphadenitis, 446
Suppurative otitis media, 992
Supraventricular arrhythmia, 174*t*–175*t*, 176*f*
Supraventricular tachycardia, 174*t*–175*t*, 176*f*
  junctional, 174*t*–175*t*
  paroxysmal, 888, 1097
  treatment of, 762–763, 880, 888, 1097
Suprax. *See* Cefixime
Surfactant therapy
  beractant (Survanta), 1072
  calfactant (Infasurf), 1072–1073
  for newborns, 500
  poractant alfa (Curosurf), 1073
Surgery
  antiemetic therapy prior to, 1056
  bacterial endocarditis prophylaxis for, 191, 192*b*, 192*t*
  cardiac, 190–191
  for hydrocephalus, 564
  for lymphadenitis, 461*t*–468*t*
  for mastoiditis, 461*t*–468*t*
  nausea and vomiting associated with, 996–997
  orthopedic, 693
  for seizures, 564
  treatment regimens, 625
  for vesicoureteral reflux, 523
Sur-Q-Lax. *See* Docusate
Survanta. *See* Surfactant
Surveillance
  developmental, 230–235
  for mental health issues, 246
Survival curves, 725
Sustol. *See* Granisetron
Sutures, infant skull, 353.e1*f*
Suturing, 65–67
  of animal bites, 94–95
  guidelines for material, size, and removal, 67*t*
  techniques, 65–67, 66*f*

Sweat, 304t
Sweat chloride test (quantitative pilocarpine ionoelectrophoresis), 654–655
Sweet Ease. See Sucrose
Symbicort. See Budesonide and formoterol
Symbols, 733t
Symmetrel. See Amantadine hydrochloride
Symmetrical tonic neck reflex (STNR), 236.e4t–236.e5t
Sympathomimetics, 22t
Synagis. See Palivizumab
Synchronized IMV (SIMV), 91
Synchronized intermittent mandatory ventilation (SIMV), 91
Syncope
 cardiogenic, 557t
 cough, 557t
 differential diagnosis of, 557t
Syndrome of inappropriate antidiuretic hormone (SIADH), 274–276
Synercid. See Quinupristin and dalfopristin
Synovial fluid, 718t
Synthetic cannabinoids, 23t–24t
Synthroid. See Levothyroxine
Syphilis, 457t–458t
 congenital, 1009, 1011
 diagnosis of, 218f
 management of, 115t–116t
 neurosyphilis, 1010–1011
 primary, 120t
 screening guidelines for sexually active adolescents, 114
 serology, 455.e2t
 treatment of, 1009–1011
Systemic lupus erythematosus, 693–696
 associated autoantibodies, 693–694, 695t
 classification criteria for, 693, 694t
 drug-induced, 696
 incomplete, 693
 neonatal, 696
 synovial fluid characteristics, 718t
 treatment of, 916
Systemic lupus erythematosus nephritis, 693, 693.e1t
Systemic-to-pulmonary artery cardiac shunts, 190, 190f
Systems review, 111
Systolic blood pressure (SBP), 165f
Systolic heart murmurs, 168b

T
T lymphocytes, 408t
t test, 724t
T wave, 167, 172, 172t
T_3 (triiodothyronine), 263t
T_4. See Levothyroxine; Thyroxine
T&A (tonsillectomy and adenoidectomy), 138
Tachyarrhythmia, 771
Tachycardia
 atrial, ectopic, 174t–175t
 atrioventricular reentrant, 174t–175t
 in poisoning, 21.e1t–21.e3t
 sinus, 174t–175t
 supraventricular. See Supraventricular tachycardia
 ventricular. See Ventricular tachycardia
Tachypnea, 21.e1t–21.e3t
Tacrolimus (Prograf, Astragraf XL, Envarsus XR, Protopic, FK506)
 for Behçet disease, 700
 formulary entry, 1074–1075
 for GVHD, 621
Taenia saginata, 1008
Taenia solium, 1008
Tagamet. See Cimetidine
Takayasu arteritis, 697t
Tall stature, 277
Tambocor. See Flecainide acetate
Tamiflu. See Oseltamivir phosphate
Tamoxifen, 385b
Tanner staging
 of breast development, 109f
 of pubic hair, 110f
Tapazole. See Methimazole
Tapeworm, 1008
Target sign, 678, 679f
Tay-Sachs disease, 345–346
Tazarotene (Avage, Fabior, Tazorac)
 formulary entry, 1075–1076
 formulations and concentrations, 216t
Tazicef. See Ceftazidime
Tazobactam, 461t–468t
Tazobactam with piperacillin (Zosyn)
 formulary entry, 1022–1023
 for sinusitis, 461t–468t
 for spinal fusion infections, 461t–468t
Tazorac. See Tazarotene
Taztia XT. See Diltiazem
TBG (thyroxine-binding globulin), 263t
TBI (total body irradiation), 619
TBI (traumatic brain injury), 82
TCAs. See Tricyclic antidepressants
Td vaccine. See Tetanus toxoid

Tdap (tetanus, diphtheria, & acellular pertussis) vaccine (Boostrix, Adacel), 426
   administration, 427
   contraindications to, 426–427
   precautions, 426–427
   in pregnancy, 424
   for pre-teens and adolescents, 124t
   recommended schedule for, 413f, 415f–418f
   routine vaccination, 426
Technetium uptake, 261
Technetium-99m (99mTc)
   hepatobiliary scintigraphy with 99mTc-iminodiacetate (HIDA), 678
   methylene diphosphonate bone scans, 682f–683f
TEE (total energy expenditure), 579
TEE (transesophageal echocardiography), 184
TEF (thermic effect of food), 579
Teflaro. See Ceftaroline fosamil
Tegretol. See Carbamazepine
Telogen effluvium, 212
Temozolomide (Temodar), 613t–615t
Temper tantrums, 233t–235t
Temperature
   conversion formulas, 708
   rectal, 493
Temporal arteritis, 697t
Tempra. See Acetaminophen
Tendon reflexes, 550–551
Tenex. See Guanfacine
Tenormin. See Atenolol
Tension pneumothorax
   signs of, 79
   treatment of, 79
Terazosin, 544t–545t
Terbinafine, 481t
Terbutaline
   for asthma, 11
   dose adjustment in renal failure, 1125t–1134t
   formulary entry, 1076
Terminal illness
   discontinuing interventions in, 632
   DNAR orders in, 632
   memory making in, 631–632
Tersi. See Selenium sulfide
Testicles
   imaging, 680
   normal size, 284t
Testosterone, 283t
TET spells, 189t, 977, 1034

Tetanus immunoglobulin (TIG)
   administration, 427
   after Ig or blood product administration, 426.e1t
Tetanus immunoprophylaxis, 95, 426–427
   in burns, 100
   contraindications to, 426–427
   after Ig or blood product administration, 426.e1t
   indications for, 428t
Tetanus toxoid (Td), 426
   administration, 427
   precautions, 426–427
Tetanus vaccines
   catch-up vaccination, 414f, 426
   diphtheria, tetanus, & acellular pertussis (DTaP), 426
      catch-up schedule for, 414f
      recommended schedule for, 413f, 415f–418f
   diphtheria/tetanus/pertussis vaccines, 426–427
   routine vaccination, 413f, 415f–418f, 426
   tetanus, diphtheria, & acellular pertussis (Tdap), 426
      catch-up schedule for, 414f
      in pregnancy, 424
      for pre-teens and adolescents, 124t
      recommended schedule for, 413f, 415f–418f
Tetany, 807
Tetracaine, 141t, 153t
Tetracycline HCl
   for acne vulgaris, 214, 217t
   derivatives, 214
   dose adjustment in renal failure, 1111t–1124t
   formulary entry, 1077
   for gastroenteritis, 461t–468t
   for oral ulcers, 700
   spectrum of activity, 451t
   for syphilis, 115t–116t
Tetrahydrocannabinol (THC). See Dronabinol
Tetralogy of Fallot, 166b, 188t–189t
6-TG. See Thioguanine
Thalassemia, 369–372
α-Thalassemia, 369–372
β-Thalassemia, 371–372
Thalassemia intermedia, 371
Thalassemia major, 372
Thalassemia minor, 371
Thalassemia trait, 371

THC (tetrahydrocannabinol). *See* Dronabinol
The Arc, 242
The Joint Commission Official "Do Not Use" List, 733*t*
Theophylline (Theo-24, Theochron, Elixophyllin)
 for asthma, 651*f*–652*f*
 formulary entry, 1077–1078
Thera-Ear. *See* Carbamide peroxide
Thermal injury, 95–100, 96*t*
Thermazene. *See* Silver sulfadiazine
Thermic effect of food (TEF), 579
Thiamine (vitamin B$_1$)
 for coma, 14
 formulary entry, 1078–1079
 in infant multivitamin drops, 588*t*
 in multivitamin tablets, 589*t*–590*t*
 recommended intakes, 586*t*
 reference values, 709*t*–716*t*
Thin glomerular basement membrane, 532*f*
Thioguanine (6-TG, 6-thioguanine)
 characteristics of, 613*t*–615*t*
 late effects of cancer, 625.e1*t*–625.e2*t*
Thiopental
 for deep sedation, 145
 for intubation, 6*f*
 for RSI, 7*t*–8*t*
Thioridazine, 1079
Thiotepa, 613*t*–615*t*
Third ventriculostomy, endoscopic (ETV), 564
Thoracentesis, 52–55, 53*f*
Thoracic trauma
 blunt, 78–80
 common injuries, 79
 laboratory studies in, 79
Thorazine. *See* Chlorpromazine
3 Ps, 224
3TC. *See* Lamivudine
Thrombin time, 377*t*–378*t*
Thrombocytopenia, 373–375, 694*t*
 in chemotherapy patients, 624
 neonatal, 374–375
 neonatal alloimmune (NAIT), 374–375
Thrombocytopenic purpura
 idiopathic (ITP), 373–375
 immune (ITP), 405, 920, 1046
 thrombotic (TTP), 375, 623
Thrombolytic therapy, 766
 indications for, 382
 for stroke, 567

Thrombosis, 379–382
 septic, 947, 952
 treatment of, 380–382
Thrombotic microangiopathy (TMA), 375, 623
Thrombotic thrombocytopenic purpura (TTP), 375, 623
Thrush (oral candidiasis), 481*t*, 841
Thumb spica splint, 71*f*, 70.e1
Thyroid gland
 adolescent examination of, 112
 function of, 261–266
 late effects of cancer treatment on, 625.e1*t*–625.e2*t*
Thyroid scan, 261
Thyroid storm, 265–266
Thyroid tests, 261
 interpretation of, 261, 262*t*
 normal values, 263*t*
Thyroiditis, Hashimoto, 265
Thyroid-stimulating hormone (TSH), 263*t*
ThyroSafe. *See* Potassium iodide
ThyroShield. *See* Potassium iodide
Thyrotoxicosis
 neonatal, 266
 treatment of, 1026, 1034
Thyroxine (T$_4$)
 mean values in infants, 263*t*
 normal values, 263*t*
Thyroxine-binding globulin (TBG), 263*t*
Ti (inspiratory time), 90–91, 91.e1
Tiagabine (Gabitril)
 formulary entry, 1079–1080
 for seizures, 562*t*
Tiazac. *See* Diltiazem
Tickborne illnesses, 470, 479*t*–480*t*
Tics/habit spasms, 557*t*
Tidal volume (V$_T$), 90
Tigan. *See* Trimethobenzamide HCL
Timed urine specimens, 523
Timolol
 for hemangioma, 207
 topical, 207
Tinactin. *See* Tolnaftate
Tinea capitis, 211–212, 481*t*
Tinea corporis, 210, 481*t*
Tinea cruris, 481*t*
Tinea pedis, 481*t*
Tinea unguium, 481*t*
Tinea versicolor, 210, 1057
Tiotropium (Spiriva HandiHaler, Spiriva Respimat), 1080
Tirosint. *See* Levothyroxine
Tissue adhesives, 68

Tissue plasminogen activator (TPA), 377t–378t
Tissue transglutaminase (TTG), 325
Tivorbex. *See* Indomethacin
TLC (total lung capacity), 641–643, 643f, 643t
TLP (tonic labyrinthine prone) reflex, 236.e4t–236.e5t
TLS (tonic labyrinthine supine) reflex, 236.e4t–236.e5t
TMA (thrombotic microangiopathy), 375
TMP-SMX (trimethoprim-sulfamethoxazole). *See* Sulfamethoxazole and trimethoprim
TOA (tubo-ovarian abscess), 680
TOBI. *See* Tobramycin
Tobramycin (Tobrex, TOBI, Bethkis, Kitabis Pak)
  dose adjustment in renal failure, 1111t–1124t
  formulary entry, 1081–1082
  spectrum of activity, 451t
Tobramycin with dexamethasone (TobraDex), 1081
Tobrex. *See* Tobramycin
α-Tocopherol. *See* Vitamin E
Toenails, ingrown, 225, 225.e5f
Tofranil. *See* Imipramine
Toilet training, 233t–235t
Tolerable upper intake level (UL), 583
Tolerex formula, 594t–602t
Tolnaftate (Tinactin), 1083
Tonic labyrinthine prone (TLP) reflex, 236.e4t–236.e5t
Tonic labyrinthine supine (TLS) reflex, 236.e4t–236.e5t
Tonic neck reflex
  asymmetrical (ATNR), 236.e4t–236.e5t
  symmetrical (STNR), 236.e4t–236.e5t
Tonic seizures, 558b
Tonic-clonic seizures, 934, 941, 1083
Tonsillectomy and adenoidectomy (T&A), 138
Tonsillitis, 774, 789, 816, 819–821, 823, 835–836
Topamax. *See* Topiramate
Topical antibacterial agents, 214, 100.e1b
Topical calcineurin inhibitors, 222
Topical corticosteroids, 222, 223t
Topical emollients, 701.e3
Topical local anesthetics, 139, 141t
Topical retinoids
  for acne vulgaris, 214, 215t
  formulations and concentrations, 216t

Topiramate (Topamax, Trokendi XR, Qudexy XR)
  formulary entry, 1083–1084
  for migraine prevention, 556t
  for seizures, 559t–560t, 562t
Topoisomerase inhibitors
  chemotherapeutic agents, 613t–615t
  late effects of, 625.e1t–625.e2t
Toprol-XL. *See* Metoprolol
Toradol. *See* Ketorolac
Torsades, 23t–24t
Total anomalous pulmonary venous return, 188t–189t
Total body irradiation (TBI), 619
Total energy expenditure (TEE), 579
Total iron-binding capacity (TIBC), 709t–716t
Total lung capacity (TLC), 641–643, 643f, 643t
Total parenteral nutrition (TPN), 625
Total parenteral nutrition (TPN)-induced cholestasis, 1089
Tourette's syndrome, 782, 911
Toxicology screens, 20–21, 21t
Toxidromes, 22t
Toxocariasis, 955
Toxoplasmosis, 457t–458t
  congenital, 1040, 1069
  imaging of, 665
  treatment of, 786, 847, 1040, 1069
TPA (tissue plasminogen activator), 377t–378t
Trachea, 184
Tracheitis, 461t–468t
Tracheoesophageal fistula, 677, 677.e1f
Traction alopecia, 212
Trained night feeding, 233t–235t
Tramadol, 138
Trandate. *See* Labetalol
Transaminase. *See* Alanine aminotransferase (ALT); Aspartate aminotransferase (AST)
Transcranial Doppler (TCD), 372t, 675
Transderm Scop. *See* Scopolamine hydrobromide
Transdermal (patch) contraceptive, 129
Transesophageal echocardiography (TEE), 184
Transferrin, 709t–716t
Transfusion reactions
  acute, 385–390
  delayed, 389–390
Transgender, 123, 285–286
Transient erythroblastopenia of childhood (TEC), 367

Transient neonatal pustular melanosis, 217–219, 218f
Transitioning into adult care, 134
Transplantation
  bone marrow. See Bone marrow transplantation (BMT)
  heart, 192b, 1074, 1091
  kidney
    allograft rejection in, 532f
    management of, 978, 1074, 1090–1091
  kidney-pancreas, 1091
  liver, 1074
  solid organ, 423
  stem cell. See Hematopoietic stem cell transplantation (HSCT)
Transposition of the great arteries, 166b, 188t–189t
Transthoracic echocardiography (TTE), 184
Transurethral catheterization, 520
Transvaginal ultrasound, 680
Trauma, 73
  abdominal, 678
    emergency treatment of, 79–80
    laboratory studies in, 79
  acute head injury, 14
  birth, 495
  blunt thoracic and abdominal, 78–80
  cervical spine, 78, 666–667
  closed head trauma (CHT), 75–78
  Focused Assessment with Sonography for Trauma (FAST), 79
  head, 14, 75–78, 665
  imaging in, 680
  intraabdominal injury (IAI), 79
  long bone, 80–81
  nonaccidental. See Child abuse
  orthopedic, 80–81
  specific injuries, 75–81
  thoracic, 79
  web resources, 73
Traumatic arthritis, 718t
Traumatic brain injury (TBI), 82
Traumatic subungal hemorrhage, 225.e1f
Travasol (amino acid 8.5%), 302t
Traveler's diarrhea, 461t–468t
Travelers' Health (CDC) (website), 412, 426
Travelers to foreign countries, 426, 429
Trazodone, 1084–1085
Treponema pallidum particle agglutination (TP-PA), 455.e2t

Tretinoin
  formulations and concentrations, 216t
  topical preparations (Retin-A, Avita, Renova, Tretin-X), 1085–1086
Tretinoin with clindamycin (Veltin, Ziagen), 1085–1086
Tretin-X. See Tretinoin
Trial elimination diets, 400
Triamcinolone
  formulary entry, 1086–1087
  injection preparations (Kenalog), 1086–1087
  nasal preparations (Nasacort Allergy 24HR, Nasal Allergy 24 Hour), 1086–1087
  potency, 223t, 271t
  topical preparations (Triderm, Kenalog, Oralone), 1086–1087
Triamterene (Dyrenium)
  dose adjustment in renal failure, 1125t–1134t
  formulary entry, 1087
  for hypertension, 544t–545t
Trichinellosis, 955
Trichomoniasis, 118t, 968
Trichophyton sudanese, 211–212
Trichophyton tonsurans, 211–212
Trichophyton violeum, 211–212
Trichostrongylus, 1037
Trichotillomania, 213
Trichuris, 955
Tricuspid atresia, 188t–189t
Tricuspid stenosis, 166b
Tricyclic antidepressants (TCAs)
  ECG effects of, 180t
  overdose, 23t–24t
Triderm. See Triamcinolone
Trifluridine (Viroptic), 1087–1088
Trigeminy, 177t
Triglycerides
  persistently high, 200
  reference values, 709t–716t
Triiodothyronine (T_3), 263t
Trileptal. See Oxcarbazepine
Trilisate. See Choline magnesium trisalicylate
TriLyte. See Polyethylene glycol (PEG) electrolyte solutions
Trimethobenzamide HCL (Tigan), 1088
Trimethoprim-sulfamethoxazole (TMP-SMX). See Sulfamethoxazole and trimethoprim
Trimox. See Amoxicillin
Triple Antibiotic. See Neomycin/polymyxin B + bacitracin
Tripod positioning, 12

Triptans, 554–555, 554t
Trisomy 13, 349
Trisomy 18, 349
Trisomy 21, 347–350
  AAP guidelines for health supervision in, 348–349
  differential diagnosis of, 278f
  dominant cardiac defects, 185t
Tri-Vi-Sol, 588t
Trizivir. See Zidovudine with abacavir and lamivudine
Trokendi XR. See Topiramate
Tromethamine, 932
Tromethamine-Iodoxamide, 397
Trousseau's sign, 307, 21.e1t–21.e3t
Trumenba (MenB-FHbp). See Meningococcal B vaccine
Trypanosomiasis, 1013
TSH (thyroid-stimulating hormone), 263t
TTE. See Transthoracic echocardiography
TTP (thrombotic thrombocytopenic purpura), 375, 623
Tube feeding: formulas for, 601t–602t
Tuberculin skin test (TST), 484, 485b
Tuberculosis (TB), 484–486
  active disease, 484–485
  immunoprophylaxis for, 439
    administration, 439.e1
    routine vaccination, 439.e1
    side effects of, 439.e1
  INH-resistant, 928
  latent infection, 484–485
  multidrug-resistant, 1066
  prophylaxis for, 928
  screening for, 123, 433, 484
  treatment of, 485–486, 882, 928, 1038, 1050, 1066
Tuberculous arthritis, 718t
Tuberous sclerosis, 352
Tuberous sclerosis complex, 561
Tubo-ovarian abscess (TOA), 680
Tubular disorders, 535b, 537–538
Tubular necrosis, 532f
Tubular reabsorption (Tx), 525
Tubulointerstitial disease, 531t
Tularemia, 1066
Tumor lysis syndrome, 616, 764
Tumor necrosis factor inhibitors
  for arthritis, 692
  for Behçet disease, 700
  for idiopathic pneumonia syndrome, 623
  toxicity, 691.e1t

Tumors, 203, 204f–205f
  brain
    associated cerebral edema, 852
    management of, 612, 852
    signs and symptoms of, 609t–611t
  gonadal, 609t–610t
  metastatic, 218f
  neuroectodermal, 611t
  neuroepithelial, 611t
  rhabdoid, 611t
  vascular, benign, 203–207
  Wilms', 532f, 609t–610t
Tums. See Calcium carbonate
Turner syndrome, 349–350
  AAFP guidelines for, 349–350
  differential diagnosis of, 278f
  dominant cardiac defects, 185t
22q11 syndrome, 356–357
24-hour urine, 526
24-hour urine protein, 534
Twinrix (HepA/Hep B combination), 442
TwoCal HN formula, 594t–600t
Two-tailed tests, 723
Tx (tubular reabsorption), 525
Ty21a (Vivotif), 439
  administration, 439
  contraindications to, 439
  precautions, 439
  routine vaccination, 439
  side effects of, 439
Tylenol. See Acetaminophen
Tympanostomy tubes, 834, 992
Type I errors, 723
Type II errors, 723
Typhim Vi (ViCPS), 439
  administration, 439
  side effects of, 439
Typhlitis, 618
Typhoid fever immunoprophylaxis, 439
Tyrosine kinase inhibitors, 613t–615t
Tyrosinemia, hereditary, 342

U

U wave, 167
UA (umbilical artery) catheterization, 45–48, 47f
UC. See Ulcerative colitis
Uceris. See Budesonide
UCSF Center of Excellence for Transgender Health, 255
UEP (upper extremity placing) reflex, 236.e4t–236.e5t
UFH. See Unfractionated heparin
UGI (upper gastrointestinal) series, 677–678

Ulcerative colitis (UC), 323
  induction of remission, 800
  mild/moderate, 914, 959
  treatment of, 959
Ulcers, 203, 209f
  corneal, 942, 992
  duodenal, 884, 939, 995, 1045, 1068
  gastric, 939, 995, 1045
  genital, 700
  NSAID-induced, 939
  oral, 694t, 699–700
  prophylaxis of, 832
  stress, 1068
  treatment of, 995
Ulipristal (UPA, Ella), 130–131
Ulipristal (UPA, Ella), 130–131
Ulnar gutter splint, 71f, 70.e1
Ultrasound (US), 663
  advantages and disadvantages of, 664t
  in biliary atresia, 678
  in bowel obstruction, 678
  estimation of gestational age with, 490.e3
  fetal, 490.e1
  head, 664
  of head, 665
  intussusception findings, 678, 679f
  kidney and bladder, 521
  in pyloric stenosis, 677–678
  renal/bladder (RBUS), 679–680
  in testicular pathology, 680
  transvaginal, 680
  in uterine and ovarian pathology, 680
  in vessel abnormalities, 675–676
Ultresa. See Pancrelipase
Umbilical artery (UA) catheterization, 45–48, 47f
  ultrasound confirmation, 47, 47.e1f
Umbilical cord blood
  reference values, 709t–716t
  serum complement levels, 408t
  serum immunoglobulin levels, 407t
Umbilical vein (UV) catheter (UVC), 492
Umbilical vein (UV) catheterization, 45–48
  ultrasound confirmation, 48, 48.e1f
Unasyn. See Ampicillin/sulbactam
Underweight, 571
Unfractionated heparin (UFH), 380–382
  dose adjustment algorithm, 381t
  dose initiation guidelines, 381t
  for thrombosis, 380–382, 381t
Uniparental disomy, 334.e1
Unithroid. See Levothyroxine

Universal Precautions, 30, 486
UPA. See Ulipristal
Upper airway obstruction, 12–13
Upper airway procedures, 815, 822, 824
Upper airway resistance syndrome, 656
Upper extremity placing (UEP) reflex, 236.e4t–236.e5t
Upper gastrointestinal (UGI) series, 677–678
Upper intake level (UL), 583
Upper motor neuron findings, 549t
Urea: fractional excretion of (FEurea), 525
Urea cycle defects, 342
Urea nitrogen, 709t–716t
Ureaplasma urealyticum, 973
Uremia, 529
Ureteral obstruction, bilateral, 527t
Ureteroscopy, 543
Urethral infections, 817
Urethral obstruction, 527t
Urethral prolapse, 532f
Urethritis, 532f, 790
Urgent neurology consultation, 567
Uric acid, 709t–716t
Uric acid nephropathy, 527t
Urinalysis, 516
  for bilirubin/urobilinogen, 518, 518t
  culture, 520–523
  dipstick test, 516
  for epithelial cells, 518
  gram stain, 518
  nitrite test, 519–520
  obtaining samples for, 519
  for proteinuria, 531–534
  for RBCs, 518
  in rheumatic disease, 704
  for sediment, 518
  spot urine, 526
  timed specimens, 523
  toxicology screens, 21t
  24-hour urine, 526
  for WBCs, 518
Urinary acidification, 774
Urinary acidification defects, 526
Urinary alkalinization, 758, 1062
Urinary bladder catheterization, 58–59
Urinary tract disease, 531t
Urinary tract infections (UTIs)
  acute, 817
  catheter-associated, 520
  complicated, 833, 942
  culture-positive, 520–523
  diagnosis of, 519–520

Urinary tract infections (UTIs) (Continued)
evaluation of, 519–523
febrile, 520, 679–680
imaging, 521–522, 679–680
initial management of, 461t–468t
lower, 520
Practice Guidelines for Children 2–24 months (AAP), 516, 519
prophylaxis of, 988, 1070
risk factors for, 519
screening for, 518
treatment of, 519–523, 817, 820, 824, 1015
uncomplicated, 833, 942
upper, 520
Urinary tract mycosis, 777
Urine
color, 516
red, 530
sugars in, 517
turbidity, 516
Urine amino acids, 336t
Urine anion gap (UAG), 537
Urine calcium, 526
Urine concentration, 526
Urine ketones, 517
Urine organic acids, 336t
Urine osmolality, 526
Urine pH, 517
Urine protein, 517, 534
Urine protein/creatinine ratio, 533–534
Urine reducing substances, 338–339
Urine specific gravity, 516–517
Urobilinogen, 518, 518t
Urolithiasis, 532f
Urology
late effects of cancer treatment, 625.e1t–625.e2t
pediatric, 523
referral to, 523
Uro-Mag. *See* Magnesium oxide
Ursodiol (Actigall, Urso 250, Urso Forte), 1088–1089
Urticaria
acute transfusion reaction, 389
food allergy, 397
treatment of, 400
U.S. Department of Agriculture (USDA): Healthy Eating Guidelines, 570
U.S. Department of Health and Human Services (HHS)
My Family Health Portrait Tool, 334
requirements for contraception benefits, 125–131
U.S. Food and Drug Administration (FDA)
drug information data sources, 732
web resources, 412
U.S. National Library of Medicine, 721.e1
U.S. Preventive Services Task Force (USPSTF), 114
Uterine bleeding, abnormal, 956
Uterine pathology, 680
UTIs. *See* Urinary tract infections
Uveitis, chronic, 689t

V

Vaccinations. *See* Immunizations
Vaccine Adverse Event Reporting System (VAERS), 412
Vaccine Education Center (CHOP), 412
Vaccine information statement (VIS), 412
Vaginal infections
candidiasis, 889
diagnostic features of, 117, 118t
management of, 118t
Vaginal ring, 130
Vaginosis, bacterial, 118t, 837, 968
Vagistat-3. *See* Miconazole
Valacyclovir (Valtrex)
dose adjustment in renal failure, 1111t–1124t
for eczema herpeticum superinfection, 222
formulary entry, 1089–1090
for herpes, 115t–116t, 471t–476t
for oncology patients, 626t
for varicella, 440, 471t–476t
Valcyte. *See* Valganciclovir
Valganciclovir (Valcyte)
for CMV, 457t–458t, 471t–476t
dose adjustment in renal failure, 1111t–1124t
formulary entry, 1090–1091
Valium. *See* Diazepam
Valproic acid (Depakene, Depacon)
formulary entry, 1091–1092
for seizures, 559t–560t, 562t
Valsartan (Diovan), 1093
Valtrex. *See* Valacyclovir
Values, 630
Vancomycin (Vancocin, First-Vancomycin, Vancomycin+SyrSpend SF PH4)
for catheter-related bloodstream infections, 461t–468t

Vancomycin (Vancocin,
   First-Vancomycin,
   Vancomycin+SyrSpend SF PH4
   (Continued)
   for cellulitis, 461*t*–468*t*
   dose adjustment in renal failure, 1111*t*–1124*t*
   formulary entry, 1093–1095
   for gastroenteritis, 461*t*–468*t*
   for mastoiditis, 461*t*–468*t*
   for meningitis, 461*t*–468*t*
   neonatal dosing, 513*t*–514*t*
   for osteomyelitis, 461*t*–468*t*
   for parotitis, 461*t*–468*t*
   for septic arthritis, 461*t*–468*t*
   for sinusitis, 461*t*–468*t*
   spectrum of activity, 452*t*
   for spinal fusion infections, 461*t*–468*t*
   for ventriculoperitoneal shunt infection, 461*t*–468*t*
Vancomycin-resistant *Enterococcus faecium* (VRE or VREF) infections, 947, 952, 1044
Vandazole. *See* Metronidazole
Vanderbilt Diagnostic Rating Scales, 237*t*–238*t*
Vanillyl mandelic acid, 287.e1*t*
Vantin. *See* Cefpodoxime
Varicella (chickenpox), 457*t*–458*t*, 471*t*–476*t*
   antimicrobial prophylaxis against, 626*t*
   diagnosis of, 218*f*
   treatment of, 761, 900, 1089
Varicella immunoprophylaxis, 406, 439–440
   administration, 440
   catch-up schedule for, 414*f*
   for children with HIV disease, 423
   after Ig or blood product administration, 426, 426.e1*t*
   postexposure, 440
   for pre-teens and adolescents, 124*t*
   recommended schedule for, 413*f*, 415*f*–418*f*
   routine vaccination, 439
Varicella-zoster immune globulin (human) (VariZig, VZIG)
   administration, 440
   formulary entry, 1095
   after Ig or blood product administration, 426.e1*t*
   postexposure, 440
   special considerations, 440

Varicella-zoster virus (VZV) vaccine (Varivax)
   administration, 440
   catch-up schedule for, 414*f*
   after chemotherapy, 625.e3
   for children with HIV disease, 423
   after HSCT, 625.e3
   after Ig or blood product administration, 426, 426.e1*t*
   MMRV combination vaccine (ProQuad), 423, 441
   for pre-teens and adolescents, 124*t*
   recommended schedule for, 413*f*, 415*f*–418*f*
VariZig. *See* Varicella-zoster immune globulin (human)
Vas deferens, 656
Vascular access, 31–48, 492
Vascular anomalies, 203–207
Vascular disease
   causes of, 531*t*
   renal lesions, 527*t*
Vascular rings, 667, 669*t*
Vascular tumors, benign, 203–207
Vasculitis, 696–701
   associated autoantibodies, 695*t*
   childhood syndromes, 697*t*
   definition of, 696
   medium-large vessel, 696, 697*t*
   small vessel, 696, 697*t*
Vasodilator therapy
   for hypertension, 544*t*–545*t*
   pulmonary, 501–502
Vasodilatory shock, 1096
Vasomotor/nonallergic rhinitis, 396
Vaso-occlusive crisis, 370*t*–371*t*
Vasopressin (Pitressin, Vasostrict), 273
   disorders of, 274–276
   formulary entry, 1096
Vasopressin test, 275, 275*t*
Vasostrict. *See* Vasopressin
Vasotec. *See* Enalapril maleate
VATER association, 496
VATER/VACTERL syndrome, 184, 185*t*
VCFS (velocardiofacial syndrome), 356–357
VCR. *See* Vincristine
VCUG (voiding cystourethrogram), 521, 679–680
V_E (minute ventilation), 92–93
Vecuronium bromide
   antidotes, 1097
   formulary entry, 1096–1097
   for RSI, 7*t*–8*t*
Veetids. *See* Penicillin V potassium
Vegetarian formulas, 601*t*–602*t*

Velban. See Vinblastine
Velocardiofacial syndrome (VCFS), 185*t*, 356–357
Veltin. See Tretinoin with clindamycin
Venereal Disease Research Laboratory (VDRL) test, 455.*e*2*t*
Venofer. See Iron, injectable preparations
Veno-occlusive disease, 622–623
  Baltimore criteria for, 623
  modified Seattle criteria for, 622
Venous blood gas (VBG), 639
Venous hum, 167*t*
Ventilation
  assist control (AC), 91
  for asthma, 11
  bag-mask, 4, 9
  high-frequency, 91–92
  high-frequency jet, 91, 90.*e*1
  high-frequency oscillatory (HFOV), 90.*e*1
  intermittent mandatory (IMV), 90
  mechanical, 971
  minute (V_E), 92–93
  noninvasive positive-pressure (NIPPV), 11, 90
  pressure support (PSV), 91
  for respiratory failure, 89, 91–92
    effects of setting changes, 92*t*
    initial settings, 91
    modes of operation, 90–91
    parameters, 90
    types of support, 89–90
  synchronized intermittent mandatory (SIMV), 91
Ventolin HFA. See Albuterol
Ventricular arrhythmias, 177*f*, 177*t*, 771–772
Ventricular conduction blocks, 179*t*
Ventricular fibrillation, 177*f*, 177*t*, 1096
Ventricular hypertrophy
  criteria for, 173*b*
  ECG findings in, 172
Ventricular septal defect (VSD), 186*t*–187*t*
  heart sounds in, 166*b*
  sports restrictions, 199.*e*1*t*
Ventricular tachycardia, 177*f*, 177*t*
  pulseless, 1096
Ventriculoperitoneal shunts
  for hydrocephalus, 564
  imaging of, 665
  infected, 461*t*–468*t*
VePesid. See Etoposide

Veramyst. See Fluticasone furoate
Verapamil (Calan, Verelan)
  dose adjustment in renal failure, 1125*t*–1134*t*
  ECG effects of, 180*t*
  formulary entry, 1097–1098
Verelan. See Verapamil
Veripred 20. See Prednisolone
Vermox. See Mebendazole
Versed. See Midazolam
Vertebral anomalies, 184
Vertex delivery, 511
Vertigo, paroxysmal, 557*t*
Very long-chain acyl-CoA dehydrogenase (VLCAD) disorders, 341
Very low-birth-weight (VLBW) infants, 493
Vesicles, 203, 204*f*–205*f*
Vesicoureteral reflux, 522–523, 522*f*
Vesiculopustular eruptions, 218*f*
Vest therapy (high-frequency chest wall compression devices), 656
Vfend. See Voriconazole
Viagra. See Sildenafil
Vibramycin. See Doxycycline
ViCPS (Typhim Vi), 439
  administration, 439
  side effects of, 439
Vigabatrin (Sabril)
  dose adjustment in renal failure, 1125*t*–1134*t*
  formulary entry, 1098–1099
  for seizures, 559*t*–560*t*, 562*t*
Vilanterol + fluticasone furoate (Breo Ellipta), 894
Vimpat. See Lacosamide
Vinblastine (BVL, vincaleukoblastine, Velban), 613*t*–615*t*
Vincristine (VCR, Oncovin), 613*t*–615*t*
Vinorelbine (Navelbine), 613*t*–615*t*
Viokace. See Pancrelipase
Violets, 21.*e*1*t*–21.*e*3*t*
Viral bronchiolitis, acute, 1063
Viral infections, 471*t*–476*t*
  perinatal, 455
  of skin, 207–208
  treatment of, 470
Viramune. See Nevirapine
Virazole. See Ribavirin
Viroptic. See Trifluridine
VIS (vaccine information statement), 412
Visceral larva migrans, 955
Visceral leishmaniasis, 1013

Vision, 625.e1t–625.e2t
Vision screening
　for adolescents, 112, 123
Vistaril. See Hydroxyzine
Vistide. See Cidofovir
Visual-motor/problem-solving skills, 229, 231t–232t
Vital formulas, 594t–602t
Vital signs
　adolescent, 112
　monitoring in procedural sedation, 148
　newborn, 493
　normal, 493
　in poisonings, 21.e1t–21.e3t
Vitamax, 589t–590t
Vitamin A (Aquasol A)
　formulary entry, 1099
　in infant multivitamin drops, 588t
　for measles, 471t–476t
　in multivitamin tablets, 589t–590t
　recommended intakes, 586t
　reference values, 709t–716t
　supplementation, 1099
Vitamin A deficiency, 1099
Vitamin B_1. See Thiamine
Vitamin B_1 deficiency, 1078
Vitamin B_2. See Riboflavin
Vitamin B_3. See Niacin
Vitamin B_6. See Pyridoxine
Vitamin B_6 deficiency, 1039
Vitamin B_{12}. See Cobalamin; Cyanocobalamin
Vitamin B_{12} deficiency, 843
Vitamin C. See Ascorbic acid
Vitamin D, 266–267
　for breastfed infants, 267, 584–585
　in infant multivitamin drops, 588t
　in multivitamin tablets, 589t–590t
　and nephrolithiasis, 543–545
　for osteopenia, 693
　RDAs, 584
　recommendations for, 267, 586t
　reference values, 709t–716t
　supplementation, 583–584, 875
Vitamin D deficiency, 267, 267t–268t, 829
Vitamin D insufficiency, 267, 268t
Vitamin D_2. See Ergocalciferol
Vitamin D_2 supplementation, 875
Vitamin D_3. See Cholecalciferol
Vitamin D–dependent rickets, 875
Vitamin D–resistant rickets, 875
Vitamin E (α-tocopherol, Aqueous Vitamin E, Nutr-E-Sol)
　formulary entry, 1100
　in infant multivitamin drops, 588t
　in multivitamin tablets, 589t–590t
　recommended intakes, 586t
　reference values, 709t–716t
Vitamin E deficiency, 1100
Vitamin K. See Phytonadione
Vitamin K deficiency, 387b
　differential diagnosis of, 386f
　treatment of bleeding in, 1020
Vitamin K_1. See Phytonadione
Vitamins
　recommended intakes, 586t
　requirements for newborns, 497
Vitrase. See Hyaluronidase
Vivonex formulas, 570, 594t–602t
Vivotif (Ty21a), 439
　administration, 439
　contraindications to, 439
　precautions, 439
　routine vaccination, 439
　side effects of, 439
VLBW (very low-birth-weight) infants, 493
VLCAD (very long-chain acyl-CoA dehydrogenase) disorders, 341
Voice disorders, 242
Voicing my choices planning guide, 632
Voiding cystourethrogram (VCUG), 521, 679–680
Volar splint, 71f, 70.e1
Volume overload, 529
Vomiting, 318. See also Nausea and vomiting
　in acute gastroenteritis, 997
　differential diagnosis of, 319t
Von Gierke disease, 343–344
von Willebrand disease, 386f, 387t–388t, 532f, 851
von Willebrand factor (vWF), 376–379
　age-specific values, 377t–378t
Voriconazole (Vfend)
　formulary entry, 1101–1102
　for oncology patients, 626t
VoSpire ER. See Albuterol
VP-16. See Etoposide
VRE or VREF (vancomycin-resistant Enterococcus faecium) infections, 947, 952, 1044
V_T (tidal volume), 90–91
Vulvovaginal candidiasis, 118t
vWF. See von Willebrand factor
Vyvanse. See Lisdexamfetamine

VZIG. *See* Varicella-zoster immune globulin (human)

W

Waist circumference, 572–574
Waist/height ratio, 572–574
Walking reflex, 236.e4t–236.e5t
Warfarin (Coumadin, Jantoven)
  for cerebrovascular accident, 618
  and coagulation tests, 382
  formulary entry, 1102–1104
  for Kawasaki disease, 198.e1t
  medications that influence, 385b
  overdose, 23t–24t, 384t
  for stroke, 567
  for thrombosis, 382, 383t
Warm (septic) shock, 87f, 86.e1t
Warts, 207–208
Water deficits, 293, 297
  assessment of, 293
  free water deficit (FWD), 297
Water deprivation test, 274–275, 275t
Water loss, insensible, 496.e1t
Water requirements, 497t
WBCs. *See* White blood cells
Web resources
  for adolescent medicine, 108
  for analgesia and procedural sedation, 136
  for burns, 73
  for cardiology, 156
  for critical care, 73
  for development, behavior, and mental health, 229
  drug information data sources, 732
  for endocrinology, 255
  for evidence-based medicine, 721
  for gastroenterology, 316
  for genetics, 333
  for hematology, 364
  for immunoprophylaxis, 412
  for neonatology, 490
  for nephrology, 516
  for neurology, 548
  for nutrition and growth, 570
  for oncology, 607
  for palliative care, 628
  for poisonings, 20
  for pulmonology, 637
  for radiology, 663
  for rheumatology, 688
  statistics resources and software, 721
  for trauma, 73
  websites for clinicians, 108
  websites for patients, 108
Wegener granulomatosis, 532f, 697t
Weight
  conversion formulas, 708
  growth charts for boys, 574f, 578f
  growth charts for girls, 572f, 576f
  healthy, 571
  overweight, 571, 658
  for preterm infants, 580f–581f
  underweight, 571
Weight loss, 658
Wenckebach phenomenon, 178f, 178t
Wernicke's encephalopathy syndrome, 1079
Wheals, 203, 204f–205f
Wheezes, 638t
Whey-based formulas, 594t–600t
Whipworm, 955
White blood cells (WBCs)
  age-specific values, 365t
  blood smears, 393
  correction for, 553b
  CSF levels, 717t
  synovial fluid levels, 718t
  urinalysis for, 518
Whiteheads, 213
WHO Solution, 302t
Whole blood, 426.e1t
Whole exome sequencing, 358t
Whole genome sequencing, 358t
Wilate, 387t–388t
Wilcoxon matched pairs test, 724t
Williams syndrome, 185t
Wilms' tumor, 532f, 609t–610t
Wilson's disease, 1106, 347.e1
WinRho-SDF. *See* RH_0 (D) immune globulin intravenous (human)
Wolff-Parkinson-White syndrome, 166b, 176f, 179t
World Health Organization (WHO)
  classification of SLE nephritis, 693.e1t
  oral rehydration salts, 603t
  web resources, 412
Wound hygiene, 94
Wound management, 428t
Wounds, animal bite, 93–95
Wycillin. *See* Penicillin G

X

Xanthoastrocytoma, 611t
Xanthochromia, 553b
Xanthogranuloma, juvenile, 218f
Xerostomia, 1021, 701.e3
X-linked adrenoleukodystrophy, 347.e1
X-linked agammaglobulinemia, 403t–404t
X-linked disease, 334.e1
Xolegel. *See* Ketoconazole

Xopenex. *See* Levalbuterol
X-rays, 664*t*
Xtampza ER. *See* Oxycodone
Xylocaine. *See* Lidocaine

Y

Yaz. *See* Oral contraceptives
Yeast infections, 470
Yellow fever immunoprophylaxis, 441
Yersinia, 691
Young women's health websites, 108
Yuzpe method, 130

Z

Zaditor. *See* Ketotifen fumarate
Zantac. *See* Ranitidine HCl
Zarontin. *See* Ethosuximide
Zaroxolyn. *See* Metolazone
Zarxio. *See* Filgrastim
Zegerid. *See* Omeprazole with sodium bicarbonate
Zellweger syndrome, 347.e1
Zembrace SymTouch. *See* Sumatriptan
Zemuron. *See* Rocuronium
Zenatane. *See* Isotretinoid
Zenpep. *See* Pancrelipase
Zenzedi. *See* Dextroamphetamine
Zestril. *See* Lisinopril
Zetonna. *See* Ciclesonide
Ziagen. *See* Tretinoin with clindamycin
Zidovudine (Retrovir, AZT)
  formulary entry, 1104–1106
  for perinatal HIV exposure, 481*t*
Zidovudine with abacavir and lamivudine (Trizivir), 1104
Zidovudine with lamivudine (Combivir), 1104
Zileuton, 652*f*
Zinacef. *See* Cefuroxime
Zinc
  in infant multivitamin drops, 588*t*
  in multivitamin tablets, 589*t*–590*t*
  recommended intakes, 591*t*
  reference values, 709*t*–716*t*
Zinc deficiency, 1106
Zinc salts (Galzin, Orazinc), 1106
Zirgan. *See* Ganciclovir
Zithromax. *See* Azithromycin
Zmax. *See* Azithromycin
Zofran. *See* Ondansetron
Zollinger-Ellison syndrome, 880
Zolmitriptan (Zomig)
  formulary entry, 1106–1107
  for migraine, 554*t*
Zoloft. *See* Sertraline
Zomig. *See* Zolmitriptan
Zonisamide (Zonegran)
  formulary entry, 1107–1108
  for seizures, 562*t*
Zosyn. *See* Piperacillin with tazobactam
Zovirax. *See* Acyclovir
Zuplenz. *See* Ondansetron
Zyloprim. *See* Allopurinol
Zymar. *See* Gatifloxacin
Zymaxid. *See* Gatifloxacin
Zyprexa. *See* Olanzapine
Zyrtec. *See* Cetirizine
Zyrtec-D 12 Hour. *See* Cetirizine + pseudoephedrine
Zyvox. *See* Linezolid

1250

1251

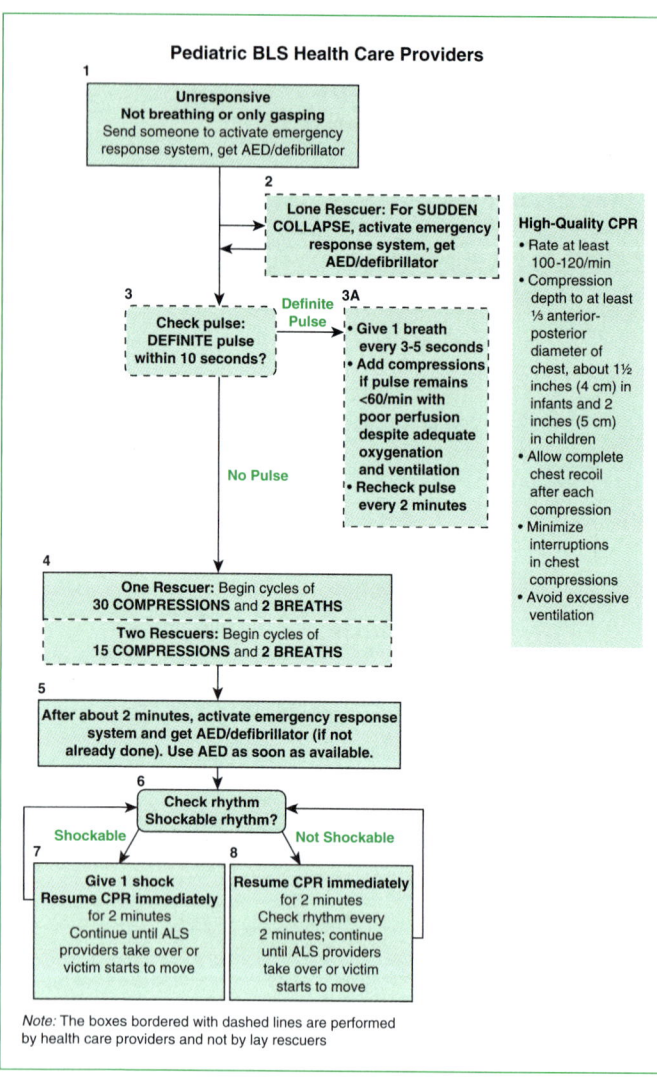

Pediatric BLS health care providers algorithm. *(Reprinted with permission. Atkins DL, Berger S, Duff JP, et al. Part 11: pediatric basic life support and cardiopulmonary resuscitation quality: 2015 American Heart Associated Guidelines Update for Cardiopulmonary Resuscitation and Emergency Cardiovascular Care. Circulation. 2015; 132(suppl 2):S519-S525.)*

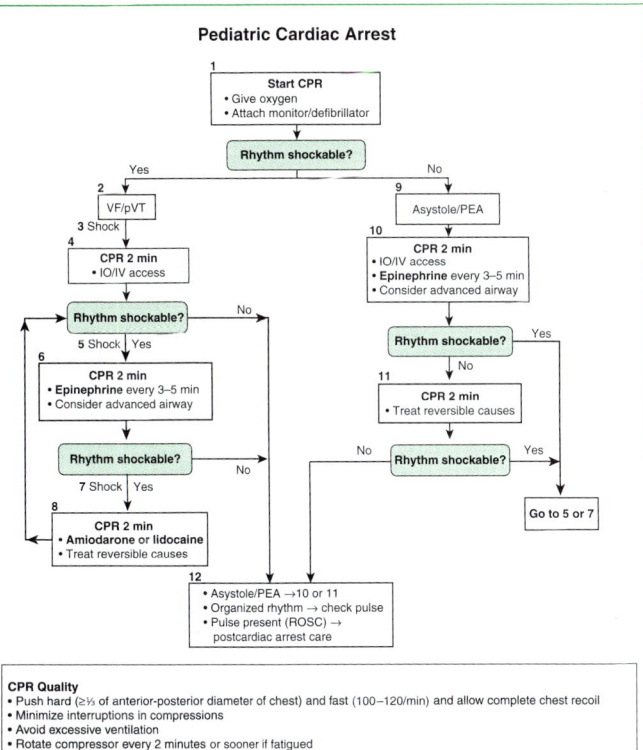

Pediatric cardiac arrest algorithm. (Reprinted with permission. de Caen AR, Berg MD, Chameides L, et al. Part 12: pediatric advanced life support: 2015 American Heart Association Guidelines Update for Cardiopulmonary Resuscitation and Emergency Cardiovascular Care. Circulation. 2015;132(suppl):S526-C542.)

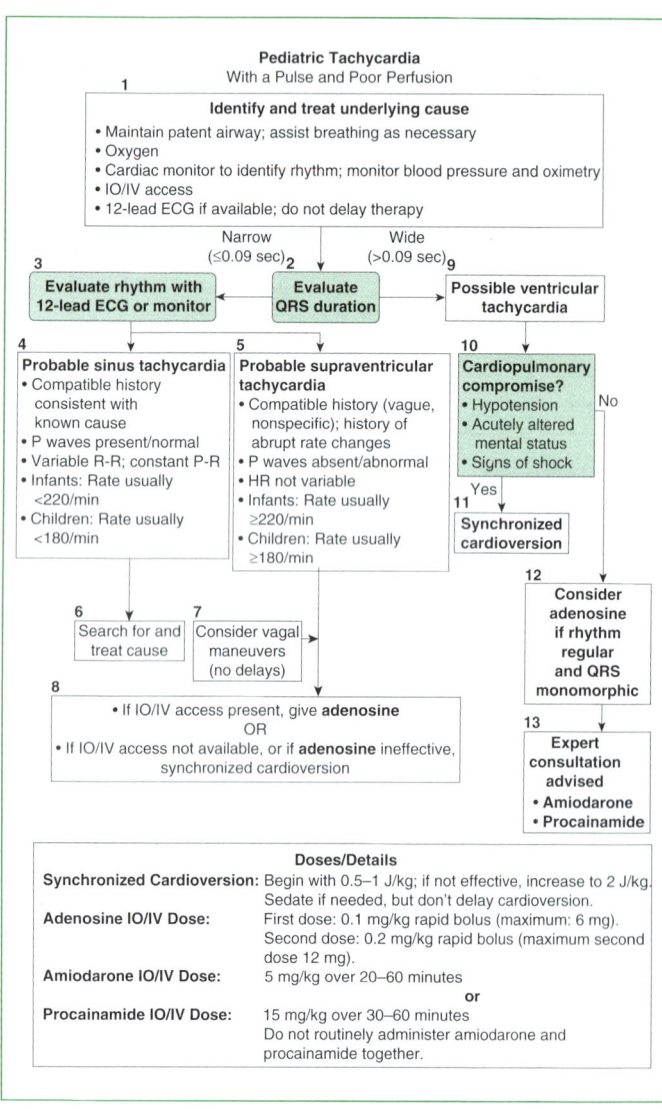

Pediatric tachycardia algorithm. *(Reprinted with permission. 2010 American Heart Association Guidelines for Cardiopulmonary Resuscitation and Emergency Cardiovascular Care. Part 14: Pediatric advanced life support. Circulation. 2010;122:S888. © 2015 American Heart Association, Inc.)*